Pharmaceutical Drug *and* Drugs Products

(With their description, medicinal preparations, administrations and therapeutic uses)

Pharmaceutical Drug *and* Drugs Products

(With their description, medicinal preparations, administrations and therapeutic uses)

A presentation of 8160 modern, non-pharmacopeal, medicinal preparations, comprising: 1878 drugs and chemicals, 535 biologicals, 860 endocrines, 1563 ampule medicaments, 209 medicinal foods, 129 mineral waters, 2344 individual and group allergens and 642 miscellaneous products.

By :

JACOB GUTMAN, M.D., Phar.D., F.A.C.P.

WILLIAM E. FITCH

Consulting Physician, Manhattan General Hospital, New York; the Riverdale, Shore Road, Williamsburg Maternity and Borough Park General Hospitals of Brooklyn; Director, Brooklyn Diagnostic Institute. Formerly Professor of Materia Medica College of Dentistry, University of State of New Jersey; Professor Clinical Chemistry Jersey City College of Pharmacy; Instructor of Medicine, New York Post Graduate Medical School and Hospital; Attending Physician Wyckoff Heights and Unity Hospitals.

Volume 1

SHREE PUBLISHERS & DISTRIBUTORS

NEW DELHI-110 002

Edition : 2008

Published by :
SHREE PUBLISHERS AND DISTRIBUTORS
20, Ansari Road, Daryaganj
New Delhi-110 002

3 Volumes Set

ISBN : 978-81-8329-255-9

Printed by :
Ruchika Printers
Delhi-110032

PREFACE

This treatise is designed to meet the demand of the progressive physicians, researchers, and pharmacy students for information concerning the most modern therapeutic agencies placed at his command by Research Laboratories. It presents without bias or comment all the popular non-pharmacopeal preparations and other remedies found useful in the treatment of disease.

The pharmaceutical concerns of America spend millions of dollars yearly for the discovery and preparation of medicinal agents of high merit. Medicine is indeed indebted to these organizations for the many epoch-making discoveries and invaluable additions to modern therapeusis made during the past few decades; most of the curative sera, vaccines, allergens, potent drugs and endocrines are the result of their researches. The physician, however, has at present no adequate means of keeping informed on all the newer additions to his armamentarium; commercial descriptions of these reach him at inopportune times and usually find their way into the waste basket, thus seldom being on hand when wanted; and except for the official publication of only Council-Accepted products, there are no authoritative sources of information embracing all the modern preparations. To provide such source is the purpose of this work.

An endeavor is here made to present without favoritism or discrimination all the non-official products-proprietary, patented, Council Accepted and others, that are popular with the medical profession. Descriptions, statements, analyses and all other data are offered without change or comment, but as found available in the numerous standard works and references consulted, or as obtained from the producers and distributors of the respective products. Every effort has been made to present the information accurately yet concisely, excluding elaborate discussions, quotations, theories and other time consuming topics of but little practical value to the clinician. The embodiment in three volumes of such a mass of material necessitated the use of phraseology as brief as was found consistent with the complete description of every important feature.

To insure ease in locating a desired preparation and to afford equal consideration to all products and producers, the arrangement throughout the book is alphabetical, by drug or distributor. Separate chapters are devoted to preparations of similar character; in each chapter like products are grouped, and preceded in each instance by a brief description with suggestions for their practical application; for each drug its various methods of administration, with dosages in the metric and U. S. systems, are presented. Incompatibilities, contraindications, strengths of solutions and methods of their preparation are given where deemed serviceable; where emphasis is desirable, italics or capitals are employed; verbiage is avoided throughout the book.

The Therapeutic Guide is intended to provide for the clinician, whether general practitioner or specialist, a wide choice of preparations of use in the numerous pathologic conditions encountered in his daily service to the sick; also to assist him in the selection of a remedy for a particular purpose. The comprehensive Index is arranged into three sections-Distributors', Drug and Therapeutic, this to assure convenience and rapidity in locating a desired drug, disease or other topic.

GLOSSARY

Definitions of the Newer Trade Terms

Alkpule: A specially treated glass vial containing chemically pure, normal 4% sodium hydroxide solution, in the exact quantity necessary to alkalize the corresponding dose of the accompanying drug.

Ambot: An ampule-bottle containing a solution for hypodermic use.

Ampacoid: A sterile, isotonic solution containing a physiologically standardized hormone of high concentration and purity.

Ampule-vial: A vial containing a sterile solution for hypodermic injection.

Aspirol: A trade name for Ampule-vial.

Bacterin: A bacterial vaccine; a suspension of killed bacteria for use in immunization.

Billet: A small tablet.

C.A.: Council or Committee Accepted (accepted by the Council on Pharmacy and Chemistry or Committee on Foods of the A.M.A., 1933).

Carpule: A glass cartridge-ampule containing in sterile solution a medicament, in definite dosage and strength.

Collosol: A suspensoid colloid with the active ingredient in the disperse phase; non-dialysable, slowly diffusible and disintegrating; is electrically charged and affected by electrolytes.

Crinogen: A preparation of glandular substance, protein and alcohol-free, in concentrated solution.

Dragee: A sugar coated pill or medicated confection.

Elixoid: A fluid preparation favorably flavored.

Emplet: An endocrine product with a protective, inert, salol-free enteric coating, insoluble in stomach but soluble in duodenal and intestinal secretions.

Enteric Coated: Specially coated to traverse the stomach intact without causing irritation, and disintegrating only in the intestines.

Enterocap: A capsule devised to protect its contents against gastric action.

Enterosol Coated: So coated as to be insoluble in gastric secretion.

Enule: A rectal suppository wrapped individually in tin foil.

Glaseptic Ampule: An ampule made of an alkali-free, non-soluble glass, assuring stability of contents.

Hypoloid: An ampule containing a solution for hypodermic injection.

Immunogen: Extraction from living bacterial culture, principally ectoplasm, free from toxic autolysates, bacterial substances, with only $\frac{1}{10}$% of the protein content of ordinary vaccines.

Isopule: An ampule containing a measured dose of a medicament.

Kapseal: A special gelatine capsule with joints hermetically sealed to keep contents airtight and prevent deterioration.

Kerakote: A keratin-composition acid resisting, coating, for carrying into the intestines medicinal products which may be impaired or destroyed in the stomach.

Keratin Coated: Coated with acid-resistant keratin, enabling contained medication to pass through the stomach unimpaired.

L.A.: Laity Advertised; popular preparations advertised to the public.

Phylacogen: A bacterial culture filtrate free from organisms.

Pulvule: A dry powdered preparation enclosed in thin walled, quickly soluble capsule of a special gelatin, assuring stability of medication.

Sanitablet: A tablet mechanically packed in cellophane to prevent contamination from handling.

Serobacterin: A bacterin or vaccine sensitized with its corresponding immune serum and of use in smaller dosage.

Soloid: A tablet of soluble ingredients for the making of solutions.

Sucret: A preparation with sucrose.

Swab-Seal: An Ampule-vial mechanically sealed for preservation of contents in sterile state.

Tabloid: A form of medicinal tablet or lozenge.

TABLE OF CONTENTS

CHAPTER V

HYPODERMIC MEDICAMENTS

CHAPTER VI

BIOLOGICALS

CHAPTER VII

ALLERGENS

CHAPTER VIII

FOODS AND BEVERAGES

CHAPTER IX

BOTTLED MINERAL WATERS

CHAPTER X

MISCELLANEOUS PRODUCTS

CHAPTER XI

THERAPEUTIC GUIDE

CHAPTER XII

CHAPTER XIII

CHAPTER XIV

CHAPTER XV

CHAPTER I

DRUGS OF KNOWN CONSTITUTION AND ACTION

This chapter presents 1,040 individual drugs and combinations of well defined composition and action, in 1,980 forms. The arrangement is alphabetical; the dosages are average and stated in both the metric and U.S. systems, approximately converted.

ABASIN (Winthrop)

Sedative

Chemical Name: Acetylbromdiethylacetylcarbamid. Brand of Acetylcarbromal.

Formula: $Br(C_2H_5)_2C.\ CO.\ NH.\ CO.\ NH.\ CO.\ CH_3$.

Description: A white crystalline odorless powder, of faintly bitter taste; sparingly soluble in water, readily soluble in alcohol.

Action: Safe efficient sedative; causes practically no depression, drowsiness or hypnosis.

Uses: In menstrual and climacteric neuroses, mild hysteria and neurasthenia; in mental irritability and nerve strain from any cause.

Supply: ABASIN—Tablets, gr 4 (0.259 Gm)—Tubes of 10—Bottles of 100.

Administration: 1–2 tablets two or three times daily, after meals; children, according to age.

Bibliography: *See Chap. XII.*

ACECOLINE (Anglo-French)

Vasodilator

Chemical Name: Acetylcholine Hydrochloride.

Formula: $(CH_3)_3NCl\ C_2H_4CO_2CH_3$.

Description: A white crystalline powder of characteristic odor and bitter-salty taste; is hygroscopic, very unstable and decomposes readily in moist air into acetic acid and choline; in form of Acecoline is made stable; is sterile, non-toxic and non-irritating.

Action and Uses: Powerfully stimulates the vagus and antagonizes the effect of epinephrin, relieving spasms, dilating peripheral arterioles and counteracting anaphylaxis. *For use* in alleviating pain and paresthesia in Raynaud's disease, endarteritis obliterans, intermittent claudication, senile and diabetic gangrene; to relieve cerebral vascular disturbances in hypertension, spasm of arteria centralis retinae, labyrinthine disorders, tinnitus, vertigo, headaches; to relieve atony of smooth musculature—bladder, stomach and intestines; used also in lead colic and tubercular hyperhidrosis.

Contraindications: Bradycardia, or its occurrence during the use of the drug.

Supply: ACECOLINE—Ampules, crystalline powder, 0.1 Gm, 0.02 Gm, 0.05 Gm, with Ampules 5 cc of distilled water—Cartons of 6 ampules.

Administration: *Subcutaneously* or *intramuscularly*, never intravenously; must be freshly prepared, each dose being dissolved in accompanying ampule of water.

Dosage: Arterial disease—0.1–0.2 Gm twice daily; lead colic—0.2 Gm every 10 min. till relieved; tubercular hyperhidrosis—0.02 Gm daily; vagus dysfunction—0.05 Gm daily.

Bibliography: *See Chap. XII.*

ACETARSONE (Abbott)

Amebacide. Spirocheticide

Chemical Name: Acetylamino-hydroxyphenyl-arsonic Acid.

Formula: $HO. CH_3CONH. C_6H_3As: O: (OH)_2$.

Composition: Is the acetyl derivative of 3-amino-4-4 hydroxyphenyl-1-arsonic acid; a pentavalent organic arsenical compound, containing about 27% of arsenic.

Description: A white, odorless powder, somewhat acid in taste; is slightly soluble in water and alcohol, readily soluble in alkalies or alkaline carbonate solutions; is stable at ordinary temperature.

Action and Uses: Antisyphilitic *for use* in general paresis and dementia paralytica; as amebacide—in the treatment of amebic dysentery.

Caution: Where gastrointestinal or cutaneous manifestations are produced because of the rather toxic arsenical content, its administration must temporarily be discontinued.

Advantages: Is often effective in cases of dementia paralytica not responding to malarial or other therapy.

Supply: ACETARSONE—Ampules, intravenous, 1 Gm and 0.5 Gm—Boxes of 25 and 100, with Alkpules of sodium hydroxide for alkalization.

ACETARSONE—Tablets (C.A.) gr 4 (0.25 Gm)—Bottles of 25 and 100.

Administration: *Orally*—2–3 tablets daily for 7–10 days.
Intravenously—Three times weekly for 7–8 weeks, in general paralysis.
Solutions are prepared by completely dissolving the contents of 1 ampule in 9 cc of normal (4%) sodium hydroxide, then adding 11 cc of sterile distilled water to make a total of 20 cc, for immediate use.

Bibliography: *See Chap. XII.*

ACETYLCHOLINE (Roche)

Vasodilator

Chemical Name: Acetylcholine Chloride.

Formula: $CH_3. CO. O. CH_2. CH_2. N(CH_3)_3. Cl$.

Composition: The acetic acid ester of choline chloride; is closely allied chemically to synthetic muscarine, the nitrous acid ester of choline chloride.

Description: Is present normally in warm blooded organisms and probably derived from choline; is perhaps identical with the vagus hormone lately disclosed in the active excised heart (Loewi).

Action: Lowers blood pressure by dilatation of peripheral vessels; relaxes spasm of smooth musculature; stimulates the parasympathetic nervous system.

Uses: In Raynaud's disease, incipient or active gangrene of extremities or amputation stumps; in endarteritis with danger of occlusion; in decubitus ulceration; in atony of smooth musculature and profuse sweats of phthisis.

Supply: ACETYLCHOLINE—Ampules, each 0.1 Gm crystalline powder, with Ampule 2 cc sterile, double distilled water—Packages of 6.

Administration: Preferably *intramuscularly*, but also given *subcutaneously;* **never** intravenously.

Dosage: 0.05–0.2 Gm daily, as a 5 % solution.

Bibliography: *See Chap. XII.*

ACETYLCHOLINE BROMIDE

Vasodilator

Chemical Name: Acetyl-ethanol-trimethyl-ammonium Hydroxide.

Formula: $(CH_3)_3N.\ Br.\ CH_2CH_2O.\ OC.\ CH_3$.

Description: A white, crystalline, deliquescent powder; is soluble in water and alcohol, forming a stable solution.

Action: Has marked spasmolytic action, dilating peripheral blood vessels, lowering blood pressure and slowing the heart; the acetyl radicle greatly intensifies the hypotensive and muscle stimulating action of choline, augmenting intestinal peristalsis and suppressing spasm of bladder, ureters and uterus; is practically free from toxicity or reaction.

Uses: In arterial hypertension, Raynaud's disease, obliterating endarteritis; in general atony of bladder, ureters and intestine; in lead colic and tubercular hyperhidrosis.

Caution: Solutions should always be prepared fresh before use.

Supply: **ACETYLCHOLINE BROMIDE**—Ampules 100 mg and 200 mg—Boxes of 6. **(Abbott)**

ACETYLCHOLINE BROMIDE—Ampules 0.1 Gm with ampule 5 cc distilled water—Bottles of 10 and 100 Gm. **(Eastman)**

Administration: In hypertension—*intravenously,* 0.1 Gm daily; *subcutaneously*—in higher dosage: first day 0.05 Gm; next day and daily for the next 10 days 0.1 Gm; then 0.2 Gm twice daily.

In intestinal and vesical atony—0.1–0.3 Gm *intravenously,* as required; *intramuscularly* with eserin; in Raynaud's disease and endarteritis obliterans—0.1–0.2 Gm daily; in lead colic—0.15–0.2 Gm every 5–10 min. until attack is relieved; in tubercular hyperhidrosis—0.02 to 0.05Gm *subcutaneously* or *intramuscularly.*

Bibliography: *See Chap. XII.*

ACIDOL **(Metz)**

Hydrochloric Acid Therapy

Chemical Name: Betaine Hydrochloride.

Formula: $N(CH_3)_3.\ CH_2CO_2.\ HCl$.

Description: Colorless crystals, freely soluble in water; contains 23.8 %, of absolute HCl; is stable in dry state, but in 1 % aqueous solution 40 % of Acidol is dissociated into free hydrochloric acid and its carrier betaine, an innocuous substance.

Action: As for fluid hydrochloric acid; is conveniently administered, palatable, easily carried about and furnishes fresh active HCl solution upon ingestion.

Uses: In all conditions where hydrochloric acid is indicated: chronic gastritis, gastric subacidity, achylia gastrica; in pernicious anemia, gastric carcinoma, gastrogenous diarrhea; in convalescence from acute febrile disease.

Supply: **ACIDOL**—Tablets, 7½ gr (0.5 Gm)—Tubes of 20.

Administration: 1 or 2 tablets after each meal.

Combinations: **ACIDOL-PEPSIN:** A combination of Acidol and pure Pepsin.

Supply: ACIDOL-PEPSIN—Tablets (Strong) containing 6 gr (0.4 Gm) Acidol, 1½ gr (0.1 Gm) Pepsin—Tubes of 20.

ACIDOL-PEPSIN—Tablets (Mild) containing ⅚ gr (0.06 Gm) Acidol, 3 gr (0.19 Gm) Pepsin—Tubes of 10.

ACIDULIN (Lilly)

Hydrochloric Acid Therapy

Chemical Name: Glutamic Acid Hydrochloride.

Formula: $COOH(CH_2)_2CH. (NH_2)COOH. HCl$.

Composition: A combination of hydrochloric acid with amino glutamic acid as its carrier.

Action and Uses: On contact with water releases free hydrochloric acid, which takes the place of absent or deficient acid in stomach and thus favorably affects hypoacidity and anacidity of pernicious anemia and gastric cancer, achylia gastrica; in gall bladder disease, chronic dyspepsia, gastrogenous diarrhea.

Advantages: Is a convenient means of administering dilute hydrochloride acid; is free from unpleasant taste and possible injury to teeth or oral mucosa.

Supply: ACIDULIN—Pulvules, each representing 10m Dil. HCl. U.S.P.—Packages of 20—Bottles of 100.

Administration: 1-2 pulvules after meals; excess of fluids to be avoided.

Bibliography: *See Chap. XII.*

ACRIFLAVINE

Antiseptic

Chemical Name: A brand of acriflavine hydrochloride: 3, 6 diamino-10-methyl-acridinium chloride hydrochloride.

Formula: $C_{14}H_{14}N_3Cl$: $HCl + H_2O$.

Description: A brownish-red, odorless crystalline powder; soluble in 3 parts of water, incompletely soluble in alcohol, nearly insoluble in ether, chloroform, liquid petrolatum, fixed and volatile oils.

Action and Uses: An antiseptic and bacteriostat, particularly to the gonococcus; *For use* in the treatment of wounds, gingivitis, gonorrheal conjunctivitis, urethritis, furunculosis, otitis media, eczema.

Supply: ACRIFLAVINE HYDROCHLORIDE—Tablets (C.A.) 0.46 gr (0.03 Gm)—Bottles of 20, 100, 1,000 and 5,000. **(Abbott)**

ACRIFLAVINE HYDROCHLORIDE—Tablets, ½ gr (0.032 Gm) enteric coated—Bottles of 100, 1,000 and 5,000. **(Abbott)**

ACRIFLAVINE HYDROCHLORIDE—Powder—Bottles 1 Gm, 5 Gm, and 1 oz. **(Abbott)**

ACRIFLAVINE "NATIONAL"—Tablets, gr 1½ (0.1 Gm)—Bottles 50 and 100. **(National Aniline)**

Administration: For urethral injection—1:1,000 to 1:10,000 in physiologic saline.
As spray—1:1,000 solution.
As antiseptic dressing—on wounds, clean and suppurating—1:10,000 in physiologic saline; as wet dressing and irrigation of wounds—same dilution; for wet packing in middle ear suppuration—1:500, in 50% alcohol.
In dental uses—gingivitis 1:1,000 solution.

Caution: Solutions may be boiled or autoclaved to 130°c without decomposition; must be stored in amber bottles; solutions over 1 week old are to be discarded.

Bibliography: *See Chap. XII.*

ACRIFLAVINE, NEUTRAL

Germicide

Chemical Name: Acriflavine base; 3, 6-diamino 10-methylacridinium chloride; or 2, 8 diamino-N-methylacridinium chloride.

Formula: $C_{14}H_{14}N_3Cl + H_2O$.

Description: A brownish red, odorless, granular powder; nearly insoluble in ether and chloroform, incompletely soluble in alcohol, soluble in about 3 parts of water; yields practically neutral solutions and may be used in higher concentrations than acriflavine hydrochloride.

Action: Antiseptic, bacteriostatic and deodorant; is comparatively free from toxicity; is non-irritating and does not interfere with phagocytic function; has specific action on gonococcus and renders alkaline urine antiseptic; is better tolerated and more effective than the hydrochloride.

Uses: In infections of the genito-urinary tract, particularly gonorrheal urethritis, cystitis, pyelitis; in burns, fissures, fistulae, chancroids; in ear, nose and throat infections; in systemic diseases: puerperal sepsis, undulant fever, influenza, endocarditis, erysipelas, Ludwig's angina; also in arthritis and dental disorders.

Supply: **ACRIFLAVINE** Neutral—Powder Bottles of 1 Gm, 5 Gm and 1 oz. **(Abbott)**

ACRIFLAVINE Neutral—Tablets (C.A.) Enteric coated, ½ gr (0.032 Gm), Bottles of 100, 1,000 and 5,000. **(Abbott)**

ACRIFLAVINE Neutral—Tablets (C.A.) Plain, 0.46 gr (0.03 Gm) —Bottles of 100, 1,000 and 5,000. **(Abbott)**

ACRIFLAVINE Neutral—Tablets—Plain, 1½ gr (0.1 Gm)—Bottles of 100, 1,000 and 5,000. **(Abbott)**

ACRIFLAVINE Neutral—Ampules (C.A.) Intravenous, 1½ gr (0.1 Gm) and 7½ gr (0.5 Gm)—Cartons of 6 ampules. **(Abbott)**

ACRIFLAVINE Neutral—Jelly (C.A.) 1:1,000, 0.1%, dissolved in Karaya gum jelly with sufficient sodium hydrate to make pH 8.5—Tubes of 1½ oz.—Jars 1 lb. **(Abbott)**

ACRIFLAVINE Neutral—Suppositories 1:2,000—Boxes of 12. **(Abbott)**

ACRIFLAVINE Neutral—Powder—Packages of 5, 10, 25 and 50 Gm. **(National Aniline)**

ACRIFLAVINE Neutral—Throat Troches (C.A.) (each 0.006 Gm)—Boxes of 30—Cartons of 12 boxes. **(National Aniline)**

ACRIFLAVINE Neutral—Ampules (C.A.)—0.5 and 1.0 Gm—Packages 5 each. **(National Aniline)**

ACRIFLAVINE Neutral—Ointment (C.A.) 1%—Tubes of 2 oz. **(National Aniline)**

ACRIFLAVINE Neutral—Tablets (C.A.) gr 1½ (0.1 Gm)—Bottles of 50 and 100. **(National Aniline)**

ACRIFLAVINE Neutral—Tablets (C.A.) gr, ½ Enteric coated—Bottles of 100. **(National Aniline)**

Administration: Irrigation—1:500 to 1:3,000 in warm physiologic saline.
Vaginal swabs or tampons—1:500 to 1:1,000 solution.
Urethral injection—1:500 to 1:1,000; irrigations—1:2,500 to 1:5,000.
Skin sterilization, pre-operative, 5% in solution of alcohol 50%, acetone 10%, water 40%.
Rectal administration—1:3,000 to 1:6,000, 1 qt.
Wet dressings, burns, etc.—1:100 to 1:500 solution.
Nose and throat—1:1,000 to 1:3,000, as spray or gargle.
Intravenously—10 to 50 cc ½% warm saline solution, freshly prepared and filtered.
Orally—1-1½ gr daily in glassful of water.

Bibliography: *See Chap. XII.*

ADALIN (Winthrop)

Sedative. Mild Hypnotic

Chemical Name: Brom-diethyl-acetyl-carbamide. Brand of Carbromal.

Formula: $(C_2H_5)_2C.\ Br.\ CO.\ NH.\ CO.\ NH_2$.

Description: A colorless and odorless powder, almost insoluble in water, readily soluble in alcohol.

Action: Sedative and hypnotic; does not affect the heart, blood pressure or respiration; is well borne by the gastro-intestinal tract; is not habit forming.

Uses: In mild neuroses, especially those of cardiac and gastric origin; in neurasthenia, hysteria, mild mental disorders; also in pertussis, asthma, climacteric and menstrual disorders.

Supply: ADALIN—Tablets (C.A.) gr 5 (0.324 Gm)—Tubes of 10—Bottles of 25.

ADALIN—Powder—Cartons of 1 oz.

Administration: As sedative—5–10 gr (0.324–0.643 Gm), two or three times daily. As hypnotic—10–20 gr (0.643–1.296 Gm), when required.

Combinations: ADALIN-LUMINAL: A combination for synergistic effect of Adalin 5 gr (0.324 Gm) and Luminal ¼ gr (0.016 Gm) per tablet. *Administration,* as sedative—1 tablet three times daily; as hypnotic—2–3 tablets, best taken in hot drink, 1 hour before retiring.

Supply: Tablets—Bottles of 25.

Bibliography: *See Chap. XII.*

ADENINE SULPHATE (Eastman)

Nucleotide Therapy

Chemical Name: Adenine Sulphate.

Formula: $C_5H_5N_5(SO_4)$.

Description: A nucleotide prepared by the hydrolysis of yeast nucleic acid with 10% sulphuric acid.

Action and Uses: Induces marked increase in number of polymorphonuclear cells and is used in nucleotide therapy of agranulocytic angina and pneumonia.

Supply: ADENINE SULPHATE—Ampules, 20 cc, 0.5 Gm in 20 cc normal saline.

ADENINE SULPHATE—Bottles 1, 3, 5 and 10 Gm.

Administration: *Intravenously,* 1 ampule twice daily.

Bibliography: *See Chap. XII.*

ADRENALIN (Parke, Davis)

Vasoconstrictor

Official Name: Suprarenin; Epinephrine.

Formula: $C_9H_{13}O_3N$.

Description: A white or cream-colored microcrystalline substance, slightly soluble in alcohol and in water, the saturated aqueous solution being somewhat alkaline to litmus; is insoluble in ether, chloroform, acetone, acids and fixed volatile oils; is freely soluble in carbonates; the chloride preparations may be sterilized by boiling without immediate impairment of activity.

Action: Constricts arterioles, especially of the cutaneous and splanchnic areas, stimulates the heart and arterial musculature and raises blood pressure; also stimulates the glycogenolytic cells of the liver, relaxes spasm of the bronchi and probably also that of the contraction ring of the uterine cervix; excessive dosage may cause cardiac fibrillation.

Uses: In shock and collapse; in serum sickness and anaphylactic reaction occurring in connection with the administration of arsphenamine, scarlet fever toxin or similar agents; in asthma and hay fever; in hemorrhages other than pulmonary and intracranial; in contraction ring dystocia; as aid to quinine in malaria; with local anesthetics to prolong their effect. Also as diagnostic agent in the Goetsch test.

Incompatibilities: Alkalies and oxidizing agents; salts of easily reduced metals, particularly iron; exposed to air, faintly alkaline solutions of adrenalin promptly lose their activity.

Supply: **ADRENALIN**—Crystals—Vials of 1 gr (0.064 Gm), for experimental use only.

ADRENALIN CHLORIDE—Solution (C.A.) Containing 1 part Adrenalin Chloride in 1000 parts of physiologic saline (with 0.5% Chloretone)—Bottles of 1 oz.; Ampules 1 cc—Boxes of 12 and 100.

ADRENALIN CHLORIDE—Dilute (C.A.)—Ampules—1½ m of 1:1,000 solution, diluted to 1 cc; Ampules—6 m of 1:1,000 solution, diluted to 1 cc—Packages of 12 and 100.

ADRENALIN—Inhalant (C.A.) Containing Adrenalin 1 part in 1,000 parts of aromatized bland oil, with 3% Chloretone—Bottles of 1 oz.

ADRENALIN—Suppositories (C.A.) Containing Adrenalin, 1 part to 1,000 parts oil of Theobroma base—Boxes of 12.

ADRENALIN AND CHLORETONE—Suppositories (C.A.) Containing Adrenalin 3/200 gr (1:1,000), Chloretone 3 gr (20%)—Boxes of 12.

ADRENALIN—Compound Suppositories—Containing Adrenalin 1/300 gr (1:6,000), Apothesine ½ gr (about 3%), Formidine 1 gr, Extract Hamamelis 1 gr—Boxes of 12.

ADRENALIN—Ointment (C.A.) Containing Adrenalin 1 part to 1,000 parts of Oleaginous base—Collapsible tin tubes ½ oz.

ADRENALIN—Tablets (C.A.)—Tablet 1, gr 3/200 and Tablet 2, gr 1/200—Tablet 1 dissolved in 15 m physiologic saline and Tablet 2 in 5 m each make 1:1,000 solution—Vials of 20.

Adrenalin Combinations:

ADREPHINE—Compound—Containing Adrenalin 1:10,000, Ephedrine sulphate 2%, Chloretone 0.5%, distilled water q.s.; combines the prompt astringent and styptic action of Adrenalin with the slower but more prolonged effect of Ephedrine—Bottles 1 oz.

ADREPHINE—Inhalant—Containing Adrenalin 1:10,000, Ephedrine hydrochloride 1%, Benzocaine 1%, Chloretone 0.5%, Alcohol 12%, Glycerin q.s.; For intranasal application—Bottles 1 oz.

ADREPHINE, ℞ *"B"*—Ampules 1 cc—Containing Adrenalin 1:2,500, Ephedrine hydrochloride 3%, Chloretone 0.5%—Boxes of 12 and 100.

ADREPHINE—Ointment—Containing Adrenalin 1:5,000, Ephedrine Hydrochloride 2%; *intranasally*, to reduce turgescence and for opening up occluded sinuses; for its styptic effect in bleeding hemorrhoids and in urethritis; topical application to bedsores or other areas of cutaneous inflammation—Tubes, collapsible, with elongated nozzle, ½ oz.

ADREPHINE—Suppositories—Containing Adrenalin 1/300 gr, Ephedrine hydrochloride ⅙ gr, Benzocaine ⅘ gr, Chloretone ½ gr—Boxes of 12.

Adrenalin Anesthetics:

ADRENALIN AND COCAINE—Tablets (C.A.)—Tubes of 20—Containing Cocaine hydrochloride ⅙ gr, Adrenalin 1/1,300 gr. For pressure anesthesia in dentistry.

ADROCAINE—Solution—Bottles 2 oz., rubber-diaphragm-capped.
A 1½% solution of Procaine containing Adrenalin 1:100,000 and Chloretone 0.5%.

ADROCAINE—Ampules, ℞ "A"—1 cc—Boxes of 12 and 100. Containing 0.02 Gm of Procaine and Adrenalin 0.00002 Gm.

ADROCAINE—Tablets, ℞ "A"—Tubes of 20—Bottles of 100. Containing Procaine ⅓ gr, Adrenalin 1/3,200 gr. To make 1 cc of a 2% procaine solution with adrenalin 1:50,000.

ADROCAINE—Tablets, ℞ "B"—Tubes of 10. Containing Procaine 4.6 gr, Adrenalin 1/200 gr. To make 1 fl. oz. of a 1% procaine solution with adrenalin 1:100,000.

APOTHESINE AND ADRENALIN—Tablets Dental (C.A.)—Tubes of 20. Containing apothesine ¾ gr, Adrenalin 1/1,600 gr; or Apothesine ⅓ gr, Adrenalin 1/2,500 gr.

APOTHESINE AND ADRENALIN—Tablets (C.A.)—Tubes of 10. Containing Apothesine 4.8 gr, Adrenalin 1/200 gr; 1 tablet makes 1 oz. of a 1% solution of apothesine and adrenalin 1:100,000.

CODRENIN—Bottles of 1 oz. Containing Cocaine hydrochloride 2%, Adrenalin 1:15,000, Chloretone 0.5%.

LOCOSTHETIC—Bottles of 1 oz. Containing Cocaine hydrochloride 0.75%, Adrenalin 1:50,000, Thymol 1:1,500, Potassium sulphate 1%, Chloretone 0.5%, Sodium chloride, q.s.

ANESTHONE CREAM—Tubes ½ oz., with elongated nozzle. Containing Adrenalin chloride 1:5,000, Ephedrine hydrochloride 2%, Benzocaine 10%.

Administration: Shock and Collapse—5 drops Adrenalin Chloride Solution in 1 oz. normal saline, intravenously, slowly: in severe instances given by centripetal arterial transfusion; in suspended animation (surgical anesthesia, drowning)—½–1 cc is injected directly into heart muscle.

Severe Hemorrhage—1 dr. Adrenalin Chloride solution 1:1,000 in pint of hot saline, given by hypodermoclysis or intravenously, slowly.

Superficial Hemorrhage—Adrenalin Chloride solution 1:1,000, for topical application by compress, for nose, mouth, throat, ear, vagina, uterus or rectum.

Hematemesis—1 dr of 1:1,000 solution, orally.

Hematuria—1 oz. of Adrenalin solution 1:5,000 to 1:10,000 instilled into bladder where kidneys are not involved.

Inflamed Mucous Membranes—1:5,000 to 1:10,000 solution, or Adrenalin Inhalant, or Adrephine Inhalant by spray or tampon, in rhinitis, chronic coryza, nasal catarrh, hay fever, pharyngitis, tonsillitis, laryngitis; also as lubricant for cystoscope, catheter or sound.

Local Anesthesia—Major operations, 5 drops of Adrenalin 1:1,000 in 1 oz. of anesthetic, i.e., 1:100,000 strength; where smaller quantities are required, 1:40,000 to 1:50,000 strengths are used. Anesthetic solution is to be sterilized first, then cooled, when the requisite number of drops of Adrenalin are added.

Asthma—2–10 m of Adrenalin 1:1,000 *subcutaneously* or *intramuscularly;* repeated if required, or site of injection is massaged to release imprisoned adrenalin.

Goetsch Test—6–8 m of Adrenalin 1:1,000, *subcutaneously;* in positive reaction the systolic pressure is increased in first 15 min. by about 10 points and pulse rate 10 beats a min., followed by a slight fall and later by a secondary rise. Heart action should be observed every 2½ min. at first, every 10 min. later. In 1½ hr, pressure becomes normal. Subjectively—tremor, pallor, heart consciousness, apprehension.

Malaria—5–8 m of the 1:1,000 solution is injected at the time quinine is administered to enhance its effectiveness; given *intramuscularly.*

Allergy—To prevent allergic reactions in the administration of arsphenamine, scarlet fever toxin, antitoxin or other agents, adrenalin ½ cc of the 1:1,000 solution is injected before or at the time the specific medication is given.

Contraction Ring Dystocia—5 m of Adrenalin Chloride solution 1:1,000 are injected.

Contraindications: Arterial hypertension, chloroform anesthesia, fibrillation.

Bibliography: *See Chap. XII.*

ADRIN SOLUTION (Sharp and Dohme

Vasoconstrictor

Composition: An Epinephrine Hydrochloride solution, 1:1,000; the blood pressure raising principle of the suprarenal gland; is biologically assayed and standardized to uniform strength.

Action and Uses: As for epinephrine; stimulates musculature of blood vessels intestines and heart; *indicated* in shock, sudden heart failure, collapse from hemorrhage, asphyxia; also in asthma and as adjunct in local anesthesia.

Supply: ADRIN—Solution—Bottles of 1 oz.

ADRIN—Solution—Ampules 1 cc—Boxes of 6 and 100.

Administration: *Orally*—5-30 m; *intravenously* and *subcutaneously*—in emergencies, in drop doses, diluted in saline; in asthma 4–8 m with frequent massage of injected area; in insulinemia—1 cc.

Locally—Is injected with anesthetics, for its blanching effect on the operative area.

Caution: Solutions are to be preserved in dark bottles; if discolored must be discarded.

AFENIL (Bilhuber-Knoll)

Calcium Therapy

Chemical Name: Calcium Chloride Urea.

Formula: $CaCl_2 . 4(NH_2)_2CO$.

Description: A standardized organic calcium preparation for intravenous administration; occurs as colorless, non-hygroscopic crystals, freely soluble in water.

Action: Corrects blood calcium deficiency, often the underlying cause of sensitivity; decreases permeability of cell wall and lessens transudation phenomena; reduces hypersensitive nerve reactivity.

Uses: In hay fever to reduce the number and severity of attacks; in vernal conjunctivitis and bronchial asthma; in eruptive skin disorders—eczema, urticaria, arsenical dermatitis and similar toxic manifestations.

Advantages: Is better tolerated than calcium chloride and more quickly diffused.

Supply: AFENIL—Ampules (C.A.) 10 cc—10% aqueous solution—Boxes of 1 ampule.

Administration: *Intravenously*—1 ampule, slowly administered, once or twice daily, or several times a week until desired results are obtained.

Caution: To prevent possible necrosis, the injection of the solution into the perivascular tissues is to be avoided.

Bibliography: *See Chap. XII.*

AGAR (Merck)

Laxative

Description: The dried mucilaginous substance extracted from Gelidium Corneum species and other closely related algae; occurs in bundles of thin translucent agglutinated membranes, of yellowish or brownish white color, brittle if dry and tough when wet; has faint odor and mucilaginous taste; is insoluble in cold water, slowly soluble in boiling water, yielding a stiff jelly on cooling.

Action: Stimulates intestinal peristalsis by its bulk; is non-irritating and non-toxic.

Uses: In constipation and diarrhea.

Supply: AGAR—Powder (C.A.)—Cartons of ¼ lb. and 1 lb.
AGAR—Shreds (C.A.)—In papers of 1 lb.

Administration: 1–4 dr. (4–15 Gm); average dose, 2 dr. (8 Gm), taken with plenty of water between meals; may be added to dough in the making of bread, biscuits, cakes.

AGAR-AGAR

Laxative

Description: A palatable form of agar-agar with a fruity taste.

Action and Uses: Stimulates peristalsis by absorbing fluid and expanding in bulk; *for use* as laxative in constipation.

Supply: AGAR-AGAR—Tins of ½ and 1 lb. (Chicago Dietetic)
AGAR-AGAR—Canisters 4 oz., 1 lb. (Schieffelin)

Administration: 1 teaspoonful to 1 tablespoonful as required; taken dry or in food.

AGOMENSIN (Ciba)

Hormone Therapy

Description: An aqueous preparation of corpus luteum, physiologically assayed on isolated smooth muscle.

Action: Induces hyperemia of female genitalia, stimulating their functional activity and increasing ovarian estrus producing hormone.

Uses: *Indicated* in cases of ovarian hypofunction, where the organs are structurally normal: In functional amenorrhea, oligomenorrhea, sterility; in various nervous manifestations associated with ovarian dysfunction.

Supply: AGOMENSIN—Tablets gr ⅓ (0.02 Gm), sugar coated—Bottles of 20 and 100.
AGOMENSIN—Ampules gr ¾ (0.04 Gm), in sterile aqueous solution—Cartons of 5 and 20 ampules.

Administration: *Oral*—1–3 tablets three times daily, supplemented by an ampule hypodermically every other day.
Subcutaneous and Intramuscular—1–4 ampules every second or third day, with 2 tablets three times daily orally on intervening days.

Bibliography: *See Chap. XII.*

AGURIN (Winthrop)

Diuretic

Chemical Name: Theobromine Sodium Acetate.

Formula: $NaC_7H_7O_2N_4 + NaC_2H_3O_2$.

Description: A white, hygroscopic, finely crystalline powder; bitter, odorless, alkaline; easily soluble in hot water, less soluble in cold; soluble in alcohol.

Action: An efficient diuretic.

Uses: In myocardial degenerative diseases, nephritis, dropsy, hepatic cirrhosis with edema.

Incompatibles: Acids, iron chloride, mercury chloride, silver nitrate, magnesia, lead acetate, tartar emetic and alkaloids.

Supply: AGURIN (C.A.)—Bottles 25 Gm.

Administration: 8–15 gr (0.5–1 Gm) in capsules, two to three times daily after meals.

Caution: Must be kept in well-stoppered bottle.

ALBOLENE (McKesson and Robbins)

Lubricant

Description: A very pure, palatable medicinal grade Russian Mineral Oil.

Action and Uses: *For use* as intestinal lubricant in spastic and other forms of chronic constipation.

Supply: ALBOLENE—Bottles 1, 4 and 16 oz.

Administration: 1–4 tablespoonfuls at bedtime.

ALLOCHRYSINE (Anglo-French)

Phthisis Therapy

Chemical Name: Double thiopropanol sulphonate of gold and sodium.

Formula: $CH_2S.\ Au.\ CHOH.\ CH_2SO_3Na$.

Composition: Contains 35% by weight of gold.

Action and Uses: Is stated to decrease fever, cough, expectoration and improve the general condition in tuberculosis; is claimed to cause no serious reactions, except an occasional erythema or pruritus.

Supply: ALLOCHRYSINE—Ampules 2 cc, containing 0.05, 0.1 and 0.2 Gm of Allochrysine, with Ampule 8 cc artificial serum—Boxes of 1 ampule of each for 1 single injection.

Administration: *Intramuscularly*—Content of 2 cc ampule mixed with 8 cc of the artificial serum, once or twice weekly for 10–15 weeks.

ALLONAL (Roche)

Hypnotic. Analgesic

Description: Allyl-isopropyl-barbituric acid, chemically fused with phenyl-dimethyl-dimethyl-amino-pyrazolon (amidopyrine U.S.P.) in proportions 1:1⅔.

Action: A non-narcotic sedative and hypnotic with the beneficial effects of morphine; in therapeutic dosage is not depressant to heart or respiration, and has no deleterious action on other organs; even in massive dosage post-hypnotic effects are transient, due to its rapid oxidation and elimination of the hypnotic component.

Uses: As sedative, hypnotic and analgesic in all conditions where such therapy is desired; in various types of insomnia, especially when due to pain; as adjunct to general, local and injection anesthesia; to counteract the by-effects of cocaine and other local anesthetics.

Supply: ALLONAL—Tablets, 2⅔ gr (0.170 Gm)—Boxes of 12 and 50.

Administration: 1 or 2 tablets in milder cases of insomnia or pain; in severer types a third tablet may be given an hour or two after the first dose; in ambulatory cases, only 1 tablet. In disturbing night cough, a tablet on retiring has a soothing effect and promotes sleep; in severely painful chronic conditions, 4 or 5 tablets a day usually suffice to give relief; still larger doses may be employed in tic douloureux, in inoperable carcinoma, in tabes.

ALPHA LOBELIN (Bischoff)

Respiratory Stimulant

Description: The hydrochloride of a crystalline alkaloid isolated from Lobelia inflata; occurs in colorless needles, readily soluble in water.

Formula: $C_{21}H_{23}NO_2$. HCl.

Action: A direct respiratory stimulant; a safe, prompt and efficient resuscitant in asphyxia.

Uses: Asphyxia neonatorum, anesthesia accidents, surgical shock, collapse, de-etherization, drowning, electrical shock, heat prostration; also in poisoning by alcohol, cyanide, cannabis indica, morphine, carbon monoxide, scopolamin, chloral, veronal, cocaine.

Supply: ALPHA LOBELIN—Ampules, 1 cc—Infant, gr 1/20 (0.003 Gm)—Boxes 6, 12 and 100.

ALPHA LOBELIN—Ampules, 1 cc—Adult, gr 3/20 (0.01 Gm)—Boxes 6, 12 and 100.

Administration: In the newborn, after clearing respiratory passages of mucus, ½-ampule is injected *intravenously* into the umbilical vein, with the infant's head downward; *intramuscularly*—1 ampule.

Adults—*Intramuscularly or subcutaneously* ¼ gr (0.015 Gm); *intravenously*—1/13-⅙ gr (0.0045-0.009 Gm).

Bibliography: *See Chap. XII.*

ALPHOZONE (Stearns)

Germicide

Chemical Name: Succinic Peroxide.

Formula: $(COOH.\ CH_2CH_2CO)_2O_2$.

Description: An organic peroxide prepared from Succinic acid and Hydrogen Peroxide; a white, fluffy, crystalline, water soluble powder; odorless and of metallic taste; stable, non-explosive.

Action: Non-corrosive, non-astringent antiseptic and disinfectant; does not coagulate albumin nor effervesce when in contact with pus.

Uses: As mouth wash, vaginal douche, irrigation and wet dressing.

Supply: ALPHOZONE—Tablets, 1 gr (0.064 Gm), Soluble—Bottles of 60.

ALPHOZONE—Powder—Vials of ½ oz.

Administration: For irrigation, douching, mouth wash or gargle, 1:1,000-1:250 solutions.

As topical antiseptic for abrasions, burns, dentures, 1:500-1:250 solutions.

As deodorant and disinfectant 1:500-1:250 solutions.

For wet dressings 1:500-1:250 solutions.

As dusting powder is mixed with talcum or boric acid, 1:20.

Caution: Solutions must be freshly prepared; 1 tablet or 1 gr (0.064 Gm) of powder in 1 oz. of water makes a 1:500 solution.

ALUCOL (Wander)

Antacid

Composition: Colloidal Aluminum Hydroxide.

Action and Uses: Adsorbs gastric hydrochloric acid and forms a colloidal gel; is soothing and protective to gastric mucosa; does not cause systemic alkalization; *For use* in gastric hyperacidity and hypersecretion, acid dyspepsia, peptic ulcer and gastric neuroses.

Supply: ALUCOL—Tablets, gr 7½ (0.49 Gm)—Boxes of 60.

ALUCOL—Powder—Boxes of 100 Gm.

Administration: 2 tablets, or 15 gr of powder, 20 min. after meals; repeated in 20 min. where necessary; tablets should be thoroughly masticated; powder may be mixed with small quantity of water.

Bibliography: *See Chap. XII.*

ALUMNOL (Metz)

Astringent. Antiseptic

Chemical Name: Aluminium Betanaphthol Disulphonate.

Formula: $Al_2[C_{10}H_5OH.\ (SO_3)_2]_3$.

Description: A fine, nearly white, non-hygroscopic powder; soluble in 1½ parts of water and glycerin, sparingly soluble in alcohol, insoluble in ether; slightly fluorescent in aqueous solution; darkens upon exposure to air.

Action: An active astringent; retards growth of pathogenic bacteria; in dilute solutions is non-irritating, in high concentrations is caustic.

Incompatibles: Is decomposed by silver and other reducible salts; by alkalies and ammoniacal compounds.

Supply: ALUMNOL (C.A.)—Powder—Bottles of 1 ounce.

Uses and Dosage: Surgery—In 0.5–3 % solutions, as mild antiseptic and irrigant; as caustic—10–20 % solutions.

Gynecology—As douche—2–5 % solutions; pessaries—5 %; gauze dressings—5 %.

Otolaryngology—Topically, in powder form or in ½ to 1 % aqueous solution, in purulent otitis; for irrigation, gargling or douche in nasopharyngeal catarrh.

Dermatology—For erosions, ulcerations, ulcus molle, abscesses, eczema, acne sycosis, favus, erythema exudativa, prurigo, either the pure powder or a mixture with equal parts of French chalk and starch up to 10 %; also as 5 % aqueous solution, 2½–10 % alcoholic solution and as 2½–20 % lanolin ointment.

ALURATE (Roche)

Hypnotic

Chemical Name: Allyl-isopropyl-barbituric acid.

Formula: $C_3H_5.\ C_3H_7.\ C.\ (CO)_2.\ (NH)_2.\ CO$.

Description: Is of high lipoid solubility and correspondingly of prompt and definite action.

Action: Induces sedation and restful recuperative sleep quickly, smoothly and with a greater degree of safety than the official barbiturates.

Uses: In insomnia and the milder forms of nervous excitation; in the more severe types of psychoses that require hospitalization; as a sedative in cough, convulsions, chorea, restlessness of fever; in spastic conditions and general nervous irritability, hysteria, menstrual and menopausal psychoses, alcoholism.

Advantages: Has about five times the hypnotic efficiency of diethylbarbituric acid, but is claimed to be relatively less toxic; is almost completely (over 80%) oxidized and the rest rapidly eliminated; because of rapid elimination, the sleep induced is not unduly prolonged nor followed on the next day by drowsiness.

Supply: ALURATE—Tablets, 1 gr (0.064 Gm), scored to permit of smaller dosage—Tubes of 12—Vials of 50.

ALURATE—Elixir—each fluidram containing ½ gr (0.032 Gm) Alurate in a palatable elixir—Bottles of 6 oz.

ALURATE—Injectable—Ampules 2.2 cc, each cc containing 0.1 Gm Alurate—Boxes of 6 ampules.

Administration: *Tablets*—In mild cases of insomnia—1 tablet at bedtime; obstinate cases, 2 tablets; taken with either a hot or cold drink.

Elixir—Sedative, ½–1 teaspoonful, three times a day in wineglassful of water; hypnotic, 2–4 teaspoonfuls. Children, according to age.

Injectable—In conditions where the value of injectable barbiturates has been definitely established, as in psychiatry and pre-anesthetic sedation in surgery and obstetrics.

ALYPIN (Winthrop)

Local Anesthetic

Chemical Name: Monohydrochloride of benzoyl 1, 3 tetramethyldiamino-2-ethyl-isopropyl alcohol. Brand of Benzopropyl.

Formula: $CH_3CH_2C(C_6H_5COO)[CH_2N(CH_3)_2]. CH_2N: (CH_3)_2. HCl$.

Description: A white, crystalline, bitter tasting powder, odorless and hygroscopic; readily soluble in water, alcohol and chloroform, insoluble in ether; is stable only in 2–4% solutions.

Action: Equally as efficient as cocaine, but less toxic and less mydriatic.

Uses: Urology—For topical application, as in cystoscopy, 1–4%.

Ophthalmology—2–4%.

Rhinolaryngology—5–10%.

Caution: Solutions should be freshly prepared; may be sterilized by boiling for 5 min.; epinephrine preparations may be added where desired.

Supply: ALYPIN (C.A.)—Tablets, ⅓ gr (0.02 Gm)—Tubes of 20.

ALYPIN (C.A.)—Powder—Bottles ¼ oz.

Advantages: Does not affect vision in eye applications.

Bibliography: *See Chap. XII.*

AMARBITAL (Kretschmar)

Hypnotic. Analgesic

Chemical Name: Dimethylaminophenyldimethylpyrazolon Diethylmalonylurea Phenylethylbarbituric acid.

Action and Uses: Sedative, hypnotic, analgesic; non-habit forming, non-depressant; *For use* in relief of headache, neuralgia, sciatica, neuritis, hysteria, eye strain; in dysmenorrhea, tabetic crises, trauma, insomnia due to pain; in pre- and postoperative dentistry.

Supply: AMARBITAL—Tablets gr 2½ (0.16 Gm)—Tubes of 12—Vials of 100.

Administration: 1–2 tablets, as required.

AMATIN (Winthrop)

Antipyretic. Analgesic

Chemical Name: Acetylmetacresotinic Acid. Brand of Metocyl.

Description: White crystals, soluble in alcohol and ether, sparingly soluble in water.

Action: As for acetyl salicylic acid but without its by-effects; is analgesic and antipyretic; is quickly eliminated and does not affect the kidneys, gastro-intestinal tract nor induce profuse sweating.

Uses: In headaches, various neuralgias, early stages of colds and influenza, fevers, tonsillitis, rheumatic affections and lumbago.

Supply: AMATIN—Tablets, 5 gr (0.3 Gm)—Tubes of 10—Bottles 100.

Administration: 1–3 tablets (5–15 gr) three times daily. Children according to age.

AMBAZIN (Farastan)

Urinary Antiseptic

Chemical Name: Sodium salt of diphenyl-disazo-ethoxyamino-phenol-aminobenzoic acid plus hydroxyquinoline sulfate.

Description: A brownish-yellow powder.

Action and Uses: Highly bactericidal and bacteriostatic; a non-irritating, non-toxic, and non-staining urinary antiseptic; *For use* in gonorrheal urethritis, cystitis, pyelitis and other affections of the urinary tract.

Supply: AMBAZIN—Capsules, 3 gr (0.2 Gm)—Boxes of 42.

Administration: 1 capsule three times daily.

Bibliography: *See Chap. XII.*

AMFETIN (Lilly)

Cell Proliferant

Description: A stable, sterile solution of a purified concentrated fraction of Bovine Amniotic Fluid; is isotonic, non-toxic, non-anaphylactic.

Action: Stimulates the defense mechanism of serous surfaces and local peritoneal factors of immunity; accelerates repair by promoting rapid formation of a plastic exudate rich in fibrin and phagocytes; hastens postoperative convalescence.

Uses: For instillation into the peritoneal cavity after abdominal operations.

Advantages: Diminishes postoperative nausea and distention; favors early return of intestinal peristalsis; reduces local tenderness and distress.

Supply: AMFETIN—Ampules, 50 cc—Packages of 6 or 25, individually packed.
AMFETIN—Bottles, rubber stoppered, 200 cc.

Administration: 50–200 cc introduced at body temperature into peritoneal cavity by syringe and catheter through last stitch before closing abdomen.

Bibliography: *See Chap. XII.*

AMINOPHYLLIN

Diuretic. Cardiotonic

Chemical Name: Theophylline Ethylenediamine.

Formula: $(CH_2.NH_2)_2C_7H_8N_4O_2 + (CH_2NH_2)_2(C_7H_8N_4O_2)_2$.

Description: A white or slightly yellow crystalline powder, of ammoniacal odor; readily soluble in water; contains about 75% Theophylline and 25% Ethylenediamine.

Action and Uses: Is more soluble than most other xanthine derivatives and thus more readily absorbed and more prompt in action; is an effective diuretic, vasodilator, cardiostimulant; increases perfusion rate of heart. *Indicated* in hypertension, in coronary disease and angina pectoris to relieve pain and dyspnea; in renal insufficiency, uremia and to promote diuresis in general.

Supply: **AMINOPHYLLIN** (C.A.)—Tablets, gr 1½ (0.1 Gm)—Tubes of 20. **(Pharmedic)**

AMINOPHYLLIN (C.A.)—Ampules, 2 cc gr. 7½ (0.48 Gm)—Boxes of 6. Ampules 10 cc (0.24 Gm), Intravenous—Boxes of 5. **(Pharmedic)**

AMINOPHYLLIN (C.A.)—Suppositories, gr 5 (0.36 Gm)—Tubes of 12. **(Pharmedic)**

AMINOPHYLLIN (C.A.)—Ampules, 2 cc gr 7½ (0.48 Gm) Intramuscular—Boxes of 6, 25 and 100. **(Searle)**

AMINOPHYLLIN (C.A.)—Ampules, 10 cc gr 4 (0.24 Gm) Intravenous—Boxes of 6, 25 and 100. **(Searle)**

AMINOPHYLLIN (C.A.)—Tablets, gr 1½ (0.1 Gm) Oral—Bottles 100—Vials 20 (6 vials to package). **(Searle)**

Administration: *Oral*—1–2 tablets in water three to four times daily after meals.
Hypodermic—1–3 ampules daily, intramuscularly or intravenously, where oral therapy is not feasible.
Rectal—2–4 suppositories daily; or 3–4 tablets, dissolved in warm water, given as retention enema.

Bibliography: *See Chap. XII.*

AMIODOXYL BENZOATE

Antiarthritic

Chemical Name: Ammonium Orthoiodoxybenzoate.

Formula: $C_6H_4(IO_2)COONH_4$.

Description: A white, crystalline, odorless powder of somewhat bitter taste; soluble in water, slightly soluble in alcohol, insoluble in ether, benzene and common organic solvents; contains about 43% iodine.

Action: A germicidal and oxidizing agent; depresses the sympathetic system and stimulates phagocytosis and immunity.

Uses: In all forms of acute and chronic arthritis, infectious, hypertrophic and gonorrheal.

Supply: **AMIODOXYL BENZOATE**—Vials, 1 Gm—Boxes of 10. **(Abbott)**

AMIODOXYL BENZOATE—Bottles 50 Gm. **(Abbott)**

AMIODOXYL BENZOATE—Vials, 1 Gm—Boxes of 6. (Burnham)

AMIODOXYL BENZOATE—Bottles of 1 oz. (Burnham)

Administration: *Intravenously*—By gravity method, 0.75–1 Gm in 100 cc sterile saline, administered slowly in from 7–12 min., and followed by saline; twice weekly for 5–10 injections.

Orally—As calcium salt, calciodoxyl benzoate, 1.5–3 Gm.

Rectally—2–3 Gm, dissolved in 3–4 oz. of water as retention enema; to be retained for 2 hr. or longer.

Caution: To avoid explosion, must not be overheated or exposed to flame; to prevent deterioration must be kept in the dark and dry.

Bibliography: *See Chap. XII.*

AMI-SALOX (Summers)

Analgesic

Chemical Name: A Pyruvic Acid derivative of Methylene-Dibenzal-Disalicyl amide.

Formula: $C_{35}H_{26}O_8N_2$.

Action and Uses: An antiseptic, analgesic and uric acid eliminant; also a cholagogue laxative; does not affect cardio-renal system. *Recommended* in infectious arthritis, rheumatism, gout and neuralgia; also as cholagogue in hepatic and gall bladder disease.

Supply: **AMI-SALOX**—Tablets, gr 5—Boxes of 100.

AMI-SALOX—Capsules, gr 5—Boxes of 100.

AMI-SALOX—Powder—Boxes of 2 oz.

Administration: 10–30 gr every 3–4 hr.

Incompatibles: Not to be used with alkaline substances.

Advantages: Insoluble in stomach, eliminating distress usually accompanying the use of salicylates.

Bibliography: *See Chap. XII.*

AMNIOTIN (Squibb)

Hormone Therapy

Description: An estrus inducing, ovarian follicular hormone, prepared from fetal fluid of cattle and physiologically standardized and tested; a stable, sterile, aqueous solution, highly purified; free from proteins, higher fats, cholesterol, phospho-lipins, pigment impurities or disagreeable odor; contains also phenol 0.5% and sodium chloride 0.8%; pH 5.5.

Action: Induces menstrual bleeding in hormonal deficiencies without affecting blood pressure; is non-toxic and non-irritating in one hundred times the usual dosage.

Uses: Indicated in cases after ovariectomy, in senile ovarian atrophy, in menopausal disturbances and arthritis, in involutional psychoses and hemophilia.

Supply: **AMNIOTIN**—Hypodermic—Vials 10 cc, each cc containing 50 rat units, in 50% ethylene or propylene glycol.

AMNIOTIN—Oral—Vials 5 cc with dropper, each cc containing 400 rat units, in corn oil, 1 drop equal to 10 units.

AMNIOTIN—Pessaries—Each pessary equals 75 rat units—Packages of 6 and 12.

Administration: In recent menopause—Amniotin Hypodermic, 1 cc, *subcutaneously*, two or three times weekly, or 10 drops Amniotin Oral twice daily, or 3 pessaries a week.

In long existing menopause—Amniotin Hypodermic, 1 to 2 cc on alternate days, or 15 drops Amniotin Oral three times daily, or 1 pessary daily.

In dysmenorrhea—Beginning 15 days before menstrual onset, 1 cc every other day for 3 to 4 doses; 10 drops twice daily or 1 pessary daily for 6–8 days.

Pessary is inserted into vagina; douching is to be avoided.

Bibliography: *See Chap. XII.*

AMPACOIDS (Reed and Carnrick)

Endocrine Therapy

Description: Sterile, isotonic, aqueous solutions of active hormonal principles prepared for hypodermic use; standardized and refined.

Action and Uses: AMPACOIDS OVARY—Each contains ovarian hormones equivalent to 15 gr of fresh ovary, associated with estrogenic hormone from prenatal urine; represents 25 rat units. *For use* in amenorrhea, dysmenorrhea, sexual neurasthenia and other forms of hypovarianism.

AMPACOIDS TESTICLE—Each cc represents 31 gr (2 Gm) fresh testicular substance. *For use* in impotence, sexual neurasthenia and other forms of hypogonadism.

AMPACOIDS PROSTATE—Each cc represents 10 gr (0.65 Gm) fresh prostatic substance. *For use* in prostatic hypertrophy, certain forms of impotence, and neurasthenia.

Supply:

AMPACOIDS OVARY 25 Units—Ampules 1 cc—Boxes of 6.

AMPACOIDS TESTICLE—Ampules 1 cc—Boxes of 6.

AMPACOIDS PROSTATE—Ampules 1 cc—Boxes of 6.

Administration: *Subcutaneously* or *intramuscularly*—1 ampule three to six times weekly; more frequently where required.

AMPULE GLUCOSE

Nutrient

Description: A dextrose preparation for intravenous use.

Action: Supplies nutrition and energy without risk of gastric upset; combats acidosis, protects the liver, conserves body tissues; reduces toxemia, promotes diuresis, corrects dehydration and low blood sugar.

Uses: In surgical acidosis or shock, toxemia of pregnancy, infectious diseases, certain diseases of the heart, skin and liver, hypoglycemia and cerebral edema.

Supply: COLLOSOL TRANSFUSION GLUCOSE—5 %, 10 %, 20 %, 50 % and 5 % in normal saline—Bottles of 20 oz. (Crookes)

AMPULE GLUCOSE (C.A.)—20 cc 10 Gm; Buffered; 1/10 % cresol as preservative—Boxes 6, 25 and 100. (Lilly)

AMPULE GLUCOSE (C.A.)—50 cc 25 Gm; Buffer ampule separate; no preservative—Boxes 6, 25 and 100 (Lilly)

AMPULE GLUCOSE (C.A.)—50 cc 25 Gm; Unbuffered; no preservative —Boxes 6, 25 and 100. (Lilly)

AMPULE GLUCOSE (C.A.)—50 cc 25 Gm; Buffered; no preservative—Boxes 6, 25, and 100. (Lilly)

AMPULE GLUCOSE (C.A.)—100 cc 50 Gm; Buffer ampule separate; no preservative—Boxes 6, 25 and 100. (Lilly)

Administration: *Intravenously*—Slowly; in dosages as indicated.

Advantages: Ready for use; keeps indefinitely; sterile; contains no pyrogen; desirable because of chemical purity and sterile state.

AMPYDIN (National Aniline)

Analgesic

Chemical Name: Dimethyl-amino-phenyl dimethyl pyrazolon. Amidopyrine.

Formula: $C_6H_5N. CO. C(N[CH_3]_2): C(CH_3). N. CH_3.$

Description: Small colorless glistening crystals; soluble in 15 parts of water, alcohol and benzene.

Action and Uses: Antipyretic and analgesic; more effective than antipyrine and free from gastro-intestinal and cardiovascular disturbances; *For use* in fevers, neuralgia, neuritis, sciatica; in intestinal spasm, migraine, headache, dysmenorrhea, gastralgia, influenza.

Supply: AMPYDIN—Tablets gr 5 (0.324 Gm)—Bottles of 10, 100, 500.

AMPYDIN—Crystals—Packages of 1 oz.

Administration: Gr 5 (0.324 Gm), repeated as frequently as necessary where pain is persistent. In fever, 1 tablet in 24 hr.

Bibliography: *See Chap. XII.*

AMYLSOL (Sutliff and Case)

Urinary Antiseptic

Formula: $C_{11}H_{16}O_2$.

Description: A derivative of resorcinol.

Action and Uses: A urinary antiseptic in urethritis, cystitis, pyelitis.

Supply: AMYLSOL—Capsules, containing, Amylsol 2 gr (0.13 Gm), Olive Oil 6 gr (0.39 Gm)—Bottles of 100, 500.

Administration: 1 capsule three times daily, with meals; increased slowly to the limit of tolerance; maximum 12 capsules daily.

Bibliography: *See Chap. XII.*

AMYTAL (Lilly)

Sedative. Hypnotic

Chemical Name: Iso-amyl-ethyl-barbituric Acid; Iso-amyl-ethyl Malonylurea.

Formula: $C_5H_{11}(C_2H_5)C(CONH)_2CO.$

Description: A white, crystalline, odorless powder of slightly bitter taste; soluble in alcohol and ether, not readily soluble in cold water; forms freely soluble salts with alkalies.

Action: Sedative, hypnotic and antispasmodic; allays restlessness, insomnia and apprehension; reduces toxicity of local anesthetics, of morphine and cocaine types.

Uses: In nervousness and simple insomnia due to worry, fatigue, alcoholism, drug addiction, pregnancy, menopause and menstrual disturbances; in hyperthyroidism, neurasthenia, acute infections and preceding operations.

Advantages: Effective with wide margin of safety; is relatively free from after effects and less cumulative than barbital or phenobarbital; is not eliminated through the kidneys.

Supply: **AMYTAL**—Tablets (C.A.) gr ¾ (0.048 Gm), gr 1½ (0.1 Gm)—Bottles of 40 and 500.

AMYTAL—Crystals—Vials of ½ oz.

Administration: As Hypnotic—1 or 2 tablets, with plenty of water or hot milk, ½–1 hour before bedtime.
As Sedative—¾–1½ gr two or three times daily.

Bibliography: *See Chap. XII.*

ANABOLIN (Harrower)

Hormone Therapy

Description: A light buff-colored powder, easily soluble in water; prepared from liver by fractional solution; is physiologically standardized, 1 gr of the extract to reduce arterial tension in a 10 Kg dog 12 mm; has traces of histamine but no choline.

Action and Uses: Reduces hypertension through its detoxication stimulus on the liver and through endocrine catalysis; increases uric acid and ammonia elimination; *For use* in toxic functional hypertension and hypertension of menopause; is of limited value in kidney sclerosis and compensating hypertension.

Caution: Contraindicated in renal insufficiency.

Supply: **ANABOLIN**—Tablets—Vials of 15—Bottles of 50.

ANABOLIN—Solution—Ampules 1 cc for intravenous injection, daily or every second day—Boxes of 5.

ANABOLIN—Solution Fortior—Ampules 1 cc double strength, for hypodermic use—Boxes of 5.

Administration: 1 tablet three times daily.

ANASTIL (Cavendish)

Expectorant

Description: Contains Guaiacol in aqueous solution; a clear, light yellow, strongly odorous liquid, of weak alkaline reaction.

Action and Uses: A deodorant expectorant and antiseptic in bronchial affections, bronchiectasis, tuberculosis, pulmonary gangrene and abscess; in grippe and pneumonia.

Contraindications: Hemoptysis and blood dyscrasias.

Supply: **ANASTIL**—Plain (containing 0.05 gr Guaiacol)—Ampules 1 cc—Boxes of 6 and 10.

ANASTIL—Reinforced (containing 0.075 gr Guaiacol)—Ampules 1 cc—Boxes of 3 and 6.

Administration: *Intramuscularly*—1 cc (with novocain) every 2 or 3 days.
Intravenously—1 cc in 3–5 cc saline, injected slowly, every 2 or 3 days.
Children 0.5 cc for 6–25 injections.

Bibliography: *See Chap. XII.*

ANAYODIN (Bischoff)

Amebacide

Chemical Name: Iodoxy-quinolin Sulphonic Acid.

Formula: $C_9H_7N. HSO_3. HI. OH.$

Description: A fine crystalline, light yellow powder, soluble in water up to 4%; iodine content—28%.

Action: Is destructive to amebae of dysentery; penetrates tissues readily; does not coagulate proteins; is well tolerated and non-irritating to kidneys, being eliminated unchanged.

Uses: In acute, chronic and relapsing amebic dysentery; also in colitis of other etiology.

Supply: **ANAYODIN**—Pills, gr 4 (0.25 Gm)—Bottles of 100.

ANAYODIN—Powder—Bottles of 25 and 100 Gm.

Administration: **Acute amebiasis**—Oral therapy only; 4 pills three times daily before meals for 8 days, followed by rest period of 10 days; course repeated until relieved, increasing to 8 pills three times daily if necessary.

Chronic amebiasis—Oral therapy preferred and administered as in acute; in protracted and more serious cases enemas are added, consisting of 200–300 cc of tepid 1½–3% solutions of Anayodin, administered after cleansing enema, for 6–8 evenings; rest period of 6 days with 3 pills orally daily during such period; course repeated where demanded.

Hospitalized cases—Are given, in addition, duodenal instillations through Rehfuss tube of 1,000 cc warm hypertonic saline, followed after 30 min. by 200–300 cc 1–2% Anayodin warm solution; given semiweekly for 4 weeks.

Colitis—1 pill three times daily for 30 days; rest period of 7 days; course repeated where demanded.

Hepatic Abscess—In combination with Activin injections.

Bacillary Dysentery—4 pills daily.

Preparation: Solution is prepared by heating the distilled water to the boiling point and allowing it to cool to 80°C or 176°F. At this temperature the required amount of Anayodin is slowly added when effervescence takes place with the evolution of carbon dioxide. After cooling to body temperature the solution is ready for use.

Bibliography: *See Chap. XII.*

ANESTHESIN

Topical Analgesic

Chemical Name: Ethyl Aminobenzoate; also known as Parathesin.

Formula: $C_6H_4. NH_2. COO. C_2H_5.$

Description: A white, crystalline powder, insoluble in water, but slightly soluble in oils, also alcohol, chloroform and ether; is odorless and tasteless.

Action: A topical analgesic like cocaine, promptly benumbing the part to which applied, exercising its superficial effect almost entirely upon peripheral nerve-endings; is non-irritating and non-toxic.

Uses: As dusting powder—for painful leg ulcers and painful postoperative wounds; as ointment in pruritus ani and vulvae and general prurigo; as suppository—in hemorrhoids, fissures and similar lesions; in oily solution—to facilitate urethral sounding, for spraying catarrhal throat and nasal passages, for earache; internally in gastric ulcer, gastralgia, vomiting of pregnancy and seasickness.

Supply: **ANESTHESIN**—Powder (C.A.)—Packages of 5 Gm and 1 oz. **(Abbott)**

ANESTHESIN—Powder—Vials 5 Gm—Bottles of 1 oz. **(Metz)**

Combinations: ANESTHESIN-CALCIDIN—Troches—for throat irritation; contains Anesthesin gr ¼ (0.016 Gm), Calcidin gr ⅓ (0.021 Gm), Licorice and Aromatics—Bottles 100 and 1,000. **(Abbott)**

ANESTHESIN AND CERIUM OXALATE COMPOUND—Tablets—Bottles 100 and 1,000. **(Abbott)**

ANESKREME—Tubes of ½ and 1 oz. **(Abbott)**

ANESPRAY—Bottles of 4 oz. **(Abbott)**

Administration: *Internally*—5–8 gr (0.324–0.512 Gm) two or three times daily after meals.

Externally—As dusting powder 10%; as ointment 4–10%; as suppository gr 3 (0.194 Gm) rectally or vaginally; as spray—3% or topically (1–2 parts of mucilage) in nose and throat applications.

ANTERI-COLE (Cole)

Hormone Therapy

Description: A solution of Anterior Pituitary sex hormones extracted from fresh gland; is physiologically standardized, each cc representing 100 mouse units (Zondek-Aschheim standardization); stable and potent for 6–9 months.

Action and Uses: Contains the follicle maturing and luteinizing hormones. *For use* in secondary amenorrhea, functional dysmenorrhea, menorrhagia, ovarian hypofunction and climacteric disturbances.

Supply: ANTERI-COLE—Ampules 5 and 15 cc—Box of 6.

Administration: 1 cc (100 mouse units) injected *subcutaneously* once or twice daily for 8–10 days following menstrual period, not during postovulation stage; in hemorrhagic states is continued until bleeding stops. In frigidity—1 injection daily for 3 or 4 days, then twice weekly for 10 doses.

ANTICOL (Mulford Colloid)

Parasiticide

Description: Occurs as lustrous, dark brown, non-hygroscopic scales, readily soluble in water; contains 20–25% of antimony.

Action and Uses: A stable, non-irritating preparation of Colloidal Antimony, easily absorbed and assimilated; germicide and parasiticide; does not cause precipitation of tissue fluids, is slowly eliminated and has prolonged action. *For use* in coccogenic infections: abscesses, boils, impetigo; also in bilharzia, leishmaniasis, kala-azar.

Supply: ANTICOL—Vials, Gm 10.

ANTICOL—Solution, 10%—Bottles of 25 cc.

Administration: *Oral*—½–5 gr (0.032 to 0.324 Gm).

Hypodermic—¼–3 cc.

ANTIDOLORIN (Hamilton)

Local Anesthetic

Chemical Name: Ethyl Chloride U.S.P.

Formula: C_2H_5Cl.

Description: A haloid ester of alcohol; at room temperature is a stable, colorless gas, of sweet ethereal odor; when cooled, condenses to a colorless mobile inflammable liquid.

Action and Uses: Evaporates rapidly and produces a freezing and benumbing effect upon the sensory nerves of applied area. *For use* as local anesthetic—by refrigeration when applied as vaporized spray, in abscesses, carbuncles, felons, subcutaneous tumors and other surgical affections; in dental extractions or minor oral procedures; as general anesthetic—by inhalation, for short operations, reducing the time required for complete anesthesia; as preliminary or adjuvant to ether or chloroform narcosis, reducing the quantities otherwise required.

Contraindications: Obstruction in air passages, valvular or myocardial disease of the heart.

Supply: **ANTIDOLORIN**—Metal Tubes 100 cc, with needle valve.

ANTIDOLORIN—Metal Automatic Tubes, 100 cc.

ANTIDOLORIN—Glass Automatic Syphon Tubes, 100 Gm.

ANTIDOLORIN—Glass Automatic Tubes 10, 30, 60, 100 Gm.

Administration: *Local*—By direct spray till part is blanched.

General—By inhalation from anesthesia mask on which the narcotic is sprayed.

ANTIFEBRIN (Burroughs Wellcome)

Antipyretic

Chemical Name: Acetanilid.

Formula: $CH_3CO.\ NH.\ C_6H_5$.

Description: A white, crystalline, sublimable solid.

Action: Antipyretic, powerful analgesic; overdosage causes toxic action on heart muscle with cyanosis and skin eruption; depresses nervous system.

Uses: To lower temperature in febrile diseases, to relieve pain in neuralgia, migraine, sciatica, dysmenorrhea and crises of locomotor ataxia.

Supply: **TABLOID ANTIFEBRIN**—Gr 5 (0.324 Gm)—Bottles of 25, 100 and 500.

Combinations: **TABLOID ANTIFEBRIN COMPOUND**—Containing Antifebrin gr 2 (0.130 Gm), Camphor Monobromate gr 1 (0.065 Gm), Caffein Citrate gr 1 (0.065 Gm)—Bottles of 100 and 500 tablets.

TABLOID QUININE COMPOUND—Containing Cinchona alkaloids gr 1 (0.065 Gm), Antifebrin gr 1⅕ (0.078 Gm), Camphor Monobromate gr ¼ (0.013 Gm), Pulv. Ipecac gr ⅛ (0.008 Gm), Ext. Cascara Sagrada gr ¼ (0.016 Gm)—Bottles of 100 and 500 tablets.

Administration: **Tabloid Antifebrin**—1 tabloid with water; average dose gr 3 (0.194 Gm).

Tabloid Antifebrin Compound—1 tabloid with little water or permitted to dissolve in mouth; repeated if necessary.

Tabloid Quinine Compound—1 tabloid each hour in early stage of colds, catarrh, infections.

Caution: Antifebrin should be administered with caution.

ANTIMONY SODIUM THIOGLYCOLLATE

(Hynson, Westcott and Dunning)

Trypanosomicide

Formula: $Sb.\ S_2CH_2(COO)_2Na\ CH_2COO$ (with a bracket linking Sb and the terminal COO)

Description: A white, odorless, faintly pinkish powder; very soluble in water, insoluble in alcohol; contains not less than 37 % of antimony; is not stable.

Action: A trypanosomicide.

Uses: Trypanosomiasis, kala azar, filariasis, granuloma inguinale.

Incompatibles: Solutions are incompatible with fixed alkalies.

Supply: ANTIMONY SODIUM THIOGLYCOLLATE (C.A.)—Ampules, 0.5%, 10 cc and 20 cc—Boxes of 12.

Administration: 1½ gr (0.1 Gm), dissolved in 10–20 cc sterile water, *intramuscularly* or *intravenously*, twice weekly for 15–25 injections.

ANTIMONY THIOGLYCOLLAMIDE

(Hynson, Westcott and Dunning)

Trypanosomicide

Chemical Name: A triamide of antimony thioglycollic acid.

Formula: $Sb(S.\ CH_2CO.\ NH_2)_3$.

Description: A white, crystalline, odorless stable powder; soluble in about 200 parts of water, slightly soluble in alcohol, insoluble in ether; contains not less than 30% antimony.

Action and Uses: As for Antimony Sodium Thioglycollate, but is less soluble and rather more toxic; *used* in trypanosomiasis, filariasis, kala azar.

Supply: ANTIMONY THIOGLYCOLLAMIDE (C.A.)—Ampules, 0.4%, 10 cc and 20 cc—Boxes of 12.

Administration: 1–2 grains (0.05–0.1 Gm), dissolved in 10–20 cc of sterile water, *intramuscularly* or *intravenously*, twice weekly for 15–25 injections.

ANTOPHYSIN

(Winthrop)

Hormone Therapy

Chemical Name: Brand of Tuitral; formerly known as Prolan.

Composition: The Anterior Pituitary hormone believed to control the development of genital organs and to regulate menstrual and gestational functions.

Description: A dry, stable powder, soluble in water, insoluble in alcohol or acetone; loses activity upon heating above 80°c or if its pH concentration is changed.

Action and Uses: Effective in ovarian hypofunction, functional amenorrhea and dysmenorrhea; in deficient lutein stimulation, menorrhagia, menopausal disorders; in sterility and infantilism.

Supply: ANTOPHYSIN—Ampules, 100 rat units—Boxes of 5, with 5 ampules of distilled water.

Administration: *Intramuscularly*—Daily, 100–300 rat units, beginning on due date of menstruation and continued for a period of 2 weeks; resumed after 2 weeks' rest.

ANTUITRIN-S

(Parke, Davis)

Hormone Therapy

Description: Is prepared from the urine of pregnant women, from which it is separated by a chemical process; is identical with the sex hormone of the anterior pituitary, as shown by animal comparative tests with glandular extracts.

Action: Induces follicle ripening, luteinization and the usual progestational uterine phenomena, i. e. development of vaginal mucosa, opening of vaginal canal and uterine hypertrophy.

Uses: In menorrhagia, metrorrhagia, functional amenorrhea, oligomenorrhea, delayed puberty and certain forms of functional sterility.

Supply: ANTUITRIN-S—Vials 10 cc, each cc standardized to contain 100 rat units.

Administration: In functional menstrual disorders and hemorrhages 50–200 rat units, *injected* daily until desired results are obtained, or for about 2 weeks; where treatment is to be continued, courses of 100 rat units three times weekly are instituted, with rest periods of several months between courses; best administered during the 10 days immediately preceding each expected menstruation. In amenorrhea and oligomenorrhea—100 rat units, injected three times a week for 2 or 3 weeks, with Theelin, optionally, between courses or simultaneously. In retarded sexual development (male or female) 6 to 8 courses, of fifteen 100 rat units (1 cc) each, may be necessary.

Bibliography: *See Chap. XII.*

AOLAN (Duke)

Non-specific Protein Therapy

Description: A sterile solution of lactalbumin in colloidal form; prepared from cow's milk, free from bacteria and toxins.

Uses: Principally as non-specific protein remedy in gonorrheal complications; in male—to relieve pain in gonorrheal epididymitis, prostatitis, seminal vesiculitis, posterior urethritis, periurethritis; in female—in gonorrheal infections of pelvic organs, salpingitis, endocervicitis and other chronic diseases of the adnexa; also used in puerperal septicemia, thrombophlebitis, gonorrheal arthritis and as provocative in the diagnosis of chronic gonorrheal infection.

Supply: AOLAN—Ampules 1, 5 and 10 cc—Boxes of 5 and 100.

AOLAN—Ampules 25 cc—Boxes of 1.

Administration: *Intradermally*—0.2–0.3 cc, sufficient for two wheals; technique must be carefully observed.

Intramuscularly—Adults 5–10 cc at intervals of 5–6 days.

As provocative—The intradermal method is used; infected areas are examined and secretions studied for the appearance of gonococci 10–24 hr. after injection.

Bibliography: *See Chap. XII.*

APOTHESINE (Parke, Davis)

Local Anesthetic

Chemical Name: Hydrochloride of gamma-diethylamino-propyl cinnamate.

Formula: $(C_2H_5)_2N. (CH_2)_3COO. CH: CH. C_6H_5. HCl.$

Description: Occurs in small, white crystals, odorless, faintly bitter taste; very soluble in water, readily soluble in alcohol, only slightly soluble in ether and acetone; solutions keep indefinitely if protected from light and air.

Action: Local anesthetic of procaine type; effective in injection anesthesia; slow in action, but equal to cocaine on neural contact and less toxic; solutions can be sterilized by boiling.

Uses: For infiltration, injection, nerve block, intraspinal and pressure anesthesia; Internally—in nausea not due to indigestion and in pain of gastric ulcer.

Supply: APOTHESINE (C.A.)—Bottles ½ oz.

APOTHESINE—Solution (C.A.)—1.5%, containing Chloretone 0.5%—Bottles 2 oz.

APOTHESINE—Tablets (C.A.) gr 1¼ (0.080 Gm), 1 tablet makes 1 fl. oz. of a 2% solution—Tubes of 20—Packages of 5 tubes—Bottles of 100.

APOTHESINE—Tablets "B" (C.A.) Hypodermic; contains Apothesine gr 4.8 (0.3 Gm), Adrenalin gr 1/200 (0.0003 Gm) to make 1 cc of a 1% solution, together with Adrenalin 1:100,000—Tubes of 10—Packages of 5 tubes.

APOTHESINE—Tablets, Dental-hypodermic; contains Apothesine gr 1/3 (0.02 Gm), Adrenalin gr 1/2,500 (0.00002 Gm) (Adrenalin 1:40,000); dissolved, 1 tablet in 1 cc of physiologic saline makes a 2% solution—Tubes of 20—Packages of 5 tubes.

APOTHESINE—Tablets, *Oral*—gr 1/2 (0.032 Gm)—Bottles of 100.

APOTHESINE AND ADRENALIN—Tablets (C.A.) Hypodermic; Apothesine gr 3/5 (0.039 Gm) Adrenalin gr 1/1600 (0.00004 Gm); to make 1 fl. dr. of a 1% solution of Apothesine with Adrenalin 1:100,000—Tubes of 20—Packages of 5 tubes.

Administration: *Subcutaneous*—0.5%–2%, with adrenalin, in sterile water or physiologic saline solution.
Spinal—2 cc of 4–6% solution.
Oral—Gr 1/2 (0.03 Gm), as necessary.

ARBUTIN

Diuretic

Official Name: Arbutinum.

Formula: $C_{12}H_{16}O_7 + \frac{1}{2}H_2O$.

Description: A glucoside obtained from leaves of Arctostaphylos Uva Ursi (Bearberry) of the Ericaceae family: occurs in long, colorless, glistening needles, or white odorless bitter-tasting powder; soluble in 8 parts of water, 16 parts of alcohol, insoluble in chloroform and ether.

Action and Uses: Urinary antiseptic and diuretic in cystitis, urethritis, effusions and edema of Bright's disease.

Supply: **ARBUTIN**—Tablets (C.A.) gr 1 (0.064 Gm)—Bottles 100, 1,000 and 5,000. **(Abbott)**

ARBUTIN—Powder (C.A.)—Bottles of 1 oz. **(Abbott)**

ARBUTIN—Powder (C.A.)—Bottles of 1 oz., 1/4 and 1 lb. **(Merck)**

ARBUTIN—Tablets gr 1/2 (0.032 Gm) and gr 1 (0.064 Gm)—Bottles of 1,000. **(Searle)**

Administration: 1 or 2 tablets every 2 hr. in water; or 15–23 gr (1.0–1.5 Gm) three to four times daily.

ARGENTIFORM (Nelson, Baker)

Antiseptic

Chemical Name: Silver Hexamethylenamine.

Description: Occurs as minute colorless crystals or snow-white crystalline powder; is sparingly soluble in water (1:500) and of metallic taste; silver content nearly 35%.

Action and Uses: Non-irritating antiseptic *for use* in genito-urinary and ophthalmic infections.

Supply: **ARGENTIFORM**—Cones, Vaginal, gr 3 (0.162 Gm)—Boxes of 12.

ARGENTIFORM—Ointment, Ophthalmic, 1/5% and 1%—Tubes, pin-point, 1 dr.

ARGENTIFORM—Ointment, Urethral, 1/5% and 1%—Tubes, collapsible, with and without applicator. Small size—2 1/8 in. long—Boxes of 12.

ARGENTIFORM—Pencils, Urethral, gr ¼ (0.016 Gm)—Boxes of 14, 30, 72—Packages of 12.

Administration: By direct application in conditions where silver is indicated.

ARGOCOL (Mulford Colloid)

Antiseptic

Description: Occurs as brilliant non-hygroscopic, black-brown scales, soluble in water; contains 20–25% metallic silver.

Action and Uses: A stable, non-irritating preparation of Colloidal Silver; a readily absorbed and assimilated antiseptic and astringent; does not cause precipitation of tissue fluids; is slowly eliminated and of prolonged action. *Used* where silver therapy is applicable: tonsillitis, conjunctivitis, catarrhal conditions of mucous membranes; in influenza, puerperal sepsis, septicemia, septic ulcers, ringworm, pustular eczema.

Supply: **ARGOCOL**—Vials 10 Gm.

ARGOCOL—Solution 10%—Bottles 25 cc.

ARGOCOL—Ointment 10%—Tubes ½ oz.—Packages of 12.

Administration: *Oral*—1–3 gr (0.064–0.194 Gm).
Hypodermic—¼–6 cc intravenously, daily.
Local—As solution or ointment.

ARGOLAVAL (Doho)

Antiseptic

Chemical Name: Silver hexamethylene-tetramine nitrate.

Formula: $AgC_6H_{12}N_5O_3$.

Action: Combines antiseptic action of silver nitrate with that of hexamethylene-tetramine; a non-irritating, painless antiseptic and astringent.

Supply: **ARGOLAVAL** Liquid (equivalent to 1% silver nitrate)—Bottles of 1 oz., 3 oz. and 1 qt.

ARGOLAVAL Ointment (equivalent to 1% silver nitrate)—Bottles of 1 oz., ½ lb.

ARGOLAVAL Eye Ointment (equivalent to 1% silver nitrate)—Bottles of 5 and 10 Gm and 3 oz.

Uses: **Ophthalmology:** In conjunctivitis, trachoma, dacryocystitis, 5–50%; alone or in combination with atropin, cocaine nitrate (not hydrochloride); the ointment also is used.

Urology: Cystitis, pyelitis; for irrigation—beginning with 1% solution and increased to 10%.

General: Wounds, ulcus cruris, furuncles, eczemas, mastitis, rhagades, fissures—applied in ointment form.

Bibliography: *See Chap. XII.*

ARGYN (Abbott)

Astringent. Antiseptic

Description: A colloidal compound of silver oxide and serum albumin; contains 19–25% silver; is soluble in water.

Action: A non-irritating, soothing and astringent silver proteinate.

Uses: **Ophthalmology**—In 10–25% solutions for conjunctivitis, trachoma, corneal ulcer and ophthalmorrhea.

Laryngology—In 5–10% solutions for douching, gargling, application in nasopharyngitis, ozena, tonsillitis;—in 10–25% solution for swabbing.

Gynecology—In 50–75% in glycerin on tampons in endometritis, cervicitis.

Proctology—1:100–1:500 in solutions for rectal fissure, hemorrhoids and ulcerative colitis.

Genito-urinary—In 10–25% solution in cystitis, vaginitis; in 10% solution as venereal prophylactic.

Supply: **ARGYN**—Tablets (C.A.) gr 6 (0.384 Gm)—Bottles of 100.

ARGYN—Powder—Bottles of 1 and 4 oz.

ARGYROL (Barnes)

Gonocide

Chemical Name: Silver Vitellin.

Composition: A preparation of colloidal silver held in suspension by a protective colloid, protein in nature; contains 20% silver.

Action and Uses: Is destructive to the gonococcus without being irritant to mucous membranes.

Urology—Is used in gonorrhea for urethral injection; in cystitis as antiseptic irrigation; in pyelitis as non-irritating medium for pelvic lavage; in chronic vesiculitis as irrigation; in vasotomy and in venereal prophylaxis.

Rhinolaryngology—In all acute infections of nose and throat, as spray, gargle or local application; in the tampon treatment of sinusitis.

Ophthalmology—In acute inflammatory conditions of the eye, especially gonorrheal ophthalmia; as prophylactic against ophthalmia neonatorum.

Gynecology—In acute gonorrhea of the urethra, cervix and duct orifices; in chronic infections, for local application and tampons.

Supply: **ARGYROL**—Crystals—Bottles of 1, 4 and 8 oz.

ARGYROL—Tablets gr 6 (0.384 Gm)—Vials of 20—Packages of 3 vials.

Administration:

In Gonorrhea—Hand injection, 3–10% solution;

In Cystitis—Irrigation, 1–500 solution;

In Vesiculitis—Injection, 5% solution;

In Pelvic Lavage—Irrigation, 5% solution;

As Venereal Prophylactic—Injection, 10% solution;

In Nose and Throat—Local application, 10–25% solution;

In Eye—Instillation, 10–50% solution;

As Eye Prophylactic—Instillation, 10–25% solution;

In Gynecology—Local application, 5–25% solution.

ARHEOL "ASTIER" (Gallia)

Urinary Antiseptic

Chemical Name: Santalol.

Formula: $C_{15}H_{26}O$.

Description: A colorless oily liquid insoluble in water, soluble in alcohol; contains the purified active principle of sandalwood oil in non-irritating form; is prepared from Santalum Album, which contains 90 % of the active principle, sesquiterpenic alcohol.

Action: Alleviates pain in dysuria, reduces inflammation, decreases frequency of micturition and relieves backache.

Uses: In affections of genitourinary tract, especially acute and chronic gonorrheal cystitis, prostatitis, urethritis.

Supply: ARHEOL—Pearls m 3 (C.A.) (0.20 Gm)—Bottles of 40 and 500.

Administration: 3–4 pearls, three times daily with meals.

ARHOVIN (Schering and Glatz)

Gonocide

Chemical Name: An addition productof diphenylamine and thymolbenzoic-acid ester.

Formula: $C_{10}H_{13}.\ C_6H_4(COO.\ C_2H_5)(C_6H_5)_2NH$.

Description: An oily, yellowish liquid of aromatic odor and cooling yet burning taste; soluble in alcohol, chloroform, ether, oils; insoluble in water.

Action and Uses: Antigonorrheic in cystitis, vaginitis, cervicitis, urethritis; also for use in uric acid diathesis.

Supply: ARHOVIN—Liquid—Bottles of 1 oz.
ARHOVIN—Capsules m 4—Tins of 50.

Administration: *Orally*—4 m (0.25 cc) in capsules, three times daily;
Locally—By vaginal tampon with liquid or oily solution 1–2 % for instillation.

ARISTOL (Winthrop)

Antiseptic. Cicatrizant

Chemical Name: Dithymol-diiodide; Brand of Thymol Iodide.

Formula: $(C_6H_2.\ OI.\ CH_3.\ C_3H_7)_2$.

Description: A red-brown, voluminous, neutral powder of characteristic, faint odor; insoluble in water and glycerin, readily soluble in ether, chloroform and fixed oils; contains 45 % iodine.

Action: Mildly antiseptic and analgesic; stimulates phagocytosis and cicatrization, diminishes secretion and renders wounds less favorable for bacterial growth.

Uses: In all dermatologic and surgical conditions where an iodine powder is useful.

Advantages: Non-irritating, non-poisonous, free from unpleasant odor; adheres to raw denuded surfaces.

Incompatibles: Alkalies, corrosive sublimate and starch.

Supply: ARISTOL—Powder (C.A.)—Bottles of 1 oz.

Administration: *As Dusting Powder*—Pure or with boric acid, equal parts.
As Spray—5–10 %, in liquid petrolatum.
As Suppository—5–15 gr (0.3–0.9 Gm), in cocoa butter.

ARSENOCOL (Mulford Colloid)

Hematinic

Description: Occurs as brilliant black, non-hygroscopic scales, readily soluble in water; contains 10 % metallic arsenic.

Action and Uses: A stable, non-irritating colloidal Arsenic; easily absorbed and assimilated; hematinic and alterative; is slowly eliminated, has prolonged action and does not cause precipitation of tissue fluids. *For use* where arsenic is indicated.

Supply: **ARSENOCOL**—Vials, Gm 10.

ARSENOCOL—Solution 10%—Bottles 25 cc.

Administration: *Oral*—½–5 gr (0.032–0.324 Gm).
Hypodermic—¼–3 cc.

ARSENOFERRATOSE (Merck)

Hematinic

Description: A palatable, aromatic vinous solution of sodium arsenoferrialbuminate (Boehringer), containing 0.3% iron and 0.003% arsenic in organic combination; alcohol 15%.

Action: Hematinic and alterative of low toxicity and non-constipating; is readily absorbed and does not stain teeth; a tonic, roborant and nervine, adapted for administration to women and children.

Uses: Anemia, chlorosis, dermatoses, chorea minor, epilepsy, general debility; functional nervous disease like neurasthenia, anorexia, malnutrition.

Supply: **ARSENOFERRATOSE**—Bottles of 8 fl. oz. Each teaspoonful represents iron, ¼ gr (0.015 Gm), arsenic, 1/400 gr (0.00015 Gm).

ARSENOFERRATOSE WITH COPPER—Bottles of 8 oz.; Containing in addition copper, gr 1/100 (0.0006 Gm) per teaspoonful.

ARSPHENAMINE

Antiluetic

Chemical Name: Diamino-dihydroxy-arsenobenzene Dihydrochloride.

Formula: $(AsC_6H_3OH.\ NH_2HCl)_2$: or $HCl.\ NH_2OH.\ C_6H_3As{:}\ AsC_6H_3OH.\ NH_2HCl$.

Description: A light yellow hygroscopic amorphous powder, readily soluble in water at room temperature, yielding a strongly acid solution; contains 30–32% Arsenic; tested chemically and biologically and of low toxicity.

Action: That of arsphenamines U.S.P.; a powerful spirillicide.

Uses: In all stages of syphilis; also in frambesia, filariasis, trypanosomiasis, malarial anemia.

Supply: **ARSPHENAMINE** (C.A). (Arsenobenzol-Billon)—Ampules, 0.1, 0.2, 0.3, 0.4, 0.5 and 0.6 Gm. **(Merck)**

ARSPHENAMINE (C.A.)—Ampules 0.1, 0.2, 0.3, 0.4, 0.5, 0.6 and 1.0 Gm. **(Mallinckrodt)**

ARSPHENAMINE (C.A.)—Ampules 0.1, 0.2, 0.3, 0.4, 0.5, 0.6, 1.0, 2.0 and 3.0 Gm—Boxes of 1—also with "Alkpule" vials of sodium hydroxide for neutralization. **(Abbott)**

ARSPHENAMINE (C.A.)—Ampules, single doses 0.1, 0.2, 0.3, 0.4, 0.5 and 0.6 Gm. **(Searle)**

ARSPHENAMINE (C.A.)—Ampules, single doses 0.1, 0.2, 0.3, 0.4, 0.5 and 0.6 Gm. **(Squibb)**

DIARSENOL (C.A.)—Ampules, 0.1, 0.2, 0.3, 0.4, 0.5, 0.6, 1, 2 and 3 Gm. **(Diarsenol)**

Administration: *Intravenously*—By gravity method only, at weekly intervals; average dose for men, 0.4 Gm; for women 0.3 Gm; increased as indicated.

Contraindications: Advanced circulatory, hepatic, renal disease; fever, hemophilia, and neural disease; active tuberculosis, alcoholism, arsenic idiosyncrasy.

Preparation of Solution: Ampule is immersed in alcohol, to detect faults in glass; after drying, end is broken off and vial rotated gently to loosen contents; the latter is dissolved in triple distilled water, 25–50 cc, according to dosage, and normal 4% sodium hydrate solution of highest chemical purity is added, 0.85 cc for each 0.1 Gm Arsphenamine (3.40 cc for 0.4 Gm); solution is filtered through sterile moistened gauze, is diluted with cool sterile distilled water or preferably 4% saline solution to make a total volume of 20 cc for each 0.1 Gm Arsphenamine; is then allowed to stand for 30 min. before use.

Bibliography: *See Chap. XII.*

ATOPHAN (Schering and Glatz)

Antiarthritic

Chemical Name: 2-phenylquinolin-4-carboxylic acid.

Formula: $C_6H_5C_9H_5N.\ COOH$.

Description: Occurs as small, needle-like, colorless, odorless crystals, or whitish powder; insoluble in cold water, soluble in hot alcohol, chloroform and ether.

Action and Uses: Analgesic, antiphlogistic, antipyretic and uricolytic; also acts as cholagogue and choleretic; *For use* in colds, influenza, gout, rheumatism, arthritis, sciatica, neuritis, uric acid diathesis.

Supply: ATOPHAN—Tablets, gr 5, gr 7½ (0.324–0.480 Gm)—Boxes of 20—Bottles of 100, 250 and 500.

ATOPHAN—Powder—Tins of 1 oz.

Combinations: ATOPHAN-UROTROPIN COMPOUND—Ampules 10 cc (containing 34% solution urotropin with gr 7½ atophan)—Boxes of 6.

ATOPHANYL (Atophan-Salicylic Acid Compound)—Intravenous—Ampules 10 cc—Boxes of 5.

ATOPHANYL (Atophan-Salicylic Acid Compound)—Intramuscular—Ampules 5 cc—Boxes of 5. Ampules ½ cc—Anesthetic—Boxes of 5.

ARCANOL Tablets (Atophan and Acetylsalicylic Acid Compound)—gr 7½ (0.480 Gm)—Bottles 25, 50, 250 and 500.

NOVATOPHAN Powder—Bottles of 1 oz.

NOVATOPHAN Tablets—Gr 7½ (0.480 Gm)—Boxes of 20.

Administration: 1 tablet or 5–10 gr powder of Atophan or any of its combinations given two or three times daily, with alkaline drinks or large amounts of water, for 3–4 days; after rest period of several days course is repeated. Ampules—intravenous or intramuscular—given as frequently as is demanded in each instance.

ATOQUINOL (Ciba)

Uricolytic. Analgesic

Chemical Name: The allyl ester of 2-phenyl-quinoline-4-carboxylate; Phenyl cinchoninic acid.

Formula: $C_9H_5N.\ C_6H_5COOC_3H_5 2:4$.

Description: A yellowish, granular, odorless powder of agreeable taste; soluble in alcohol, ether, acetone, benzene and fatty oils; almost insoluble in water.

Action and Uses: Increases renal permeability for uric acid, induces its elimination and thus decreases uricacidemia; is analgesic and antirheumatic; effective in uricacidosis, gout, rheumatic fever, arthritis-acute and chronic; also in neuralgia, myalgia and dermatoses associated with uric acid diathesis (eczematous dermatitis, psoriasis).

Caution: As in the administration of all phenyl cinchoninic acid derivatives, attention must be given to the condition of the liver.

Supply: ATOQUINOL (C.A.) Tablets gr 4 (0.25 Gm), sugar coated—Tubes of 20—Bottles of 100.

Administration: In acute conditions of moderate severity, 4–8 tablets during 24 hr., with a liberal supply of water; in the presence of severe pain, the dose may be increased to 8 tablets every 3–4 hr. for 3 doses; in chronic cases and in prolonged administration, it is essential to omit medication during 3 days out of each week.

Bibliography: *See Chap. XII.*

AUBROMID (McNeil)

Antispasmodic

Composition: A brown tablet triturate containing Auric Bromide (Bromauric Acid) gr 1/20 (0.003 Gm).

Action and Uses: Sedative and antispasmodic, *for use* in whooping cough.

Supply: AUBROMID—Tablets—Bottles of 100 and 500.

Administration: Infants—1/2 tablet in water three times daily. Children—1 or 2 tablets, according to age and condition.

AUROCOL (Mulford Colloid)

Alterative

Description: Occurs as brilliant purple scales readily soluble in water; contains 8–10 % pure metallic gold in colloid form.

Action and Uses: Is stable, non-irritating, readily absorbed and assimilated; is slowly eliminated and of prolonged action; does not cause precipitation of tissue fluids. *For use* in arthritis and in treatment of malignancy.

Supply: AUROCOL—Packages 10 and 60 Gm.
AUROCOL—Solution, 10 %—Bottles 25 cc.

Administration: *Orally*—1/40–1/10 gr (0.001–0.006 Gm).
Hypodermically—1/8–1 cc of Solution

AUROL (Hille)

Alterative. Tonic

Description: A colloidal gold preparation containing gr 1/30 (0.002 Gm) pure gold per cubic centimeter.

Action and Uses: Alterative, promoting repair and correcting disordered function; stimulates heart and raises blood pressure. *Used* in the treatment of debility, neuroses, carbuncular and other infections and in inoperable cancer.

Administration: *Orally*—15 m three times daily.
Intravenously or Intramuscularly—1–5 cc three times weekly.

Supply: AUROL—Oral—Bottles of 1 and 4 oz.
AUROL—Intravenous and intramuscular—Vial 20 cc and 60 cc.

Bibliography: *See Chap. XII.*

AVERTIN (Winthrop)

Rectal Anesthetic

Chemical Name: Tribromethanol. Brand of Ethobrome.

Formula: $CBr_3.CH_2OH$.

Description: A white, crystalline substance, soluble up to 3.5% in water at 40°c.

Action and Uses: Introduced rectally, is rapidly absorbed; produces unconsciousness quickly and quietly; abolishes conjunctival and corneal reflexes, slightly decreases blood pressure, relaxes musculature; affects bronchial and salivary secretion only slightly. Narcosis lasts 1½–2 hr., being most profound during first 30–45 min. *Used* in surgery as basal anesthetic; is occasionally supplemented by general or local anesthesia; in obstetrics—to ease delivery, to reduce convulsions in eclampsia; in tetanus—to relieve opisthotonos and convulsive seizures; in psychopathic cases—to induce somnolence and restfulness.

Advantages: Offers rapid and satisfactory basal anesthesia of adequate duration; is easily administered like an enema.

Contraindications: Severe organic liver disease, serious bilateral kidney affections, rectal lesions, acidosis, blood dyscrasias and cachexia.

Supply: **AVERTIN**—Fluid—A solution containing per cubic centimeter 1 Gm Avertin and 0.5 Gm amylene hydrate solvent—Bottles of 25 and 100 cc.

Administration: **Preoperative Preparation**—The evening before operation a mild hypnotic is administered and cleansing enema given; before operation the customary hypodermic of morphine and atropine may be used or omitted. *Dosage:* Maximum 1/10 cc (100 mg) per kilogram (2.2 lb.) of body weight; total amount not to exceed 6–8 cc for women, 9–10 cc for men; in debilitated, cachectic, dehydrated or very obese persons dosage should not be more than 0.08 cc (80 mg) per kilo; Children tolerate normal dosage.

Preparation of Solution—A solution, 2½%, is made of the determined dosage by first heating the distilled water in Erlenmeyer flask to 40°c, then adding the Avertin Fluid dosage, stoppering the flask, inverting and shaking it vigorously until all globules have disappeared; is then preserved at body temperature until used and not permitted to precipitate while cooling, which necessitates the discarding of solution.

Manner of Use—Before use solution must be tested with 1 or 2 drops of 1:1,000 aqueous (non-alcoholic) Congo-red solution when a pure orange-red color should develop; when the color is blue or violet, solution must be discarded; is used by slowly injecting into rectum, like an enema, at body temperature, 20–30 min. before operation.

Caution: Must be preserved in tightly stoppered bottles, protected against light and air; must not be exposed to open flame; the dilution must be made in water of moderate temperature, 95–140°F, to avoid splitting off of hydrobromic acid and the formation of dibromacetaldehyde, which irritates and causes necrosis of tissues.

Bibliography: *See Chap. XII.*

BACILLUS ACIDOPHILUS MILK

Acidophilus Therapy

Description: A milk culture prepared from specially selected strains of B. Acidophilus, re-isolated from the intestinal contents as frequently as necessary to insure their adaptability for intestinal implantation.

Action: Suppresses or replaces putrefactive bacteria in the intestines, reducing absorption of toxic products and favoring intestinal antisepsis; is palatable and well tolerated.

Uses: In constipation, intestinal infections, arthritis and other conditions associated with toxin absorption; also in mucous colitis, diarrhea and intestinal toxemia.

Supply: **BACILLUS ACIDOPHILUS MILK** (C.A.)—Each cubic centimeter containing not less than 250,000,000 bacilli at time of manufacture—Bottles 400 cc. **(Cheplin)**

BACILLUS ACIDOPHILUS MILK (C.A.)—Each cubic centimeter containing not less than 50,000,000 viable B. Acidophilus—Bottles 200 cc (marked with expiration date). **(Fairchild)**

BACILLUS ACIDOPHILUS MILK (C.A.)—Each cubic centimeter containing not less than 200,000,000 viable B. Acidophilus, at time of manufacture and not less than 100,000,000 at expiration date—Bottles of 8 oz.—Packages of 6—Bottles, 1 qt.—Packages 3. **(Lederle)**

Administration: Implantation may be assisted by preliminary catharsis.

CHEPLIN'S MILK—1 qt. daily during first week, then 2–3 glasses for 6–10 weeks continued with 3 glasses daily thereafter.

FAIRCHILD'S MILK—1–2 bottles daily in single or divided doses.

LEDERLE'S MILK—4–6 glassfuls first few days, then dosage graded in accordance, 1–6 daily.

Rectally—High enemas of 1 part milk to 3 or 4 parts of water.

Children—Dosage in proportion.

Caution: Diet to be low in proteins and other putrefaction inducing foods.

Bibliography: *See Chap. XII.*

BEFSAL (Summers)

Antiarthritic. Uricolytic

Chemical Name: Di-ethyl-amino-benzyl-ether of methylene disalicylamide.

Formula: $C_{24}H_{40}O_8N_4R_2$ (R = represents Pyruval Group).

Description: The Pyruvic acid derivative of the organic compound of benzyl ethyl formaldehyde and salicyl groups.

Action: A synthetic systemic antiseptic, antiarthritic and uric acid solvent; facilitates elimination of waste products; inhibits intestinal bacterial growth, relieves articular pain and disability.

Uses: Recommended in articular rheumatism and infectious arthritides; as prophylactic against rheumatoid arthritis, arthritis deformans, gout and other uratic manifestations.

Supply: **BEFSAL**—Tablets, gr 5 (0.324 Gm)—Boxes of 100—Bottles 1000.

BEFSAL—Capsules, gr 5 (0.324 Gm)—Boxes of 100.

BEFSAL—Powder—Boxes of 2 oz.

Administration: 2–3 dr. daily, or 4–6 tablets four times daily.

Combinations: **IODO-BEFSAL**—An iodine derivative of Befsal, witn alterative antiseptic and catalytic properties, *for use* in above mentioned diseases;
Supply—Capsules and tablets of 5 gr each (0.324 Gm)—Coxes of 100—Powder—Boxes of 2 oz.;
Dosage—60–120 gr daily, in divided doses.

Advantages: Insoluble in stomach, and thus produces no distress often caused by salicylates.

Incompatibles: Should not be used with alkaline substances.

Bibliography: *See Chap. XII.*

BELLAFOLINE (Sandoz)

Antispasmodic

Description: Contains the levorotatory alkaloids of belladonna leaves in pure and stable form; in doses of equal therapeutic potency is only half as toxic as atropine; is non-narcotic.

Action: Acts directly upon the parasympathetic nervous system depressing the vagus, relieving spasm and pain and decreasing secretions.

Uses: In gastralgia, gastrosuccorrhea and pylorospasm; in ureteral and gallstone colic, spastic constipation, muco-membranous colitis; in bronchial asthma, hay-fever, coryza, dysmenorrhea, enuresis, seasickness, Parkinsonism, night sweats of phthisis.

Supply: **BELLAFOLINE**—Oral—Tablets, 1/250 gr (0.00025 Gm)—Bottles of 20, 100 and 250.

BELLAFOLINE—Oral—Solution: 1:2,000 (10 drops equivalent to 1 tablet)—Bottles of 10 cc and 100 cc.

BELLAFOLINE—Injection—Ampules, 1 cc, each 1/125 gr (0.0005 Gm)—Boxes of 6 and 20.

Administration: *By Mouth*—1–2 tablets or 10–20 drops of solution, three times daily. *By Injection*—½ cc to 2 cc per day.
Children—1 drop of solution for each year of age, three times daily (maximum 10 drops three times daily).

Bibliography: *See Chap. XII.*

BENZENE (BENZOL) MEDICINAL (Merck)

Leucocyticide

Chemical Name: Benzol Crystalline. Phenyl Hydride.

Formula: C_6H_6.

Description: A colorless mobile liquid of strong, characteristic, disagreeable odor and burning taste; is insoluble in water, soluble in 90% alcohol and carbon disulphide; miscible with alcohol, ether, chloroform and oils.

Action: Antispasmodic, antiseptic and narcotic; in therapeutic doses induces transient leucocytosis followed by persistent leucopenia and reduces the spleen when enlarged; in excessive dosage produces a burning sensation in the stomach, vertigo, delirium, toxic convulsions and unconsciousness; ingestion of 1 oz. has been found to be fatal.

Uses: Principally in leukemia, especially lymphatic; also in Hodgkin's disease, polycythemia; in intestinal infestation, trichinosis.

Supply: **BENZENE (BENZOL) MEDICINAL** (C.A.)—Bottles of ¼ and 1 lb.

Administration: *Oral*—2–10 m (0.12–0.6 cc) every 3 hr., as emulsion, on sugar or in capsules; in leukemia—8 m (0.5 cc) gel. capsule as initial dose, slowly increased to 15 m (1 cc) until 60–75 m (3–4 cc) are given each day; maximum single dose 45 m (3 cc).
Rectal Enema—3–8 gr in 500 cc water, in pin and tapeworm infestations.
Externally—Pure or as ointment in scabies, pediculosis, pityriasis.

Caution: **In Leukemia**—Repeated blood examinations are to be made during course of administration, which is to be terminated before final reduction to normal cell count.

In Poisoning—Fresh air, emetics, gastric lavage and stimulants are to be given.

BENZOSOL (Metz)

Antiseptic

Chemical Name: Guaiacol Benzoate.

Formula: $(C_6H_4OCH_3O)_2CO$.

Description: A colorless, odorless, almost tasteless crystalline powder, practically insoluble in water, soluble in hot alcohol and benzine, ether, chloroform.

Action and Uses: As antiseptic expectorant in incipient pulmonary tuberculosis; as intestinal antiseptic in fermentation diarrhea, typhoid, diabetes mellitus; as urinary antiseptic in cystitis, pyelitis.

Supply: **BENZOSOL (C.A.)**—Bottles 1 oz.

Administration: Gr 3–10 (0.2–0.6 Gm), as powder, pill or in emulsion, three to four times daily.

BENZYL ALCOHOL (Seydel)

Local Anesthetic

Chemical Name: Phenmethylol.

Formula: $C_6H_5CH_2OH$.

Description: A colorless liquid of faint aromatic odor and sharp burning taste; is slightly soluble in water, more soluble in alcohol, chloroform and ether.

Action and Uses: A non-irritating, non-toxic local anesthetic for injection and local application to mucous membranes; also as analgesic in pruritus.

Supply: **BENZYL ALCOHOL (C.A.)**—Bottles of 1, 4, 8 and 16 oz.

Administration: *Subcutaneous*—1–4% solution in water or saline; *topically*, as 10% ointment or as lotion with equal parts of alcohol and water.

BENZYL BENZOATE

Antispasmodic

Chemical Name: Benzylis Benzoas; the benzyl alcohol ester of benzoic acid.

Formula: $C_6H_5COO.\ C_6H_5CH_2$.

Description: A colorless liquid of faint aromatic odor and burning taste; soluble in alcohol, chloroform, ether; insoluble in water or glycerine.

Action: Antispasmodic; lowers tone of unstriped musculature; is non-narcotic, non-habit forming.

Uses: In all painful conditions due to non-striated muscle spasm; in renal, biliary, uterine and intestinal colic; in urolithiasis, vesical spasm, bronchial spasm, pylorospasm; in hypertension, asthma, angina pectoris, aortitis; in dysmenorrhea; hiccough, pertussis, bacillary dysentery and lead poisoning.

Supply: **BENZYL BENZOATE**—Tablets, gr 2 (0.130 Gm). **(Abbott)**

BENZYL BENZOATE—Elixir—Containing benzyl benzoate 20% with 70% of 95% ethyl alcohol. **(Abbott)**

BENZYL BENZOATE—Bottles 1, 4 and 8 oz. and 1 and 5 lb. **(Fritzsche)**

BENZYL BENZOATE—Miscible, 20%—Bottles of 2 oz. **(Hynson, Westcott and Dunning)**

BENZYL BENZOATE AND BENZALDEHYDE—Solution—20% and 5% respectively—Bottles 2 oz. **(Hynson, Westcott and Dunning)**

BENZYL BENZOATE—Globules, 5 m— (Hynson, Westcott and Dunning) Tubes of 25.

BENZYL BENZOATE—Ampules 1 cc (Hynson, Westcott and Dunning) containing 0.5 cc Benzyl Benzoate, for intramuscular use—Boxes of 10.

BENZYL BENZOATE—Containers 5 lb. (Mallinckrodt)

BENZYL BENZOATE—Bottles of 1 oz., ¼ and 1 lb. (Merck)

Administration: *Orally*—5–7 m (0.3–0.5 cc) increased to 20–30 m, or 3–6 globules, or 1–2 teaspoonfuls of 20% solution or elixir per dose, repeated in half to one hour if not relieved.

Hypodermically—Ampules, where rapid action is desired.

Externally—In skin affections in 25% solution in castor oil, or as ointment.

Bibliography: *See Chap. XII.*

BENZYL FUMARATE (Abbott)

Antispasmodic

Chemical Name: Dibenzyl Fumarate.

Formula: $C_6H_5CH_2OOC.\ CH{:}\ CH.\ COO.\ CH_2C_6H_5$.

Description: A white crystalline, odorless, almost tasteless solid, practically insoluble in water, soluble in alcohol, ether and chloroform; contains not less than 99% of benzyl fumarate.

Action and Use: Antispasmodic; lowers tone of unstriped muscle; is non-narcotic. *Useful* in affections accompanied by spasm; in hypertension, asthma, biliary and renal colic.

Supply: BENZYL FUMARATE—Tablets, gr 5 (0.3 Gm)—Bottles of 100, 1,000 and 5,000.

Administration: 1–4 tablets, as necessary.

Advantages: Solid in form with less taste than benzyl benzoate.

Bibliography: *See Chap. XII.*

BENZYL SUCCINATE

Antispasmodic

Chemical Name: Dibenzyl Succinate Medicinal.

Formula: $C_6H_5CH_2OOC.\ CH_2CH_2COO.\ CH_2C_6H_5$.

Description: A white or faintly yellowish-white, crystalline powder, odorless, almost tasteless and permanent in air; is insoluble in water, soluble in alcohol, ether and chloroform; also soluble in fixed and volatile oils.

Action: Lowers tonus of smooth muscle; is non-toxic, non-habit forming; effective in disturbances accompanied by spasm.

Uses: In dysmenorrhea, angina pectoris, intestinal colic; in hypertension, asthma, renal, uterine and biliary colic; in excessive intestinal peristalsis, singultus.

Supply: BENZYL SUCCINATE—Tablets, gr 5 (Hynson, Westcott and Dunning) (0.3 gm.)—Tubes of 40.

BENZYL SUCCINATE—Bottles, 1 oz., ¼ and 1 lb. (Merck)

Administration: *Dosage*—5–15 gr (0.3 to 1 Gm), as necessary.

Benzyl compounds may also be advantageously administered in form of the water soluble and tasteless Benzycin, Sodium Benzyl Succinate or Benzyphos, Sodium Dibenzyl Phosphate.

BETA-EUCAINE HYDROCHLORIDE

Local Anesthetic **(Schering and Glatz)**

Chemical Name: Trimethylbenzoxypiperidine Hydrochloride.

Formula: $C_5H_7N(CH_3)_3(C_6H_5COO)HCl$.

Description: A white, crystalline, odorless powder, soluble in water, alcohol and chloroform.

Action and Uses: Local anesthetic, of slow action and irritating to the skin; *used* principally in dentistry and ophthalmology; also used in cystoscopy, nose and throat work, in the treatment of hemorrhoids and sciatica.

Incompatibilities: Salicylates.

Supply: BETA-EUCAINE HYDROCHLORIDE—Bottles ⅛ oz.

Administration: Cystoscopy—0.2 % solution.

Rhinolaryngology—5–10 % solution.

Dentistry—2–3 % solution; infiltration anesthesia 4–5 % solution.

Ointment (*Rectal*)—5–10 % with menthol 2 %.

Subcutaneous—in sciatica, 1 % solution 70–100 cc injected perineurally.

Dosage: Average—gr ⅛, gr ½.

BETA-EUCAINE LACTATE (Schering and Glatz)

Local Anesthetic

Chemical Name: Betacaine.

Formula: $C_5H_7N(CH_3)_3(C_6H_5COO).\ C_3H_6O_3$.

Description: A white crystalline powder, soluble in water and alcohol.

Action and Uses: Local anesthetic *for use* in ophthalmology, dentistry, rhinology, otology and urethral examination.

Supply: BETA-EUCAINE LACTATE—Bottles ½ oz.

Administration: In Ophthalmology, Dentistry and Urethral Uses—2–3 % solution.

In Rhino-Otology—10–15 % solution.

In Regional Anesthesia—2–5 % solution.

In Infiltration Anesthesia—0.12 % solution.

Dosage: Average—gr ⅛–½.

BETAINE HYDROCHLORIDE (Roche)

Hydrochloric Acid Therapy

Official Name: Betainae Hydrochloridum. Lycine Hydrochloride. Acidol.

Formula: $C_5H_{11}NO_2.HCl$.

Description: Occurs as colorless, monoclinic crystals, freely soluble in water, less soluble in 90 % alcohol, insoluble in chloroform, ether.

Action and Uses: Liberates 23.8 % of absolute hydrochloric acid in stomach; *is used* in anacidity, hypoacidity; in achylia of gastric carcinoma.

Supply: BETAINE HYDROCHLORIDE (C.A.)—Bottles of 1, 10 and 100 Gm.

Administration: 8 gr, equivalent to 18 m of HCl dilute, dissolved in water, after meals.

BETANAPHTHOL-BENZOATE (Merck)

Germicide

Chemical Name: Benzonaphthol, Medicinal.

Formula: $C_{10}H_7.\ C_6H_5CO_2$.

Description: Colorless needles or white tasteless crystalline powder, of faintly aromatic odor; almost insoluble in water, freely soluble in alcohol and ether, soluble in chloroform, fixed oils, olive oil and alkaline hydroxide solutions.

Action: Antiseptic, parasiticide, germicide, anthelminthic; not affected by gastric juice; is split up in the intestines, there to become effective as antiseptic.

Uses: *Internally*—Typhoid, chronic diarrhea, gastric dilatation; intestinal dyspepsia, cholelithiasis, diarrhea, dysentery; in hyperidrosis and as vermifuge in ankylostomiasis.

Externally—Chloasma, pediculosis, prurigo, herpes, favus, chilblains, hyperidrosis, scabies, alopecia, psoriasis, eczema.

Supply: BETANAPHTHOL BENZOATE (C.A.)—Cartons of 1 oz. and 1 lb.

Administration: *External*—2–10% ointment;

Internal—3–8 gr (0.2–0.5 Gm); average dose, 4 gr (0.25 Gm); maximum dose, 15 gr (1 Gm) single, or 45 gr (3 Gm) daily.

Incompatibles: Antipyrine, camphor, phenol, ferric chloride, menthol, potassium permanganate.

BICARBONATE OF SODA (ARM AND HAMMER)

(Church and Dwight)

Antacid

Description: A sodium bicarbonate of superior chemical purity to U.S.P. requirements; an opaque, white powder, permanent in air, odorless, of cooling saline taste and slightly alkaline reaction; soluble in 12 parts of water, insoluble in alcohol; is decomposed by hot water and converted into normal sodium carbonate.

Formula: $NaHCO_3$.

Analysis:

Carbonic acid gas	52.310
Alkali	36.890
Bicarbonate of soda	99.786
Carbonate of soda	0.115
Salt (sodium chloride)	0.100
Difference	0.089

Action and Uses: Antacid, both direct and indirect; laxative, gastric sedative, mucus solvent, antipruritic and detergent. *Used* in the treatment of acidosis; to maintain the normal hydrogen-ion concentration and acid base equilibrium of body fluids; in pre-operative preparation and post-operative care; as alkalizer in colds, influenza, hyperchlorhydria, colitis, urinary infections, rheumatism, pylorospasm, gastric and duodenal ulcer. In 2–5% solution is used locally in eczema and itching skin affections; as soda paste in superficial burns; as enema in 2–5% solution, for relief of colic in children; as 2% solution as mouth wash in stomatitis, as nasal douche in chronic rhinitis; as 5–10% solution to remove impacted cerumen; may be used *intravenously* in cases of extreme acidosis.

Incompatibles: Acids.

Supply: BICARBONATE OF SODA—Packages ½ and 1 lb.

Administration: *Dosage*—Gr 10–40 (average gr 20); much larger doses may be given in acidosis; as much as 2 oz. may be administered daily, as 4% solution by "drop enema." For intravenous injections, 2–6% sterile solution, 1,000 cc. Solutions should be made with cold water.

Bibliography: *See Chap. XII.*

BICHLORACETIC ACID (Kahlenberg)

Keratolytic

Description: A bichloracetic acid of practical purity.

Formula: $CHCl_2COOH$.

Action and Uses: A powerful keratin solvent; *used* in the removal of corns, warts and calluses.

Supply: BICHLORACETIC ACID—Bottles with glass applicators, ½ oz.

BICHLORACETIC ACID—Packages with petrolatum and camel's hair brush.

Administration: Applied locally at intervals of several days; 1–4 applications.

Bibliography: *See Chap. XII.*

BILEIN (Abbott)

Cholagogue

Chemical Name: Sodium Glyco-taurocholate "Boris."

Composition: Mixture of essential bile salts.

Action and Uses: As for bile salts.

Supply: BILEIN (C.A.)—Tablets, gr ¼ and gr 1—Bottles of 100.

Administration: ¼–1 gr two to three times daily after meals.

BILE SALTS (Lederle)

Cholagogue. Laxative

Description: A preparation from ox bile; contains highly purified sodium taurocholate and sodium glycocholate in equal proportions; is free from undesirable inactive substances, as mucin, bile pigment.

Action: As for biliary salts: is mildly antiseptic and laxative; emulsifies and favors fat absorption, stimulates liver activity, increases bile secretion and relieves constipation, causes no griping or other discomfort.

Uses: In postoperative gall bladder fistulae; in prevention of biliary calculi by dissolving toxic products of liver metabolism; in constipation, gastric dyspepsia and amebic dysentery.

Supply: BILE SALTS PLAIN—Tablets 1 gr (0.65 Gm)—Bottles of 100, 500 and 1,000;

COMBINATION BILE SALTS—Tablets—Containing bile salts 1 gr (0.65 Gm), extract of cascara ½ gr (0.33 Gm), phenolphthalein ½ gr (0.33 Gm)—Bottles of 100, 500 and 1,000.

Administration: 1–4 tablets daily before meals; dosage reduced with improvement.

BILIPOSOL (Ulmer)

Antiluetic

Chemical Name: Basic-alpha carbox-ethyl-beta-methyl-nonoate of Bismuth.

Description: A lipo-soluble bismuth in clear, homogeneous oily solution; contains 80 mg of bismuth per ampule of 2 cc.

Action and Uses: Antisyphilitic in all stages of the disease; is stated to be rapidly effective, non-irritating, readily absorbed and slowly eliminated.

Supply: BILIPOSOL (C.A.)—Ampules 2 cc—Boxes of 12, 50 and 100.

Administration: *Intramuscularly*—1 ampule every second day for first week, thereafter twice weekly until 12 treatments are administered; after a rest period of 1 month one or more series are given; continued with 1 or 2 series yearly thereafter. Children—Dosage in accordance with age.

BILIVAL (Bischoff)

Cholagogue

Official Name: Sodium Lecithino-Cholicum.

Description: A chemical combination of lecithin and sodium cholate.

Action: The cholic acid constituent is a physiologic cholagogue; its action is enhanced by the colloidal lecithin which aids the bile in inhibiting the precipitation of cholesterol and formation of calculi.

Uses: In hepatic insufficiency, biliary stasis, catarrhal jaundice, cholelithiasis, chronic constipation with bilious headache.

Supply: BILIVAL—Pills-gr 2½ (0.16)—Bottles of 100.

Administration: Acute Conditions—2–4 pills three times daily after meals, reduced to 3 pills daily.

Chronic Conditions—1 pill three times daily, during part of each month.

Contraindications: Acute and chronic empyema of the gall bladder, phlegmonous cholecystitis, impaction of stone or tumor of gall bladder.

Bibliography: *See Chap. XII.*

BI-NA-GLUCONATE (Drug Products)

Antiluetic

Chemical Name: Bismuth Sodium Gluconate, Colloidal.

Description: A soluble bismuth salt in colloidal solution; alkaline, stable, sterile, protein free, chemically and biologically tested.

Action: Antiluetic; causes less renal irritation than arsenicals.

Uses: Used in tertiary and congenital syphilis; in interstitial keratitis.

Supply: BI-NA-GLUCONATE—Ampuls Hyposols, 2 cc, (0.1 Gm) representing 25 mg metallic bismuth with 2% benzylic alcohol as local anesthetic—Boxes of 12, 25 and 100.

Administration: *Intraglutcally*—1 ampul every 5 days.

BISMARSEN (Abbott)

Antisyphilitic

Chemical Name: Sulpharsphenamine Bismuth; Bismuth Arsphenamine Sulphonate.

Formula: $C_{21}H_{21}O_{12}As_3Na_3S_3N_3Bi_2$.

Composition: The sodium salt of a bismuth derivative of arsphenamine methylene sulphonic acid.

Description: A brownish yellow amorphous powder, easily soluble in water, forming a slightly alkaline solution; arsenic content 13–15%, bismuth—23–25%; is somewhat slower in action than sulpharsphenamine and neoarsphenamine, and more rapid than bismuth.

Action: Presents the combined effectiveness of bismuth and arsenic.

Uses: In early and congenital syphilis, in cardiovascular and cerebrospinal syphilis and in tabes dorsalis.

Advantages: Convenient administration, causes little cutaneous irritation, is well tolerated.

Supply: **BISMARSEN**—Ampules (C.A.) 0.1 and 0.2 Gm—Boxes of 10 and 100.

Administration: Initial dose, 0.1 Gm, dissolved in ampule of 1 cc of sterile, distilled water with 2–3 drops of a 2% solution of butyn; used weekly, later biweekly, administered *intramuscularly.*

Bibliography: *See Chap. XII.*

BISMO-CYMOL (Abbott)

Antiluetic

Chemical Name: Basic Bismuth Camphorcarboxylate.

Formula: $(C_{10}H_{15}O.\ COO)_2Bi.\ OBi.\ OH.\ OOCO.\ C_{10}H_{15}$.

Description: A solution in olive oil of a basic bismuth derivative of campho-carboxylic acid; contains 5% elemental bismuth or 50 mgm per cc of the liposoluble compound.

Action and Uses: Antisyphilitic; is slowly absorbed and of prolonged action; is non-irritating and of low toxicity. *For use* in congenital syphilis, in cardiovascular and neural lesions.

Supply: **BISMO-CYMOL** (C.A.)—Ampules 1 and 2 cc, each 2 cc ampule containing 100 mg bismuth—Boxes of 12 and 100—Bottles—30 cc.

Administration: *Intramuscularly*—2 cc twice weekly for 6–8 weeks; after a rest period of 4 weeks another course may be given.
Infants—0.1–0.2 cc twice weekly, for 12 injections; where the treatment is combined with Arsphenamine—one injection weekly suffices.
Children, 2½–11 yr., 1 cc twice weekly for 12–16 weeks.

Contraindications: As for arsphenamine: sepsis, nephritis, insanitary mouth; in poisoning with foul breath, blue gingival line, blue spots on tongue and buccal mucosa administration must be discontinued.

Bibliography: *See Chap. XII.*

BISMOGENOL (Tosse)

Antisyphilitic

Formula: $C_6H_4OH.\ COO.\ BiO$.

Description: Bismuth Salicylate in oily suspension; is germicidal and non-toxic in therapeutic dosage; injections are quite painless.

Action and Uses: Antisyphilitic, *for use* in all stages of lues.

Supply: **BISMOGENOL**—Ampules 1 cc, equivalent to 0.06 Gm metallic bismuth—Boxes of 12, 50 and 100.

BISMOGENOL—Bottles of 30, 100 cc and 500 cc; *Strong* containing 0.1 Gm, *Weak*—0.06 Gm per cc.

Administration: *Intramuscular*—After warming ampule or bottle, 1 cc (Weak) infected twice weekly, for 30 injections; or 1 cc (Strong) once weekly.

Bibliography: *See Chap. XII.*

BISMOID (Lilly)

Antiluetic

Description: A stabilized suspension of finely divided bismuth metal in sterile aqueous medium.

Action and Uses: Spirocheticidal and alterative; is readily absorbed and non-irritating; *For use* in syphilis and its manifestations, especially in arsenic-fast cases.

Supply: BISMOID—Ampules 1 cc, containing ⅜ gr (0.025 Gm) of bismuth—Boxes of 6.

BISMOID—Vials, rubber capped, 30 cc.

Administration: *Intramuscularly*—1 ampule every 5 days for 12–15 injections; course is repeated after a rest period of 1 month.

BISMUTHOIDOL "ROBIN" (Fougera)

Antiluetic

Description: Colloidal metallic bismuth in concentrated, isotonic, sterile aqueous solution; is readily absorbed without causing local reaction.

Action: Antiluetic.

Uses: In all stages of syphilis; may be combined with arsenical therapy.

Supply: BISMUTHOIDOL "ROBIN"—Ampules, 2 cc, containing ⅛ gr (0.008 Gm) metallic bismuth—Boxes of 10 and 50.

Administration: *Intramuscularly*—1 injection every 2–3 days for 5–6 weeks, with rest period after each course.

BISMUTH SALICYLATE (Parke, Davis)

Antiluetic

Description: An insoluble bismuth preparation, suitable in supplementing soluble bismuth therapy or of arsenicals.

Action and Uses: A powerful spirocheticide; insures protracted bismuth effect; especially useful in neurosyphilis.

Supply: BISMUTH SALICYLATE (C.A.)—Ampules containing bismuth salicylate, gr 2 (0.13 Gm) in 1 cc olive oil with 3% chloretone—Packages of 12 and 100.

BISMUTH SALICYLATE (C.A.)—In oil, 0.13 Gm per cc—Bottles of 2 oz.

Administration: *Intramuscularly Only;* Technic—that of other insoluble intragluteal injections.

Dosage: Average dose, gr 2 (0.13 Gm) or 1 cc, twice a week, avoiding supersaturation.

Advantages: Minimum toxicity; effective in Wassermann-fast cases and those intolerant of arsenicals.

Bibliography: *See Chap. XII.*

BISMUTH SODIUM TARTRATE (Searle)

Antiluetic

Formula: $C_4O_{11}H_3Bi_4Na$.

Description: A white, finely divided, tasteless and odorless powder; its aqueous solution when buffered with 25% sucrose is non-irritating on injection and readily absorbed; is stable and permanent in air; represents 74% metallic bismuth; soluble in 3 parts of water, leaving a light residue which is soluble in sodium hydroxide.

Action and Use: Antiluetic of low toxicity and prolonged therapeutic action; especially effective in neurosyphilis and Wassermann-fast cases.

Supply: **BISMUTH SODIUM TARTRATE** (C.A.)—Ampules 2 cc 1.5% solution—Boxes 12, 25 and 100.

BISMUTH SODIUM TARTRATE (C.A.)—Vials 60 cc—Package of 6 vials.

BISMUTH SODIUM TARTRATE (C.A.)—Solution, 1½%, Glycerinated—containing per cubic centimeter Bismuth Sodium Tartrate, 0.03 Gm, Benzyl Alcohol, 0.04 Gm, Sucrose, 0.50 Gm.

Administration: 1 ampule twice weekly for 6–10 weeks; followed by a course of arsphenamine after 3–4 weeks rest; given *intramuscularly.*

Bibliography: *See Chap. XII.*

BISMUTH VIOLET (Table Rock)

Germicide

Composition: A loose combination of bismuth with the triphenyl-methane dye, hexamethyl-triamin-triphenyl-carbinol-chlorid.

Action and Uses: Antiseptic, germicidal and analgesic; stimulates epithelization; is non-poisonous and non-irritating to mucous membranes; *used* in the treatment of wounds, suppurations, skin affections and eye diseases; also in dental practice.

Supply: **BISMUTH VIOLET**—Liquid, 0.4% of dye—Vials ½ and 6 oz.

BISMUTH VIOLET—Ointment, 1%, in lanolin base—Jars 1 oz., 4 oz. and 1 lb.

Administration: Liquid—in 10% aqueous-glycerine dilution is used in diseases of eye, nose, sinuses (conjunctivitis, sinusitis, oral affections) and for skin grafting; Ointment—in impetigo, ringworm, burns, scabby crusty wounds.

Bibliography: *See Chap. XII.*

BISMUTOSE (Winthrop)

Antacid. Intestinal Astringent

Chemical Name: Bismuth Albuminate.

Description: A bismuth-albumin combination in powder form; is tasteless and odorless; contains about 22% of bismuth and 66% albuminoid; absorbs two to three times its volume of fluid, thus covering a large surface area.

Action: Reduces gastric hyperacidity; exerts mild astringent effect and favors intestinal antisepsis; its conversion into bismuth oxide imparts a black color to the stools.

Uses: In inflammatory and ulcerative conditions of the gastrointestinal tract; in gastritis, gastric and duodenal ulceration; in subacute and chronic intestinal catarrh of children.

Supply: **BISMUTOSE**—Powder, in cartons 1 oz.

Administration: ½ to 1 or more teaspoonfuls three times daily. Children 15–30 gr (0.9–1.9 Gm) and over; given in gruel, milk or water.

BISOCOL (Mulford Colloid)

Antiluetic

Description: Occurs as brilliant black non-hygroscopic scales, readily soluble in water; contains 20–25% metallic bismuth.

Action and Uses: A stable, non-irritating, readily absorbed and assimilated Colloidal Bismuth; is slowly eliminated and does not cause precipitation of tissue fluids. Is antiluetic in all stages of syphilis.

Supply: BISOCOL—Vials Gm 10.

BISOCOL—Solution—Ampule-vial, 25 cc.

Administration: 2–20 gr (0.130–1.296 Gm).

BISOCOL—Solution ¼–2 cc.

BOROCAINE (Sharp and Dohme)

Local Anesthetic

Chemical Name: Ethocaine Borate.

Formula: $C_{13}H_{20}O_2N_25HBO_2$.

Description: A stable, white, crystalline powder, freely soluble in cold water, normal saline, isotonic glucose and Ringer's solution without bicarbonate.

Action: A local anesthetic, non-irritating, non-narcotic and non-toxic.

Supply: BOROCAINE—Powder—Bottles of 1, 5 and 20 Gm.

BOROCAINE—Tablets, Hypodermic, ⅓ gr (0.02 Gm)—Tubes of 20—Bottles of 100.

BOROCAINE—Tablets, Hypodermic, 1½ gr (0.1 Gm)—Tubes of 20—Bottles of 100.

BOROCAINE—Tablets ⅓ gr (0.02 Gm) and Epinephrine 1/1,300 gr (0.00005 Gm) —Tubes of 20—Bottles of 100.

BOROCAINE—Tablets 1½ gr (0.1 Gm) and Epinephrine 1/260 gr (0.00025 Gm) —Tubes of 20—Bottles of 100.

BOROCAINE—For Dental Use—¾ gr (0.05 Gm) and epinephrine 1/800 gr (0.00008 Gm)—Tubes of 20—Bottles of 100.

Administration: Dentistry—Root canal work, 1–2 cc 2%; infiltration anesthesia—½–1%.

Surgery—Tonsillectomy, ½–1%; nerve block 1–2%.

Topical—2–10%, in accordance with location and severity of condition.

BROMETONE (Parke, Davis)

Sedative

Chemical Name: Tri-brom-tertiary-butyl alcohol.

Formula: $C.\ Br_3.\ COH.\ (CH_3)_2$.

Description: A product of interaction of bromoform and acetone; contains 77% of bromine; occurs as fine, white prismatic crystals, of camphor odor and taste; is slightly soluble in water, soluble in alcohol, ether, benzene and most organic solvents.

Action and Uses: A sedative like bromides; does not affect the gastrointestinal tract; *for use* in severe headache, cough, epilepsy, chorea and other neurotic disturbances.

Supply: BROMETONE (C.A.)—Bottles of 1 oz., ¼ lb.

BROMETONE (C.A.)—Capsules, gr 5 (0.324 Gm)—Bottles of 100.

Administration: 5 gr two to three times daily.

Advantages: Better tolerated than the bromides.

BROMINOL (Abbott)

X-Ray Contrast Medium

Composition: Brominized olive oil, containing about 33 % Bromine.

Action: Is radio-opaque, stable and of constant composition; produces shadows of ample density.

Uses: Especially valuable in Roentgen diagnosis of respiratory tract, nasal sinuses, in localization of spinal cord tumors and obstructions; in uterine, fallopian tube and blood vessel injections.

Advantages: Is stable, distinctly but not severely irritable and cannot cause iodism; is easily instilled and drained off.

Supply: BROMINOL—Heavy—containing 85 % brominized oil and 15 % brominized olive oil esters, in wide mouth containers of 10 and 25 cc.

BROMINOL—Light—of low viscosity, with 33 % brominized olive oil esters, in wide mouth containers of 10 and 25 cc.

Administration: 20 cc, warmed (35–40°c) slowly injected by catheter or syringe.

Bibliography: *See Chap. XII.*

BROMIPIN 10% (Merck)

Sedative

Description: A 10 % brominized vegetable oil; a product of sesame oil, containing 9.8–11.2 % of bromine in organic combination; a yellow oily fluid, of purely oleaginous taste.

Action: Nervine and sedative; an efficient substitute for bromides, rarely causing bromism.

Uses: Epilepsy, neurasthenia, cardiac neuroses; in convulsive cough, insomnia, chorea; neuralgia, muscular twitching; migraine, headache, neuritis; sea-sickness.

Supply: BROMIPIN 10 % (C.A.)—Bottles of 25 Gm.

Administration: Average dose—1 teaspoonful, three or four times per day. Epilepsy—in adults, ½–2 tablespoonfuls, three or four times daily; in children—2–4 teaspoonfuls per day, in emulsion with peppermint water and syrup, or pure, or flavored with oil of peppermint. As enema, children under 1 yr., 15 m (1 cc) for each month of age; 1–4 yr., 3–4 fl. dr. (12–15 cc); over 4 yr., 4–5 fl. dr. (15–20 cc); still older children 6–8 fl. dr. (25–30 cc), in milk or flaxseed tea.

BROMIPIN 33% (Merck)

X-Ray Contrast Medium

Description: 33 % Brominized Vegetable Oil.

Action and Uses: As for Bromipin 10 %; also as a contrast medium in bronchography in tuberculous subjects; is especially adapted for hypodermic use.

Supply: BROMIPIN 33 % (C.A.)—Bottles of 25 Gm.

Administration: In *bronchography*, 2½–8 fl. dr. (10–30 cc), the average quantity being 6 fl. dr. (25 cc), warmed to 37–40°c before or during injection. *Internally*—in epilepsy 20 m (1.3 cc), increased to 40–160 m (3–10 cc). *Rectally*, as enema, for adults 4–10 fl. dr. (15–40 cc). *Externally*—equal parts 33 % Bromipin and castor oil to relieve irritation in frost bites.

BROMOCOL (Mulford Colloid)

Sedative

Description: Occurs as brilliant black non-hygroscopic scales, readily soluble in water; contains 20–25 % bromine.

Action and Uses: A stable, non-irritating, readily absorbed and assimilated colloidal bromine; is slowly eliminated and does not cause precipitation of tissue fluids. *For use* where bromides are indicated.

Supply: BROMOCOL—Vials 10 Gm.

Administration: 2–10 gr (0.130–0.384 Gm).

BROMSULPHALEIN

(Hynson, Westcott and Dunning)

Liver Function Diagnosis

Chemical Name: Disodium Phenoltetrabromphthalein Sulphonate.

Formula: O. CO. C_6Br_4C $[C_6H_3(OH)SO_3Na]_2$.

Description: A white, crystalline powder, containing 37 % of bromine; soluble in water, insoluble in alcohol and acetone.

Action: When intravenously introduced about 85 % is eliminated from the circulation in about 1 hr., provided the liver is functioning normally; where liver function is deficient, the dye is retained in the blood for a longer period and in greater concentration.

Uses: As liver function test, determined colorimetrically from blood after intravenous injection.

Supply: BROMSULPHALEIN (C.A.)—Ampules 3 cc, sterile 5 %—Boxes of 6.

Administration: *Intravenous Injections*—0.002 Gm per kilogram of body weight, undiluted; determination is made from 4–5 cc of blood obtained in ½ and 1 hr. from the other arm; the serum is separated by centrifugation and examined colorimetrically by comparison with established standard.

BROMURAL (Bilhuber-Knoll)

Sedative. Hypnotic

Chemical Name: Alpha mono-brom-iso-valeryl carbamide; is neither a bromide nor a barbiturate.

Formula: $(CH_3)_2CH$. CHBr. CONHCO. NH_2.

Description: A white, almost tasteless crystalline powder, soluble in alcohol, ether, alkalies and hot water; insoluble in cold water.

Action: A quickly acting somnifacient, inducing restful sleep for 5–6 hr. and longer; an efficient sedative in nervous hyperactivity, allaying hyperexcitation and irritability; is non-cumulative, non-habit forming.

Uses: As sedative in circulatory neuroses, neurasthenia, menopausal hypertension; in asthma, whooping cough and for preliminary sedation in anesthesia; as hypnotic in various types of insomnia.

Supply: BROMURAL (C.A.)—Tablets gr 5 (0.32 Gm)—Tubes of 10—Bottles of 100.
BROMURAL (C.A.)—Powder—Cartons of 1 oz.

Administration: *As Sedative*—1 tablet, several times daily.
As Hypnotic—2–4 tablets at bedtime.
Children in proportion.

Bibliography: *See Chap. XII.*

BROVALOL (Schering and Glatz)

Sedative

Chemical Name: Bornyl Bromovalerate.

Description: A colorless, oily liquid, soluble in alcohol, chloroform, ether; insoluble in water.

Action and Uses: Sedative in states of excitation where bromides or valerates are indicated.

Supply: BROVALOL—Pearls, 4m—Tin of 30.

Administration: 1–3 pearls, several times daily.

BULBOCAPNINE HYDROCHLORIDE (Merck)

Antispasmodic

Official Name: Bulbocapnine Hydrochloride.

Formula: $C_{19}H_{19}NO_4$. HCl.

Description: An alkaloid from tubers of Bulbocapnus cavus (Cordyalis cava); a white, crystalline powder, soluble in water.

Action and Uses: Exerts a pronounced influence upon spasmodic conditions of muscles accompanying some diseases of the nervous system; has proven of benefit in the treatment of tremors of various etiology, especially of paralysis agitans and chorea; in ataxic conditions of tremulous character.

Supply: BULBOCAPNINE HYDROCHLORIDE—Tablets 1½ gr (0.1 Gm)—Tube of 10.

BULBOCAPNINE HYDROCHLORIDE—Ampules 1 cc—Box of 5.

Administration: *Dose Single*—1½ gr (0.1 Gm), internally, subcutaneously or intramuscularly; per day 1½–3 gr (0.1–0.2 Gm).
Maximum Dose—3 gr (0.2 Gm).

Bibliography: *See Chap. XII.*

BUTESIN (Abbott)

Local Anesthetic

Chemical Name: n-butyl-p-amino-benzoate.

Formula: $C_6H_4NH_2COO(C_4H_9)$.

Composition: The normal butyl ester of para-amino-benzoic acid.

Description: A white, crystalline odorless and tasteless, powder; almost insoluble in water, freely soluble in alcohol, ether, benzene, vegetable and animal oils.

Action: A powerful local anesthetic; is slowly absorbed producing lasting effect; is non-irritating and non-toxic.

Uses: Wherever it is desired to deaden pain: in surface wounds, skin and malignant ulceration, tonsillitis, sore throat, earache; in minor surgery and dental operations.

Supply: BUTESIN—Powder (C.A.)—Bottles of 5 Gm and 1 oz.

Administration: Used pure as dusting powder; also used in suppositories, troches and ointment.

Combinations: EPHEDRINE BUTESIN—Spray—Contains Butesin 1% with Ephedrine 1%—Bottles of 1, 4, 16 oz. *For use* in painful turgescence of nasal mucosa, for relief in hay fever, asthma, coryza.

EPHEDRINE BUTESIN—Jelly—Contains Butesin ⅜ % with Ephedrine 1 % in soothing, bland jelly base with no aromatics; for use in the relief of nasal obstruction, in coryza, hay fever, asthma—Collapsible tubes of ½ oz. for home use.

BUTESIN COMPOUND—Suppositories—containing Butesin, 2½ gr, Ext. Hydrastis, ⅛ gr, Ext. Hamamelis, 1 gr; for rectal use—Boxes of 12.

BUTESIN PICRATE (Abbott)

Analgesic. Protective

Chemical Name: Dinormalbutyl-p-amino Benzoate Trinitrophenol.

Formula: $(C_6H_4NH_2COO.\ C_4H_9)_2C_6H_2(NO_2)_3OH$.

Description: A yellow, odorless, amorphous powder of slightly bitter taste; has the anesthetic qualities of Butesin with the tissue fixing properties of picric acid.

Action: Relieves pain, combats suppuration and stimulates granulation in affected area.

Uses: In all abrasions, ulcers, extensive burns and other destructive external injuries.

Supply: **BUTESIN PICRATE**—Ointment (C.A.)—1 %, in white wax, paraffin, petrolatum, water and sodium borate—Jars 1 and 2 oz., 1 and 5 lb.

BUTESIN PICRATE EYE—Ointment (C.A.) 1 %, in petroleum base—Tubes ⅛ oz.—Jars 3½ oz.

BUTESIN PICRATE—Powder (C.A.) 5 %, with sodium stearate 95 %—Bottles of 1 oz.

Administration: For local application.

Bibliography: *See Chap. XII.*

BUTOLAN (Winthrop)

Vermifuge

Chemical Name: Carbaminic acid-ester of paraoxydiphenylmethane. Brand of Carphenol.

Formula: $C_6H_4CH_2C_6H_5O.\ CO.\ NH_2$.

Description: A white, tasteless, almost odorless crystalline powder; insoluble in water, soluble in hot alcohol, benzol and acetic acid.

Action: A prompt efficient vermifuge in oxyuriasis, causing death of organisms in dilutions of 1:4,000 in 5 min.

Uses and Administration: *Dosage*—Adults and older children, 1 tablet three times daily; children below age of 10—¼–½ tablet; to be taken for about 1 week and then followed by a purgative, as castor oil or calomel; in obstinate cases a second course of treatment may be necessary. During and after treatment, enemas should be given of 1 tablespoonful of liquor aluminis acetatis to the quart of water or of limewater; scrupulous cleanliness of patient's hands with frequent change of underclothing is essential; irritation of the anal region may be relieved by white precipitate ointment.

Advantages: Is practically tasteless, free from undesirable by-effects and easily administered.

Supply: BUTOLAN—Tablets 7½ gr (0.5 Gm)—Tubes of 20.

Bibliography: *See Chap. XII.*

BUTYL-CHLORAL HYDRATE

Sedative. Hypnotic

Chemical Name: Trichlorbutylidene; "Croton" Chloral Hydrate.

Formula: $CH_3CHCl. CCl_2CH(OH)_2$.

Description: Nearly white trimetric laminae, of an acrid, nauseating taste and pungent odor; soluble in about 50 parts of water, in its own weight of 90% alcohol and glycerine and slowly in 20 parts of chloroform.

Action and Uses: Analgesic, hypnotic, teniafuge; is similar to chloral, but more active, less depressing and of greater analgesic power; *used* in neuralgias, tic douloureux, toothache, tabetic pains; in stenocardia, spasms, insomnia of heart disease.

Supply: **BUTYL-CHLORAL HYDRATE** (C.A.)—Bottles of 1 oz., ¼ lb., 1 lb. **(Merck)**

Administration: *Dose*—Hypnotic—5–18 gr (0.3–1.2 Gm); analgesic—1½–5 gr (0.09–0.3 Gm) at 1 dose, in pill, or in mixture of water, alcohol and glycerin.
Maximum Dose—30 gr (2 Gm) single, 60 gr (4 Gm) daily.
Externally—With equal parts of phenol.

Combinations: **TABLOID BUTYL CHLORAL HYDRATE et GELSEMIUM**, **(Burroughs Wellcome)** containing Butyl chloral hydrate, 3 gr (0.194 Gm), Gelsemium hydrochloride, 1/200 gr (0.00032 Gm)—Bottles of 25, 100 and 500.
Dosage—1 to 3 tabloids dissolved in half glass of water; repeated when necessary.

Antidotes: Picrotoxin, atropine, strychnine, caffeine, artificial respiration, stomach siphonage.

BUTYN **(Abbott)**

Local Anesthetic

Chemical Name: P-aminobenzoyl-gamma-dinormalbutylamino-propanolsulphate.

Formula: $[NH_2C_6H_4, COO(CH_2)_3N. (C_4H_9)_2]H_2SO_4$.

Description: A crystalline, colorless, odorless synthetic compound; soluble in water, very soluble in alcohol, acetone, chloroform; insoluble in ether.

Action: A local anesthetic effective through intact mucosa like cocaine; is as powerful as phenacaine (holocaine) and more efficient than cocaine or eucaine of similar dilutions; is non-irritating.

Uses: **Ophthalmology**—For removal of foreign bodies, relief of pain, abrasions of cornea and all eye operations, including cataract.

Rhinology—In submucous resection, radical accessory sinus work, antrum puncture, turbinectomy and ordinary nasal examinations; in tonsillectomy and various laryngological procedures.

Genitourinary Surgery—Intraurethral and endovesical examinations and operations.

Dentistry—Various dental procedures necessitating anesthesia.

Infiltration Anesthesia—In numerous operations: appendectomy, herniotomy, thyroidectomy, hemorrhoidectomy.

Advantages: Anesthesia is more rapidly induced, more efficient, longer lasting; does not dilate the pupil, cause drying of conjunctivae, affect accommodation or ocular tension; does not influence blood vessels; is non-narcotic and not affected by boiling.

Supply: **BUTYN**—Powder (C.A.)—Bottles 5 Gm and 1 oz.

BUTYN—Eye Ointment 2%—Tubes—Box of 12.

BUTYN—Solution 2% (C.A.)—Bottles 1 oz.

BUTYN—Tablets, gr 3 (C.A.) (0.2 Gm)—Vials of 10 and 100.

BUTYN—Tablets (C.A.) Hypodermic, gr 1/6 (0.01 Gm) with Epinephrine 1/2,000 gr (0.032 mg)—Bottles of 100, 1,000 and 5,000.

BUTYN-EPHEDRINE—Solution, Butyn 1%, Ephedrine 1%—Bottles of 1, 4 and 16 fl. oz.

BUTYN AND EPINEPHRINE CHLORIDE—Solution—Ampule, 2 cc—Box 12 and 100.

Solutions: One 3 gr tablet dissolved in 20 cc distilled water makes 1% solution; one tablet Butyn with Epinephrine, dissolved in 1 cc distilled water makes 1% solution.

Water must be boiled before adding tablet; it is then gently heated until tablet is dissolved. Plain sterile distilled water only should be used for making solution.

Incompatibles: Any chloride, including normal saline, bromides and Ringer's solution.

Caution: Is to be used in smaller quantities than cocaine; excepting in dentistry, where 3/4% is permitted, no hypodermic injection stronger than 1/4% solution is to be administered.

Administration and Dosage: **Eye**—2% solution, for topical use or instillation; for profound anesthesia—up to 5%; operation to begin not later than 10 min. after last instillation.

Nose—2% for topical use; Butyn Ephedrine solution is here recommended.

Throat—2% topically; for infiltration in tonsillectomy 1/10–1/4%.

Genitourinary—For examination, 4 cc of 1% solution, applied topically with cotton pledget, for 3 min., a few minutes before examination.

Proctology—In pruritus 1/2% solution injected around anus; infiltration anesthesia—1/10–1/4%, maximum 1/2% solutions.

Bloodless Surgery—Tablets of Butyn with Epinephrine are to be employed.

Bibliography: *See Chap. XII.*

B VITAMINS (Burroughs Wellcome)

Nutrient

Composition: An extractive of B vitamin fractions from brewer's yeast; free from the presence of yeast cells.

Action and Uses: Provides Vitamins B_1 and B_2 (F and G); promotes normal nutrition, restores appetite and intestinal tonus; *used* in conditions of disturbed nutrition where B vitamin deficiency is suspected.

Supply: **B Vitamins**—Tabloid—Yeast Concentrate gr 1 3/4 (0.112 Gm)—Bottles of 100 and 500.

Administration: 1–3 tabloids after meals.

Bibilography: *See Chap. XII.*

CADECHOL (Bischoff)

Cardiotonic

Chemical Name: Camphor-choleic Acid.

Formula: $C_{24}H_{40}O_4$—$C_{10}H_{16}O$.

Composition: A definite chemical combination of pure Japanese camphor (about 28%) and choleic acid; not a mixture or synthetic product.

Description: A white, odorless crystalline powder having a slight taste of camphor.

Action: The desoxy-choleic acid in itself is not therapeutically active, but makes the camphor content soluble in the intestinal tract and promotes its absorption; is a cardiac stimulant and tonic.

Uses: Chronic cardiac insufficiency; enuresis in children.

Advantages: Lacks almost entirely the disagreeable camphor taste.

Supply: CADECHOL—Tablets 1½ gr—Packages of 20 and 100.

CADECHOL—Powder—Packages ½ and 1 oz.

Administration: 1–2 tablets four or five times a day; in enuresis 1–2 tablets on retiring.

Bibliography: *See Chap. XII.*

CALCIUM BENZIODOXYL (Searle)

Antiarthritic

Chemical Name: Calcium salt of Ortho-iodo-oxybenzoic Acid.

Formula: $C_{15}H_9O_{10}I_2Ca$.

Description: As a salt of ortho-iodoxy-benzoic acid is claimed to possess better palliative action than the salicylates and iodides; is a white crystalline silken powder, enclosed in capsules for oral administration; is well tolerated.

Action and Uses: Reduces joint swellings, eliminates muscular spasm, shortens progress of disease and hastens restoration in function in various forms of arthritis.

Supply: CALCIUM BENZIODOXYL—Capsules gr 7½ (0.5 Gm)—Bottles of 25.

Administration: 1 capsule every 1–2 hr., with water on empty stomach, for 3–4 doses; repeated every 3–4 days for 6 weeks; after rest period of 2 weeks course is repeated.

Bibliography: *See Chap. XII.*

CALCIUM GLUCONATE

Calcium Therapy

Composition: Normal calcium salt of gluconic acid; an oxidation product of glucose.

Formula: $(C_6H_{11}O_5COO)_2CaH_2O$.

Description: Occurs as white, odorless, tasteless crystals or as light amorphous powder; soluble in boiling water, 1:30 in cold water, insoluble in alcohol and fat solvents; is completely oxidized, more palatable than calcium chloride and non-irritating.

Action: Increases blood calcium; affects transudation phenomena and is essential for rhythmic excitation of heart muscle.

Uses: In all calcium deficiencies: in tetany-parathyreopriva, maternal, idiopathic, infantile; in allergic manifestations, asthma, hay fever, urticaria, angioneurotic edema, moist itching dermatoses, diarrhea; preoperatively to shorten blood coagulation time.

Supply: CALCIUM GLUCONATE—Ampules 10 cc, 10%—Boxes of 6, 25 and 100 for intravenous and intramuscular use. (Abbott)

CALCIUM GLUCONATE—Wafoids, segmented, gr 5 (0.324 Gm) combined with aromatics—Bottles 100 and 1,000. (Drug Products)

CALCIUM GLUCONATE—Tablets, segmented, gr 10 (0.643 Gm) combined with aromatics—Bottles 100 and 1,000. (Drug Products)

CALCIUM GLUCONATE—Tablets, gr 15—Bottles of 100. (Lafayette)
Powder—Bottles of 1 oz. ¼ and 1 lb.

CALCIUM GLUCONATE—Bottles of 4 oz. (Mallinckrodt)

CALCIUM GLUCONATE—Powder—Bottles of ¼ lb. (Squibb)
Tablets 22 gr (1½ Gm)—Bottles of 50.

Administration: *Oral*—1 dr. in powder or tablet form, three times daily after meals, best given with Viosterol 250D and parathyroid hormone.
Intravenous and Intragluteal—1 ampule daily or every other day.

Bibliography: *See Chap. XII.*

CALCIUM LEVULINATE (Crookes)

Calcium Therapy

Description: An aqueous solution of calcium levulinate, containing 1.31% calcium, equivalent to 1.82% calcium oxide.

Action: As for calcium; not being supersaturated has no tendency to solidify; has prolonged action.

Uses: Where calcium is desirable; in tetany, calcium deficiency diseases, anaphylactic disturbances, preoperatively.

Advantages: Has high content of calcium, nearly 50% higher than calcium gluconate; causes no reactions even in subcutaneous extravasation during intravenous injection.

Supply: **CALCIUM LEVULINATE**—Ampules 10 cc, Intravenous and intramuscular—Boxes of 6.
CALCIUM LEVULINATE—Ampules 2 cc Intramuscular only—Boxes of 6.

Administration: *Intravenously*—10–20 cc, warmed to body temperature, injected slowly as often as is demanded.
Intramuscularly—As may be necessary.

CALCIUM PEROXIDE

(Roessler and Hasslacher)

Antacid. Antiseptic

Chemical Name: Calcium Peroxide; Calcium Superoxide.

Formula: $CaO_2 + 8H_2O$.

Composition: A mixture of the Calcium salt of Hydrogen Peroxide, with Hydroxide and Carbonate of Calcium; contains 13.3% available oxygen in about 60–75% of Calcium Peroxide.

Description: A light, cream colored, tasteless and odorless powder; is slightly soluble in water, decomposing into calcium hydroxide and peroxide of hydrogen with evolution of oxygen.

Action and Uses: Antacid, antiseptic and germicidal; is preferable to hydrogen peroxide because of its slow evolution of oxygen and prolonged action; is a strong oxidizer, destroyer of microorganisms.

Advantages: *Used* instead of milk of lime in acid dyspepsia and in summer diarrhea of infants; as a convenient means for the sterilization of water.

Supply: **CALCIUM PEROXIDE**—Cases of 100 lb.

Administration: 1–5 gr (0.06–0.3 Gm) in water or with sodium bicarbonate, two or three times daily.

CALCIUM PHOSPHATE TRIBASIC (Merck)

Calcium Therapy

Official Name: Calcii Phosphas Tribasicus.

Formula: $Ca_3(PO_4)_2$.

Description: Occurs as white, tasteless and odorless powder; is insoluble in water, readily soluble in dilute mineral acids.

Action and Uses: Reconstructive *for use* in disturbances of nutrition, and in repair of bone tissue; also *used* in peptic ulcer, as antacid.

Supply: CALCIUM PHOSPHATE TRIBASIC (C.A.)—1 lb. or 5 lb. cartons.

Administration: *Dose*—8–20 gr (0.5–1.3 Gm); in peptic ulcer 10–25 gr (0.6–1.6 Gm) average dose 15 gr (1 Gm) every hour. Children, ¾–1½ gr (0.05–0.1 Gm) for every year of age.

CALCIUM THIOCYANATE (Sutliff and Case)

Vasodilator

Chemical Name: Calcium Thiocyanate.

Action and Uses: Vasodilator in arterial hypertension, arteriosclerosis, luetic aortitis, endarteritis and gout.

Supply: CALCIUM THIOCYANATE—Tablets, enteric coated, gr ¾ (0.048 Gm)—Bottles 100, 500 and 1,000.

Administration: 1 tablet three times daily after meals for 6–8 weeks; in stubborn cases 4 tablets daily, for 1 or 2 weeks.

CALCOL (Mulford Colloid)

Calcium Therapy

Description: Occurs as greyish white scales, readily soluble in water; contains 20–28% Calcium.

Action and Uses: A stable, non-irritating, readily absorbed and assimilated colloidal calcium; is slowly eliminated, of prolonged action and does not cause precipitation of tissue fluids. *For use* in calcium deficiency, acidosis, excessive gastric acidity.

Supply: CALCOL—Packages 10 and 60 Gm.
CALCOL—Capsules gr 5 (0.324 Gm)—Bottles 100.
CALCOL—Solution 10%, 25 cc.

Administration: *Orally*—2½–15 gr (0.162–0.972 Gm).
Intravenously—¼–10 cc.
Internally—1–5 cc.

CALCREOSE (Maltbie)

Expectorant

Chemical Name: Calcium Creosotate.

Description: A loose chemical combination of equal parts by weight of Creosote and hydrated Calcium Oxide; a dark brown powder of sharp taste, partly soluble in water.

Action and Uses: As for creosote, but with little or no gastric irritation; an expectorant and antiseptic in coughs, colds, bronchial affections and tuberculosis; an intestinal antiseptic in diarrhea and enteritis.

Supply: CALCREOSE—Powder (C.A.) 50%—Packages of 1 lb.

CALCREOSE—Tablets gr 1 (0.06 Gm) Aromatic, for use in children—Bottles of 100, 500 and 1,000.

CALCREOSE—Tablets (C.A.) gr 4 (0.26 Gm) Enteric coated, for intestinal affections—Bottles of 100, 500 and 1,000.

CALCREOSE—Solution (C.A.)—Bottles of 1 pt. and 1 gal.

Administration: 1–2 teaspoonfuls or 4–8 tablets in water several times daily.

Combinations: COMPOUND SYRUP OF CALCREOSE (C.A.)—Each ounce represents: Calcreose solution, ♏ 160 (9.58 cc), Wild cherry bark, gr 20 (1.27 Gm), Alcohol, ♏ 24 (1.48 cc), Chloroform, ♏ 3 (0.18 cc), Aromatics and Syrup q.s. *For use* as expectorant in stubborn coughs.
Supply—Bottles of 4 oz., 1 pt. and 1 gal.
Administration—1–2 teaspoonfuls every 2 or 3 hr.

CALCREOSE COMPOUND 2—Contains: Calcreose, gr 4 (0.26 Gm), Reduced Iron, gr ½ (0.03 Gm), Arsenic Trioxide, gr 1/150, Strychnine, gr 1/150. *For use* alone or alternately with plain Calcreose tablets (1–4 gr) when larger doses of Calcreose are desired with the addition of arsenic, iron and strychnine.
Supply—Tablets—Bottles of 100, 500 and 1,000.

CALCREOSE COMPOUND 3—Contains: Calcreose, gr 2 (0.13 Gm), Reduced Iron, gr ¼ (0.016 Gm), Arsenic Trioxide, gr 1/300, Strychnine, gr 1/300. *For use* in children, as above.
Supply—Tablets—Bottles of 100, 500 and 1,000.

CALCREOSE EUPHORBIA COMPOUND—Contains: Calcreose, gr 3 (0.19 Gm), ext. Euphorbia pilulifera, gr 1 (0.06 Gm), Tinct. Lobelia, ♏ 3 (0.18 cc). *For use* in asthma.
Supply—Tablets—Bottles of 100, 500 and 1,000.
Administration—1 tablet every hour until relieved, then 1 every 2–3 hr.

CALCREOSE WITH IODINE—Contains: Calcreose, gr 4 (0.26 Gm), Iodine gr 1/30 (0.002 Gm).
Supply—Tablets—Bottles of 100, 500 and 1,000.
Administration—1–3 tablets with a glass of water every 2–4 hr.; is started with small doses and increased as necessary.

CREODIDE—Tablets, Plain—Contains: Calcreose, gr ½ (0.03 Gm), Iodine gr 1/20 (0.003 Gm). *For use* in croup, tonsillitis and bronchitis in children.
Supply—Tablets—Bottles of 100, 500 and 1,000.
Administration—1 tablet crushed, in teaspoonful of hot water every 10 min., for 3–4 doses until relieved.

CREOMINT—Lozenges—Contains: Calcreose, gr 1 (0.064 Gm), Elm bark, gr 2 (0.130 Gm), Cubeb powder, gr ½ (0.032 Gm), Balsam tolu, gr ⅕ (0.012 Gm), Benzocaine, gr 1/50 (0.0013 Gm), Menthol, gr 1/35 (0.002 Gm), Oil peppermint, ♏ 1/50 (0.0013 Gm). *For use* in acute and subacute inflammations of the pharynx and larynx.
Supply—Lozenges—Bottles of 100, 500 1,000.
Administration—To be slowly dissolved in the mouth.

CALGLUCON (Sandoz)

Calcium Therapy

Chemical Name: Normal Calcium Gluconate.

Formula: $[HOCH_2.CH(OH)CH(OH)CH(OH)CH(OH)COO_2]Ca. H_2O$.

Description: Occurs as white, odorless, tasteless granules; insoluble in alcohol and fat solvents, soluble in cold water (1 in 30), in boiling water (1 in 4–5); contains 13% CaO, corresponding to 9% calcium ion.

Action: Has been shown to lessen transudation phenomena, to influence nervous, glandular and muscular activity, to relieve smooth muscle spasm, to increase phagocytosis and reinforce body defenses against infection. Is superior to other calcium salts because less toxic, better tolerated and well absorbed; is non-irritant to tissues; is therefore suitable for intravenous and painless intramuscular injections; is well tolerated orally.

Uses: In conditions where calcium is indicated to meet an increased physiologic demand or correct a deficiency, as in pregnancy, lactation, fractures, rickets, dental caries, tetany. Is *used* also in hemorrhage, itching and oozing dermatoses, arsphenamine dermatitis, angioneurotic edema, anaphylaxis, serum disease, asthma, urticaria, mucous and ulcerative colitis, diarrhea; in epididymitis, salpingitis, prostatitis, gonorrheal arthritis, jaundice and tuberculous enteritis.

Supply: CALGLUCON—Powder (C.A.)—Cartons of 100 and 500 Gm.

CALGLUCON—Ampules (C.A.) 10% and 20% solution, 10 cc—Boxes of 5, 20, 100.

CALGLUCON—Ampules (C.A.) 10% and 20% solution, 5 cc—Boxes of 10, 50 and 150.

CALGLUCON—Ampules (C.A.) 10% solution, 2 cc—Boxes of 3, 10 and 50.

CALGLUCON—Tablets (C.A.)—Chocolate flavored, 1.5 Gm—Tins 30, 150 and 1,000.

CALGLUCON—Tablets (C.A.)—Effervescent, 4 Gm.—Tins of 12 and 66.

Administration: Effervescent tablets: one twice daily; children ⅓–1; in water.

Chocolate tablets: 1 or 2 chewed, three times daily; children ⅓ to 1 tablet.

Powder: 1 heaping teaspoonful, three times daily; children 1 level teaspoonful three times daily.

Injection: *Intramuscularly* and *intravenously*, 10 cc or more, every 1–3 days; children 2–5 cc daily.

Bibliography: *See Chap. XII.*

CALOMELOL (Heyden)

Antiluetic

Official Name: Hydrargyri Chloridum Mite Colloidale.

Description: A preparation of Calomel in combination with an Albuminate, in colloidal form; is a grayish, odorless, tasteless powder consisting of 80% Mercury salt and 20% Protein; is soluble in water giving an opalescent suspension; is insoluble in alcohol, ether and benzene.

Action: As for mercurous chloride, but is more rapid, more effective and non-irritating.

Uses: By inunction—in secondary syphilis; as dusting powder—for syphilitic ulceration; as 2% dressing—on wounds.

Incompatibles: Same as Calomel.

Supply: CALOMELOL—Ointment (C.A.) containing 45 parts Calomelol in lard—Tubes of 2 oz.

CALOMELOL—Powder—Vials of 1 oz.

Administration: *Internal*— In dosages same as calomel.
External—Inunction of ointment, 1½ dr. daily for 30 days.

CAMPIODOL SOLUTION (Abbott)

X-Ray Contrast Medium

Description: Chlor-iodized rape seed oil diluted with olive oil esters; is non-irritating, non-toxic, stable and thoroughly radiopaque.

Action and Uses: *Used* as diagnostic medium for radiologic study of respiratory tract, spinal canal, cerebral ventricles, nasal sinuses, uterine adnexae.

Supply: CAMPIODOL—Solution—Bottles of 20 cc.

CAMPIODOL (C.A.)—Emulsion—Ampules 20 cc—Boxes of 6.

Administration: In quantities in accordance with the type of radiographic examination and method of administration.

CAPROKOL (Sharp and Dohme)

Urinary Germicide

Chemical Name: Hexylresorcinol.

Formula: $C_6H_3(OH)_2(C_6H_{13})$.

Description: A heavy resinous yellowish fluid, of pungent odor and astringent taste; solidifies at room temperature; is very soluble in water, soluble in ether, chloroform and benzene.

Action: Non-toxic, non-irritating, stable, readily absorbed and excreted in the urine; active in dilution of 1:1,000; phenol coefficient over 70.

Uses: As urinary antiseptic in infections due to bacillus coli, bacillus pyocyaneus and staphylococcus. *Used* in cystitis, pyelitis and urethritis; in gonorrheal disease and chronic prostatitis; preoperatively—to relieve strangury and postoperatively—pain in genitourinary surgery, in gynecologic and obstetric procedures.

Supply: CAPROKOL—Solution (C.A.), 2½% in olive oil, 0.1 Gm hexylresorcinol per dram—Bottles of 4 oz.

CAPROKOL—Capsules (C.A.)—Boxes of 25, 50 and 100.

Administration: 2–4 capsules, three times daily after meals; continued for 2 weeks after the urine has become bacteria-free.

Children, 1 teaspoonful of solution (well tolerated by children) every 4 hr.; increased to 3–6 teaspoonfuls, according to age.

Caution: All diuretics, citrates and bicarbonates are to be avoided during Caprokol therapy.

Bibliography: *See Chap. XII.*

CARBARSONE (Lilly)

Amebacide

Chemical Name: P-Carbamino-phenyl Arsonic Acid.

Formula: $H_2O_3As.\ C_6H_4NH.\ CO.\ NH_2$.

Description: A white, crystalline, odorless stable powder of slightly acid taste; is practically insoluble in water, soluble in carbonate or bicarbonate solutions; contains about 28.85% arsenic.

Action: Destroys mobile amebae, eliminates cysts and gives symptomatic relief; is clinically efficient and non-toxic in therapeutic dosage.

Uses: In the treatment of amebiasis (Entameba histolytica).

Contraindications: Liver or kidney disease, amebic hepatitis, intolerance of arsenic.

Supply: CARBARSONE—Pulvules, gr 3¾ (0.25 Gm)—Bottles 20 and 500.

CARBARSONE—Vials, Gm 2—Box of 6, for retention enema.

Administration: 1 pulvule, twice daily after meals, for 10 days; after a 10-day interval, a second course may be given. In severe instances, in addition, retention enemas, 2 Gm of vial dissolved in 200 cc of warm bicarbonate solution, injected slowly and preceded by alkaline cleansing enema; administered every other night, five times. Diet should be low in starch and high in vitamin values.

Bibliography: *See Chap. XII.*

CARBON DIOXIDE-OXYGEN MIXTURES

(Ohio Chemical)

Anesthetic Gases

Composition: Mixtures of the two gases, Carbon Dioxide and Oxygen supplied in the following proportions, with carbon dioxide content accurate to the extent indicated.

	Per Cent		Per Cent	Tolerance	Per Cent
Oxygen.......	95	Carbon Dioxide......	5	plus, minus,	0.5
"	95.5	" "	4.5	" "	0.5
"	93	" "	7	" "	0.5
"	90	" "	10	" "	0.8
"	85	" "	15	" "	0.8
"	80	" "	20	" "	0.9
"	75	" "	25	" "	0.9
"	70	" "	30	" "	1.0

Action and Uses: The mixture of carbon dioxide with oxygen enables the anesthetist to exercise better control over the anesthetized than with oxygen alone; induction is more rapid, excitement stage is lessened or eliminated, respiration is deeper and relaxation more pronounced, elimination of anesthetic at conclusion of anesthesia is quicker; it also aids in overcoming the shallow respiration and weak pulse which may result from an overdosage of ether and lessens likelihood of post-operative pneumonia. *Useful* in general anesthesia; in starting respiration in the new born infant; in resuscitation of persons overcome by carbon monoxide or other poisonous or asphyxiating gases.

Supply: CARBON DIOXIDE-OXYGEN MIXTURES—In steel cylinders.

Administration: By passing the gas mixture into an inhalation apparatus as used for general anesthesia, or by an apparatus especially designed for the purpose.

Bibliography: *See Chap. XII.*

CARBON TETRACHLORIDE

Parasiticide

Chemical Name: Benzinoform; Tetrachlormethane.

Formula: CCl_4.

Description: A heavy, clear, colorless, non-inflammable liquid, of characteristic odor; soluble in about 2,000 parts of water; miscible with alcohol, ether, benzene.

Action and Uses: Anthelmintic and vermicide; *useful* in hookworm disease; also in oxyuris vermicularis, ascaris lumbricoides and trichocephalus dispar, but less effective.

Supply: CARBON TETRACHLORIDE (C.A.)—Capsules 20 m— **(Parke, Davis)** Vials 12 and 100.

CARBON TETRACHLORIDE (C.A.)—Capsules 0.3 and 1 cc—Boxes of 12 and 100. **(Sharp and Dohme)**

Administration: Single dose only—Adults 30–45 m; Children—2 m per year up to 15 yr. of age; given in water, milk or gelatin capsules, on empty stomach, followed in 3 hr. by dose of Epsom salts; or is given with the salt.

Caution: Not to be administered to alcoholics; not to be repeated within 3 weeks; in the constipated is to be preceded by a laxative 3 days before administration.

CARDYSATE (Bischoff)

Digitalis Therapy

Description: A stable, uniformly active, fresh extract, dialyzed from fresh digitalis leaves and free from inert matter.

Action and Uses: Is stated to be non-cumulative, of quick action, rapid absorption and elimination and to produce no disagreeable secondary effects. *For use* as cardiac stimulant and diuretic in all conditions where digitalis therapy is indicated.

Supply: CARDYSATE—Bottles 15 cc.

Administration: 5–15 m as needed.

CARGENTOS (Sharp and Dohme)

Antiseptic

Chemical Name: Silver Protein, Mild.

Composition: A Colloidal Silver and modified Casein preparation, containing 20–25% of silver; is non-hygroscopic and readily soluble; does not precipitate chlorides or proteins.

Action: A deeply penetrating and non-irritating germicidal agent.

Uses: In hyperemia and infections of the mucous membranes of eye, ear, nose and throat, urethra, vagina: in urethritis, vaginitis, purulent and catarrhal conjunctivitis, corneal ulcers, otitis media, chronic pharyngitis.

Supply: CARGENTOS—Scales (C.A.)—Vials of ½ and 1 oz.

CARGENTOS—Capsules (C.A.) gr 3—Bottles of 50.

CARGENTOS—Ointment 5% (C.A.)—Tubes ½ oz., with elongated tip, for urethral use.

CARGENTOS—Ointment 10% (C.A.)—Tubes ⅛ oz., with tip, for eye application.

CARGENTOS—Suppositories (C.A.) gr 2—Boxes of 12, for urethral use.

Administration:

Oral—In gastrointestinal inflammation and ulceration—2–5 gr, two to three times daily.

Eye: In simple conjunctivitis—solutions 25%, in purulent or gonorrheal conjunctivitis—ointment 10%, in corneal ulcers—50%, ophthalmia neonatorum prophylaxis—25%; before operations, for several days—25%.

Nose and Throat—As spray—10–20%; for swab—25–50%.

Surgery—In wounds and ulcers—as solution or ointment 1–10%.

Urology—In Neisserian infections: acute injections—3–10%, chronic—10–20%; urethral irrigation 0.1%, urethral suppositories—2 gr; in cystitis—5 cc of 20–50% or 30 cc of 10–25%.

Gynecology—Solutions—10–25%; tampons, in glycerin—25%; suppositories—5 gr.

Rectal—Irrigation 0.1–1%; injection 10%; suppositories 2 gr.

CARITOL (S.M.A.)

Vitamin Therapy

Description: A red colored 0.3% solution of Carotene (primary vitamin A) in vegetable oil; is claimed to be the only product containing primary vitamin A alone; has no fishy taste.

Action and Uses: Provides carotene (primary vitamin A), an essential food factor in important bodily requirements and in the synthesis of secondary vitamin A by the liver; possesses growth-promoting, hemoglobin regenerative and anti-infection properties. *Recommended* in the prevention of infections of the upper respiratory tract, of common colds and sinus disease.

Supply: CARITOL—Bottles, dropper top, 15 and 50 cc, in special cartons.

Administration: 3–5 drops daily for infants and young children; 5–10 drops daily for adults; administered orally, alone or with cod liver oil, haliver oil or viosterol.

Bibliography: *See Chap. XII.*

CASEOSAN (Heyden)

Non-specific Protein Therapy

Description: A sterile 5% Casein solution of constant composition.

Action: Stimulates the organism in the formation of antibodies and in overcoming infection.

Uses: In low grade and post-partum pelvic infections, parametritis, torpid adnexal tumors; in furunculosis, adenitis, periostitis, erysipelas; in arthritis deformans, muscular and acute gonorrheal rheumatism, sciatica; in bubo, prostatitis, epididymitis, gonorrheal conjunctivitis, keratitis parenchymatosa; in dentistry—for root infection, severe gingivitis, focal neuralgia.

Supply: CASEOSAN—Ampules 1 cc—Boxes of 10.

CASEOSAN—Ampules 10 cc—Boxes of 5. Ampules 5 cc—Boxes of 6.

Administration: Intravenous, intramuscular, subcutaneous, intracutaneous. Dose is varied in accordance with the individual case, but be sufficient to produce a moderate general reaction and a distinct but not too violent local reaction. *Average Dosage—Intramuscular and subcutaneous,* 0.5–2.0–3 cc (to 5 cc); *intravenous,* 0.25–2.0 cc (to 3 cc) *intracutaneous,* 0.3–1 cc; administration—at 1–3 day intervals.

Bibliography: *See Chap. XII.*

CELLASIN "BARR" (Cellasin)

Oral Diabetotherapy

Description: A powerful sugar and starch splitting ferment prepared from fungi; is active in alkaline medium and not affected by natural enzymatic activity or gastric acidity; converts starches, cane sugar and glucose at 75–115°F into lactic acid and carbon dioxide; emulsifies fats with formation of fatty acids and sodium soaps.

Action and Uses: Is stated to increase the carbohydrate tolerance of the organism and to be useful in diabetes mellitus; locally is effective on diabetic wounds and gangrenous sores.

Supply: CELLASIN "BARR" 1—Tablets containing Cellasin, gr 7 (0.45 Gm); Sodium bicarbonate gr 3 (0.19 Gm)—Bottles of 200, 500 and 1,000.

CELLASIN "BARR" 2—Tablets containing Cellasin, gr 3½ (0.23 Gm); Sodium bicarbonate gr 1½ (0.09 Gm)—Bottles of 200, 500 and 1,000.

Administration: 12–15 tablets daily (4–5 tablets taken 1–2 hr. after meals) till urine is sugar free; thereafter dosage is gradually reduced, but continued 4–6 tablets daily for long period.

CEREVISINE "CHAPELLE" (Fougera)

Yeast Therapy

Official Name: Saccharomyces Cerevisiae.

Composition: Contains in active concentrated form enzymes, nuclein and nucleinic acid of the yeast plant.

Action: Stimulates phagocytic power in infections; is also laxative.

Uses: Internally—in pustular skin eruptions, furunculosis, acne, carbuncles, styes; in intestinal indigestion, chronic constipation; locally in vaginitis, cervical erosions, leukorrhea.

Supply: CEREVISINE "CHAPELLE"—Tablets, ½ and 1 Gm—Bottles of 75 and 150.

CEREVISINE "CHAPELLE"—Tablets, chocolate—Bottles of 75.

CEREVISINE "CHAPELLE"—Granulated—Vials 3 oz.

Administration: *Internally*—1 tablet every hour.

Locally—In form of paste, made with water; also applied as poultice.

CHAULMESTROL (Winthrop)

Leprosy Therapy

Chemical Name: Brand of Ethyl Chaulmoograte; a mixture of ethyl esters of the unsaturated acids of chaulmoogra.

Description: A thin, light, oily fluid, of neutral reaction, faint odor and not unpleasant taste; insoluble in water but miscible in all proportions with alcohol and ether.

Action: Its therapeutic properties are ascribed to the optically active, unsaturated fatty acids of the chaulmoogric series, chiefly chaulmoogric acid ($C_{18}H_{32}O_2$) and hydnocarpic acid ($C_{16}H_{28}O_2$).

Uses: In leprosy and tuberculosis.

Advantages: Is preferable to chaulmoogra oil because it is free from disagreeable taste and odor, is better adapted for prolonged use, is more rapid and reliable in action and does not cause gastro-intestinal disturbances.

Supply: CHAULMESTROL—Bottles 1 oz., ¼ and 1 lb.

CHAULMESTROL (C.A.)—Ampules 1 cc and 3 cc—Boxes of 10.

Administration: Leprosy—*Orally*—In gradually increasing doses, from 1 cc to 5 cc and more daily, after meals, in warm milk or hot tea; *intramuscularly* and *intravenously*, once weekly, beginning with 1 cc and increasing by 1 cc every second and third injection until 3–5 cc is reached.

Tuberculosis—*Intramuscularly* ½–6 cc every fifth day; *intravenously* in smaller doses.

Bibliography: *See Chap. XII.*

CHINIOFON

Amebacide

Chemical Name: Sodium Iodoxyquinolinesulphonate.

Formula: C_9H_6ONIS.

Description: A canary-yellow, odorless powder, of bitter taste, but distinct sweetish after-taste; soluble from 3–10 % in water with effervescence resulting from the uncombined remainder of sodium bicarbonate and iodohydroxyquinoline-sulphonic acid; insoluble in alcohol, ether, chloroform and organic solvents; iodine content about 26.5 %; stable even in hot climates if kept dry in amber bottles.

Action: Is destructive to Entameba dysenteriae histolytica and certain other protozoan organisms; supplies substances inimical to the growth of the amoebae in the body and in vitro; it probably affects the encysted ameba in the intestinal wall after absorption into the blood stream; is eliminated in the urine and causes no iodism.

Supply: **CHINIOFON** (C.A.)—Tablets, Plain and Enteric coated, 4 gr—Bottles of 100—Vials of 20, Plain only—Packages of 6. **(Searle)**

CHINIOFON—Tablets, Keratin coated, 4 gr—Bottles of 50. Powder—Bottles of 1 oz. **(Winthrop)**

Administration: **Acute Amebic Dysentery:**

Oral—1 tablet three times daily the first day, after meals; increased to 2 tablets on the second to fifth days; then 3 tablets on the sixth and seventh days, if well tolerated.

Rectal—A solution is prepared by sprinkling the quantity of Chiniofon to be used, evenly, on the surface of warm water (176°F) in a clean vessel; after effervescence has subsided the solution is cooled to body temperature and administered; injections are given daily for 4 days only.

To Prevent Relapse—3 tablets administered daily on 3 consecutive days, followed by an interval of 4 days; this sequence being repeated for 3 weeks; special diet regulation is not required.

Chronic Amebic Dysentery—The same method as for acute dysentery, except that rectal injections are given, after a cleansing enema, every evening. The strength of solutions is gradually increased: first day 1 Gm in 200 cc of water, second day 2 Gm in 300 cc, third, fourth and fifth days 3 Gm in 400, 500 and 600 cc of water respectively. If well tolerated the same dosage is repeated on the sixth and seventh days.

Enemas should be high and retained for 6–8 hr.; where retention is difficult 25–30 drops of tincture of opium is added or the quantity of water reduced. Where the higher parts of the colon are affected, oral administration is preferable.

After treatment—For 3 weeks injections of 2 or 3 Gm of Chiniofon in 300–500 cc of water given on 3 successive days with intervals of 3–4 days.

In Ulcerative and Membranous Colitis following amebic dysentery; injections alone or in conjunction with oral therapy is employed.

In Hepatitis and Liver Abscess—combined treatment with emetine is indicated.

In Bacillary Colitis and Mucous Colitis—rectal enemas are advisable in addition to internal therapy.

Bibliography: *See Chap. XII.*

CHLORAMINE (Squibb)

Dakin Antiseptic

Chemical Name: Sodium-paratoluene-sulphon-chloramide.

Formula: $CH_3 . C_6H_4SO_2NNaCl$.

Description: A white, almost odorless, crystalline powder containing 11.5–13 % available chlorine; is freely soluble in water, forming a stable solution of alkaline reaction; is non-irritating, non-toxic.

Action and Use: A safe powerful disinfectant for irrigation of all wounds by the Carrel-Dakin technic, in 2% solution; *useful* for eye, nose, and throat antisepsis and in infections of other organs.

Supply: CHLORAMINE—Tablets (C.A.), 4.6 gr (0.3 Gm) (2 tablets make 2% solution in 1 oz. of water)—Bottles of 10, 100, 500, 1,000.

CHLORAMINE—Powder (C.A.)—Bottles of 1 and 5 lb.

Administration: **Eye**—1/10% solution in physiologic saline.

Mouth, Nose, Throat—½% solution.

Urethra—½–2% solution.

Wounds—As dry powder or irrigation—2%.

CHLORAZENE (Abbott)

Dakin Antiseptic

Chemical Name: Chloramine-T. (Chloramine, U.S.P.)

Formula: $C_6H_4(CH_3)(SO_2N.\ NaCl) + 3H_2O$.

Composition: Contains active chlorine, from 11.5 to 13%.

Description: A white, crystalline substance of faintly chlorous odor, slightly bitter taste; freely soluble in water, insoluble in alcohol.

Action: Deodorant, antiseptic and disinfectant; decomposes bacterial toxins, is stable, non-toxic and slightly irritant.

Uses: Externally only—as antiseptic in the treatment of infected wounds; as disinfectant in obstetrics, gynecology and urology; as gargle and mouth wash in various oral affections.

Incompatibles: Oils, fats, acids and organic substances in general.

Caution: Slowly stains and tarnishes metal.

Supply: CHLORAZENE—Tablets (C.A.) 4.6 gr (0.3 Gm)—Tubes of 24—Bottles of 100, 1,000; 1 tablet in 1 oz. of water makes a 1% solution.

CHLORAZENE AROMATIC—Powder (C.A.)—Containing Chlorazene 5%, Sodium bicarbonate 5%, Eucalyptol 2%, Saccharin 1%, Sodium chloride 87%—Bottles of 2 and 4 oz.

CHLORAZENE—Surgical Powder—Cans, sprinkler top 1 oz.

CHLORAZENE—Surgical Cream (C.A.) 1% in sodium stearate and watery base—Jars of 2 oz. and 1 lb.

CHLORAZENE—Surgical Gauze (C.A.) 5%—Rolls of 1 and 5 yd.

Administration: *In Surgery*—1% solution; stronger where indicated.
For Irrigation of bladder, urethra, vagina—1/10%, increased as indicated.
As Gargle, Spray or Douche—¼% solution.

CHLORBUTANOL (Merck)

Local Anesthetic

Chemical Name: Trichlortertiary-Butylalcohol.

Formula: $CCl_3.\ C(OH).\ CH_3.\ CH_3$.

Description: A white crystalline volatile compound, of camphoraceous odor and taste; soluble in water (8 in 1,000), glycerin, alcohol, ether, benzin, acetone, chloroform, glacial acetic acid.

Action and Uses: A local anesthetic, sedative and antiseptic; is readily absorbed from the alimentary tract and somewhat depressant to cardiovascular and respiratory systems; is non-habit forming. *For use* in insomnia, vomiting, spastic conditions; as local anesthetic in dentistry and nose and throat disorders; as preservative for hypodermic solutions; for pre-anesthetic sedation.

Supply: CHLORBUTANOL—Hydrous (C.A.)—Boxes of ¼ and 1 lb.

CHLORBUTANOL—Anhydrous (C.A.)—Boxes of ¼ and 1 lb.

Administration: 0.3–1.3 Gm (5–20 gr), dry or in capsules.

Hypodermically—As saturated aqueous solution for local anesthesia.

CHLORETONE (Parke, Davis)

Hypnotic. Antinauseant

Chemical Name: Acetone Chloroform. Chlorbutanol.

Formula: $C_4H_7OCl_3$.

Description: A white, crystalline, volatile compound of camphoraceous taste and odor; dissolves freely in alcohol or ether, but only to the extent of about 0.7% in water; is stable in the presence of dilute acids.

Action and Uses: Is absorbed unchanged from the alimentary tract and acts on the cerebral reflexes; is non-toxic and non-habit forming; is antinauseant, antiseptic and hypnotic. *For use* in insomnia, chorea, pertussis, persistent hiccup, delirium tremens; for the control of tetanic convulsions in addition to serum treatment; as a preventive of mal-de-mer and of operative and post-operative nausea; as sedative and recuperative agent in prolonged and painful labor; as a preservative of alkaloidal and other solutions.

Supply: CHLORETONE (C.A.)—Vials 1 oz.—Bottles ¼ lb.

CHLORETONE (C.A.)—Capsules gr 3–5 (0.194–0.324 Gm)—Bottles of 100 and 500.

Administration: As Hypnotic—Gr 10 (0.643 Gm) repeated in ½ hr.

Antispasmodic—Gr 3–30 (0.194–1.944 Gm), repeated as necessary.

Preoperative—Gr 10–20 (0.643–1.296 Gm).

In Tetanus—Gr 40–60 (2.592–3.888 Gm) in olive oil as enema.

In Dystocia—Gr 10 (0.643 Gm) during first stage, then gr 5 (0.324 Gm) as required.

In Seasickness—Gr 5–20 (0.324–1.296 Gm), in single or divided doses.

Combinations: **CHLORETONE EMOLLIENT**—Contains Chloretone 1 Gm per 100 Gm of Liquid petrolatum, with Camphor and Menthol in proportion; *used* as dressing for burns and wounds.

Supply: Bottles, 16 oz. and 1 gal.

CHLORETONE INHALANT—Each 100 Gm contains Chloretone 1.0 Gm; Camphor 2.5 Gm; Menthol 2.5 Gm; Oil cinnamon 0.25 Gm; refined Liq. petrolatum 93.75 Gm; antiseptic and emollient; *used* by spray in rhinitis, laryngitis, pharyngitis or bronchitis; as protective is applied directly to fissured nipples, minor cuts, abrasions, burns and insect bites.

Supply—Bottles of 2, 4, 16 oz. and 1 gal.

CHLORINE GAS "ROEHLING" (Lakeside)

Inhalant. Antiseptic

Description: Highly purified Chlorine gas for inhalation therapy.

Action: A strong bactericidal and antiseptic agent in respiratory diseases; a safe, dependable method of administering chlorine gas.

Uses: In the prevention and treatment of colds, influenza, bronchitis and pneumonia.

Supply: CHLORINE GAS "ROEHLING"—Ampules 10 cc, containing 0.85 Gm chlorine.

Administration: By inhalation; 1 ampule for each 700 cu. ft. of room space is placed on flat saucer 5 ft. from patient, windows and doors being tightly closed to insure maintenance of concentration; ampule is then opened near center, emptied two-thirds and inhaled; the remainder is added in 30 min.; administered once daily, as necessary.

Caution: Room must be free from exposed water, wet surfaces, wet towels or any moist articles; ampule should be clean and dry and not too near patient.

CHLORINE-SODA AMPULES

(Johnson and Johnson)

Antiseptic

Composition: Contains in a sealed glass tube 4.8 Gm of almost 100 % pure Chlorine and in separate paper container Sodium Carbonate Monohydrated 21.3 Gm; the solution of the two in 1,000 cc of water yields a preparation similar to U.S.P. surgical chlorinated soda.

Action and Uses: As for chlorinated soda.

Supply: CHLORINE-SODA AMPULES (C.A.)—Package of 2 above containers.

Administration: The monohydrated sodium carbonate is placed in a 3 qt. vessel containing 1,000 cc of water. The liquid chlorine tube is then suspended from a rubber stopper, inserted into the vessel holding the dissolved carbonate, and then shaken for several minutes to break the glass tube; the mixture is strained to remove the broken glass and is then ready for use.

CHLOROXYL

(Lilly)

Uricolytic

Chemical Name: Cinchophen Hydrochloride.

Formula: $C_6H_5C_9H_5N. COOH. HCl.$

Description: A yellow, crystalline powder, of somewhat bitter and astringent taste; slightly soluble in alcohol, insoluble in water, chloroform and ether.

Action and Uses: Flushes uric acid from the organism through increased kidney elimination; reduces uricacidemia; is rapid analgesic, antipyretic, antiphlogistic. *Useful* in gout, acute articular rheumatism, arthritis; in neuralgia, neuritis, lumbago, sciatica, hemicrania; in iritis, episcleritis and in pyorrhea alveolaris.

Contraindications: Liver and kidney diseases, pregnancy, malnutrition, iodiosyncrasy.

Supply: CHLOROXYL—Tablets (C.A.), gr 5 (0.3 Gm)—Boxes of 20 and 100.

CHLOROXYL—Powder (C.A.)—Bottles of 1 oz.

Administration: 5–15 gr *orally*, repeated as indicated.

CHOLE-CYSTO-COL

(Abbott)

X-Ray Contrast Medium

Composition: Colloidal Tetraiodophenolphthalein in stabilized emulsion.

Action and Uses: Is rendered soluble in the intestine and is absorbed; is neutral, non-irritating and free from nausea or laxative-producing effects.

Used as cholecystographic medium in X-ray diagnosis of gall bladder affections.

Supply: CHOLE-CYSTO-COL—Bottles 2 Gm, single dose—Cartons of 12.

Administration: 1 dose 2 Gm, administered in water or grape juice or ginger-ale; exposures are made in 12 hr. and after.

Bibliography: *See Chap. XII.*

CHOLEVAL (Merck)

Gonocide

Official Name: Colloidal Silver-Sodium Cholate.

Description: Contains 10% Silver with Sodium Cholate as protective colloid; a dark brown, almost black, lustrous, odorless powder, readily soluble in water.

Action: Antiseptic, bactericidal, antigonorrhoeic; the sodium cholate attacks the pus cells, liberates contained bacteria, exposing these to the destructive action of the silver; solutions are non-astringent and seldom irritating.

Supply: CHOLEVAL—Powder—Bottles ⅛ and 1 oz.

CHOLEVAL—Tablets gr ¼ (0.016 Gm)—Bottles of 50—Tubes of 10.

Uses and Administration: In anterior urethritis as injections, in 0.25% solution, three to four times daily; gradually increased to 1.5%, then decreased; as irrigation, in 1:1,000–1:500 solution.

In acute and chronic cholangitis, cholecystitis, and other inflammatory complications of the biliary tract including residual typhoid infection or hepatic abscess, *intravenously*—1½ gr (0.1 Gm) in 10 cc sterile distilled water, daily if necessary; in severe cases 3 gr (0.2 Gm) in 10 cc of water. Solutions are made by sprinkling the Choleval on the surface of the water in a sterile porcelain dish and slowly dissolving.

Bibliography: *See Chap. XII.*

CINCHOPHEN

Analgesic. Uricolytic. Eliminant.

Chemical Name: Phenyl-quinoline-carboxylic Acid. Phenylcinchoninic Acid.

Formula: $C_6H_5C_9H_5N.COOH$.

Description: A white or almost white odorless powder of exceedingly bitter taste; nearly insoluble in cold water, slightly soluble in cold alcohol; soluble in glycerol, hot alcohol and benzene; forms soluble salts with alkalies.

Action: Analgesic, relieving pain particularly in joints and bones; is uric acid eliminant by increasing kidney permeability; is moderately antipyretic and rapidly effective.

Uses: In gout, acute and chronic arthritis, rheumatic fever, neuralgia, neuritis, lumbosacral disease, sciatica; iritis, episcleritis.

Supply: CINCHOPHEN (C.A.)—Tablets, gr 5, 7½ (0.3 and 0.5 Gm) each—Bottles of 100 and 1,000. (Abbott)

CINCHOPHEN (C.A.)—Tablets, gr 7½ (0.5 Gm)—Packages 20, 100 and 1,000. (Calco)

CINCHOPHEN (C.A.)—Powder, in multiples of 1 oz. (Calco)

CINCHOPHEN (C.A.)—Powder—Bottles 1 oz., ¼ and 1 lb. (Squibb)

CINCHOPHEN (C.A.)—Tablets, gr 5, 7½ (0.3 and 0.5 Gm) each—Packages of 100 and 1,000.

Administration: 5–15 gr—three or four times daily; continued in acute cases for 2–5 days; in chronic—same dosage but followed by rest periods of several days every 5 days; may be prescribed with sodium bicarbonate tablets to be powdered before use.

Contraindications: Renal calculi, nephritis, thyrotoxicosis, active infection of the biliary tract, major abdominal operations, idiosyncrasy.

Caution: Total dosage not to exceed 150 gr during 1 course. Danger of occasional acute yellow liver atrophy and other toxic symptoms; occurrence of nausea, anorexia, urticaria point to discontinuance of drug.

Bibliography: *See Chap. XII.*

CITRIN (Table Rock)

Hypotensor

Description: A glucoside saponin, Cucurbocitrin, prepared from the seed of watermelon, Cucurbita citrullus; is an aqueous extract of the active principle and free from proteoses, peptones and histamin.

Action and Uses: Hypotensive and thus decreases irritability, dizziness and dyspnea, symptoms associated with arterial hypertension, particularly of moderate intensity, where it is most indicated; is non-toxic, non-cumulative and does not depress the heart. *For use* in arterial hypertension.

Supply: **CITRIN**—Capsules 50 mg Cucurbocitrin—Bottles of 30 and 100.

Administration: 1–5 capsules daily, before meals.

Bibliography: *See Chap. XII.*

CLYMOCOL (Merck)

Germicide

Chemical Name: Mono-chlor-methyl-isopropyl-phenol.

Formula: $Cl. CH_3. C_3H_7. C_6H_2OH$.

Description: A 6% colloidal suspension of Chlorthymol; a clear, light amber, slightly aromatic, stable liquid, miscible with water.

Action: A concentrated, non-toxic germicide of phenol coefficient (F.D.A.) not less than 4; does not attack tissue, metal or rubber and has no solvent action on catgut or silk ligatures; is non-irritating and does not impair tissue repair.

Uses: In all surgical procedures for antiseptic and germicidal purposes.

Supply: **CLYMOCOL**—Bottles of 4, 16 oz. and 1 gal.

Administration: Standard solution in general surgery for topical application, irrigation or wet dressing—2% (2½ dr. to the pint of water); increased where indicated to 5 and 10%; for bladder irrigation, vaginal douching, instillation into body cavities—0.5%; for operating room and instrument disinfection—2–5%.

COAGULEN (Ciba)

Hemostatic

Description and Action: A non-toxic, non-irritating powder prepared from blood platelets; coagulates blood because of contained thromboplastic substance or thrombokinase; is soluble in water.

Uses: Indicated in all hemorrhages, external and internal, due to deficiency of thrombokinase.

Externally—In various surgical hemorrhages, tonsillectomy, hemorrhoidectomy, dental extraction and oozing wounds of any kind.

Internally—In hemophilia, purpura hemorrhagica, hemorrhagic disease of the newborn; in gastric, uterine, pulmonary and intestinal hemorrhages; in pemphigus.

Supply: COAGULEN—Powder—Bottles of 2.5 Gm, 5 Gm and 10 Gm.

COAGULEN—Ampules 1.5 cc and 5 cc, 3 % sterile solution—Carton of 5.

COAGULEN—Ampules 20 cc, 3 % sterile solution, 1 in carton.

Administration: *Oral*—5–10 Gm, dissolved in ¼ to 1 full glass of water, sipped slowly.

Subcutaneously and Intramuscularly—1.5–5 cc as preoperative prophylactic; *Postoperatively*—May be given up to 20 cc.

Intravenously—2–3 cc of ampule content, several times daily.

Locally—To prevent hemorrhage, is applied topically, or is injected simultaneously with the local anesthetic, 1 or 2 small ampules.

Bibliography: *See Chap. XII.*

CODAMINES TABLETS (Stearns)

Vitamin Therapy

Description: A chocolate coated, pleasant tasting tablet of Cod Liver Oil Concentrate, containing not less than 250 vitamin A and 100 vitamin D units per tablet; prepared in an atmosphere of carbon dioxide to prevent oxidation of the vitamin A active portion.

Action and Uses: As for cod liver oil; each tablet is equivalent to ½ teaspoonful of high grade cod liver oil.

Supply: CODAMINES—Tablets—Bottles of 100.

Administration: Adults—2–4 tablets three to four times daily.

Children and Infants—1–3 tablets crushed in milk, one to three times daily.

Bibliography: *See Chap. XII.*

COD LIVER OIL CONCENTRATES

Vitamin Therapy

Description: Concentrates prepared from Cod Liver Oil, of definite vitamin potency, in tablet and liquid form.

Action and Uses: As for cod liver oil; *For use* in rickets, malnutrition, delayed dentition; in pregnancy, convalescence and other conditions where vitamin therapy is indicated.

Supply: COD LIVER OIL CONCENTRATE (C.A.)—Prepared from the **(Clinadol)** non-saponifiable fraction of Norwegian cod liver oil, in oil of maize, with oil of cassia and 3/1,000 % of gluside; has an assayed vitamin A potency of not less than 5,500 units Vitamin D, 1,428 units (A.D.M.A.) per gram of oil—Bottles of 10 and 60 cc. *Dosage:* 10–40 drops daily, 6 drops being equivalent to 1 teaspoonful of cod liver oil of 500 "A" units.

COD LIVER OIL "White's" Tablets (C.A.)—Each contains **(Health Products)** not less than 685 units vitamin A and 450 vitamin D equivalent to ½ dr. of cod liver oil—Bottles of 100, 240 and 1,000 tablets coated against oxidation. *Dosage:* 2–4 tablets three times daily; infants, 1 mo., 1 tablet daily; 1 yr. 1 tablet three times daily, crushed in milk or orange juice.

VITAMIN CONCENTRATE OF COD LIVER OIL **(McKesson and Robbins)** (C.A.)—Contains 5,500 units vitamin A and 146 units vitamin D per gram; pleasantly flavored—Bottles of 11 cc. *Dosage:* 3–6 drops three times daily.

VITAMIN CONCENTRATE TABLETS OF COD **(McKesson and Robbins)** LIVER OIL (C.A.)—Contains per tablet not less than 1,000 units of vitamin

A and not less than 250 vitamin D (Int.), with 1 gr dicalcium phosphate; chocolate coated—Bottles of 85. *Dosage:* 2 tablets after meals.

COD LIVER OIL CONCENTRATE—Tablets—Each contains vitamin A 1000, vitamin D 100 units:—Bottles of 80. *Dosage:* 2–4 three times daily; infants 1 tablet, children 3 tablets daily, crushed, after meals. (Merrell)

TABLETS, VITAMINS A AND D—Each contains 1,200 U.S.P. vitamin A units and 600 A.D.M.A. vitamin D units—Tins of 15—Bottles of 70. *Dosage:* 4 tablets daily yielding at least 4,800 vitamin A and 2,400 vitamin D units. (Scott and Bowne)

Bibliography: *See Chap. XII.*

COD LIVER OIL

Nutrient. Vitamin Therapy

Description: A fixed oil obtained from fresh livers of Gadus morrhua and other species of Gadus; is of light, clear, straw color, high purity and fresh bland taste; saturated with CO_2 gas to preserve vitamin A content; physiologically standardized to contain 1,250 vitamin A and 50 units vitamin D, per gram.

Action: Fortifies against infection, maintains normal calcium and phosphorus metabolism; assists in bone calcification and in delayed union of fractures, in formation of denture and prevention of dental decay.

Uses: As dietary supplement for infants, especially after weainng; for expectant and nursing mothers; for convalescents and adults on restricted diets; as prophylactic in tuberculosis, as antiinfective in furunculosis, styes, keratomalacia, mastoiditis; as antixerotic and antirachitic.

Supply: **COD LIVER OIL**—Containing per ounce vitamin A, 14,000 units, vitamin D, 7,000 units—Bottles of 8, 16, 32 oz. and 1 gal. (Hance)

COD LIVER OIL—Capsules, m 10, m 20—Boxes of 12 and 100. (Hance)

COD LIVER OIL—Capsules, 2½ Gm—Boxes of 100. (Hance)

COD LIVER OIL AND CREOSOTE—Capsules, containing cod liver Oil m 19, creosote m 1—Boxes 12 and 100. (Hance)

COD LIVER OIL—Flavored (C.A.)—Containing more than 150 vitamin D and more than 1,000 vitamin A units per gram—Bottles, 4, 12 and 16 oz. (Patch)

COD LIVER OIL—Plain (C.A.)—Bottles of 4 and 12 fl. oz. (Squibb)

COD LIVER OIL—Mint Flavored (C.A.) (with 0.67 % oil of spearmint); has a content of not less than 1250 U.S.P. units of vitamin A and an antirachitic potency of not less than 750 A.D.M.A. units per gram—Bottles 4 and 12 fl. oz. (Squibb)

Administration: Infants—8–30 m three times daily. Children—½ teaspoonful three times daily. Adults—1 teaspoonful three times daily. Administered best before meals, in fruit juices or followed by pinch of salt.

Bibliography: *See Chap. XII.*

COD LIVER OIL (S.M.A.)

Nutrient. Vitamin Therapy

Description: A high grade Cod Liver Oil fortified with Carotene (primary vitamin A) and containing both primary and secondary vitamin A and natural vitamin D; is three times as potent in vitamins; 1 teaspoonful is equivalent to 3 teaspoonfuls of standard cod liver oil.

Action and Uses: Wherever a more palatable concentrated cod liver oil is indicated; only one-third the dosage is required.

Supply: **COD LIVER OIL**—Bottles 4 oz., protected, in special cartons.

Administration: 1 teaspoonful daily for the average individual.

Bibliography: *See Chap. XII.*

COD LIVER OIL "KEPLER"

(Burroughs Wellcome)

Nutrient. Vitamin Therapy

Action: As for cod liver oil.

Uses—As dietetic adjunct in the treatment of disturbed nutrition, simple anemia, loss of weight; to provide vitamin "B."

Supply: KEPLER COD LIVER OIL—Bottles 4, 8 and 16 oz.

Combinations: KEPLER COD LIVER OIL WITH MALT EXTRACT.

KEPLER COD LIVER OIL WITH MALT EXTRACT AND CREOSOTE—Contains—Creosote m 4 (0.246 cc) per ounce.

KEPLER COD LIVER OIL WITH MALT EXTRACT AND HYPOPHOSPHITES—Contains in addition, per ounce: Calcium hypophosphite gr 4 (0.259 Gm); Potassium hypophosphite gr 2 (0.130 Gm); Sodium hypophosphite, gr 2 (0.130 Gm).

KEPLER COD LIVER OIL WITH MALT EXTRACT AND IRON IODIDE—Contains in addition Iron Iodide gr 2 (0.130 Gm) per ounce.

KEPLER COD LIVER OIL WITH MALT EXTRACT AND PHOSPHORUS—Contains in addition per ounce—Phosphorus gr 1/64 (0.001 Gm).

KEPLER HAEMOGLOBIN WITH MALT EXTRACT AND COD LIVER OIL (B vitamines fortified); Contains in addition per fluid ounce—Haemoglobin. Wellcome Brand 4⅗ gr with concentrated extract from Brewers' Yeast 3⅗ gr.

Supply—Of all combinations—Bottles of 9 and 18 oz.

Administration—1–2 dessertspoonfuls three times daily before or after meals for all the above preparations.

COD LIVER OIL "NEWFOUNDLAND"

(Mead Johnson)

Nutrient. Vitamin Therapy

Description: Prepared from fresh cod livers; is biologically assayed for potency of vitamins A and D and is low in fatty acids.

Action: Fortifies against infections of mucous membranes; aids in calcium and phosphorus utilization. Food value—250 calories per ounce.

Uses: Wherever vitamins A and D are useful: in xerophthalmia, xerosis, hemeralopia, rickets, tetany, osteomalacia, allergies, tuberculosis.

Supply: COD LIVER OIL "NEWFOUNDLAND" (C.A.) Plain or Flavored.—Bottles 4, 8 and 16 oz.

Administration: Twice daily; infants up to 1 mo.—½ teaspoonful; children 1–6 mo.—1 teaspoonful twice daily; 2 mo. and over —1½ teaspoonful three times daily.

Bibliography: *See Chap. XII.*

COD LIVER OIL "PETER MOLLER'S" (Schieffelin)

Nutritive. Vitamin Therapy

Description: A standardized preparation of Norwegian Cod Liver Oil without disagreeable taste, after-taste or odor; is of light color and hydroxyl-free; each ounce contains 14,150 units Vitamin A and 7,075 units Vitamin D.

Action: Antirachitic, growth promoting, food-tonic.

Uses: In all conditions where cod liver oil is indicated.

Supply and Administration: MOLLER COD LIVER OIL—Plain—Bottles of 4 and 8 oz. *Dosage*—1 teaspoonful–1 tablespoonful three times daily; children ½–1 teaspoonful three times daily.

MOLLER COD LIVER OIL—Flavored—containing per ounce 28,300 Vitamin A units and 8,490 Vitamin D units. *Supply*—Bottles 4, 8 oz. *Dosage*—1 teaspoonful–1 tablespoonful two or three times daily; children ½ dosage.

MOLLER COD LIVER OIL—Super Strength—containing per ounce 28,300 Vitamin A units and 14,150 Vitamin D units. *Supply*—Bottles 4 oz. *Dosage*—1 teaspoonful–1 tablespoonful one to two times daily; children 1 teaspoonful doses.

Combinations: MOLLER A-B-C-D VITAMIN FOOD—A combination of Cod Liver Oil with Malt Extract and concentrated orange juice; a palatable emulsion without oily taste, odor or appearance. Contains per ounce: Vitamin A—11,320 units; vitamin B—5.66 rat units; vitamin C—28.3 international guinea pig units; vitamin D—3,396 units.
For use as nutrient, antirachitic, anti-xerophthalmic, anti-scorbutic, antineuritic and pellagra preventive. *Supply*—Jars of 15 oz. *Dosage*—1–2 teaspoonfuls three times daily, as adjunct to diet; infants ½ teaspoonful three times daily.

Bibliography: *See Chap. XII.*

COLLARGOL (Heyden)

Antiseptic

Official Name: Argentum Colloidale.

Composition: Contains Colloidal Silver and Silver Oxide formed by reduction and stabilized by derived egg albumin with which it is partly combined; has an equivalence of 78% metallic silver.

Description: Occurs as small, hard, bluish-black, scale-like brittle pieces, soluble in 20 parts of water and forming a colloidal suspension; is stable and not precipitated by acids or alkalies in the presence of albumin.

Action and Uses: Intravenously induces non-specific therapy reaction with leucocytosis, fever and chills; locally is antiseptic and effective in all conditions where silver is employed.

Supply: COLLARGOL (C.A.)—Granules—Bottles of ½ and 1 oz.—Tubes of 1 Gm.
UNGUENTUM CREDÉ (C.A.)—Containing 15% of collargol.—Jars of ½ oz.—Packages of 2.

Administration: *Intravenously*—10–20 cc of a sterile 2% aqueous suspension, carefully filtered, but not boiled;
Internally—1 gr (0.064 Gm) dosage.
Locally—In 0.02–1% solutions.
As Ointment—15%, 2–4 Gm rubbed thoroughly into the skin.
As Dusting Powder—As a 5% mixture with finest clay.
Bougies—3 gr (0.194 Gm).
Vaginal Suppositories and Tampons—¾ gr (0.048 Gm).

COLLENE (Collene)

Colloidal Antiseptic

Description: A colloidal solution, containing 0.05% ionic Silver.

Action and Uses: An odorless, stable, non-irritating, non-staining antiseptic and mild astringent, of slightly metallic taste; is not affected by boiling: *For use* in infections of the eye, ear, nose, throat, bladder; in wounds, ulcers, abscesses and for colonic irrigation.

Supply: COLLENE—Bottles of 1½ oz., 8 oz. and 64 oz.

Administration: By swab, tampon, spray, gargle, instillation and wet dressing;
In eye, nose, throat conditions—applied full strength.
In ears, urethra, vagina—half strength.
For bladder irrigation, ulcerations, dressings—30 % dilution.
For colon irrigation—25 % dilution.

COLLOIDAL MERCURY SULPHIDE (Hille)

Antiluetic

Official Name: Hydrargyri Sulphidum Colloidale-Hille.

Formula: HgS.

Description: A stable, potent, black solution; odorless, tasteless and non-irritating; contains 86.22 % Metallic Mercury and 13.78 % Sulphur with 2 % as colloidal Mercury Sulphide.

Action and Uses: A mercurial for the treatment of syphilis in all stages.

Supply: COLLOIDAL MERCURY SULPHIDE 1 % (C.A.)—Oral—Bottles 1 and 12 oz.

COLLOIDAL MERCURY SULPHIDE 2 % (C.A.)—Hypodermic—Bottles of 20, 60 and 360 cc.

Administration: 2–5 cc *intramuscularly* twice weekly.

Incompatibilities: Tannin, concentrated acid solutions, alkalies and salts.

Bibliography: *See Chap. XII.*

COLLOSOL ANTIMONY (Crookes)

Parasiticide

Composition: A colloidal suspension of Antimony Sulphide Sb_2S_3 1:2,500, or 0.04 %, in suitable emulsoid.

Action and Uses: A parasiticide in leishmaniasis, ulcus molle serpiginosum, granulomr pudendi, sleeping sickness, bilharziasis, leprosy; lately applied also in tuberculosis.

Supply: COLLOSOL ANTIMONY—Ampules 0.5 cc, 1 cc, 2 cc, 5 cc, 10 cc—Boxes of 6.

COLLOSOL ANTIMONY—For injection—Bottles 30 cc.

COLLOSOL ANTIMONY—Oral—Bottles 4 oz., 8 oz., 16 oz., 80 oz.

Administration: *By Injection*—2 cc, increased to 10 cc, one or two times weekly.
Oral—½–1 cc two to three times daily.
In Tuberculosis—0.5–1 cc weekly, by special method.

COLLOSOL ARGENTUM (Crookes)

Antiseptic

Official Name: Collosol Argentum Liquidum.

Description: A colloidal suspension of Metallic Silver, 1:2,000 or 0.05 %; is isotonic, non-irritant, free from caustic properties, does not stain tissues and may be boiled without precipitation.

Uses and Administration: Is applicable where silver preparations without caustic action are desired; is soothing, healing and applied as paste, ointment or in pure solution.

Dermatology—As ointment or wet dressing undiluted in impetigo contagiosa, acne, ringworm, tinea versicolor, pustular eczema of hairy parts, chronic eczema, carbuncles, follicular impetigo, pruritus ani.

Otology—Either pure or diluted with warm normal saline, in otitis media suppurativa, earache, labyrinthine suppuration in children.

Ophthalmology: As instillation, 2–3 drops of the undiluted liquid two to three times daily; as injection, diluted with 5–6 parts of warm saline, without previous cocaine instillation; in wounds of cornea, sclera and conjunctiva; in interstitial keratitis, blepharitis and dacryocystitis; in ophthalmia neonatorum, gonorrheal or other purulent ophthalmia.

Rhinolaryngology—In form of spray or gargle, either undiluted or diluted with 2–4 parts of warm saline; also as cotton plugs soaked in the liquid; in septic and follicular tonsillitis, Vincent's angina, postnasal catarrh, sinusitis, rhinitis.

Genito-Urinary—Undiluted or diluted 1–2–4 parts of warm water; also as pessaries and suppositories; in gonorrheal and chronic cystitis, epididymitis, urethritis, vaginitis, prostatitis; in pruritus ani, hemorrhoids, fissure.

Medical—*Intravenously or Intramuscularly*—1 ampule twice or thrice weekly in septicemia, pyemia, puerperal sepsis and meningitis complicating middle ear disease.

Supply: **COLLOSOL ARGENTUM**—Injection—Bottles, rubber-capped, 30 cc—Boxes of 1 and 4.

COLLOSOL ARGENTUM—Injection—Ampules, 2 cc, 5 cc, 10 cc and 20 cc—Boxes of 6.

COLLOSOL ARGENTUM LIQUIDUM—Bottles 1, 4, 8, 16 and 80 oz.

COLLOSOL ARGENTUM BETA—0.25% solution, or five times the strength of the Liquid; a stock preparation, for dilution with warm water or normal saline for immediate use. Bottles 8 and 16 oz.

COLLOSOL ARGENTUM OPHTHALMIC—½ oz. pipettes, Packages of 12 and 100.

PASTA COLLOSOL ARGENTUM—0.25%—Jars 1, 3 and 16 oz.

UNGUENTUM COLLOSOL ARGENTUM—1%—Jars 1, 3, 8 and 16 oz.

COLLOSOL ARGENTUM Soap—Boxes of 3 Tablets.

COLLOSOL ARGENTUM Bougies—Box of 12.

COLLOSOL ARGENTUM Oil—Bottles of 1, 4 and 8 oz.

COLLOSOL ARGENTUM Dentifrice—Tubes—Packages of 12 Tubes.

COLLOSOL ARGENTUM Tampons—Box of 3.

PESSARIES AND SUPPOSITORIES—0.25%—Boxes of 6 and 12; also children's size.

Bibliography *See Chap. XII.*

COLLOSOL ARSENIC (Crookes)

Spirillicide

Composition: A Colloidal Arsenious Sulphide, As_2S_3 1:1,000, each cc containing approximately 0.0013 Gm Arsenious acid, or 1 dr.—1/15 gr.

Action and Uses: A mild, non-irritating agent *for use* in trypanosomiasis, blackwater fever and parasitic skin affections; also as hematinic in anemia.

Supply: **COLLOSOL ARSENIC**—Ampules 1 and 2 cc—Boxes of 6.

Administration: *Intramuscularly*—1 cc twice weekly, 10 doses as one course.
Orally—½–1 teaspoonful in water two or three times daily after meals; increased slowly.

COLLOSOL AURUM (Crookes)

Gold Therapy

Description: An aqueous colloidal suspension of Metallic Gold, 0.05%.

Uses: In infections: septicemia, typhoid fever, septic bronchopneumonia, influenza; in some nervous and skin diseases: lupus, tuberculides, psoriasis; in the Lange Colloidal Gold Test.

Supply: **COLLOSOL AURUM**—Oral (1:2,000)—Bottles 4 oz.

COLLOSOL AURUM—Hypodermic—Ampules 1 cc (1:8,000), 2 cc (0.01%)—Boxes of 6.

COLLOSOL AURUM—For Lange Colloidal Gold Test—Bottles 2, 4, 8 and 20 oz.

Administration: *Oral*—1 teaspoonful three times daily, well diluted in water.
Intramuscular—1 ampule every 2–4 days.

COLLOSOL BROMIDE (Crookes)

Sedative

Composition: Prepared by bromination of protein; contains Bromine 8% in a highly buffered solution of Hydrogen Bromide.

Action and Uses: A nerve sedative in epilepsy, nervous disorders and excessive excitability.

Supply: **COLLOSOL BROMIDE**—Oral—Bottles 4, 8, 16, 80 oz.

Administration: 1–2 teaspoonfuls three times daily in water; or 2–4 teaspoonfuls at bedtime.

COLLOSOL CALAMINE LOTION (Crookes)

Astringent

Composition: A 10% colloidal suspension of Calamine.

Action and Uses: In localized skin affections, as astringent and soothing application.

Supply: **COLLOSOL CALAMINE LOTION**—Bottles of 3, 6, 12 and 80 oz.

Administration: Applied locally with sponge and allowed to dry.

COLLOSOL CALCIUM (Crookes)

Calcium Therapy

Description: An aqueous 0.85% colloidal suspension of Calcium Oleate, with calcium content of 0.05%.

Action: As for calcium salts and non-specific protein therapy.

Uses: In the treatment of dental caries, tuberculosis; as prophylactic in hay fever and erythromelalgia; as hemostatic in hemoptysis and postoperative hemorrhage; as corrective in calcium deficiency diseases in general.

Supply: **COLLOSOL CALCIUM**—Oral—Bottles of 4, 10, 20 and 80 oz.

COLLOSOL CALCIUM—Hypodermic—Ampules ½, 1 and 2 cc—Boxes of 6.

COLLOSOL CALCIUM—Hypodermic—Bottles of ½ and 1 oz, rubber-capped—Boxes of 1 and 4.

Administration: *Intramuscularly*—In tuberculosis—0.3 cc–0.7 cc every 7 days or more frequently; in hemoptysis—½ cc once or twice weekly.

Orally—1 dr. three times a day in water.

In Calcium Deficiency—1 cc, two or three times weekly, by injection.

To Prevent Postoperative Hemorrhage—1 cc, 12 and 6 hr. before operation, then immediately after operation and 6 hr. later.

Combinations: COLLOSOL CALCIUM WITH LECITHIN—Contains collosol calcium with lecithin 1%; *For use* where the effect of both is desired: in nervous debility, neurasthenia, emotional disturbances. *Supply*—Ampules ½ cc, 1 and 2 cc—Boxes of 6—Bottles (injection) ½ oz. and packages of four 1 oz. bottles—Bottles, Oral 4, 10, 20, 80 oz. *Administered—Intramuscularly or Subcutaneously* —0.5–2 cc daily.

Orally—As for collosol calcium.

COLLOSOL CALCIUM WITH VITAMIN D—Contains colloidal calcium salts of fatty acids, 1%, with 250 International units Vitamin D in the form of Irradiated Ergosterol, per teaspoonful; is equivalent in Vitamin D potency to ½ teaspoonful of cod liver oil. *For use* where cod liver oil is indicated; administered in same dosage.

Supply—Bottles, Oral 4, 10, 20, 80 oz.

Bibliography: *See Chap. XII.*

COLLOSOL CHLOR-CARVACROL (Crookes)

Antiseptic

Composition: Contains 5% Chlor-Carvacrol, a combination of a thymol like substance, Carvacrol, with Chlorine; has a phenol coefficient 144.

Action and Uses: Is strongly bactericidal and effective against mouth bacteria, even in the presence of serum; *For use* as antiseptic gargle, spray, mouth wash in septic sore throat, dental sepsis and decay.

Supply: COLLOSOL CHLOR-CARVACROL—Bottles 1, 4, 8 and 16 oz.

Administration: 5–10 drops in wineglassful of water as spray, gargle, mouth wash, whenever desired.

COLLOSOL CHRYSAROBIN (Crookes)

Parasiticide

Composition: Colloidal Chrysarobin, 1:500.

Action and Uses: A non-staining parasiticide *for use* in psoriasis and other skin affections.

Supply: COLLOSOL CHRYSAROBIN—External—Bottles 0.2%—4, 8, 16, 80 oz.

COLLOSOL CHRYSAROBIN—Oral—Bottles 0.2%—4, 8, 16, 80 oz.

COLLOSOL CHRYSAROBIN—Intravenous—Bottles 1 oz.

COLLOSOL CHRYSAROBIN—Intravenous—Ampules 1:1,000—Boxes of 6.

Administration: By topical application to the affected area, as necessary.

Oral—½–1 teaspoonful in water two to three times daily.

Intramuscularly or Intravenously—1–3 cc weekly.

Bibliography: *See Chap. XII.*

COLLOSOL CUPRUM (Crookes)

Cancer Therapy

Description: An aqueous 0.05% colloidal suspension of Copper.

Action: Is claimed to be of value in ameliorating pain, decreasing discharges and improving the general health in malignant disease; is also hematinic.

Uses: In epithelioma, gastric carcinoma, cancer of breast, uterus and rectum; in secondary anemias in combination with iron or other hematinics; in ophthalmia, where its application is painless and non-irritating.

Supply: COLLOSOL CUPRUM—Oral—Bottles 1, 4, 8, 16 oz.

COLLOSOL CUPRUM—Hypodermic—Bottles, rubber capped, 1, 4, 8, 16 oz.

COLLOSOL CUPRUM—Ampules 1, 2, 3 and 5 cc—Boxes of 6.

COLLOSOL CUPRUM—Ophthalmic—Bottles, eye-dropping, ½ oz.

COLLOSOL CUPRUM—Paste—Jars 1 oz.

COLLOSOL CUPRUM—Suppositories—Boxes of 12.

Administration: **In Malignancies**—3 cc *intramuscularly* on the first, fourth, seventh and twelfth days; then weekly until symptoms improve; thereafter once monthly for a year.
Oral—1 teaspoonful, freely diluted with water.
Ophthalmic—As instillation.

Combinations: COLLOSOL CUPRUM ET FERRUM—Containing Copper 1:20,000.
Supply—Ampules 1, 2 cc—Boxes of 6; Bottles (injection), rubber-capped—30 cc; Bottles (oral)—4, 8, 16, 80 oz.

COLLOSOL CUPRUM ET FERRO-ARSENICUM—Containing Copper 1:20,000.
Supply—Ampules 1, 2 cc—Boxes of 6; Bottles (injection), rubber capped—30 cc; Bottles (oral)—4, 8, 16, 80 oz.

COLLOSOL CUPRUM ET FERRO-MANGANESE—Containing Copper 1:20,000.
Supply—Ampules 1, 2 cc—Boxes of 6; Bottles (injection), rubber-capped—30 cc; Bottles (oral)—4, 8, 16, 80 oz.

Bibliography: *See Chap. XII.*

COLLOSOL FERRUM (Crookes)

Hematinic

Composition: Colloidal Ferric Hydroxide, $Fe(OH)_3$, 1:2,000.

Action and Uses: *For use* in chlorosis, anemia, debility, and after infections; in hastening resolution in cellulitis and erysipelas; and in syphilis.

Supply: COLLOSOL FERRUM—Ampules 1 cc, 2 cc—Boxes of 6.

COLLOSOL FERRUM—Bottles—Injection 1 oz.

COLLOSOL FERRUM—Bottles—Oral 4, 8, 16, 80 oz.

Administration: *Intramuscularly*—2 cc one to two times weekly
Orally—1 teaspoonful in water three times daily.

COLLOSOL HYDRARGYRUM (Crookes)

Antiluetic

Composition: A colloidal suspension of Mercury.

Action and Uses: As for mercury in syphilis. *For use* locally on luetic ulcers; for sub-conjunctival injection—in sympathetic ophthalmia, iritis, choroiditis, choroidoretinitis, retrobulbar neuritis; hypodermically—in locomotor ataxia, luetic meningitis, general paralysis, cerebral syphilis, gonorrheal arthritis.

Supply: COLLOSOL HYDRARGYRUM—Ampules 1 %, 3 cc—Boxes of 6.

COLLOSOL HYDRARGYRUM—Injection, 1 %—Bottles of 30, 120 cc.

COLLOSOL HYDRARGYRUM—Oral, 0.05 %—Bottles of 4, 8, 16 and 80 oz.

COLLOSOL HYDRARGYRUM—Cream 5 %—For inunction—Jars of 1, 3 and 16 oz.

Administration: *Orally*—1 teaspoonful three times daily after meals
Intramuscularly—3 cc, three times weekly.
Subconjunctival Injection—As indicated.
Locally—Applied as frequently as indicated.

COLLOSOL ICHTHYOL (Crookes)

Antiseptic

Description: Ichthyol in colloidal form; miscible in all proportions with water, glycerine and alcohol.

Action and Uses: Mild antiseptic and emollient in eczema, psoriasis, acne, chronic ulcers; in gynecologic and surgical inflammations.

Supply: COLLOSOL ICHTHYOL—Bottles 2, 4, 8, 16 oz.

COLLOSOL ICHTHYOL—Capsules gr 2½—Bottles of 50, 100 and 200.

COLLOSOL ICHTHYOL—Ointment 10 %—Jars 1, 3, 16 oz.

COLLOSOL ICHTHYOL—Ointment with Resorcin—Jars 1, 3, 8, 16 oz.

COLLOSOL ICHTHYOL—Ointment with Resorcin and Chrysarobin—Jars 1, 3, 8, 16 oz.

COLLOSOL ICHTHYOL—Pessaries—Boxes of 6.

COLLOSOL ICHTHYOL—Soap—Boxes of 3 tablets.

COLLOSOL ICHTHYOL—Suppositories—Boxes of 12.

COLLOSOL ICHTHYOL—Tampons—Boxes of 3.

COLLOSOL ICHTHYOL GLYCERINE—50 %—Bottles of 4, 8, 16, 80 oz.

COLLOSOL ICHTHYOL SODIUM—Granular—Bottles of 1 oz.

Administration: Ointment or lotion—10 %, locally.
Internally—5 to 10 gr in capsules.

Combination: COLLOSOL ICHTHYOL-CALCIUM—Contains equal parts of Calcium Lactate and Sodium Ichthyolate; *For use* in skin diseases. *Supply*—Capsules gr 2½, equivalent to gr ½ elemental calcium—Bottles of 50, 100 and 200. *Administration*—1–3 capsules three times daily after meals.

Bibliography: *See Chap. XII.*

COLLOSOL IODINE (Crookes)

Alterative

Description: A combination of Iodine with colloidal and semi-colloidal decomposition products of protein, readily separated into hydriodic acid and iodine; is rendered isotonic with sodium chloride; contains 0.02 % of iodine.

Action: As for iodine preparations.

Uses: In goitre, hypothyroidism, thyroidal obesity, some cases of hyperthyroidism; in lead and mercurial poisoning, rheumatoid arthritis, inflamed glands and joints; in fibrositis, skin affections; in syphilis, to minimize intolerance to salvarsan, in puerperal sepsis.

Advantages: Minimum risk of iodism, prolonged activity, freedom from disagreeable taste, irritation or staining.

Supply: **COLLOSOL IODINE**—Oil—containing approximately 1% free iodine. Bottles, 1, 4, 8, 16 and 80 oz.

COLLOSOL IODINE—Oil with Methyl Salicylate—Bottles of 1, 4, 8, 16 and 80 oz.

COLLOSOL IODINE—Aqueous 0.2%—For oral use—Bottles 4, 10, 20 and 80 oz;—For intravenous or intramuscular use—Bottles, rubber-capped, 4 oz.

COLLOSOL IODINE—Intramuscular—Ampules 1 cc 1%—Boxes of 6—Bottles rubber-capped 30 cc.

COLLOSOL IODINE—Ampules 0.2%—Bottles 5 cc, 10 cc, 20 cc and 25 cc—Boxes 6.

COLLOSOL IODINE—Ampules 0.4% (C.I.N.S.) 10 cc—Boxes of 6—Bottles, rubber-capped, 30 cc.

COLLOSOL IODINE—Ampules 0.8%, 1 cc—Boxes of 6—Bottles, rubber-capped, 30 cc.

COLLOSOL IODINE—Paste—Jars 1 and 3 oz.

COLLOSOL IODINE—Pessaries—Box of 6.

COLLOSOL IODINE—Pigmentum—Bottles of 1 and 2 oz.

COLLOSOL IODINE—Suppositories—Boxes of 12.

COLLOSOL IODINE—Pastilles, Iodine gr 1/6 in soft base—Boxes of 24 and 48.

COLLOSOL IODINE—Pastilles, Iodine gr 1/10, and Black Currant, in hard base—Tins of 2 oz.

Administration: *Oral*—1–3 teaspoonfuls of Collosol Iodine, Oral, three times daily after meals.

Intramuscular—1 cc, ampule 1%, every fourth day.

Intravenous—0.2% solution 20–100 cc. 0.8% solution 5–10 cc according to the occasion.

Local—The aqueous Collosol undiluted as spray or douche; Collosol Iodine Oil or Ointment for gentle massage through the skin.

Bibliography: *See Chap. XII.*

COLLOSOL KAOLIN (Crookes)

Adsorptive

Chemical Name: Colloidal Aluminum Silicate.

Formula: $Al_2Si_2O_7 + 2H_2O$.

Description: A neutral non-irritating powder, insoluble in water.

Action: Adsorbs certain alkaloidal substances and bacterial toxins, preventing their absorption into the organism and favoring their elimination; changes the intestinal flora from predominantly proteolytic to an aciduric type in 10–35 days; eliminates bacillus Welchii and renders harmless the toxins of Vibriocholera; passes the intestinal tract unchanged.

Uses: In mucous and ulcerative colitis, bacillary dysentery and chronic diarrheas; also in rheumatoid arthritis and other affections where checking of putrefactive absorption is desirable.

Supply: **COLLOSOL KAOLIN**—Tins 6 and 16 oz. and 2½ lb.

COLLOSOL KAOLIN WITH PHENOLPHTHALEIN—Tins 6 and 16 oz. and 2½ lb.

Administration: 1 dessertspoonful to 1 oz. of water, mornings and evenings; for colonic irrigation, 1–2 heaping tablespoonfuls in about a gallon of warm water.

Bibliography: *See Chap. XII.*

COLLOSOL LACTALUMINA (Crookes)

Antacid

Composition: Aluminium Hydroxide in colloidal suspension.

Action and Uses: Antacid without causing gas evolution; *For use* in gastric hyperacidity and resulting symptoms; as astringent and soothing mouth wash and gargle in ulcerated conditions of the mouth and throat.

Administration: *Internally*—1–4 teaspoonfuls in water, ½ hr. before meals or 1 hr. after meals.

Gargle—1–2 teaspoonfuls in wine-glassful of water, when necessary.

Supply: COLLOSOL LACTALUMINA—Bottles of 6, 12 and 80 oz.

Combinations: COLLOSOL LACTALUMINA LAXATIVE—Contains in addition a small amount of Phenolphthalein; *For use* in intestinal stasis—Bottles of 6, 12 and 80 oz.

COLLOSOL LACTALUMINA WITH BISMUTH—Contains in addition Bismuth; *For use* in recurrent diarrhea with intermittent griping pains—Bottles 6, 12 and 80 oz.

COLLOSOL LACTOMAGNESIA (Crookes)

Antacid

Composition: Colloidal Magnesium Hydroxide, gr 43 (10%) per ounce.

Action and Uses: Antacid and laxative; *For use* in hyperacidity, gastric ulcer, infantile disorders; locally—as mouth wash and in dental practice.

Supply: COLLOSOL LACTOMAGNESIA—Bottles of 4, 8, 80 oz.

Administration: *Internally*—Adults—1–2 teaspoonfuls; children—¼–1 teaspoonful in water, two or three times daily; infants—1 teaspoonful in pint of milk, or ½ teaspoonful per bottle.

As Mouth Wash—2 teaspoonfuls in ½ glass water.

COLLOSOL MANGANESE (Crookes)

Bactericide

Description: Contains Manganese 0.25% in an emulsoid colloid medium, preventing its precipitation in the presence of blood plasma.

Action: Like other manganese products it enhances antibody formation and is protective against endotoxins of septic bacteria: tubercle bacilli, streptococci, staphylococci, pneumococci and other microorganisms; is also hematinic.

Uses: In acne, suppurative and vulgaris; in furuncles, boils and other deep seated coccogenic infections; in psoriasis in addition to other remedies; in sycosis, impetigo contagiosa and other staphylococcic infections.

Supply: COLLOSOL MANGANESE—For oral use—Bottles of 4, 8, 16 and 80 oz.

COLLOSOL MANGANESE—"Single Sol"—For injection—Ampules ½, 1 and 2 cc—Boxes of 6.

COLLOSOL MANGANESE—"Double Sol"—For injection by mixing in the syringe just prior to use—Bottles, of ½ and 1 oz., rubber-capped.

Administration: *Oral*—1 teaspoonful in water three times daily, after meals.

Intramuscular—½–1 cc every 2 or 3 days until 6–8 cc have been administered according to condition.

Bibliography: *See Chap. XII.*

COLLOSOL PALLADIUM (Crookes)

Gonocide

Composition: Colloidal Metallic Palladium, 1:2,000.

Action and Uses: In gonorrheal and other coccogenic infections; lately used in epilepsy.

Supply: **COLLOSOL PALLADIUM**—Ampules ½, 1 cc—Boxes of 6.
COLLOSOL PALLADIUM—Injection—Bottles 30 cc.
COLLOSOL PALLADIUM—Oral—Bottles 4, 8, 16, 80 oz.

Administration: *Intramuscularly*—0.5–1 cc.
Orally—1 teaspoonful in water two or three times daily, after meals.

Bibliography: *See Chap. XII.*

COLLOSOL SELENIUM (Crookes)

Cancer Therapy

Description: An 0.05% solution of Selenium, in colloidal form.

Uses: Is regarded as a useful palliative in the treatment of malignant diseases, especially inoperable cancer; also used in the prevention of recurrences after removal.

Supply: **COLLOSOL SELENIUM**—Ampules 1 cc, 5 cc and 10 cc—Boxes of 6.
COLLOSOL SELENIUM—Hypodermic—Bottles, rubber-capped, 30 cc.
COLLOSOL SELENIUM—Oral—Bottles, 1, 4 and 8 oz.

Administration: *Intramuscular*—5 cc twice weekly for 2 weeks, then once weekly for 10 additional weeks.
Intravenous—5 cc first and third day, 10 cc fifth, eighth, tenth and twelfth days; after 1 month's rest—10 cc twice weekly for 5 weeks, till a total of 100 cc have been injected.
Oral—1 dr. in water three times daily, between meals.

Bibliography: *See Chap. XII.*

COLLOSOL STANNUM (Crookes)

Antiphlogistic

Composition: A colloidal Stannum Oleate 1:2,000.

Action and Uses: In furunculosis.

Supply: **COLLOSOL STANNUM**—Ampules 1, 2 cc—Boxes of 6.

Administration: 1 cc every 2 or 3 days, *intramuscularly.*

COLLOSOL SULPHUR (Crookes)

Antiseptic. Laxative

Description: A 0.1% sulphur solution in colloidal state.

Action and Uses: Recommended in cases of sulphur deficiency; in intestinal toxemia accompanying arthritis; in skin diseases and painful joint affections.

Supply: **COLLOSOL SULPHUR**—Ampules 1 cc, 2 cc, 5 cc and 10 cc—Boxes of 6.
COLLOSOL SULPHUR—Oral—Bottles of 8, 16, 32 and 80.
COLLOSOL SULPHUR—External—Bottles 4 and 80 oz. (baths and lotion).

COLLOSOL SULPHUR—Oil—Bottles 2, 4, 8 and 16 oz.

COLLOSOL SULPHUR—Cream—Jars 1, 3, 8 and 16 oz.

COLLOSOL SULPHUR—Pessaries—Boxes of 6.

COLLOSOL SULPHUR—Pigmentum—Jars 1 and 2 oz.

Administration: *Oral*—1 teaspoonful three times daily, in water, after meals.
Intramuscular—1–2 cc, twice weekly.
External—For sulphur baths: 4 oz. of Collosol Sulphur to 20 gal. of warm water; immersion for 10–15 min. offers full therapeutic effect.
For general use—Collosol Sulphur External—undiluted or diluted ten to twenty times in skin and joint affections, topically.

Bibliography: *See Chap. XII.*

COLLOSOL TRIMINE (Crookes)

Antiseptic

Description: A combination of Colloidal Iron, Manganese Hydroxide and Zinc Hydroxide.

Action and Uses: *For use* in a variety of venereal conditions, acute and subacute, and in gonorrheal ophthalmia.

Supply: COLLOSOL TRIMINE—Ampules 1 cc—Boxes of 6.

COLLOSOL TRIMINE—Bottles of 1 and 4 oz.

Administration: 0.5–1.5 cc *intramuscularly*, repeated in 3 days and continued till a total of 6 cc have been injected.
Oral Use—Teaspoonful three times daily after meals, as hematinic.

COLLOSOL ZINC (Crookes)

Astringent

Composition: A *neutral* solution of Colloidal Zinc Hydroxide, 0.05%.

Action and Uses: *For use* in various ophthalmic infections where acid-zinc solutions are undesirable.

Supply: COLLOSOL ZINC—Bottles 1, 4 oz.

COLLOSOL ZINC—Pipette Bottle, double solution for instantaneous mixing—½ oz.

Administration: By ophthalmic pipette.

COLSUL (Crookes)

Pyrexia Therapy

Composition: A 1% solution of Elementary Sulphur in water and in olive oil.

Action and Uses: To induce pyrexia and thus leukocytosis in the treatment of mental disorders and arthritis; chills produced are light, reactions moderate; is applicable to all ages and apparently safe.

Supply: COLSUL—Oily—Ampules 1, 2, 5, 10 cc—Boxes of 6; Bottles 30 cc.

COLSUL—Aqueous—Ampules 1, 2, 5, 10 cc—Boxes of 6; Bottles 30 cc.

Administration: Initial dose ½ cc *hypodermically*, increased by ½ cc to maximum dosage of 5 cc or until the desired degree of pyrexia is obtained; may be used up to 10 and 12 cc.

CONCENTRATED LIVER EXTRACT (Armour)

Hematopoietic

Description: A water soluble extract from fresh liver, containing in stable form the fraction active in blood regeneration; each tablespoonful represents ¼ lb. fresh liver substance; alcohol 20%.

Action and Uses: Hematopoietic; effective in pernicious anemia.

Supply: CONCENTRATED LIVER EXTRACT (C.A.)—Bottles of 16 oz.

Administration: *Oral*—1 tablespoonful three times daily, with milk, orange juice and any other beverage.

Combination: **CONCENTRATED LIVER EXTRACT WITH IRON**—A combination with iron ammonium citrate gr 12 (0.768 Gm) or 128 mg of metallic iron per teaspoonful; is sugar free and contains 20% alcohol. *For use* in various forms of secondary anemia. *Supply*—Bottles of 8 oz. *Administration*—1–2 teaspoonfuls, two to three times daily, in milk or fruit juices. Infants—1–2 drops, increased to 5–10 drops, in sweetened water after feeding.

Bibliography: *See Chap. XII.*

CORAMINE (Ciba)

Cardio-respiratory Stimulant

Chemical Name: Pyridine-beta-carbonic acid Diethylamide.

Formula: 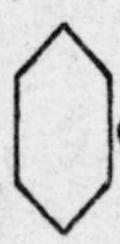 CO. $N(C_2H_5)_2NC_5H_4COH(C_2H_5)_2$.

Description: A yellow syrupy liquid, with faintly bitter rather pungent taste; is freely soluble in water and marketed in 25% aqueous solution; for oral administration is rendered more palatable by the addition of lactic acid.

Action: Stimulates cardiovascular system; increases blood flow by stimulation of the heart, improves coronary circulation; stimulates the respiratory center directly when depressed by drugs or toxins.

Advantages: Compared to digitalis its action is more prompt, becoming manifest in 15–30 min. after oral administration and almost immediately upon intravenous injection; is not as cumulative as digitalis, nor does it affect auriculoventricular conductivity; it enhances the coronary flow and potentiates the therapeutic action of digitalis; large doses intravenously are comparatively safe.

Uses: In acute circulatory failure in pneumonia, influenza, diphtheria and other infections; in chronic myocardial failure and surgical conditions; in poisoning by cresol, phenol, chloral and other drugs; in respiratory failure during anesthesia; in morphine, barbital and illuminating gas poisoning; in asphyxia neonatorum.

Supply: CORAMINE—Liquid—For oral use—Bottles of ½ and 3 oz.

CORAMINE—Ampules—1.1 cc—Cartons of 5, 20, 100 and 500; Ampules 5.5 cc, Cartons of 3 and 12.

Administration: *Oral*—15–30 m (1–2 cc) in water, three or four times daily.
Subcutaneously, Intramuscularly or Intravenously—1 or 2 ampules usual dosage; in severe cases the dose may be materially increased and as much as 15 cc may be injected. In children large doses are tolerated.

Bibliography: *See Chap. XII.*

COREINE "DANIEL-BRUNET" (Fougera)

Laxative

Composition: A pure, non-medicated preparation of Mucilage, absorbing 40–50 times its own volume of water.

Action: Is chemically inert, harmless, non-irritating; absorbs fluids and swells in volume thus acting as mechanical stimulus to intestinal peristalsis and as aperient.

Uses: In constipation, colitis, fermentative diarrheas, proctitis, sigmoiditis.

Supply: **COREINE "DANIEL-BRUNET"**—Granules—Tins of 4 oz.
COREINE "DANIEL-BRUNET"—Flakes—Tins of 4 oz.

Administration: Adults—1–2 dr. in water, milk, after meals; maintenance dose—1–2 dr., once after breakfast.
Children—½–1 dr. twice daily.
In Colitis with Diarrhea—2–3 dr. four to six times daily.
In Proctitis and Sigmoiditis—Enemas, 2 tablespoonfuls to a pint of warm water.

CORYFIN (Winthrop)

Local Anodyne

Chemical Name: Ethylglycolic acid ester of menthol. Brand of Colmenthol.

Formula: $C_{10}H_{19}O—COCH_2OC_2H_5$.

Description: A colorless oily fluid of faint menthol odor; easily soluble in alcohol, almost insoluble in water; readily miscible with olive oil and liquid petrolatum.

Action: As for menthol but more prolonged, better tolerated, less irritating and free from decided odor; is cooling and analgesic relieving local discomfort; is mildly astringent; internally is carminative.

Uses and Administration: **In Nasal Catarrh**—Painted lightly on mucous membranes, full strength or mixed with liquid petrolatum, using brush or cotton pledget which may be left in the nostrils for a short time; as spray in 10–30 % solution.
Pharyngitis—Used as above; also 3–4 drops on sugar dissolved slowly in the mouth.
Laryngitis—As inhalant, 10 drops to a pint of boiling water.
Other Uses—As superficial application, like other menthol products, in headaches, neuralgia, pruritus, in earache and ear furunculosis.
Internally—For flatulence, colic, singultus—using several drops on a lump of sugar, as mentioned above.

Supply: **CORYFIN**—Bottles of 1 oz.

CREOSOTAL (Winthrop)

Phthisis Therapy

Chemical Name: Creosote Carbonate.

Description: A clear, yellow, honey-like, almost odorless liquid; is miscible with alcohol, ether and fixed oils, insoluble in water.

Action: As for creosote; is non-irritating to the stomach, being disintegrated chiefly in the intestines; is slowly absorbed and is practically free from toxicity and kidney irritation; is antiseptic, alterative.

Uses: In chronic bronchitis, phthisis pulmonalis, pneumonia and similar pulmonary affections; also in intestinal fermentation, typhoid fever, dysentery.

Supply: CREOSOTAL (C.A.)—Bottles of 1 oz., ¼, ½ and 1 lb.

Administration: Adults, ½–4 dr. (2.0–16.0 Gm) daily, in divided doses. Children, ¼–1 dr (1.0–4.0 Gm) daily; administered either pure, in capsules, in emulsion, or in milk, coffee and wine, or mixed with cod liver oil; also by inunction.

CRESATIN (Sharp and Dohme)

Antiseptic

Chemical Name: Metacresyl Acetate.

Formula: $CH_3C_6H_4O(CH_3CO)$.

Description: A colorless, oily liquid of characteristic odor and low volatility; practically insoluble in water, soluble in organic solvents, in oils and in petrolatum liquidum, 5%.

Action and Uses: Antiseptic and analgesic, free from toxic effects; *useful* in rhinolaryngological practice: naso-pharyngitis, tonsillitis, ethmoiditis; in purulent otitis media, auditory furunculosis.

Supply: CRESATIN (C.A.)—Bottles of 1 oz.

CRESATIN—Spray—Containing Metacresyl acetate, 5%; Methyl salicylate, 2%; Camphor, ½%; Methyol, 1%; Oil base—Bottles of 4 oz.

CRESATIN—Suppositories, Rectal, 10%—Boxes of 20.

CRESATIN—Suppositories, Vaginal, 10%—Boxes of 20.

Administration: As spray for nasopharyngeal application, in atomizer or nebulizer; applied in full strength or diluted with oil or alcohol.

CRYOGENINE (Anglo-French)

Antipyretic

Chemical Name: Phenylsemicarbazide.

Action and Uses: Analgesic and antipyretic; does not disturb the gastro-intestinal, respiratory and cardio-vascular systems. *For use* in headache, migraine, neuralgia, sciatica, lumbago, rheumatism, gout, influenza, colds; in all fevers.

Supply: CRYOGENINE—Tablets 0.5 Gm—Tubes of 10.

CRYOGENINE—Tablets 0.25 Gm—Tubes of 10.

Administration: *As Antipyretic*—Gr 4–30 (0.25–2 Gm) daily.
As Analgesic—Gr 15–45 (1–3 Gm) daily.
Children: ½ dose.

CRYSTALLINE ÇAROTENE (S.M.A.)

Vitamin A Therapy

Description: Crystalline Carotene (primary vitamin A), of definite vitamin potency and absolute purity; 1 Gm of pure Carotene supplies 2,000,000 Sherman units of vitamin A.

Action and Uses: For vitamin A research.

Supply: **CRYSTALLINE CAROTENE**—Tubes 100 mg, sealed in vacuum.

Administration: *Orally*—In oil solution. It has been shown that carotene satisfies the minimal vitamin A requirements of the rat when fed at a level of ½ gamma (0.0000005 Gm) daily.

Bibliography: *See Chap. XII.*

CUPRICOL (Mulford Colloid)

Hematinic

Description: Occurs as lustrous, dark brown, non-hygroscopic scales, readily soluble in water; contains 20–25 % of copper.

Action and Uses: A stable, non-irritating Colloidal Copper, a readily absorbed and assimilated hematinic; is slowly eliminated and of prolonged action; does not cause precipitation of tissue fluids. *For use* in anemias where copper is beneficial.

Supply: **CUPRICOL**—Vials, Gm 10.

CUPRICOL—Solution, 10 %, 25 cc.

Administration: *Orally*—½–5 gr (0.032–0.324 Gm).
Hypodermically—½–3 cc. For intravenous use where indicated.

CYMARIN (Winthrop)

Cardiotonic. Diuretic

Formula: $C_{30}H_{46}O_8COOCH_3$.

Description: The active principle of Apocynum; chemically pure, colorless, heavy prismatic crystals of bitter taste; slightly soluble in cold water, more so in hot water, easily soluble in acetone, alcohol and chloroform.

Action: As official strophanthin; is similar to digitalis in action on heart and kidneys but is less readily absorbed from the gastro-intestinal tract and causes emesis if taken in large doses.

Uses: In chronic valvular disease, chronic myocarditis, pneumonia and similar instances where cardiac stimulation and diuresis is desired.

Supply: **CYMARIN** (C.A.)—Tablets of 1/200 gr (0.3 mg)—Bottles of 50.

CYMARIN (C.A.)—Ampules 1/60 gr (0.9 mg) solution for hypodermic use—Boxes of 10.

Administration: *Orally*—1 or 2 tablets; daily dose, 1/60–1/30 gr.
Intravenously or Intramuscularly—Single dose 1 or 2 ampules; to be replaced by digitalis after 5–6 days treatment.

CYPRESS OIL "SCHIMMEL" (Fritzsche)

Antispasmodic

Official Name: Oleum Cupressi.

Description: An oil distilled from Cupressus Sempervirens; a yellowish liquid of pleasant cypress odor; soluble in 2–7 parts of 90 % alcohol.

Action and Uses: Is antispasmodic; *recommended* in whooping cough to reduce the number and severity of attacks, thus lessening the incidence and gravity of complications.

Supply: **CYPRESS OIL "SCHIMMEL"** (C.A.)—Bottles 1, 4 and 8 oz.—1 and 5 lb.

Administration: Is sprayed for inhalation on bed sheets, pillows and underwear of children, in dilutions of 1 in 4 parts of alcohol; repeated once or twice during the night if paroxysms are severe.

D.C.P. 340 (Parke, Davis)

Calcium Therapy

Chemical Name: Dicalcium Phosphate.

Formula: $CaHPO_4 + 2H_2O$.

Description: A combination of purified Calcium and Phosphorus, finely powdered, in the proportions present in milk; is readily soluble in gastric juice and freely absorbed.

Action and Uses: To assist bone metabolism, prevent or check dental caries, supply calcium for growth and the maintenance of health; in pregnancy to prevent osteomalacia in mother or rickets in child; as a sedative agent in spastic conditions in children or adults.

Supply: D.C.P. 340—Bottles, wide mouth, 4 oz. and 1 lb.

Administration: *Oral*—½–¾ level teaspoonful or 20–30 gr (1.296–1.944 Gm) daily, ½ hr. before or 2 hr. after meals; may be increased to gr 80 (5.184 Gm) daily. Infants—given with milk feedings.

DECHOLIN (Riedel-de Haen)

Choleretic

Chemical Name: Dehydrocholic Acid.

Formula: $C_{20}H_{33}(CO)_3COOH$.

Description: An oxidation product of cholic acid derived from natural bile acids; occurs as a fine, colorless, crystalline powder, of bitter taste and sparingly soluble in glacial acetic acid and alcohol. **DECHOLIN-SODIUM** is the sodium salt of dehydrocholic acid, is soluble in alcohol and water, forming a stable, slightly alkaline solution and is, therefore, used for intravenous injection.

Action: Is a rapidly effective choleretic and cholagogue, relatively non-toxic; in therapeutic doses, either preparation does not affect cardiovascular, nervous or hematopoietic systems; compared with normal bile constituents its toxicity is 1/10 that of sodium taurocholate, 1/13 of sodium glycocholate and 1/22 of sodium cholate; upon intravenous injection is followed in 15–20 min. by a profuse flow of bile lasting 1–1½ hr., effecting excretion of bilirubin, cholesterin, pigment; is diuretic in hepatic engorgement with edema.

Uses: In liver insufficiency with biliary tract engorgement; to outline bile ducts at operation and to relieve postoperative symptoms; in cardiac decompensation with hepatic cirrhosis, dysfunction, ascites and similar complications; in cholecystography to test distensibility of gall bladder, to hasten the appearance of a gallbladder shadow and the elimination of previously administered gallbladder dye; lately used in melancholia, schizophrenia, biliary migraine, and arsphenamine poisoning.

Caution: Not to be employed in mechanical obstruction of gallbladder tract and cautiously in acute yellow atrophy of liver, acute hepatitis and progressing jaundice.

Supply: DECHOLIN—Tablets (C.A.) (0.25 Gm), For Oral use—Boxes of 18, 100 and 500.

DECHOLIN SODIUM—Ampules (C.A.) 10 cc, 5%, For Intravenous use—Boxes of 3 and 20.

DECHOLIN-SODIUM—Ampules (C.A.) 10 cc, 20%, For Intravenous use—Boxes of 3 and 20.

Administration: *Orally*—1–2 tablets, two to three times daily after meals, for 3–5 weeks when dosage may be diminished.

Intravenously—1 ampule of 20% solution, slowly injected on 3 successive days; first day 5 cc, second and third day 10 cc; when less intensive effect is desired or at end of treatment the weaker ampules (5%) are used.

Bibliography: *See Chap. XII.*

DEXTROSE. GLUCOSE

Nutrient

Description: Dextrose preparations for intravenous use; chemically pure and sterile.

Action: As for dextrose; combats acidosis, reduces toxemia, corrects dehydration and nutrition; food value: 1 Gm yields 4.1 calories.

Uses: In numerous instances where the administration of dextrose is desired; in lowered blood sugar states, in starvation, hyperinsulinemia, postoperatively, toxemia of pregnancy, cerebral edema. (Abbott)

Supply: **DEXTROSE** (C.A.)—Ampules 50 cc containing in solution, 25 Gm of Dextrose—Boxes of 6, 25 and 100.

Ampules 20 cc, containing Dextrose 10 Gm in distilled water—Boxes of 6, 25 and 100.

Ampules 10 cc, containing Dextrose 5 Gm, in distilled water—Boxes of 6, 25 and 100.

Ampules 100 cc, containing Dextrose 50 Gm, in distilled water to make 500 cc—Boxes of 6, 25 and 100.

DEXTROSE (C.A.)—Ampules 20 cc containing 10 Gm dextrose. (Lakeside)

GLUCOSE (C.A.)—Ampules 20 cc, 10 Gm Glucose, 1/10% Cresol; (Lilly) buffered—Boxes of 6, 25 and 100.

Ampules 50 cc, 25 Gm Glucose, no preservative; buffer separate—Boxes of 1, 6, 25 and 100.

Ampules 50 cc, 25 Gm Glucose, no preservative; unbuffered—Boxes of 1, 6, 25 and 100.

Ampules 50 cc, 25 Gm Glucose, no preservative; buffered—Boxes of 1, 6, 25 and 100.

Ampules 100 cc, 50 Gm Glucose, no preservative; buffer separate—Boxes of 1, 6, 25 and 100.

DEXTROSE (C.A.)—Ampules 10 cc, 5 Gm—Boxes of 6 and 50. (Miller)

Ampules 20 cc, Dextrose 10 Gm—Boxes of 6 and 50.

Ampules 50 cc, Dextrose 25 Gm—Boxes of 6 and 50.

Ampules 100 cc, Dextrose 50 Gm—Boxes of 6 and 50.

Ampules 50 cc, Dextrose 25 Gm—Boxes of 6 and 50; ampule double-ended, rubber-capped.

GLUCOSE (C.A.)—Ampules 20 cc, Glucose 10 Gm—Boxes (Parke, Davis) of 6 and 25.

Ampules 50 cc, Glucose 25 Gm—Boxes of 1, 6 and 25.

Ampules 100 cc, Glucose 50 Gm—Boxes of 1, 6 and 25.

GLUCOSE (C.A.)—Ampules 20 cc, Glucose 10 Gm—Boxes (Sharp and Dohme) of 6 and 25.

Ampules 50 cc, Glucose 25 Gm—Boxes of 1, 6 and 25, with ampule buffer solution, of disodium hydrogen phosphate and potassium biphosphate.

GLUCOSE (C.A.)—Ampule 50 cc, Glucose 25 Gm, Double- (Sharp and Dohme) end vial, with ampule of above buffer solution—Boxes of 1, 6 and 25.

Ampule 100 cc, Glucose 50 Gm with ampule of buffer solution of above content—Boxes of 1, 6 and 25.

Administration: *Intravenously*, slowly—in quantities as required.

Advantages: Ready for immediate use, keeps indefinitely, is sterile.

DEXTROSE-RINGER'S CONCENTRATE (Abbott)

Nutrient

Composition: Each 100 cc contains Dextrose 25% by weight in concentrated Ringer's solution; when diluted with distilled water to 500 cc, forms a 5% dextrose in ordinary Ringer's solution.

Action and Uses: For prevention and treatment of surgical shock, in sepsis and following hemorrhage; to maintain nutrition and afford rest to the gastro-intestinal tract.

Supply: DEXTROSE-RINGER'S CONCENTRATE (C.A.)—Ampules 100 cc—Boxes 6, 25 and 100.

Administration: *Intravenously*, slowly, as 5% solution, 500 cc per hour, then diminished to 100 cc per hour; continued several days if necessary; in shock, given 200 cc per hour.

Bibliography: *See Chap. XII.*

DIAL (Ciba)

Hypnotic. Sedative

Chemical Name: Diallylmalonylurea. Diallylbarbituric Acid.

Formula: $(C_2H_5)_2CCONHCONHCO$.

Description: A fine, white crystalline powder of slightly bitter taste; soluble in alcohol and ether, practically insoluble in water or in paraffin hydrocarbons; differs from barbital in that both of the ethyl groups of the latter are replaced by allyl groups.

Action: Sedative and hypnotic; affects the higher nervous centers and does not depress the circulation or respiration; is completely decomposed in the tissues and excreted in the urine only in very small proportions; causes no renal irritation even in large doses.

Uses: As sedative—in migraine, whooping cough, chorea, cardiac neuroses, hyperthyroidism, neurasthenia.

As hypnotic—in simple insomnia or that of cardiac disease, head injuries.

Postoperatively—as substitute for morphine to allay restlessness and sleeplessness not due to actual pain; in cases with pain, is used in conjunction with other analgesics, the action of which it potentiates. Also valuable in the insane, in drug addicts, strychnine poisoning, tetanus, eclampsia and obstetrics.

Advantages: Is more active than barbital, more prompt and efficient.

Supply: DIAL—Tablets (C.A.) ½ gr (0.03 Gm)—Cartons of 24—Bottles of 100 and 1,000. Tablets 1½ gr (0.09 Gm)—Tubes of 12—Bottles of 100 and 1,000.

DIAL—Elixir (C.A.) each dram containing ¾ gr (0.04 Gm) of Dial—Bottles of 2 and 6 oz. and 1 gal.

DIAL—Ampules (C.A.) 1 cc, each cc containing 1½ gr (0.09 Gm) of Dial and 6 gr (0.35 Gm) Urethane—Cartons of 5.

DIAL—Ampules (C.A.) 2.3 cc—Cartons of 5, 20 and 100.

DIAL—Powder (C.A.)—Bottles of 10 gr and 1 oz.

Administration: *As Sedative*—1 tablet ½ gr (0.03 Gm) or ½ teaspoonful elixir, one to four times daily.

As Hypnotic—1–3 tablets 1½ gr each, or 2–6 teaspoonfuls of elixir, or 1–2 ampules, ½–1 hr. before sleep is desired; usually 1 dose suffices.

Preoperative—1–3 tablets 1½ gr each or 2–6 dr. of elixir the night preceding and 1 or 2 hr. just before operation; where profound effect is desired larger doses may be employed.

In Obstetrics—As sedative or for semi-narcosis, 2–4 cc, *intramuscularly;* or 2–4 tablets or equivalent of elixir orally, repeated in 2 or 3 hr. if necessary; maximum 24 hr. dose in obstetrics—9 gr.

Bibliography: *See Chap. XII.*

DIASTASE

Starch Digestant

Description: A diastatic enzyme prepared from hog pancreas.

Action and Uses: 1 part will convert 250 parts of starch into dextrose in 3 hr. *Used* for predigestion of starches and relief of flatulence in intestinal indigestion of carbohydrate origin.

Supply: DIASTASE—Powder—Bottles of 1 oz. **(Armour)**

DIASTASE—In strengths of 1:125, 1:200, 1:300—Packages of 1 oz., ¼ and 1 lb. and other quantities desired. **(Stearns)**

Administration: 2 or 5 gr (0.130 or 0.324 Gm) three times daily, as required.

DIBROMIN (Parke, Davis)

Germicide

Chemical Name: Dibrom-malonyl-ureide. Dibrombarbituric Acid.

Formula: $C_4Br_2N_2H_2O_3$.

Description: A white crystalline almost odorless powder of slightly astringent taste; is soluble in water up to 3–4%; also soluble in glycerin, alcohol and ether; insoluble in oils; contains about 56% Bromine.

Action: Powerfully germicidal; action is analogous to that of Dakin's solution; does not coagulate blood or tissue albumins; is practically non-irritating in therapeutic concentration.

Uses: For topical use in ulcers, abscesses, infected wounds or sinuses, vaginitis, cervicitis, cystitis, urethritis, leucorrhea, endometritis, osteomyelitis, fistulae.

Incompatibles: Alkalies and reducing agents.

Supply: DIBROMIN—Capsules (C.A.). gr 6 (0.38 Gm)—Bottles of 50.

Administration: As wet dressing, irrigation, instillation, wet pack, gargle, tampon or dusting powder in dilutions ranging in strength from 1:500–1:10,000; for gonorrheal hand injections 1:500–1:800, irrigations 1:1,250–1:2,500; in vaginitis or cystitis, 1:5,000; in pharyngitis or tonsillitis 1:10,000.

Preparation: All solutions of less than 1% should be freshly prepared. 1 Capsule dissolved in 1 pt. of water makes 1:1,250 solution; in 1 gal. a 1:10,000 solution.

Bibliography: *See Chap. XII.*

DI-CITURIN (Chemico-Biologic)

Hypotensor

Chemical Content: Potassium Acetyl Citrate with Magnesium Salicylate.

Action and Uses: Is stated to be non-depressant on the heart, non-irritating to the kidneys and to cause no digestive disturbances; *For use* in hypertension and symptoms induced by hypertension; in renal and arthritic disturbances.

Supply: DICITURIN—Tablets gr 5—Bottles of 100.

Administration: Gr 60 daily, or 6 doses of gr 10 each, every 3 hr.; in hypertension with nephritis—Gr 15 every 3 hr., 6 doses daily.

DIGALEN "CLOETTA" (Roche)

Digitalis Therapy

Description: Contains all the beneficial cardioactive principles of digitalis leaves, as isolated by Cloetta; is freed from inert and injurious constituents of the leaf to favor its quick and complete absorption.

Action and Uses: As for digitalis.

Supply: DIGALEN "CLOETTA" (C.A.)—Oral Tablets, ½ cat and 1 cat unit potency, sugar coated, readily soluble—Vials of 25 tablets; 4 vials to carton.

DIGALEN (C.A.)—Oral Solution—Vials of 30 cc, each cubic centimeter equals 1 cat unit.

DIGALEN (C.A.)—Injectable—Ampules 2.1 cc; 2 cc equals 1 cat unit—Boxes of 6 and 12 ampules.

Administration: Average dose ½–1 cc of Oral Solution; or Oral Tablets, ½ cat unit, 1–2 three times daily; or 1 cat unit tablet, 1 or more tablets daily.

DIGIFOLINE (Ciba)

Digitalis Therapy

Description: An odorless, colorless, amorphous powder; soluble in water, methyl and ethyl alcohol; insoluble in ether; contains all the active glucosides of digitalis, free from extractives, digitonin (saponin), coloring and inert matter; standardized by the frog method of Focke.

Action and Uses: As for digitalis; is of uniform activity, rapidly absorbed from alimentary canal or subcutaneous tissue.

Supply: DIGIFOLINE—Ampules (C.A.) 1.1 cc—Cartons of 5, 20, 100 and 500.

DIGIFOLINE—Ampules (C.A.) 5.0 cc—Cartons of 1.

DIGIFOLINE—Liquid (C.A.)—Bottles of 1 oz. (approximately 30 cc).

DIGIFOLINE—Tablets (C.A.) each equivalent to 1½ gr (0.09 Gm) of digitalis leaves—Tubes of 25—Bottles of 100 and 500.

Administration: *Orally*—1 tablet or 1 cc of Liquid four times daily until desired effects are obtained.

Massive Dosage—Initial dose 11 gr (0.7 Gm) of tablets or 2 fl. dr. (7.7 cc) of liquid per 100 lb. of body weight; if clinically unimproved and no toxic symptoms appear, ½ the amount may be given at the end of 6 hr., and repeated every 6 hr. until desired therapeutic action is effected or toxic symptoms occur, or until total dosage reaches 22 gr (14.0 Gm) of tablets or 4 dr. of liquid per 100 lb. of body weight—each dose being ½ that immediately preceding it.

Subcutaneously or Intramuscularly—1 cc ampule one to four times daily as the severity of case demands.

Intravenously—½ m of contents of ampule (approximately 0.03 cc) per pound of body weight, provided patient has received no digitalis medication during preceding 2 weeks; at end of 2 hr., in absence of desired therapeutic effects or toxic symptoms, ⅛ m per pound of body weight may be administered at 2 hr. intervals until improvement is obtained or toxic symptoms occur, or a total dosage of 1 m per pound of body weight has been reached; this total should not be exceeded.

Maintenance Dosage—Once digitalization has been effected after any method of administration, 1½ gr daily as tablet or 16 m of the liquid will suffice to maintain the average patient, although individual variations are encountered.

Bibliography: *See Chap. XII.*

DIGIFORTIS (Parke, Davis)

Digitalis Therapy

Description: A fat-free Digitalis preparation of high purity and potency; prepared from especially grown and selected leaves of Digitalis purpurea and standardized to 150 % the activity of the U.S.P. tincture; alcoholic content 65 %.

Action and Uses: Stimulates cardiac rhythm with prolongation of the diastolic pause; increases contraction of ventricular walls, with lessened relaxation and increased cardiac tone.

Supply: DIGIFORTIS—Bottles, 1 fl. oz.

DIGIFORTIS—Tablets Compressed, ½ and 1 gr (0.032–0.647 Gm) of powdered standardized leaf—Bottles of 50.

DIGIFORTIS—Kapseals, containing 1 gr (0.647 Gm) of powdered leaf—Bottles of 100 and 500.

Administration: *Orally or Rectally*—After digitalization by any method average dose 0.5 cc (8 m) or one 1 gr (0.647 Gm) tablet or kapseal.

Bibliography: *See Chap. XII.*

DIGIGLUSIN (Lilly)

Digitalis Therapy

Description: Contains all the active glucosides of digitalis leaves; tested and standardized; in stable form.

Action and Uses: As for digitalis.

Administration: As for digitalis.

Supply: DIGIGLUSIN—Tablets, gr 1½ (0.1 Gm)—Bottles of 40 and 500.

DIGIGLUSIN—Liquid, each cubic centimeter = 1 cc of potent tincture—Bottles of 1 and 4 oz., 1 pt.

DIGIGLUSIN—Ampules, each cubic centimeter equivalent to 15 m of potent tincture—Boxes of 6.

DIGINUTIN (Burroughs Wellcome)

Digitalis Therapy

Composition: A solution of total glucosides of Digitalis leaf, free from inert matter; is potent, miscible with water and stable also in warm climate; standardized to be equivalent to freshly prepared Tr. Digitalis, 1 cc or 17 m to equal 1 cat unit.

Action and Uses: As for digitalis.

Supply: DIGINUTIN—Bottles of 1 and 8 oz.

Administration: As for digitalis.

DIGIPOTEN (Abbott)

Digitalis Therapy

Description: A mixture of Digitalis glucosides, free from saponins and standardized by admixture of milk sugar; is a pale green powder, of bitter taste; soluble in water and 25 % alcohol.

Action: That of high quality digitalis leaves, of constant concentration and potency; *used* in all conditions where digitalis therapy is indicated.

Supply: DIGIPOTEN—Tablets (C.A.) gr ½ (0.03 Gm)—Bottles of 100 and 1,000.

Administration: As for digitalis therapy in general.

DIGISMITH AND DIGILUTEA PREPARATIONS

(Upsher Smith)

Description: **DIGISMITH** preparations are made from Digitalis Purpurea.

DIGILUTEA preparations are prepared from Digitalis Lutea. Both are produced from especially cultivated and carefully selected leaves; standardized in International Units.

Action and Uses: As for Digitalis.

Supply: **DIGISMITH**—Tincture 1 International Unit per cubic centimeter (25% stronger than U.S.P. unit)—Bottles of 1 oz.

DIGISMITH—Capsules—1 International Unit (equivalent to about 2 gr (0.130 Gm) of U.S.P. Digitalis Powder)—Bottles 24, 500 and 1,000.
¾ International Unit = 1½ gr (0.09 Gm)—Bottles 24, 500 and 1,000.
⅓ International Unit = ⅔ gr (0.04 Gm)—Bottles 24, 500 and 1,000.

DIGISMITH—Tablets—1 International Unit (equivalent to about 2 gr (0.130 Gm) of U.S.P. Digitalis Powder)—Tubes of 24.
¾ International Unit = 1½ gr (0.09 Gm)—Tubes of 24.
½ International Unit = 1 gr (0.06 Gm)—Tubes of 24.

DIGILUTEA—Tincture—1 International Unit in 1 cc (25% stronger than U.S.P. unit)—Bottles of 1 oz.

DIGILUTEA—Capsules—1 International Unit equivalent to about 2 gr (0.130 Gm) of U.S.P. Digitalis Powder—Bottles 24, 500 and 1,000.
⅓ International Unit = ⅔ gr (0.04 Gm)—Bottles 24, 500 and 1,000.

DIGILUTEA—Tablets—1 International Unit equivalent to about 2 gr (0.130 Gm) of U.S.P. Digitalis Powder—Tubes of 24.

Advantages: Digilutea is less nauseating; is especially indicated in the intolerant for digitalis.

Administration: Same methods of digitalization as with U.S.P. preparations, but taking into consideration the fact that ¾ International Unit (tablet or capsule) is equivalent to 1 cat unit.

Dosage: In calculating dosage in International Units, it may be suggested, that the patient's body weight in pounds be divided by 12; the obtained number affords a safe indication as to the number of International Units needed for physiological saturation. This total dose may be effectively distributed over a period of 3 days. Thus a 144 lb. patient would require for digitalization 12 International Units, given in the form of Capsules Digismith 1 International Unit, 1 capsule four times a day for 3 days. Maintenance dose would be about 1–2 International Units given in 1 daily dose.

Bibliography: *See Chap. XII.*

DIGITABS

(Fraser)

Digitalis Therapy

Description: Enteric coated tablets, each containing m 5 of Tr. Digitalis, prepared from selected digitalis leaves.

Action and Uses: As for digitalis.

Supply: DIGITABS—Tablets gr 5 (0.324 Gm)—Bottles 100 and 1,000.

Administration: One or more tablets as required.

DIGITALIN (Amorphous) (Burroughs Wellcome)

Digitalis Therapy

Description: A white amorphous powder, prepared from Digitalis seeds, containing crystalline glucoside Digitalin with a large proportion of Saponins.

Action and Uses: As for digitalis.

Supply: DIGITALIN—Tabloid—*Hypodermic*—gr 1/100 (0.00065 Gm)—Tubes of 20, 50—Packages of 500.

DIGITALIN—Tabloid—*Oral*—gr 1/100 (0.00065 Gm)—Bottles of 100 and 500.

Administration: Tabloid—*Hypodermic*—1–2 tabloids, maximum 3 tabloids gr 1/30 (0.00216 Gm) as required.

Tabloid—*Oral*—1–3 tabloids daily; maximum gr 1/60 (0.00108 Gm) per dose.

DIGITALIN (Crystalline) (Burroughs Wellcome)

Digitalis Therapy

Description: A crystalline glucoside prepared from Digitalis leaves; similar to or identical with Digitoxin; is very active but more irritant.

Action and Uses: As for Digitalis.

Supply: HYPOLOID DIGITALIN—1 cc, gr 1/140 (0.001 Gm)—Boxes of 10.

TABLOID DIGITALIN—Gr 1/250 (0.00026 Gm)—Bottles of 25 and 100.

Administration: 1 ampule or 1 tabloid when necessary; both with great caution.

DIGITALINE "NATIVELLE" (Fougera)

Digitalis Therapy

Formula: $C_{34}H_{54}O_{11}$.

Composition: The crystallized, active principle of Digitalis.

Description: Occurs as thin, colorless, odorless, rectangular leaflets, slightly soluble in water and ether, easily soluble in alcohol and chloroform.

Action: As for digitalis but with more prolonged action on the heart; is gastro-intestinal irritant and may cause disturbances.

Supply: DIGITALINE "NATIVELLE"—Granules, 0.1 mg (gr 1/600)—Bottles of 60. (Each granule is equivalent to 1 cc fresh digitalis tincture or to gr 1½ (0.1 Gm) powdered leaves.)

DIGITALINE "NATIVELLE"—Solution, 1:1,000, 5 drops containing 0.1 mg (gr 1/600).

DIGITALINE "NATIVELLE"—Ampules, 1 cc Intramuscular, containing 0.25 mg (gr 1/240) digitaline in oil.

DIGITALINE "NATIVELLE"—Ampules, 1 cc Intravenous, containing 0.2 mg (gr 1/300).

Uses and Administration: In mild ventricular insufficiency—0.1 mg or 5 drops of solution for 5 days of each 10 days; double dosage for moderate insufficiency for first 5 days, followed during next 5 days by theobromine salts; in severe decompensation—0.2 mg or 10 drops of solution for first 5 days, then 0.1 mg or 5 drops daily; if needed, an ampule daily for 3–4 days. Similar dosage in other cardiac conditions, but not to exceed 0.001 Gm (1/60 gr); if toxic symptoms appear, must immediately be stopped.

Advantages: Is a definite chemical entity, of unvarying composition and activity, rigorously pure, and thus of constant therapeutic effect.

Antidotes: Emetics, nitroglycerin, tannin, morphine, camphor, alcoholic stimulants.

DIGITALIS (Lederle)

Digitalis Therapy

Description: Dried Digitalis Leaf of 1 cat unit potency to 1½ gr of the powdered leaf; standardized by the Hatcher method.

Action and Uses: As for digitalis; is of uniform and accurate potency, easily and conveniently administered; is readily absorbed, stable and does not deteriorate for 5 yrs.

Supply: DIGITALIS—Tablets—Tubes of 20 each—Packages of 5 tubes, of ¾ gr (½ cat unit); 1½ gr (1 cat unit) and 3 gr (2 cat units).

Administration: Digitalization—First Day: ¼ of total calculated dose, 4 units; then 2 units at intervals of 6 hr., or a total of 10 units in first 24 hr.;
Second Day; 2 units three times at 6 hr. intervals.
Third and subsequent days: 1 or 2 units in one administration as maintenance dose.

Caution: The above applies only if no digitalis has been given for 10 days previously; if in doubt, 1 unit is administered three to four times a day and toxic symptoms watched for.

DIGITALIS "DUO-TEST" (McNeil)

Digitalis Therapy

Description: Defatted Digitalis, doubly standardized and tested by the U.S.P. frog method and Reed-Vanderkleed guinea-pig method.

Action and Uses: As for digitalis. Cardiac stimulant and diuretic in various heart diseases.

Supply: DIGITALIS "DUO-TEST"—Capsules (C.A.)—Each equivalent to gr 1 standardized powdered digitalis leaves—Bottles of 100, 500, 1,000, 5,000.

TINCTURE DIGITALIS "DUO-TEST" (C.A.) 10%—Bottles of 1 oz., with dropper.

Administration: 1 capsule two or three times daily as required; tincture—5–15 m three times daily.

DIGITALIS PREPARATIONS

Supply: PULVOIDS DIGITALIS FOLIUM—Pulvoids, gr. ¾ (0.048 Gm) ½ cat unit—Bottles 100, 1,000. **(Drug Products)**
Gr. 1½ (0.09 Gm) 1 cat unit—Bottles 100, 1,000.
Gr ½ (0.032 Gm) ⅓ cat unit—Bottles 100, 1,000.

DIGIPIT—Bottles of 1 oz. **(Harvey Pittenger)**

DIGICARDIUM—Bottles of 1 oz. **(Rorer)**

DIGITALIGEN—Tablets, Gr ⅓ (0.02 Gm), Gr. 1 (0.06 Gm)—Bottles of 1,000. **(Searle)**

DIGITALIGEN—Tincture—Bottles of 1 oz., 1 pint.

DIGITALIS LEAVES—Powdered—Capsules 1 gr (0.06 Gm) representing 1 m fluid extract or 10 m tincture—Bottles of 1,000.

DIGITORA—Tablets, gr 1½—Vials of 30—Tablets, scored—Vials of 40. **(Upjohn)**

DIGINFUSE—Tablets—Tubes of 12. **(Upjohn)**

DIGI-CARDALIS—Tablets (enteric coated)—Bottles of 100, 500 and 1,000. **(Westerfield)**

Uses: As for digitalis.

DIGITAN **(Merck)**

Digitalis Therapy

Description: A purified, physiologically standardized extract of Digitalis made by the original Digipuratum process; contains the active glucosides in natural proportions, obtained from selected leaves of Digitalis purpurea and free from inert matter, saponins and digitonin; is a greenish, odorless, bitter tasting powder, standardized to equalize the official U.S.P. preparations; insoluble in water and dilute acids, soluble in weak alkali.

Action: Is promptly absorbed, rapidly eliminated; its uniformity of composition permits accurate dosage and avoidance of cumulative effect or intoxication.

Uses: Cardiac disease, heart failure; nephritis, arteriosclerosis, arterial hypertension; to support heart action in pneumonia, emphysema, epilepsy, gastric dilatation.

Supply: DIGITAN—Powder—Bottles ⅛ oz.

DIGITAN—Ampules (C.A.) 1 cc—Boxes of 6.

DIGITAN—Ampules (C.A.) (Rectal) 15 cc—Boxes of 1.

DIGITAN—Tincture (C.A.)—Bottles of 12 cc and 1 fl. oz.

DIGITAN—Tablets (C.A.) gr 1½—Tubes 12—Bottles of 100.

Administration: 1½ gr (0.1 Gm) as required.

DIGITOS **(Sharp and Dohme)**

Digitalis Therapy

Description: A standardized aqueous preparation of the glucosides of Digitalis leaves, free from chlorophyl, fat, tannin and other inert matter of the crude drug, differing physically and chemically from digitoxin and true digitalin; a clear, yellow or slightly opalescent fluid, containing not more than ½ % of solids; alcohol 7%.

Action and Uses: As for digitalis. For intramuscular and intravenous use only.

Supply: DIGITOS (C.A.)—Ampules 1 cc—Boxes of 12.

DIGITOS (C.A.)—Ampules 5 cc—Boxes of 4.

Administration: Same as Tincture Digitalis, 5–60 m or more at intervals of 24–48 hr.

DIGITOXIN **(Merck)**

Digitalis Therapy

Chemical Name: Digitaline Cristalliseé (Nativelle)

Formula: $C_{42}H_{66}O_{13}$ (Windaus); $C_{34}H_{54}O_{11}$ (Kiliani).

Description: The active glucoside present in leaves of Digitalis purpurea; occurs as thin, colorless rectangular anhydrous leaflets, odorless and of bitter taste; slightly soluble in water, ether and fatty acids; easily soluble in alcohol and chloroform.

Action and Uses: A prompt, reliable and powerful heart tonic of uniform therapeutic activity; *useful* in valvular lesions, myocarditis, congestive period of pneumonia and in pneumonia following operations.

Supply: DIGITOXIN (C.A.)—Vials, 1 Gm.

Administration: *Oral* 1/240–1/60 Gr (0.00025–0.001 Gm) three times daily, with 3 m (0.2 cc) chloroform, 60 m (4 cc) alcohol, and 1½ fl. oz. (45 cc) water.
Enema—1/80 Gr (0.0008 Gm) with 10 m (0.6 cc) alcohol, and 4 fl. oz. (120 cc) water, one to three times daily.
Maximum Dose—1/30 Gr (0.002 Gm) single; 1/20 Gr (0.003 Gm) daily.
Antidotes—Emetics, stomach syphon, tannic acid, nitroglycerin, morphine early, strophanthin later, stimulants, camphor, mustard plaster.

DI-HYDRANOL (Sharp and Dohme)

Germicide

Chemical Name: Heptyl Resorcinol; 2–4 Dihydroxyphenyl n-Heptane.

Composition: A 5% solution of Heptyl Resorcinol in olive oil.

Action: Is stated to be powerfully germicidal, especially against pathogenic intestinal flora; is one hundred times more effective than phenol; is non-toxic if used in strengths of therapeutic efficiency.

Uses: In fermentative dyspepsia and intestinal infections.

Supply: DI-HYDRANOL—Solution—Bottles, 4 oz.
DI-HYDRANOL—Capsules—Elastic soluble, each 0.15 gr—Boxes of 50.

Administration: 2-3 capsules or 1 or 2 fl. dr. three to four times daily.

DILAUDID (Bilhuber-Knoll)

Sedative. Narcotic

Chemical Name: Dihydromorphinone Hydrochloride.

Formula: $C_{17}H_{19}O_3$. HCl.

Description: A white, crystalline powder derived from morphine; is readily soluble in water.

Action and Uses: As for morphine; a powerful analgesic, sedative and narcotic.

Supply: DILAUDID—Tablets—gr 1/24—Tubes of 10; gr 1/16, 1/20—Tubes of 20 and 100.
DILAUDID—Suppositories—gr 1/24 (0.0025 Gm) in Ol. theobromatis—Boxes of 6.
DILAUDID—Ampules—1 cc—gr 1/32 (0.002 Gm) in saline—Boxes of 6.
DILAUDID—Tablets—hypodermic—gr 1/32 (0.002 Gm)—Tubes of 20; also gr 1/20, gr 1/16.
DILAUDID—Powder—Vials gr 15.

Administration: *Oral*—gr 1/24 (0.0025 Gm); initial dose gr 1/48 (0.0013 Gm) increased when necessary to gr 1/24 or 1/16 (0.0025–0.004 Gm).
Hypodermic—Gr 1/32 (0.002 Gm) effect begins in 15 min. and lasts for 6 or 8 hr.

Advantages: Well tolerated, non-nauseant and non-constipating; quickly active, readily soluble.

Bibliography: *See Chap. XII.*

DIMAZON (Heilkraft)

Cell Proliferant

Chemical Name: Diacetyl Amido Azotoluene.

Formula: $CH_3C_6H_4N: NC_6H_3(CH_3)N(CH_3CO)_2$.

Description: An orange colored, crystalline powder, soluble in alcohol, ether, chloroform, benzene, acetone, oils, fats, petrolatum; insoluble in water.

Action: Stimulates proliferation of epithelial cells and promotes healing.

Uses: In indolent varicose ulcers, sluggish, non-granulating wounds, eczema, intertrigo, severe burns, ulcus cruris, erythrodermia, conjunctivitis, keratitis.

Advantages: Odorless, non-staining and non-irritating.

Supply: **DIMAZON**—Ointment (C.A.)—2% in petrolatum 98%—Tubes of 1 oz.

DIMAZON—Powder (C.A.)—5% in talcum 95%—Boxes of 1 oz.

DIMAZON—Oil (C.A.)—2% in mineral oil 98%—Bottles of 1 oz.

Administration: **Dermatology**—Applied as ointment-dressing every day; may be alternated with the powder or Anesthesine, Orthoform, if an anesthetic effect is desired.

Ophthalmology—Gentle massage of cornea daily with ointment and instillation of scopolamine.

Bibliography: *See Chap. XII.*

DIMOL (Anglo-French)

Intestinal Antiseptic

Description: A compound of Dimethylomethoxyphenol with Tri- and Tetramethylophenol.

Formula: $C_6H_2(CH_3)_2(OCH_3)OH$.

Action and Uses: An intestinal disinfectant; destroys intestinal bacteria without producing toxic effect and passes unchanged in the feces. *For use* in acute gastro-enteritis, fermentative diarrhea, infantile disorders, auto-intoxication, intestinal putrefaction, non-amebic dysentery, acute and chronic colitis; also in rheumatism and arthritis accompanied by intestinal toxicosis.

Supply: **DIMOL**—Pulverettes—sugar coated, gr 1 (0.064 Gm)—Bottles of 50.

DIMOL—Pulverettes—keratin coated, gr 1 (0.064 Gm)—Bottles of 50.

DIMOL—Syrup—For children, dr. 1, equivalent to gr 0.3 (0.018 Gm) of Dimol—Bottles of 4 and 16 oz.

Administration: 2–4 pulverettes, after meals, with water.
Children—1½–3 dr. (6–18 Gm) four to five times daily.
Infants—½–1½ dr. (2–6 cc).

Bibliography: *See Chap. XII.*

DIONIN (Merck)

Sedative. Narcotic

Official Name: Ethyl Morphine Hydrochloride.

Formula: $C_{17}H_{17}(NO)(OH)(OC_2H_5).HCl + 2H_2O$.

Description: White, crystalline faintly bitter powder, soluble in about 8 parts water.

Action and Uses: Sedative, antispasmodic and narcotic; cough sedative, ocular lymphagogue and analgesic; effective in the treatment of painful affections; produces no constipation, nausea, lassitude or habituation; may be used instead of morphine in most of the indications for that alkaloid, except where it is desired to check secretion and in cases of severe pain; does not produce as frequently disagreeable after-effects as morphine; is particularly effective in aborting acute coryza and alleviating the distressing symptoms of hay fever.

Internally—*Used* in checking irritation in phthisis, chronic bronchitis, emphysema, asthma; to "abort coryza," morphiomania; to relieve painful affections, insomnia, laryngitis, influenza, pneumonia, enteritis, colic, cardialgia, whooping cough; in gynecological operations and also prior to chloroform anesthesia.

Externally—In corneal affections, iritis, glaucoma, interstitial keratitis, dry and chronic conjunctival catarrh, opacity of vitreous humor, atrophic rhinitis.

Supply: DIONIN—Powder—Bottles ⅛ oz. and 1 oz.—Vials 1 Gm.

DIONIN—Tablets—Gr ¼ (0.016 Gm)—Bottles 50 and 100. Gr 1 (0.064 Gm) (for hypodermic and ophthalmic use)—Bottles 100—Tubes 25.

Administration: *Internally and Subcutaneously*—⅙ to 1 gr (0.01 to 0.06 Gm), two or three times daily, in tablet, pill or solution; as *hypnotic*, at evening, ½–¾ gr (0.03–0.05 Gm); average dose ¼ gr (0.015 Gm)—*Injection* in morphinism, 1 or 2 gr (0.06–0.12 Gm) single dose; 3–15 gr (0.2–1 Gm) per day.

Externally—(Eye diseases), 1–2 drops of 5–10% solution, or pure to produce chemosis; 2 drops of an 0.5–2% solution four times per day as analgesic; in gynecology, ⅔ gr (0.04 Gm) in vaginal suppositories. Maximum dose (except in morphinism) 1⅓ gr (0.08 Gm) single; 5 gr (0.3 Gm) daily.

Antidote: Same as for morphine and codeine.

Bibliography: *See Chap. XII.*

DIOXOGEN (Oakland)

Antiseptic

Chemical Name: Hydrogen Dioxide.

Formula: H_2O_2.

Description: A solution of Hydrogen Peroxide; uniform, stable, free from impurities and of neutral reaction; supplies 12.5 volumes of nascent active oxygen.

Action and Uses: Is non-irritating antiseptic, destroying bacteria and their spores; does not precipitate albumen, devitalize tissue or inhibit activity of enzymes; *For use* in sterilizing drinking water and milk, as surgical and general antiseptic and to stimulate granulations and repair of tissues; also *used* in acute indigestion, ptomaine poisoning, dysentery, diarrheas and peptic ulcer; in pyorrhea and oral affections, as mouthwash.

Supply: DIOXOGEN—Bottles of 2, 4 and 8 oz.

Administration: Topically, freely, in full strength; to sterilize water, 3 dr. of a 3% solution per gallon; internally, 15–30 drops in 2 oz. of water, repeated every 15–30 min. till relieved.

DIURETIN (Bilhuber-Knoll)

Diuretic. Cardiac Stimulant

Description: A double sodium salt of Salicylic Acid and Theobromine; a white, hygroscopic powder, freely soluble in water.

Action: Diuretic and cardiac stimulant; dilates renal blood vessels and improves kidney circulation.

Uses: Nephritis with albuminuria or anasarca; in angina pectoris to relieve left ventricle and dilate coronaries; in angina abdominis, vascular spasm and arteriosclerotic disorders for vasodilation.

Incompatibles: Incompatible with acids and ammonia bases.

Advantages: A powerful, prompt diuretic with lasting effects; a chloride eliminant; readily absorbed.

Supply: DIURETIN—Tablets gr 8 (0.5 Gm)—Tubes of 20—Vials of 50.

DIURETIN—Powder—Cartons of 1 oz.

Administration: *Average Dose*—8–16 gr (0.5–1.0 Gm), or 1–2 tablets three or four times daily after meals. In arteriosclerosis—up to 24 gr daily. As diuretic—up to 80 gr daily. In angina pectoris—24–60 gr daily.

Bibliography: *See Chap. XII.*

DUOTAL (Winthrop)

Phthisis Therapy

Chemical Name: Guaiacol Carbonate.

Formula: $CO_3(C_6H_4OCH_3)_2$.

Description: A white, almost tasteless and odorless powder, insoluble in water; contains 90.5% of pure guaiacol.

Action: As for guaiacol carbonate, U.S.P.

Uses: Chronic bronchitis, pneumonia and tuberculosis; as intestinal antiseptic in typhoid and intestinal infections.

Supply: DUOTAL—Tablets (C.A.)—5 gr—Tubes of 10.
DUOTAL—Powder (C.A.)—Carton, 1 oz.

Administration: Adults; 5–15 gr (0.3–1.0 Gm), children, 2–8 gr (0.12–0.5 Gm), three times daily.

ELARSON (Winthrop)

Alterative. Hematinic

Chemical Name: Chlor-arseno-behenolate of Strontium. Brand of Arsoben.

Description: An almost odorless powder, containing about 13% of Metallic Arsenic and 6% of Chlorine; insoluble in water and practically insoluble in alcohol, ether and olive oil.

Action: As for other organic arsenicals; is better tolerated by the gastrointestinal tract than arsenous acid or Fowler's solution and is adapted for prolonged administration.

Uses: In various anemias, skin diseases, chorea, malaria, neuralgias and other conditions where arsenic is indicated.

Supply: ELARSON—Tablets, each equivalent to 1/96 gr (0.0006 Gm) arsenous acid—Bottles of 60.

Administration: Adults, 2 tablets, three to five times daily.
Children, 1 tablet, two or three times daily; dosage may progressively be increased.

Combinations: FERRO-ELARSON—Brand of Ferarsoben. Each tablet contains the equivalent of 1/96 gr (0.0006 Gm) arsenous acid and ½ gr (0.03 Gm) of reduced iron. *Supply*—Tablets—Bottles of 60. *Administration*—Adults 1 tablet three times daily, gradually increased to three. Children 1 tablet daily, after meals.

EMPIRIN (Burroughs Wellcome)

Antipyretic

Composition: A pure form of Acetyl Salicylic Acid, containing no free acids, neither salicylic nor acetic.

Action and Uses: As for aspirin; analgesic and antipyretic; is more toxic than sodium salicylate but less irritant.

Supply: TABLOID EMPIRIN—Gr 1 (0.065 Gm) and gr 5 (0.324 Gm)—Bottles of 100 and 500.

Administration: As antipyretic, 1–3 tabloids, either strength, as required, with water, two to three times daily; as analgesic—15 gr initial dose, 10 gr at intervals for 3–4 doses.

Combinations: TABLOID EMPIRIN COMPOUND—Contains Empirin gr 3½ (0.227 Gm), Acetphenetidine gr 2½ (0.162 Gm), Caffein gr ½ (0.032 Gm). *Dose*—1 or 2 tabloids taken with water—Bottles of 100 and 500.

TABLOID EMPIRIN COMPOUND—Contains Empirin gr 3½ (0.227 Gm), Acetphenetidin gr 2½ (0.162 Gm), Caffein gr ½ (0.032 Gm), Codein Phosphate gr ⅛ (0.008 Gm).
Dose—1 or 2 tabloids taken with water—Bottles of 100 and 500.

EPHEDRINE

Vasoconstrictor

Chemical Name: Alpha-hydroxy-beta-methylamino Propylbenzene.

Formula: $C_6H_5.\ CHOH.\ CH(NHCH_3).\ CH_3$.

Description: The active principle of Ma Huang, Ephedra equisetina (Bunge); is similar to Epinephrine chemically; occurs as almost colorless needles, soluble in water, alcohol, chloroform and liquid petrolatum; insoluble in ether; does not deteriorate if exposed to light, air or boiling.

Action: Excites the sympathetic nervous system similarly to epinephrine, but its effects are more prolonged though less intense; is effective when orally administered. Is mydriatic, vasoconstrictor and cardio-respiratory stimulant; relieves bronchial spasm, stimulates central nervous system, stimulates uterine muscle, contracts capillaries and arterioles reducing hyperemia and swelling raising blood pressure; is non-habit forming. In large doses depresses the heart and may cause glycosuria.

Uses: In all instances where epinephrin is employed: in rhinitis, sinusitis, colds, conjunctivitis; in hay fever, asthma, bronchitis, whooping cough; in surgical and other shock, anesthesia accidents, spinal anesthesia; in various hemorrhages, in mydriasis.

Supply: EPHEDRINE—Inhalant (C.A.) 1%, in light mineral oil—Bottles of ½ oz. (Abbott)

EPHEDRINE—Nasal Ointment, 1%—Tubes of 1 oz.—Boxes of 12. (Abbott)

EPHEDRINE—Inhalant, 1% solution, in light mineral oil, tinted and perfumed with oil of rose—Bottles 1 oz. (Lederle)

EPHEDRINE INHALANT COMPOUND (C.A.)—Containing Ephedrine 1 Gm, Menthol 0.02 Gm, Camphor 0.66 Gm, Oil of thyme 0.31 cc, in Paraffin oil q.s. 100 cc—Bottles of 1 oz. and 1 pt. (Lilly)

EPHEDRINE INHALANT PLAIN (C.A.)—Contains Ephedrine 1 Gm, Cinnamic aldehyde and Benzaldehyde, in aromatized Paraffin oil 100 cc—Bottles 1 oz. and 1 pt. (Lilly)

EPHEDRINE COMPOUND (C.A.)—Ointment—Contains Ephedrine 1%, Menthol 0.65%, Camphor 0.65%, Oil of thyme 0.375% in Petroleum base—Nasal tip tubes, ½ oz. (Lilly)

EPHEDRINE—Inhalant, Plain, contains Ephedrine 1% in liquid petroleum base—Bottles of 1 and 16 oz. (Parke, Davis)

EPHEDRINE—Inhalant, Compound, contains Ephedrine 1%, Menthol 0.6%, Camphor 0.6%, Geraniol 0.32%, Liquid petrolatum base—Bottles 1 and 16 oz. (Parke, Davis)

Administration: For topical application or inhalation, in nose and throat by swab, spray, dropper.

Advantages: Is stable, does not deteriorate in solution and is not destroyed by boiling; is effective if orally administered with action persisting for several hours; has wide margin of safety between therapeutic and toxic dosage; does not cause secondary vasomotor dilatation.

Bibliography: *See Chap. XII.*

EPHEDRINE HYDROCHLORIDE

Vasoconstrictor

Chemical Name: A-hydroxy-b-methylamino-3, 4-dihydroxyethylbenzene hydrochloride.

Formula: $C_6H_5CHOH. CH(CH_3NH). CH_3HCl.$

Description: White needle-like crystals containing 80–82.5 % of the active principle of Ma-Huang.

Action and Uses: As for Ephedrine.

Supply: **EPHEDRINE HYDROCHLORIDE**—Tablets (C.A.) ¼, ½ gr (0.016–0.032 Gm)—Vials of 20 and 40. **(Abbott)**

EPHEDRINE HYDROCHLORIDE—Capsules (C.A.) ⅜ gr (0.0025 Gm), ½ gr (0.0324 Gm) ¾ gr (0.05 Gm)—Bottles of 40 and 500. **(Abbott)**

EPHEDRINE HYDROCHLORIDE—Ampules (C.A.) 1 cc, ¾ gr (0.005 Gm)—Boxes of 6 and 100. **(Abbott)**

EPHEDRINE HYDROCHLORIDE—Solution (C.A.)—Bottles of 1 oz. and 1 pt. **(Abbott)**

EPHEDRINE HYDROCHLORIDE—Syrup (C.A.) containing ⅛ gr (0.008 Gm) per dram—Bottles of 4 oz., 1 pt. and 1 gal. **(Abbott)**

EPHEDRINE HYDROCHLORIDE—Syrup (C.A.) Double Strength gr ¼ (0.016 Gm)—Bottles of 4 oz., 1 pt. and 1 gal. **(Abbott)**

EPHEDRINE—Elixir, Containing Ephedrine Hydrochloride, gr ⅛ per dram; alcohol 10 %—Bottles 4 oz., 1 pt. and 1 gal. **(Abbott)**

EPHEDRINE HYDROCHLORIDE—Solution 3 %—Bottles of 1 and 16 oz. **(Burroughs Wellcome)**

EPHEDRINE HYDROCHLORIDE—Tabloid—Gr ½ (0.032 Gm)—Tubes of 6—Bottles of 25 and 100. **(Burroughs Wellcome)**

EPHEDRINE HYDROCHLORIDE—Hypoloid—1 cc, gr ½ (0.032 Gm)—Boxes of 10. **(Burroughs Wellcome)**

EPHEDRINE COMPOUND—Elixoid—Containing per dram Ephedrine hydrochloride gr ¼, Syrup Tolu m 15, Tr. Pruni Virginianae m 2, Chloroform m ⅛—Bottles of 1 and 16 oz. **(Burroughs Wellcome)**

EPHEDRINE HYDROCHLORIDE—Capsules, (C.A.) gr ½, ¾ and ⅜—Bottles of 40 and 100. **(Gane, Ingram)**

EPHEDRINE HYDROCHLORIDE—Solution 3 %, with 0.5 % chlorbutanol as preservative—Bottles 1 oz. **(Lederle)**

EPHEDRINE HYDROCHLORIDE—Tablets—gr ¼, gr ½, gr ¾, 100 tablets (5 tubes of 20) in each size. **(Lederle)**

EPHEDRINE HYDROCHLORIDE—Crystalline (C.A.)—Vials gr 30 (1.94 Gm)—Bottles ¼ oz. **(Lilly)**

EPHEDRINE HYDROCHLORIDE (C.A.)—Tablets, Hypodermic, gr ¼ (0.016 Gm) and gr ½ (0.03 Gm)—Tubes of 20—Bottles of 100. **(Lilly)**

EPHEDRINE HYDROCHLORIDE—Pulvules, gr ⅜ (0.024 Gm) and ¾ (0.048 Gm)—Bottles 40 and 500. **(Lilly)**

EPHEDRINE HYDROCHLORIDE (C.A.)—Solution 3%—Bottles of 1 oz. and 1 pt. **(Lilly)**

EPHEDRINE HYDROCHLORIDE (C.A.)—Syrup—Each fluid ounce containing 1 gr or 0.22 Gm per 100 cc—Bottles of 1 pt. and 1 gal. **(Lilly)**

EPHEDRINE HYDROCHLORIDE—Alkaloid—Vials of 30 gr, ¼ and 1 oz. **(Parke, Davis)**

EPHEDRINE HYDROCHLORIDE (C.A.)—Capsules, gr ⅜ (0.024) and gr ¾ (0.048 Gm)—Bottles of 40 and 500. **(Parke, Davis)**

EPHEDRINE HYDROCHLORIDE (C.A.)—Tablets, gr ¾ (0.048 Gm)—Vials of 25—Bottles of 100. **(Squibb)**

EPHEDRINE HYDROCHLORIDE (C.A.)—Tablets gr ⅜ (0.024 Gm)—Vials of 25—Bottles of 100. **(Squibb)**

AMPULE EPHEDRINE HYDROCHLORIDE—Ampules 1 cc—Boxes of 6. **(Zemmer)**

SOLUTION EPHEDRINE HYDROCHLORIDE 3%—Bottles 1 and 4 oz. and 1 pt. **(Zemmer)**

Administration: *Orally*—Gr ⅜ (0.024 Gm), increased if necessary to gr ¾ (0.048 Gm), every 4–8 hr; Syrup—1–2 teaspoonfuls, every 3–4 hr.
Subcutaneously—1–2 ampules, as indicated.
Intravenously and Intramuscularly—⅙ gr (0.01 Gm) or ½–1 ampule. In eye therapy—3% solution, with or without atropine.

Advantages: Is stable, does not deteriorate in solution and is not destroyed by boiling; is effective if orally administered, with action persisting for several hours; has wide margin of safety between therapeutic and toxic dosages; does not cause secondary vasomotor dilatation.

Caution: Care should be exercised in the use of ephedrine preparations in heart disease and hyperthyroidism.

Bibliography: *See Chap. XII.*

EPHEDRINE SULPHATE

Vasoconstrictor

Chemical Name: Ephedrine Base-alpha hydroxy-beta methylamino-propyl benzene.

Formula: $[C_6H_5.\ CHOH.\ CH(NHCH_3).\ CH_3.]_2H_2SO_4$.

Description: White odorless fine crystals, easily soluble in water and hot alcohol, less soluble in cold alcohol.

Action and Uses: As for Ephedrine.

Supply: EPHEDRINE SULPHATE—Solution—Containing Ephedrine Sulphate 3%, Chlorbutanol ½% in distilled water—Bottles 1, 4 oz. and 1 pt. **(Fraser)**

EPHEDRINE SULPHATE (C.A.)—Capsules, gr ½, ¾ and ⅜—Bottles 40 and 100. **(Gane, Ingram)**

EPHEDRINE SULPHATE (C.A.)—Ampules, 1 cc, gr ¾ (0.048 Gm)—Boxes of 6. **(Lilly)**

EPHEDRINE SULPHATE CRYSTALLINE (C.A.)—Vials gr 30 (1.94 Gm)—Bottles ¼ oz. **(Lilly)**

EPHEDRINE SULPHATE—Elixir (C.A.)—Each fluid ounce containing gr 2 (0.13 Gm) or 0.44%—Bottles of 1 pt. and 1 gal. **(Lilly)**

EPHEDRINE SULPHATE (C.A.)—Tablets, Hypodermic, gr ¼ (0.016 Gm) and gr ½ (0.03 Gm)—Tubes of 20—Bottles of 100. **(Lilly)**

EPHEDRINE SULPHATE—Jelly (C.A.) 1%, contains Eucalyptol 0.1% and aromatics in water-soluble base—Tubes nasal tip, ½ oz. (Lilly)

EPHEDRINE SULPHATE—Pulvules, (C.A.) gr ⅜ (0.024 Gm) and ¾ (0.048 Gm)—Bottles 40 and 500. (Lilly)

EPHEDRINE SULPHATE—Solution 3% (C.A.) Bottles of 1 oz. and 1 pt. (Lilly)

EPHEDRINE SULPHATE—Syrup (C.A.)—Each fluid ounce containing 1 gr or 0.22 Gm per 100 cc—Bottles of 1 pt. and 1 gal. (Lilly)

EPHEDRINE SULPHATE—Syrup (C.A.)—Each fluid ounce containing 2 gr or 0.44 Gm per 100 cc—Bottles of 1 pt. and 1 gal. (Lilly)

EPHEDRINE SULPHATE—Alkaloid—Vials of 30 gr, ¼ and 1 oz. (Parke, Davis)

EPHEDRINE SULPHATE (C.A.)—Ampule, gr ¾ (0.048 Gm) in 1 cc distilled water. (Parke, Davis)

EPHEDRINE SULPHATE (C.A.)—Capsules, gr ⅜ (0.024) and gr ¾ (0.048 Gm)—Bottles of 40 and 500. (Parke, Davis)

EPHEDRINE SULPHATE (C.A.)—Solution, 3%—Bottles of 1 and 16 oz. (Parke, Davis)

Administration: Dose gr ¾–1½ (0.045–0.9 Gm) for adults, one to three times daily; maximum daily dose—gr 4½ (0.3 Gm); may be given orally, subcutaneously, intramuscularly; topically in 1–3% solution; is compatible with colloidal silver preparations.

Combinations: **EPHEDRINE-MERTHIOLATE**—Solution contains Ephedrine sulphate 1%, Merthiolate 1:5,000; *For use* in naso-pharyngeal inflammation, sinusitis; as decongestive and germicidal soothing agent. (Lilly)

Supply—Bottles 1 oz., 1 pt.; Jelly—½ oz. nasal-tip tubes. *Administration*—By spray, dropper, swab and topically.

Bibliography: See *Chap. XII.*

EPINEPHRIN HYDROCHLORIDE (Lederle)

Vasoconstrictor. Cardiac Stimulant

Description: A sterile solution of the active principle of Suprarenal Medulla; physiologically standardized; strength—1:1,000, for injection.

Action and Uses: For use in shock resulting from the use of specific protein therapy, serum shock, urticaria; in cardiac or vasomotor failure during spinal or other anesthesia; to check paroxysms in bronchial asthma.

Supply: **EPINEPHRIN HYDROCHLORIDE** (C.A.)—Vial 5 cc rubber-stoppered, sterile.

EPINEPHRIN HYDROCHLORIDE (C.A.)—Ampules 1 cc—Box of 12.

EPINEPHRIN HYDROCHLORIDE—Vials 1 oz.

Administration: Dose 3–10 m *intramuscularly,* massaging site of injection to aid absorption.

EPININE (Burroughs Wellcome)

Vasoconstrictor

Chemical Name: 3-4-dihydroxyphenylethylmethylamine.

Description: A synthetic product of the Epinephrine group of sympathomimetic amines; is more stable in slightly acid condition; does not readily deteriorate and is boilable.

Action and Uses: As for epinephrine; 1:100 solution Epinine is equivalent in potency to 1:1,000 solution epinephrine.

Supply: EPININE—Solution 1:100—Bottles 25 cc.

TABLOID OPHTHALMIC—Epinine HCl. gr 1/8 (0.0075 Gm)—Tubes of 10. One tabloid in 10 m of water, forms a 1:100 solution for ophthalmic use.

Administration: One tabloid placed on conjunctiva where it is immediately dissolved and effective; or several drops of solution.

Combinations: EPININE COMPOUND TABLOID—Contains Epinine HCl, gr 1/1,000 (0.00065 Gm), pulv. ipecac gr 1/50 (0.0013 Gm), acid benzoic gr 1/40 (0.0016 Gm), oil gaultheriae m 1/30 (0.002 cc)—Bottles of 25, 100, 500; *Administration*—dissolved in mouth every 1 or 2 hr.; *For use* by public speakers.

EPININE HYDROCHLORIDE—Hypoloid—1 cc of 1:100 solution—Boxes of 10; *Dosage*—5–15 m *hypodermically; Intravenously*—1 cc in 500 cc saline.

EPININE HYDROCHLORIDE—Enule—gr 1/6, (0.012 Gm) 1:100 solution—Boxes of 12; One enule repeated as necessary.

EPININE—Nasal Jelly—Contains 1/2 % Epinine and 1 % each of camphor and menthol, in a water soluble base. *For use* as application to nasal passages to relieve congestion. *Supply*—Collapsible tubes with nasal tip.

EPISOL (Crookes)

Sclerosing Agent

Composition: A "Treves-Barber" Sodium Morrhuate preparation.

Action and Uses: *For obliteration* of varicose veins.

Supply: EPISOL—Ampules 5 cc—Boxes of 6.

EPISOL—Bottles 30 cc.

Administration: 1/2–1 cc, maximum 10 cc, injected at each sitting.

ERGAMINE (Burroughs Wellcome)

Secretory Stimulant

Chemical Name: 4 beta-amino-ethylglyoxaline. Histamine.

Description: An organic base derived from ergot.

Action and Uses: Stimulates gastric secretion, uterine contractions; *used* in gastric analysis.

Supply: TABLOID HYPODERMIC ERGAMINE ACID PHOSPHATIC—Ergamine gr 1/64 (0.001 Gm)—Tubes of 20, 50—Packages of 500.

Administration: 1 tabloid *hypodermically* or *intramuscularly;* dosage increased with great caution.

ERGOT ASEPTIC (Parke, Davis)

Uterine Stimulant

Description: A liquid extract of Ergot, assayed by the cock's comb method, of the potency of fluid extract of ergot U.S.P.; potency guaranteed for 1 yr.

Action and Uses: As for ergot.

Supply: ERGOT ASEPTIC (C.A.)—Ampule 1 cc—Box of 6.

Administration: 1–2 ampules, *intramuscularly.*

ERGOTOXINE (Burroughs Wellcome)

Uterine Stimulant

Description: An alkaloid of Ergot.

Action and Uses: Causes tetanic contraction of unstriped musculature, particularly of the uterus, beginning ¼–½ hr. after administration and lasting 12 hr. or longer; is more effective on the pregnant uterus and one nearing term, but is most powerful on the puerperal uterus; also raises blood pressure.

Supply: **ERGOTOXINE**—Tabloid—Hypodermic—Containing Ergotoxine gr 1/100 (0.00065 Gm)—Tubes of 20 and 50—Packages of 500.

ERGOTOXINE ET STRYCHNINAE SULPHATIS—Tabloid—Hypodermic—Containing Ergotoxine gr 1/100 (0.00065 Gm) and Strychnine Sulphate gr 1/20 (0.0032 Gm)—Tubes of 20 and 50—Packages of 500.

Administration: 1 or 2 tabloids, with or without strychnine, dissolved in water and injected *subcutaneously* or *intramuscularly.*

ERYTHGEN LIVER EXTRACT (Carnrick)

Hematopoietic

Description: A highly purified protein-free fraction of liver extract, of brown color and water soluble; contents of 1 ampule is equivalent to 50 Gm fresh liver; 1 part of powder to 40 of fresh liver; 1 oz. of liquid to 5 oz. of liver.
For use in pernicious anemia.

Supply: **ERYTHGEN LIVER EXTRACT**—Ampules 2½ cc—Boxes of 6.

ERYTHGEN LIVER EXTRACT—Capsules—Bottles of 100.

ERYTHGEN LIVER LIQUID—Bottles of 8 oz.

Administration: *Intramuscularly*—2 ampules daily for 3 or 4 days, followed by a rest period of 1 week; then 2 ampules weekly.
Orally—1–4 teaspoonfuls, or 6 capsules, three times daily.
Maintenance Therapy—1–2 ampules once weekly.

ERYTHROL TETRANITRATE (Merck)

Vasodilator

Chemical Name: Tetranitral.

Formula: $CH_2(ONO_2).(CH.ONO_2)_2.CH_2(ONO_2)$.

Description: Colorless, crystalline scales, insoluble in cold water, soluble in alcohol; like nitroglycerine explodes on percussion.

Action: A powerful vasodilator, lowering the tone of arterial musculature and causing prompt fall in blood pressure; acts like amyl nitrite but action is slower and more prolonged, lasting 3–4 hr.; relieves the heart of excessive resistance and lessens cardiac dyspnea.

Uses: Aneurysm, aortitis, arteriosclerosis, cardiac insufficiency with dyspnea; in angina as prophylactic, when premonitory symptoms appear; in asthma and vascular diseases with muscular spasm; in arterial hypertension and chronic nephritis; in pneumonia, neuritis, uremia.

Supply: **ERYTHROL TETRANITRATE** (C.A.)—Tablets gr ¼ (0.016 Gm)—Bottles of 50.

ERYTHROL TETRANITRATE (C.A.)—Tablets gr ½ (0.032 Gm)—Tubes of 24—Bottles of 100.

Administration: Gr ¼–1 (0.03–0.06 Gm) every 4–6 hr.

Caution: Because of explosive tendency on percussion is marketed in tablet form only, chocolate coated.

Bibliography: *See Chap. XII.*

ESCHATIN (Parke, Davis)

Hormone Therapy

Description: A fairly stable extract of Suprarenal Cortex (Swingle-Pfiffner), standardized in dog units, 1 cc to represent 30 Gm fresh beef cortex; contains practically none of the medullary hormone Adrenalin (only 1 part to 3,000,000); is sensitive to heat and thus must not be subjected to heat sterilization.

Action and Uses: Specific in Addison's disease and of service in other states of hypoadrenia.

Supply: **ESCHATIN**—Vials 10 cc—rubber diaphragm capped.

Administration: In extreme collapse, 20 cc daily, *intravenously*, in individual doses of 10 cc. In cases of moderate severity, 1–5 cc *subcutaneously;* repeated in accordance with symptoms.

Bibliography: *See Chap. XII.*

ESSENCE OF PEPSIN (Armour)

Digestant. Vehicle

Description: Prepared from the glandular layer of fresh animal stomach; contains gastric enzymes in palatable, stable liquid form; alcohol content about 12%.

Action and Uses: Assists protein digestion, 1 teaspoonful digesting 12 oz. of hard-boiled disintegrated egg-white; relieves discomfort in insufficiency of peptic secretion; *For use* in dyspepsia and gastric atony; also as vehicle.

Supply: **ESSENCE OF PEPSIN**—Bottles of 1 pt.—Jugs of 1 or 5 gal.

Administration: 1–2 teaspoonfuls after meals.
For making junket and whey—1 teaspoonful in ½ pt. lukewarm (112°F) milk, stirred and cooled.

Combination: **ELIXIR OF LACTATED PEPSIN**—Has same proteolytic power as essence of pepsin, and is used as vehicle and tonic in digestive tract disturbances.
Supply—Bottles 1 pt.—Jugs of 1 or 5 gal.
Administration—2 teaspoonfuls to 1 tablespoonful after meals.

ESTEROL (Stearns)

Antispasmodic

Chemical Name: Benzyl Succinate, Medicinal.

Formula: $C_6H_5CH_2.OOC(CH_2)_2COO.CH_2C_6H_5$.

Description: A white, crystalline powder, tasteless and odorless.

Action: Is non-narcotic, non-toxic antispasmodic; relieves pain from spastic contraction of unstriped muscle.

Uses: In sin6ultus, spastic headache, hypertension, asthmatic states; in biliary and ureteral colic, diarrhea with cramps, spastic constipation, mucous colitis; in dysmenorrhea and excessive labor pains.

Supply: **ESTEROL**—Tablets gr 5 (0.3 Gm)—Vials of 500.

Administration: Dysmenorrhea—3–4 tablets, after 1 hr. 1–4 tablets, in hot water.

Hiccough—5 tablets; after 1 hr. 4 tablets; after 2 hr. 3 tablets, and gradually reduced.

Colics—4 tablets, followed by 2 every hour till relieved; in severe cases hourly administration.

Other Conditions—2–4 tablets three to four times daily.

Contraindications: Hypotension, atony and atonic constipation.

ETHIDOL (Burroughs Wellcome)

Iodine Therapy

Chemical Name: Ethyl Iodo Ricinoleate.

Composition: A preparation containing iodine 20 % in organic combination.

Action and Uses: Antiseptic and absorbent; promotes resolution of inflammatory induration; *For use* externally in muscle and joint trauma, enlarged glands, myalgia, lumbago and orchitis.

Supply: **ETHIDOL**—Bottles of 4 oz.

Administration: *Externally*—Rubbed lightly into part affected until absorbed, or spread on dressing and applied.
Injection—½–1 cc, *intraglandularly*, on alternate days.

ETHYL IODIDE (Burnham)

Iodine Therapy

Description: A volatile organic liquid of ethereal odor and high specific gravity; specially purified for inhalation.

Formula: C_2H_5I.

Action and Uses: When inhaled is absorbed by the blood and there largely hydrolyzed; presents a convenient method for the introduction of the iodide ion into the blood stream in asthma, spasmodic dyspnea, mycotic skin infections and similar conditions where iodides are indicated.

Supply: **ETHYL IODIDE**—Bottles of 1, 6 and 16 oz.

Administration: Administered by *inhalation* of the vapor. Initial dose 1½ cc, average dose 3 cc, maximum 5 cc, increased by ½ cc daily. About 10 min. should be allowed for the inhalation of each cubic centimeter: treatments omitted every third or fourth day.

Bibliography: *See Chap. XII.*

ETHYL SALICYLATE

Analgesic

Official Name: Aethylis Salicylas.

Formula: $C_6H_4OH.COO.C_2H_5$.

Description: A salicylic ether; a transparent, colorless, very refractive volatile liquid of pleasant characteristic odor and taste; insoluble in water, soluble in alcohol and ether.

Action and Uses: Analgesic, counter-irritant and antipyretic. *For use* in conditions where methyl salicylate is employed, but the ethyl is less toxic and less irritant.

Supply: **ETHYL SALICYLATE (C.A.)**—Bottles 1 oz. (Merck)
SAL-ETHYL (C.A.)—Capsules m 5—Bottles 50 and 500. (Parke, Davis)

Administration: 5–10 m (0.3–0.6 cc) three to four times daily.

Caution: To be kept in dark, air-tight bottles; becomes yellow or brown on exposure to air.

EUPHTHALMINE HYDROCHLORIDE

Mydriatic

Chemical Name: Phenyl-glycoly-methyl-vinyl-diaceton-alkamine Hydrochloride.

Formula: $C_5H_6N(CH_3)_4(C_6H_5CHOH. COO)HCl$.

Description: A mandelic ester related to eucaine; occurs as a white, granular, odorless powder, permanent in air; soluble in water, alcohol, chloroform; insoluble in ether; solution is clear, colorless, neutral in reaction; also known as Eucatropine.

Action and Uses: A non-irritating mydriatic; does not increase intraocular tension and has no effect on accommodation; its systemic effects are similar to atropine. *For use* where mydriasis is required.

Supply: **EUPHTHALMINE HYDROCHLORIDE**—Tabloid Ophthalmic gr 1/40 (0.0016 Gm)—Tubes of 12. **(Burroughs Wellcome)**

EUPHTHALMINE—Vials—½, 1 Gm. **(Schering and Glatz)**

Administration: 1 tabloid placed on conjunctiva, or 2 or 3 drops of 5–10% solution instilled into eye; repeated in 20 min. if necessary.

EUQUININE **(Merck)**

Antipyretic

Official Name: Quinine Ethyl Carbonate, U.S.P.X.

Formula: $OC_2H_5. CO. OC_{20}H_{23}N_2O$.

Description: A white conglomeration of needles, containing approximately 82% quinine; is tasteless, readily soluble in alcohol and ether, almost insoluble in water.

Action and Uses: Presents the characteristic quinine action, but, being practically tasteless, is readily taken by children, and others; does not derange stomach or intestines, nor give rise to bitter eructations, nausea or vomiting; causes cinchonism more rarely and less intensely than the soluble salts of quinine. Is *indicated* in malaria, febrile infectious diseases, neuralgia, and particularly in whooping cough; is most *useful* in quinine idiosyncrasy and as prophylactic for malaria where it is used extensively.

Supply: **EUQUININE**—Cartons ½ and 1 oz.

Administration: May be administered in larger doses than quinine because of greater freedom from unpleasant effects; ordinarily, 4–8 gr (0.259–0.512 Gm) are given to adults, two to three times daily; Children 1–3 gr (0.064–0.194 Gm) according to age.

Incompatibles: To be given in tablet or powder form, or mixed with milk, soups, cocoa, sherry, but never in solution with an acid which develops a bitter taste.

Bibliography: *See Chap. XII.*

EURESOL **(Bilhuber-Knoll)**

Antiseptic

Chemical Name: Resorcinol Monoacetate; m-hydroxyphenyl Acetate.

Formula: $C_6H_4OH(OOC. CH_3)$.

Description: A synthetic organic compound; a transparent, pale yellow, faintly aromatic oil; soluble in alcohol and acetone, insoluble in water; miscible with ointment bases.

Action: Astringent, stimulant, antiseptic, readily penetrating and non-irritating.

Uses: In the treatment of acne, eczema, dandruff, alopecia, itching dermatoses, seborrhea, psoriasis, urticaria, sycosis.

Incompatibles: Alkalies.

Advantages: Action is more prolonged and more penetrating than resorcin; is also less irritating and less toxic.

Supply: EURESOL (C.A.)—Vials 1 and 8 oz.
EURESOL PRO CAPILLIS (C.A.)—Scented—Vials 1 and 8 oz.

Administration: Scalp—Euresol pro capillis, as inunction, in alcoholic solution 2–5%; if dry, scalp is rubbed with small amount of olive oil.
Other conditions—Euresol, as ointment 5–50%; applied every other day for 1–3 weeks; then once weekly.

Bibliography: *See Chap. XII.*

EXTRACTUM PANCREATIS (Fairchild)

Digestant

Description: An extract of the pancreas having an enzyme activity of Pancreatin, U.S.P.

Action and Use: Digesting agent; in presence of alkalies digests all proteins, converts starches into sugar and emulsifies fats; *used* in assisting digestion especially of starches and fats.

Supply: EXTRACTUM PANCREATIS—Bottles 1 oz., ¼, ½ and 1 lb.

Administration: 7½ gr (0.5 Gm) 2 hr. after meals, preceded by full dose of alkali to insure alkaline medium for action.

FARASTAN (Farastan)

Antiarthritic

Chemical Name: Mono-Iodo-Cinchophen.

Action and Uses: Analgesic, antipyretic and antiarthritic; is particularly suitable in the treatment of chronic arthritis, neuritis, sciatica, gout.

Supply: FARASTAN—Capsules 3¾ gr (0.25 Gm)—Boxes of 48.

Administration: 1–2 capsules three times daily after meals, with much water.

Caution: As for all cinchophen preparations.

Bibliography: *See Chap. XII.*

FERRIC AMMONIUM CITRATE (Lederle)

Hematinic

Official Name: Ferri et Ammonii Citratis.

Description: Faintly astringent, extremely hygroscopic powder, soluble in water; marketed in capsules for protection against light, to prevent injury to teeth, and to avoid unpleasant taste; is readily absorbed.

Action and Uses: Hematinic, favorably affecting hemoglobin percentage; *For use* in chlorosis, anemia and similar conditions where iron is indicated.

Supply: FERRIC AMMONIUM CITRATE (C.A.)—Capsules 7 gr (0.5 Gm), equivalent to 1.25 gr (0.08 Gm) of metallic iron—Bottles of 100.

Administration: 2–4 capsules, three times daily.

FERROCOL (Mulford Colloid)

Hematinic. Bactericide.

Description: Occurs as lustrous dark brown non-hygroscopic scales, readily soluble in water; contains 25% Ferric Hydrate and 0.1% Colloidal Copper.

Action and Uses: A stable, non-irritating, readily absorbed and assimilated Colloidal Iron; is slowly eliminated, of prolonged action and does not cause precipitation of tissue fluids. Is locally bactericidal, in erysipelas, cellulitis, nasal catarrh, pharyngitis and laryngitis. Colloidal copper is added as catalyst, to increase action of colloidal iron.

Supply: FERROCOL—Vials, Gm 10.
FERROCOL—Solution, 10%—Ampule—Vial 25 cc.

Administration: *Orally*—1–5 gr (0.064–0.324 Gm) ¼–2 cc.
Intravenously—Where indicated.
Locally—As wet dressing or by dropper.

Combination: VITACOL—(Liquor Ferrocol Compound) for oral administration; each teaspoonful contains—gr 1 (0.064 Gm) Colloidal iron and gr ⅛ (0.008 Gm) colloidal manganese and gr 1/64 (0.001 Gm) Colloidal copper.
Dosage—1 teaspoonful three times daily.

FERROPHYTINE (Ciba)

Hematinic

Chemical Name: The Iron salt of Inosit Hexaphosphoric Acid.

Formula: $C_6H_{12}O_{27}P_6Fe_6$.

Description: Contains about 7½% of iron and 6% vegetable phosphorus; is insoluble in gastric juice, but in the intestine is converted into a soluble and assimilable ferric hydroxide.

Uses: In conditions in which iron and phosphorus are indicated.

Supply: FERROPHYTINE—Pills containing 2½ gr (0.16 Gm) of Ferrophytine and Extract of Gentian 1½ gr (0.09 Gm)—Bottles of 100.

Administration: 1–2 pills three times a day after meals.

Bibliography: *See Chap. XII.*

FERRO-SAJODIN (Winthrop)

Iodine Therapy

Chemical Name: Basic Iodobehenate of Iron. Brand of Ferioben.

Formula: $Fe(OH)(C_{21}H_{42}ICOO)_2$.

Description: A reddish-brown, odorless, tasteless powder; insoluble in water or alcohol, slightly soluble in chloroform, ether and warm fatty oils; contains at least 5% iron and about 24.5% iodine.

Action: As for iodine, but without gastric irritation; is gradually absorbed and slowly excreted.

Uses: In all conditions where internal iodine therapy is indicated; arteriosclerosis, syphilis, arthritis, goitre, glandular enlargement, asthma, scrofula and anemia.

Supply: **FERRO-SAJODIN (C.A.)**—Chocolated tablets, 8 gr (0.51 Gm)—Tubes of 20.

Administration: Adults, 1–3 tablets three times daily, thoroughly chewed or crushed. Children ½–1½ tablets.

Advantages: Does not injure the teeth; is not constipating.

Bibliography: *See Chap. XII.*

FIBROLYSIN (Merck)

Cicatrix Resolvent

Description: Sterile solution of a compound comprising 2 molecules of Thiosinamine and 1 molecule Sodium Salicylate.

Formula: $CS(NH_2)NHC_3H_5 + \frac{1}{2}(C_6H_4OHCOON_a) + H_2O$.

Action and Uses: Softens fibrous tissue; is cicatricial resolvent with selective action for pathologic connective tissue; is *indicated* in conditions in which scar tissue is producing mechanical disability or pain; is most useful where assisted by suitable mechanical therapy, as massage, stretching, dilating. *For use* in the treatment of scars, adhesions, strictures (rectal, urethral and esophageal); in chronic fibrositis and middle-ear deafness.

Supply: FIBROLYSIN—Ampules 2.3 cc—Boxes of 10.

Administration: *Intramuscularly* usually, also *subcutaneously* or *intravenously*, 1 ampule, or smaller dosage given every second or third day, for 20–50 injections.

Contraindications: Not to be used where old fibrous tissue acts as support to important structures, or when in active inflammatory state or in latent inflammation; in the aged with arteriosclerosis; in otorrhea, or where the discharge has recently ceased.

Caution: Solution is unstable if exposed to light and air.

Bibliography: *See Chap. XII.*

FLUMERIN-H

(Hynson, Westcott and Dunning)

Antiluetic

Chemical Name: Disodium-2-hydrox Mercuri-fluorescin.

Formula: $NaOOC.\ C_6H_4.\ C.\ C_6H_4(HgOH)(ONa):\ C_6H_3O.$

Description: A red, odorless powder, slightly hygroscopic; soluble in water, insoluble in alcohol, chloroform and ether.

Action: A powerful antisyphilitic; permits the administration of larger dosage of mercury without endangering the general system or renal apparatus.

Uses: In all stages of syphilis, particularly first and second.

Incompatibles: Alkaline salts, acids, halogens.

Supply: **FLUMERIN-H (C.A.)**—Tubes 0.15, 0.20, 0.25, 0.30 Gm.
FLUMERIN-H (C.A.)—5 Gm, Ampule, for hospital use.

Administration: *Intravenously*—0.002–0.005 Gm per Kilogram of body weight, in 2% solution of sterile (not saline) water, every 3 or 4 days; solution will keep for 3 days if preserved in dark, well stoppered bottles.

FLUORESCEIN

Diagnostic Dye

Chemical Name: Resorcinolphthalein; Dioxyfluorane.

Formula: O: $(C_6H_3OH)_2$: C. C_6H_4. COO.

Description: An orange red powder, insoluble in water, ether, chloroform, benzol; soluble in boiling alcohol and glacial acetic acid.

Action and Uses: For detection of foreign bodies imbedded in the cornea; to define limits of corneal ulcers and other corneal lesions; in diagnosing an impervious nasal duct.

Supply: **FLUORESCEIN**—Tabloid Ophthalmic, gr 1/250 (0.00026 Gm)—Tubes of 12 and 25. **(Burroughs Wellcome)**

FLUORESCEIN (C.A.)—Bottles 1/8 and 1 oz. **(Merck)**

Administration: Eye—1 tabloid is placed on conjunctiva, or the solution is instilled with dropper; in nasal duct obstruction, Fluorescein gr 8, Sodium bicarbonate gr 15, in water q.s. 1 fl. oz., is used.

FOLLUTEIN (Squibb)

Hormone Therapy

Description: A sterile, glycerine solution of female sex-stimulating pro-hormone of the anterior pituitary gland; prepared from the urine of pregnant women; contains no proteins, fats, phospholipins or cholesterol; is physiologically standardized and free from growth promoting pituitary hormones and amniotin; potent for 6 mo.

Action: Dependent upon the time of administration, it either stimulates the formation of graafian follicles and greater production of estrus-inducing hormone, or induces ovulation and luteinization with formation of hemorrhagic spots and pseudo-pregnant endometrial changes.

Uses: *For use* in functional primary amenorrhea, scanty irregular menses, frigidity, sterility with migraine, obesity of secondary amenorrhea.

Supply: **FOLLUTEIN**—Vials of 5 cc, each cubic centimeter containing 250 rat units equal, to 50 Aschheim-Zondek mouse units; with syringe and vial of distilled water.

Administration: Primary Amenorrhea—5–10 cc or 1,250 to 2,500 rat units injected daily for 5 days; if menstruation fails to appear in 15–16 days, course is repeated in 3 weeks.

Secondary Amenorrhea (in absence of Folliculin)—3–5 cc or 750–1,250 units injected daily for 5 days, 2 days after supposed cessation of flow; repeated for several consecutive months if necessary.

Sterility—1 injection 3–5 cc or 750–1,250 rat units on the fifteenth day of cycle; repeated for several consecutive months if necessary.

Premature Menopause—1,250 to 2,500 units injected in 5 days.

Functional Menorrhagia—125–350 rat units daily until next period, regardless of cessation of bleeding.

Caution: Vial content must be thoroughly mixed with diluent and not be used after 3 weeks when diluted; must be preserved in refrigerator.

Bibliography: *See Chap. XII.*

FORMALIN (Schering and Glatz)

Antiseptic

Chemical Name: Oxymethylene.

Formula: HCOH.

Description: Solution of formaldehyde; a clear, colorless liquid, of pungent odor and caustic taste; its vapors are intensely irritating to mucous membranes.

Action and Uses: Antiseptic, disinfectant, antihidrotic; *used* in surgical wounds, abscesses and for fumigation; in respiratory affections—by inhalation; in oral and pharyngeal infections, in pelvic disease, gonorrhea, dermatoses.

Supply: **FORMALIN** (C.A.)—Liquid—Bottles 1/4, 1/2, 1 and 5 lb.

FORMALIN—Pastils, gr 5—Tin of 60—1 Gm—Tin of 20, 100, 250 and 500.

FORMALIN—Disinfector with lamp, without pastils.

FORMALIN—Sterilizer without lamp, with pastils.

PARAFORM—Powder—Bottles 1 oz., 1 lb.

Administration: *Locally*—1.5–2 % solution, in irrigation of body cavities.
Intravenously—1:5,000 solution in 500–750 cc of normal saline, for sepsis.
By Inhalation—In 6 % solution.
As Spray—2 % solution.

FORMIN (Merck)

Antiseptic

Chemical Name: A brand of Methenamine; Hexamethylene Tetramine, U.S.P.

Formula: $(CH_2)_6N_4$.

Description: A white, crystalline powder, soluble in water and alcohol.

Action: A systemic antiseptic liberating formaldehyde in acid medium; is strongly antiseptic in acid urine.

Uses: As genito-urinary antiseptic, diuretic, uric acid solvent—in uric acid diathesis, disinfection of urinary passages, pyelitis, cystitis (also gonorrheal), prostatic hypertrophy, postoperative anuria, enuresis; in encephalitis epidemica and lethargica and meningitis; in acute biliary infections, acute coryza, acute and chronic bronchitis, typhoid; scarlatinal nephritis; in infectious enteritis, typhus (intravenously), trypanosomiasis.

Supply: **FORMIN**—Powder—Boxes 2 oz. and 1 lb.

FORMIN—Tablets, (C.A.) gr 5 (0.324 Gm)—Bottles 50, 100, 500 and 1,000.

FORMIN—Tablets, (C.A.) gr 7 1/2 (0.480 Gm); 20 in tube—Bottles of 70, 500 and 1,000.

Administration: 5–15 gr (0.3–1 Gm) two or three times daily, with large quantities of water; is best alternated with sodium biphosphate, in doses of 15–20 gr (1–1.3 Gm) in sweetened water, frequently repeated till urine is acid; in colds and bronchitis 10 gr (0.6 Gm) four times per day.
Intravenously—In typhoid, pneumonia, nephritis, liver diseases and broncho-pneumonia, 4–30 gr (0.25–2 Gm), only in 25 % solution.

FORTOSSAN (Ciba)

Phosphorus Therapy

Chemical Name: Sodium Inosithexaphosphate and Lactose.

Formula: $C_6H_{12}O_{27}P_6Na_2 + 35H_2O$ and Lactose.

Description: Is readily soluble in milk and unaffected by boiling; palatable and suitable for use in infants and young children.

Uses: Indicated in conditions where an increase of phosphorus is desired: in rickets, delayed union of fractures, nervous disorders, metabolic diseases, anorexia.

Supply: **FORTOSSAN**—Powder—Packages of 3 oz., with measure (10 gr) for convenience in dosage.

Doses: For Infants—under 2 mo.—1 measure—10 gr (0.65 Gm) four times daily. 2-6 mo.—2 measures—20 gr (1.3 Gm) four times daily. 6-12 mo.—3 measures—30 gr (2.0 Gm) four times daily.
For Children—1-2 yr.—4 measures—40 gr (2.5 Gm) four times daily.

Bibliography: *See Chap. XII.*

GASTRIC MUCIN "FOGELSON" (Stearns)

Gastric Sedative

Description: A fine straw colored non-hygroscopic powder, prepared from hog stomach; with water forms a viscous mucilaginous mixture possessing a high combining power; is purified with ethyl alcohol to remove histamin and other secretogogues; pH 6.5-6.75.

Action: 1. Adsorptive—Combines with excess acid in the stomach; (1 Gm of gastric mucin will adsorb 12-15 cc of N/10 HCl).
2. Protective—Covers the gastric mucosa with a viscid tenacious coating, inhibiting irritation of digestive juices on ulcerated and diseased mucosa.

Uses: *Especially indicated* in peptic ulcer, both gastric and duodenal.

Supply: **GASTRIC MUCIN**—Jars, amber glass, ½ lb.

Administration: *Massive Treatment*—1-2 tablespoonfuls in warm water or malted milk, ½ hr. before meals followed by milk; in severe cases, repeated hourly.
Small Dose Treatment—1 teaspoonful in small amount of cold water, well stirred, swallowed before a mass forms and followed by drinking of warm water; repeated hourly if necessary.

Bibliography: *See Chap. XII.*

GENTIAN VIOLET MEDICINAL

Germicide

Composition: A mixture of penta- and hexa-methyl pararoseaniline chlorides; a brand of gentian violet medicinal N.N.R.; a dark green powder of metallic lustre, soluble in 10 parts of water, alcohol and chloroform, insoluble in ether.

Action and Uses: Antiseptic and germicidal, especially effective against staphylococcus; *For use* principally in staphylococcus infections of joints, pleural cavity, in osteomyelitis, pyelitis and cystitis; also in staphylococcus septicemia, intravenously.

Supply: **GENTIAN VIOLET MEDICINAL** (C.A.)—10 Gm, 25 Gm and 100 Gm packages. **(Coleman and Bell)**

GENTIAN VIOLET MEDICINAL "CHURCHMAN" (C.A.) **(National Aniline)**
—Tablets, gr ½ (0.324 Gm) Plain and Enteric Coated—Bottles of 100 and 500.

Administration: *Intravenously*—1-5 mg per kilogram of body weight, administered cautiously and slowly, in 0.5% dilution.
Externally—On wounds, ulcers, mucous membranes in dilution of 1-1,000.

Caution: In the feeble, or if cyanosis occurs during intravenous injection cardiac stimulants must be administered.

Bibliography: *See Chap. XII.*

GLYCINE (Eastman)

Diuretic

Chemical Name: Aminoacetic Acid; Glycocoll.

Formula: $NH_2.\ CH_2COOH$.

Description: Occurs as colorless, sweet crystals; easily soluble in water, very slightly soluble in ether.

Action and Uses. Diuretic in nephritis, hepatic disease with oliguria and cardio-hepatic stasis; also found *useful* in pseudo-hypertrophic muscular dystrophy.

Administration: 75 gr (5 Gm) dissolved in 150 cc water, daily.

Supply: GLYCINE—Bottles of 100 Gm.

Caution: Is not to be confused with photographic **Glycin** for non-medicinal use.

Bibliography: *See Chap. XII.*

GLYCOTAURO

(Hynson, Westcott and Dunning)

Cholagogue

Description: A purified concentrated ox bile, containing 50% of the natural bile salts, sodium glycocholate and taurocholate, with other therapeutic constituents of ox-gall; standardized, 1 Gm to represent 15 cc of fresh ox-bile.

Action: A natural cholagogue, hepatic stimulant and intestinal digestion activator.

Uses: In hepatic insufficiency, cholelithiasis, jaundice; postoperatively in gall bladder surgery; in enhancing the efficiency of resinous cathartics. In children—in persistent constipation.

Supply: GLYCOTAURO—Tablets (C.A.) Enteric, Salol coated, gr 2 (0.130 Gm) 2 tablets are equivalent to 1 dr. ox-gall—Tubes of 72.

GLYCOTAURO—Capsules (C.A.) gr 5 (0.324 Gm)—Boxes of 36.

GLYCOTAURO—Capsules (C.A.) gr 2½ (0.150 Gm)—Boxes of 48.

Administration: Adults, 5 gr (0.324 Gm), children 2½ gr (0.150 Gm), three times daily for 8 days; reduced to 2 doses daily for 12 days and a single dose for 24 days; rest intervals, where necessary, before repeating course of treatment.

Combination: GLYCOTAURO WITH CASCARA AND PHENOLPHTHALEIN—Contains per tablet: glycotauro, 2½ gr (0.150 Gm); extract cascara, ½ gr (0.032 Gm); phenolphthalein, ½ gr (0.032 Gm). A stronger laxative, indicated in cases with pronounced constipation. *Supply*—Tablets—Tubes 50. *Administration*—Adults—1-3 tablets at night or when desired; may be combined with 2 doses of simple Glycotauro tablets daily. Children—According to age.

Bibliography: *See Chap. XII.*

GOLD SODIUM THIOSULPHATE

Lupus Therapy

Official Name: Sodii et Aurii Thiosulphas.

Formula: $Na_3Au(S_2O_3)_2 + 2H_2O$.

Composition: A complex salt comprising 1 molecule of gold thiosulphate and 3 molecules of sodium thiosulphate; contains about 37.4% gold.

Description: Occurs as white, glistening, prismatic or needle-like crystals, freely soluble in water, forming a colorless solution; is very slightly soluble in alcohol, ether and chloroform.

Action and Uses: Very effective in lupus erythematosus; *also used* in lichen scrofulosorum and certain types of pulmonary tuberculosis.

Supply: GOLD SODIUM THIOSULPHATE (C.A.)—Ampules 0.01, 0.025, 0.05, 0.1 and 0.25 Gm—Boxes of 6, 25. **(Abbott)**

GOLD SODIUM THIOSULPHATE (C.A.)—Ampules 1 cc—10 mg, 2 cc—25 mg, 5 cc—50 mg of salt. **(Searle)**

Administration: To be used with great caution, *intravenously* or *intramuscularly*—initial dose 1/6 gr (0.01 Gm), prepared with 2–5 cc of sterile distilled water; subsequent doses increased by 0.01 Gm, at weekly intervals, with frequent rest periods. Maximum doses: Male—100 mg, Female—75 mg.

Contraindications: Albuminuria, renal dysfunction, pregnancy, enteritis, stomatitis, liver disease; in severe reaction, must be discontinued.

Bibliography: *See Chap. XII.*

GUPHEN (Gane-Ingram)

Analgesic

Chemical Name: Phenyl-Cinchoninic Acid-Guaiacol Ester.

Description: An agreeable, non-irritating, tasteless, odorless definite chemical compound.

Action and Uses: Decongestive, analgesic, antipyretic, antiseptic; *For use* in acute and chronic bronchitis, angina, influenza, colds, pleurisy, pneumonia; also in arthritis, rheumatism, lumbago and local infections.

Supply: GUPHEN—Tablets, gr 7½ (0.5 Gm)—Packages 20—Bottles 100.

Administration: 1–2 tablets three or four times daily.

GYNERGEN (Sandoz)

Uterine Stimulant

Chemical Name: Ergotamine Tartrate.

Formula: $(C_{33}H_{35}N_5O_5)_2 \cdot H_2C_4H_4O_6$.

Description: A specific alkaloid of ergot in pure and stable form; occurs as colorless, rhombic crystals, soluble with difficulty in water (1:5,000) and in ethyl alcohol (1:5,000); solution is practically tasteless.

Action: Induces prompt, steady, strong contractions of the uterus, more prolonged than those caused by pituitary preparations; also inhibits the functions of the sympathetic nervous system and is indicated in conditions associated with sympathicotonia; is more stable and effective than ergot.

Uses: *For use* in prevention and treatment of postpartum uterine atony and hemorrhage, in Cesarean section, incomplete abortion; in menorrhagia and metrorrhagia; also in migraine and pruritus of renal and hepatic origin, and in Graves' disease.

Supply: GYNERGEN—Ampules (C.A.) 1 cc (0.0005 Gm)—Boxes 6, 12, 50 and 100.

GYNERGEN—Ampules (C.A.) 0.5 cc (0.00025 Gm)—Boxes of 6 and 50.

GYNERGEN—Tablets (C.A.) 0.001 Gm—Bottles of 15, 100 and 500.

GYNERGEN—Liquid (C.A.) solution ergotamine tartrate 1 in 1,000—Bottles of 15 cc and 100 cc.

Administration: *Intramuscularly*—Average effective dose: 0.5 cc, maximum—1 cc; in emergencies injection may be repeated after interval of at least 20 min.

Orally—In less urgent cases and in "follow-up" treatment—1 tablet (or 15 drops of the liquid) two to four times a day.

In Pruritus—1 tablet three or four times daily for 3 days; in severe itching 0.5–1 cc *intramuscularly.*

In Graves' Disease—1 tablet three times daily, diminished progressively; after 2–3 weeks treatment—intermission of 1–3 weeks.

In Migraine—0.25 cc to 1 cc *intramuscularly* to cut short attacks; as preventive 2 or 3 tablets daily for periods of one week and intervals of 7–10 days.

Bibliography: *See Chap. XII.*

HALAZONE

Disinfectant

Chemical Name: Para-sulphone Dichloramido Benzoic Acid.

Formula: $C_6H_4(SO_2N. Cl_2)COOH$ 1: 4.

Description: White powder, of strong chlorine odor; slightly soluble in water and chloroform, more soluble in glacial acetic acid, benzene and alkaline hydroxide solutions.

Action: A powerful disinfectant; like free chlorine will sterilize polluted water in high dilutions, 1:200,000–1:500,000.

Uses: As disinfectant for numerous purposes; for sterilization of water (1–2 tablets per liter), making doubtful or contaminated water potable, especially for campers, explorers, military units.

Supply: **HALAZONE** (C.A.)—Tablets—Containing 4 mg—Bottles of 100 and 1,000. **(Abbott)**

HALAZONE (C.A.)—Tablets—0.004 Gm each—Bottles of 100 and 1,000. **(Monsanto)**

Bibliography: *See Chap. XII.*

HALIBUT LIVER OIL (COLLOSOL BRAND) (Crookes)

Vitamin Therapy

Composition: Vitamin A concentrate prepared from halibut liver oil and fifty times as potent as standard cod liver oil; has also high content of Vitamin D.

Action and Uses: In all conditions where vitamin therapy is indicated.

Supply: **HALIBUT LIVER OIL**—Vials 5, 30 cc.

HALIBUT LIVER OIL—Capsules—Bottles of 25, 100.

Administration: 1–3 m in milk three times daily, or 1 capsule daily.

HALIVER OIL PLAIN

Vitamin Therapy

Description: The expressed oil from fresh halibut livers; standardized by bio-assay and contains at least one hundred times the amount of vitamin A, 50,000 units per gram, and ten to thirty times the amount of vitamin D as standard cod liver oil; 3 m, or 10 drops, or 1 capsule is equal in vitamin A content to more than 4 teaspoonfuls of cod liver oil.

Action and Uses: Anti-infective and rich source of vitamin A; is growth promoting and disease resisting; *For use* in all disorders where cod liver oil is indicated.

Supply: HALIVER OIL PLAIN—Bottles 10 cc and 50 cc. (Abbott)

HALIVER OIL PLAIN—Capsules 3 m—Boxes of 50. (Abbott)

HALIVER OIL, PLAIN—Capsules 3 m—Boxes of 50. (Parke, Davis)

HALIVER OIL, PLAIN—Vials 10 and 50 cc with dropper. (Parke, Davis)

Administration: Adults—10–20 m daily.
Children—10 drops daily.
Infants—2–3 drops, three times daily.

Bibliography: *See Chap. XII.*

HALIVER OIL WITH VIOSTEROL 250D

Vitamin Therapy

Description: A halibut liver oil blended with a pure, wholesome vegetable oil to insure a vitamin A potency of 30,000 U.S.P. units, or at least sixty times that of high grade cod liver oil, and supplemented with Viosterol to possess a vitamin D potency of 3,333 Steenbock units per gram, or equal to that of Viosterol 250D. 1 m (3 drops) equals 1 teaspoonful of cod liver oil in vitamin A potency and exceeds it in vitamin D units.

Action and Uses: As for cod liver oil; is especially valuable for those intolerant of larger dosage of cod liver oil in the treatment of vitamin deficiencies, nutritional disorders, rickets, osteomalacia, malnutrition and expectant mothers.

Supply: HALIVER OIL WITH VIOSTEROL 250D (C.A.)—Containers 5 cc and 50 cc, with special dropper. (Abbott)

HALIVER OIL WITH VIOSTEROL 250D (C.A.)—Capsules, soft elastic, 5 m each containing 3 m of the oil—Boxes 25 and 100. (Abbott)

HALIVER OIL WITH VIOSTEROL 250D (C.A.)—Capsules, 3 m—Packages of 25 and 100. (Parke, Davis)

HALIVER OIL WITH VIOSTEROL 250D (C.A.)—Vials 5 cc and 50 cc, with dropper. (Parke, Davis)

Administration: Normal infants—10 drops by special dropper or one 5 m capsule; for the premature and rapidly growing infants—15 drops; older children—10–20 drops or in capsules; adults 20 drops or more, capsules in proportion.

Bibliography: *See Chap. XII.*

HEGONON (Schering and Glatz)

Gonocide

Chemical Name: Silver Nitrate Ammonio-Albumose.

Description: A light brown powder, containing 7% silver, organically combined; slightly soluble in water.

Action and Uses: Antiseptic and astringent in gonorrhea.

Supply: HEGONON—Bottles ½ oz.

Administration: *Urethral Injection*—0.25% solution.
Irrigation—1:2,000–1:6,000 solution.

HELMITOL (Winthrop)

Urinary Antiseptic

Chemical Name: Methenamine Anhydromethylene Citrate. Brand of Citramin.

Formula: $C_7H_8O_7.\ (CH_2)_6N_4$.

Description: A white crystalline powder of agreeable acidulous taste; soluble in 10 parts of water, forming a neutral solution; is almost insoluble in alcohol and ether.

Action: A genitourinary antiseptic, through liberation of formaldehyde; is especially valuable where urine is alkaline; is eliminated by the kidneys and does not affect the gastro-intestinal tract.

Uses: In all types of cystitis, chronic prostatitis, urethritis and pyelitis; in scarlatinal and typhoid infections and other conditions where methenamine is indicated.

Advantages: Easily administered, well tolerated, suitable for prolonged use.

Supply: **HELMITOL**—Tablets 5 gr—Bottles of 25 and 100.

HELMITOL—Tablets 7½ gr—Tubes of 20.

HELMITOL—Powder—Bottles 1 oz.

Administration: 10–15 gr (0.6–1 Gm) three or four times daily, dissolved in water.

Bibliography: *See Chap. XII.*

HEMOSTATIC SERUM (Parke, Davis)

Hemostatic

Description: Consists principally of prothrombin and thrombokinase in physiologically balanced solution; a clear, light-amber or colorless liquid; a refined product, containing not more than one-third as much protein as normal horse serum; also known as Hemoplastin.

Action: Controls hemorrhage in defective coagulability of the blood; standardized on dogs to reduce the blood clotting time by two-thirds; has no coagulating effect on the circulating blood; serum sickness rarely follows its use; never—when administered orally.

Uses: Before or after surgical operations; to control hemorrhage and oozing after bone surgery; in purpura hemorrhagica, bleeding of the newborn, intestinal hemorrhages and indolent ulcers.

Supply: **HEMOSTATIC SERUM**—Bulb 2 cc and 5 cc, rubber-diaphragm-capped—Vial 5 cc, rubber-stoppered—for oral use.

Administration: *Prophylactic*—Oral—5 cc, 3–6 hr. prior to operation; in bad risks, several doses at 6 hr. intervals previous to operation; given in fruit juices, water or cracked ice.

Intravenous—2–5 cc, preferably the larger dose, before or after operation; repeated if necessary.

HEPATI-COLE (Cole)

Hematopoietic

Description: A physiologically standardized solution of liver extract, each cubic centimeter representing 20 Gm fresh liver tissue.

Action and Uses: In pernicious anemia for parenteral use and quick action.

Supply: **HEPATI-COLE**—Ampules 5 cc—Boxes of 6.

Administration: *Intramuscularly*—1–2 cc daily during relapse. Maintenance dose 1 cc once or twice weekly, guided by blood picture.

HEXALET (Riedel)

Urinary Antiseptic

Chemical Name: Sulfosalicylic Hexamethylenamine.

Formula: $(CH_2)_6N_4SO_3H.C_6H_3(OH)COOH$.

Description: A white crystalline substance of pleasant acid taste and readily soluble in water.

Action and Uses: Antiseptic and astringent to inflamed mucous membranes of the urinary passages. *Useful* in acute and chronic cystitis, gonorrheal urethritis, pyelitis, pyelonephritis, renal and vesical uric acid concretions.

Supply: HEXALET—Tablets—gr 7½ (0.5 Gm)—Bottles of 20 and 50.

HEXALET—Powder—Bottles 1 oz.

Administration: 15 gr, three to six times daily after meals; dissolved in water before use.

Bibliography: *See Chap. XII.*

HEXYL-RESORCINOL SOLUTION S.T. 37 (Sharp and Dohme)

Germicide

Official Name: Liquor Hexylresorcinolis.

Formula: $C_6H_3(OH)_2(C_6H_{13})$.

Description: A stable non-toxic, non-irritating 1:1,000 solution of hexylresorcinol in 30% glycerin and 70% water; active in the presence of organic matter; colorless, odorless and non-staining.

Action and Uses: A rapid, powerful and penetrating germicide. *Used* in abrasions and bruises, abscess cavities, granulating surfaces, affections of the mucous membranes of the nose, throat, mouth, urethra, bladder and renal pelvis.

Supply: HEXYL-RESORCINOL SOLUTION S.T. 37 (C.A.)—Bottles 5 and 12 oz.—Applicator bottles—½ oz.

HEXYL-RESORCINOL SOLUTION S.T. 37—Sucrates, 2½ mg of hexylresorcinol, as lozenges—Boxes of 24.

HEXYL-RESORCINOL SOLUTION S.T. 37—Tooth Paste—Collapsible tubes, 2 oz.

Administration: *Topically*—By swab, applicator, wet dressing, in full strength.
For Irrigation of Nose, Urethra, Bladder—Diluted with 3–4 parts of water.
For Dental Use—After brushing teeth, undiluted.

Bibliography: *See Chap. XII.*

HEPATRAT (Kretschmar)

Hematopoietic

Composition: A liver extract for parenteral use.

Action and Uses: An antianemic principle; is free from protein and does not produce anaphylaxis; 3 cc are equivalent to 500 Gm of liver; *For use* in pernicious and other severe anemias, as infantile; in lead, bismuth and salvarsan intoxication; in convalescence.

Supply: HEPATRAT—Ampules, 2 cc—Boxes of 3 and 10.

Administration: *Intramuscularly*—2 cc, in severe cases 6 cc daily, for 6–8 weeks, then replaced by oral therapy.

HISTAMINE (Roche)

Vagotropic

Chemical Name: B-imidazolyl-ethylamine Dihydrochloride. Imido "Roche."

Formula: $C_5H_9N_3 . 2HCl$.

Composition: A biogenous amin found in almost all animal tissues and produced by the action of about 30 types of putrefactive bacteria, among them the Bacillus coli.

Action: Primarily a stimulator of the autonomic nervous system, and as such exerts a most pronounced effect upon smooth musculature; also acts as a vasodilator, thereby lowering blood pressure considerably; some veins and capillaries, as those of the lung and liver, are constricted by histamine; stimulates gastric, salivary and bronchial secretions.

Uses: Principally for diagnostic purposes in differentiation of types of gastric achylia.

Supply: **HISTAMINE DIHYDROCHLORIDE**—Vials of 1 Gm.

HISTAMINE DIHYDROCHLORIDE—Ampules 1.1 cc, solution 1:1,000, known as Imido "Roche" for subcutaneous and intramuscular use—Boxes of 6 and 50.

Administration: *Diagnostic—Subcutaneously or Intramuscularly*—1 ampule (1 cc or 1 mg) as necessary.

Injection is followed by withdrawal of gastric contents at stated intervals for determination of hydrochloric acid concentration.

Caution: Toxic effects such as marked fall of blood pressure, nausea, increased gastric peristalsis, may be checked by injections of epinephrine.

HOLOCAIN (Metz)

Ocular Surface Anesthetic

Chemical Name: Ethenyl-diethoxydiphenylamidine Hydrochloride. Brand of Phenacaine.

Formula: $C_{17}H_{22}O_2N_2HCl$.

Description: A white crystalline powder, soluble up to 2%, in boiling water forming a neutral solution.

Action: Produces rapid and prolonged surface anesthesia, without injury to the cornea, without producing mydriasis or increasing intraocular tension.

Uses: As surface anesthetic in most minor and many major eye operations; *for the relief* of pain in conjunctivitis, corneal ulcer, keratitis, glaucoma and blepharospasm.

Supply: **HOLOCAIN (C.A.)**—Powder—Vials 1 and 5 Gm—Bottles of 1 oz.

HOLOCAIN—Solution 1%—Bottles 1 oz.

Administration: 1% solution is dropped into the eye or applied to the lids with cotton-wrapped probe.

Incompatibles: Alkalies, alkaline carbonates and common alkaloidal reagents.

Caution: Stock solution need not be boiled, but should be filtered from time to time; must be prepared with distilled water, in porcelain or alkali-free glass receptacle, and not mixed with any other substance.

Bibliography: *See Chap. XII.*

HOMATROPINE HYDROCHLORIDE

Mydriatic

Official Name: Homatropinae Hydrochloridum.

Formula: $C_{16}H_{21}NO_3$. HCl.

Description: A condensation product of tropin and mandelic acid; occurs as small white crystals, soluble in water and alcohol.

Action and Uses: Is mydriatic like the hydrobromide salt of homatropine; its effect in 1 % solution upon the eye is more transitory than that of atropine; internally is *used* in night sweats of phthisis and as sedative.

Supply: **HOMATROPINE HYDROCHLORIDE** (C.A.)—Vials 5 and 15 gr. **(Merck)**

HOMATROPINE HYDROCHLORIDE (C.A.)—Bottles 1/8, 1/2, 1 oz. **(Roche)**

Administration: *Internal*—Average dose—1/120–1/60 gr (0.0005–0.001 Gm).
Maximum daily dose—1/20 gr (0.003 Gm).
External—(to eye) in 1–2 % solution.

Caution: In case of poisoning—emetics or stomach siphon; then tannin and animal charcoal; emetic again followed by castor oil; artificial respiration, heat, stimulants, where necessary.

HOMOCAMFIN **(Winthrop)**

Cardio-Respiratory Stimulant

Chemical Name: 3-Methyl-5-isopropyl-2-cyclohexenon, in aqueous sodium salicylate solution. Brand of Cyclosal.

Formula (of Cyclosal): CH_3. C: CH. CO. CH_2. CH. (CH[CH_3]$_2$)CH.

Description: A yellowish oil of pleasant odor and bitter taste; sparingly soluble in water; soluble in alcohol, ether and benzene.

Action: Is two to four times as stimulating as camphor and almost instantaneously effective when given intravenously, with maximum effect within 10 min.; when injected intramuscularly, its greatest effect occurs in 15–30 min.; stimulates exhausted nerve centers of the heart and respiratory apparatus; increases force of pulse and depth and frequency of breathing; is eliminated as glycuronic acid by the kidneys.

Uses: In cardiovascular failure, myocarditis, surgical shock, pneumonia, narcotic poisoning.

Supply: **HOMOCAMFIN**—Ampules, Intravenous (C.A.), 1 cc (1 %)—Boxes of 5.

HOMOCAMFIN—Ampules, Intramuscular (C.A.), 2 cc (10 %)—Boxes of 5.

Administration: *Intramuscularly*—Adults 1½–2 cc, children 2–12 yr., 0.5–1 cc;
Intravenously—(In emergency only) adults 1 cc, children 2–12 yr., 0.3–0.5 cc, cautiously; increased if necessary.

Caution: Ampules *amber colored* for intramuscular use only; *white ampules* for intravenous.

Bibliography: *See Chap. XII.*

HYDRASTININ **(Winthrop)**

Hemostatic. Uterine Stimulant

Chemical Name: Methylenedioxy-n-methyl-dihydroisoquinolin Hydrochloride.

Formula: $C_{10}H_8O_2N(CH_3)$. HCl.

Description: A yellowish-white, odorless, bitter, crystalline powder, easily soluble in water and alcohol; a synthetic product, free from the impurities of the natural alkaloid.

Action: Causes constriction of the uterine arteries and to a lesser extent of the blood vessels of the general circulation; controls hemorrhage, induces contraction of the uterine muscle, raises lowered blood pressure, causes no cardiac depression.

Uses: In uterine subinvolution, menorrhagia, metrorrhagia, menopausal bleeding, endometritis and hemoptysis.

Advantages: Frequently effective when cotarnin and ergot fail; more efficient and safer than natural hydrastinin.

Supply: LIQUOR HYDRASTININ—Bottles of 25 Gm.
HYDRASTININ—Tablets ½ gr—Tubes of 15.

Administration: Liquor, 20–40 drops three to four times daily, in sweetened water. Tablets, 1—three or four times daily.

ICHTHALBIN

Intestinal Antiseptic

Chemical Name: Ichthyol albuminate.

Description: A sulphur preparation, comprising ichthyol and albumin; an odorless, almost tasteless grayish brown powder, insoluble in water and weak acids, including gastric fluid; soluble in alkaline intestinal fluids.

Action: Is intestinal antiseptic, decreasing putrefaction and enhancing the assimilation of food; is non-irritating and well tolerated; applied externally, reduces inflammatory exudative processes with vascular dilatation.

Uses: *Internally*—In subacute and chronic gastrointestinal catarrh; in tubercular enteritis, peritonitis and typhoid fever; in rheumatism and sciatica with intestinal toxicosis.
Externally—In skin affections: moist infantile eczema, scrofula, urticaria, rosacea, congestive dermatoses, acne vulgaris, seborrhoeic disorders, lichen strophulus; in boils and ulcers; in gynecologic diseases.

Supply: ICHTHALBIN—Tablets, gr 5 (0.3 Gm)—Bottles of 100. (Bilhuber-Knoll)
ICHTHALBIN—Powder—Boxes of 1 oz. (Bilhuber-Knoll)
ICHTHALBIN—Tablets, gr 5 (0.3 Gm)—Bottles of 100. (Merck)
ICHTHALBIN—Powder—Cartons of 1 oz. (Merck)

Administration: 10–30 gr (0.6–2 Gm) two or three times daily, before meals, in powder or in tablets; children, 2–10 gr (0.12–0.6 Gm) according to age.
Externally—Applied as dusting powder on ulcers and as tampon in pelvic affections.

Bibliography: *See Chap. XII.*

ICHTHARGAN (Merck)

Gonocide

Description: A brown, odorless, slightly hygroscopic powder, easily soluble in water, glycerin, dilute alcohol; contains 30 % silver.

Action: Astringent, antiphlogistic, bactericide.

Uses: *Externally*—In gonorrhea, for urethral hand injection, or as Janet's wash in posterior urethritis;
Topically—In furunculosis, trachoma and in female pelvic infections.

Incompatibles: Soluble chlorides.

Supply: ICHTHARGAN—Powder—Bottles of 1/8 and 1 oz.

Administration: Genitourinary—Hand injections 1:1,000 in distilled water; urethral irrigations 1:3,000; in posterior urethritis—3% topically; for chronic urethritis—ointment 5% with yellow wax 10% in cocoa butter.

In Furunculosis—5–10% ointment.

In Trachoma—0.5–3%.

In Gynecology—Tampons 1:5:100 in glycerin; lotions 1:1,000 glycerin.

Caution—Solutions must be preserved in dark bottles.

ICHTHYMALL (Mallinckrodt)

Antipruritic

Description: Prepared by sulphonation of crude oil obtained by the distillation of bituminous Tyrolean shale; a thick, viscid fluid of dark brown color, containing organically combined sulphur; is soluble in water, glycerine, alcohol and miscible with ointment bases.

Action: Antiseptic, soothing and antipruritic.

Uses: In acute dermatitis, erythema nodosum, acne, eczema, erythema, chilblains and various indurations.

Supply: ICHTHYMALL—Bottles of 1 oz., 1/4 lb., 1 lb.

ICHTHYMALL—Tubes, collapsible, 1 oz., 1/4 lb.

Administration: Applied locally either as ointment or by painting with solution, as often as necessary.

ICHTHYNAT (Heyden)

Emollient

Official Name: Ammonium Sulfoichthynatum.

Description: An aqueous solution of ammonium compounds, containing sulphur as sulphones, sulphonates and sulphides; a brown-black syrupy liquid of burning taste and empyreumatic odor.

Action and Uses: As antiseptic in minor surgical and gynecological affections, externally.

Supply: ICHTHYNAT (C.A.)—Bottles of 1/4, 1/2, 1, 5 lbs.

Administration: Applied locally on tampon, or by painting, as necessary.

ICHTHYOL (Merck)

Antiphlogistic

Chemical Name: Ammonium Ichthyol-Sulphonate; Ammonium Sulphoichthyolate.

Description: A soluble, sulphonated hydrocarbon prepared from the oily distillate obtained from a mineral deposit found in Tyrol; a thick, brown liquid of bituminous odor, soluble in water, and in a mixture of equal volumes of water, alcohol and ether; is partly soluble in pure alcohol or ether and miscible with glycerin and fats.

Action: Antiphlogistic, mildly antiseptic and soothing to inflamed mucous membranes, upon which it also exerts a vasoconstrictor effect.

Uses: *Internally*—For its assimilable sulphur in skin diseases, scrofula and intestinal toxemia.

Externally—As ointment or 5–50 % solution in scarlet fever; in 5–10 % lanoline ointment in mastitis, epididymitis, synovitis, parotitis, lumbago; in acne and other skin diseases, insect bites and stings; also used to promote absorption of swellings and effusions, to relieve pain in inflammation, burns, scalds, hemorrhoids; in gout, rheumatism and neuralgia, abscesses, vernal conjunctivitis, carbuncles, chilblains, urticaria.

As 10 % solution in glycerin, or tampons, or as vaginal suppositories in uterine and vaginal inflammation; in 1–3 % solutions in urethral infections in gonorrhea; in ivy poisoning—undiluted.

Incompatibles: Potassium iodide, hydrastis, resorcinol, mercury bichloride; acids precipitate it into a dark, resinous mass; alkaline hydroxides or carbonates decompose it; with alkaloids or their salts compounds are formed of much firmer consistency and far less solubility.

Supply: ICHTHYOL—Bottles 1 oz., ¼ and 1 lb.—Tubes 1 oz., and ¼ lb.

Administration: *Locally*—By painting, tampon, suppository; as rectal irrigation 5 %, vaginal douche 2 %.

Tampons—10–25 % in glycerine.

Suppositories—10 %.

Internally—3–30 m (0.2–2.0 cc) in pill or capsule form.

Bibliography: *See Chap. XII.*

ICTEROSAN (Schering and Glatz)

Cholagogue

Composition: A sterile, standardized, neutral 10 % aqueous solution of the Sodium salt of Atophan, with 0.16 Gm Beta-Eucain Hydrochloride added.

Action and Uses: A cholagogue and choleretic; *useful* in catarrhal jaundice, cholangitis, cholecystitis, cholelithiasis, biliary stasis.

Supply: ICTEROSAN—Ampules 5 cc—Boxes of 6.

Administration: 1 ampule, warmed, injected *intravenously*, very slowly daily; also *intramuscularly*.

IDOCOL (Mulford Colloid)

Iodine Therapy

Description: Light brown lustrous, non-hygroscopic scales, readily soluble in water; also available for external use in water-insoluble form, which in the presence of traces of alkalies is converted into the soluble form; contains 20–25 % iodine.

Action and Uses: A stable, non-irritating, readily and completely absorbed and assimilated preparation of Colloidal Iodine; is slowly eliminated, of prolonged action and does not cause precipitation of tissue fluids; does not produce iodism; *For use* locally as antiseptic; internally as systemic alterative in pyemia and in syphilis.

Supply: IDOCOL—Vials Gm 10.

IDOCOL—Solution—10 %—Bottles 25 cc.

IDOCOL—Soluble Capsules—gr 2½ and gr 5 (0.162–0.324 Gm)—Bottles of 100 each.

Administration: 1–5 gr (0.064–0.324 Gm), in capsules.

Orally—Solution, ¼–4 cc (⅜–6 gr).
Locally—5–25 % solution.
Intravenously—10 % solution.

ILETIN (Lilly)

Insulin Therapy

Description: The active principle derived from the islet tissue of animal pancreas; stable, non-irritating, non-toxic and of uniform strength.

Action and Uses: To control level of blood sugar in diabetes mellitus, to improve nutrition and increase weight.

Supply: **ILETIN (C.A.)**—Vials of 5 cc U-10, U-20, U-40, containing respectively 50, 100, 200 units—Vials of 10 cc U-10, U-20, U-40, U-80, containing respectively 100, 200, 400, and 800 units.

Administration: *Subcutaneously*—Dosage regulated in accordance with conditions presented, blood sugar level, glycosuria, nutritional state and acidosis.

INFUNDIN (Burroughs Wellcome)

Oxytocic. Vasoconstrictor

Chemical Name: Extract of Pituitary, Posterior Lobe.

Description: A stable, sterile preparation.

Action and Uses: As for pituitary extract; has oxytocic and pressor action, affecting uterus, bladder, intestines and arterial smooth muscle; checks polyuria; *useful* in uterine inertia, post-partum hemorrhage; surgical shock, intestinal atony and paresis; in post-operative urine retention, diabetes insipidus.

Supply: **INFUNDIN**—Hypoloid 0.5 and 1 cc (5 International units per cubic centimeter)—Boxes of 6 and 100.

INFUNDIN—Hypoloid 0.5 and 1 cc (10 International units per cubic centimeter —Boxes of 6 and 100.

Administration: 5–10 International units, injected *intramuscularly* or given rectally in saline;

Obstetrics—2 International units ante-partum; 10–15—post-partum.

INSULIN

Insulin Therapy

Description: An aqueous solution of the active principle of the islet tissue of beef pancreas; accurately standardized, uniformly potent, and stable; has low nitrogen content and is free from reaction-producing substances.

Action and Uses: Lowers blood sugar; makes possible carbohydrate utilization in a normal manner; each unit assists in the average utilization of 2 Gm of carbohydrate; *used* as adjunct to diet in the treatment of diabetes mellitus and in all its complications; also in undernutrition.

Supply:

INSULIN (C.A.)—Vials, 5 cc of 10, 20 and 40 units per cubic centimeter. **(Sharp and Dohme)**

INSULIN (C.A.)—Vials, 5 cc containing 10, 20, 40 units per cubic centimeter or 50, 100, 200 units per vial. **(Squibb)**

INSULIN (C.A.)—Vials, 10 cc containing 10, 20, 40, 80, 100 units per cubic centimeter or 100, 200, 400, 800, 1,000 units per vial. **(Squibb)**

INSULIN (C.A.)—Vials, 5 cc—of 10, 20, 40 units per cc. **(Stearns)**

INSULIN (C.A.)—Vials, 10 cc—100 units per cubic centimeter. **(Stearns)**

Administration: *Subcutaneously* 15–30 min. before meals. Dosage is calculated in each instance in accordance with the glycemia or glycosuria, calory requirement, nutritional state, the presence of acidosis or infection.

Bibliography: *See Chap. XII.*

IODEIKON

X-Ray Contrast Medium

Chemical Name: Sodium Tetraiodophenolphthalein.

Formula: $C_{20}H_8I_4O_4Na_2$.

Description: A bluish, odorless, hygroscopic powder; soluble in water and alcohol.

Action and Uses: Upon absorption is eliminated by the liver with the bile into the gall bladder; the latter then becomes radiographically opaque and visualized; *used* for x-ray study of the gall bladder.

Supply: **IODEIKON** (C.A.)—Capsules, Keratin coated, 0.25 Gm—Bottles of 100. **(Abbott)**

IODEIKON (C.A.)—Vials ½ oz., for 1 dose—Boxes of 12. **(Abbott)**

CHOLEMULSION—Bottles, for 1 dose. **(Lafayette Pharmacal)**
An emulsion of Iodeikon containing colloidal and other substances.

CHOLEPULVIS—Powder form—Bottles for 1 dose. **(Lafayette Pharmacal)**

IODEIKON—Capsules, Enterocap coated, gr 5—Bottles of 100 with 100 capsules of prepared sodium carbonate gr 7. **(Lafayette Pharmacal)**

IODEIKON—Pulvules, Enteric coated, 0.25 Gm—Bottles of 100, 500. **(Lilly)**

IODEIKON—Ampules 3.5 Gm—Boxes of 5. **(Mallinckrodt)**

IODEIKON—Bottles of 25 and 100 Gm. **(Mallinckrodt)**

IODEIKON—Capsules, Enterocap, 0.25 Gm—Bottles of 100. **(Lafayette)**

Administration: *Oral Method*—3½–4 Gm of Iodeikon dissolved in 1 or 2 oz. of water and mixed with half glass of grape juice is taken at appointed time; or 10–15 capsules or pulvules, or 6 capsules each containing Iodeikon 12 gr, agar 2 gr, soda bicarbonate, 2 gr, are taken half an hour after a light, non-fatty evening meal. Cholecystography in 12, 14, 16–18 hr.

Intravenous Method—55 mg per kilogram of body weight, total not to exceed 3½ Gm; dissolved in 1 oz. of freshly distilled water, filtered, sterilized for 15 min. over water bath, diluted to 200 cc with Ringer's or normal saline solution and injected slowly for 15 min. with needle through rubber tube, by the gravity method, and followed with diluent alone; or injected directly by syringe in concentration less than 8%, allowing 10 min. for injection; solutions must be isotonic. Radiographs taken 4, 8 and 12 hr. after administration.

Fatty meal where desired; plates taken 1 or 2 hr. later.

Contraindications: Myocardial insufficiency, hypotension, jaundice and uremia.

Bibliography: *See Chap. XII.*

IODICIN **(Burroughs Wellcome)**

Iodine Therapy

Description: The Calcium salt of Iodo-Ricinoleic Acid.

Action and Uses: Is tasteless, odorless, easily absorbed, non-irritating and slowly excreted; *For use* in goitre prophylaxis.

Supply: IODICIN—Capsules gr 3 (0.194 Gm), representing 1 gr organic iodine—Boxes of 50.

TABLOID IODICIN—gr ½ (0.03 Gm), representing ⅙ gr organic iodine—Bottles of 25, 100 and 500.

Administration: 1–3 tabloids, three to four times daily; may be used to replace potassium iodide on all occasions. In simple goitre prophylaxis, 1 tabloid weekly; in treatment of simple goitre, 2–3 tabloids weekly.

IODIPIN 40% (Merck)

X-Ray Contrast Medium

Official Name: Iodized Vegetable Oil, 40%.

Description: A product containing 40%, iodine, firmly held in organic combination with fatty acids; is free from irritant action.

Action and Uses: Is opaque to the X-ray, and *used* in diagnosis of pulmonary, spinal cord and urologic lesions; in the demonstration of intrathoracic cavities; in the diagnosis of bronchiectasis, pulmonary abscess, tumors, tuberculosis and pneumothorax; of fistulous tracts, foreign bodies, stenoses; in the location of tumors of the spinal cord.

Supply: IODIPIN 40%—Ampules 2 cc—Bottles 25 Gm.

IODIPIN 40%—Tablets of 50.

Administration: In bronchography, 15–20 cc for each lung; in myelography, 2 cc; in pyelography and ureterography of both sides, 15–20 cc.

IODO BISMUTHATE OF QUININE "FRAISSE" (Fougera)

Antiluetic

Description: A stable, non-toxic, non-irritating preparation containing Bismuth, Iodine and Quinine.

Action and Uses: A rapidly absorbed antiluetic; *For use* in neurosyphilitic conditions except paresis; in cases intolerant of arsenic.

Supply: IODO BISMUTHATE OF QUININE "FRAISSE"—Ampules 4 cc, 0.2 Gm, in olive oil—Boxes of 6 and 25.

IODO BISMUTHATE OF QUININE "FRAISSE"—Ampules 3 cc, 0.3 Gm, in olive oil—Boxes of 6 and 25.

IODO BISMUTHATE OF QUININE "FRAISSE"—Bottles of ampular concentrations, 60 Gm.

Administration: *Intramuscularly*—0.2 Gm every 3 days, 20 injections in all; second course 0.3 Gm every 5 days, total of 15 injections; course alternated with arsenicals.

IODO-BISMUTH OF QUININE (Huxley)

Antiluetic

Composition: A suspension of Iodo-Bismuth of Quinine in lanolin-oily base; contains 0.04 cg metalloid bismuth per cubic centimeter.

Action and Uses: An insoluble bismuth, *for use* in the treatment of syphilis.

Supply: IODO-BISMUTH OF QUININE—Ampules, 2 cc—Boxes of 10 and 100.

IODO-BISMUTH OF QUININE—Vials 10 cc and 30 cc.

Administration: 2 cc (0.08 cg) three times weekly for 20 injections, *intramuscularly.*

Bibliography: *See Chap. XII.*

IODOCHLOROL (Searle)

Radiopaque Medium

Description: An iodized peanut oil containing Iodine 27 %, Chlorine 7.5 % in chemical combination with the fatty acids of the oil; each cubic centimeter represents 0.332 Gm Chlorine and 0.929 Gm Iodine.

Action and Uses: A radiopaque medium for X-ray diagnosis; has stability, pleasant taste, fine flavor, high radiopacity; *used* in gynecologic, sinus and bronchial radiography; also in iodine therapy.

Supply: **IODOCHLOROL**—Bottles of 20 cc.

Administration: *Radiography*—5–15 cc in accordance with requirements.
Internally—1–2 teaspoonfuls, two to three times daily.

Combinations: **IODOCHLOROL EMULSION**—1 part of Iodochlorol emulsified with 3 parts of potassium oleate; has low viscosity, is miscible with water and is non-irritating; *For use* in retrograde pyelography; *Supply*—Bottles of 20 cc.

Bibliography: *See Chap. XII.*

IODOMUTH (Summers)

Astringent. Antiseptic

Chemical Name: Bismuth-oxy-iodid-methylene-dimethyl Gallate.

Description: A combination of Bismuth, Gallic Acid, Iodine and Formaldehyde; occurs as fine reddish-brown, odorless, tasteless powder, insoluble in water and gastric juice.

Action and Uses: Orally administered is but slowly disintegrated and affects every part of gastrointestinal tract, producing a soothing, protecting, stimulating antiseptic and deodorant effect. *Used* in peptic ulcer, ulcerative colitis, tubercular diarrhea, dysentery; topically in burns, ulcers, luetic sores, ozena, varicose ulcers.

Supply: **IODOMUTH**—Tablets—gr 5—Boxes of 100.
IODOMUTH—Powder—Boxes of 2 oz.

Administration: Gr 10–30 every 2–3 hr.
Locally—As dusting powder or as 40 % ointment.

Incompatibles: Incompatible with acid and alkaline substances.

Bibliography: *See Chap. XII.*

IODOSTARINE (Roche)

Iodine Therapy

Chemical Name: Diiodotariric Acid.

Formula: $C_{18}H_{32}I_2O_2$.

Composition: An iodine addition product of tariric acid, derived from the fruit of a species of Picramnia; contains 47.5 % of iodine.

Description: A white crystalline solid, odorless and tasteless; insoluble in water, slightly soluble in cold alcohol, soluble in warm alcohol, chloroform, benzene and carbon disulphide; is stable on exposure to air.

Action: Has the advantage over inorganic iodides of being longer retained and therefore better utilized; is well borne and causes no gastric or intestinal irritation.

Uses: In the prevention and treatment of simple goiter, especially in regions where goitre is endemic.

Supply: IODOSTARINE (C.A.)—Tablets—Chocolate (each representing 10 mg of iodine)—Boxes of 50.

Administration: For goitre prevention: 1 tablet per week during school year; during pregnancy 1–2 tablets per week throughout the term; for treatment: 2–3 tablets per week.

Bibliography: *See Chap. XII.*

IODOSYL (Nelson, Baker)

Antiseptic

Formula: $C_6H_3I(OI)COOH$.

Description: An amorphous, garnet colored, velvety soft powder, of slight odor and taste; insoluble in water and oils, sparingly soluble in ether, chloroform.

Action and Uses: Local antiseptic and alterative; has therapeutic qualities analogous to iodoform, but is non-toxic, non-irritating and odorless; *For use* in goitre, glandular enlargement, intestinal infections, ulcers, wounds, ophthalmic and urethral diseases.

Administration: As dusting powder and in other forms for external use; Internally, 1 capsule as indicated.

Supply: IODOSYL—Duster tins, ½ and 1 oz.

IODOSYL—Powder Blower—Bottles ⅓ oz.

IODOSYL—Capsules gr 2—Bottles of 50.

IODOSYL—Nasal-points, small suppositories for nasal application, containing Iodosyl, 56 parts; Sodium Chlorate, 112 parts; Sodium Borate, 56 parts; Eucalyptol, 9 parts; Menthol, 4½ parts; Cacao Butter, 762½ parts—Boxes of 30, 144.

IODOSYL—Ointment 6% Aseptic, for surgical uses—Tubes collapsible; sizes—trial, small, medium, large—Jars 1 lb.

IODOSYL—Ointment—Ophthalmic 2 and 6%—Tubes pinpoint, 1 and 6 dr.

IODOSYL—Ointment—Urethral 6%—Tubes, with and without applicator.

IODOSYL—Ointment Compound—Hemorrhoidal tubes, collapsible with rectal applicator.

IODOSYL—Ointment Compound, Urethral—Tubes with and without applicator Contains Iodosyl, 50 parts; Zinc Phenolsulphonate, 2½ parts; Mercuriform, 1¼ parts; Alum, 12½ parts; Sodium Borate, 12½ parts; Petrolatum, 921¼ parts.

IODOSYL—Pencils (Gonorrheal)—Boxes of 14, 30 and 72.

Contains Iodosyl, 50 parts; Sodium Borate, 12½ parts; Alum, 12½ parts; Zinc Phenol sulphonate, 5 parts; Mercuric Oleate, 2½ parts; Cacao Butter, 917½ parts.

IODOSYL—Pencil (Milder formula) same composition except ½ proportions of zinc phenol-sulphonate and mercuric oleate—Boxes of 14, 30 and 72.

SUPPOSITORIES COMPOUND IODOSYL—Hemorrhoidal—Boxes 12, 48. Contains Iodosyl, 50 parts; Tannin, 50 parts; Alum, 25 parts; Atropine sulphate, ¼ part; Cacao Butter, 874¾ parts.

OINTMENT ATROPINE AND IODOSYL 1—(Regular) Ophthalmic containing Atropine, 1 per cent; Iodosyl, 2 per cent— Tubes, pinpoint, 1 dr.

OINTMENT ATROPINE AND IODOSYL 3—(Special) Ophthalmic containing Atropine, 0.5 per cent; Iodosyl, 6 per cent—Tubes, pinpoint, 1 dr.

IOTHION (Winthrop)

Iodin Therapy

Chemical Name: Diïodohydroxypropane. Brand of Iopropane.

Formula: $C_3H_5I_2OH$.

Description: A yellowish, oily liquid of faint and not unpleasant odor; insoluble in water, easily soluble in alcohol, ether, chloroform and oils; contains 77–80% iodine.

Action: Is absorbed by the intact skin and excreted through the kidneys, in the urine; is non-irritating in concentrations ordinarily employed and non-staining.

Uses: In glandular enlargement, various arthritides, parenchymatous goiter, tertiary syphilis, skin diseases, like ringworm of scalp or sycosis barbae; also in trachoma, blepharitis, pannus; in chronic salpingitis and endometritis.

Supply: **IOTHION (C.A.)**—Bottles 1 oz.

Combination: **IOTHION-OIL** (C.A.), containing Iothion 10 parts, chloroform, 10 parts, olive oil 80 parts—Bottles 1 oz.

Administration: Externally only—Iothion-Oil, representing the average strength for skin application, is chiefly used; if desired may further be diluted with pure olive oil, or used in solution with alcohol and glycerin, or as 5–20% ointment with petrolatum; parts treated should not be heavily covered or bandaged.

IPRAL CALCIUM (Squibb)

Sedative. Hypnotic

Chemical Name: Calcium Ethyl Isopropyl Barbiturate.

Formula: $Ca(C_2H_5C_3H_7C. CO. NH. CO. N. CO.)_2 + 2H_2O$.

Description: A crystalline powder of white or faintly yellow color and slightly bitter taste: soluble in 40 parts of water at 25°c.

Action: Is sedative and hypnotic, acting on the central nervous system, with selective effect on the higher centers; in therapeutic dosage produces sleep similar to normal, without after effects or drowsiness; does not depress the circulation and is non-narcotic.

Uses: Recommended in combating restlessness, irritability, sleeplessness; in preoperative preparation and post operative sedation.

Supply: **IPRAL CALCIUM**—Tablets (C.A.) gr 2 (0.12 Gm)—Vials of 10—Bottles of 100, 1,000.

IPRAL CALCIUM—Tablets (C.A.) gr ¾ (0.048 Gm)—Vials of 10 —Bottles of 100, 1,000.

Combination: **IPRAL AMIDOPYRINE**—Tablets gr 4⅓ (0.28 Gm); contains Ipral gr 2 (0.13 Gm) with Amidopyrine 2⅓ gr (0.15 Gm) per tablet, for additional analgesia in insomnia with pain—Vials of 10—Bottles of 100, 1,000.

Administration: *Sedative*—1–2 tablets followed by hot drink.

Hypnotic—2–3 tablets followed by hot drink; repeated in 6–12 hr. as indicated.

Bibliography: *See Chap. XII.*

IRON CITRATE GREEN (Parke, Davis)

Hematinic

Formula: $FeC_6H_5O_7 + 3H_2O$.

Description: Green transparent scales, very soluble in water, unstable if exposed to light; contains an equivalent of 16% Iron and 8.1% of Ammonium.

Action and Uses: Hematinic in anemia, chlorosis.

Supply: IRON CITRATE GREEN (C.A.)—Ampules, gr ¼, ¾ and 1½ Iron and Ammonium Citrate, each with Quinine and Urea Hydrochloride 0.005 Gm—Boxes 6 and 12.

Administration: Gr ¼ (0.015 Gm) to 1½ gr (0.097 Gm), *intramuscular* or *subcutaneous*, as needed.

IRON LACTATE (Merck)

Hematinic

Official Name: Ferrum Lacticum.

Formula: $Fe(C_3H_5O_3)_2 + 3H_2O$.

Description: Occurs in pale, greenish-white flakes comprising numerous needle shaped crystals of peculiar odor and sweetish ferruginous taste; is slowly soluble in 40 parts of cold and 12 parts of boiling water; insoluble in alcohol, freely soluble in alkalies.

Action and Uses: Hematinic, tonic and alterative. *For use* in all types of secondary anemia, chlorosis, and other conditions where organic iron in palatable form is desired.

Supply: IRON LACTATE (C.A.)—Bottles 1 oz., ¼ and 1 lb.

Administration: *Dose*—2–10 gr (0.12–0.6 Gm), several times daily; average dose 5 gr (0.3 Gm).

Caution: To be kept from air and light.

ISACEN (Roche)

Laxative

Chemical Name: Diacetyldioxyphenylisatin.

Formula: $C_{24}H_{19}O_5N$.

Composition: The diacetyl derivative of dihydroxyphenylisatin.

Description and Action: A white crystalline, odorless, tasteless powder, insoluble in dilute acids and thus passing through the stomach unchanged; under the influence of the alkaline contents of the intestine a gradual splitting off of the laxative component, dioxyphenylisatin, takes place which becomes effective; is not absorbed and is excreted entirely through the feces, none appearing in the urine; is non-toxic.

Uses: As laxative or purgative, in all chronic cases of constipation.

Advantages: Does not enter the circulation and can not injure the kidneys, liver or skin; is harmless even in nephritis, dermatoses and during pregnancy and lactation.

Supply: ISACEN—Tablets (C.A.), 1/13 gr (0.005 Gm)—Vials of 40.

ministration: *Dose*—1–2 tablets, more in obstinate cases, taken at bedtime.

ISAROL (Ciba)

Antipruritic. Antiseptic

Official Name: Bitumen Sulphonatum.

Description: A reddish-brown to brownish-black syrupy liquid of strong empyreumatic odor; soluble in water or glycerine, miscible with fixed oils or fats; partly soluble in alcohol or ether.

Action: Mildly irritant and antiseptic, producing moderate rubefacience; is antipruritic; if taken internally in large doses, is gastric irritant and purgative; its therapeutic effect is due to the organically combined sulphur.

Uses and Administration: **Dermatology**—In conditions where sulphur is indicated; in ointment form, 5–50% incorporated with lanolin, petrolatum, zinc oxide ointment, castor oil or glycerin.

Surgery—As antiseptic and irritant in indolent ulceration and similar lesions.

Gynecology and Proctology—In form of tampons and ointment, either pure or in combination with other drugs, in pelvic infections, rectal fissure, ulcers, pruritus ani.

Internally—Where ammonium sulphoichthyolate is employed, as in intestinal putrefaction and secondary anemia; 5–30 m in capsules.

Supply: ISAROL (C.A.)—Bottles of 1 and 4 oz. and 1 lb.

ISAROL (C.A.)—Tubes of ¼ lb. and 1 oz.

Bibliography: *See Chap. XII.*

ISO-IODEIKON (Mallinckrodt)

Radiopaque Medium

Chemical Name: Phentetiothalein Sodium; Phenoltetraiodophthalein Sodium.

Formula: $C_{20}H_{6}O_{4}I_{4}Na_{2}$.

Description: Occurs as bronze purple, odorless granules, soluble in water and alcohol.

Action and Uses: On intravenous injection in normal liver function the dye is excreted with the bile into the gall bladder in sufficient concentration to present a radiographic shadow; in abnormal functioning the dye is retained in the blood and its concentration there determines the extent of liver damage; causes little toxicity; is better tolerated, more informative and applicable in smaller dosage than Iodeikon. *Used* in cholecystography and as liver function test.

Supply: ISO-IODEIKON (C.A.)—Ampules 2.5 Gm—Boxes of 5.

ISO-IODEIKON (C.A.)—Bottles of 10 and 25 Gm.

Administration: 40 mg per kilogram of body weight, total dose not to exceed 2.5 mg; solution is prepared by dissolving the determined dosage in 1 oz. of freshly distilled water, sterilizing over boiling water bath for 15 min. and diluting with about 150 cc of Ringer's or normal saline; is injected by gravity method, during a period of at least 15 min.; where the syringe method is used, the concentration must not exceed 8%, the time not to be less than 15 min. Radiography in 4, 8 and 12 hr. after administration; fatty meal where desired given after the 8 hr. observation and radiographed 1 or 2 hr. after.

Caution: Solution to be strictly isotonic; clean glassware and pure distilled water only must be employed.

Liver Function Test: 8 cc of blood is obtained ½–1 hr. after injection of dye for analysis and colorimetric study.

Contraindications: Myocardial insufficiency, uremia; in jaundice to be used with discrimination.

Bibliography: *See Chap XII.*

KAYLENE (Fougera)

Detoxicant

Description: A colloidal Kaolin derivative.

Action: Is protective to gastric mucosa; affects the intestinal flora, reducing intestinal toxemia, flatus and foetor by absorption.

Uses: As detoxicant in chronic intestinal stasis, colitis, diarrhea, dysentery, food poisoning, arthritis; as protective in gastritis and peptic ulcer.

Supply: KAYLENE—Cartons of 10 oz.

KAYLENE-OL—An emulsion of Kaylene and heavy liquid petrolatum—Bottles of 16 oz.

KAYLENE-OL WITH PHENOLPHTHALEIN, 0.5 %—Bottles of 16 fl. oz.

Administration: 1 tablespoonful in water, ½ hr. before meals or once at bedtime.

KELENE (Merck)

Anesthetic

Chemical Name: Ethyl Chloride; Monochlorethane.

Formula: C_2H_5Cl.

Description: A colorless, highly volatile liquid of agreeable odor and sweetish burning taste.

Action and Uses: Produces anesthesia by refrigeration. *Used* topically—for minor operations; by inhalation—for operations of short duration, or preliminary to ether anesthesia; in dental surgery, for tooth extraction; *Used* also in neuralgia, sciatica, neuritis, rodent ulcer; is sprayed locally in lupus, trichophytosis, skin transplantation, condylomata, herpes zoster; in aphonia of singers and public speakers.

Caution: To be kept cool and away from an open flame; is highly inflammable.

Supply: KELENE (C.A.)—Pure ethyl chloride, in automatically closing and plain-cap tubes adapted for spraying; in 10, 30, 60 and 100 Gm and in 3 cc and 5 cc tubes.

Administration: *As Spray*—Heat of hand forces stream of anesthetic from container; tube is held 6–10 in. from the thoroughly cleansed surface to be anesthetized; is applied until sprayed area is refrigerated and anesthetized. *In inhalation anesthesia*—is employed by the usual open cone method.

KEPHALIN (Armour)

Hemostatic

Description: A phosphatid extract from the brain tissue of cattle; essentially a brain lipoid; is an amorphous, yellowish powder of characteristic odor and taste; readily soluble in chloroform and ether, slightly soluble in alcohol; forms an opalescent emulsion in neutral aqueous solution; may be sterilized by boiling without affecting its hemostatic qualities; contains little protein.

Action and Uses: Hemostatic; checks capillary oozing; *for use* in all surface hemorrhages.

Supply: **KEPHALIN (C.A.)**—Bottles of 10 Gm.

Administration: 0.1 %–0.2 % saline suspension, applied on gauze sponges or direct to bleeding area; for coating catheters in catheterization after prostatectomy—in same strength For convenience, dilutions may be made from a 5 % ether stock solution.

Caution: Not to be used in those sensitive to beef protein.

KERAPHEN (Picker X-Ray)

Radiopaque Medium

Description: A peppermint flavored bluish powder, containing principally Sodium Tetraiodophenolphthalein; turns white when thoroughly stirred in water; is palatable and stable.

Action and Uses: Being insoluble in acid medium, is non-irritating to gastric mucosa; is absorbed only in small intestine in alkaline fluid; is radiopaque and thus *used* as diagnostic agent in oral cholecystography.

Supply: **KERAPHEN "A"**—For shadows of average density; Single dose bottles, dye 3 Gm—Packages of 12.

KERAPHEN "B"—For denser shadows or heavier individuals; Single dose bottles, dye 4 Gm—Packages of 12.

Administration: Light evening meal is taken at 6 P.M.; within the next hour the contents of one bottle is dissolved in 1/4 glass of water, thoroughly stirred until its color is changed and administered best with lemonade, orange juice or grape juice; no food or cathartics, only fluids are permitted until after x-ray the next morning, 12, 15, 18 and 24 hr. after dye administration.

KRESIVAL (Winthrop)

Expectorant. Anticatarrhal

Chemical Name: Calcium Cresolsulphonate.

Description: A palatable syrupy fluid containing calcium salts of cresolsulphonic acids 6 %; by a special process of sulphonation, the 40 % of cresols from creosote are rendered non-irritating and non-toxic.

Action: As for creosote and calcium; stimulates fluid secretion from nose and upper respiratory passages and relieves cough; is slightly sedative and antispasmodic; is practically non-irritating to gastrointestinal and genitourinary organs and of agreeable taste.

Uses: In acute and chronic bronchial affections; in laryngitis, influenza, tuberculosis, measles, pneumonia and pertussis.

Supply: **KRESIVAL**—Bottles of 8 oz.

Administration: Adults, 2–4 teaspoonfuls, three to four times daily. Children, 1 teaspoonful, mixed with equal parts of water.

Combination: **KRES-LUMIN**—A combination of Kresival with Luminal, 1/16 gr to the teaspoonful, for additional sedation; an expectorant and cough sedative without after-effects. *For use* to replace opiates in relief of cough. *Dosage* same as for Kresival. *Supply*—Bottles of 4 and 8 oz.

Bibliography: *See Chap. XII.*

LAC-PROTEINATE (National Drug)

Non-specific Protein Therapy

Description: A sterile colloidal solution of the protein-protogen and lactalbumin in milk, combined with protein-albuminoid substances; is bacteria and toxin-free.

Action and Uses: For non-specific protein treatment; to stimulate leucocytosis and increase antibody formation in various infections.

Supply: LAC-PROTEINATE—Ampule-Vials 1 cc, 5 cc, 10 cc and 25 cc—Packages of 12 and 100.

Administration: *Initial Dose*—½–2 cc, increased by 1–2 cc until 5–10 cc are injected; given every 12–72 hr.

LACTIGEN (Abbott)

Non-specific Protein Therapy

Description: A lipo-protein antigen prepared from sterilized milk of tuberculin-tested cows; is toxin-free and biologically standardized.

Action and Uses: A foreign protein agent stimulating cells in resisting disease, increasing their enzymic activity, stimulating the function of the hematopoietic system, leukocytosis and anti-body production; *For use* in acute and chronic infections—iritis, arthritis, epididymitis, influenza, eczema, gonorrhea and similar infections.

Supply: LACTIGEN—Ampules 5 cc—Boxes of 6, 25 and 100.

LACTIGEN—Ampules 10 cc—Boxes of 6, 25 and 100.

Administration: *Intramuscularly*—Dosage depending upon the individual's reactivity and the character of the affection, beginning with small doses and increasing up to 10 cc; administered every 3–5 days, after reaction from previous injection has subsided.

Contraindications: Pulmonary tuberculosis, diabetes, cardiac decompensation, alcoholism.

Bibliography: *See Chap. XII.*

LAR-IO-BEN (Marvell)

Antiseptic

Chemical Name: Iodobenzol Gallate.

Composition: Combines the action of phenol, iodine and gallotannic acid, in solution.

Action: Antiseptic, antizymotic, deodorant, astringent.

Uses: As spray or gargle in the prophylaxis of nose, mouth and throat infections; is especially applicable in dentistry and dental affections.

Supply: LAR-IO-BEN—Bottles 4 and 8 oz., 1 pt., 1 qt. and 1 gal.

Administration: In dilutions up to 50%.

LAROCAINE (Roche)

Surface Anesthetic

Chemical Name: The hydrochloride of 1-p-aminobenzoyl-2.2-dimethyl-3-diethyl-amino-propanol.

Formula: $H_2N.C_6H_4.COO.CH_2.C(CH_3)_2.CH_2N(C_2H_5)_2HCl$.

Description and Action: Occurs as a white crystalline powder; is an unusually safe and effective substitute for cocaine in surface and local anesthesia; its action is prolonged, lasting from 3–5 hr. and less epinephrine is needed in its use than with procaine; is rapidly detoxified and when used in the usual therapeutic concentration is non-irritant.

Uses: **Ophthalmology**—For corneal and conjunctival anesthesia, in 2–5 % solutions.

Otorhinolaryngology—5–10 % solution.

Urology—For vesical anesthesia, 30–50 cc of ¾–1 % solution.

General Surgery—¼–2 % solutions; ordinarily, ½–1 % solutions.

Advantages: Is not irritant to cornea and is non-mydriatic; is non-narcotic and non-habit forming.

Supply: LAROCAINE—Powder—Vials ⅛, ¼, ½, 1 oz.

Directions: Stock solutions should be kept in dark bottles; solutions are made with distilled water or physiological saline and sterilized by boiling for 10 min.; epinephrine is added just prior to administration.

LEAD SELENIDE (Anglo-French)

Cancer Therapy

Chemical Name: Colloidal Lead Selenide "British Royal Infirmary."

Description: A stable and comparatively non-toxic, brown to black fluid.

Uses: In inoperable carcinoma.

Supply: LEAD SELENIDE—Ampules 5, 10 and 15 cc.

Administration: *Intravenously*—Initial dose 5 cc, increased gradually to 15 cc; preceded and followed at each injection by 5 % glucose solution; given weekly for 8–12 weeks; after rest period of 3 mo., may be repeated as required.

Caution: In severe reaction, epinephrin is to be administered; complications of lead poisoning must be guarded against.

LENIGALLOL (Bilhuber-Knoll)

Antiseptic

Chemical Name: Triacetyl Pyrogallol.

Formula: $C_6H_3(CH_3CO_2)_3$.

Description: A white crystalline powder, insoluble in water and alcohol.

Action: Is strongly reducing and mildly caustic; favors normal keratinization of non-nuclear epidermal tissues; relieves hyperemia, exudation and itching.

Uses: In eczema, mycosis between toes and fingers, dermatophytosis, psoriasis and other dermatologic disturbances.

Advantages: Is free from toxic reactions of pyrogallic acid.

Supply: LENIGALLOL—Zinc ointment 6 % (C.A.)—Tubes of ½ oz.

LENIGALLOL—Powder (C.A.)—Bottles of ¼ oz., 1 oz.

Administration: As 1–6 % ointment, applied generally once or twice daily; in mycosis ¼–½ %; in eczema 1–20 % ointment, usually combined with zinc oxide. Ointment is to be applied fresh daily, after area is cleaned and crusts removed with olive oil; water is to be avoided; treated area to be covered by bandage.

Bibliography: *See Chap. XII.*

LENNOX ETHYLENE (Ohio Chemical)

Anesthetic Gas

Chemical Name: Ethylene.

Formula: C_2H_4.

Description: A colorless gas of characteristic odor and taste, somewhat lighter than air (Sp. Gr. = 0.97, A = 1); is solid below minus 169.4°c, and boils at minus 103.9°c; is inflammable and explosive when a mixture of the gas and oxygen or air is brought into contact with a flame or static spark; 1 volume of the gas dissolves in about 4 volumes of water at 0°c and in 7 volumes of water at 20°c, in about ½ volume of alcohol at 25°c; is soluble in ether.

Action: A mixture of 90% ethylene and 10% oxygen has a direct anesthetic action on the nervous system, abolishing all motor reflexes; the undiluted gas produces asphyxia phenomena, which the addition of oxygen overcomes.

Uses: *For induction* of deep surgical anesthesia.

Supply: **LENNOX ETHYLENE (C.A.)**—In compressed state, in steel cylinders.

Administration: By passing the gas into an inhalation apparatus, from which it is inhaled after admixture with the required amount of oxygen.

Advantages: Rapid and more pleasant induction, satisfactory relaxation without cyanosis or sweating, and prompt post-anesthetic recovery.

Bibliography: *See Chap. XII.*

LIANTRAL (Duke)

Antiseptic

Description: A purified coal tar extract containing 2.1% phenols and free from undesirable elements; a brown, thick liquid, readily soluble in benzol, partly soluble in ether, alcohol, oils, fats; miscible with ointment bases.

Action and Uses: Antiseptic and stimulant in lichen planus, lichenoid eczemas, neurodermatitis and similar diseases.

Supply: **LIANTRAL**—Bottles of 2 and 4 oz.

Administration: Applied locally twice daily and dusted freely with cornstarch.

Combination: **LIANTRAL CASEIN OINTMENT 5%**—Has a non-fatty base removable with water; particularly effective in seborrhea of the scalp. *Supply*—Collapsible tin tubes, 50 Gm.

LIPOIODINE (Ciba)

Iodine Therapy

Chemical Name: Ethyl Diiodobrassidate.

Formula: $C_{21}H_{39}I_2COO(C_2H_5)$.

Description: A white, odorless, tasteless, crystalline powder; insoluble in water, slightly soluble in alcohol, very soluble in fatty oils, liquid petrolatum, ether and benzine; is decomposed by direct sunlight; contains approximately 41% iodine in organic combination.

Action: Is of neutral reaction and non-irritating locally. Administered orally, is almost completely absorbed unchanged and gradually decomposed in the tissues with the liberation of the iodine ions; causes no digestive disturbances; unlike alkali iodides it penetrates all tissues including nervous and fatty.

Uses: In all diseases where iodides are used internally: lues, asthma, cardiorenal disease, arteriosclerosis, chronic bronchitis, arthritis, chronic plumbism, goitre, hypothyroidism.

Supply: LIPOIODINE—Tablets (C.A.) Plain and Sugar coated, 4½ gr (0.3 Gm)—Bottles of 30 and 100.

Administration: In prolonged iodine therapy, 2 tablets are given 1 day, with one on the next day during the course of treatment.
In goitre prophylaxis—2–4 tablets daily for a period of 10 days yearly; in dysthyroidism where iodine is employed—2–6 tablets daily as required.

Advantages: Pleasant taste, freedom from gastrointestinal irritation; general distribution to all organs; steady, prolonged action; convenience of administration.

Bibliography: *See Chap. XII.*

LIPOIODINE DIAGNOSTIC (Ciba)

X-Ray Contrast Medium

Description: A 60% solution of Lipoiodine in purified sesame oil, a solvent most resistant to rancidity.

Action: Is radiopaque; its slow absorption permits repeated x-ray exposures at various intervals; is non-irritating, causes no inflammatory reaction and does not become encysted being completely absorbed in 1–2 weeks; contains no free iodine and is not affected by heat, light or moisture; on injection penetrates easily into every recess.

Uses: For the localization of bronchial and pulmonary lesions; for uterosalpingography; as a diagnostic aid in gynecology; in the detection of urethral strictures and delineation of cavities; in sinus diagnosis and numerous other instances. Therapeutically, by intratracheal injection, is of great value in bronchiectasis, and chronic bronchitis.

Contraindications: None; intratracheal injections must be given cautiously; should not be used in the presence of advanced circulatory complications, as angina pectoris, aneurysm or cardiac decompensation.

Supply: LIPOIODINE—Ampules (C.A.) 5 cc—Cartons of 1 and 5; each ampule contains 3 gr lipoiodine and 2.7 cc sesame oil.
LIPOIODINE—Solution (C.A.)—Bottles of 10 cc, when liquefied.

Administration: The quantity used varies from 5–20 cc, and is determined by the extent of the field under investigation; x-ray exposures are made shortly after the injection. Before use, the required number of ampules or vials are placed in a hot water bath and contents heated to approximately body temperature; the oil retains the desired heat and remains liquid at average room temperature over a sufficiently long period to permit its proper application.

Caution: Specimens that have become dark brown in color should be discarded.

Bibliography: *See Chap. XII.*

LIPIODOL "LAFAY" (Fougera)

Contrast Medium. Iodine Therapy

Composition: A stable combination of about 40% pure iodine with poppy seed oil.

Description: Is a thick viscous, oily liquid of an alliaceous odor and taste; insoluble in water.

Action and Uses: Is radiopaque and thus used in the x-ray study of soft organs and cavities; also employed internally where prolonged iodine medication is indicated; is very slowly absorbed, non-irritating and well tolerated. *Used* in radiography by intratracheal injection of pulmonary affections in the diagnosis of cerebrospinal tumors, the study of fistulae, accessory nasal sinuses, lacrymal ducts, in uterosalpingography, in the genitourinary tract; internally in circulatory diseases, emphysema, asthma, chronic bronchitis, goitre, syphilis, glandular swellings.

Supply: LIPIODOL "LAFAY"—Ampules (C.A.) 1, 2, 3 and 5 cc—Boxes respectively of 12, 8, 6 and 4.

LIPIODOL "LAFAY"—Aluminum Flasks (C.A.) 20 cc.

LIPIODOL "LAFAY"—Capsules (C.A.) 0.5 Gm, equivalent to 0.2 Gm iodine—Flasks of 50.

LIPIODOL "LAFAY"—Tablets (C.A.), chocolated, equivalent to 0.04 Gm iodine—Boxes of 50.

Administration: *Radiography*—After previously warming to 104°F, is injected in quantities of 1–5 cc or over, in accordance with type of examination.

Internally—2–5 tablets or capsules daily, with meals.

Combinations: ASCENDANT LIPIODOL "GUERBERT"—Contains 11 cg of pure iodine per cubic centimeter and used where a medium of lesser density is desired, as in subarachnoid diagnosis; in 1–2 cc dosage.

DESCENDANT LIPIODOL "GUERBERT"—Contains 54 cg of pure iodine per cubic centimeter and used in the diagnosis of intradural tumors; dosage of 2 cc.

LIVER EXTRACT

Hematopoietic

Description: A palatable, standardized, concentration of the antianemic principle of fresh liver, for oral and intramuscular administration; a brownish, granular, hygroscopic powder, free from coagulable proteins and lipoids; miscible with water, milk, soup, orange and lemon juice or other liquids.

Action and Uses: Stimulates the hematopoiectic function of the bone marrow, promoting reticulocytosis and erythrocytosis; a specific in pernicious anemia, in continuous treatment and in relapses.

Supply: LIVER EXTRACT (C.A.)—Boxes of 20 vials, each vial represents 100 Gm fresh liver. **(Fairchild)**

LIVER POWDER (C.A.)—*For oral use*, each vial is equivalent to 100 Gm fresh liver—Packages 24 vials. **(Lederle)**

SOLUTION LIVER EXTRACT (C.A.)—*Oral*—Bottles 8 oz., equal to 2,400 Gm (5.3 lb.) of liver; 10 cc equals 100 Gm, ¼ lb. liver; alcohol 20% as preservative. **(Lederle)**

SOLUTION LIVER EXTRACT (C.A.)—*Parenteral*—Refined and concentrated, for intramuscular use—Vials 3 cc—Packages of 3; each vial equivalent to 100 Gm active liver substance. **(Lederle)**

LIVER EXTRACT—Capsules—each capsule equivalent to 10 Gm of fresh liver—Bottles of 100. **(National Drug)**

LIVER EXTRACT (C.A.)—Ampules 2 cc, equivalent to 10 Gm of liver—Packages of 6. **(Parke, Davis)**

LIVER EXTRACT (C.A.)—Vials, approximately 2 Gm each—Packages of 24 vials. **(Parke, Davis)**

LIVER CONCENTRATE—Autolized (C.A.)—Containing 88% concentrate and 12% cocoa; each gram represents 20–30 Gm antianemic potency of fresh liver; Vials of 1 Gm. **(Squibb)**

Dosage—4–6 teaspoonfuls daily for 10 days; maintenance dose 1–2 dr. daily.

LIVER EXTRACT—*Intramuscular*—Vials 5 cc, each vial equivalent to 100 Gm fresh liver—Boxes of 1. **(Stoddard)**

LIVER EXTRACT—*Oral*—Vials, each equivalent to 100 Gm fresh liver—Packages of 24. **(Stoddard)**

Administration: In dosages graded in accordance with the red cell count.

Initial Dose—In relapse; 300–400 Gm of liver equivalent, orally, in powder, solution or parenterally—intramuscularly and subcutaneously; powder may be taken in orange juice, cocoa, chocolate, buttermilk, milk, soup or water; continued for about 10 days, or until desired blood count is obtained.

Maintenance Dose—200–300 Gm of liver equivalent, daily, checked by hemoglobin and red cell count.

Severe Cases—300–500 Gm of liver equivalent, as massive initial dose, by stomach tube or intravenously if necessary.

LIVER EXTRACT 343 (Lilly)

Hematopoietic

Description: A water soluble non-protein extract obtained from mammalian liver; standardized so that 3–4 Gm represent 100 Gm of fresh liver; is insoluble in ether and precipitated by acetone and strong alcohol.

Action and Uses: Stimulates blood regenerating tissues and erythrocytosis; a specific in the treatment of pernicious anemia; also *useful* in anemia of sprue, dibothryocephalus infestation and pellagra.

Supply: **LIVER EXTRACT 343** (C.A.)—Powder Vials—Boxes of 24, for oral use.

LIVER EXTRACT 343 (C.A.)—Ampules, rubber-capped, 10 cc, for intramuscular use—Boxes of 1 ampule.

Administration: *Orally*—3 vials daily in water, orange juice or other liquids; in some cases up to 6 and 8 vials, in accordance with blood response.

Intramuscularly—2 cc daily.

Bibliography: *See Chap. XII.*

LIVER EXTRACT E-29 (Valentine)

Hematopoietic

Description: An aqueous liver extract, in concentrated form and free from coagulable proteins; 1 oz. represents in potency 240 Gm of raw liver; contains both fractions, the Cohn-Minot and Whipple, and vitamin B Complex (chiefly the antipellagric factor).

Action and Uses: Hematopoietic, *For use* in primary pernicious anemia.

Supply: **LIVER EXTRACT E-29**—Bottles of 8 oz.

LIVER EXTRACT E-29 WITH IRON—Containing 31 gr (2 Gm) of ferric ammonium citrate per ounce, with traces of liver copper, *For use* in secondary anemia.

Supply—Bottles of 8 oz.

Administration: 1–2 tablespoonfuls three times daily, increased or decreased in accordance with blood picture.

LIVER EXTRACT FRACTION, A-5

(Sharp and Dohme)

Hemopoietic

Description: A brownish hygroscopic powder of slightly, disagreeable taste; fairly soluble in water; 1 Gm represents 20 Gm of whole raw liver.

Action and Uses: As for liver extracts.

Supply: **LIVER EXTRACT FRACTION, A-5**—Vials, representing 100 Gm of liver—Packages of 2 dozen.

LIVER EXTRACT FRACTION, A-5—Capsules, ½ Gm each, representing 10 Gm fresh liver—Boxes of 10 and 1,000.

Administration: Contents of 1 vial, three times daily; or 8–15 capsules, or their contents removed and taken with hot water, orange or tomato juice or other palatable fluids.

Bibliography: *See Chap. XII.*

LIVER EXTRACT 100X—CONCENTRATED (Stearns)

Hematinic

Description: Prepared from fresh, prime, mammalian livers, freed from proteins and fats.

Action and Uses: Hemopoietic in pernicious anemia.

Supply: **LIVER EXTRACT 100X**—Capsules—Bottles of 40 and 500. 5 capsules contain the extract of ½ lb. liver.

Administration: Dosage regulated in accordance with blood picture.

LIVER EXTRACT, PLAIN (Stearns)

Hematopoietic

Description: Prepared from fresh, prime mammalian livers, freed of protein and fats.

Action and Uses: Hematopoietic in pernicious anemia.

Supply: **LIVER EXTRACT PLAIN**—Capsules—Bottles of 100. 45 capsules contain the extract from 1 lb. of liver.

Administration: Dosage regulated as indicated by blood conditions.

LIVER EXTRACT, ORAL (Chappel)

Hematopoietic

Description: A crystal clear, golden yellow concentrate of the antipernicious anemia fraction from the livers of horses; is free from nauseating and unpleasant taste, inert solid residues.

Action and Uses: Hematopoietic in pernicious anemia; is well tolerated by those in whom ordinary liver extract is nauseating; a high purity permits long continued, daily administration without objections and reactions.

Supply: **LIVER EXTRACT, ORAL** (C.A.)—Bottles of 8 and 16 oz., each bottle containing the extract from 4,800 Gm of liver (100 Gm of whole liver are refined to less than 1.8 Gm of solid extract).

Administration: *Orally*—½ oz. three times daily during remission period; ½ oz. daily for maintenance therapy.

Bibliography: *See Chap. XII.*

LIVER EXTRACT, SUBCUTANEOUS (Chappel)

Hematopoietic

Description: A crystal clear, golden yellow concentrate of the anti-pernicious anemia fraction from the livers of horses; prepared for administration by subcutaneous injection; is non-irritating and free from reaction producing substances, its hematopoietic potency is controlled by clinical tests.

Action and Uses: In pernicious anemia; is especially useful in the treatment of those who have an aversion to liver orally, who are unable to assimilate it because of gastrointestinal conditions; is adapted for use in the uncooperative, stuporous, comatose and careless; being highly refined it permits in these routine, hazardless subcutaneous injections instead of deep intramuscular or intravenous.

Advantages: Is relatively pure, free from lipoidal and protein residue and is free from unpleasant reactions.

Supply: LIVER EXTRACT SUBCUTANEOUS (C.A.)—Ampules 2½ cc, containing condensed principle from 25 Gm liver—Boxes of 12.

Administration: 2½ cc daily *subcutaneously* during remission period; same dosage weekly for maintenance therapy.

Bibliography: *See Chap. XII.*

LUMINAL (Winthrop)

Sedative. Antispasmodic. Hypnotic

Chemical Name: Phenylethylmalonylurea. Brand of Phenobarbital.

Formula: $(C_6H_5)_2(CO)_3(NH)_2C$

Description: White, odorless, somewhat bitter powder, almost insoluble in cold water, readily soluble in organic solvents and dilute alkalies.

Action: In small doses offers marked sedative and antispasmodic effect, in larger doses is one of the more powerful true hypnotics.

Uses and Administration: In many disturbances requiring sedative or hypnotic therapy.

Epilepsy—Adults, in the average case, 1½ gr (0.09 Gm) at night, but when seizures occur during the day, given in divided doses, morning and night, or three times daily. In more severe cases, 3 gr (0.19 Gm) or more a day. Bromides are continued during the first week in decreasing doses. During menstrual and climacteric periods, temporary increase of dose may be necessary.
Children: 7–15 yr., ¼–¾ gr (0.01–0.04 Gm) daily, gradually increased up to 1½ gr (0.09 Gm) if necessary. Where Luminal is to be discontinued, dosage is gradually decreased and bromides substituted in increasing amounts.

Insomnia—1½–3 gr (0.09–0.19 Gm) in ordinary cases; 5 gr (0.32 Gm) or more in severe psychoses, with effects closely watched.

Eclampsia—3–6 gr (0.19–0.38 Gm) (or Luminal-Sodium subcutaneously).

Other Conditions—Migraine, ¾–1 gr (0.04–0.06 Gm) two or three times daily; vomiting of pregnancy, ½ gr (0.03 Gm)–1½ gr (0.09 Gm) every 4–6 hr. (if oral administration is not tolerated, Luminal-Sodium is given by injection); in hypertension and hyperthyroidism, ½–1 gr (0.03–0.06 Gm) two or three times daily; chorea, pertussis, cardiac neuroses, gastric neuroses, dysmenorrhea, preoperative and postoperative cases, ¼–½ gr (0.016–0.03 Gm) two or three times a day.

Supply: LUMINAL—Tablets ¼ gr (C.A.) (0.016 Gm) and ½ gr (0.03 Gm)—Bottles of 100.

LUMINAL—Tablets, 1½ gr (C.A.) (0.09 Gm)—Bottles of 50.

LUMINAL—Capsules 1½ gr (C.A.) (0.09 Gm)—Bottles of 50.

LUMINAL—Elixir—A palatable mixture containing ¼ gr (0.016 Gm) Luminal to teaspoonful of elixir; stable, unvarying in composition, convenient of administration; should be given without admixture of other drugs. Dosage, 1–2 teaspoonfuls three or four times daily.

Bibliography: *See Chap. XII.*

LUMINAL SODIUM (Winthrop)

Sedative. Hypnotic

Chemical Name: Luminal Sodium. Brand of Phenobarbital Sodium.

Formula: $(C_6H_5)(C_2H_5)$: C: CONH. CON. NaCO.

Description: The monosodium salt of Luminal; a white crystalline, hygroscopic powder, very soluble in water and suitable for hypodermic medication.

Action and Uses: A sedative and hypnotic, particularly adapted for subcutaneous and rectal administration when quick sedative effect is required, as in eclampsia, tetanus, status epilepticus, cocaine intoxication, dementia, drug addiction.

Supply: **LUMINAL SODIUM** (C.A.)—Tablets, gr 1½ (0.09 Gm)—Bottles of 50.

LUMINAL SODIUM (C.A.)—Ampules, gr 2 (0.13 Gm)—Boxes of 5.

LUMINAL SODIUM (C.A.)—Powder—Bottles ½ oz.

Administration: As for Luminal. As enema or suppository 3–6 gr (0.19–0.38 Gm). Solutions must be freshly prepared from the ampule and distilled water.

Bibliography: *See Chap. XII.*

LUNOSOL (Hille)

Antiseptic. Astringent

Official Name: Argenti Chloridum Colloidale Saccharatum.

Description: A preparation of colloidal silver chloride 10% and sucrose 90%; a white, granular powder, soluble in water, forming an opalescent colloidal solution; has a sweetish metallic taste.

Action and Uses: Is strongly antiseptic and germicidal; does not irritate the skin nor mucous membrane; does not coagulate albumin nor stain tissues; colloidal silver nitrate is equal in antiseptic potency to that of silver nitrate; *useful* in diseases of the eye, urethra, bladder, rectum and vagina.

Supply: **LUNOSOL** (C.A.)—Bottles of 1, 4, and 16 oz.

Administration: For urethra, 1% solution; bladder, 0.1–1% solution; rectum, 0.25%; vagina, 0.25%; nose, throat, ear, 5%; tampon, 10%; and cervix, 10% solution.

Preparation of Solution: 1 Teaspoonful (gr 90–100) in 2 oz. water or 6 gr to 1 dr. makes a 10% solution.

1 Teaspoonful (gr 90–100) in 1 qt. water offers a 0.1% or 1:1,000 solution.

Bibliography: *See Chap. XII.*

MAGNESIUM PEROXIDE (Roessler and Hasslacher)

Antacid. Antiseptic.

Composition: Contains Magnesium Peroxide 15%; available Active Oxygen 4.3%.

Description: A white tasteless powder consisting of magnesium peroxide and magnesium hydroxide; in water suspension liberates oxygen.

nor mucous membrane; does not coagulate albumin nor stain tissues; is equal in antiseptic potency to that of silver nitrate; *useful* in diseases of the eye, urethra, bladder, rectum and vagina.

Action and Uses: Mildly laxative, disinfectant, and antacid; is converted by gastric juices into magnesium salts and H_2O_2; *used* in rheumatism, gout, gastric hyperacidity, tonsillitis, pyorrhea.

Supply: **MAGNESIUM PEROXIDE**—In Bulk.

Administration: *Externally*—As dusting powder; locally in dentifrices; *Orally*—5–20 gr in Keratin coated capsules; Children 2–4 gr.

MAGNESIUM PHOSPHATE TRIBASIC (Merck)

Antacid

Official Name: Magnesii Phosphas Tribasicus.

Formula: $Mg_3(PO_4)_2$.

Description: A white odorless tasteless powder, almost insoluble in water, readily soluble in dilute mineral acids.

Action: Neutralizes gastric acidity without producing systemic alkalization.

Uses: As antacid in gastric hyperacidity and ulcer; as laxative in constipation.

Supply: **MAGNESIUM PHOSPHATE TRIBASIC (C.A.)**—Cartons, ¼ and 1 lb.

Administration: 15–75 gr (1.0–5.0 Gm) two to three times daily after meals.

MALLOPHENE (Mallinckrodt)

Urinary Antiseptic

Chemical Name: Beta phenyl-azo-alpha alpha diamino pyridine Hydrochloride.

Formula: $C_6H_5.\ N:N.\ C_5H_2N.\ NH_2NH_2.\ HCl$.

Description: A non-irritating, highly penetrating antiseptic dye; also known as Azophene.

Action: Is bacteriostatic toward staphylococci, streptococci, B. coli and gonococci; stimulates cellular function, favors regeneration of injured tissue; soothes mucous membranes, reduces complications; is eliminated through the kidneys, coloring the urine orange red; is active in acid and alkaline urine.

Uses: In prostatitis, pyelitis, cystitis, renal complications; in dental cases as gingivitis, socket work, trench mouth.

Supply: **MALLOPHENE**—Tablets, 0.1 Gm (gr 1½), sugar coated—Bottles of 25, 50, 500.

MALLOPHENE—Soluble Discs, 0.1 Gm (1½ gr)—Bottles of 50—Tubes of 10—Boxes of 5 tubes.

MALLOPHENE—Powder—Bottles of 5 Gm.

Administration: 2 or more tablets, three times daily during initial treatment; dosage then decreased.
In Prophylaxis, prior to cystoscopy and catheterization—2 tablets repeated in 3–4 hr.; maximum effect produced in 4–8 hr.
Urethral Injection—0.5% solution.
Instillation and Douching—0.25%.
Topically and as Dusting Powder—0.25%.
In Dentistry—In paste form with glycerin.

Preparation: 1 Disc in 100 cc of boiling water forms a 0.1% solution.

MALTINE PLAIN (Maltine)

Nutrient Tonic

Composition: A concentrated extract of malted barley, wheat and oats with all their soluble nutritive elements; contains water soluble vitamins and starch digesting enzymes; 1 Gm of Maltine converts in 30 min. at 40–42°c. 5–7 Gm of starch into maltose and dextrins; contains 70 units per oz. of antineuritic vitamin B and 36 units (9 units per ounce) of antipellagra vitamin B_2 or G; alcohol 3.88 %.

Action and Uses: An easily digestible carbohydrate food; bone producing, tissue building and nutrient; *useful* in malnutrition and anemia, as supplement in infant feeding, pregnancy and nursing mothers; as appetite stimulating nutrient and digestant vehicle.

Supply: MALTINE PLAIN (C.A.)—Bottles of 1 pt. and 1 gal.—Jars of 1 lb.

Administration: 1 dessert to 1 tablespoonful three times daily; children—according to age.

Combinations: 1. MALTINE WITH CASCARA SAGRADA—Contains with Maltine 45 gr Cascara Sagrada and 3.9 % Alcohol per fluid ounce; *For use* as tonic-laxative in constipation. *Supply*—Bottles 1 pt.—Jars 1 lb. and 1 gal. *Administered*—Teaspoonful or more as required; children in proportion.

2. MALTINE WITH MINERAL OIL AND CASCARA SAGRADA (C.A.)—Contains by volume Maltine 60 %, Mineral oil 40 %, Cascara sagrada (non-bitter) 10 gr per fluid ounce; Alcohol 1.9 %; *indicated* in spastic constipation accompanying conditions in which maltine is useful. *Supply*—Bottles 1 pt.—Jars 1 lb. and 1 gal. *Administered*—Dessertspoonful mornings and before retiring; children teaspoonful daily or as needed.

3. MALTINE WITH COD LIVER OIL (C.A.)—Contains Maltine 70 %, Cod liver oil 30 %, Alcohol 1.9 %, comprising per ounce 450 units vitamin A (U.S.P.), 100 units of Vitamin D (A.D.M.A.); is rich in Vitamin B and contains some Vitamin G; is palatable and easily assimilable. *Useful* in rickets and other deficiency diseases. *Supply*—Bottles of 1 pt.—Jars 1 lb. 1 gal; *administered* 2–4 teaspoonfuls three times daily; children in proportion.

4. MALTINE WITH COD LIVER OIL AND IRON IODIDE (C.A.)—Contains Cod liver oil 30 %, Maltine 70 %, Alcohol 1.9 %, with Iron iodide 2 gr per ounce comprising 450 units (U.S.P.) vitamin A, 100 units (A.D.M.A.) vitamin D per gram; is rich in Vitamin B and has some Vitamin G. *Used* in some types of goitre with malnutrition. *Supply*—Bottles 1 pt.—Jars, 1 lb. and 1 gal. *Dosage*—2–4 teaspoonfuls three times daily; children in proportion.

5. MALTINE WITH IRON IODIDE—Contains 2 gr Iron Iodide to the ounce of Maltine. *Supply*—Bottles 1 pt.—Jars 1 lb., and 1 gal. *Dosage*—2–4 teaspoonfuls three times daily; children in proportion.

6. MALTINE WITH CREOSOTE—Contains Maltine with 4 ♏ of creosote per ounce, alcohol 1.9 %; *For use* where creosote medication is desired. *Supply*—Bottles 1 pt.—Jars 1 lb., and 1 gal. *Administered* 2–4 teaspoonfuls three times daily; children in proportion.

7. MALTINE FERRATED—Contains Maltine with 8 gr soluble Ferric Pyrophosphate to the ounce; Alcohol 3.9 %. *Administered* where a nutrient and haematinic is desired. *Supply*—Bottles 1 pt.—Jars 1 lb. and 1 gal. *Dosage*—2–4 teaspoonfuls three times daily; children in proportion.

8. MALTINE WITH HYPOPHOSPHITES—Contains Maltine with Calcium hypophosphite 3 gr; Sodium hypophosphite 3 gr; Iron hypophosphite 2 gr per fluid ounce; Alcohol 3.9 %; *indicated* in all cases in which hypophosphites are generally employed. *Supply*—Bottles 1 pt.—Jars 1 lb., 1 gal. *Dosage*—2–4 teaspoonfuls three times daily; children in proportion.

9. MALTINE WITH IRON, QUINIA AND STRYCHNIA—Contains Maltine, 4 gr Iron pyrophosphate, 1 gr Quinine sulphate, $\frac{2}{45}$ gr Strychnia, per fluid ounce;

For use as nerve and general tonic. *Supply*—Bottles 1 pt.—Jars 1 lb., 1 gal. *Dosage*—2–4 teaspoonfuls three times daily; children in proportion.

10. **MALTO-YERBINE**—Contains Maltine with extract Yerba Santa, 30 gr per ounce, Alcohol 3.9%; *For use* in children's coughs and in the colds of the aged and of convalescents. *Supply*—Bottles 1 pt.—Jars 1 lb., 1 gal. *Dosage*—Tablespoonful three times daily; children teaspoonful or two, repeated as often as necessary.

11. **MALTINE AND COD LIVER OIL CONCENTRATE**—Contains Maltine and Cod liver oil, each tablet representing vitamin A—1,200 U.S.P. units vitamin D—300 units (A.D.M.A.). *For use* in vitamin deficiency and malnutrition, convalescence, invalids, expectant and nursing mothers. *Supply*—Tablets—Boxes of 12.

12. **MALTINE WITH SPLEEN MARROW AND IRON**—Contains Maltine with Spleenmarrow concentrate (Wilson) m 10, Iron and ammonium citrate gr 10 with traces of copper and cod liver oil concentrate and vitamin A, B, D and G, per ounce. Alcohol 5%, *For use* as hematopoietic stimulant in anemia. *Supply*—Bottles 1 pt.—Jars 1 lb., 1 gal. *Dosage*—2–4 teaspoonfuls three times daily with meals; children according to age; taken plain, with milk, cocoa or fruit juices.

Bibliography: *See Chap. XII.*

MANGACOL (Mulford Colloid)

Germicide

Description: Occurs as lustrous black-brown, non-hygroscopic scales, readily soluble in water; contains 20–25% metallic manganese.

Action and Uses: A stable, non-irritating, easily absorbed and assimilated preparation of Colloidal Manganese; is slowly eliminated, has prolonged action and causes no precipitation of tissue fluids. *For use* as germicide in coccogenic diseases, abscesses, boils, impetigo, furunculosis, eczema, folliculitis.

Supply: MANGACOL—Vials, Gm 10.

MANGACOL—Solution 10%, Ampule-Vial 25 cc.

Administration: ¼–1 gr (0.016–0.064 Gm); *intramuscularly;* used also *locally* and *intravenously.*

MANGANESE BUTYRATE (Crookes)

Non-specific Therapy

Description: A neutral, isotonic, non-colloidal solution of Manganese Butyrate; rapid in action and effective.

Action and Uses: Stimulates resistance in acute streptococcal infections.

Supply: MANGANESE BUTYRATE—Ampules 1 cc—Boxes of 6.

MANGANESE BUTYRATE—Bottles, Injection 15, 30 cc.

Administration: By *intramuscular* injection, in dosages 0.5–1 cc.

MANGANESE DIOXIDE (Govett)

Hematinic

Description: Contains in colloidal suspension 0.05% Manganese Dioxide; is practically tasteless, easily absorbed, non-toxic and non-irritating.

Action and Uses: That of manganese dioxide to stimulate oxidation processes; *For use* in furunculosis, anemia.

Supply: MANGANESE DIOXIDE—Bottles of 8 oz., containing ½ mg of drug per cubic centimeter.

Administration: 2–4 teaspoonfuls in half glass of water three times daily ½ hr. before meals.

MAN-NA-GLUCONATE (Drug Products)

Non-specific Therapy

Composition: A colloidal solution of Manganese Sodium Gluconate.

Action and Uses: Affects coccus infections, stimulates antibody formation in suppurative conditions; is non-irritating and stable; *For use* in furunculosis, carbuncle, acne, sycosis, chronic ulcers, gonorrhea.

Supply: MAN-NA-GLUCONATE—Hyposols, 1 cc for Intravenous use—containing 0.003 Gm metallic manganese and 2 % benzylic alcohol as anesthetic—Boxes of 12, 25 and 100.

Administration: Boils—Beginning with 0.5 cc increased to 2.0 cc, every fourth day, 6 injections.

Acne—12 injections, 1 every fourth day, beginning with 0.5 cc, increased by 0.5–1.5 cc.

Gonorrhea—1 cc every fourth day—2 doses, then once weekly.

MEDINAL (Schering and Glatz)

Hypnotic

Chemical Name: Sodium salt of Diethylmalonylurea; Barbital Sodium.

Formula: $(C_2H_5)_2C$: (CON. Na. CONH): CO.

Description: White crystalline powder, of somewhat bitter taste; is readily soluble in water (1:5).

Action and Uses: Sedative and hypnotic; is easily absorbed and quickly eliminated, causing no after effects. *For use* in insomnia and nervousness.

Supply: MEDINAL—Tablets, gr 5 (0.324 Gm)—Boxes of 12—Bottles 50, 100 and 500.

MEDINAL—Powder—Bottles of ½ oz.

MEDINAL—Suppositories, gr 10 (0.643 Gm)—Boxes of 6.

MEDINAL—Elixir—Bottle of 6 oz.

Administration: *Oral*—5–15 gr (0.324–0.972 Gm) of powder or 1–2 teaspoonfuls of elixir at bedtime.
Rectal—5–10 gr (0.324–0.643 Gm), in form of suppository.
Subcutaneously—7½ gr (0.480 Gm).

MELUBRIN (Metz)

Analgesic, Antipyretic

Chemical Name: Phenyl-dimethyl-pyrazolon Amino-methane-sulphonate.

Formula: $C_{11}H_{11}N_2O$. NH. CH_2SO_3. Na.

Description: A white, odorless almost tasteless crystalline powder, easily soluble in water forming an unstable solution; is slightly soluble in alcohol.

Action and Uses: Powerful antipyretic and analgesic; in ordinary dosage is non-toxic and non-depressant to cardio-vascular and respiratory systems; *Used* to relieve pain in neuralgia, neuritis, sciatica, rheumatism; as febrifuge in febrile conditions.

Supply: **MELUBRIN**—Tablets gr 15 (C.A.)—Tubes of 10.

MELUBRIN—Powder (C.A.)—Bottles of 1 oz.

Administration: 15–30 gr (1–2 Gm) every 3 or 4 hr.; maximum dose to 150 gr (10 Gm) daily.

MENTHOL-Y (N.Y. Quinine)

Synthetic Menthol

Chemical Name: Methylpropylphenyl Hexahydride.

Formula: $C_{10}H_{19}OH$.

Description: Has same chemical constitution as Japanese menthol; occurs as colorless acicular crystals, of strong odor and peppermint taste; slightly soluble in water, freely soluble in alcohol, chloroform, ether, petrol benzene.

Action: As for menthol; analgesic, antiseptic, anesthetic and stimulant.

Uses: As Japanese menthol substitute, in all instances where the latter is indicated.

Supply: **MENTHOL-Y**—Bottles of 1, 4 and 16 oz.—Tins of 5 and 25 lb.

Administration: *Average Dose*—1 gr.

In Vomiting—1/6–3 gr, as indicated.

Dental—Crystals applied in cavity.
Externally—1:5 in oil, 1:10 in ointment base.

ME-OX-OL (Tucker Pharmacal)

Disinfectant

Composition: Methylchlor Oxybenzol. Chlor-cresol.

Description: A germicidal agent against micrococcus aureus destroying the organism in 2% solution in 5 min.; also effective against bacillus coli, typhosus, pyocyaneus; is readily soluble in water, forming a clear, non-irritating, penetrating, cleansing and non-poisonous solution; does not attack tissue, metal or rubber.

Action and Uses: Indicated as germicide and antiseptic in wounds, abscesses, burns, cuts, abrasions; as deodorant gargle, douche and in obstetrical practice.

Supply: **ME-OX-OL**—Bottles, 2 fl. oz.

Administration: *As Disinfectant*—4 cc to pint of water;
As Antiseptic—4 cc to 1/2 pt. of water;
For Sterilization of Instruments—9 cc to 1/2 pt. of water;
As Douche—8–16 cc to each quart of water.

MERCIOL (Mulford Colloid)

Antiluetic

Description: Occurs in lustrous red-brown non-hygroscopic scales, readily soluble in water; contains 20% Mercuric Iodide.

Action and Uses: A stable, non-irritating Colloidal Mercuric Iodide, readily absorbed and assimilated; is slowly eliminated and of prolonged action; does not cause precipitation of tissue fluids; is antiluetic *for use* in all stages of syphilis.

Supply: **MERCIOL**—Vials, Gm 10.

MERCIOL—Capsules Soluble, gr 1 and gr 2—Bottles of 100.

MERCIOL—Ointment 5%—Tubes of ½ oz.

Administration: *Dosage*—⅙–½ gr (0.012–0.032 Gm).
Locally as ointment.

MERCURETTES

Antiluetic

Description: Oblong cakes or briquettes of cacao butter, delicately perfumed, containing 50 gr (3.25 Gm) of metallic mercury, minutely subdivided and uniformly distributed throughout the mass.

Action and Uses: As for metallic mercury; is readily absorbed and permits accurate dosage; can conveniently be halved or quartered with a sharp knife, without being touched by the fingers; *used* in syphilis; also in parasitic skin diseases.

Supply: **MERCURETTES (C.A.)**—Packages of 6, 50 and 100 cakes. **(Parke, Davis)**

MERCURIAL CREAM, BLUE—Containing 10% **(Burroughs Wellcome)** Metallic Mercury in Creocamphor base; *Intramuscular* injection m 16, gr 1½; *Supply*—Bottles of 2 oz.

CALOMEL CREAM—Containing 5% Calomel in Creocamphor base; *Intramuscular* injection m 16, gr ¾; **(Burroughs Wellcome)**

Supply—Bottles of 2 oz.

Administration: Mercurettes should be vigorously rubbed or slapped into the skin two to three times weekly; the creams—*intramuscularly* twice weekly.

Caution: Signs of mercurialism should be guarded against during administration.

MERCURIC OXYCYANIDE **(Abbott)**

Antiluetic

Official Name: Hydrargyri Oxycyanidum.

Formula: $Hg(CN)_2HgO$.

Description: A white or nearly white, fine powder, containing 51.7–56% mercuric cyanide and 44.3–48% of mercuric oxide; is soluble in about 80 parts of water.

Action and Uses: An antiseptic more powerful but less irritating than mercuric chloride; does not corrode metals; *used* in the treatment of syphilis.

Supply: **MERCURIC OXYCYANIDE**—Ampules (C.A.) 5 cc, containing gr ⅛ (0.008 Gm) of mercuric oxycyanide—Boxes 6, 25 and 100.

MERCURIC OXYCYANIDE—Ampules (C.A.) 5 cc, containing gr ¼ (0.016 Gm) of mercuric oxycyanide—Boxes 6, 25 and 100.

MERCURIC OXYCYANIDE—Ampules (C.A.) 5 cc, containing gr ⅙ (0.01 Gm) of mercuric oxycyanide—Boxes of 6, 25 and 100.

Administration: *Intravenously*—With great caution, one to two times weekly.

MERCURIC SALICYLATE

Antiluetic

Official Name: Hydrargyri Salicylas.

Composition: A compound of Mercury and Salicylic Acid containing not less than 54% nor more than 59.5% of Mercury.

Description: An odorless, white, slightly yellowish or slightly pinkish powder; practically insoluble in water and in alcohol.

Action and Uses: Antiluetic. *For use* in the treatment of syphilis.

Supply: **MERCURIC SALICYLATE** (C.A.)—Ampules—Sterile, 1 cc, containing in suspension Mercuric Salicylate gr 1 with Butyn 0.6 %, Camphor 10 %, Eugenol 1 %, in neutral vegetable oil—Boxes of 12 and 100. **(Abbott)**

HYPOLOID MERCURY SALICYLATE—1 cc–gr 1½ (0.097 Gm); *Administration*—1 cc weekly, *intramuscular* injection; *Supply*—Boxes of 10 and 100. **(Burroughs Wellcome)**

MERCURY SALICYLATE CREAM—20 and 10 %; *Administration*—1 cc weekly, *intramuscular* injection; *Supply*—Jars of 2 oz. **(Burroughs Wellcome)**

MERCURY SALICYLATE (C.A.)—Ampules, Sterile—of 3 strengths gr 1, gr 1½, gr 2, with a mixture of vegetable fats, liquid at body temperature—Boxes of 12 each. **(Hynson, Westcott and Dunning)**

MERCURY SALICYLATE (C.A.)—Ampules Glaseptic—gr 1, gr 2 of Mercuric salicylate, Apothesine 0.01 Gm; in olive oil 1 cc—Boxes of 12. **(Parke, Davis)**

Administration: After warming ampule in warm water until liquefied, is injected *intramuscularly* only, at 3–5 day intervals.

MERCUROCHROME

Antiseptic

Chemical Name: The disodium salt of 2:7-dibromo-4-hydroxy mercurifluorescein.

Formula: $NaOOC.C_6H_4C:C_6H_2OBr:OC_6HBr(ONa)(HgOH) + 3H_2O$.

Composition: Contains 24–26 % of Mercury.

Description: Occurs in irridescent green scales and granules; odorless, permanent in air, freely soluble in water, insoluble in chloroform and ether; aqueous solutions are cherry red, stable and do not precipitate blood serum.

Action: Potent and efficient germicide; destroys bacillus coli and staphylococcus aureus in the urine in dilution of 1:1,000 in 1 min.; causes no systemic ill effects.

Uses: *For use* in urethritis, cystitis, pyelitis; in ophthalmia neonatorum and other eye and ear affections; in abscesses, septicemia and infections of all types.

Supply: **MERCUROCHROME** (C.A.)—Tablets 4.6 gr (0.294 Gm)—Bottles 30 and 100. **(Hynson, Westcott and Dunning)**

MERCUROCHROME (C.A.)—Sealed tubes 7½ gr (0.480 Gm) for hypodermic use—Boxes of 6. **(Hynson, Westcott and Dunning)**

MERCUROCHROME (C.A.)—Powder—Bottles of 10 and 100 Gm. **(Hynson, Westcott and Dunning)**

MERCUROCHROME (C.A.)—Ampules 10 and 20 cc of 1 % solution, stabilized with 0.18 % of ammonium hydroxide—Boxes of 6, 25, 100. **(Searle)**

Administration: **In Dentistry**—3–5 %, for sterilization of root canals, in gingivitis, stomatitis, aphthae.

Gonorrheal Urethritis and Cystitis—1–2½ % solution, as injection and irrigation.

Ophthalmia—0.5–2.5 % solutions.

For Local Use—0.5–5 % solutions; greater concentrations in special conditions.

Ureteral Catheterization—1 %, in kidney pelvis infections.

Intravenously—0.4 %, prepared directly from the drug, in freshly distilled water and not boiled; dosage—1–5 mg per kg body weight.

Caution: Intravenous injection may be followed by transient vomiting, diarrhea, elevation of temperature, prostration, mercurial stomatitis.

Incompatibles: Acids, alkaloidal salts and local anesthetics. Fresh made stains, may be removed with acidulated alcohol; fixed stains by Labaraque solution or any other hypochlorite, followed by dilute acid; stained linen is soaked for 2 min. in 20% chlorinated soda solution, then in added ¼ volume of 5% acetic acid, agitated and mixed.

Bibliography: *See Chap. XII.*

MERCUROCHROME, COLLOSOL BRAND (Crookes)

Germicide

Description: Irridescent green scales or granules, readily soluble in water; contains 26.8% mercury; prepared by the action of mercuric acetate on dibromo-fluorescein.

Action and Uses: Antiseptic; non-colloidal germicide; *For use* in numerous conditions where antiseptic and germicidal action is desired.

Supply: MERCUROCHROME—Scales (for preparing solutions) Gm 10, 25, 50, 100.

MERCUROCHROME—Solution, Aqueous: 2% Topical—Bottles 1, 4, 8, 16 oz.

MERCUROCHROME—Solution, Aqueous: 2%, Topical—Bottle, 5 cc.

MERCUROCHROME—Solution, Alcoholic: 5% (in 50% alcohol)—Bottles ½ oz. with dropper.

MERCUROCHROME—Solution, Alcoholic: 5% (in 50% alcohol)—Bottles 1 oz.

MERCUROCHROME—Solution, Isotonic: 2% with ophthalmic pipette—Bottles ½ oz.

MERCUROCHROME—0.4% Intravenous Set—25 cc, containing Scales 0.1 Gm, Isotonic glucose solution 25 cc, for 1 injection.

MERCUROCHROME—Pessaries—Boxes of 6.

MERCUROCHROME—Pigmentum: 1, 2 oz.

MERCUROCHROME—Tampons—Boxes of 3.

Bibliography: *See Chap. XII.*

MERCUROCOL (Mulford Colloid)

Antiluetic

Description: Occurs as greyish black lustrous non-hygroscopic scales, readily soluble in water; contains 10–12% Metallic Mercury.

Action and Uses: A stable, non-irritating, readily absorbed and assimilated form of Colloidal Mercury; is slowly eliminated, has prolonged action, does not cause precipitation of tissue fluids and is less toxic than non-colloid mercurials; *For use* in syphilis and relapsing malaria.

Supply: MERCUROCOL—Vials, Gm 10.

MERCUROCOL—Solution 1%, Ampule-vial 25 cc.

MERCUROCOL—Ointment 10%—Tubes ½ oz.

Administration: ⅛–½ gr (0.008–0.032 Gm); Solution—¼–6 cc; Ointment—topically; *Intravenously*, as indicated.

MERCUROL (Parke, Davis)

Antiluetic

Official Name: Hydrargyri Nucleinas.

Description: A compound of mercury with nucleinic acid derived from yeast; is a brownish white powder soluble in warm water, insoluble in alcohol; contains 20% metallic mercury, and is available only in combination with Iodalbin.

Action and Uses: As for soluble mercurial compounds; has marked antisyphilitic and bactericidal power; is active in the presence of serum; *For use* as antisyphilitic and as local antiseptic.

Supply: **MERCUROL (C.A.)**—Tablets—Containing Iodalbin gr 5 (0.324 Gm) and Mercurol gr 1 (0.064 Gm)—Bottles of 100.

Administration: 1 or 2 tablets, as required.

MERCUROPHEN (Sharp and Dohme)

Germicide

Chemical Name: Sodium Oxymercury-oxinitrol-phenolate.

Description: An odorless, brick red powder, freely soluble in water, of somewhat metallic taste and slightly staining; is stable but forms sediment when exposed to air or CO_2; is superior to phenol or mercuric salts; contains 50% mercury.

Action and Uses: A mercurial germicide used for disinfection of instruments, catheters, surgeons' rubber gloves; also of skin, sputum, urine, pus and for similar purposes; as germicide in gonorrheal urethritis, pneumococcus conjunctivitis, pyogenic skin infections,—impetigo, sycosis, furunculosis.

Supply: **MERCUROPHEN**—Powder—Vials of 10 Gm.

MERCUROPHEN—Tablets 1 gr—Bottles of 100.

Administration: Sterilization of instruments, catheters, gloves—1:5,000 solution; of urine, feces, pus, utensils—1:2,000; in diseases of skin—1:1,000 solution for 1 minute only; for application to mucous membranes—1:5,000–1:15,000 solution.

Bibliography: *See Chap. XII.*

MERCUROSAL (Parke, Davis)

Antiluetic

Chemical Name: Di-sodium-hydroxy-mercuri-salicyl-oxy-acetate.

Formula: $C_6H_3COONa. OCH_2COONa. HgOH$.

Description: A synthetic compound of mercury; a white amorphous powder, freely soluble in water, faintly alkaline to phenolphthalein; contains 43.85% by weight of metallic mercury.

Action and Use: Antisyphilitic; compared with bichloride on the basis of contained mercury is only one-fourth as toxic; does not precipitate blood serum; can be injected intramuscularly with a minimum of discomfort, but the intravenous method is preferable, the tolerated dose is larger and repeated injections cause no material injury to vein.

Supply: **MERCUROSAL (C.A.)**—For Intramuscular Use—0.05 Gm in sealed glass tube—Packages of 12 and 100; also packages of 50 tubes, 10 doses in each tube.

MERCUROSAL (C.A.)—For Intravenous Use—0.1 Gm in sealed glass tube—Packages of 12 and 100; also packages of 50 tubes, 10 doses in each tube.

MERCUROSAL (C.A.)—Solution—For Intravenous Use—Ampules containing 3 gr (0.1 Gm) in 5 cc of distilled water—Boxes of 6, 25 and 100.

MERCUROSAL (C.A.)—For Intravenous or Intramuscular Use—Bottles, rubber-diaphragm-capped, 50 cc, containing 0.1 Gm Mercurosal in each 4 cc.

Administration and Dosage: Usual intravenous dose 0.1 Gm, daily or every other day, for 15–20 injections.
Intramuscular dose 0.05 Gm or more, at intervals of 3 or 4 days.

Caution: During a course of Mercurosal treatment, iodides if used should be administered with very great caution, to avoid the risk of mercuric iodide formation. Incompatible with acids and strong reducing agents.

MERCURY BENZOATE (Abbott)

Antisyphilitic; Gonocide

Official Name: Hydrargyrum Benzoicum.

Formula: $Hg(C_6H_5COO)_2 + H_2O$.

Description: The mercuric salt of benzoic acid; a white crystalline powder, slightly soluble in water, more soluble in salines, insoluble in alcohol and ether.

Action: As for mercurials; antiluetic and gonocidal.

Uses: In syphilis and locally in gonorrhea.

Supply: **MERCURY BENZOATE**—Ampules, 1 cc, 2 % solution containing gr 1/3 of mercury benzoate in 2½ % sodium chloride solution per ampule—Boxes of 12 and 100.

Administration: Lues—1 ampule, *intramuscularly*, every second day.
Gonorrheal Urethritis—As irrigation with equal parts of sodium chloride, in 1:2,000–1:1,000 solutions.

MERCURY CYANIDE (Merck)

Germicide

Official Name: Hydrargyrum Cyanatum.

Formula: $Hg(CN)_2$.

Description: White or colorless, odorless prismatic crystals, of bitter metallic taste and exceedingly poisonous; soluble at 15°c in about 13 parts of water and 15 parts of alcohol; more soluble in boiling water and boiling alcohol; very slightly soluble in ether.

Action and Uses: An alterative, antiseptic, antisyphilitic; like mercuric chloride is a powerful antiseptic and germicide but less irritating to the skin and mucosa. Internally *used* as diuretic in cardiac disease; externally—in ophthalmic and rhinologic affections, diphtheria, croup, pelvic infections.

Supply: **MERCURY CYANIDE** (C.A.)—Bottles 1 oz. ¼ and 1 lb.

Administration: *Orally*—1/16–1/8 gr (0.004–0.008 Gm) per diem.
Externally—1:4,000 or 1:2,000 solution.
Hypodermically—25–35 m (1.5–2.1 cc) of 1 % solution, intramuscularly also intravenously.
Tampons—0.04 % solution, in membranous rhinitis.
Gargle—0.01 % solution, in diphtheria or croup.

MERCURY SUCCINIMIDE

Antiluetic

Official Name: Hydrargyri Succinimidum.

Formula: $Hg[(CH_2CO)_2N]_2$.

Description: The mercuric salt of Succinic Acidimide; a white crystalline powder, soluble in about 5 parts of hot and 20 parts of cold water, in 300 parts of alcohol.

Action: As for mercurials; is non-irritating, stable, effective; antisyphilitic, alterative, antiseptic.

Uses: *For use* in luetic conditions where mercurials are indicated; also in infections: acute miliary and pulmonary tuberculosis, typhoid, broncho-pneumonia.

Supply: **MERCURY SUCCINIMIDE** (C.A.)—Ampules 1 cc, containing Mercury Succinimide gr 1/4 (0.016 Gm), with Butyn 0.6%—Boxes of 12, 100—Bottles of 60 cc. **(Abbott)**

HYDRARGYRI SUCCINIMIDI—Hypodermic Tabloids Gr 1/5 (0.013 Gm) soluble, intramuscular—Tubes 12, 50 and 500. **(Burroughs Wellcome)**

MERCURY SUCCINIMIDE (C.A.)—Bottles of 1 oz., 1/4 lb., 1 lb. **(Merck)**

MERCURY SUCCINIMIDE (C.A.)—Glaseptic Ampules 1/6 gr (0.01 Gm), each cubic centimeter containing 0.01 gr Mercury Succinimide, 0.005 gr Apothesine, in saline—Boxes of 12, 100. **(Parke, Davis)**

MERCURY SUCCINIMIDE (C.A.)—Ampules, each cubic centimeter containing 1/6 gr (0.01 Gm)—Boxes of 12. **(Sharp and Dohme)**

MERCURY SUCCINIMIDE (C.A.)—Tablets, Hypodermic 1/10 gr (0.006 Gm) and 1/5 gr (0.012 Gm)—Tubes of 20—Bottles of 100. **(Sharp and Dohme)**

Administration: *Intramuscularly*—1 ampule or gr 1/6–1/4 (0.01–0.016 Gm), once daily or every other day.
Subcutaneously—8–15 m (0.5–1 cc) of an 2.5% aqueous solution, which does not precipitate albumen.
Orally—Gr 1/6–1/4 (0.01–0.016 Gm) daily.

Caution: Urine and gums are to be watched for signs of mercurial irritation.

MEROXYL (Hynson, Westcott and Dunning)

Antiseptic

Composition: A mixture of the sodium salt 2, 4-dihydroxy-3, 5-dihydroxy-mercuri benzophenone-2'sulphonic acid, 50%, with ammonium 2, 4-dihydroxybenzophenone 2 sulphonate, sodium acetate and water.

Description: Occurs as pink colored powder, easily soluble in water.

Action and Uses: A local antiseptic; *For use* as wet dressing in wounds, ulcers, abrasions; as irrigation of infected wounds, bladder, in acute gonorrhea, abscess, carbuncle and other inflammations; as douche in vaginitis, endocervicitis.

Supply: **MEROXYL**—Tablets (C.A.) 2.3 gr (0.147 Gm)—Boxes of 30.

Administration: As wet dressing and irrigation—0.1% solution; for other applications—in strengths of 0.5% and over.

Bibliography: *See Chap. XII.*

MERTHIOLATE (Lilly)

Antiseptic. Germicide

Chemical Name: Sodium Ethyl Mercuri Thiosalicylate.

Formula: $C_2H_5.\ HgS.\ C_6H_4COONa$.

Description: A mercurial solution of high germicidal potency; in dry state occurs as light cream colored, odorless, orthorhombic, crystalline powder, containing 49% mercury; is readily soluble in water and saline, miscible with soap and alcohol.

Action: Bactericidal and antiseptic; potent in the presence of organic matter; non-toxic, non-irritating, non-staining and stable in solution; is not affected by heat, cold or dilution.

Uses: *Useful* as rapid and effective surface antiseptic and germicide, on skin and mucous membranes; in eye, nose, throat, genitourinary practice; for disinfection of instruments and similar uses.

Incompatibles: Strong acids, iodine, salts of heavy metals, boric acid preparations.

Advantages: High germicidal activity, sustained antiseptic effect, freedom from irritation, stability.

Supply: **MERTHIOLATE**—Solution 1:1,000 (C.A.), containing 1 Gm Merthiolate, ¼ Gm Sodium Borate and Sodium Chloride for isotonicity per 1,000 cc of water—Bottles 4 oz. and 1 pt.

MERTHIOLATE—Tincture, 1:1,000 (C.A.), Alcohol-acetone-water soluble—Bottles 4 oz. and 1 pt.

MERTHIOLATE—Ointment 1:2,000 (C.A.)—Jars 1 oz. and 1 lb.

MERTHIOLATE—Jelly 1:1,000 (C.A.), containing Merthiolate 0.1%, Eucalyptol 0.016%, Eugenol 0.016% in water-soluble base—Tubes ½ oz.

MERTHIOLATE—Ophthalmic Ointment, 1:5,000 (C.A.); 1 dr.—Collapsible tubes with pin point nozzle.

Administration: For skin disinfection the tincture is indicated; in septic infected wounds, in nose and throat conditions the aqueous solution, 1:1,000; for eyes 1:5,000 solution; for bladder irrigation 1:5,000 to 1:10,000; for instrument disinfection 2:1,000 solution.

Bibliography: *See Chap. XII.*

MESOTAN (Winthrop)

Antiarthritic. Analgesic

Chemical Name: Methyloxymethyl Ester of Salicylic Acid. Brand of Salmester.

Formula: $C_6H_4OH.\ CO.\ O.\ (CH_2O.\ CH_3)$.

Description: A clear, yellowish, faintly aromatic oily fluid, slightly soluble in water, readily soluble in fixed oils and alcohol.

Action: Predominantly local; is readily absorbed from the skin, requiring no inunction, relieving pain and swelling; is an active counterirritant, free from disagreeable odor; valuable as auxiliary to internal salicylate therapy.

Uses: In all types of muscular and articular rheumatism; in gout, lumbago, sciatica and neuralgia.

Supply: **MESOTAN** (C.A.)—Bottles of 1 oz.

Administration: Is mixed ordinarily with olive or cottonseed oil, 1 part of Mesotan to 2, 3 or 4 parts of oil; applied gently without rubbing and covered with light permeable dressing; to avoid irritation, the site of application should be changed, and intervals of a day or two allowed before using the same site; applications usually made twice daily.

MESUROL (Winthrop)

Antiluetic

Chemical Name: Basic Bismuth-methoxy-hydroxy-benzoate. Brand of Benzobis.

Formula: $C_6H_3.\ OCH_3.\ COO.\ OH.\ Bi(OH)_2$.

Description: A yellowish-gray powder, insoluble in water and most organic solvents; contains 54–57 % of bismuth; remains sterile when freely exposed to air for long periods.

Action and Uses: As for bismuth preparations; being well tolerated permits the use of large dosage; injections are painless, absorption prompt, toxicity rather slight. *Used* in secondary, tertiary and congenital syphilis.

Supply: MESUROL—Powder—Bottles of 15 Gm.

MESUROL—Ampules (C.A.) 1 cc (a 20 % emulsion in sesame oil, each cubic centimeter containing ¾–1 gr of bismuth in synthetic combination)—Boxes of 10.

Administration: Deep intramuscular injections, once or twice weekly, beginning with 0.5 cc, increased to 1 cc for 8–12 doses.

Children, dosage in proportion; infants, from 0.05–0.1 cc.

Caution: Care of the mouth and examinations of the urine are advisable during treatment.

Bibliography: *See Chap. XII.*

METAPHEN (Abbott)

Germicide. Antiseptic

Chemical Name: The anhydride of 4-nitro-5-hydroxy-mercuri-ortho cresol.

Formula: $C_2H_2.\ CH_3ONO_2Hg$.

Composition: Contains from 56–57 % of Mercury in organic combination.

Description: A yellow, odorless and tasteless powder, insoluble in water, almost insoluble in methyl alcohol.

Action: A germicide more powerful than mercuric chloride; is relatively non-irritating to mucous membranes or skin and without corroding effect on metallic instruments or rubber.

Supply and Uses: METAPHEN—Tincture (C.A.), a 1:200 alcohol-acetone-aqueous solution—Bottles 1–4 oz. and 1 gal.; *For use*—as skin sterilizer, disinfectant.

METAPHEN in Oil-A, a 1:5,000 solution in neutral olive oil with 3 gr of Menthol per ounce—Bottles 16 oz. and 1 gal.; *For use*—in irrigation of acute and chronic gonorrheal and other infections of the urinary tract; in diseases of the eye, ear, nose, throat and chronic skin affections.

METAPHEN in Oil-C—A 1:1,000 solution for ear, nose and throat therapy.

METAPHEDRIN—Inhalant, an aqueous solution of Ephedrine 1 % with Metaphen 1:5,000—Bottles of 4, 16 oz., 1 gal.; *For use*—in colds, hay fever, sinus and nasal infections.

METAPHEN INHALANT 99—Containing Metaphen 1:2,500, Ephedrine 1 % and mineral oil made compatible by special process—Bottles 1, 4 and 16 oz.; *For use* as ephedrine solutions—in coryza, hypertrophic rhinitis, sinusitis.

METAPHEN 2,500 (C.A.)—A solution of 1:2,500 in water, with ⅓ % Sodium Bicarbonate and Sodium Hydroxide; for disinfecting and sterilizing surgical instruments, rubber goods; in colds, skin affections—Bottles of 1 and 4 oz.

METAPHEN C—Sterilization solution (84 % alcohol); for colds, sterilization of instruments—Bottles 1 qt. and 1 gal.

METAPHEN AQUEOUS—An aqueous solution of 1 % Ephedrine in Metaphen 1:5,000; for sinus irrigation, tonsillar and pharyngeal infections—Bottles 1 and 4 oz. and 1 pt.

METAPHEN—Ampules 10 cc (C.A.), 1:1,000, for intravenous use in septicemia, prostatitis, cystitis—Boxes of 6, 25 and 100.

METAPHEN—Ointment 1:5,000, for scabies, pediculosis, ringworm, sycosis and other cutaneous eruptions of parasitic or bacterial origin—Tubes 2 oz.

METAPHEN—Eye Ointment 1:3,000—Tubes of ⅛ oz.

METAPHEN—Suppositories (*Vaginal*) 1:2,000—Boxes of 12.

METAPHEN—Liquid soap 1:1,000, as cleanser and disinfectant—Bottles 4 oz.

METAPHEN—Antiseptic Bar Soap 1:500 for office use, prophylaxis.

Bibliography: *See Chap. XII.*

METAPHYLLIN (Hurst)

Cardiotonic. Diuretic

Chemical Name: Aminophyllin. Theophyllin-Ethylenediamine; also called Euphyllin.

Formula: $(NH_2CH_2CH_2NH_2)_2(C_7H_8N_4O_2)_3$.

Description: A crystalline powder freely soluble in water.

Action and Uses: Cardiotonic, vasodilator and diuretic in edema of cardio-renal origin, in cardiac insufficiency and in angina pectoris.

Supply: **METAPHYLLIN (C.A.)**—Tablets 0.1 Gm—Tubes 20—Bottles 100 and 250.

METAPHYLLIN (C.A.)—Suppositories 0.36 Gm—Packages of 10.

METAPHYLLIN (C.A.)—Ampules 2 cc, 0.48 Gm; Intramuscular—Boxes 6.

METAPHYLLIN (C.A.)—Ampules 10 cc, 0.24 Gm, Intravenous—Boxes 5.

METAPHYLLIN (C.A.)—Powder—Vials 5, 10 and 25 Gm.

Administration: 1–2 tablets, three to four times daily, in water; or 2–4 suppositories daily.

Intramuscularly, or Intravenously—1–3 ampules daily.

Combinations: **METAPHYLLIN WITH CALCIUM**—For intravenous, oral, or rectal use in cardiac insufficiency, edemas of cardiorenal origin, coronary sclerosis, angina pectoris, cardiac and bronchial asthma, arteriosclerosis, hypertension. *Supply*—Tablets—Tubes 20—Bottles 100 and 250. Ampules 10 cc, intravenous—Boxes of 5. Suppositories—Boxes of 10.

Administration—As for Metaphyllin.

METAPHYLLIN WITH CALCIUM AND IODINE—Has the additional advantages of Iodine.

Supply—Tablets—Tubes of 20—Bottles of 100 and 250; Suppositories—Cartons of 10; Ampules, 10 cc intravenous—Cartons of 5.

Administration—Of Metaphylin with Calcium—1 tablet three times daily. Suppositories 2 daily.

Ampules 2–3 injections weekly.

Bibliography: *See Chap. XII.*

METHATROPIN (Pharmedic)

Antispasmodic

Chemical Name: Methyl Homatropine Bromide.

Formula: $C_{16}H_{21}NO_3CH_3Br$.

Description: A white powder, easily soluble in water, soluble with difficulty in alcohol, insoluble in ether.

Action: That of atropin, but is said to be 30 to 50 times less toxic; affects strongly the parasympathetic system, relaxes non-striated musculature, relieves spasm, reduces secretions, and is mydriatic.

Uses: To relieve pain and spasm in biliary colic, pylorospasm, intestinal hyperperistalsis; to check hyperhidrosis and gastric hypersecretion; used also in cardiac irregularities, bronchial asthma, bladder irritation, nocturnal enuresis, and as sedative in alcoholic excitation periods.

Supply: METHATROPIN—Tablets 0.0025 Gm—Tubes of 20—Bottles of 100.
METHATROPIN—Powder—Vials 1 Gm.

Administration: *For internal uses*—1 to 2 tablets three times daily.
As mydriatic—2%; to paralyze accommodation—3%.

METHYLENE BLUE

Antidote

Chemical Name: Methylthionine Chloride U.S.P.

Formula: $C_{16}H_{18}N_3ClS. + 3H_2O$.

Description: A sterile, standardized 1% solution of methylene blue.

Action and Uses: A chemical antidote in poisoning with carbon monoxide or cyanide. Theory of action is that of activation of oxygen by methylene blue, when aerobic oxidation is interfered with, as in above conditions. On intravenous injection is rapidly reduced to colorless leuco-compounds; is excreted in the urine and feces (traces in the sweat and sputum), partly unchanged and partly as methylene azure; raises blood pressure by cardiac stimulation and vasoconstriction and stimulates respiration; large doses are depressant. Its action is antagonistic to drugs that stimulate the vagus.

Supply: METHYLENE BLUE—Ampules 50 cc—Packages of 1, 6, 25, 100. (Loeser)
METHYLENE BLUE—Ampules 50 cc—Packages of 1 and 6. (Rorer)

Administration: *By Intravenous Injection*—50-100 cc of 1% solution, given warmed as soon after exposure as possible, and repeated as necessary.

METRAZOL (Bilhuber-Knoll)

Cardiotonic

Chemical Name: Pentamethylenetetrazol.

Formula: $C_5H_{10}N_4$.

Description: A white tasteless crystalline chemically neutral substance; stable, sterilizable and soluble in water.

Action: A promptly acting circulatory and respiratory stimulant, its effect lasting ½-2 hr.; stimulates central nervous system and vasomotor and respiratory centers; is compatible with other cardiac drugs.

Uses: Is *used* in sustaining circulation in chronic cardiac insufficiency and depression in infectious diseases, in relieving congestion and promoting diuresis; in sudden circulatory failure and cardiovascular collapse, in respiratory distress and heart failure; in shock, asphyxia neonatorum, drug depression.

Advantages: Is quickly effective even if subcutaneously injected or orally administered; is not excitant as is caffeine; may be used in conjunction with digitalis and ephedrine.

Supply: METRAZOL—Ampules (C.A.), 1 cc, gr 1½ (0.1 Gm)—Boxes of 6 and 20.
METRAZOL—Tablets (C.A.), gr 1½ (0.1 Gm)—Tubes of 10—Bottles of 100.
METRAZOL (C.A.)—Powder—Vials of 5 and 25 Gm.
METRAZOL—Solution (C.A.), 10% aqueous—Vials of 10 cc.

Administration: Ampules 1 or 2, several times daily, *subcutaneously*.
Powder—gr 1½-3, or solution—gr 1½-3, several times daily, *orally*.

Bibliography: *See Chap. XII.*

METYCAINE (Lilly)

Local Anesthetic

Chemical Name: Hydrochloride of gamma-(2-methyl piperidino)-propyl benzoate; formerly known as Neothesin.

Description: An odorless, white, crystalline powder, easily soluble in water, alcohol and chloroform; insoluble in ether and olive oil; is stable in solution and unaffected by heat or light.

Action and Uses: A local anesthetic producing prompt diffusible profound anesthesia on mucous membranes or other surfaces; is especially *useful* in eye, ear, nose and throat work; also in urology, surgery and dentistry.

Supply: METYCAINE—Tablets gr 2½ (0.15 Gm)—Tubes of 10.

METYCAINE—Solution 2%—Bottles of 1 oz.

METYCAINE—Powder—Bottles of ½ oz.

METYCAINE—Ampules 1 cc, 1%—Boxes of 6.

Combination: METYCAINE AND ADRENALIN—Ampules 1 cc (metycaine 2%, adrenalin 1:25,000)—Boxes of 6. Ampules 2.5 cc (metycaine 2%, adrenalin 1:50,000)—Boxes of 6.

Administration: By topical application, instillation or infiltration.

In Urology—2–4%.

In Ophthalmology—2%.

In Nasolaryngology—2%.

In Dentistry—2–4%.

Bibliography: *See Chap. XII.*

MOOGROL (Burroughs Wellcome)

Leprosy Therapy

Chemical Name: Ethyl Chaulmoograte.

Composition: A mixture of ethyl esters of the unsaturated acids, chaulmoogric and hydnocarpic of chaulmoogra oil.

Description: An oily liquid, almost colorless, limpid, of faint odor and not unpleasant taste.

Action and Uses: *For use* in leprosy.

Supply: MOOGROL—Bottles of 25 and 100 cc.

Administration: *Intramuscularly*—1 cc once weekly; increased by 1 cc to a maximum of 3–5 cc weekly.

Orally—1–5 cc daily, in increasing doses.

Bibliography: *See Chap. XII.*

NAIODINE "LOGEAIS" (Fougera)

Iodine Therapy

Description: A 1% aqueous solution of Sodium Iodide, stabilized, non-toxic, non-irritating.

Action and Uses: An antispasmodic and general sedative; is readily assimilated; *For use* in herpes zoster, lumbago, sciatica, intercostal and trigeminal neuralgia, rheumatic iritis; in spasmodic affections—dyspnea, angina pectoris, asthma, emphysema; in inflammatory conditions—acute articular rheumatism, chronic arthritis, orchitis, otitis, sinusitis, chest pains in pneumonia or pleurisy.

Supply: NAIODINE "LOGEAIS"—Ampules, 5 cc, 10 cc, 20 cc, each cubic centimeter containing gr 1/6 of Sodium Iodide—Boxes of 6.

Administration: *Intensive Treatment*—20–40 cc in accordance with severity of case; injected *intramuscularly*, two or three times daily.
Maintenance Dose—5–10 cc daily.

NASON'S PALATABLE COD LIVER OIL

(Tailby-Nason)

Nutrient

Composition: Cod Liver Oil of a potency of 1,000 vitamin A and 150 vitamin D units per gram; is made palatable by the addition of 0.5 % of essential oils as flavoring agent.

Action and Uses: As for cod liver oil.

Supply: NASON'S PALATABLE COD LIVER OIL (C.A.)—Bottles 4 oz. and 12 oz.

Administration: 1/2–1 teaspoonful three times daily.
Children 1/4–1/2 teaspoonful.

NATURAL SALICYLATES (Merrell)

Antiarthritic

Description: Prepared from genuine natural oil of birch; not a synthetic product.

Action and Uses: Analgesic, antiarthritic; is less irritating to the gastrointestinal tract; is better tolerated especially in massive dosage. *Indicated* in all conditions where salicylates are used: colds, tonsillitis, influenza, neuralgia, rheumatism, arthritis.

Supply:

ACID SALICYLIC—(Fine crystals) (C.A.)—Vials 1 oz.—Bottles 1/4 and 1 lb.

SODIUM SALICYLATE—Tablets (C.A.)—gr 5 (lettered "M")—Bottles of 100, 500 and 1,000.

SODIUM SALICYLATE—Powder (C.A.)—Bottles 1 oz., 1/4 and 1 lb.

SODIUM SALICYLATE—Ampules 10 cc (20 %) Intravenous—Boxes 6 and 25.

SODIUM SALICYLATE WITH SODIUM IODIDE—15 1/2 gr each—Ampules 20 cc Intravenous—Boxes 6 and 25.

Administration: 1 gr Natural Sodium Salicylate per pound of body weight, for 24 hr., then 15 gr a day; treatment is best accompanied by thorough alkalinization.

NATURAL VITAMIN D (S.M.A. Corp.)

Vitamin Therapy

Description: A highly potent extract of the antirachitic principle of cod liver oil; is neither a concentrate nor an irradiation product; 10 drops are equivalent to 3 teaspoonfuls of standard, potent cod liver oil; a natural Vitamin D product prepared by the "Zucker Process."

Action and Uses: For the prevention or cure of rickets.

Supply: NATURAL VITAMIN D—Bottles, dropper top, 5 cc and 50 cc, in special cartons.

Administration: Average prophylactic dose—10 drops daily; curative 15–30 drops daily, depending on the severity of the case.

Bibliography: *See Chap. XII.*

NEOARSPHENAMINE

Antiluetic

Chemical Name: Neosalvarsan. Arsphenamine-S. 3-diamino-4-dihydroxyarseno-mono-methylene sulphoxylate sodium.

Formula: $NH_2OH. C_6H_3As: AsC_6H_3. OH. NH(CH_2O)OSNa.$

Description: A combination of arsphenamine with formaldehyde-sulphoxylate; a yellow hygroscopic powder, readily soluble in water, yielding a clear neutral solution; contains 19–20% arsenic.

Action and Uses: Is highly toxic against spirochetes and trypanosomes; *For use* primarily in syphilis, especially primary and secondary; also in other spirilla infections.

Supply: **NEOARSPHENAMINE** (C.A.)—Ampules 0.15, 0.3, 0.45, 0.6, 0.75, 0.9, 1.5, 3.0, 4.5 Gm—Boxes of 1 Ampule—Packages of 10 ampules with 10 ampules distilled water, in above strengths. **(Abbott)**

NEODIARSENOL (C.A.)—Ampules 0.15, 0.3, 0.45, 0.6, 0.75, 0.9. **(Diarsenol)**

NEOARSPHENAMINE (C.A.)—Ampules 0.15, 0.3, 0.45, 0.61, 075, 0.9 and 1.5 Gm. **(Mallinckrodt)**

NEOARSPHENAMINE (C.A.)—Ampules 0.15, 0.3, 0.45, 0.6, 0.75, 0.9 Gm with ampules of 10 cc distilled water—Packages for 1 dose and 10 doses. **(Merck)**

NEOARSPHENAMINE (C.A.)—Ampules 0.15, 0.30. 0.45, 0.60 Gm. **(Searle)**

NEOARSPHENAMINE (C.A.)—Ampules 0.15, 0.30, 0.45, 0.60, 0.75, 0.9, 3.0, 4.5 Gm, with 10 cc ampule of distilled water. **(Squibb)**

Administration: *Intravenously* by syringe method, occasionally *intramuscularly.* Injections usually given at weekly intervals; in early stages of disease twice weekly. Dosage regulated according to individual requirements; treatment alternated with or followed by courses of mercury, bismuth or both, with or without rest periods after each course.

Dosage—Initial—Males, 0.3 Gm followed by 0.4, etc.; females, smaller dosage; children, average doses, from 3–9 mo. 0.3 Gm.

Intramuscularly—0.1–0.15 Gm; from 1–2 yr.—0.2 Gm; from 2–3 yr.—0.25 Gm; from 3–5 yr. 0.3 Gm.

Caution: Is contraindicated in advanced circulatory disease, neural affections, cachexias, and in those with idiosyncrasy for arsenic.

Preparation: For solution of the Neoarsphenamine, triple glass-distilled water supplied with ampules, or freshly distilled water at room temperature, or sterile 4% saline solution from chemically pure sodium chloride is to be used; ampule is immersed in alcohol for sterilization and detection of flaws in glass; if powder becomes discolored due to alcohol entering the ampule, contents must be discarded. 10 cc of water are used for the total dose in the intramuscular method; powder is sprinkled on the surface of the water and allowed to dissolve without stirring, heating or the addition of alkalis; when completely dissolved solution is filtered through sterile moistened gauze. Neoarsphenamine solutions should not be allowed to stand more than 20 min. before use; left over portions of powder or solution should be discarded.

NEO BORNYVAL **(Riedel)**

Palatable Valerian

Chemical Name: Isovaleryl Glycolate.

Formula: $(CH_3)_2CH. CH_2COO. CHCOO. C_{10}H_{17}.$

Description: A colorless, almost odorless, tasteless oily liquid; soluble in alcohol, ether and benzene, insoluble in water.

Action: That of valerianates, but free from disagreeable odor and gastric irritation; induces effective sedation and analgesia with little discomfort.

Uses: *For use* in hysteria, nervous insomnia, cardiovascular and other neuroses, morbid and emotional states, hypochondria, neurasthenic anaphrodisia, menopausal disturbances.

Supply: NEO BORNYVAL—Pearls m 4—Bottles of 25.

Administration: 1–3 pearls two to four times daily after meals.

NEOCAINE (Anglo-French)

Local Anesthetic

Chemical Name: Para-aminobenzoyl Diethylaminoethanol Hydrochloride.

Formula: $NH_2. C_6H_4. COO. C_2H_4. N(C_2H_5)_2HCl$.

Description: Colorless crystals or powder, soluble in water and alcohol, insoluble in ether.

Action and Uses: A local anesthetic of low toxicity and maximum relaxation. *Used* principally for spinal anesthesia; also for local and regional work.

Supply: NEOCAINE—(Spinal) Ampules 0.05, 0.08, 0.10, 0.12, 0.15, 0.20, 0.30 Gm—Boxes of 12.

NEOCAINE—(Local and Regional) 0.50 Gm—Boxes of 12 tubes, each tube containing 2 capsules.

NEOCAINE—(Local and Regional) Capsules 0.05 Gm—Bottles of 20, 100.

NEOCAINE SURRENINE—Ampules ½ % and 1 % solution—Boxes of 12.

NEOCAINE—Pure (without Surrenine)—Ampules ½ %, 1 % and 2 % solution—Boxes of 12.

NEOCAINE—Pure (without Surrenine)—Vials rubber-capped 10 cc, ½ %, 1 % and 2 % solution—Boxes of 6.

Administration: *Spinal*—The spinal fluid is allowed to drop directly into the ampule, dissolving the pure crystals; this solution is then slowly injected, aspirated and reinjected.

Bibliography: *See Chap. XII.*

NEOCINCHOPHEN

Uricolytic. Analgesic

Chemical Name: Ethyl ester of methyl-phenyl-quinolin-carboxylic-acid; also known as Novatophan.

Formula: $CH_3C_9H_4N. C_6H_5COOC_2H_5$, 6: 2: 4.

Description: A pale, yellow powder, odorless and tasteless; nearly insoluble in water and dilute alkalies, freely soluble in ether and chloroform.

Action: Is analgesic, antipyretic, uric acid eliminant and cholagogue; increases permeability of kidneys for uric acid and excretion of urates; decreases uricacidemia.

Uses: In all conditions associated with uricacidosis; acute rheumatic fever, gout, arthritis, neuralgia, sciatica; before intraocular operations.

Caution: Large doses may cause albuminuria, acid eructation, diarrhea, scarlatinal rash, cardiac distress, dysuria.

Advantages: Is devoid of gastric irritation, low in toxicity and almost tasteless.

Supply: NEOCINCHOPHEN (C.A.)—Tablets, gr 5 (0.324 Gm) gr 7½ (Abbott) (0.480 Gm)—Boxes of 20—Bottles 100 and 1,000.

NEOCINCHOPHEN (C.A.)—Powder—Packages of 1 and 4 oz. (Abbott)
NEOCINCHOPHEN (C.A.)—In bulk, in quantities desired. (Benzol)
NEOCINCHOPHEN (C.A.)—Cartons ¼–1 lb. (Merck)

Administration: 1–2 tablets (7½–15 gr) three or four times daily or oftener, after meals, with abundance of water; continued intermittently for periods of 3 or 4 days.

Bibliography: *See Chap. XII.*

NEO-ERGOT (Abbott)

Uterine Stimulant

Description: A solution of purified Ergot Alkaloids of standardized potency and free from non-specific amines, inert and toxic matter; is palatable.

Action and Uses: A uterine muscle stimulant and hemostatic; more stable and more dependable than ordinary fluid extract of ergot; *used* in menorrhagia and metrorrhagia.

Incompatibles: Alkalies or oxidizing agents.

Supply: NEO-ERGOT—Vials 1 oz.

Administration: *Orally*—15–30 m after labor; in post-partum hemorrhage—30–60 m; in menorrhagia and metrorrhagia—10–30 m.

Bibliography: *See Chap. XII.*

NEOFOSFAN (Winthrop)

Phosphorus Therapy

Chemical Name: Sodium salt of Dimethylaminomethylphenylphosphinous Acid; Brand of Phosodyl.

Formula: $N(CH_3)_3.\ P.\ OH.\ ONa. + 3H_2O$.

Description: A white crystalline substance, readily soluble in water; contains about 11% phosphorus in combination.

Action: Possesses distinct tonic properties, improves the appetite and increases weight and strength; is relatively non-toxic; is excreted as ethyl sulphuric acid in the urine causing but little renal irritation; therapeutic action is probably exerted before disintegration of the compound has occurred.

Uses: Neurasthenia, psychoneuroses, convalescence from acute infections and surgical operations, in early pulmonary tuberculosis.

Supply: NEOFOSFAN—Ampules 1 cc (1%)—Boxes of 10.

Administration: 1 ampule *intramuscularly* or *subcutaneously*, daily or at intervals of several days; 20–40 injections constitute a course.

NEO-IOPAX (Schering)

Radiopaque Medium

Chemical Name: Disodium salt of 3.5 diiodo-4-pyridoxyl-N-methyl-2.6-dicarboxylic acid; also known as Uroselectan-B, abroad.

Formula: $C_8H_3O_5NI_2Na_2$.

Description: A pyridine derivative containing 51.5% iodine; is extremely soluble, dissolving 100 Gm in 100 cc of water; in ampules the sterilized solution remains stable, not changing chemically.

Action and Uses: For the visualization of kidneys and ureters by the intravenous method; to study strictures, bladder disease, fistulae, urinary hemorrhages, enlarged prostate, ureteral deformities; also as functional test in determining the capacity of the kidneys by their rate of elimination.

Supply: NEO-IOPAX (C.A.)—Ampules 20 cc (containing 15 Gm of Neo-Iopax dissolved in 20 cc of a 10% solution of invert sugar, a mixture of equal quantities of dextrose and levulose).

NEO-IOPAX—(Retrograde) (C.A.)—Ampules 10 cc—Bottles 50 cc.

Administration: *Intravenous Method*—One ampule is first warmed to body temperature in water bath; the fluid is then slowly injected into the cubital vein, with an ordinary 20 cc syringe; children are given correspondingly smaller doses.
Single Exposures—Made in 20–30 min. after injection;
Series of Exposures—First is made in 10 min., second—in 30 min., third—in 50 min. after injection; bladder is emptied before second and third exposures. In normally functioning kidneys, the best pyelograms may be obtained in 2–5 min.
Retrograde Method—After warming solution to body temperature, is injected into ureters; as excretion takes place immediately the X-rays are ordinarily also taken immediately.

Contraindications: Care should be exercised in its use in cases of acute and chronic uremia; in severe systemic diseases accompanying disorders of the urinary tract; in hepatic disease.

Bibliography: *See Chap. XII.*

NEONAL (Abbott)

Hypnotic. Sedative

Chemical Name: N-butyl ethyl barbituric acid; -N-butyl ethyl-malonylurea.

Formula: $nCH_9(C_2H_5)CCONH.\ CONH.\ CO$ (ring closure between C and CO)

Description: A white crystalline, odorless powder, of slightly bitter taste; readily soluble in alcohol (1 in 5), ether (1 in 10); very slightly soluble in cold water.

Action: As sedative and hypnotic is about three times as effective as barbital and thus given in correspondingly smaller dosage.

Uses: In nervous tension, neuroses and similar states; in insomnia and psychasthenia; in preoperative sedation; in whooping cough, alcoholism.

Supply: NEONAL—Tablets (C.A.) 1½ gr (0.1 Gm)—Bottles of 10, 100 and 1,000.

NEONAL—Powder (C.A.)—Bottles of 1 and 4 oz.

Administration: From ¾–6 gr (0.5–0.4 Gm) in divided doses; maximum dose in 24 hr. 6 gr.

NEO-RIODINE "ASTIER" (Gallia)

Alterative

Chemical Name: Sodium Iodo-propanol-sulfanate.

Formula: $C_3H_6O_4ISNa$.

Composition: A 10% aqueous solution of an organic sodium salt of Iodine, containing 44% iodine; each cubic centimeter represents 0.10 Gm Iodo-propanol Sulfanate of Sodium or about 38–40 mg iodine.

Description: Neutral, colorless solution, slowly soluble in water.

Action and Uses: As alterative in angina pectoris, coronary sclerosis, hypertension, arteriosclerosis; in asthma, emphysema, syphilis; in acute and chronic rheumatism and lymphatism.

Contraindications: Myocardial degeneration, pulmonary edema, tuberculosis.

Supply: NEO-RIODINE "ASTIER"—Ampules 5 cc—Boxes of 10, 50.

Administration: *Intramuscularly*—Beginning with 1 cc increased to 2, 3 and 5 cc, three or four times weekly, in courses of 8–10 injections and repeated where necessary; may also be administered intravenously.

NEOROBIN (Abbott)

Chrysarobin Therapy

Description: A derivative of Chrysarobin extracted from Goa powder, derived from the Araroba tree of Brazil.

Action: Is five times as powerful as chrysarobin and 50% more active as a reducing agent; produces more vigorous hyperemia and desquamation with less staining.

Uses: Psoriasis, parapsoriasis, dermatitis seborrhoeica, dandruff, pityriasis rosea and other dermatologic conditions where a stimulant and roborant effect is desired.

Supply: NEOROBIN—Vials, 1 gr, 25%—Packages of 6.

Administration: *Externally*—1–5 gr per ounce of petrolatum.

Caution: To prevent oxidation it should not be exposed to air for any prolonged period; ointment must be prepared immediately upon opening vial and dispensed in collapsible tubes.

Bibliography: *See Chap. XII.*

NEOSALVARSAN (Metz)

Antiluetic

Chemical Name: Sodium 3-diamino-4-dihydroxyarsenobenzene Methanol Sulphoxylate. Brand of Neoarsphenamine.

Formula: $NH_2. OH. C_6H_3. As: As. C_6H_3. OH. NH. (CH_2O)OSNa.$

Description: A yellow powder, readily soluble in water at room temperature, yielding a clear neutral solution.

Action and Uses: That of all arsenical preparations; is a powerful antiluetic; *used* in syphilis in all stages.

Supply: NEOSALVARSAN—Ampules (C.A.) Single dosage 0.15, 0.3, 0.45, 0.6, 0.75 and 0.9 Gm. with or without one 10 cc ampule of triple glass-distilled water.

NEOSALVARSAN—Ampules (C.A.) Multiple dosage; 1.5, 1.8, 3.0 and 4.5 Gm.

Administration: *Intravenously*—By syringe or by the gravity method; also intramuscularly. Dosage regulated according to case and indications; Males, initially 0.3 Gm followed by 0.4 and 0.6 Gm; Females, slightly smaller doses. Children, *intramuscularly*, average dose from 3–9 mo., 0.1–0.15 Gm; 1–2 yr., 0.2 Gm; 2–3 yr., 0.25 Gm; 3–5 yr., 0.3 Gm.

Injections are given at weekly intervals; in the early stages of the disease, 2 injections a week may be given; is generally alternated or followed by courses of mercury or bismuth or both, either by the continuous method or intermittently with a period of rest after each course.

Contraindications: Advanced neurologic and circulatory disease of non-syphilitic origin; fetid bronchitis; actively progressing tuberculosis; idiosyncrasy for arsenic.

Preparation of Solution: Water at room temperature, either supplied in ampules or other fresh triple distilled water, or 0.04% sterile saline prepared from chemically pure sodium chloride is utilized for dilution; 10 cc of the diluting fluid for each 0.1 Gm of Neosalvarsan is used in the intravenous gravity method; a total of

10–20 cc in the intravenous syringe method, and 5–10 cc in the intramuscular. The ampule containing drug is immersed in alcohol for sterilization; where the powder becomes discolored because of a defect in the glass ampule, the contents must not be used; the powder is sprinkled on the surface of the diluting fluid without stirring, heating or the addition of alkali. When completely dissolved, is filtered through sterile moistened gauze; must not be permitted to stand more than 20 min. before using; left over portions of powder or solution should be discarded.

NEO-SILVOL (Parke, Davis)

Antiseptic

Description: A colloidal combination of silver iodide, 20%, with a soluble protein base; occurs as cream colored, glistening granules, soluble up to 50% in water, slowly soluble in glycerin and insoluble in oil; aqueous solutions are opalescent by reflected light and milky by transmitted light; is not precipitated by sodium chloride, nor by urine, either acid or alkaline; is not affected by light; its solutions do not darken on drying.

Action and Uses: Antiseptic; is twenty times as active in affecting the gonococcus as is carbolic acid; is non-irritating to inflamed mucosa; *For use*—in all conditions where silver protein is employed.

Supply: NEO-SILVOL—Powder—Bottles 1 oz. and ¼ lb.

NEO-SILVOL—Capsules (C.A.) gr 6 (0.384 Gm) for preparing solutions—Bottles of 50 and 500.

NEO-SILVOL—Ointment (C.A.) 5%, in collapsible tin tubes with elongated nozzle.

NEO-SILVOL—Suppositories Vaginal (C.A.) 5%, in glycero-gelatin base, enclosed in soft tin—Boxes of 12.

Administration: Genitourinary—In urethritis, by irrigation or injection, 1–15%; in cystitis, 5–10 cc of 10% solution or weaker solutions in larger quantities; in vaginitis, cervicitis, 5–50% by irrigation or tamponade.

Eye, Nose, Throat—In blepharitis, simple and purulent conjunctivitis, gonorrheal ophthalmia, rhinitis and pharyngitis, 10–50%, according to conditions; following tonsillectomy in 10% solution by swab.

Dentistry—In dental caries, 20% solution, on cotton swab; for erosions and exposed roots, 50% solution; infected sinus, 5%, by irrigation; pyorrhea, 10% solution to flood roots.

Urography—Ureterally, 20% solution.

Bibliography: *See Chap. XII.*

NEOSKIODAN (Winthrop)

Radiopaque Medium

Chemical Name: 3.5 diiodo-4-pyridon-N-acetic acid diethanolamine. Brand of Neomethiodal; now known as DIATRAST.

Description: A white, odorless powder, readily soluble in water, and very stable even when boiled.

Action and Uses: Gives exceptionally clear roentgenograms; causes no local or systemic reaction; *For use* in intravenous urography.

Contraindications: Serious bilateral impairment of renal function, renal insufficiency, uremia.

Supply: NEOSKIODAN—Ampules 10 and 20 cc (35% by volume).

Administration: The usual dose 1 ampule (20 cc) given *intravenously;* if administered rapidly optimum time for exposure of the x-ray film is within 10–20 min. after injection; when the rate of injection is slow, the densest shadows usually appear after 15–30 min.

NEOSTAM (Burroughs Wellcome)

Parasiticide

Chemical Name: Stibamine Glucoside; nitrogen glucoside of sodium-p-aminophenylstibinate.

Description: An organic antimony compound, 1/20 as toxic as sodium antimony tartrate.

Action and Uses: A parasiticide in kala-azar, filiariasis, bilharziasis.

Supply: **NEOSTAM**—Vials of 0.05, 0.1 Gm, 0.2 Gm, 0.5, 1 Gm.

Administration: *Intravenously*—0.1 Gm per 100 lb. of body weight, administered as 4% solution in distilled water, on alternate days, until 3 Gm per 100 lb. of weight have been given.

NEO-SYNEPHRIN (Stearns)

Vasoconstrictor

Chemical Name: Levo-meta Hydroxyphenylethanolmethylamine Hydrochloride.

Formula: $C_6H_4OH.\ CHOH.\ CH_2.\ NH.\ CH_3HCl.$

Description: A white, crystalline substance, soluble in water and alcohol.

Action and Uses: A vasoconstrictor with prolonged action; affects muscle tissue directly and not through the myoneural junction; is not as effective as epinephrine, but less toxic; raises blood pressure, dilates coronary arteries, relaxes bronchial tubes and intestinal musculature, dilates pupil; raises tone of uterine muscle, relieves hyperemia and congestion; *used* in reducing nasal swelling in infections, in allergy, asthma; in cardiac weakness and hypotension; also in local anesthesia, minor surgery and dental operations.

Supply: **NEO-SYNEPHRIN**—Solution 1/4%, Aqueous, with 0.1% Sodium Benzoate, *For use* as vasoconstrictor—Bottles of 1 oz.

NEO-SYNEPHRIN—Solution 1%, Aqueous, with 0.1% Sodium Benzoate for making local anesthesia solutions—Bottles of 1 oz.

NEO-SYNEPHRIN-PROCAINE—Tablets, for local anesthesia; 1 Tablet dissolved in 1 cc of distilled water yields an isotonic solution of Procaine Hydrochloride 2%, Neo-Synephrin Hydrochloride 0.03%, Sodium Chloride 0.7%, Potassium Sulphate 0.4%—Bottles 100 tablets.

EMULSION NEO-SYNEPHRIN—Plain, 1/4% with Oil of Sesame and Sodium Benzoate 0.4%—Bottles 1 oz.

EMULSION NEO-SYNEPHRIN—Compound 1/4% with Camphor, Menthol and Oil Red Thyme, with Oil of Sesame, Sodium Benzoate 0.4%—Bottles 1 oz.

ELIXIR NEO-SYNEPHRIN—1/10%. *Supply*—In bulk.

NEPHRITIN (Reed and Carnrick)

Hormone Therapy

Description: A specially prepared extract from the cortex and convoluted tubules of kidney from young, normal animals; contains hormones thought to be associated with control of kidney function and metabolism.

Action: Induces diuresis without causing irritation of kidney parenchyma; increases urea elimination, decreases cylindruria, hematuria and edema.

Supply: **NEPHRITIN**—Tablets—Bottles of 80, 500 and 1,000.

Uses and Dosage: In acute nephritis—4 tablets four to eight times daily.
In chronic nephritis—4 tablets three to four times daily.
In uremia—4 tablets every 2 hr. throughout attack.
In albuminuria of pregnancy, and eclampsia—15–30 tablets daily.
As prophylactic against kidney complications in infectious diseases—2 tablets three times daily.

Bibliography: *See Chap. XII.*

NEUTRALON. LUDOSAN (Schering)

Antacid

Composition: A synthetic Aluminum Silicate combined with 12 % Sodium Silicate, now know as **Ludosan.**

Description: A fine, white, odorless, tasteless powder; the aluminum silicate is insoluble in water, the sodium silicate is soluble; the latter is also soluble in gastric hydrochloric acid.

Action and Uses: Is antacid and astringent; in the stomach, the sodium silicate portion readily dissolves to form sodium chloride and insoluble silicic acid, while the aluminum silicate forms a chloride and silicic acid; thus free acidity is reduced by both constituents and the gastric mucosa is covered by a protective coating; *used* in hyperacidity, peptic ulcer, duodenal ulcer.

Supply: LUDOSAN—Box of 100 Gm.

Administration: 1 teaspoonful in water, three times daily, before meals.

Combination: **BELLADONNA-LUDOSAN**—Contains Neutralon with 0.6 % Extract Belladonna; used in excessive vagus irritability and hypersecretion. Boxes of 100 Gm.
Dosage—1 teaspoonful in water, three times daily before meals.

Bibliography: *See Chap. XII.*

NIAZO (Schering)

Genitourinary Antiseptic

Chemical Name: 2 Butyloxy-2.6′-diamino 5.5′ azopyridin; also known as Neotropic.

Formula: $C_{14}H_{18}ON_6$.

Description: A micro-crystalline powder of slightly reddish tinge, forming a light yellow solution in water.

Action and Uses: A genitourinary antiseptic; is readily absorbed, highly penetrating and eliminated through the kidneys; relieves irritation in cystic tumor, gonorrheal infections; *used* in bacteriuria, cystitis, pyelitis, pyelonephritis and as post-operative urinary antiseptic.

Supply: **NIAZO**—Tablets, gr 1½ (0.097 Gm)—Bottles of 24 and 48.

Administration: 2 tablets three times daily for several weeks.

Bibliography: *See Chap. XII.*

NIZIN (Burroughs Wellcome)

Astringent. Antiseptic

Composition: A Zinc salt of Sulfanilic Acid.

Formula: $(NH_2.\ C_6H_4.\ SO_3)_2Zn$.

Action and Uses: Astringent and antiseptic; is non-irritating, non-staining, non-toxic and readily soluble in water; *For use* in gonorrheal vaginitis, urethritis, cystitis; in conjunctivitis, trachoma; in sluggish ulcers and moist eczema.

Supply: NIZIN—Soloid gr 2 (0.130 Gm)—Bottles of 100 and 500.

NIZIN—Soloid gr 20 (1.296 Gm)—Bottles of 25.

NIZIN—Bottles of 1, 4 and 16 oz.

Administration: *For Urethral or Vaginal Injection*—2 gr to 1 oz. water.
Vaginal Douche—1 teaspoonful to 1 qt. of warm water.
Topically—6 gr to 1 oz.
Eye Lotion and for Bladder Irrigation—1 gr to 1 oz.

NORMOLACTOL (Bischoff)

Antiseptic

Chemical Name: Calcium-Sodium Lactate.

Composition: A lactic acid and its calcium salt buffer mixture of hydrogen ion concentration 3.7.

Action and Uses: Is *used* in leukorrhea of any origin; for its buffer effect to reestablish the normal reaction and flora of vagina.

Supply: NORMOLACTOL—Tablets—Boxes 20 and 250.

Administration: 1 tablet inserted into vaginal canal each evening for 3 days.

Bibliography: *See Chap. XII.*

NORMAL HORSE SERUM

Hemostatic

Description: A clear blood serum obtained from healthy horses.

Action: Contains thrombokinase, which converts blood prothrombin into thrombin and interacts with fibrinogen to form fibrin; stimulates intestinal production of coagulen ferment.

Uses: In burns—to coagulate exuding tissue plasma, encourage normal epithelization, prevent infection, minimize absorption of toxins and scar formation; in hemorrhages of hematopoietic origin: melena neonatorum, hemophilia, purpura hemorrhagica; also in uterine hemorrhage, gastro-duodenal ulcer, bleeding from wounds and persistent epistaxis.

Supply: NORMAL SERUM (C.A.)—Cresol preserved—Packages 1 syringe container 10 cc—Bottles 25 and 100 cc. (Cutter)

NORMAL HORSE SERUM (C.A.)—With and without tricresol ¼%—Package of 1 syringe 10 cc—Vials 10 and 25 cc. (Gilliland)

NORMAL HORSE SERUM (C.A.)—Syringes 10 cc—Vials of 30 and 100 cc. (Lederle)

CONJUNCTIVAL TEST (C.A.)—For diagnosis of hypersensitiveness to horse serum protein—Vials 1:10 dilution, for 5–10 tests. (Lederle)

NORMAL HORSE SERUM (C.A.)—Package syringe 10 cc—Vials 20 cc. (Lilly)

NORMAL HORSE SERUM (C.A.)—With preservative, syringes of 10 and 20 cc—Packages of double end vial 50 cc with intravenous outfit—Bottles of 100 cc. (Mulford)

NORMAL HORSE SERUM (C.A.)—Syringes 10 cc—Packages 1 and 2—Package of 1 intravenous outfit 50 cc—Ampules 25 cc. (National Drug)

NORMAL HORSE SERUM (C.A.)—Package of 1 syringe 10 cc—Vials, rubber diaphragm, 10 and 30 cc. (Parke, Davis)

NORMAL HORSE SERUM (C.A.)—Syringes 10 cc 1 or 2 in package—Vials 20 and 50 cc. (Squibb)

THYROIDECTOMIZED HORSE SERUM—*For use* in hyperthyroidism—Vials, rubber stoppered, 30 cc. (Parke, Davis)

Dosage—Hypodermic, 1–2 cc every 2–3 days.

Oral—25 drops three times daily, increased by 1 drop until symptoms subside; then gradually reduced.

Administration: *Topically*—By pressure with gauze or cotton saturated with serum.

Burns—After area is bathed in normal saline for ½–3 hr. and devitalized tissue is removed, is sprayed with serum, covered with rubber dam; applied twice daily for 5–10 days.

Uterine Bleeding—Applied as packing.

Orally—30–100 cc repeated in 12–24 hr. intervals, as necessary.

Subcutaneously or Intramuscularly—10–20 cc daily repeated until 100 cc are administered.

Precautions: Ephinephrin and atropine must be on hand for possible horse serum anaphylaxis, shown by the appearance of an urticarial rash, swelling of mucous membranes, of joints and in more severe reactions also rapid pulse, lowered temperature, occasionally convulsions. In individuals with history of asthma or related protein anaphylactic conditions special caution must be exercised in the administration of horse serum.

NORWEGIAN COD LIVER OIL

Nutrient. Vitamin Therapy

Description: A fully refined, high grade oil, prepared from fresh livers of cod fish; is of light color, clear transparency and of high vitamin potency.

Action and Uses: As for cod liver oil; is the largest natural source of growth-promoting and infection-resisting vitamin A and antirachitic vitamin D.

Supply: **NORWEGIAN COD LIVER OIL**—Bottles of 8 and 16 oz. and gallons of 1 and 5. (McKesson and Robbins)

Dosage—Desertspoonful three times daily after meals.

Children: ½–2 teaspoonfuls.

SCOTT'S NORWEGIAN COD LIVER OIL (C.A.)—Containing vitamin A 1,000 (U.S.A.) units, vitamin D 250 (A.D.M.A.) units, per gram. Plain and Flavored—Bottles of 3, 6½ and 14 oz. (Scott and Bowne)

Administration: 2 teaspoonfuls daily, equivalent to 7,360 units vitamin A, 1,840 units vitamin D.

Combinations: **SCOTT'S EMULSION OF COD LIVER OIL** (C.A.)—Contains vitamin A 140 (U.S.P.) units and vitamin D, 70 (A.D.M.A.) units per gram; is prepared from 27.9 % (30 % by volume) plain cod liver oil, 12½ % glycerin, 1.56 % acacia 1.46 % tragacanth, 0.15 % flavoring and 0.13 % agar—Bottles of 8 and 16 oz. *Administration*—3 tablespoonfuls daily, containing 6,300 units vitamin A and 3,450 vitamin D units. (Scott and Bowne)

NOSTAL (Riedel-de Haen)

Hypnotic

Chemical Name: Isopropyl-bromallyl-malonylurea; also known as Noctal.

Formula: $C_{10}H_{13}O_3N_2Br$.

Description: Colorless, odorless, slightly bitter crystals; easily soluble in alcohol and acetone, soluble with difficulty in water, chloroform, benzine.

Action: Hypnotic, affecting the higher cerebral centers and inducing refreshing sleep resembling normal, for 6–8 hr.; is non-narcotic, non-habit forming and does not affect cardiovasculo-renal systems; is rapidly absorbed and four times as powerful as barbital.

Uses: In insomnia not due to pain, as that from overwork, nervousness, and in neurasthenia.

Supply: NOSTAL—Tablets, 1½ gr (0.097 Gm) (C.A.)—Packages of 10—Bottles of 50.

Administration: *As Hypnotic*—Adults 1–2 tablets; in severe cases 2–4 tablets, in hot water, milk or tea.
As Sedative—And in children, ½–1 tablet.

Bibliography: *See Chap. XII.*

NOVASPIRIN (Winthrop)

Antiarthritic

Chemical Name: Methylene-citryl Salicylic Acid. Brand of Salicitrin.

Formula: $(CH_2COO)_2(C_6H_4.\ COOH)_2C.\ COO.\ O.\ CH_2$.

Description: A grayish-white, odorless, crystalline powder of faintly acidulous taste; almost insoluble in water, easily soluble in alcohol, less soluble in ether and chloroform and stable in air; contains 62% of salicylic acid.

Action: As for salicylic acid, but is well borne even by the sensitive stomach, produces no tinnitus, cardiac depression nor sweating; is of agreeable taste and can be given for prolonged period.

Uses: In all rheumatic affections: acute articular rheumatism, muscular rheumatism, rheumatoid arthritis; also in influenza, colds, tonsillitis, various types of neuralgia.

Supply: NOVASPIRIN—Tablets (C.A.), 5 gr (0.3 Gm)—Bottles of 100.
NOVASPIRIN—Powder—Cartons 1 oz.

Administration: Adults, 10 to 15 gr (0.6–1.0 Gm), several times daily, increased to 30 gr (2.0 Gm) in severe cases if necessary.
Children, 2½–5 gr (0.15–0.3 Gm).

Bibliography: *See Chap. XII.*

NOVASUROL (Winthrop)

Diuretic

Chemical Name: Double salt of Sodium Mercurio-chlorphenoxylacetate with Diethylbarbituric Acid. Brand of Merbaphen.

Formula: $(NaOOCCH_2O)Cl.\ C_6H_3HgCO{:}\ NCO.\ C(C_2H_5)_2.\ CONH.$ (CO and NH joined by a bond)

Description: A white, crystalline, odorless powder, soluble in cold water with slight alkaline reaction; contains 33.9% of mercury in complex non-ionizable combination.

Action: Probably has direct action upon the tissues, abstracting water and salts held in colloidal combination; also has a direct effect upon the kidneys; diuresis begins 1–3 hr. after injection and lasts for 12–24 hr., occasionally 48 hr.

Uses: In all conditions where profuse and rapid diuresis is demanded; very valuable in cardiac dropsy, cardiorenal edema, nephroses, hepatic cirrhosis.

Supply: NOVASUROL—Ampules 1.2 cc (C.A.), 10% neutral sterile solution—Boxes of 5.

Administration: Ordinarily *intramuscularly*, but also given *intravenously;* first dose to determine tolerance, 0.5 cc, other injections 1 and 2 cc; repeated once or twice weekly; effect is heightened by the simultaneous oral administration of ammonium chloride or ammonium nitrate, 90–150 gr daily. Never administered subcutaneously.

Caution: Because of its high percentage of mercury, is contraindicated in acute nephritis and in chronic renal disease with marked tubular and glomerular changes; in susceptible individuals transient symptoms—headache, nausea, vertigo, stomatitis, vomiting, skin eruptions may occur.

Bibliography: *See Chap. XII.*

NOVATROPIN (Kretschmar)

Antispasmodic

Chemical Name: Homatropine Brommethylate; Homatropine Methyl Bromide.

Formula: $C_{16}H_{21}. NO_3. CH_3Br$.

Description: A white crystalline powder, readily soluble in water and in dilute alcohol; insoluble in ether.

Action and Uses: As for atropine, but fifty times less toxic; is mydriatic, antispasmodic and diminishes secretions in ptyalism, hyperchlorhydria, gastric ulcer, hyperhidrosis; relieves spasm in colic: biliary, ureteral, pyloric; in asthma, arteriosclerosis; also used in colds, cardiac irregularities and dental affections.

Supply: NOVATROPIN—Tablets (0.0025 gr)—Tubes of 20.

NOVATROPIN—Solution 0.2% (10 drops = 0.001 gr)—Bottles of 20 gr.

NOVATROPIN—Ampules (0.0025 gr)—Boxes of 3, 6.

NOVATROPIN—Powder, in bulk.

Administration: *Daily Dosage*—Adults 0.005–0.05 gr, children 0.001–0.01 gr; Ampules, one to three daily, *subcutaneously*. Tablets, 1 or 2 three times daily. Solution, 10 drops three to five times daily.

In Ophthalmology—2–5% solution, in accordance with duration of mydriasis desired.

Bibliography: *See Chap. XII.*

NOVIFORM (Heyden)

Antiseptic

Chemical Name: Tetrabrompyrocatechin Bismuth.

Formula: $Bi(C_6Br_4O_2)OH$.

Description: A finely divided yellow, odorless, tasteless powder; slightly soluble in alcohol and ether, insoluble in water; contains 30% of bismuth oxide.

Action: Antiseptic, astringent, deodorant; is easily spread over surface, adherent and sterilizable.

Uses: Surgery—In minor affections: furunculosis, carbuncles, abscesses, tubercular fistulae; in 10% oily solution—for injection into tubercular joints.

Dermatology—In condylomata, chancre, balanitis, intertrigo.

Gynecology—In vaginal fistula, after laparotomy.

Ophthalmology—As ointment in blepharitis, blennorrhagia.

Rhinolaryngology—After removal of polyps, septum operations, turbinectomy.

Dentistry—Tamponing abscesses, after extraction, on ulcerated gums, in osteomyelitis.

Supply: NOVIFORM—Powder—Bottles 1 oz.

Administration: Used in powder form, pure or with talcum; as bougies or ointment.

Bibliography: *See Chap. XII.*

NOVOCAIN (Metz)

Local Anesthetic

Chemical Name: Para-aminobenzoyl Diethylaminoethanol Hydrochloride. Brand of Procain Hydrochloride.

Formula: $NH_2C_6H_4COO.\ CH_2CH_2N(C_2H_5)_2CHl$.

Description: Colorless crystals or white crystalline, odorless powder; soluble in equal parts of cold water, less soluble in cold alcohol; the aqueous solution is neutral, not affected by prolonged or repeated boiling and may be autoclaved to 12 lb. pressure.

Action: A highly efficient local anesthetic, one of the safest and least toxic; virtually free from untoward effects on the respiratory and circulatory systems; does not affect the pupil.

Incompatibles: Caustic alkalies and their carbonates, iodine and iodides, picric and tannic acids, mercurous chloride and silver salts.

Supply: NOVOCAIN—Crystals (sterile)—Ampules of 50, 100, 120, 150, 200, 300, 500 mg—Boxes of 10—Vials, 5 Gm and 1 oz.

NOVOCAIN—Solution, 1% (C.A.)—Ampules 2 and 5 cc—Boxes of 10.

NOVOCAIN—Solution 20% (C.A.)—Ampules, 1½ cc and 5 cc—Boxes of 10.

NOVOCAIN—Tablets (C.A.)—1 gr (0.06 Gm)—Bottles of 100.

NOVOCAIN—Tablets, (F) (C.A.)—0.05 Gm—Tubes of 20—Bottles of 100.

NOVOCAIN—Tablets, (D) (C.A.)—Novocain 0.2 Gm, Sodium chloride 0.06 Gm—Tubes of 10—Bottles of 100.

"NOVOCAIN-SUPRARENIN SOLUTIONS (N.S.)" (C.A.)—Solution (Isotonic) "E," Novocain 2%, Suprarenin 1:20,000.
Ampules 1 cc—Boxes of 20.
Ampules 3 cc—Boxes of 10 and 100.
Ampules 6 cc—Boxes of 10.
Solution (Isotonic) "K," Novocain 1%, Suprarenin 1–50,000.
Ampules 2 cc and 6 cc—Boxes of 10.
Solution (Isotonic) "T," Novocain 2%, Suprarenin 1–50,000; (used when smaller quantity of Suprarenin than in "E" solution is desired).
Ampules 1 cc—Boxes of 20.
Ampules 3 cc—Boxes of 10 and 100.
Concentrated, Novocain 20%, Suprarenin 1–9,000.
Ampules 1½ cc and 5 cc—Boxes of 10.

"NOVOCAIN-SUPRARENIN TABLETS (N.S.)" (C.A.)—

"A"	Novocain	0.125	Gm,	Suprarenin	0.000125	Gm—	Tubes	of 10—	Bottles	of	100.
"B"	"	0.1	"	"	0.00025	" —	"	" 10—	"	"	"
"C"	"	0.05	"	"	0.000083	" —	"	" 50—	"	"	"
"E"	"	0.02	"	"	0.00005	" —	"	" 20—	"	"	"
"H"	"	0.06	"	"	0.00006	" —	"	" 15—	"	"	"
"K"	"	0.08	"	"	0.00006	" —		" 15—	"	"	"
"T"	"	0.02	"	"	0.00002	" —	"	" 20—	"	"	"
Pluglets		0.01	"	"	0.00002	" —	"	" 20—	"	"	"

Uses and Administration: General Surgery—Infiltration, ¼–½ %, according to volume required; for nerve block 1 %; for spinal anesthesia, Novocain crystals (100–300 mg), dissolved in spinal fluid. *Used* in all minor surgical operations, boils, carbuncles, abscesses, circumcision, removal of lipomas, warts, moles, foreign bodies, wound suturing, rectal surgery.

Rhinolaryngology—For injection 0.5–1 % with Suprarenin (1:1,000) in concentration of 3–5 m to the ounce.

Ophthalmology—For conduction and infiltration anesthesia 3 to 5 cc of 2 % solution usually suffice.

Urology—3 % for urethral anesthesia.

Bibliography: *See Chap. XII.*

NUPERCAINE (Ciba)

Local Anesthetic

Chemical Name: Alpha-butyl-oxycinchoninic Acid; Diethyl-ethylene-diamide Hydrochloride.

Formula: $C_9H_5N.\ OC_4H_9(2)CONH(CH_2)_2N(C_2H_5)_2HCl(4)$.

Description: A white crystalline powder easily soluble in water; is unaffected by heat up to 120°c.

Action: Local anesthetic. Is non-narcotic and many times more powerful than cocaine or procaine with more lasting effect; is suitable for any type of local anesthesia.

Supply: NUPERCAINE—Ampules (C.A.) 2 cc; Containing 1:200 Nupercaine in buffered salt solution for Spinal Anesthesia—Cartons of 10.

NUPERCAINE—Ampules (C.A.) 5 cc; Containing 1:1,000 Nupercaine in physiologic salt solution, for Injection Anesthesia other than spinal—Cartons of 10—Ampules 25 cc in individual cartons.

NUPERCAINE—Solution 1:50 (C.A.) Nupercaine in physiologic salt solution for topical use in Nose and Throat only—Bottles of 1 oz.

NUPERCAINE—Tablets 0.05 Gm (C.A.) (approx. ⅚ gr) each—Tubes of 20.

NUPERCAINE—Powder—Bottles of 1 and 5 Gm.

NUPERCAINE—Ointment, Nupercaine 1 % in neutral ointment base—Tubes 1 oz.—Jars 1 lb.

NUPERCAINE—Ampules 2 cc (C.A.); Containing 1:1,000 Nupercaine with 1:100,000 Epinephrine, for Injection Anesthesia other than spinal—Cartons of 5.

NUPERCAINE—Ampules 5 cc (C.A.); Containing 1:1,000 Nupercaine with 1:100,000 Epinephrine, for Injection Anesthesia other than spinal—Cartons of 10.

Uses and Administration:

Infiltration and Nerve Block—1:2,000–1:1,000 in physiologic sodium chloride solution, with 0.1–0.5 cc of epinephrine hydrochloride 1:1,000 to each 100 cc.

Caudal Anesthesia—30–35 cc of 1:1,000 or 20–25 cc of 1:500 solution in physiologic sodium chloride.

Spinal Anesthesia—7.5–10 mg (1.5 cc–2.0 cc) of 1:200 Nupercaine (hydrochloride) in buffered salt solution, or 5–15 cc of 1:1,500 in 0.5 % sodium chloride solution.

Surface Anesthesia—In nose and throat procedures, 1–2½ %.

Topical Application—In burns, sunburn, eczema, ulcers, carcinomatous lesions, for the relief of pain and prurigo in 1 % ointment or 1:4,000–1:1,000 aqueous solution; in pruritus ani, hemorrhoidal discomfort, rectal ulcers and fissures in 1 % ointment.

In Rhinitis, Pharyngitis, Hay Fever—As spray in 1:500–1:200 solution in combination with epinephrine or ephedrine.

In Pain of Tuberculous Laryngitis or Neoplasm of Larynx—1–2.5 % in physiologic salt solution with epinephrine.

In Ophthalmology—In 1:1,000–1:200 solution.

In Genitourinary Tract—In 1:1,000–1:500 solution.

Caution: Aqueous solutions should be slightly on the acid side of neutrality (Optimum pH 6.2–6.5); the water should be distilled, the sodium chloride chemically pure; where solution is slightly alkaline and base is liberated, a drop or two of dilute HCl, but not in excess, may be added and solution shaken until precipitate disappears.

Bibliography: *See Chap. XII.*

OLEO-BI (Roche)

Antiluetic

Composition: An injectable Bismuth Oleate in very fine suspension in Olive Oil, with an equivalent of 0.05 Gm of Bismuth to each cubic centimeter.

Uses: For the treatment of syphilis, especially its late manifestations; *used* either alone, or alternated with other antiluetic remedies.

Supply: **OLEO-BI**—Ampules (C.A.), 2 cc, equivalent to 0.1 Gm Bismuth—Cartons of 12.

Administration: Contents of 1 ampule (2 cc) injected deep into the gluteal muscle, two or three times a week in a course of 12–20 injections, followed by 1 mo. of rest before repetition.

OPTOCHIN BASE (Merck)

Pneumococcicide

Chemical Name: Ethylhydrocupreine Base; Numoquin Base.

Formula: $C_6H_{28}N_2O_2$.

Description: A faintly yellowish-white bitter powder; insoluble in water, soluble in alcohol, oils, fats and acid gastric juices.

Action and Uses: Specific for pneumococcus infections; powerful pneumococcicide even in high dilutions; is fully active in 1:400,000 serum.
Internally—In specific therapy of pneumonia (including postoperative); also as prophylactic against pneumonia in severe or prolonged exposure to cold.
Externally—To prevent pneumococcus infection following operations for cataract, in serpiginous corneal ulcer.

Supply: **OPTOCHIN BASE**—Powder (C.A.)—Vials ⅛ oz.

OPTOCHIN BASE—Tablets (C.A.) gr 2 (0.13 Gm)—Bottles of 30.

Administration: **In Pneumonia**—4 gr (0.25 Gm) administered with 5 fl. oz., (150 cc) milk (no other food), 5 times daily, day and night, for 3 days only; treatment should begin preferably on the first, but not later than the third day following onset of disease. In infections not due to the pneumococcus or where the treatment in pneumococcus pneumonia is begun later than the third day, no results are obtainable.
Externally—Applied in 1–2 % ointment or oily solution in serpiginous ulcer of the eye.

Caution: *For internal use*, Optochin Base *only* should be employed; if administered as above outlined, no serious visual or auditory disturbances are likely, but if mild disturbances do occur, the drug is suspended for a day, and then resumed in smaller dosage.

Bibliography: *See Chap. XII.*

OPTOCHIN HYDROCHLORIDE (Merck)

Pneumococcicide

Chemical Name: Ethylhydrocupreine Hydrochloride. Numoquin Hydrochloride.

Formula: $C_{21}H_{28}N_2O_2$. HCl.

Description: An alkaloid synthetized from and allied to quinine; a white, faintly yellowish, bitter crystalline powder; soluble in 2 parts warm water, 5 parts of alcohol, very soluble in chloroform; insoluble in ether and petroleum benzene.

Uses: *Used* as spinal injection in pneumococcus meningitis; also for injection in empyema of children. Externally, in corneal serpiginous ulcer and as prophylactic in occupational eye injuries from splinters of stone, wood, particles of steel and sand.

Supply: **Optochin Hydrochloride (C.A.)**—Vials gr 15.

Administration: In pneumococcic meningitis, spinal injection of 15 m (1 cc) of a 1:1,000 solution in sterile saline for about each 2 kilos of body weight; given twice daily for 4–5 days and at least 1 injection daily as long as living pneumococci are present in spinal fluid; in empyema of children after aspiration of pus, ¼–½ gr (0.015–0.03 Gm) per kilo of body weight, is injected as a 5 % solution.

Application: In corneal serpiginous ulcer, a 1–2 % solution (or ointment), with or without 2 % atropine sulphate, is applied on a pledget of cotton two or three times daily; to maintain the effect, a few drops of a 1 % solution is instilled every hour during the day and a 1–2 % ointment applied at night. The first application is painful, subsequent ones are not, because of local anesthetic effect.

Caution: It should be remembered that Optochin Hydrochloride should *not* be given internally; for internal use Optochin Base *only* should be employed.

ORIDINE (Lilly)

Iodine Therapy

Composition: The Calcium salt of the Iodized Fatty Acids of cotton seed oil; contains 23–25 % organic Iodine.

Description: A light brown powder, tasteless and quite odorless; almost insoluble in cold alcohol, ether, benzene; slightly soluble in chloroform.

Action and Uses: As for organic iodine compounds; is better utilized because of low solubility and protracted retention in the organism; *indicated* in conditions where iodine therapy is useful.

Supply: **ORIDINE**—Tablets (C.A.) each equivalent to 0.01 Gm of iodine—Boxes of 40.

Administration: **In Goitre Prophylaxis**—1–3 tablets daily for 40 days; in **Other Diseases**—dosage in accordance, 1 Gm of Oridine being equivalent to gr 5 of potassium iodide.

ORPHOL (Schering and Glatz)

Antiseptic

Chemical Name: Bismuth Betanaphthol.

Formula: $Bi_2O_2(OH). C_{10}H_7O$.

Description: A brownish or grayish, odorless, tasteless, amorphous powder, insoluble in water.

Action and Uses: Antiseptic and astringent in diarrheas of tuberculosis, dysentery, intestinal fermentation, gastritis; locally on wounds, ulcers.

Supply: **ORPHOL** (C.A.)—Bottles 1 oz., 1 lb.

Administration: *Locally*—As dusting powder.
Orally—Gr 8–15, three times daily; children ½ dosage; in tuberculous diarrhea, 60–120 gr daily.

ORTAL SODIUM (Parke, Davis)

Hypnotic

Chemical Name: Sodium Hexyl-ethyl-barbiturate.

Formula: $C_{12}H_{19}O_3N_2.Na$.

Description: A white, stable powder, readily soluble in water.

Action: A rapidly effective hypnotic, inducing quiet, restful sleep, safely, pleasantly and without after-effects; does not unduly depress blood pressure or respiration; preoperatively, reduces the amount of anesthetic required; tends to prevent toxic reactions from cocaine or procaine.

Uses: Indicated in insomnia, nervousness, migraine, epilepsy, acute alcoholism and drug addiction; for preoperative sedation in surgery and obstetrics; as antidotal prophylactic in local anesthesia; as sedative in gastrointestinal neuroses, chorea, pertussis, hypertention and menopausal disorders.

Supply: **ORTAL SODIUM**—Capsules gr 3 (0.2 Gm)—Bottles of 25, 100 and 500.

Administration: Average dosage—1 or 2 capsules, repeated as required.
In epilepsy—2–3 capsules daily.
In preoperative obstetrical sedation—gr 6 when active labor has begun, repeated in 3 hours if necessary.
In preoperative surgical sedation—gr 3 four hours and gr 6 one hour before administration of general anesthetic.
In alcoholism and drug addiction—gr 3 every 4–6 hours for restlessness; gr 3–6 for allaying excitement and discomfort due to withdrawal of habit-forming drug.

Bibliography: *See Chap. XII.*

ORTHOFORM (Metz)

Analgesic

Chemical Name: Methyl m-amino-para-oxybenzoate.

Formula: $C_6H_3(NH_2)(OH)COO.\ CH_3$. 3: 4: 1.

Description: A white crystalline non-hygroscopic powder, odorless and tasteless; almost insoluble in water, soluble in 5–6 parts of alcohol and 50 parts of ether and in collodion.

Action: A surface anesthetic; because of poor solubility penetrates tissues very slowly, and offers prolonged action; causes no local irritation and is practically non-toxic.

Uses: In gastric ulcer and gastralgia; as analgesic in burns, varicose ulcers, tuberculous and syphilitic affections, corneal ulcers, conjunctivitis, pharyngitis, rhinitis, hemorrhoids.

In Dentistry—In preparation of cavities before filling, packing of sockets, after extraction.

Incompatibles: Silver nitrate, formaldehyde, potassium submanganate, antipyrin, bismuth subnitrate, organic silver proteins.

Supply: **ORTHOFORM**—Vials (C.A.) of 5 Gm—Bottles of 1 oz.

ORTHOFORM—Troches 1/4 and 1/2 gr (0.016 and 0.032 Gm)—Bottles of 100.

Administration: *Internal*—8–15 gr (0.51–0.97 Gm) in emulsion.

External—Plain, as dusting powder; mixed with milk sugar, for insufflation; as ointment incorporated with lanolin; may also be combined with mercury chloride, carbolic acid, tincture of iodine, iodoform, zinc oxide, Europhen, Aristol, calomel and salicylic acid. Troches are dissolved on the tongue in painful mouth and throat diseases.

OSCODAL (Metz)

Vitamin Therapy

Composition: A biologically standardized Cod Liver Oil Concentrate in tablet form, containing Vitamin A not less than 25,000 units, and Vitamin D 1,330 units per gram: each tablet (0.02 Gm) is equivalent in vitamin potency to 1/2 teaspoonful of cod liver oil.

Action and Uses: As for cod liver oil in general.

Advantages: Is devoid of nauseating fishy odor, does not become rancid, may be used in warm or cold climate, is conveniently administered and well tolerated.

Supply: **OSCODAL**—Tablets (C.A.), Sugar coated—Bottles of 42 and 100.

Administration: Adults, 2 or 3 tablets, three times daily before meals. Children 1–2 tablets.

Bibliography: *See Chap. XII.*

OUABAIN

Cardiac Stimulant

Chemical Name: G-Strophanthin Thoms; Crystallized Strophanthin.

Formula: $C_{30}H_{46}O_{12} + 9H_2O$.

Description: Colorless quadratic crystals, of bitter taste; soluble in hot water, in 100 parts of cold water, 30 parts of cold absolute alcohol, 30 parts of amyl alcohol; slightly soluble in ether and chloroform.

Action: Cardiac stimulant of strophanthin type, but more active, more powerful; is more rapidly eliminated and less cumulative than digitalis; is poorly absorbed from gastrointestinal tract and thus not suitable for oral administration.

Uses: Generally in emergencies, not in continuous therapy; in cardiac dilatation, broken compensation of chronic interstitial myocarditis and valvular disease, with edema and dyspnea.

Supply: **OUABAIN**—Ampules (C.A.) 0.5 mg (**Hynson Westcott and Dunning**)—Boxes of 4.

OUABAIN—Ampules (C.A.) gr 1/128 (0.0005 Gm) in 2 cc of buffered sterile normal solution—Boxes of 12. **(Lilly)**

OUABAIN (C.A.)—Vials 5 and 15 gr. **(Merck)**

Administration: *Intravenously*—0.5 mg or 1 ampule in physiologic saline, only once in 24 hr.; solution must be freshly prepared and used immediately.

Intramuscularly—1/2–1 mg or 1 ampule daily.

Maximum dosage—1/10 gr (0.006 Gm) daily.

Caution: Where digitaline or strophanthin have been previously given care should be taken not to administer Ouabain within 24 hr.

OUABAINE "ARNAUD" (Fougera)

Cardiotonic

Chemical Name: Crystallized Strophanthin.

Formula: $C_{30}H_{46}O_{12} + 9H_2O$.

Description: A glucoside obtained by Arnaud from Acocanthera ouabaio; occurs in the form of colorless bitter quadratic crystals, easily soluble in hot water, in 100 parts of cold water and 30 parts of cold absolute alcohol; slightly soluble in ether and chloroform.

Action and Uses: A cardiac stimulant; *useful* in acute heart failure, in cardiac arrhythmia, nephritic heart and similar cardiac conditions.

Advantages: Is more powerful than strophantin, more rapidly effective, less cumulative, and sooner excreted.

Supply: **OUABAINE "ARNAUD"**—Tablets, gr 1/60 (1 mg)—Bottles of 40.

OUABAINE "ARNAUD"—Tablets, gr 1/240 (0.25 mg)—Bottles of 40.

OUABAINE "ARNAUD"—Ampules—Intravenous, 1 cc, gr 1/240 (0.25 mg)—Bottles of 6.

OUABAINE "ARNAUD"—Ampules—Intramuscular, 2 cc, gr 1/120 (0.50 mg)—Bottles of 6.

OUABAINE "ARNAUD"—Solutions 4:1,000 (Drops) or 1:1,000 (Solubaine)—Bottles of 10 cc.

Administration:

Intravenously—1–2 ampules (1/4–1/2 mg) daily, for 3–5 days, beginning with 1/2 ampule (1/8 mg) where necessary; administered in 4,000–8,000 parts of normal saline, freshly prepared; is not to be repeated within 24 hr.

Orally—Solution 4:1,000, 35–50 drops daily in divided doses for 4–5 days.

Tablets—2–4 (1 mg each) daily, in divided doses, for 3–5 days.

Solubaine (1:1,000 solution), 15–50 drops daily in divided doses, for 5–10 days.

OVARIALHORMON FOLLICULIN MENFORMON

Hormone Therapy

Description: An aqueous solution of Ovarian Folliculin hormone free from proteins; standardized to contain 40 mouse units with less than 0.1 mg of solid substance per cubic centimeter; chloretone and sodium chloride are added for osmotic and sterile purposes.

Action and Uses: That of folliculin; in amenorrhea and sterility; lately also favorably employed in retinitis pigmentosa.

Supply: **FOLLICULIN (OVARIAN HORMONE)**—Crinogen Ampules **(Colwell)** 1 cc—Boxes of 12.

OVARIALHORMON FOLLICULIN MENFORMON—Ampules **(Kretschmar)** 1 cc—Boxes of 3.

OVARIALHORMON FOLLICULIN MENFORMON—Dragees **(Kretschmar)** 100 mouse units—Packages of 10 and 25.

OVARIALHORMON FOLLICULIN MENFORMON—Solution— **(Marvell)** Ampules 1 cc—Boxes of 3.

OVARIALHORMON FOLLICULIN MENFORMON—Dragees 100 **(Marvell)** mouse units—Boxes of 10.

Administration: *Subcutaneously*, *Intramuscularly* or *Intravenously*—1–2 ampules daily for 30 injections, or 1–2 dragees orally.

OVOGAL (Riedel)

Cholagogue

Chemical Name: Albumin Cholate.

Description: A combination of bile acids and egg albumin; a yellowish green powder, insoluble in water, acids, ether, benzol, chloroform, alcohol, fats; soluble in alkaline media with re-formation of glycocholic and taurocholic acids and albumin.

Action and Uses: A cholagogue, liver stimulant and intestinal antiseptic. *Useful* in dyspepsia, intestinal catarrh, fatty stools, chronic constipation, acute and chronic hepatic and biliary disease and biliary colic.

Supply: OVOGAL—Capsules (C.A.) 7½ gr (0.480 Gm)—Boxes of 50.

Administration: 2 capsules, three times daily after meals with water.

OXO-ATE (Smith, Kline and French)

Antiarthritic

Chemical Name: Ammonium Ortho-iodoxybenzoate; Amiodoxyl-benzoate.

Formula: $C_6H_4(IO_2)COO.\ NH_4$.

Action: A highly germicidal agent against the staphylococcus and streptococcus; stimulates phagocytosis and the formation of agglutinins and of specific hemolysins.

Supply: OXO-ATE—Vials, 1 Gm—Boxes of 6.

Administration: *Intravenously*—1 Gm thoroughly dissolved in 100 cc freshly distilled, sterile water or saline; given by gravity method, at body temperature, slowly during 10 min.; twice a week, 8–10 doses; initial dose 0.5 Gm in 50 cc water. *Rectally*—After cleansing enema, 1 Gm in 50 cc water injected high into the rectum twice a week, for 3–4 weeks.

Caution: If overheated, will explode; need not be sterilized; injection of normal saline preceding and following the intravenous administration of the drug is advisable; magnesium sulphate pack over site of injection is helpful in preventing thrombosis. Untoward effects as malaise, slight nausea, stinging sensation in nose, lachrymation and sneezing—are transitory.

Bibliography: *See Chap. XII.*

OXO-ATE "B" (Smith, Kline and French)

Antiarthritic

Chemical Name: Calcium Ortho-iodoxybenzoate. The Calcium salt of O-Iodoxybenzoic Acid.

Formula: $[C_6H_4(IO_2)COO]_2Ca + 8H_2O$.

Action and Uses: Analgesic and antirheumatic; *used* in arthritis and rheumatoid conditions, as lumbago, sacroiliac disease, and as adjunct in intravenous therapy of Oxoate.

Advantages: Small doses twice weekly; obviates massive dosage of salicylates and iodides.

Supply: OXO-ATE "B"—Tablets—0.5 Gm—Tubes of 24.
OXO-ATE "B"—Capsules—Bottles of 24.

Administration: *Orally*—Initial dose 1 tablet or capsule; then given three to four times daily, with glassful of water, after meals.

Bibliography: *See Chap. XII.*

OXYL-IODIDE (Lilly)

Antiarthritic

Chemical Name: Hydriodide of Phenylcinchoninic Acid.

Formula: $C_{16}H_{11}O_2NHI$.

Description: An organic iodine and cinchoninic acid combination; a golden yellow powder, insoluble in gastric juice, soluble in alkaline intestinal secretion.

Action: Analgesic, antirheumatic, antineuritic; favors elimination of uric acid.

Uses: In gonorrheal rheumatism, neuralgia, gout, myalgia, myositis.

Supply: OXYL-IODIDE—Tablets 3 gr (0.194 Gm)—Bottles of 40 and 500.

Administration: 2 Tablets after meals, with plenty of water.

Contraindications: Hepatic and biliary dysfunctions, pregnancy, alcoholism.

Precautions: Frequent interruptions during administration of the drug and a high carbohydrate diet with abundant fluids are advisable.

Combination: OXYL-IODIDE COMPOUND—Contains oxyl-iodide with an equal quantity of phenyl-cinchoninic acid; represents 1 part of iodine to 5 parts of phenyl cinchoninic acid, 2 parts of which are in chemical union with the iodine.

Supply—Pulvules gr 6 (0.384 Gm)—Bottles 40 and 500; Powder—Packages 1 and 4 oz.; *Dosage* and uses—as for Oxyl-Iodide.

OXYNTIN (Fairchild)

Hydrochloride Acid Therapy

Description: Contains 10% by weight of absolute Hydrochloric Acid in combination with Albumin, the acid being loosely bound to the protein; each grain represents 1 m of dilute hydrochloric acid.

Action and Uses: In all cases of hypoacidity and achylia gastrica.

Supply: OXYNTIN—Powder—Bottles of 30 Gm.

OXYNTIN—Capsules—Gr 5—Bottles of 50 capsules.

OXYNTIN WITH PEPSIN—Gr 5—Bottles of 50 capsules.

OXYNTIN WITH NUX VOMICA—Gr 5—Bottles of 50 capsules.

Administration: 5–15 gr powder or capsules ½–1 hour after meals.

OXYQUINOLIN SULPHATE (Benzol)

Antiseptic

Chemical Name: Oxyquinolin.

Formula: $(C_9H_7NO_2)_2H_2SO_4$.

Description: A yellow crystalline powder of burning taste and saffron like odor; soluble in water, insoluble in ether, soluble with difficulty in alcohol.

Action: A powerful antiseptic, more effective than corrosive sublimate; does not injure the skin or mucous membranes and does not coagulate serum and proteins; is analgesic and non-toxic.

Uses: In all conditions where an antiseptic is employed.

Administration:

	Solution
For wounds, ulcers, burns	1:1,000
As nasal douche	1:3,000
As gargle	1:2,000
As vaginal douche and rectal irrigation	1:1,000–1:100

Internally—Gr 5 (0.3 Gm) three times daily after meals.

Supply: OXYQUINOLIN SULPHATE—In bulk, in quantities desired.

PANOPSIN (Spicer)

Digestive

Description: Pancreatic amylopsin, prepared from the acinous cells of the pancreas; stable and of high amylolytic capacity.

Action: Will convert five hundred times its weight of starch into sugar essential for absorption.

Uses: In fermentative disturbances and defective starch digestion.

Supply: PANOPSIN—Tablets, flavored, gr 2½ (0.160 Gm)—Bottles of 50.

Administration: 1–2 tablets, before meals.

PANTERIC TABLETS AND CAPSULES (Parke, Davis)

Digestant

Description: Triple Strength Pancreatin, U.S.P., in enteric coated tablets and enteric coated granules, enclosed in gelatin capsules.

Action and Uses: That of the contained pancreatic enzymes—amylopsin, trypsin and steapsin, but unimpaired by contact with the gastric juice. *Indicated* in intestinal indigestion and its sequelae, as food asthma, urticaria, malnutrition; often of service in diabetic cases, but not a substitute for insulin.

Supply: PANTERIC—Tablets Enteric and Chocolate coated, 5 gr (0.324 Gm)—Bottles of 100 and 500.

PANTERIC—Capsules, containing Enteric-coated Granules, 5 gr (0.324 Gm)—Bottles of 100 and 1,000.

Administration: Adults, 1 or 2 tablets or capsules three times daily, after meals. Children according to age; any desired dose may be taken from the capsules.

Combination: PANTERIC COMPOUND—Tablets—Each tablet contains

	Gr	Gm
Pancreatin, triple strength U.S.P.	4	0.259
Sodium Glycocholate	¾	0.048
Sodium Taurocholate	¾	0.048

Action and Uses—Lessens putrefaction in the intestinal tract; in intestinal indigestion has same effect as Plain Panteric Tablets. *For use* in catarrhal jaundice, enterotoxicosis and chronic constipation; as cholagogue in cholecystitis or cholelithiasis.

Supply—Tablets Enteric and Chocolate coated—Bottles of 100 and 500.

Administration—1 or 2 tablets three times daily, 1 hr. after meals.

PANTHESINE (Sandoz)

Anesthetic. Antipruritic

Chemical Name: N-diethyl-leucinolester of p-aminobenzoic Acid.

Formula: $C_{17}H_{28}O_2N_2$.

Description: A synthetic product, soluble in water, forming a stable solution; is sterilizable by heat.

Action and Uses: Local anesthetic, of equal potency but ⅓ toxicity of cocaine; is non-irritating. *For use* as local anesthetic in all surgical procedures.

Supply: PANTHESINE—Bottles of 1, 5, 25 and 100 Gm.

Administration: Surgery—*Infiltration* and *Conduction*—0.2% solution with 10 to 20 drops epinephrine, 1:1,000, to 100 cc of solution; *Lumbar*—5–6 cc 0.5% solution diluted with spinal fluid to make 10 cc; *Surface* application—10% solution.

Rhinolaryngology—*Infiltration*—0.2% solution; *Surface* application—10% solution.

Ophthalmology—*Instillation*—4–10 drops of 2% solution; *Infiltration*—0.5% solution with 2 drops epinephrine, 1:1,000, per cc.

Dentistry—*Infiltration* and *Conduction*—0.5% solution with ½ drop epinephrine, 1:1,000, per cc.

Combinations: PANTHESINE OINTMENT—Containing 5% panthesine in vegetable emollient base; *For use* in numerous superficial lesions—paronychia, furuncles, herpes zoster, pruritus, sunburn, arthritis, lumbago; blepharitis, corneal erosions, aphthae; also in nasal catarrh, pyorrhea, gingivitis and hemorrhoidal inflammation. *Administration*—is gently rubbed into the painful area in quantities varying in size from a pea to a teaspoonful; repeated two to four times daily, oftener if necessary; *Supply*—Tubes of 10, 20 and 100 Gm.

Bibliography: *See Chap. XII.*

PANTOCAIN (Winthrop)

Local Anesthetic

Chemical Name: P-butyl-amino-benzoyl-dimethyl-amino-ethanol Hydrochloride.

Formula: $CH_3.(CH_2)_3NH$ 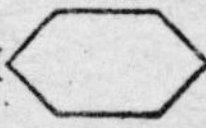 $COO.(CH_2)_2N(CH_3)_2.HCl$.

Description: Small, colorless and odorless crystals, freely soluble in water and physiologic salt solution, yielding a neutral reaction; is resistant to prolonged boiling.

Action: Produces rapid surface anesthesia and is a satisfactory substitute for cocain; can be applied in all forms of local anesthesia, affording the desired effect even in high dilution; anesthesia sets in rapidly and is of long duration.

Uses: In spinal anesthesia, urology, otolaryngology and ophthalmology, surgery.

Supply: PANTOCAIN—Ampules, 2 cc, 1% Solution (Spinal)—Boxes of 10.

PANTOCAIN—Bottles of 1 oz., 2% Solution (Surface Anesthesia).

Administration: Spinal anesthesia, 1% solution, the adult dose ranging from 1–2 cc; surface and mucosa anesthesia, ¼, ½, 1, 2% solution, with or without Suprarenin.

Directions: Solutions for surface anesthesia are prepared by diluting, if necessary, the 2% solution, sterilizing by boiling for short period, cooling and adding Suprarenin.

PANTOPON (Roche)

Sedative Narcotic

Description: Contains the total alkaloids of opium in the form of soluble hydrochlorides, in proportions existing naturally in gum opii, but freed from resins and all inert matter.

Action: An injectable opium producing the beneficial effects of total opium, but devoid of its ballast; is absorbed more promptly and is free from the nauseant odor and taste of the ordinary opium preparations. In efficiency, 1 gr of Pantopon is equal to 4.5 gr of powdered opium, and contains ½ gr of anhydrous morphine.

Uses: Wherever an opiate is indicated; takes the place of morphine or codeine or their derivatives, since it makes immediately available the smooth beneficial effects of total opium. *Used* in surgery for the control of pre- and post-operative pain, and as an aid to anesthesia; in obstetrics is used alone or in conjunction with scopolamine in more difficult labor cases.

Advantages: Causes less nausea, excitation, and respiratory depression; exerts greater sedative and analgesic action than morphine.

Supply: PANTOPON—Powder—Vials of ⅛, ¼, ½ and 1 oz.

PANTOPON—Tablets, Oral, ⅙ gr—Vials of 20.

PANTOPON—Tablets, Hypodermic, ⅓ gr—Tubes of 20.

PANTOPON—Ampules 1.1 cc (⅓ gr per cubic centimeter)—Cartons of 6 and 12.

Administration: *As Sedative*—1/24–1/12 gr.
In Cough Mixtures—1/24 gr per dose, in place of codeine.
As Analgesic—⅙–⅓ gr, the latter replacing ¼ gr of morphine.

PAPAIN (Burroughs Wellcome)

Digestant

Description: A digestive ferment obtained from the fruit of Carica Papaya (Papaw tree); an enzyme similar to pepsin; a grayish white, slightly hygroscopic powder; digests about two hundred times its weight of coagulated albumin in an alkaline medium in 5 hr.

Action and Uses: Chiefly proteolytic, converting proteins into peptones; does not require acid medium for action; *useful* in gastric atony and hypochlorhydria.

Supply: PAPAIN—Tabloid—Gr 2 (0.130 Gm)—Bottles of 100.

Administration: 1 or 2 tabloids taken with little water, two to three times daily, ½ hr. before meals.

PAPAVERINE

Antispasmodic

Chemical Name: The hydrochloric acid and sulphuric acid salts of papaverine, an alkaloid of opium.

Formula: Papaverine Hydrochloride $C_{20}H_{21}O_4N.\ HCl$.
Papaverine Sulphate $(C_{20}H_{21}O_4N)_2H_2SO_4$.

Composition: The sulphate contains not less than 85% of papaverine, the hydrochloride not less than 88% of the alkaloid.

Description: Both salts occur as fine white crystalline powders, odorless and of bitter taste; both are soluble in alcohol, sparingly soluble in water, freely soluble in chloroform, insoluble in ether; the hydrochloride is stable in air, the sulphate is hygroscopic.

Action: Antispasmodic and analgesic; relaxes smooth musculature of all organs to various degrees; is effective in all hypertonic states; is a local anesthetic and central analgesic, non-narcotic and non-toxic.

Uses: In angina pectoris, arteriosclerosis, cerebral congestion; in gastric ulcer, pylorospasm, spastic constipation, cholelithiasis, biliary colic, infantile diarrhea; in chloroform narcosis, eclampsia, hemoptysis; in bronchial or cardiac asthma; in uremic convulsions; in whooping cough, seasickness; in abortion, dysmenorrhea, vomiting of pregnancy; in tabetic vascular crises.

Supply: PAPAVERINE HYDROCHLORIDE (C.A.)—Vials 15 gr— Bottles ⅛ and 1 oz. (Merck)

PAPAVERINE SULPHATE (C.A.)—Ampules 1.1 cc (⅔ gr)—Cartons of 6. (Roche)

PAPAVERINE HYDROCHLORIDE (C.A.)—Powder—Vials 1 Gm Tablets, Oral, gr ¼. (Roche)

Administration: *Orally*—Adults, ¾–1⅓ gr (0.05–0.08 Gm) single dosage; maximum dosage—up to 4 gr (0.259 Gm) daily; in gastric ulcer ¾ gr (0.048 Gm) with 1/120 gr (0.0005 Gm) atropine sulphate per day, increased gradually to double this dose.
Children, 1/12–¾ gr (0.005–0.05 Gm) three times daily.
Intravenously—1/12–⅙ gr (0.005–0.012 Gm) up to ⅔ gr (0.042 Gm); to reduce blood pressure, 1⅓ gr (0.085 Gm).

PARATHESIN (Metz)

Surface Anesthetic

Chemical Name: Brand of Ethyl Aminobenzoate. Anesthesin.

Formula: $COOC_2H_5(1).C_6H_4.NH_2(4)$.

Description: A fine, white, crystalline powder, odorless and tasteless; almost insoluble in cold, sparingly soluble in hot water; soluble in alcohol up to 20%, chloroform—to 50%, ether—to 25%, fatty oils 2–3%; may be incorporated in animal fats and petrolatum.

Action: Renders denuded surfaces insensitive; relieves pain, produces prolonged anesthesia; is practically non-toxic and non-irritating.

Uses and Administration: Surgery—As dusting powder, or in oily solution or ointment, 5–20%—in the treatment of wounds, burns, ulcers, bed-sores, suppurating buboes, cracked nipples, moist eczema and excoriated skin lesions.

Rhinology—In oily or alcoholic solution, 3–20%, as swab, spray or as paratroches, in ulcerative stomatitis, rhinitis, otalgia.

Urology—As suppositories and bougies, 3–8 gr, in vesical tenesmus, cystitis, and urethritis.

Proctology—As ointment, 5–20%, in hemorrhoids, fissures, pruritus ani and vulvae.
Internally—For relief of pain in gastric ulcer and cancer, 3–5 gr, before meals.

Supply: PARATHESIN—Powder—Vials of 5 Gm—Bottles 1 oz.

PARA-TROCHES—1 gr (0.06 Gm)—Bottles of 100.

PARA-THOR-MONE (Lilly)

Hormone Therapy

Description: A hormone extract (Collip), accurately standardized in the raising of blood calcium content in the animal organism; contains in stable aqueous solution the active principles of the Parathyroid Gland and is extremely potent.

Action and Uses: Raises blood calcium, with highest response 15 hr. after injection; is specific in prevention and treatment of tetany; is *used* in rickets, spasmophilia, urticaria, certain types of nephritis; in chronic ulcers, tuberculosis, delayed blood coagulability; in eclampsia, radium poisoning and angioneurotic edema.

Supply: PARA-THOR-MONE (C.A.)—Vials 5 cc, rubber capped, 20 units per cubic centimeter (R 20).

PARA-THOR-MONE (C.A.)—Ampules 1 cc—Boxes of 6.

Caution: To be kept at a temperature between 35 and 45°F.

Administration: *Intramuscularly, subcutaneously and intravenously.*

In Tetany—28–60 units daily; infants 18–20 units.

In Hemorrhage—38–40 units; dosage controlled by requirements.

In Other Conditions—Is graded in accordance with blood calcium content.

Bibliography: *See Chap. XII.*

PAROIDIN (Parke, Davis)

Hormone Therapy

Description: Parathyroid Extract (Hanson); prepared from fresh bovine parathyroids and physiologically standardized on parathyroidectomized dogs; each cubic centimeter contains 150 Hanson units, calculated in terms of calcium mobilization; 100 units increase the calcium content of the dog's blood by 1 mg per 100 cc.

Action: Raises blood calcium content by mobilization.

Uses: *For use* in controlling tetany, due to defective parathyroid function; in certain forms of menorrhagia; in conjunction with vitamin D to equalize the physiologic distribution of calcium in numerous other pathologic disorders.

Supply: PAROIDIN (C.A.)—Bottles 5 cc, rubber-diaphragm-capped.

Administration: *Subcutaneous or Intramuscular* (not intravenous)—0.2–0.4 cc (30–60 units), every 12 hr. for 5 or 6 days; rest period of a week or two, repeated if necessary.

Children—0.1–0.2 cc at similar intervals.

Bibliography: *See Chap. XII.*

PAROLEINE (Burroughs Wellcome)

Mineral Oil

Composition: Pure Liquid Paraffin; is colorless, tasteless, odorless and of neutral reaction.

Action and Uses: As for other mineral oils; is *used* as intestinal lubricant in chronic obstipation and as dressing for burns and ulcerations.

Supply: PAROLEINE—Bottles of 4 and 16 oz.

Administration: 1–3 teaspoonfuls before meals as laxative.

Externally—In full strength or in combination with other medicaments.

Combinations: PAROLEINE—Spray Compound—Contains Menthol, gr 5 (0.324 Gm); Chlorbutol, gr 6 (0.389 Gm); Eucalyptia, m 5 (0.9 cc); Paroleine, q.s. 29.5 cc. *For use* as spray in laryngeal and nasal affections. *Supply*—Bottles of 1 and 16 oz.

LAXAMEL—Contains Paroleine 80%. A palatable jelly for *internal use*. *Supply*—Glass jars of 4 oz.

PAROXYL (SPIROCID) (Metz)

Amebacide

Chemical Name: 4-Oxy-3-acetylamino-phenylarsonic Acid.

Formula: C_6H_3. OH. NH. $COCH_3$. AsO_3H_2.

Description: A white, odorless, crystalline powder, soluble with difficulty in water and alcohol, easily soluble in caustic soda, sodium carbonate and ammonium solutions.

Action and Uses: Affects certain protozoa, such as the ameba, frambesia, trypanosome and similar intestinal parasites; *used* principally in amebic dysentery and for eradicating dysentery cysts and encysted flagellates; also helpful in prophylaxis and treatment of congenital syphilis in children.

Supply: PAROXYL—Tablets, 4 gr (0.259 Gm)—Bottles of 30.

Administration: Adults, 1 tablet three times daily for a period of 1 week; where required, the course may be repeated after a 10-day rest interval.
Children—Dosage in proportion, according to age.

PELLETIERINE TANNATE (Burroughs Wellcome)

Anthelminthic

Composition: The insoluble Tannate of Pomegranate root bark.

Action and Uses: Anthelminthic for tapeworm, hookworm, taenia solium.

Supply: PELLETIERINE TANNATE—Tabloid gr 2 (0.130 Gm)—Bottles of 25.

Administration: 1–4 tabloids on empty stomach; after 2 hr. 1 oz. of castor oil, repeated in 4 hr.

PENTNUCLEOTIDE (Smith, Kline and French)

Leucocyte Proliferant

Description: A mixture of the Sodium Salts of Pentose Nucleotides.

Action: It is assumed that nucleotides have chemotactic, initiatory and maturation stimulating powers for neutrophilic myelocytes, when the basic mesenchymal tissues from which they arise are in a condition to respond to a stimulus; where effective, it causes a fall in temperature and increase in leucocytes, total count and polymorphonuclears.

Uses: In agranulocytic angina, malignant neutropenia; in infections accompanied by a low white blood cell count; in leucopenia from chronic benzol poisoning; is *not indicated* in infections *without* leucopenia.

Supply: PENTNUCLEOTIDE—Ampules (C.A.) 10 cc—Boxes of 12.

Caution: Must be kept at room temperature and in the dark; must not be used if turbid or precipitated. Reactions as shown by dyspnea, bradycardia, sweats, chills, fever, etc., may be prevented by initial hypodermic injection of atropine gr $1/150$.

Advantages: Is almost a specific in several hitherto uncontrollable affections.

Administration: 10 cc injected *intragluteally* twice daily until a definite rise in cell count is obtained; then once daily until the count is normal for 3 days; repeated, if no improvement is obtained after the usual 5 days. In desperate cases, 20 cc twice daily for 4 days, then 10 cc twice daily until the cell count is normal for 3 days; injections are given at least 2 hr. after meals.

Bibliography: *See Chap. XII.*

PENTOBARBITAL-SODIUM (Abbott)

Sedative. Hypnotic

Chemical Name: Sodium Ethyl (1-methyl-butyl) Barbiturate; formerly named Nembutal.

Formula: $NaC_2H_5[CH_3CH_2CH_2(CH_3)CH]C\ CONHCO:NCO.$

Description: The monosodium salt of ethyl (1-methyl butyl) barbituric acid; occurs as a white, crystalline, odorless powder of slightly bitter taste; is very soluble in water, freely soluble in alcohol, practically insoluble in ether.

Action and Uses: Is more effective than barbital but its action is of relatively shorter duration; is *used* as sedative, particularly prior to local, general or spinal anesthesia; as antispasmodic and hypnotic to produce sleep of short duration; to control nausea from any cause, also convulsions in tetanus, strychnine poisoning, mania and similar conditions.

Advantages: Rapid action, small dosage, prolonged sedation and short hypnotic effect.

Supply: PENTOBARBITAL-SODIUM (C.A.)—Capsules, gr ½ and gr 1½ (0.032 Gm and 0.097 Gm)—Bottles of 24, 100, 1,000.

PENTOBARBITAL-SODIUM (C.A.)—Sterile Powder, gr 7½ (0.480 Gm) in Ampules for intravenous use.

Administration: *Preoperative*—For preanesthetic sedation—1½–3 gr, with or without ⅙ gr morphine and 1/300 gr atropine, or of morphine and hyoscine.
As Hypnotic—1½ gr; more when required.
For Children—Infants up to 1 yr.—½ gr; up to 3 yr.—1 gr, dissolved in a few cubic centimeters of water and administered rectally.
For Adults—Rectal administration by retention enema, 2½% solution; or by direct introduction of soluble capsules into rectum.

Caution: Solutions decompose on standing.

Bibliography: *See Chap. XII.*

PEPTONE SOLUTION

Non-specific Protein Therapy

Description: Prepared by hydrolysis from lean muscle; contains primary and secondary proteoses and peptones.

Action and Uses: A non-specific protein therapy agent for immunization and desensitization in bronchial asthma, angioneurotic edema, anaphylaxis, skin and other allergies; is non-irritating.

Supply: PEPTONE SOLUTION—Ampules 1 cc and 2 cc—5% sterile, isotonic solution—Boxes of 12, 50 and 100. **(Armour)**

PEPTONE SOLUTION—5% sterile Ampule-Vials 1 cc and 5 cc—Packages of 12 and 100. **(National Drug)**

PEPTONE SOLUTION—5% sterile Ampule-Vials 30 cc—Packages of 12. **(National Drug)**

Administration: Initial dose 0.5 cc *intramuscularly*, increased twice weekly by 0.5–1 cc till 4 or 5 cc are given, guided by reaction and symptoms; *may also be used intravenously.*

Bibliography: *See Chap. XII.*

PERALGA (Schering and Glatz)

Analgesic

Chemical Name: Amidopyrine Diethylbarbiturate.

Formula: $C_{34}H_{46}N_8O_5$.

Description: A yellow powder easily soluble in hot water; a compound of 2 molecules of amidopyrine and 1 molecuie of veronal.

Action and Uses: Antipyretic, analgesic and sedative; *effective* in various painful affections such as dysmenorrhea, migraine, neuralgia, arthritis, earache, neuritis, toothache, trauma.

Supply: PERALGA—Tablets gr 6 (0.384 Gm)—Boxes of 6 and 12—Bottles of 50, 100 and 500.

PERALGA—Powder—Bottles of ½ and 1 oz.

Administration: 1 tablet or 5–10 gr of powder, repeated as necessary.

PERISTALTINE (Ciba)

Laxative

Description: A preparation of water soluble Glucosides of Cascara Sagrada, physiologically standardized, suitable for oral and hypodermic use.

Action: Taken orally or injected hypodermically, produces a laxative effect in 8–10 hr., without undue irritation or disturbance of the digestive tract.

Uses: In all types of chronic constipation; as prophylactic in intestinal stasis to avoid distention before or after laparotomy.

Supply: PERISTALTINE—Tablets—Gr 1½ (0.097 Gm) sugar coated—Bottles of 15.

PERISTALTINE—Ampules—Gr 2½ (1.5 cc)—Cartons of 5 and 20.

Administration: *Oral*—For chronic constipation, 1 or 2 tablets at bedtime; in obstinate cases, same dosage two to three times daily.

Hypodermic—In prophylaxis of intestinal stasis, 1 ampule *subcutaneously* or *intramuscularly* repeated in 12 hr., if passage of flatus or stool does not occur. In known obstinate cases of constipation an ampule may be injected mornings and evenings for several days prior to operation, with or without the oral administration of tablets.

Advantages: Is the only cascara preparation physiologically standardized and in ampule form *for hypodermic use;* is of definite composition, of uniform and constant action.

Bibliography: *See Chap. XII.*

PERNOSTON (Riedel-De Haen)

Hypnotic

Chemical Name: Sodium secondary Butyl-beta-bromallyl Barbiturate.

Formula: $C_{11}H_{14}O_3N_2Br.\ Na$.

Description: Occurs as a white crystalline, odorless powder of slightly bitter taste; is freely soluble in water.

Action: Intravenous injection produces sleep in 2-3 min.; intramuscular, in about ½ hr.; sleep lasts from 5–8 hr., in obstetrical cases about 3 hr., after operation 1–4 hr., according to dosage; the action is that of a hypnotic and not an anesthetic and in therapeutic doses merely eliminates consciousness; is rapidly broken down in the organism and is thus a short acting hypnotic; recovery from sleep is relatively quick, prolonged nursing care unnecessary.

Uses: **Psychiatry**—In restlessness and severe insomnia, given *intramuscularly;* in the treatment of drug addicts for continued sleep of several days during withdrawal of the habit forming drug is given first *intravenously* and later continued with *intramuscular* injections.

Surgery and Gynecology—As pre-anesthetic or pre-operative hypnotic, to quiet the patient prior to anesthesia; also as a means of reducing from 50–80% of the inhalation anesthetic, often a very desirable feature.

Obstetrics—For the alleviation of pain in childbirth and to produce so-called twillight sleep; in post-partum eclampsia, where slow intravenous injection of 4–5 cc will almost instantly ward off an attack; in tetanic and other convulsions.

Contraindications: Severe kidney disease with urine retention or uremic symptoms.

Caution: Intravenous injection is to be given slowly, at most 1 cc per minute as controlled by the watch; injection is interrupted as soon as sleep is produced; where morphine also is desired prior to an operation, it is given in one-half the usual dosage; atropine may be given instead of morphine in doses of 0.4–0.6 mg (1/150–1/100 gr) ½ hr. before the administration of Pernoston.

Dosage: 1 cc per 12½ kg (27½ lb.) of body weight.

Supply: PERNOSTON—Ampules 1.1 cc (10%)—Boxes of 10
PERNOSTON—Ampules 2.2 cc (10%)—Boxes of 10
PERNOSTON—Ampules 2.2 cc (10%)—Boxes of 50
} 1 cc of the solution in ampule contains 0.1 Gm (1½ gr) of Pernoston.

Bibliography: *See Chap. XII.*

PEROXOIDS (Merck)

Antacid

Chemical Name: Magnesium Superoxol.

Formula: MgO_2.

Description: A white, odorless, tasteless powder, containing 25% of Magnesium Peroxide of high purity; is insoluble in water, but readily dissolves in acids with the production of hydrogen peroxide.

Action: Antifermentative, antacid and mildly laxative. By the action of the acid gastric juices, it is converted into mildly laxative magnesium salts and magnesium oxide, which act as an antacid; hydrogen peroxide is also formed, which in turn liberates active oxygen, effective in inhibiting fermentation and putrefactive processes; stimulates peristalsis and the secretion of alkaline gastric mucus; is non-toxic.

Uses: In disorders of the stomach and intestines, particularly with faulty digestion and fermentation; in hyperacidity, pyrosis, flatulence, intestinal autointoxication, excessive putrefaction and decomposition; in nausea, habitual constipation; also found *useful* in the alleviation of diseases with intestinal toxemia, in angina pectoris, gastric ulcer, pylorospasm, systemic acidosis, gout and diabetes.

Supply: PEROXOIDS—Tablets, gr 5 (0.3 Gm)—Tubes of 15—Bottles of 50 and 250.

Administration: 2 or 3 tablets or ½–1 teaspoonful stirred in a little water, as required.

Incompatibles: Acids and alkalies.

Advantages: Free from harmful or toxic effect.

PHANODORN (Winthrop)

Hypnotic

Chemical Name: Cyclohexenylethylbarbituric Acid. Brand of Cyclobarbital.

Formula: $(CH_2)_4(CH)\overline{C(C_2H_5)C}: (CONH)_2: CO.$

Description: A white, crystalline powder, of bitter taste; is sparingly soluble in water, more easily soluble in alkaline solution, readily soluble in alcohol, less soluble in ether.

Action: Hypnotic, of a potency midway between Veronal and Luminal; is fairly well absorbed, prompt in action and produces only moderate respiratory depression without initial excitation; the sleep produced is of normal character.

Uses: Nervous insomnia, neurasthenia, insomnia associated with hysteria, psychoses and cardiac disorders.

Supply: PHANODORN—Tablets (C.A.) 3 gr (0.194 Gm)—Tubes of 10—Bottles 100.

Administration: *Average Dose*—1 tablet, in obstinate cases 2 tablets, given at bedtime with a large cup of hot milk, weak tea or other warm drink.

Bibliography: *See Chap. XII.*

PHENACETIN (Winthrop)

Antipyretic. Analgesic

Chemical Name: Acetylparaphenetidin. Brand of Acetphenetidin.

Formula: $C_6H_4. O. C_2H_5. NH. CO. CH_3.$

Description: A white, odorless, tasteless, glistening, crystalline powder, soluble with difficulty in cold water, more readily soluble in hot water and easily soluble in alcohol.

Action: Analgesic, sedative, antipyretic and antispasmodic; in large doses is cardiac depressant and may produce hemolysis; in average doses is free from injurious effects.

Uses: As analgesic in headache, neuralgia, sciatica; as antipyretic in tonsillitis, pneumonia, typhoid, rheumatism and other febrile conditions.

Supply: PHENACETIN (C.A.)—Tablets, 5 gr—Bottles of 25 and 100.
PHENACETIN (C.A.)—Powder—Cartons of 1 oz.

Administration: Adults, 5–10 gr (0.3–0.6 Gm); children in proportion.

PHENOBARBITAL-SODIUM

Hypnotic

Chemical Name: Sodium Phenylethylbarbiturate.

Formula: $(C_6H_5)(C_2H_5): C: CONH. CONNa: CO.$ or $Na(C_{12}H_{11}N_2O_3).$

Description: A white crystalline hygroscopic powder, freely soluble in water.

Action and Uses: Is particularly indicated when quick sedation is desired, as in eclampsia, tetanus, status epilepticus, cocaine intoxication, dementias, drug addiction.

Supply: PHENOBARBITAL-SODIUM—In bulk, in quantities desired. (Benzol)

PHENOBARBITAL-SODIUM (C.A.)—Tablets gr 1½—Bottle of 50, 100, 500 and 1,000. (Gane-Ingram)

PHENOBARBITAL-SODIUM (C.A.)—Powder—Bottles ½, 1 and 4 oz. (Gane-Ingram)

PHENOBARBITAL-SODIUM (C.A.)—Boxes of ½ oz, ¼ and 1 lb. (Merck)

Administration: *Orally* 1½–5 gr (0.097–0.324 Gm); smaller dosage in the feeble. women and tubercular.
Rectally—20% solution; boiled, cooled and administered.
Hypodermically—20% solution, 1½–5 gr (0.097–0.324 Gm), as required.

PHENOLSULPHONPHTHALEIN

(Hynson, Westcott and Dunning)

Renal Function Test

Chemical Name: Phenolsulphonphthalein.

Formula: $(C_6H_4OH)_2CO.\ C_6H_4SO_2$.

Description: A crystalline, bright to dark red powder, stable in air; soluble in 1:300 parts of water and 350 parts of alcohol.

Action: Injected into tissues is readily absorbed and, except for small traces, is almost completely excreted in the urine, beginning 5–10 min. after injection and being almost totally eliminated (60–80%) within 2 hr.

Uses: Valuable in determining functional renal capacity; pre- and postoperatively; in nephritis, acute and chronic; in cardiorenal disease, uremia or impending uremia; in urinary obstruction to determine efficiency of each kidney.

Supply: PHENOLSULPHONPHTHALEIN (C.A.)—Ampules 1 cc, containing 6 mg of drug in sterile solution—Boxes of 10.

Administration: With bladder empty, 1 cc is injected *intravenously* or *intramuscularly;* this is preceded ½ hr. by the drinking of ½–1 glassful of water, to facilitate the excretion of the dye and urine; where injected intramuscularly—urine is collected after 70 min. and again 1 hr. later; an estimate of the total dye excreted is made by colorimetric determination. Normal: 1 hr.—50%, 2 hr.—85% elimination.
Where intravenously administered—urine is collected after 15 min., 30 min. and 1 hr. Normal elimination: 15 min.—35–45%, 30 min.—50–65%, 1 hr. 65–80%.

Caution: Exactly 1 cc, must be carefully injected.

Bibliography: *See Chap. XII.*

PHENOLTETRACHLORPHTHALEIN

(Hynson, Westcott and Dunning)

Liver Function Test

Official Name: Phenoltetrachlorphthaleinum.

Formula: $(C_6H_4OH)_2CO.\ C_6Cl_4CO$.

Composition: A dibasic dye formed by the condensation of phenol and tetrachlorphthalic acid or its anhydride.

Action and Uses: Is *used* for the determination of liver function; the test is based upon the fact that the dye, introduced intravenously, is normally eliminated by the liver from the venous circulation in 1 hr. and is absent from the venous blood in that time; if present, the liver is functioning improperly.

Supply: PHENOLTETRACHLORPHTHALEIN (C.A.)—Ampules, 2 cc of the disodium salt in solution; each cubic centimeter is equal to 50 mg of Phenoltetrachlorphthalein—Boxes of 8.

Administration: *Rosenthal Method*—5 mg per kilogram of body weight, or 0.05–0.4 Gm of the disodium salt is injected *intravenously;* after 1 hr. the blood is colorimetrically tested for the presence of dye; in diseases of the liver, the percentage of dye still circulating in the blood represents a quantitative index of the degree of impairment of hepatic function.

Bibliography: *See Chap. XII.*

PHLORIDZIN (Merck)

Renal Function Test

Chemical Name: Phlorhizin.

Formula: $C_{21}H_{24}O_{10} + 2H_2O$.

Description: A glucoside obtained from the roots of fruit trees: apple, pear, cherry, plum and others; occurs as small crystals of silky texture, pinkish color; at first, of bitter then of sweetish taste and no odor; is freely soluble in hot water and alcohol, sparingly soluble in ether.

Action: Produces renal glycosuria and polyuria; destroys malarial parasites; is also antipyretic.

Uses: In remittent and intermittent fever, but dangerous to use, large doses cause severe glycosuria; is of doubtful value as test of renal inadequacy; assurance of the absence of glucose from urine must first be had before applying the test.

Supply: PHLORIDZIN (C.A.)—Bottles, 1 oz.

Administration: *Renal Function Test*—1/12 gr (0.005 Gm) is dissolved in 15 m (1 cc) of a 0.5% solution of sodium carbonate and injected hypodermically just after the bladder has been emptied. If the kidneys are adequate, glucose appears in the urine in 1/4–1/2 hr.

Internal Dose—5–10 gr (0.3–0.6 Gm), as antipyretic.

PHYLLICIN (Bilhuber-Knoll)

Diuretic

Chemical Name: Theophylline-Calcium Salicylate.

Formula: $C_7H_3N_4O_2C_6H_4CO_2$. Ca. + $2H_2O$.

Description: A white crystalline powder, slightly soluble in water.

Action and Uses: Diuretic and cardiac stimulant; reduces edema in congestive heart failure and relieves dyspnea; increases cardiac blood supply, ameliorates anginal pain in coronary disease and increases heart efficiency.

Advantages: Permits larger dosage and extended therapy without disturbing the gastro-intestinal tract or irritating the kidneys.

Supply: PHYLLICIN—Tablets gr 4 (0.25 Gm)—Tubes of 20—Bottles of 100.

PHYLLICIN—Powder—Bottles of 1/2 oz.

Administration: 1 tablet or gr 4 of powder two to four times daily after meals.

Bibliography: *See Chap. XII.*

PHYTINE (Ciba)

Calcium-Phosphorus Therapy

Chemical Name: Calcium Magnesium Inosithexaphosphoric Acid.

Description: Contains 12% calcium, 22% phosphorus, 1.5% magnesium in organic combination; is fully absorbed and non-toxic.

Uses: Indicated wherever calcium and phosphorus in a readily assimilable form is desired; in rickets, osteomalacia, delayed union of fractures; in asthma, vasomotor rhinitis, urticaria, tetany, spasmophilic expressions in young children; also *useful* in nervous affections, convalescence, tuberculosis, pregnancy and lactation.

Supply: PHYTINE—Tablets—4 gr (0.259 Gm)—Bottles of 40.

Administration: Adults—1–4 tablets daily, with meals.
Children—2–6 yr.—1 or 2 tablets daily; 6–10 yr.—2 or 3 tablets daily.

Bibliography: *See Chap. XII.*

PIPERAZINE (Winthrop)

Uricolytic

Chemical Name: Diethylenediamin.

Formula: $NH(CH_2)_2:(CH_2)_2NH$.

Description: Transparent, hygroscopic crystals of alkaline reaction, freely soluble in water.

Action: A uric acid solvent, twelve times as powerful as lithium carbonate; is oxidized in the organism only partly and in part is eliminated unchanged; is thought to form with the uric acid of the organism a soluble urate which is readily excreted and thus to reduce hyperuricemia.

Uses: Uricacidemia, gout, chronic rheumatism, rheumatoid arthritis, renal calculi, uratic tophi and other disturbances of uratic origin.

Supply: PIPERZINE—Powder, ½ oz. in bottles.

Administration: 15–20 gr (1.0–1.2 Gm) daily, given with abundance of alkaline mineral water.

PITOCIN (Parke, Davis)

Hormone Therapy

Chemical Name: Alpha-Hypophamine.

Description: Is the oxytocic principle of the Pituitary Gland, biologically standard ized to contain 10 international units of oxytocic activity per cubic centimeter.

Action: Stimulates uterine contraction in labor; shortens coagulation time in hemorrhage; does not increase blood pressure.

Uses: In uterine inertia in cases where Pituitrin is contraindicated on account of its blood pressure raising action; to hasten delivery in protracted labor without physical impediment; in exhaustion of uterine contractility; in eclamptic or preeclamptic cases, where it is preferable to pituitary extract or Pituitrin.

Contraindications: Those of Pituitrin in obstetrics, except that high blood pressure is not a contraindication.

Supply: PITOCIN—Ampules (C.A.)—½ cc and 1 cc—Boxes of 6 and 100.

Administration: 0.2–0.5 cc (3–8 m) *intramuscularly;* repeated if necessary at intervals of 20–30 min.

Bibliography: *See Chap. XII.*

PITRESSIN (Parke, Davis)

Hormone Therapy

Chemical Name: Beta-Hypophamine.

Description: Contains the pressor and antidiuretic principle of the Pituitary Gland; standardized to contain 20 pressor units per cubic centimeter, or double the activity of Pituitrin.

Action: Stimulates heart and blood-vessels by peripheral action, producing a more gradual rise in blood pressure and longer lasting than that produced by adrenalin; stimulates intestinal musculature and increases peristalsis; prevents excessive loss of water from body tissues.

Uses: In urticaria, angioneurotic edema; in postoperative or paralytic flatulence and intestinal atony, atonic constipation, ischuria paradoxa; in hypotension of shock, pneumonia or diphtheria; in nocturnal enuresis and diabetes insipidus.

Contraindications: Epilepsy, nephritis with hypertension, arteriosclerosis, goitre with cardiac complications, angina pectoris, coronary sclerosis.

Supply: PITRESSIN—Ampules 1 cc (C.A.)—Boxes of 6 and 100.

PITRESSIN—Nasal Jelly—Tubes of 3 Gm—Boxes of 6.

Administration: *Hypodermic*—3–5 m.
Intranasal—By spray, pledget or jelly.

PITUITARY EXTRACT (Lederle)

Vasoconstrictor

Description: Is prepared from standard Post-Pituitary powder, in 3 strengths per cubic centimeter—5 units (mild obstetrical), 10 units (regular obstetrical and surgical) and 20 units (surgical).

Uses and Administration: Obstetrics:

For Induction of Labor—In castor oil and quinine technique.
Intramuscularly—2–4 units every 2 hr. for 3 doses.

First Stage of Labor—Only in marginal placenta praevia with incomplete dilatation of the cervix and ruptured membranes—2 units.

Second Stage of Labor—To stimulate contractions in secondary uterine inertia, not due to mechanical causes, and where the fetal head is on the pelvic floor—2–4 units; repeated only when the effect of the previous dose has worn off.

Third Stage of Labor—To prevent hemorrhage and to complete expulsion of the placenta—5 units.

Postpartum—As prophylactic against uterine relaxation and hemorrhage—5–10 units with ergot; in postpartum hemorrhage—10 units; in Cesarian section—10 units injected into uterine muscle immediately before incision, as prophylactic against excessive hemorrhage.

Contraindications—Contracted pelvis, nephritis, myocarditis, arteriosclerosis, threatened uterine rupture.

Surgical Shock—To raise blood pressure—20 units; intravenously, if necessary, in emergencies.

Intestinal Stasis—20 units immediately after operation, and repeated every 6 hr. for 4 doses, where demanded.

Diabetes Insipidus—Beginning with 3–4 units, increased daily until an intestinal reaction is produced; in infants—half units.

Vesical Atony—For incontinence of urine—10–20 units, children 2 units, gradually increased.

Supply: PITUITARY EXTRACT—Ampules 1 cc (white), 5 international units—Cartons of 6 and 100.

PITUITARY EXTRACT—Ampules 1 cc (yellow), 10 international units—Cartons of 6 and 100.

PITUITARY EXTRACT—Ampules 1 cc (red), 20 international units—Cartons of 6 and 100.

PITUITARY LIQUID (Armour)

Vasoconstrictor

Description: A sterile, isotonic solution of the active principles of Posterior Pituitary.

Action and Uses: Checks uterine atony and hemorrhage by stimulating uterine musculature; promotes intestinal peristalsis and raises arterial tension. *Used* in uterine inertia during second stage of labor; in post-partum hemorrhage after placental expulsion; in surgical prophylaxis against postoperative intestinal paresis and urinary suppression.

Supply: PITUITARY LIQUID—Obstetrical (C.A.)—Ampules 0.5 and 1 cc—Hypodermic—Boxes 6, 50 and 100.

PITUITARY LIQUID—Surgical—Ampules 1 cc (Double strength) Hypodermic—Boxes 6, 50, 100.

PITUITARY LIQUID—Surgical and Obstetrical—Ampules 1 cc—Hypodermic—Boxes 6, 50 and 100.

Administration: Induction of Labor—Watson technic; Castor oil at 6 P. M., quinine gr 10 (0.65 Gm) 7 P. M., soapsuds enema at 8 P. M., quinine again gr 10 (0.65 Gm) at 9 P. M. and 10 P. M.; following morning ½ cc pituitary liquid; repeated every ½ hr. for 6 doses.

Surgical—1–2 cc 4 hr. after operation as prophylactic; same dosage in paralytic ileus, sudden heart failure.

Medical—In diabetes insipidus and arterial hypotension—*hypodermically* or *intranasally*, 0.5–1 cc; increased if necessary.

PITUITARY SOLUTION

Vasoconstrictor

Official Name: Solutio Hypophysis.

Description: A sterile, aqueous solution of Postpituitary, physiologically standardized; includes the oxytocic, pressor and diuretic principles.

Action: Vasoconstrictor, powerful stimulant of smooth musculature; oxytocic and hemostatic.

Uses: In uterine inertia, induction of labor and slow labor, threatened eclampsia, prevention of post-partum hemorrhage, lateral placenta praevia; also in intestinal paresis, urinary retention, vesical incontinence; as hemostatic—in uterine hemorrhage from fibroids, uterine appendages and ovarian cyst; in menorrhagia, metritis, endometritis, post-partum curettage; in pulmonary hemorrhage; in diabetes insipidus, shock.

Supply: LIQUOR PITUITARII U.S.P.—Ampules 1 cc, 10 units—Boxes 5. (Harrower)

PITUITARY SOLUTION—Obstetrical (C.A.)—Ampules 1 cc, 5 units—Boxes of 6 and 100. (Squibb)

PITUITARY SOLUTION—Surgical (C.A.)—Ampules 1 cc, 20 units—Boxes of 6 and 100. (Squibb)

Administration: *Subcutaneously or Intramuscularly*—3–10 units obstetrical, 3–30 units surgical; repeated in ½–1 hr. if necessary.

Contraindications: Nephritis, myocarditis, arteriosclerosis, first stage of labor, contracted pelvis, twin pregnancy.

PITUITRIN (Parke, Davis)

Vasoconstrictor

Composition: An aqueous extract of the posterior lobe of the Pituitary Gland, physiologically standardized for pressor and oxytocic activity.

Action and Uses: Tones up the vascular system; is of great value in the prevention of surgical shock; has prompt effect on both vesical atony and excessive diuresis. Stimulates the contractility of the sensitized uterus, being thus of great service, when carefully used, in protracted labor due to uterine inertia.

Supply: PITUITRIN—Ampules (C.A.) 0.5 cc—Boxes of 6 and 100.

PITUITRIN—Ampules Surgical (C.A.) 1 cc—Boxes of 6 and 100.

Administration: *Hypodermic;* also *intranasal:*

Obstetrics—For weak pains in the second stage of labor or toward the end of the first stage, when the cervix is dilated or freely dilatable, membranes ruptured and presenting part well engaged; dose—0.2—0.5 cc (3–8 m), *hypodermically;* repeated if necessary in 20–30 min.; in the third stage, after placental delivery to induce uterine involution, in postpartum hemorrhage from atony and in the late puerperal hemorrhages—same dosage.

Surgery—In failing blood pressure, atonic hemorrhage, postoperative intestinal stasis, tympanites, ischuria paradoxa—1 cc (16 m) every 3 or 4 hr. If Pituitrin "S" is used, the dose is halved.

Nocturnal Enuresis—0.2–0.5 cc (3–8 m) on retiring; repeated if required.

Diabetes Insipidus—0.5–1 cc (8–16 m) as often as required.

Cardiac Failure of Pneumonia, Diphtheria, Peritonitis and Other Infections—0.5–1 cc.

Contraindications: Hypertension, nephritis, hyperthyroidism with cardiac complications, arteriosclerosis, epilepsy, eclampsia, pre-eclampsia, irregularity of fetal heart beat, contracted pelvis, fetal malposition, tumor, complete uterine inertia. uterine scars from previous Caesarian section.

Bibliography: *See Chap. XII.*

PIXALBOL (Bilhuber-Knoll)

Antiseptic

Description: A purified colorless tar without sticky or ill-smelling qualities; a thin, pale yellow liquid, miscible with alcohol and petrolatum.

Action: Antiparasitic, antipruritic, stimulating; relieves itching, reduces infiltration, promotes epithelization.

Uses: In all conditions where tar is employed, in eczema, pruritus, urticaria, strophulus, hyperhidrosis, alopecia.

Supply: PIXALBOL—Bottles 1 and 8 oz.

Administration: *Used* as paint or ointment, or in alcoholic solution.

Advantages: Is non-staining and free from inert and irritant terpenes

Bibliography: *See Chap. XII.*

PLASMOCHIN (Winthrop)

Antimalarial

Chemical Name: N-diethylamino-isopentyl-8-amino-6-methoxyquinolin. Brand of Aminoquin.

Description: A tasteless, granular, bright yellow stable powder, freely soluble in alcohol, almost insoluble in water.

Action: Rapidly destroys the sexual forms (gametes) of malarial parasites, controls the fever and other symptoms and prevents relapses; the Plasmochin base is broken off in the gastrointestinal tract and is readily absorbed.

Uses: In malaria, all types—tertian, quartan, subtertian; also in blackwater fever.

Supply: PLASMOCHIN—Tablets, ⅓ gr (0.021 Gm)—Bottles of 25.

PLASMOCHIN COMPOUND—Tablets ⅙ gr (0.012 Gm), containing 2 gr (0.130 Gm) of quinine sulphate—Bottles of 50.

Administration: Plasmochin—Adults—1 tablet three times daily; infants and children, in proportion.

Plasmochin Compound—Adults, 2 tablets three times daily; infants, 1 tablet daily; children, 1 tablet one to four times daily. Treatment may be continuous, when full dosage is given for 2 weeks and then reduced during the succeeding 4 weeks; or intermittent, where the drug is given 5–7 days followed by an interval of 4 days after each course.

Caution: Plasmochin Compound is not to be administered to pregnant women and those with marked quinine idiosyncrasy; in these only Plasmochin (plain) is to be used. Untoward effects are shown by cyanosis, methemoglobinemia, abdominal pain, epigastric tenderness, headache, giddiness, nausea, clammy sweats.

Bibliography: *See Chap. XII.*

PLESTRIN SOLUTION (Harrower)

Hormone Therapy

Description: A clear standardized solution of the estrus producing hormone identical with Folliculin but prepared from placenta; standardized to contain 50 rat units per cubic centimeter.

Action and Uses: Will induce estrus in ovariectomized animals; *For use* in organic ovarian insufficiency, infantilism, maldevelopment of uterus and ovaries, primary amenorrhea or sterility.

Supply: PLESTRIN SOLUTION—Ampules 1 cc—Boxes of 5.

PLESTRIN—Capsules, 5 gr, equivalent to 5 rat units—Boxes of 40.

Administration: 1 ampule *intramuscularly* daily or every other day for several months, particularly during 10 days preceding menstruation; 1–3 capsules three times daily as supplement to Plestrin Solution therapy.

PLUMBICOL (Mulford Colloid)

Lead Therapy

Description: Occurs in greyish white lustrous scales, fairly soluble in water; contains 20% lead.

Action and Uses: A stable, non-irritating, readily absorbed and assimilated preparation of Colloidal Lead; is slowly eliminated and of prolonged action; does not cause precipitation of tissue fluids. *For use* in the treatment of malignancy.

Supply: PLUMBICOL—Vials 10 and 60 Gm.

PLUMBICOL SOLUTION—10% Ampule—Vial 25 cc.

Administration: *Orally*—½–2½ gr (0.032–0.162 Gm).
Hypodermically—¼–2 cc.

POTASSIUM BISMUTH TARTRATE (Abbott)

Antiluetic

Official Name: Potassii Bismuthi Tartras cum Butyni.

Formula: $C_4H_2O_9Bi_3K.\ 4H_2O$.

Composition: A basic potassium bismuth tartrate, containing from 64% to 69% of bismuth.

Description: Occurs as a finely granular white odorless powder, of sweetish taste and permanent in air; is soluble in water, insoluble in alcohol, chloroform and ether, completely soluble in alkalies and decomposed by acids.

Uses: As adjuvant to arsenicals in the treatment of syphilis; is especially indicated in cases resistant to or intolerant of arsenicals and mercury.

Contraindications: Sepsis, severe nephritis, oral infection.

Supply: **POTASSIUM BISMUTH TARTRATE WITH BUTYN** (C.A.), Ampules 2 cc, containing Potassium Bismuth Tartrate 0.1 Gm, with Butyn 0.012 Gm, suspended in almond oil—Boxes of 10 and 100 ampules.

POTASSIUM BISMUTH TARTRATE WITH BUTYN (C.A.)—Ampules 2 cc, containing Potassium Bismuth Tartrate 0.2 Gm, with Butyn 0.012 Gm, suspended in almond oil—Boxes of 10 and 100—Bottles 20 cc—Box of 6.

POTASSIUM BISMUTH TARTRATE WITH BUTYN (C.A.)—Ampules 10%, each cubic centimeter containing Potassium Bismuth Tartrate 0.1 Gm, Butyn 0.6% and Metaphen 0.01%, suspended in expressed almond oil—Boxes of 6.

Administration: 0.1–0.2 Gm *intramuscularly only*, at intervals of 4–7 days, until a total of 2.4 Gm–3.0 Gm is administered.

Caution: Should never be injected intravenously.

POTASSIUM MERCURIC IODIDE (Abbott)

Germicide. Antiluetic

Official Name: Potassii Hydrargyri Iodidi; Mercury Biniodide.

Formula: K_2HgI_4.

Description: Yellow crystals, deliquescent in air; soluble in alcohol and in 1 part of water; contains 25.5% of mercury.

Action and Uses: An effective germicide; does not coagulate albumin; *used* externally in various skin affections, for irrigation, disinfection of instruments and excreta; internally in syphilis.

Advantages: Is more soluble than ordinary mercuric oxide; safer than mercuric chloride and only half as toxic.

Supply: **POTASSIUM MERCURIC IODIDE**—Ampules (C.A.)—1 cc, containing gr ¼ (0.0016 Gm) of the drug in 0.01 Gm of potassium iodide solution—Boxes of 12 and 100.

Administration: *Externally*—1:100–1:1,000 solution in 0.9% saline for irrigation, disinfection.
Internally—1 ampule *intramuscularly*, every 3–4 days.

PROCAINE (Abbott)

Anesthetic

Chemical Name: Procaine Hydrochloride; Para-amino-benzoyl-diethylaminoethanol Hydrochloride.

Formula: $NH_2(C_6H_4CO)OC_2H_4N(C_2H_5)_2HCl$.

Description: Small colorless, odorless, stable crystals or white crystalline powder.

Action: A powerful local anesthetic, less toxic than cocaine or its substitutes.

Administration and Uses: **Dental**—Conductive anesthesia—2% solution for intra- or extra-nerve block. Infiltration anesthesia—1–2% solution for contact and high pressure infiltration, intraosseous, peridental, subperiosteal and in ionization.

Medical—Infiltration anesthesia—For nerve block ½–1% solution; direct and perineural—5% solution; spinal 5–10% solution; urethral—5%.

Supply: **PROCAINE**—Tablets (C.A.) gr ⅓ (0.021 Gm)—Tubes 20, 5 tubes to box—Bottles of 100.

1 tablet in 1 cc makes 2% solution.

PROCAINE—Tablets (C.A.) gr ¾ (0.048 Gm)—Tubes of 20, 5 tubes to box—Bottles of 100.

1 tablet in 2½ cc makes a 2% solution.

PROCAINE—Tablets (C.A.) gr 3 (0.194 Gm)—Tubes of 10—Bottles of 100, 1,000.

1 tablet in 10 cc makes a 2% solution.

PROCAINE—Tablets (C.A.) A-P 1—Containing Procaine gr ⅓ (0.021 Gm), Epinephrine gr 1:2,500 (0.00002 Gm) and Sodium Chloride sufficient for isotonicity—Bottles 100, 1,000.

1 tablet in 1 cc makes a 2% solution.

PROCAINE—Tablets (C.A.) A-P 2—Containing Procaine gr ⅓ (0.021 Gm), Epinephrine gr 1/1,500 (0.00004 Gm) and Sodium Chloride sufficient for isotonicity—Bottles 100, 1,000.

1 tablet in 1 cc makes a 2% solution.

PROCAINE—Spinal (C.A.)—Ampule, 100, 120, 150 and 200 mg crystals—Cartons of 1.

Caution: In preparing solutions from tablets containing epinephrin, the distilled water should first be boiled before these are added; no Ringer's or saline need be used.

PROCAINE BORATE AND EPINEPHRIN (Searle)

Local Anesthetic

Chemical Name: Procaine Borate.

Formula: $C_{13}H_2ON_2O_25HBO_2$.

Description: A white amorphous powder, freely soluble in water; most useful in 2% concentrations in dental work and in ½–1% in surface anesthesia in eye or other fields.

Action and Uses: Is fourteen times less toxic than cocaine and two and one half times less toxic than novocaine; causes immediate anesthesia lasting for an hour and a quarter; *used* for local and surface anesthesia, in medicine and dentistry.

Supply: **PROCAINE BORATE AND EPINEPHRIN**—Tablets (C.A.) 0.05 gr—Bottles of 100.

PROCAINE BORATE—Powder—Bottles 15½ gr (1 Gm) (1 Gm in 100 cc distilled water makes a 1% solution).

Bibliography: *See Chap. XII.*

PROFLAVINE

Antiseptic

Chemical Name: 3.6 Diaminoacridinium Monohydrogen Sulphate.

Formula: $C_{13}H_{12}N_3 . HSO_4$.

Description: A reddish brown, odorless, crystalline powder, soluble in water and alcohol, almost insoluble in chloroform, ether and petroleum.

Action and Uses: Is a strong antiseptic *for use* in wounds, ulcers, abscesses and other infections.

Supply: **PROFLAVINE** (C.A.)—Bottles of 1 Gm, 5 Gm, 1 oz. **(Abbott)**

PROFLAVINE (C.A.)—Bottles of 5 Gm, 10 Gm. **(National Aniline)**

Administration: For topical application by swab, syringe or on gauze, in 1:1,000 physiologic saline solution; also as 1% ointment. In gonorrheal infections, for injection—1:1,000, for irrigation—1:4,000.

PROGYNON **(Schering)**

Hormone Therapy

Composition: Standardized female sex hormone including lipoids from placenta and ovaries freed from the follicular element.

Action and Uses: *For use* in female sex deficiencies, menopausal disturbances, ovarian dysfunction, amenorrhea, dysmenorrhea, nausea and vomiting of pregnancy; in sterility due to uterine underdevelopment.

Supply: **PROGYNON**—Tablets—each 45 Allen-Doisy Units—Bottles of 30 and 60.

PROGYNON—Tablets—each 200 Allen-Doisy Units—Bottles of 30.

PROGYNON—Ampules—1 cc, each 25 Allen-Doisy Units—Boxes of 12.

PROGYNON—Ampules in oil 2,000 Units (absorbed over 14 days)—Boxes of 1 and 3.

Administration: *Menstrual Disturbances*—1 tablet three times daily or 1 ampule daily for 10 days prior to the expected menstrual period.

Menopausal Disorders—1 tablet three times daily until symptoms are ameliorated, then dosage is decreased.

Bibliography: *See Chap. XII.*

PROPOSOTE **(Parke, Davis)**

Expectorant

Chemical Name: Creosote Phenylpropionate.

Description: An amber colored, oily liquid of creosote-like odor and slightly bitter taste; insoluble in water, soluble in alcohol, ether and fatty oil; contains 50% of creosote.

Action and Uses: An expectorant; does not affect the stomach but is decomposed in the intestines and its components are eliminated through the kidneys; *For use* in all conditions where creosote is helpful: chronic bronchitis, tuberculosis.

Supply: **PROPOSOTE**—Capsules (C.A.) 5 m and 10 m—Boxes of 12 and 100.

Administration: 5–10 m three times daily; children—5 m per dose.

PROSTIGMIN (Roche)

Intestinal Peristaltic

Chemical Name: Dimethyl-carbamic ester of 3-oxyphenyl-trimethyl-ammonium methyl sulphate.

Formula: $C_{13}H_{22}O_6N_2S$.

Description: A synthetic compound resembling physostigmine but differing from it chemically by its less complicated molecular structure, and pharmacologically by a more powerful action on peristalsis, less pronounced miotic effect and almost complete absence of cardiac by-effects; is a white powder, fully soluble in water and to a lesser degree in alcohol.

Uses: An *injectable* intestinal peristaltic for use whenever intestinal function is imperative, as in major post-operative cases; here an injection is given the day following the operation; in intestinal paralysis from any cause; also in the bed-ridden requiring catharsis.

Supply: PROSTIGMIN—Ampules, 1.1 cc (0.05% solution)—Boxes of 6.

Administration: Contents of 1 ampule is injected *subcutaneously* or *intramuscularly* and followed in 30 min. by a glycerin enema, 150–200 cc; if no evacuation occurs after 4 or 5 hr. the injection can be safely repeated.

Caution: Should not be used in asthmatics because of its physiologic stimulation of the parasympathetic system and contraction of smooth musculature.

PROTAN (Sharp and Dohme)

Intestinal Astringent

Chemical Name: Tannin Caseinate.

Description: A chemical combination of Casein with about 50% of Tannic Acid; a light brown powder, tasteless, odorless and partly insoluble in water; does not coagulate albumin nor affect pepsin and peptones.

Action: Passes through the stomach unchanged and without affecting it; is soluble in the alkaline secretions of the intestine where its astringent effect is produced on the entire bowel.

Uses: Indicated in all types of enterocolitis with thin and watery stools: cholera morbus, acute intestinal catarrh, chronic diarrhea; especially valuable in these diseases of children.

Supply: PROTAN—Powder (C.A.)—Boxes of 1 oz.

PROTAN—Tablets (C.A.) gr 5—Bottles of 100 and 1,000.

Combination: PROTAN COMPOUND—Tablets—Bottles of 100, contains: Protan, 2 gr; Bismuth subnitrate, 1/4 gr; Zinc Sulphocarbolate, 1/8 gr; Opium powdered, 1/50 gr; Calomel, 1/40 gr; Pepsin, 1/8 gr; Pancreatin, 1/8 gr; Powdered Ginger, 1/16 gr; Guaiacol, 1/20 gr; Oil anise, q.s.

Administration: 5–10 gr every 1 or 2 hr.; in infants and children, as demanded; in chronic diarrhea—10–30 gr every 1 or 2 hr. until effect is obtained.

PROTARGOL (Winthrop)

Antiseptic. Gonocide

Chemical Name: Silver Albumose. Brand of strong Silver Protein.

Description: An organic silver derivative; a fine yellowish powder, soluble up to 50% in water; contains 8.3% silver in organic combination.

Action: Powerful antigonorrhoeic, non-irritating in strengths ordinarily used; is efficient even in weak solutions.

Uses and Administration: Urology—Acute urethritis, solutions of ½–1%; in chronic gonorrhea 2–5%; as prophylactic, 2%.

Gynecology—Infections of female genitals, endometritis, vaginitis, vulvovaginitis, endocervicitis, from 2–10%.

Rhinolaryngology—½–10% for topical application in nose and throat.

Ophthalmology—Ophthalmia neonatorum prophylaxis, 2%; acute and chronic conjunctivitis and blepharitis, ½–2%; trachoma—up to 20 or 25%.

Surgery—For ordinary wounds and ulcers, from 1–10%; for rectal irrigation, in colitis and proctitis, 2%.

Supply: PROTARGOL—Powder (C.A.), Bottles 1 oz.

PROTARGOL—Granules (C.A.); containing ⅓ of Protargol combined with ⅔ of Urea for greater solubility—Bottles 1 oz.

Caution: Solutions should be freshly prepared without heating and preserved in dark colored bottles; Protargol stains, if fresh, may be removed with soap and water; if old—with peroxide and ammonia.

Bibliography: *See Chap. XII.*

PSYLLIUM SEED

Laxative

Official Name: Semen Psyllii.

Description: Seeds of Plantago Psyllium and related species; are of ovoid shape, about 3 × 1.5 mm in size, convex on one side, concave on other; dark brown color, tasteless and odorless.

Action: Mixed with equal parts of water forms a mucilaginous bulky mass which acts as direct stimulant to the intestine and produces a laxative effect.

Uses: Where laxative action is desired, particularly in spastic constipation with small stools.

Supply: PSYLLIUM SEED—Bottles of 10 oz. (Lilly)

PSYLLIUM (PLANTAGO SEED)—Cans of 12 oz., and 5 lb. (MacDowell)

Administration: 1–4 dr. (4–15 Gm) mixed with fruit juices, hot water, as jelly or with other food; one to three times daily after meals.

P-THIOCRESOL (Eastman)

Epithelial Proliferant

Description: A product of substitution of the SH (sulphydryl) radicle for the OH group in cresol; soluble in alcohol, nearly insoluble in water.

Formula: $CH_3C_6H_4SH$.

Action and Uses: Stimulates cell proliferation and production of granulation tissue in chronic ulceration and slow healing wounds; produces new skin of greater thickness.

Supply: P-THIOCRESOL—Crystalline solid—Bottles 10 Gm, 100 Gm.

Administration: Applied in 1:10,000 solution every 48 hr., using saline wet dressings between applications.

Bibliography: *See Chap. XII.*

PYRAMIDON (Metz)

Analgesic. Antipyretic

Chemical Name: Dimethylaminophenyldimethylpyrazolon. Brand of Amidopyrine.

Formula: $C_6H_5.\ N.\ CO.\ C(N[CH_3]_2):C(CH_3).\ N.\ CH_3.$

Description: A white, faintly bitter crystalline powder, readily soluble in alcohol and in 10–15 parts of water.

Action: Similar to that of antipyrine but more effective, relief from pain being more prompt and more prolonged; is comparatively harmless to cardiovascular and renal systems and seldom causes gastric disturbances.

Uses: Influenza, colds, neuralgia, migraine, rheumatic pains and febrile diseases, especially measles.

Supply: PYRAMIDON—Tablets (C.A.), 1½ gr (0.09 Gm)—Bottles of 25 and 100.

PYRAMIDON—Tablets (C.A.) 5 gr (0.32 Gm)—Tubes of 10—Bottles of 100.

PYRAMIDON—Tablets (C.A.) in 1 oz. cartons.

PYRAMIDON—Elixir (C.A.)—Bottles of 4 oz.; very agreeable and palatable, each dram containing 2½ gr Pyramidon; best given alone to avoid possible chemical incompatibility; *Dosage*—1–2 teaspoonfuls.

PYRAMIDON SALICYLATE—Tablets 0.25 Gm each—Bottles of 25.

Administration: Adults—3–5 gr, repeated if necessary in 3 or 4 hr.
Children—1 gr per year of age; maximum 5 gr every 4 hr.

Bibliography: *See Chap. XII.*

PYRIDIUM (Merck)

Genito-Urinary Antiseptic

Chemical Name: Phenylazo-2-6-diamino-pyridine mono-hydrochloride. The monohydrochloride of an azo dye of the pyridine series.

Formula: $C_6H_5N:NC_5H_2N(NH_2)_2(2)(6)HCl.$

Description: Occurs as red, odorless, microcrystalline powder of somewhat bitter taste; is only slightly soluble in cold water (about 0.3:100), more soluble in boiling water (about 5:100), poorly soluble in alcohol and soluble in glacial acetic acid; is insoluble in oils, acetone, benzene, chloroform, ether and toluene. The aqueous solution (1 in 500) is red and is distinctly acid in reaction; contains 28% of nitrogen.

Action and Uses: A non-toxic, non-irritating, deeply penetrating antiseptic; is bactericidal in vitro in aqueous solution against staphylococci, streptococci, gonococci, colon and diphtheria bacilli; in the urine, whether acid or alkaline, is bacteriostatic; internally, is non-toxic and non-irritating and has considerable penetrative power; is excreted by the kidneys in 45 min. to 1 hr., staining the urine red; its antibacterial properties are relative to the dosage ingested and the fluid intake. *Useful* in gonococcus as well as colon bacillus and mixed infections —in cystitis, pyelitis of adults or children, in pyelitis of pregnancy.

Supply: Pyridium—Tablets 1½ gr (0.1 Gm), Sugar coated—Bottles of 50, 500, 1,000—Tubes of 12.

PYRIDIUM—Solution (1%), with 10% Dextrose added—Bottles of 100 and 1,000 cc.

PYRIDIUM—Ointment (10%) Jars 25 Gm.

PYRIDIUM—Powder—Vials 2, 5 and 10 Gm.

Administration: *Internally—Prophylactic*—Adults—1 tablet or 1 dr. (0.4) of solution four times daily.
Therapeutic—2 tablets or 2 dr. of solution three times daily before meals.

Children: Up to 3 mo.—3 m of solution four times daily.

3– 6 mo.	6 "
6– 9 "	9 "
9–12 "	12 "
1– 3 yr.	24–30—twice daily
3– 6 "	30–40 " "
6– 9 "	40–50 " " (or ½ tablet)
9–12 "	50–60 " " (½ tablet three times daily)
12–15 "	1 tablet or 1 dr. three times daily.

Externally—Urethral injection—1:3,000 to 1:1,000; bladder irrigation—1:6,000 to 1:1,000; kidney lavage—1:10,000; to 1:1,500; topical application—1:400 to 1:100; *Topically*—the powder mixed with water or glycerin to a paste, and the ointment are used in appropriate conditions.

Contraindications: Nephritis, uremia, chronic gastrointestinal disorders, hyperacidity.

Incompatibilities: Mercury bichloride, silver nitrate, sulphur compounds and strong mineral acids; also chlorine, iodine and all alcoholic solutions.

Bibliography: *See Chap. XII.*

QUINICARDINE "NATIVELLE" (Fougera)

Cardiac Rhythm Normalizer

Description: Gluten coated tablets of Quinidine Sulphate, gr 3 (0.194 Gm).

Action: Checks fibrillation; decreases auricular irritability, slows heart rate, lengthens auriculo-ventricular conduction time.

Uses: *Effective* in fibrillation, arrhythmia, tachycardia.

Supply: QUINICARDINE "NATIVELLE"—Tablets 3½ gr (0.227 Gm)—Bottles of 20.

Administration: Course consists of 10 days; first day 1 tablet is given to determine idiosyncrasy to drug and if no susceptibility is shown is repeated in 2 hr. Regular administration is begun the next day with 6–8 tablets daily, maximum dose 15–30 gr (1.0–2.0 Gm), until normal rhythm is established; continued till tenth day and then followed by digitalis therapy for 4–6 weeks; another course of 10 days is repeated if necessary.

Contraindications: In cardiac insufficiency with bradycardia and in auricular thrombosis and embolism.

QUINIDINE

Cardiac Rhythm Regulator

Chemical Name: Conchinine; Quinidina; N.F.V. Chinidine.

Formula: $C_{20}H_{24}N_2O_2 + 2H_2O$.

Description: An alkaloid obtained from Cinchona bark; occurs as white crystals or amorphous white powder; is odorless, intensely bitter; very slightly soluble in water and petroleum benzin; soluble in alcohol, ether, chloroform.

Action: Decreases irritability and conductivity of heart muscle and prolongs auricular diastole, thus reestablishing normal rhythm in the fibrillating heart;

slows the pulse rate, increases its force and tone; is a protoplasm poison, affecting protozoa, though less powerfully than quinine; has no cumulative effect, being quickly eliminated.

Uses: Antiperiodic, antipyretic, antiseptic and tonic; *most effective* in auricular fibrillation, recent and paroxysmal; is employed in other conditions instead of quinine but is somewhat weaker in action; its salts are less agreeable to take, but more promptly effective.

Supply: QUINIDINE (C.A.)—Bottles of 1 oz.—Tins of 5 oz. (Merck)

QUINIDINE (C.A.)—Bottles of 1 oz.—Tins of 5, 25, 50 and 100 oz. (N. Y. Quinine)

Administration: *Dose*—Tonic—½–3 gr (0.03–0.2 Gm); average dose 1½ gr (0.1 Gm).

Antiperiodic—20–30 gr (1.3–2 Gm). Average dose 15 gr (1 Gm) per day.

Colds—5–10 gr (0.3–0.6 Gm), in syrup, capsule or pill.

Auricular Fibrillation—3 gr (0.2 Gm) as preliminary dose to determine possible idiosyncrasy; if none is present, then 6 gr (0.36 Gm) four to five times daily until normal rhythm is established, and continued as maintenance dose as frequently as conditions demand. *Maximum Dose*—15–30 gr (1–2 Gm).

Contraindications: Auricular thrombosis, ventricular tachycardia, ventricular extrasystole, acute or recurrent endocarditis, angina pectoris, quinine idiosyncrasy.

Caution: Causes sometimes, particularly in susceptible people, unpleasant or even dangerous symptoms (nausea, vomiting, convulsions, palpitation, headache, fainting, rapid idioventricular rhythm).

Bibliography: *See Chap. XII.*

QUININE AND UREA HYDROCHLORIDE

(Burroughs Wellcome)

Local Anesthetic

Composition: A combination of Quinine and Urea Hydrochloride.

Action and Uses: Produces local anesthesia slowly (in 10–30 min.) but of prolonged duration; is desirable in nerve block and infiltration therapy, in pruritus ani or vulvae.

Supply: QUININE AND UREA HYDROCHLORIDE—Soloid—Gr ¾ (0.05 Gm), 1 soloid dissolved in 200 cc forms a solution of 1:400 or ¼%—Tubes of 25.

Administration: Sufficient solution is injected until tissue at site of injection is infiltrated.

QUININE AND UREA HYDROCHLORIDE SOLUTION, 5%

(Parke, Davis)

Sclerosing Agent

Description: An aqueous solution of Quinine and Urea Hydrochloride.

Action and Use: Has a sclerosing effect upon hemorrhoidal veins when injected into the hemorrhoid or submucously in the rectal lumen. *Used* for painless non-surgical treatment of internal hemorrhoids.

Supply: QUININE AND UREA HYDROCHLORIDE SOLUTION, 5%—Ampules 2 cc (0.1 Gm in 2 cc of distilled water)—Boxes of 12.

Administration: If injected into the hemorrhoidal vein, a few minims will suffice for each injection; if injected externally to the vein 2 cc or even more may be necessary for a single injection; given deeply, so that distention of tissues follows; repeated at weekly intervals until the hemorrhoidal enlargement is completely reduced.

Contraindications: Ulceration, severe inflammation or irreducible prolapse.

Bibliography: *See Chap. XII.*

QUINIOBINE (Spicer)

Antiluetic

Chemical Name: Quinine Bismuth Iodide.

Formula: $C_{20}H_{24}N_2O_2I_4Bi$.

Description: A clear red-brown liquid, containing per cubic centimeter Bismuth, 0.030 Gm, Iodine, 0.075 Gm, Quinine, 0.03 Gm, Lecithin, 0.22 Gm, in olive oil.

Action and Uses: Is non-irritating and readily absorbed; *For use* in all stages of syphilis, especially tertiary; in visceral with cardiac involvement, in lues of central nervous system and of the eyes.

Supply: QUINIOBINE—Ampules (C.A.) 2 cc—Boxes of 6.

QUINIOBINE—Liquid—Bottles of 25 and 100.

Administration: *Intragluteal injections*—Adults, first day—1 cc; fourth day—2 cc; second week, 1½–2 cc twice; continued for 12–14 semiweekly injections.

In visceral lues and in the feeble, 1 cc; repeated as necessary; in cardiac and neural syphilis—0.1 cc, increased by 0.1 cc.

Infants, 0.05–0.1 cc increased by 0.05 cc semiweekly; total quantity for infants, 3 cc.

Intervals between courses—6 weeks.

Bibliography: *See Chap. XII.*

QUINISAL (Merck)

Antipyretic

Chemical Name: Quinine Bi-salicylosalicylate.

Formula: $C_{20}H_{24}N_2O_2(OH. C_6H_4. CO. OC_6H_4. COOH)_2$.

Description: A white fluffy odorless, crystalline powder, slightly bitter in taste; practically insoluble in water, soluble in acid gastric juice.

Action and Uses: Antipyretic, antiseptic, analgesic: offers the combined effects of salicylates and quinine where these are indicated; particularly useful in painful or febrile diseases: in malarial headache, neuritis, rheumatism, lumbago, pericarditis amenorrhea. Very effective as a prophylactic to abort a "cold," in tonsillitis, coryza, bronchopneumonia.

Supply: QUINISAL—Tablets, gr 4 (0.259 Gm)—Each 4 gr yielding the approximate equivalent of quinine gr 2 (0.130 Gm) and salicylosalicylic acid gr 2½ (0.162 Gm)—Tubes of 10—Bottles of 20, 250 and 1,000.

QUINISAL—Powder—Vials of 1 oz.

Administration: 1–2 tablets, 4–8 gr (0.259–0.512 Gm) every 2 hr.

Bibliography: *See Chap. XII.*

RADIUM SALTS (Radium Chemical)

Radiation Therapy

Description: Derived from Radium, a bivalent metallic element, forming soluble salts—Radium Bromide and Radium Chloride, and insoluble salts—Radium Carbonate and Radium Sulphate.

Action: The therapeutic value of radium is due to its radioactivity, a property of spontaneous emission of radiations which have the power of discharging electrified bodies. All the radioactive elements disintegrate spontaneously; the transformation of the atom is accompanied by the emission of so-called "rays"—alpha and beta particles and gamma rays, this process continuing at a regular rate irrespective of the physical or chemical state of the radioactive substance. The activity of these preparations is measured by U.S. Bureau of Standards methods. The quantity of radiation is roughly proportional to the amount of Radium C^1, C_1, C_2, present; the efficacy of the treatment is due to the beta and gamma rays.

Uses: For implantation into malignant growths without removal of radium container; *For use* in carcinoma of uterine cervix, of the breast, penis, vulva, vagina, lip, tongue, tonsils, prostate, oesophagus, rectum, cheek, urinary bladder, skin; for irradiation in benign uterine bleeding, fibromyoma uteri, and some dermatoses.

Supply: **RADIUM BROMIDE—RADIUM BELGE** ($Ra\ Br_2$) (C.A.)—A mixture of radium bromide and barium bromide, containing 90 % or more of radium salt, with gamma ray activity due to substances other than radium (mesothorium, radiothorium) not to exceed 0.2 %.

RADIUM CARBONATE—RADIUM BELGE ($RaCO_3$) (C.A.)—A mixture of radium carbonate and barium carbonate, containing 90 % or more of radium salt, with gamma ray activity due to substances other than radium (mesothorium, radiothorium) not to exceed 0.2 %.

RADIUM SULPHATE—RADIUM BELGE ($RaSO_4$) (C.A.)—A mixture of radium sulphate and barium sulphate, containing 90 % or more of radium salt, with gamma ray activity due to substances other than radium (mesothorium, radiothorium) not to exceed 0.2 %.

RADIUM—Needles of Monel Metal, Gold, Platinum 1–12.5 mg.

RADIUM—Tubes of Glass, Silver, Platinum 10–100 mg.

RADIUM—Plaques of Monel Metal, 2.5 mg, 5 mg, 10 mg, brass screen.

Administration: By filtration with a suitable metallic or other screen, the length of time of application and the amount of radium to be used varying with the pathological conditions. The metals used are irridium, platinum, gold, lead, steel alloy, nickel-copper alloy. Dosage is expressed in milligram hours. Where direct application of the radium to the tissue is feasible, screening is unimportant. For direct implantation, 1–10 mg; for cavity work, 25 mg; for surface work, 2.5, 5, 10 plaques.

Bibliography: *See Chap. XII.*

RADON

Radiation Therapy

Description: A gaseous element, radon, created during the disintegration of the radium atom and the expulsion of an alpha particle; belongs to the group of inert gases; has a period of maximum decay—133.3 millicurie hours per initial millicurie; of half decay—3.85 days; 99.5 % of activity is lost in 30 days.

Action and Uses: In the process of disintegration of the atom, energetic beta and gamma rays are released, which are of therapeutic value in irradiation therapy.

Used for treatment of malignant growths: carcinoma of cervix uteri; breast, penis, vulva, vagina, uterine body, lip, tongue, tonsils, prostate, esophagus, rectum, cheek, urinary bladder, skin; *also used* for irradiation in benign uterine bleeding, fibromyoma uteri and similar conditions.

Supply: **RADON** (C.A.)—In seeds of gold and platinum, **(Radium Emanation)** permanent and removable, containing definite specified, 1–5 millicuries of radon in accordance with demand in each case, with applicators, filters and instruments, where desired.

RADON (C.A.)—In tubes containing the desired millicuries, **(Radon Co.)** of radon, from 10 upwards; are glass capillary, 15 mm long, encased in container of gold, platinum or other specified metal.

RADON (C.A.)—Implants containing 1–5, usually 1–2 millicuries, **(Radon Co.)** and made of 24 karat gold, 0.3 mm wall thickness, 0.75 mm outside diameter, 4 mm length; sealed mechanically.

Administration: By implantation into various types of tumor masses and tissues, by special technic; also externally in dermatologic diseases—*Tubes*—By topical application. Instruments may be obtained with preparations.

Bibliography: *See Chap. XII.*

RED MERCURIC IODIDE

Antiluetic

Official Name: Hydrargyri Iodidum Rubrum. Mercury Biniodide.

Formula: HgI_2.

Description: A scarlet red amorphous powder, odorless and stable in air; soluble in 115 parts of alcohol, insoluble in water.

Action and Uses: Antiseptic and antisyphilitic in the treatment of lues.

Supply: **MERCURY BINIODIDE** (C.A.)—Ampules 1 cc, containing **(Abbott)** gr 1/6 in oil—Boxes of 12 and 100.

MERCURIC POTASSIUM IODIDE—Ampules 1 cc, containing **(Abbott)** gr 1/4 (Mercury Biniodide)—Boxes of 12 and 100.

RED MERCURIC IODIDE (C.A.)— **(Hynson, Westcott and Dunning)** Ampules 1 cc containing 1/6 gr (0.01 Gm), in neutral fatty oil—Boxes of 10.

Administration: *Intramuscularly*—1/4–1 cc, repeated at 1–5-day intervals.

RESORCINOL MONOACETATE (Eastman)

Antiseptic

Chemical Name: Resorcin Acetate; Meta Acetyloxyphenol.

Formula: $C_6H_4(OH)OOCCH_3$.

Description: Is a lemon yellow, viscous liquid; soluble in alcohol, acetone and most organic solvents; sparingly soluble in water.

Action: As for Resorcinol, being only gradually liberated its action is more prolonged and milder.

Uses: In acne, sycosis, alopecia, seborrhea and similar dermatologic diseases.

Supply: RESORCINOL MONOACETATE (C.A.)—Bottles of 1,000 Gm.

Administration: In 5–20% ointment or in acetone solution; in alopecia—3–5% alcoholic solution.

RIODINE "ASTIER" (Gallia)

Iodine Therapy

Formula: $(C_{18}H_{33}O_3)_3(IH)_2C_3H_5$.

Description: A 66% solution in oil of an Iodized Glyceric Ether of Ricinoleic acid; contains 17% of iodine; is an oleaginous liquid, of light amber color and faintly alkaline reaction; is insoluble in water, soluble in alcohol, chloroform or ether.

Action: Is absorbed gradually and retained longer, assuring slow steady absorption of iodine without danger of iodism.

Uses: In arteriosclerosis, cardiorenal disease, bronchial asthma, chronic bronchitis, pulmonary emphysema; in chronic rheumatoid arthritis, lead poisoning and latent syphilis; in hypothyroidism, simple goitre and obesity.

Supply: **RIODINE**—Capsules (C.A.) gr 3.1 (0.20 Gm) equivalent to ½ gr of iodine—Bottles of 50 and 300.

Administration: 2–6 capsules daily after meals.

RIVANOL (Metz)

Antiseptic

Chemical Name: Ethoxydiamino-acridin. Brand of Ethodin.

Formula: $C_2H_5O.\ C_{13}H_6.\ N(NH_2)_2.\ CH_3.\ CHOH.\ CO_2H$.

Description: A fine yellow crystalline powder, slowly soluble in about 15 parts of cold water, 9 parts of boiling water and about 110 parts of alcohol; aqueous solutions are unaffected by boiling; is supplied for use as lactate.

Action: Has marked antiseptic and germicidal properties; is relatively non-toxic and non-irritating to tissues; is not inhibited in action in the presence of serum.

Uses and Administration: **Surgery**—On wounds, abscesses in solution of 1:1,000 to 1:500; in purulent arthritis 10–15 cc of 1:1,000 or 1:500 dilution is injected into the joint.

In pleural empyema, after evacuation of pus, 50–200 cc, 1:500 solution is injected into pleural cavity and repeated three to four times, at intervals of a few days.

Urology—In gonorrhea—as irrigation, 1:4,000 to 1:3,000, in accordance with the acuteness of inflammation; in cystitis, 30–50 cc of 1:5,000 to 1:1,000 solution introduced into the bladder; in pyelitis, the renal pelvis is irrigated with 1:2,000 solution.

Ophthalmology—In acute conjunctivitis—instillations of 1:500, two to three times daily.

Rhinolaryngology—In purulent rhinitis, as spray—1:1,000 solution; in tonsillitis and pharyngitis—sprays of 1:2,000.

Dermatology—In eczema and impetigo contagiosa, in 1% petrolatum ointment or 5–10% in a paste with zinc oxide, talcum, glycerin and water.

Gynecology—In puerperal sepsis is administered *intravenously*, 1:1,000 Rivanol 1 part and dextrose 2 parts.

Supply: **RIVANOL**—Lactate, Tablets 1½ gr (0.1 Gm)—Tubes of 20;

RIVANOL—Lactate, Powder—Bottles of 5 Gm and 1 oz.

RIVANOL WITH DEXTROSE—Capsules containing Rivanol Lactate 1½ gr (0.1 Gm) Dextrose 3 gr (0.2 Gm)—Bottles of 25; is more soluble and less irritating than Rivanol alone; thus used in slightly stronger solutions.

Bibliography: *See Chap. XII.*

SABROMIN (Winthrop)

Bromine Therapy

Chemical Name: Calbromen. Calcium Dibrombehenate.

Formula: $Ca(H_{21}H_{41}Br_2. COO)_2$.

Description: A white, odorless, tasteless powder of neutral reaction; insoluble in water and alcohol, soluble in ether, chloroform, acetone, benzene and carbon tetrachloride; contains 29% bromine and 3.8% calcium.

Action and Advantages: Being a synthetic fatty compound and lipoid-like body this bromide is better utilized and more slowly absorbed and eliminated than other bromides; does not disturb the gastrointestinal tract; liberates calcium of assistance in nerve regulation.

Uses: Wherever bromides are indicated: nervous excitation, nervous tachycardia, neurasthenia, gastric neuroses, insomnia and similar conditions; is especially indicated where prolonged bromide therapy is desired without fear of inducing gastric disturbances or bromism.

Supply: SABROMIN—Tablets (C.A.), 8 gr (0.51 Gm)—Tubes of 20.

SABROMIN—Powder—Bottles of 1 oz.

Administration: 5–20 gr (0.32–1.29 Gm) three to four times daily, 1 hr. after meals thoroughly chewed before swallowing.

SAJODIN (Winthrop)

Iodine Therapy

Chemical Name: Calcium Iodobehenate. Brand of Calioben.

Formula: $Ca(C_{22}H_{42}IO_2)_2$.

Description: An odorless, tasteless, whitish powder; insoluble in water, alcohol, ether and acetone, soluble in chloroform and benzol; contains 24.5% iodine.

Action: That of iodine but without causing gastric irritation; is gradually absorbed and slowly excreted, appearing in the urine 1–2 hr. after administration and requiring 4 days in elimination.

Uses: In all conditions where internal iodine therapy is indicated; arteriosclerosis, syphilis, arthritis, goiter, glandular enlargement, asthma, and others.

Supply: SAJODIN—Tablets (C.A.), 1 gr (0.06 Gm)—Bottles of 24.

SAJODIN—Tablets (C.A.), 8 gr (0.51 Gm)—Tubes of 20.

SAJODIN—Powder—Bottles of 1 oz.

Administration: 5–15 gr (0.3–1.0 Gm) three or four times daily, 1 hr. after meals; tablets to be chewed before swallowing.

For Goitre—1 gr (0.06 Gm) tablets daily, in accordance with individual case.

Advantages: Freedom from gastrointestinal distress and iodism; palatability, adaptability for prolonged use.

Bibliography: *See Chap. XII.*

SAL-ETHYL CARBONATE (Parke, Davis)

Analgesic

Chemical Name: Salicylic Ethyl Ester Carbonate.

Formula: $(C_6H_4)_2(COO. C_2H_5)_2CO_3$.

Description: A salicylic acid compound; is insoluble in water and the gastric secretions, but is decomposed in the small intestine and slowly eliminated in the urine.

Action and Uses: Antirheumatic, antiarthritic, analgesic and cholagogue; reduces inflammation and pain; is helpful in arthritis, gout, tonsillitis, neuritis, sciatica, influenza and grippe; for its cholagogue effect in cholecystitis and catarrhal jaundice.

Supply: SAL-ETHYL CARBONATE—Bottles of ¼ and 1 lb.

SAL-ETHYL CARBONATE—Tablets (C.A.) gr 1 (0.064 Gm)—Bottles of 100 and 500.

SAL-ETHYL CARBONATE—Tablets (C.A.) gr 5 (0.324 Gm)—Bottles of 100 and 500.

SAL-ETHYL CARBONATE WITH AMIDOPYRINE (C.A.)—Compressed tablet containing Sal-Ethyl Carbonate (0.23 Gm (gr 3½) with Amidopyrine 0.11 Gm (gr 1½)—Bottles of 100 and 500.

Administration: Gr 5–15 (0.32–0.97 Gm) as required; as much as 60–120 gr daily may be given without disturbing the stomach.

SALIHEXIN (Abbott)

Genito-Urinary Antiseptic

Chemical Name: Hexamethylenetetramine-acetylamino-salicylic acid.

Formula: $(CH_2)_6N_4.\ C_6H_3(COOH)(OH)(NHCOCH_3)$.

Description: A chemical combination of acetylamino-salicylic acid and hexamethylene tetramine; is readily soluble in water, quickly absorbed and eliminated; is ten times less toxic than sodium salicylate.

Action and Uses: Antipyretic, antiseptic, analgesic of low toxicity, not injurious to heart or gastrointestinal tract. *Used* in urinary infections, pyelitis, cystitis, nephritis; in neuralgia, arthritis, meningitis.

Supply: SALIHEXIN—Capsules gr 2½—Bottles of 100 and 1,000.

SALIHEXIN—Ampules 10 cc—Boxes 6, 25 and 100.

Administration: *Oral*—2 capsules every 3 or 4 hr.
Intravenous—1 ampule injected slowly every 2 days, or daily if necessary, for 15 injections.

Bibliography: *See Chap. XII.*

SALIPYRIN (Riedel)

Antipyretic. Anodyne

Chemical Name: Antipyrine Salicylate.

Formula: $C_{11}H_{12}N_2OC_6H_4OHCOOH.\ C_{18}H_{18}N_2O_4$.

Description: A chemical combination of antipyrine and salicylic acid; a white, coarsely-granular, odorless, somewhat sweet powder; soluble in 200 parts of cold water, more soluble in alcohol and ether; is decomposed by acids.

Action and Uses: Anodyne, antipyretic, antirheumatic. *For use* in infections of the upper respiratory passages and influenza; in rheumatic conditions, neuralgia, lumbago, migraine and pains in general; also in dysmenorrhea, menorrhagia and similar menstrual disorders.

Supply: SALIPYRIN—Powder—Packages of 1 oz.

SALIPYRIN—Tablets (C.A.), gr 7½ (0.480 Gm)—Bottles of 20 and 50.

Administration: 7½–15 gr (0.480–0.972 Gm) on empty stomach, followed by water; best with some digestive vehicle, taken several times daily.

Bibliography: *See Chap. XII.*

SALIT (Heyden)

Antiarthritic

Chemical Name: Borneol Salicylate.

Formula: $C_{10}H_{17}O.\ CO.\ C_6H_4OH$.

Description: Is a salicylic acid ester of an alcohol of the camphor group; an oily, reddish brown liquid of slight odor and taste; soluble in alcohol, ether, oils; insoluble in water; contains about 70% borneol salicylate.

Action: Is absorbed from the skin when rubbed in, appearing in the urine in about 2 hr. and continuing to be excreted for 25–48 hr.; applied externally gives an agreeable warm sensation to the skin shortly after application.

Uses: Where it is desired to administer salicylates without burdening the stomach or where not tolerated; in rheumatic disorders, muscular rheumatism, lumbago, gout, arthritis, neuritis; also in general inflammatory conditions.

Supply: SALIT—Oil—Bottles 1 oz.

SALIT—Cream—Tubes.

SALITUM PURUM—Bottles of 25 Gm.

Administration: After washing the skin with soap and water and drying, Salit Oil or Salit Cream is rubbed in, twice daily; in chronic cases the cream is to be preferred; where local irritation appears the medication should be washed off with alcohol and discontinued.

Bibliography: *See Chap. XII.*

SALOPHEN (Winthrop)

Antiarthritic. Analgesic

Chemical Name: Salicylic Acid Ester of Acetyl Para-amidophenol. Brand of Phenetsal.

Formula: $(C_6H_4OH.\ CO)O.\ C_6H_4NH.\ CO.\ CH_3$.

Description: A whitish, crystalline powder, odorless, tasteless, of neutral reaction; almost insoluble in cold water, somewhat more soluble in hot water, easily soluble in alcohol and ether.

Action: As for salicylates; being insoluble in acid fluids, passes the stomach unchanged and does not affect it; in the intestines, where it is absorbed, it is split into nascent salicylic acid and acetylpara-amidophenol ester and acts as antirheumatic, analgesic and intestinal disinfectant

Uses: Rheumatism, tonsillitis, coryza, influenza, pharyngitis, neuralgias; in intestinal putrefaction.

Supply: SALOPHEN—Tablets (C.A.) 5 gr (0.324 Gm)—Bottles of 25 and 100.

SALOPHEN—Powder—Cartons of 1 oz.

Combinations: SALOPHEN-PHENACETIN—Tablets containing Salophen, 3½ gr; Phenacetin, 1½ gr—Bottles of 25.

SALOPHEN-PHENACETIN QUININE—Tablets containing Salophen, 3 gr; Phenacetin, 1 gr; Quinine, 1 gr—Bottles of 25.

Administration: Adults, 15 gr (0.972 Gm) or 2–3 tablets three or four times daily. Children, 3–8 gr (0.194–0.512 Gm).

SALVARSAN (Metz)

Antiluetic

Chemical Name: Diamino-dihydroxy-arsenobenzene Dihydrochloride. Brand of Arsphenamine.

Formula: $As_2C_{12}H_6(OH)_2(NH_2.HCl)_2$.

Description: A light-yellow powder, readily soluble in water at room temperature yielding a strongly acid solution.

Action: As for arsphenamines.

Uses: In all stages of syphilis and its complications.

Contraindications: Advanced circulatory and neural disease, active tuberculosis, arsenical idiosyncrasy.

Supply: SALVARSAN (C.A.)—Ampules of Single dosage: 0.1, 0.2, 0.3, 0.4, 0.5, 0.6 Gm
SALVARSAN (C.A.)—Ampules, Multiple doses: 1, 1.2, 2.0 and 3.0 Gm.

Administration: *Intravenously*—By gravity method only, at weekly intervals.
Males, 0.4 Gm maximum 0.6 Gm.
Females, 0.3 Gm, maximum 0.4 Gm.

Preparation of Solution: The ampule is immersed in alcohol for disinfection and detection of leakage; after breaking off its end the ampule is rotated gently, the contents loosened and dissolved in 25 to 50 cc triple distilled water, without stirring. Normal 4% sodium hydrate solution of highest chemical purity, is then added in amounts necessary to produce neutral or slightly alkaline reaction, using 0.84 cc for 0.1 Gm to 5.04 cc for 0.6 Gm Salvarsan. The solution is filtered through sterile moistened gauze, diluted with cool sterile distilled water or preferably 4% saline solution to make a total volume of 20 cc for each 0.1 Gm Salvarsan. It should stand for 30 min. before being administered; left over portions should be discarded.

SALVARSAN GLUCOSE SOLUTION (Metz)

Salvarsan Therapy

Description: A 5% aqueous Glucose solution of Salvarsan Base.

Action: As for Salvarsan.

Uses: Externally in Vincent's angina and pyorrhea alveolaris.

Supply: SALVARSAN GLUCOSE SOLUTION—Ampules—3 cc—Boxes of 10.

Administration: The affected mucous membrane is previously cleansed with hydrogen peroxide swabs, the mouth rinsed with water, the lesions dried and then completely covered with the Salvarsan Glucose Solution, using a cotton-wrapped applicator; left in contact with the tissues as long as possible; no fluids should be allowed for at least 30 min. after application; treatment should be administered daily.

SALYRGAN (Metz)

Diuretic

Chemical Name: Mercury salicylallylamide-o-acetate of sodium.

Formula: $NaOOC.CH_2O.C_6H_4.CONH.CH_2CH(O.CH_3)CH_2.HOH$.

Description: A white, crystalline, odorless powder of bitter taste; is fully soluble in water with an alkaline reaction to litmus, readily soluble in alcohol, insoluble in ether; contains not less than 37.6% of mercury in non-ionizable form; is available only in 10% aqueous solution.

Action: Possesses spirocidal properties but is chiefly used for its strong diuretic action, effected (1) by the extraction of fluids and salts from their colloidal state in which they exist in the tissue cells; and (2) through direct stimulation of the secretory function of the kidneys.

Uses: Is very *effective* in hepatic ascites, cardiac and cardiorenal edema, nephroses; also beneficial in hydrothorax, tuberculous peritonitis, pericardial effusion and general anasarca.

Supply: SALYRGAN (C.A.)—Ampules 1 cc—Boxes of 5.

SALYRGAN (C.A.)—Ampules 2 cc—Boxes of 10.

Administration: *Only intravenously or intramuscularly, never* subcutaneously beginning with 0.5 cc (half an ampule); if this is well tolerated a full ampule is administered the following day and repeated every 3 or 4 days; in severe cases 2 cc ampules are given; *more effective* if ammonium chloride or ammonium nitrate, from 90–150 gr daily, in enteric coated pills, is administered orally as auxilliary.

Advantages: Produces profuse and prompt diuresis; injections are painless and free from by-effects.

Contraindications: Acute nephritis and advanced chronic nephritis.

Bibliography: *See Chap. XII.*

SALYSAL (Merck)

Analgesic

Chemical Name: Salicylsalicylic Acid; Salicyl Salicylate; Diplosal.

Formula: OH. C_6H_4COO. C_6H_4COON.

Description: A colorless, odorless and tasteless crystalline powder; insoluble in water and dilute acids; soluble in dilute alkaline solutions, alcohol, ether.

Action and Uses: Antipyretic, analgesic. *Useful* in conditions where salicylates are indicated; in acute and chronic articular rheumatism, tonsillitis, neuralgia, lumbago, influenza; in cystitis, pyelitis.

Supply: SALYSAL—Powder—Vials 1 oz.

SALYSAL—Tablets gr 5 (0.324 Gm)—Tubes of 10—Bottles of 50, 250.

Administration: 1–3 tablets, 5–15 gr (0.324–0.972 Gm), three times daily in water.

SANDOPTAL (Sandoz)

Hypnotic

Chemical Name: Isobutylallyl Barbituric Acid. Isobutylallylmalonylurea.

Formula: iso-$C_4H_9(C_3H_5)$C CONH CONH CO.
|______________|

Action and Uses: Quickly induces peaceful sleep of natural intensity and duration and followed by a feeling of well-being on awakening; also augments the action of analgesics for the relief of pain, especially of neuralgic character; *used* in insomnia with or without pain.

Supply: SANDOPTAL—Tablets (C.A.)—Sugar coated, 3 gr (0.2 Gm)—Tubes of 10—Bottles of 100.

Administration: For mild insomnia, 1 tablet, in obstinate cases 2–4 tablets, half an hour before retiring.

Bibliography: *See Chap. XII.*

SANTYL (Bilhuber-Knoll)

Urinary Sedative

Chemical Name: Neutral Salicylic Ester of Santalol.

Formula: $C_6H_4OHCOO(C_{15}H_{23})$.

Description: A thin, pale yellow oil of slight odor and taste; insoluble in gastric juice and thus non-irritant to gastric mucosa.

Action and Uses: Is slowly split in the intestines into santalol and salicylic acid; acts as sedative and analgesic in urinary affections, allaying tenesmus, dysuria and strangury; decreases urethral discharge. *Used* in gonorrheal urethritis, cystitis, prostatitis; also in non-gonorrheal diseases in women; postoperatively in bladder surgery.

Incompatibles: Alkalies and substances incompatible with salicylates and sandalwood oil.

Advantages: Has no unpleasant odor; does not irritate kidneys or stomach and causes no eructations; permits more intensive treatment.

Supply: SANTYL (C.A.)—Liquid—Bottles ½ oz.

SANTYL—Capsules (C.A.), 6 m (0.35 cc)—Boxes of 30 and 100.

Administration: 25–50 m, 4–8 capsules, (1.5–3.0 cc) three times a day after meals.

Bibliography: *See Chap. XII.*

SARCOPTOL (Anglo-French)

Antipruritic

Description: A preparation of Colloidal Sulphur.

Action: Antiseptic, antiparasitic, antipruritic, analgesic; non-toxic, non-irritating and readily penetrating because of physical state and ultramicroscopic size of its particles.

Uses: In acne and seborrhea to diminish and restore normal sebaceous secretion; in eczema and prurigo to allay itching, exudation and scaling; in scabies, ringworm and pediculosis to destroy causative organisms; in pityriasis to check branny scale formation.

Supply: SARCOPTOL—Bottles 4 oz.

Administration: Applied locally or painted with a brush; in scabies—is rubbed in thoroughly till absorbed; in dandruff—used diluted with 4–5 parts of olive oil.

SCARLET R SALVE "BIEBRICH"

Cell Proliferant

Chemical Name: Toluyl-azo-toluyl-azo-beta-naphthol; "Biebrich" Scarlet Red Medicinal.

Formula: $CH_3C_6H_4N:NC_6H_3CH_3N:N.\ C_{10}H_6OH$.

Description: A dark brownish-red powder, almost insoluble in water, slightly soluble in cold alcohol, benzene and acetone, easily soluble in 15 parts of chloroform, fats, oils, hot alcohol, petrolatum and paraffin.

Action: Has antiseptic and desiccating properties; promotes granulation and epithelial growth.

Uses: *Useful* in burns, skin grafts, wounds, ulcus cruris, decubitus ulcers, lupus, skin suppuration, soft chancre.

Supply: SCARLET R SALVE (C.A.)—Containing 8% Scarlet Red Medicinal, 2% Eucalyptol, 90% Petrolatum—Jars of 1 oz. **(Heilkraft)**

SCARLET RED MEDICINAL "BIEBRICH" (C.A.)—Bottles of 1 oz., ¼ lb., 1 lb. **(Merck)**

SCARLET RED MEDICINAL "BIEBRICH" (C.A.)—Bottles of 10, 25, 50 Gm. **(National Aniline)**

SCARLET RED SULPHONATE EMULSION (C.A.)—4%—Bottles of 1 oz. **(Parke, Davis)**

SCARLET RED SULPHONATE OINTMENT—"A," (C.A.)—5% sulphonate, 95% petrolatum and wax—Collapsible tubes of 1 oz. **(Parke, Davis)**

SCARLET RED SULPHONATE OINTMENT—"B," (C.A.)—10% sulphonate, 90% petrolatum and wax—Jars of ½ lb. **(Parke, Davis)**

Administration: Wound is thoroughly cleansed with boric acid or salt solution and dried (peroxide, silver nitrate or iodine may be used if desired); for about 1 cm around the defect or wound edge the skin is anointed with some bland ointment, the wound is then covered with the scarlet ointment or liquid, spread on gauze; dressed every 24-48 hr., alternating with some bland ointment; where desired Scarlet Red salve may be combined with Balsam of Peru, Blue Ointment or Iodoform Ointment.

SCILLAREN **(Sandoz)**

Cardiodiuretic

Official Name: Glucosidum e Scilla Totum.

Composition: Contains the pure, total glucosidal principles of squill (Urginea maritima) comprising 2 parts of Scillaren A, a slightly soluble crystalline powder of the chemical formula $C_{36}H_{52}O_{13}$, and 1 part of Scillaren B, an amorphous glucosidal substance; is assayed to contain 1,200 frog doses per milligram; Scillaren B is adapted for intravenous use and assayed to contain 1,600 frog doses per milligram.

Action: Slows the rhythm and augments the amplitude of the heart beat; produces a more efficient systole and prolonged diastole, thus affording rest to the heart and improving the circulation in general; also increases the output of urine; at times is effective when other agents have failed.

Uses: In valvular lesions, edema of cardiac origin, chronic myocarditis, aortic insufficiency; of special service in cases refractory to digitalis.

Supply: SCILLAREN—Tablets (C.A.), 1/80 gr (0.0008 Gm)—Tubes of 20—Bottles 100 and 250.

SCILLAREN—Solution (C.A.) (for oral use) 1/80 gr (0.0008 Gm) per cubic centimeter—Bottles of 20 cc and 200 cc.

SCILLAREN "B"—Ampules (C.A.), 1 cc 1/130 gr (0.0005 Gm) per cubic centimeter—Boxes of 6, 12 and 50.

Administration: To secure diuresis or to establish compensation: treatment is begun with massive doses, 2 tablets, or 40 drops oral solution three to four times daily; in urgent cases, or in those refractory to oral therapy, *intravenous* injections of Scillaren B, not to exceed a total of 1 cc per day, are used. When diuresis and compensation have been secured, treatment is continued with progressively decreasing doses orally for as long as necessary. Maintenance dose when compensation has been obtained, or for support of a weak myocardium, 1 tablet or 20 drops oral solution two to four times daily.

Bibliography: *See Chap. XII.*

SCOPOLAMINE STABLE (Roche)

Cerebral Sedative

Chemical Name: Scopomannit.

Formula: $C_{17}H_{21}NO_4$.

Description: An aqueous solution of pure Scopolamine Hydrobromide U.S.P. with 10% of Mannite to prevent decomposition; the salt is colorless and odorless, freely soluble in water, less soluble in alcohol, slightly soluble in chloroform and insoluble in ether.

Action: Does not materially affect respiration, circulation or blood pressure and is twice as effective upon the peripheral organs as is the optically inactive drug; is excreted by the kidneys.

Uses: **In Obstetrics**—For production of "twilight sleep"; the first injection, gr 1/200, is given when the cervix is dilated at least two fingers' width and labor pains recur every 5-10 min.; further injections to be made, if necessary, at intervals of 2 hr. To obtain optimal effect it is best to give Pantopon, 1/3 gr, with the first injection; the opiate is not to be repeated.

In Surgery—Preliminary to anesthesia to reduce the dosage of narcotics, gr 1/100, with or without Pantopon or morphine.

In Psychiatry—As cerebral sedative in acute mania, delirium tremens, drug addiction, alcoholism, tetanus and similar disturbances, gr 1/100–1/50, repeated cautiously.

Supply: **SCOPOLAMINE STABLE (C.A.)**—Ampules 1.2 cc, of 2 strengths, gr 1/100, surgical, and gr 1/200, Obstetrical—Cartons of 12.

SEDORMID (Roche)

Sedative

Chemical Name: Allyl-isopropyl-acetyl-carbamide.

Formula: $(CH_3)_2.\ CH.\ [CH_2.\ CH.\ CH_2].\ CHCONHCONH_2$.

Description: Is a definite chemical substance, neither a bromide nor a barbiturate; is almost tasteless, slightly soluble in water, somewhat more soluble in organic solvents.

Action: An effective sedative, more potent and more rapid in action than bromides, yet not as powerful as barbiturates; is very quickly and almost completely (98%) oxidized in the body, only traces being found in the urine even after large dosage.

Uses: Is *indicated* in all the milder conditions of nervousness and excitation; for daytime use by those who require small doses of a non-narcotic sedative at regular intervals.

Advantages: Does not affect the heart rate, blood pressure, respiration, kidney or other functions.

Supply: **SEDORMID**—Tablets, 4 gr—Boxes of 10—Bottles of 100.

Administration: Tablets are scored, and 2 or 3 half-tablets per day will allay nervousness and excitability; at night, in the milder cases of insomnia 1 or 2 tablets may be given before bedtime although not as an hypnotic in the strict sense.

SELENCOL SOLUTION (Mulford Colloid)

Selenium Therapy

Description: Contains 10% Colloidal Selenium.

Action and Uses: In arthritis and in malignancy.

Supply: SELENCOL SOLUTION—10%, Ampule-Vial 25 cc.
Administration: *Hypodermically*—¼–2 cc.

SERENIUM (Squibb)

Genito-Urinary Antiseptic

Chemical Name: Hydrochloride of 2-4-diamino-4'ethoxy-azo-benzene.

Description: An organic azo dye of high bacteriostatic power; is excreted in the urine coloring it red.

Action: A powerful urinary antiseptic, most active in acid medium; is non-toxic, and non-irritant in ordinary doses.

Uses: Acute and chronic pyelitis, cystitis, gonorrhea; in urinary infections of infants and children.

Supply: SERENIUM—Tablets 1½ gr (0.1 Gm)—Bottles of 25, 50, 500.

Administration: *Dosage*—Children 3–12 yr.—¼ tablet three times daily.
Infants up to 3 yr.—½ tablet three times daily.
Adults—2 tablets three times daily; is administered for 4–5 days a week, and for 2 weeks after symptoms have subsided.

SHADOCOL (Davies, Rose)

X-ray Contrast Medium

Composition: Contains Sodium Tetraiodophenolphthalein.

Formula: $NaO. O: C. C_6H_4. C: C_6H_2I_2OC_6H_2I_2ONa$.

Description: A dark blue, somewhat hygroscopic, odorless, crystalline powder; soluble in water and alcohol, insoluble in acid medium.

Action and Uses: Is radiopaque, non-irritating to gastric mucosa, and absorbed only in small intestine in alkaline medium. *For use* in oral cholecystography.

Supply: SHADOCOL—Bottles of 1 oz. for 1 administration.

Administration: Contents of 1 bottle are stirred in half glass of water until mixture turns white; is taken at 9 P.M. about 3 hr. after light evening meal, and followed by drinking of water during next 2 hr.; no food or drink to be allowed subsequently; radiography—16 hr. later.

SILOSAN (Ciba)

Analgesic

Chemical Name: Acetyl-salicylic acid.

Formula: C_6H_4COOH.

Description: An acetyl salicylic acid of high purity, containing no free acid; is not affected by gastric juices and is thus non-irritating to the stomach; is fully absorbed in the intestines.

Action and Uses: As for salicylic acid and salicylates; is analgesic, antipyretic, antirheumatic. *For use* in acute rheumatic fever, myalgia, headaches, colds, malaise, sciatica and other painful or febrile affections.

Supply: SILOSAN—Tablets, 5 gr (0.324 Gm), Chocolate coated—Bottles of 100.
SILOSAN—Powder—Cartons of 1 oz.

Administration: 1–3 tablets or 5–15 gr (0.324–0.972 Gm) of powder in water; repeated when necessary.

Combination: SILOSAN COMPOUND—Each tablet represents acetylsalicylic acid gr 3½ (0.227 Gm) acetphenetidin gr 2½ (0.162 Gm) caffeine, gr ½ (0.032 Gm). *Supply*—Tablets, Chocolate coated—Bottles of 100. *Administration*—1 or 2 tablets with water, repeated at 3–4 hr. intervals if necessary.

SILVER LACTATE (Merck)

Astringent

Official Name: Argenti Lactas.

Formula: $AgC_3H_5O_3 + H_2O$.

Description: Occurs as white or slightly gray granular masses or crystalline needles, soluble in about 15 parts of water; contains 50–51.5% of metallic silver.

Action and Uses: *Used* as powerful astringent and active antiseptic; 1 in 300 and 500 aqueous solution is said to be equal in disinfecting power to a 1 in 1,000 solution of mercuric chloride; is irritating if applied in substance to wounds; *For use* in sore throat, tonsillar disease, gonorrheal infections.

Supply: SILVER LACTATE (C.A.)—Bottles 1 oz.

Administration: 1:100–1:2,000 solution; in dentistry in 1:500 for washing foul root abscesses.

Caution: Should be kept in dark bottles.

SILVER NITRATE SOLUTION

Antiseptic

Description: A 1% solution of silver nitrate in *wax capsules* lined with paraffin.

Action and Uses: An antiseptic in convenient form for use in the prevention of gonorrheal ophthalmia in the new-born.

Supply: SILVER NITRATE SOLUTION (C.A.)—Ampules—Boxes of 12. (Cutter)
SILVER NITRATE SOLUTION (C.A.)—Ampules—Boxes of 12. (Lederle)
SILVER NITRATE SOLUTION (C.A.)—Capsules—Package of 12—Boxes, containing 2 capsules. (Parke, Davis)

Administration: Capsule is pierced with needle, solution is expelled a drop at a time by pressure with thumb and finger; 2 drops of the preparation are to be instilled into each eye.

SILVER-SALVARSAN (Metz)

Antiluetic

Chemical Name: Sodium salt of Silver-diamino-dihydroxy-arseno-benzene.

Formula: $Ag_2O.\ 2[NH_2(ONa)C_6H_3As]$.

Description: A brownish-black powder, readily soluble in water, yielding a clear dark-brown solution of alkaline reaction; is approximately 2 times as trypanocidal as salvarsan and 3 times as potent as neosalvarsan; contains 20–21% arsenic, 13–14% silver.

Action and Uses: As for Salvarsan; preferably *used* in neurosyphilis and Wassermann-fast cases.

Supply: SILVER-SALVARSAN (C.A.)—Ampules of single dosages: 0.1, 0.15, 0.2, 0.25, 0.3 Gm.

SILVER-SALVARSAN (C.A.)—Ampules for multiple dosage: 0.6 Gm.

Administration: Adults: initial dose, 0.1 Gm, gradually increased every 4 days or longer to 0.2 Gm in female, 0.3 Gm in male.

Preparation of Solution: Same as that of Salvarsan.

Caution: In serious nervous disorders, aneurysm, liver, kidney and heart diseases, or headaches of non-syphilitic origin, dosage employed should be small, and the drug given with caution.

SILVOGON (Bischoff)

Antiseptic

Chemical Name: Silver Potassium Cyanide-Potassium Choleate.

Formula: $C_{24}H_{39}O_5KAg(CH_2)K$.

Description: An organic silver, soluble in water, forming a clear stainless stable solution; silver content 16.7 %.

Action: A mucous membrane antiseptic penetrating deeply into crypts and glandular ducts and destroying local organisms; is non-irritating and does not coagulate albumen or serous discharges.

Uses: **Surgical**—For wounds, ulcers, irrigations—1:1,000; wet dressings—1:10,000.

Otolaryngology—In infections, wounds and ulcers of the eye, ear, nose and throat—1:2,000.

Genitourinary—Gonorrheal urethritis, male and female, vaginitis—1:2,000; cervicitis—1:500.

Supply: SILVOGON—Tablets, gr ⅖ (0.03 Gm)—Bottles 50 and 100.

SILVOGON—Powder—Packages of ¼ and ½ oz.

Solutions: 2 tablets in 4 oz. of water make a 1:2,000 solution. 1 tablet in 10 oz. of water makes a 1:10,000 solution.

Bibliography: *See Chap XII.*

SILVOL (Parke, Davis)

Antiseptic. Astringent

Description: Mild silver protein; a finely subdivided silver combined with an alkaline protein; standardized to contain 20 % of silver; added to water forms a stable suspension, practically a solution.

Action and Uses: Antiseptic. *For use* as topical application in all conditions where silver protein is employed; in gonorrheal affections, conjunctivitis, pelvic disease.

Supply: SILVOL—Bottles of 1 oz. and ¼ lb.

SILVOL—Capsules, gr 6 (0.384 Gm)—Bottles of 50 and 500. (1 capsule in 1 fl. dr. of water makes a 10 % solution.)

SILVOL—Bougies (C.A.) 5 % Silvol in a cacao-butter base—Packages of 25 and 100, with introducer.

SILVOL—Suppositories—Vaginal (C.A.) 5 % Silvol in a glycero-gelatin base —Boxes of 12.

SILVOL—Ointment (C.A.)—5 % Silvol in petrolatum, lanolin and white wax.

Administration: **As Gonorrheal Prophylactic**—3–10 % solution; for urethral irrigation—1:1,000; in pelvic infection, as tampon—25 % solution in glycerin. **In Ophthalmia**—As 25 % solution or 10 % ointment.

SIOCOL (Mulford Colloid)

Antiseptic

Description: Occurs as lustrous, grey, non-hygroscopic scales, readily soluble in water; contains 20–25 % Silver Iodide.

Action and Uses: A stable, non-irritating, readily absorbed and assimilated preparation of Colloidal Silver Iodide; is slowly eliminated and of prolonged action; does not cause precipitation of tissue fluids. *For use* as fungicide and antiseptic in infections of eye, ear, nose, throat; *internally* in septicemia, influenza, suppurative wounds, abscesses; *locally*—in cystitis, leukorrhea, prostatitis.

Supply: SIOCOL—Vials 10 Gm.

SIOCOL—Solution 10 % Ampule—Vials 25 cc.

SIOCOL—Ointment 10 %—Tubes of ½ oz.—Packages of 12.

Administration: *Orally*—1–3 gr (0.064–0.162 Gm).
Hypodermically—(Siocol Solution) ¼–2 cc (intravenously where indicated).
Locally—5–25 % solution or undiluted.

SISTOMENSIN (Ciba)

Hormone Therapy

Description: Is the ovarian hormone in lipoid form, standardized by the Allen-Doisy and Herrmann method; is a light viscid oil, comprising carbon, 81.33 %–81.62 %, hydrogen, 11.32 %–11.49 % and oxygen, 6.89 %–7.35 %; injected into mature castrated female rats, induces oestrus reaction; in immature female rabbits causes rapid growth of vagina, ovaries, uterus and mammae; brings about the regeneration of cells in the ganglia of uterine cervix after these have undergone chromatolysis following oophorectomy.

Uses: Indicated in all ovarian hormone deficiencies, genital bleeding of ovarian origin, menorrhagia, metrorrhagia, ovarian dysmenorrhea, in hemorrhage and other disturbances of menopause.

Supply: SISTOMENSIN—Tablets ⅕ gr (0.015 Gm), Sugar coated—Bottles of 40 and 100.

SISTOMENSIN—Ampules 1.1 cc, containing 0.05 Gm Sistomensin in sterile oily solution—Cartons of 5 and 20.

Administration: *Oral*—1–3 tablets three times daily; is supplemented by intramuscular injections 1 cc thrice weekly.
Intramuscular—1–2 ampules three times weekly, accompanied by 6 tablets orally on intervening days.

Advantages: Being lipoid in form is claimed to be more stable than aqueous preparations of the ovarian hormone and more readily absorbed from the alimentary tract; where injected intramuscularly the injection area serves as a depot from which the hormone is gradually absorbed.

Bibliography: *See Chap. XII.*

SKIAGENOL (Parke, Davis)

Radiopaque Medium

Description: A vegetable oil containing 20 % Iodine in true chemical combination.

Action and Uses: A radiographic medium for outlining the bronchial tree, nasal sinuses, uterus and fallopian tubes, intrapleural spaces or any directly accessible cavity or duct: does not enter the circulatory system; is non-irritating, soothing and sterile; is decomposed by a temperature of 140°F.; its viscosity is such that a return drainage by gravity occurs readily.

Used in the diagnosis of bronchiectasis or other bronchial and pulmonary conditions, to outline empyemic areas after drainage, to visualize the form and position of the uterus and fallopian tubes and in the study of suspected cavities.

Supply: SKIAGENOL Bottles—of 30 cc.

Administration: By direct instillation, after warming the oil to body temperature and in accordance with the usual technic employed in the study of a particular organ.

SKIODAN (Winthrop)

Radiopaque Medium

Chemical Name: Mono-iodo-methane Sulphonate of Sodium. Brand of Methiodal.

Formula: CH_2. I. SO_3Na.

Description: Contains 52% of iodine in firm organic combination; the iodine is not liberated or absorbed in the organism, and thus no free iodine is found in the blood or urine, and no iodism or other symptoms are produced; is non-toxic, non-irritating and causes no local or systemic reaction.

Uses: In intravenous urography, retrograde pyelography; also arteriography.

Supply: SKIODAN—Solution (C.A.), 40%, sterile—Bottles of 50 cc (20 Gm).

SKIODAN—Powder—Bottles of 20 Gm.

Dosage: **Intravenous Urography**—Standard dose for adults—50 cc of 40% solution; children—according to weight, 5 cc for every 15 lb., or according to age: up to 1 yr. 10 cc, 2–4 yr. 10–20 cc, 5–7 yr. 20–25 cc, 8–10 yr. 20–30 cc, 11–13 yr. 30–35 cc, 14–16 yr. 35–40 cc.

Retrograde Pyelography—In thin individuals 10% solutions are generally used; in ordinary persons—15 or 20% concentrations.

Administration: Skiodan solution should be warmed to body temperature and slowly injected in the usual manner, allowing 2–3 min. for introduction of the total dose. The first exposure is usually made in 5 min., the second in 15 min. after injection; in some cases exposures as early as 2 min. and as late as 2½ hr. are necessary, depending upon kidney function.

Caution: If entire bottle is not used at one time, the remaining portion may safely be employed later but must first be sterilized in boiling water.

Bibliography: *See Chap. XII.*

SOAMIN (Burroughs Wellcome)

Parasiticide

Chemical Name: Sodium p-aminophenylarsenate.

Composition: A pentavalent organic arsenical containing 22.8% arsenic.

Action and Uses: As parasiticide in trypanosomiasis and syphilis.

Supply: SOAMIN—Bottles 5 and 25 Gm.

TABLOID SOAMIN—Gr 1 (0.065 Gm)—Bottles of 100 and 500.

TABLOID SOAMIN—Gr 3 (0.194 Gm)—Bottles of 25, 100 and 500.

Administration: *Subcutaneously or Intramuscularly*—On alternate days, gr 1–3 (0.065–0.194 Gm), dissolved in sterile water.
Oral—Gr ¼–1 (0.016–0.065 Gm), dissolved in water, two or three times daily after meals; maximum dose not to exceed gr 3.

Caution: Solution must be used immediately upon preparation.

Bibliography: *See Chap. XII.*

SODIUM-AMYTAL (Lilly)

Sedative

Chemical Name: Sodium Iso-amyl Ethyl Barbiturate.

Formula: $NaC_5H_{11}(C_2H_5)CCONHCO:NCO$.

Description: White hygroscopic, slightly bitter granular powder, more soluble than amytal; is soluble in water, less soluble in alcohol, insoluble in ether; for oral, rectal, intramuscular and intravenous use.

Action: Sedative, hypnotic and anticonvulsant; reduces toxicity of local anesthetic agents of the cocaine group; is antispasmodic.

Uses: In sedation before general anesthesia; in obstetrical sedation to relax lower uterine segment; for control of convulsions in tetanus, rabies, status epilepticus, meningitis, eclampsia; to relieve pain in renal and biliary colic.

Contraindications: Vascular depression in the elderly.

Advantages: Not eliminated through the kidneys and therefore does not irritate these organs.

Supply: SODIUM-AMYTAL (C.A.)—Pulvules gr 3 (0.19 Gm)—Bottles of 40 and 500; ampules—0.25, 0.5 and 0.1 Gm—Boxes of 1.

Administration: **Surgical**—1 pulvule orally, the night before and 2 or 3 pulvules 2 hr. preceding operation; *rectally*—same dosage; children—up to 1 pulvule orally.

Obstetrical—1 pulvule when cervix is dilated 26 mm, and 1 after 1–4 hr.

Medical—1 or 2 pulvules orally every 6 hr.

In Tetanus—2 or 4 pulvules till convulsions are controlled.

Bibliography: *See Chap. XII.*

SODIUM DIARSENOL (Diarsenol)

Antiluetic

Chemical Name: Sodium Arsphenamine.

Formula: $NaO.NH_2C_6H_3As:AsC_6H_3NH_2ONa$.

Description: The sodium salt of 3-diamino-4-dihydroxy-1-arsenobenzene; contains 19% of arsenic. A bright yellow powder, very unstable in air; is readily soluble in water, forming a yellow-orange solution of alkaline reaction.

Action and Uses: As for arsphenamine; does not require alkalization.

Supply: SODIUM DIARSENOL (C.A.)—Ampules 0.15, 0.3, 0.45, 0.6, 0.75, 0.9 Gm.

Administration: 0.45 to 0.9 Gm for adults, using 20 cc of sterile distilled water to each 0.1 Gm, for solutioen; childrn in proportion.

SODIUM MORRHUATE, COLLOSOL BRAND (Crookes)

Sclerosing Agent

Composition: The Sodium salt of a particular fraction of the Fatty Acids of cod liver oil with a high iodine content; strength 5%.

Action and Uses: As sclerosing agent for varicose veins and hemorrhoids; is slightly toxic, causes little bruising with less possibility of sloughing and is more rapid in action.

Supply: **SODIUM MORRHUATE, COLLOSOL BRAND**—Ampules 5%—2 cc, 15 cc—Boxes of 6—Bottles 30 cc.

SODIUM MORRHUATE, COLLOSOL BRAND—Ampules 10%—2 cc, 15 cc—Boxes of 6—Bottles 30 cc.

Administration: ½–1 cc for each puncture, up to a total of 10 cc at 1 treatment, either directly into the vein or in cases of hemorrhoids, into surrounding mucous membrane for strangulation.

Bibliography: *See Chap. XII.*

SODIUM PERBORATE

(Roessler and Hasslacher)

Antiseptic

Formula: $NaBO_3 + 4H_2O$.

Description: A white granular or crystalline powder, slightly soluble in water, and dissociating into an alkaline solution containing hydrogen peroxide and borates; contains 91.4% of perborate with available active oxygen 9.5%.

Action and Uses: An oxidizing agent and antiseptic *used* in the preparation of dental and mouth washes, tooth powders, in dental surgery and Vincent's angina; also employed in acne vulgaris, infected wounds, chronic ulcers, diabetic gangrene; as hemostatic in epistaxis and other local hemorrhages; as ear, nose and throat deodorant.

Supply: **SODIUM PERBORATE**—In bulk.

Administration: *Locally*—As dusting powder or as wash in the conditions enumerated; *as medical bath*—10 oz. with ½ oz. manganese borate as catalyzer, in cardiac decompensation, neurasthenia, tachycardia, functional neuroses, nephritis, arteriosclerosis.

SODIUM PEROXIDE

Antiseptic

Official Name: Sodii Peroxidum.

Formula: Na_3O_2.

Description: A yellowish-white, somewhat granular, hygroscopic powder, stable at ordinary temperature; is readily soluble in water with development of heat, the formation of sodium hydrate and evolution of 20.5% of available oxygen.

Action and Uses: Powerful oxidizer and bleaching agent; is applied as soap or paste in the treatment of indurated comedones.

Supply: **SODIUM PEROXIDE (C.A.)**—Bottles of 1 oz.—Containers of ¼ lb.—Cartons of 5 lb. (Merck)

SODIUM PEROXIDE—Tins of 10 and 20 lb. (Roessler and Hasslacher)

Administration: *Externally*—In the form of a paste, prepared with liquid paraffin, or as a soap; not used internally.

Combination: **SODIUM DIOXIDE—Dental—A (Roessler and Hasslacher)** brand of sodium peroxide containing 96% and over of sodium peroxide, and not more than 0.006% of iron; *For use* in bleaching discolored teeth with dead pulps and disinfection of root canals.

SODIUM THIOSULPHATE (Searle)

Detoxicant

Chemical Name: Sodium Thiosulphate.

Formula: $Na_2S_2O_3 + 5H_2O$.

Description: A white hygroscopic crystalline powder, easily soluble in water.

Action and Uses: Is *used* in the treatment of mercurial, arsenical, bismuth and other metallic poisonings; is indicated in the toxic reactions encountered in the treatment of syphilis with metals (especially in exfoliative dermatitis); if injected locally at the site of the previous arsenical injection, is helpful in allaying the intense local reaction in cases of unintentional extravascular injection of the arsenic. Also used as adjunct in the treatment of Wassermann-fast syphilis. and in lupus vulgaris.

Supply: **SODIUM THIOSULPHATE**—5 cc ampules 10%—Boxes of 6, 25 and 100.
SODIUM THIOSULPHATE—10 cc ampules 10%—Boxes of 6, 25 and 100.

Administration: 5–10 cc *intravenously*, repeated 4–8 hr. later; then 1 injection daily till symptoms have subsided and no metallic poison is found in excretions.

SOLARGENTUM (Squibb)

Antiseptic. Gonocide

Description: Occurs as brownish-black odorless, lustrous granules of no unpleasant taste; soluble in distilled water and glycerine, insoluble in alcohol and oils; contains not less than 20% metallic silver in colloidal state; is free from inorganic salts and slightly hygroscopic.

Action: Antiseptic, mildly astringent; non-irritating in any concentration and not affected by serous discharges and chlorides in urine.

Uses: In gonorrhea, for prophylaxis and treatment; in cystitis, vaginitis, cervicitis; in dysentery and cholera infantum; in purulent conjunctivitis, nose and throat practice and ophthalmia neonatorum; in pyelography and as substitute for bismuth paste.

Supply: **SOLARGENTUM**—Packages of 1 oz., ¼ and 1 lb.

SOLARGENTUM—Tablets (C.A.), gr 4.6—Bottles of 100 and 500. (1 tablet dissolved in 1 oz. of water makes a 1% solution.)

Administration: **Gonorrhea**—For urethral injection 10%; as irrigation 1:1,000; in cystitis, instillation of 5 cc 20–50% solution.

Ophthalmology—25% solution.

Rhino-Laryngology—As spray 10–20%; topical application 25–50%.

Gynecology—25% in glycerine for tampons.

Pyelography—In 2% solution.
Intestinal Irrigation—1:1,000 solution.
As substitute for bismuth paste—200 gr is mixed with heavy petrolatum and lanolin, to make 4 oz.

Preparation: Cold water only to be used for making solution; this to be discarded after 3 mo.

SOLARSON (Winthrop)

Tonic. Alterative

Chemical Name: Ammonium Heptenchlorarsonate. Brand of Chlorarsenol

Formula: $CH_3(CH_2)_4CCl$: CH. AsO. OH. ONH_4.

Description: A 1% sterile solution of chlorarsenol, rendered isotonic by the addition of sodium chloride; contains per cubic centimeter 0.01 Gm of chlorarsenol, corresponding to 1/16 gr (0.004 Gm) of arsenous acid.

Action and Advantages: As for arsenical compounds, with the advantage that it is better utilized than cacodylates; the injections are almost painless, better tolerated and do not impart a garlicky odor to the breath.

Uses: Anemia, chlorosis, skin diseases, malaria, neuroses and tuberculosis.

Supply: SOLARSON—Ampules 1 cc (C.A.)—Boxes of 10.

Administration: *Subcutaneously or Intramuscularly*—1 ampule daily or every second or third day, with weekly intervals between courses of 10–12 injections.

Bibliography: *See Chap. XII.*

SOL-BI "FRAISSE" (Fougera)

Antiluetic

Description: A solution of Tricamphocarbonate of Bismuth in oil; contains 4% metallic bismuth; standardized, readily absorbed and non-irritating.

Action and Uses: An effective spirocheticide and antiluetic.

Supply: SOL-BI "FRAISSE"—Ampules, 2 cc, (0.08 Gm each)—Packages 6 and 25.

Administration: First week 3 intramuscular injections, then twice weekly until 12 injections are administered, followed by a rest period of 1 mo.; then a second series of 12 injections with another rest period of 1 mo.; after which a third series with a rest period of 3 mo. is given; it is advisable to give 2 series of injections each year for several years.

SOLVOCHIN (Spicer)

Quinine Therapy

Description: A 25% Quinine Solution.

Action: Is stable, non-irritating, alkaline (pH:7.2), concentrated and free from after effects; permits painless intramuscular injection of quinine; is specific for pneumococcus pneumonia.

Use: As quinine therapy in croupous or lobar pneumonia; also in malaria and in uterine inertia to induce labor.

Supply: SOLVOCHIN—Ampules—2.2 cc—Boxes of 3 and 12.

SOLVOCHIN—Ampules—Hospital package of 50.

Administration: Pneumonia—2 cc *intramuscularly* for 3 successive days, given as early as possible.

Obstetrics—½–1 cc intramuscularly at ½ hr. intervals.

Malaria—2 cc twice a day for 14 days; continued 1 cc daily for 14 more days.

Inoculation Malaria—2 cc three times daily on the first and third days.

Bibliography: *See Chap. XII.*

SORICIN (Merrell)

Detoxifying Agent

Composition: Purified Sodium Ricinoleate.

Action and Uses: Is said to act in testinal detoxicant and to neutralize absorption of toxins; administered orally is useful in mucous and ulcerative colitis, intestinal toxemia, spastic colon, intestinal tuberculosis, chronic constipation and chronic appendicitis; also employed for relief of symptoms in eczema, urticaria and migraine of systemic origin; applied externally has same action.

Supply: SORICIN—Capsules, Enteric coated gr 10—Boxes of 20 and 100.

SORICIN—Capsules, Enteric coated gr 5—Boxes of 40 and 100.

Administration: 40–60 gr daily, with ice water, 20 min. before meals and on retiring; continued for 2 weeks then reduced to 20 gr daily; later 15–20 gr daily for 6 weeks to 6 months.

Combination: **SORICIN SURGICAL 32%.** Physiologically standardized solution for the treatment of external infections, ulcers, burns, douching and colon irrigation. *Supply*—Bottles of 2 and 8 oz. *Administration*—Wet dressings—2–4%; *Colonic Irrigation*—¼% gradually increased to 2% solutions, after preliminary cleansing of intestines; *Vaginal Douche*—1–5% solution; *Abdominal Infections*—2% in saline solution.

Bibliography: *See Chap. XII.*

SPIROFORM (Bischoff)

Antiarthritic. Uricolytic

Chemical Name: Acetyl Phenylsalicylate.

Formula: $C_6H_4O. CH_3CO. COOC_6H_5$.

Description: A white crystalline powder, practically tasteless and of faint aromatic odor; soluble in alcohol, insoluble in water.

Action: Analgesic, antipyretic and intestinal antiseptic; passes through the stomach practically unchanged, reaches the small intestine where it is broken up and its disinfectant and therapeutic influence is exerted; stimulates heart and respiration; large doses may be administered and salicylic acid saturation obtained without unpleasant by-effects or profuse diaphoresis.

Uses: In rheumatism, neuralgia, migraine, influenza.

Supply: SPIROFORM—Powder—Boxes of 1 oz.

SPIROFORM—Tablets—gr 7½—Boxes of 50.

Administration: *As Antirheumatic*—15–20 gr in tablet or powder form, three or four times daily.

As Antipyretic and Intestinal Antiseptic—1–2 tablets three times daily.

SPIROSAL (Winthrop)

Analgesic

Chemical Name: Monoglycol Ester of Salicylic Acid. Brand of Glysal.

Formula: $C_6H_4OH. CO. O. (CH_2. CH_2. OH)$.

Description: An almost colorless, odorless oily fluid; easily soluble in alcohol, ether and chloroform, soluble in about 110 parts of water and 8 parts of olive oil.

Action: Its external application relieves pain and inflammation and is attended with but little irritation even when thoroughly rubbed in; its absorption occurs more readily than that of oil of wintergreen, solutions in alcohol being almost completely absorbed; does not stain tissues.

Uses: For its local effect in rheumatism, lumbago, rheumatoid arthritis, torticollis and gout; as adjuvant to the internal administration of salicylates.

Supply: SPIROSAL (C.A.)—Bottles of 1 oz.

Administration: Dilutions with 2–3 parts of alcohol, or with olive oil, 1 dr. to the ounce, are applied externally, thoroughly rubbed in and the part covered with a bandage or flannel.

STANNOXYL (Anglo-French)

Staphylocide

Composition: A preparation containing Metallic Tin 42.5 % and Tin Oxide 7.5 %.

Action and Uses: Raises natural resistance against staphylococcus infections and favors increased leukocytosis; *For use* in the prophylaxis and treatment of boils, styes, pustular acne, suppurating wounds, chronic osteomyelitis, mastitis, mixed tubercular infections.

Supply: STANNOXYL—Tablets, gr 3—Vials of 80.

STANNOXYL—Ampules, 1 cc, intramuscular, 2 mg each—Boxes of 8.

STANNOXYL—Liquid—concentrated—Bottles of 2½ oz.

STANNOXYL—Gauze, sterile, impregnated.

STANNOXYL—Ointment, in tubes.

STANNOXYL—Glycerine—Jars of 2 oz.

Administration: Tablets, 4–8 daily, with water after meals.
Ampules, 1–2 *intragluteally*, daily.
Liquid, on tampons soaked with 1–2 % solution.
Stannoxyl bath—in generalized furunculosis.

Bibliography: *See Chap. XII.*

STEARODINE (Parke, Davis)

Iodine Therapy

Chemical Name: Calcium Iodostearate.

Formula: $Ca[CH_3(CH_2)_7CHI(CH_2)_8CO_2]_2$.

Description: Is a cream colored, almost odorless solid; soluble in chloroform, ether, benzene, insoluble in water; contains 26–28 % iodine in organic combination.

Action and Uses: An acceptable form of iodine element for systemic use, in the prevention of goitre or for its treatment in the early stages.

Supply: STEARODINE (C.A.)—Chocolate tablets, equivalent to gr ⅙ (0.01 Gm) of organically combined iodine—Bottles of 100 and 500.

Administration: 1 tablet each week, as long as required; or twice a week for 2 mo. in spring and fall.

STOVARSOL (Merck)

Amebacide

Chemical Name: Acetylamino Hydroxy Phenyl Arsonic Acid.

Formula: $HO.\ CH_3CONH.\ C_6H_3As{:}\ O{:}\ (OH)_2$.

Description: A white, odorless powder of somewhat acid taste; is slightly soluble in water and alcohol, readily soluble in alkalies and alkaline carbonates; is stable at ordinary temperature; contains 27.28% arsenic.

Action and Uses: In the treatment of amebic dysentery, for eradicating cysts and encysted flagellates; useful also as arsenical in syphilis, especially congenital in infants and children.

Supply: STOVARSOL—Tablets (C.A.) gr 4 (0.25 Gm)—Bottles of 25 and 500.

STOVARSOL—Tablets gr 1.5 (0.10 Gm)—Bottles 50 and 500.

Administration: Amebic Dysentery—1 tablet two to three times daily for 7 days.

Syphilis—Usual dosage of arsenicals, 1–2 tablets daily.

Caution: On the appearance of toxic symptoms, gastrointestinal irritation, urticaria, erythema, hemorrhagic eruptions, medication must immediately be discontinued.

STRONTIUM PEROXIDE

(Roessler and Hasslacher)

Antiseptic

Formula: SrO_2.

Composition: Contains Strontium Peroxide 80%; available active Oxygen 10.7%.

Description: An impalpable white, odorless, tasteless powder consisting of strontium peroxide and strontium hydroxide, stable in dry air, but gradually decomposed with liberation of oxygen.

Action and Uses: As oxidizing agent and antiseptic in dentifrices and as ointment in minor surgical affections; as deodorant.

Supply: STRONTIUM PEROXIDE—Cases 100 lb.

Administration: Locally as dusting powder or ointment.

STYPTICIN

(Merck)

Astringent. Hemostatic

Official Name: Cotarnine Hydrochloride U.S.P.X.

Formula: $C_{12}H_{13}NO_4HCl$.

Description: A hydrochloride oxidation product of cotarnine; a yellow, hygroscopic, bitter, crystalline powder, easily soluble in water and in alcohol.

Action and Uses: An effective styptic and hemostatic; is neither escharotic nor toxic in medicinal doses; given internally, is *useful* in profuse menstruation, endometritis, climacteric hemorrhage, threatened abortion; also in hemoptysis, vesical and ureteral hemorrhages. Externally is of service in dental, nasal and parenchymatous bleeding.

Supply: STYPTICIN—Powder—Bottles ¼ and ⅛ oz.—Vials of 25 gr (1.6 Gm).

STYPTICIN—Tablets ¾ gr (0.048 Gm)—Tubes 200—Bottles 100.

STYPTICIN—Tablets (Hypodermic and Dental) ¾ gr (0.048 Gm)—Tubes of 10—Boxes of 4 tubes.

Administration: Gr ½–4 (0.03–0.25 Gm) as required, four to five times per day, in gelatin capsules, or sugar coated tablets; in menorrhagia, ¾ gr (0.05 Gm) four to five times per day.

Subcutaneously, in urgent cases, 1½–4 gr (0.1–0.25 Gm) in 10% solution.

Externally—As styptic, pure or in strong solution, or as 30% on gauze or cotton.

SUBLAMINE (Schering and Glatz)

Antiseptic

Chemical Name: Mercury Ethylene Diamine Sulphate.

Formula: $HgSO_4$, $2(CH_2 NH_2)_2 + 2H_2O$.

Description: Occurs as white crystals, containing 44% Mercury; is freely soluble in water.

Action and Uses: Antiseptic, disinfectant and antiluetic; *used* in syphilis, skin diseases, gynecology, ophthalmology, otology.

Supply: SUBLAMINE—Powder—Bottles ½ oz.

SUBLAMINE—Tablets, 1 Gm—Tubes 20—Bottles 100.

Administration: Dermatoses—1:1,000 solution. *Vaginal Douche*—1:500–1:1,000 solution.
Collyria—1:3,000–5,000 solution.
Irrigation—1:5,000 solution.
Intramuscularly—in syphilis, 3–4% solution.

SUFROGEL (Heyden)

Sulphur Therapy

Description: A sterile milky white, stable 0.3% suspension of finely divided Sulphur, in gelatin.

Action: On absorption it acts as systemic oxidizer, increasing nitrogen, sulphur and urobilin excretion; as non-specific protein therapy agent stimulates leucocytosis and favorably influences joint cartilages.

Uses: In chronic rheumatism, arthritis deformans, chronic sciatica; also in bronchial asthma and skin diseases, as acne rosacea, acne vulgaris, psoriasis.

Supply: SUFROGEL—Ampules 1 cc and 5 cc—Boxes of 3.

Administration: 1 injection of 0.2–0.4 cc every 8 days, *intragluteally*, for 6 doses only; in a few cases 0.5–1.0 cc may cautiously be employed; overdosage is to be avoided; ampules must be warmed and well shaken before use; should be kept in a cool place when not in use.

Bibliography: *See Chap. XII.*

SULFACTOL (Metz)

Sulphur Therapy

Chemical Name: Sodium Thiosulphate.

Formula: $Na_2S_2O_3 . 5H_2O$.

Description: Colorless, odorless chemically pure crystals; freely soluble in water, alcohol and ether; slightly deliquescent in moist air and liquefy at 50°c; are partly decomposed at boiling temperature.

Action: Counteracts toxic effects, such as dermatitis occurring during arsenical treatment of syphilis; liberates the arsenic or other heavy metals deposited in tissues and promotes their elimination.

Uses: In the prevention and treatment of toxic reactions during arsenic, bismuth and mercury administration, and in poisoning by these metals; also in eczema.

Supply: SULFACTOL—Ampules, sterile crystals, 10 gr (0.6 Gm) and 15 gr (1.0 Gm) —Boxes of 10.

SULFACTOL—Combination Package, 5 ampules of crystals, 15 gr (1.0 Gm) and 5 ampules of sterile triple distilled water, 10 cc.

SULFACTOL—Tablets, Enteric coated, 8 gr (0.5 Gm)—Bottles of 100 and 1,000.

Administration: *Intravenously*—10–15 gr dissolved in 10 cc of distilled water, once daily until the desired effect is obtained; then at longer intervals.
Orally—1–2 tablets three times daily before meals, as supplement to intravenous therapy.

SULFAX (Boericke and Tafel)

Antiseptic

Chemical Name: Oxyquinoline Sulphate.

Formula: $(C_9H_7ON)_2 . H_2SO_4$.

Action and Uses: Non-irritating, soothing, healing, antiseptic; *For use* in nasal infections, oral hygiene, eye diseases, pelvic infections, surgical conditions; also in burns, plant dermatitis and pyorrhea alveolaris.

Supply: SULFAX—Tablets, gr 1 (0.064 Gm)—Bottles of 1, 7 and 20 oz.
SULFAX—Dusting Powder—Cans of ½, 4 and 16 oz.
SULFAX—Vaginals—Boxes of 12.

Administration: *Gargle*—1:2,000 solution.
Douche—In 1:3,000 solution.
Wet Dressing—1:1,000 solution.
Irrigation—1:1,000 solution, increased if necessary.

Incompatibles: Soap, alkalies, salts of iron and mercury.

SULFIDAL (Heyden)

Sulphur Therapy

Description: A yellowish white powder, containing 75% sulphur and 25% albumin; is soluble up to 10% in water, forming a slightly cloudy solution, bluish white in color and sedimenting upon standing.

Action and Uses: As for colloidal sulphur; compared to precipitated and sublimated sulphur its particles are distinctly smaller and the surface effect accordingly greater. *For use* where sulphur is indicated: seborrhea, alopecia seborrhoeica and other skin diseases; internally, in constipation, mercurial poisoning, rheumatism, respiratory catarrh, chlorosis.

Supply: SULFIDAL—Powder—1, 4 and 8 oz.—Bottles 1 lb.

Administration: **Acne Rosacea**—On face, 10% with Lassar's paste; on back, 10%.
Scabies and Prurigo—20–25% ointment.
Seborrhea or Alopecia—2–5% or 10% solution four times daily.
Sulphur Baths—25–50 Gm of Powder dissolved in 500–1,000 parts of glycerine per bath.
Orally—2–5 gr one or two times daily.

Bibliography: *See Chap. XII.*

SULFONAL (Winthrop)

Sedative. Hypnotic

Chemical Name: Diethylsulfondimethylmethane. Brand of Sulphonmethane.

Formula: $(CH_3)_2 . C. (SO_2)_2(C_2H_5)_2$.

Description: White, odorless, tasteless crystals; sparingly soluble in cold water (1–500 parts), more soluble in warm water, readily soluble in alcohol and ether.

Action: Induces sleep in the absence of pain or marked mental excitation; in ordinary doses does not affect the cardiovascular system and is well tolerated by the stomach; its habitual use, especially in anemic women, may cause hematoporphyrinuria.

Uses: In simple insomnia and insomnia of mental diseases.

Supply: SULFONAL—Tablets, 5 gr (0.3 Gm)—Bottles 25 and 100.

SULFONAL—Powder—Cartons 1 oz.

Administration: 15–30 gr (1.0–2.0 Gm) dissolved in hot fluid or followed by warm drink.

Caution: During prolonged use of Sulfonal, alkalies or alkaline carbonated waters should be taken liberally and the bowels kept open by saline laxatives.

SULPHARSPHENAMINE

Antisyphilitic

Chemical Name: Disodium 3, 3′-diamino-4, 4′-dihydroxyarsenobenzene-N-dimethylene-sulphonate.

Formula: $NaOSO_2CH_2NH.\ OH.\ C_6H_3As{:}\ As.\ C_6H_3OH.\ NH.\ CH_2.\ O_2SO.\ Na.$

Description: Yellowish powder of peculiar sulphur odor, readily soluble in water at room temperature; when kept in solution decomposes gradually.

Action and Advantages: An antisyphilitic, especially adapted for intramuscular use in those whose veins are not readily accessible, as in children and the obese.

Uses: In syphilis and most of its manifestations, especially neurosyphilis.

Supply: SULPHARSPHENAMINE (C.A.)—Ampules—Single doses 0.2, 0.3, 0.4, 0.6 Gm. **(Abbott)**

SULFARSENOL (C.A.)—Ampules—Single doses 0.06, 0.12, 0.18, 0.30, 0.42, 0.60 Gm. **(Anglo-French)**

SULPHARSPHENAMINE (C.A.)—Ampules—Single doses 0.15, 0.3, 0.45, 0.75, 0.9, 1.5 Gm. **(Mallinckrodt)**

SULPHARSPHENAMINE (C.A.)—Ampules—Single doses—0.1, 0.2, 0.3, 0.4, 0.5, 0.6 Gm. **(Merck)**

SULPHARSPHENAMINE (C.A.)—Ampules—Single doses—0.1, 0.15, 0.3, 0.45, 0.6, 0.75, 0.9 Gm with or without one 10 cc ampule of triple distilled water. **(Metz)**

Ampules—For multiple doses, 3.0 Gm.

SULPHARSPHENAMINE (C.A.)—Ampules—Single doses 0.10, 0.20, 0.3, 0.4, 0.5, 0.6 Gm. **(Searle)**

SULPHARSPHENAMINE (C.A.)—Ampules—Single doses 0.1, 0.2, 0.3, 0.4, 0.5, 0.6, 0.9, 3.0 Gm with **(Squibb)**

Ampules—5 cc, sterile and double distilled water.

Administration: *Intramuscularly*—Beginning with 0.15 Gm gradually increased to 0.6; injections given once or twice weekly. The drug is dissolved in 2–4 cc of distilled water; where intravenously employed is dissolved in 10–20 cc of distilled water.

Dosage: Infants 3–8 weeks—0.05–0.15 Gm; 2–6 mo.—0.1 Gm.
Children ½–1 yr.—0.15 Gm, 1–2 yr.—0.15–0.2 Gm.
Adults—Usual dosage.

Caution: Solution should never be injected unless freshly prepared, filtered and perfectly clear.

SULPHOCOL (Mulford Colloid)

Sulphur Therapy

Description: Occurs in lustrous, yellow-white, non-hygroscopic scales, readily soluble in water; contains 20–25 % elemental Sulphur.

Action and Uses: A stable, non-irritating, readily absorbed and assimilated preparation of Colloidal Sulphur; is slowly eliminated and thus of prolonged action; does not cause precipitation of tissue fluids; increases tolerance for mercury. Is *used* in disturbed sulphur metabolism and liver impairment, in intestinal toxemia, rheumatism, arthritis, neuritis; also as sulphur baths.

Supply: SULPHOCOL—Vials 10 Gm.

SULPHOCOL—Solution 10 %, Ampule-vials 25 cc.

SULPHOCOL—Capsules Soluble, gr. 5—Bottles of 100.

SULPHOCOL—Ointment 10 %—Tubes ½ oz.—Packages of 12.

Administration: *Orally*—½–3 gr (0.032–0.194 Gm) several times daily.
Hypodermically—¼–5 cc (½–10 gr).

SUPER D COD LIVER OIL (Upjohn)

Vitamin Therapy

Description: A standardized preparation containing not less than 30,000 U.S.P. units Vitamin A, and a minimum of 10,000 units Vitamin D (McCollum line test) per fluid ounce; is palatable, uniform and readily assimible.

Action and Uses: That of cod liver oil with high vitamin content; is anti-rachitic, anti-infective bone and muscle building, and tonic; *used* in conditions of vitamin deficiency, is nutritional endurances.

Supply: SUPER D COD LIVER OIL—Bottles 3, 8 and 16 oz.

Administration: 1–4 teaspoonfuls three times daily.
Children ¼–1 teaspoonful, three times daily.

Combinations: SUPER D COD LIVER OIL CONCENTRATE: 2 m being equivalent to 1 teaspoonful of Super D Cod Liver Oil. 1 cc contains: Vitamin A 30,000 U.S.P., Vitamin D: 10,000 units.
Dosage—3–6 drops three times daily after meals, in orange juice—Bottles of 5 cc, with dropper.

SUPER D CONCENTRATE—Perles; each perle is equivalent to 3 teaspoonfuls of standard cod liver oil. *Supply*—Bottles of 30. *Administration*—1–2 perles daily.

SUPRARENALIN (Armour)

Vasoconstrictor

Chemical Name: Epinephrine.

Formula: $C_6H_3(OH)_2CHOH.\ CH_2.\ NH.\ CH_3$.

Description: The active principle of suprarenal medulla; a watery, clear, stable, non-irritating isotonic fluid, unaffected by boiling.

Action and Uses: Contracts blood vessels, raises blood pressure, slows and stimulates the heart; is *used* in arresting capillary hemorrhage, in eye, nose, throat and other operations; to relieve asthma, urticaria and other allergic conditions; in shock, anesthesia accidents and in combination with local anesthetics.

Supply: SUPRARENALIN—Crystals (C.A.)—Vials 1 gr (0.064 Gm).

SUPRARENALIN—Solution (C.A.)—Containing suprarenalin sulphate equivalent to 1:1,000 epinephrine—Bottles 1 oz.

SUPRARENALIN—Ampules (C.A.) 1 cc—1:1,000 and 1:10,000 solution—Boxes of 6, 50 and 100.

SUPRARENALIN—Ointment (C.A.)—1:1,000 in petrolatum base—Collapsible tubes ⅝ oz.

Administration: *General Dosage*—5–30 m (0.3–2 cc) every 2–3 hr. if necessary.

In Shock—*Hypodermic*—10–15 m (0.06–1 cc) of 1:1,000 solution or 1–5 cc of 1:10,000 solution in 500 cc of isotonic saline, by *hypodermoclysis.*

In Asthma—5–10 m of Solution, *intramuscularly;* also by spraying the throat and larynx.

In Urticaria—10–20 m, *intravenously,* given slowly, repeated if necessary.

In Local Anesthesia—To intensify and prolong effect of the anesthetic, 5–15 m per cubic centimeter of anesthetic solution.

Topical Application—1:15,000–1:1,000 solution.

SUPRARENIN (Metz)

Vasoconstrictor. Hemostatic

Chemical Name: Bitartrate of dioxy-phenyl-ethanol-methyl-amine. Brand of Epinephrin (Synthetic).

Formula: $C_6H_3(OH)_2$. CHOH. CH_2NH. CH_3.

Description: Synthetic epinephrine, the active principle of the suprarenal gland; nearly white, finely granular, odorless, crystalline powder, soluble in water, yielding an acid reaction; stable for an indefinite period if protected from light, heat and moisture.

Action and Uses: Has same physiological action as the natural epinephrine obtained from the adrenal gland; stimulates vasoconstrictors, raises blood pressure, slows the heart and directly stimulates its muscle. *Used* extensively with local anesthetics, in shock, hemorrhage, asthma, hay fever, mucosal hyperplasia and in heart failure.

Incompatibles: Alkalies and oxidizing agents (iodine, potassium permanganate, hydrogen peroxide); is rapidly destroyed by formaldehyde.

Advantages: Is claimed to be preferable to the natural epinephrine because of its definite composition, freedom from soluble or insoluble protein matter and greater stability.

Supply: **SUPRARENIN**—Solution (C.A.), 1:1,000—Bottles 1 oz.

SUPRARENIN—Ampules (C.A.) 1 cc—Boxes of 20.

SUPRARENIN—Tablets (C.A.), 1 mg—Tubes of 20; 1 tablet dissolved in 1 cc of sterile water or salt solution makes 1:1,000 dilution.

Administration: *Externally*—Is applied plain, on gauze or cotton to bleeding area. *Internally*—Is given—*subcutaneously,* 4–8 m in asthma; *intravenously*—30 m to a pint of physiologic saline or glucose in shock; *intramuscularly*—5–15 m of 1:1,000 solution; for direct injection into the heart—not more than 2 cc should be used.

SURGICAL MAGGOTS (Lederle)

Necrotic Tissue Digestant

Description: A species of fly larvae preserved in a liver-agar medium.

Action and Uses: Removes necrotic tissue and offensive odors, destroys bacterial putrefaction, stimulates drainage, and hastens healing; is easily applied. *For use* in osteomyelitis, suppurating wounds, decubitus ulcers and tendon sloughs.

Supply: SURGICAL MAGGOTS (C.A.)—1 Sterile package, glass enclosed, containing 1 therapeutic dose.

Administration: *Applied locally* with adhesive straps, exposing wound to open end of container; wire gauze cage covers the opening to prevent maggots from leaving the wounds; allowed to remain for 5 days; then flushed out with saline and reapplied fresh; repeated for 6–10 weeks.

SYNEPHRIN TARTRATE (Stearns)

Vasoconstrictor

Chemical Name: Hydroxyphenylmethylaminoethanol Tartrate; P-Methylaminoethanolphenol Tartrate.

Formula: $(HOC_6H_4CHOHCH_2NHCH_3)_2C_4H_4O_6$.

Description: A white, crystalline substance, soluble in water and alcohol.

Action and Uses: A vaso-constrictor of prolonged action, affecting muscle tissue directly and not through the myoneural junction; is not as effective as epinephrine, but less toxic; raises blood pressure, dilates coronary arteries, relaxes bronchial tubes and intestinal musculature, dilates the pupil; raises the tone of uterine muscle, relieving hyperemia and congestion. *Used* in reducing swelling in nasal affections, in allergy, asthma, cardiac weakness and hypotension; also in local anesthesia, minor surgery and dental operations.

Supply: SYNEPHRIN TARTRATE—Solution, 3% (C.A.)—Contains Synephrin Tartrate 3%, Sodium Benzoate 0.2%, Sodium Chloride 0.8% in distilled water—Bottles of ½, 1 oz.

SYNEPHRIN TARTRATE—Solution, 5% (C.A.)—Contains Synephrin Tartrate 5%, Sodium Benzoate 0.2%, Sodium Chloride 0.8% in distilled water—Bottles 1 oz.

SYNEPHRIN TARTRATE EMULSION, COMPOUND (C.A.)—Contains Synephrin Tartrate 2.5%, Sodium Benzoate 0.4%, Camphor 0.07%, Menthol 0.052% and oil of Red Thyme 0.17% in emulsion of Oil of Sesame and Acacia with distilled water—Bottle ½ oz.

Administration: *Dosage*—Gr 1½–3 (0.1–0.2 Gm) three times daily; is administered *orally, hypodermically* or the emulsion; *topically* by application to mucous membranes of the nose, throat or the eyes.

Bibliography: *See Chap. XII.*

TAKA-DIASTASE (Parke, Davis)

Starch Digestant

Description: A vegetable diastase in powder form, obtained from Aspergillus oryzae, grown on sterilized wheat bran; liquefies three hundred times its weight of starch in 10 min.

Action and Uses: Converts starchy foods into the soluble starches, dextrins, maltose and even traces of dextrose; acts to best advantage in neutral or slightly acid medium, and should therefore be taken with meals or immediately after. By freeing the starches from the proteins in the stomach, it assists in the disposition of the latter while it prepares the starches for ultimate conversion into dextrose and levulose in the intestine. *Indicated* in all conditions of faulty starch digestion.

Supply: TAKA-DIASTASE—Bottles ½, 1, 4 oz., and 1 lb.

TAKA-DIASTASE—Capsules gr 2½ (0.15 Gm)—Bottles 25, 100 and 500.

TAKA-DIASTASE—Tablets gr 2½ (0.15 Gm)—Bottles 50, 100 and 500.

LIQUID TAKA-DIASTASE—Each dram contains 2½ gr (0.15 Gm) of Taka-Diastase in solution—Bottles of 8, 16 oz. and 1 gal.

Administration: Gr 2½–5; may be added to children's food for predigestion.

Combinations:

TAKA-DIASTASE AND PANCREATIN—Tablets—Chocolate coated, containing Taka-Diastase, 2 gr (0.13 Gm); Pancreatin, U.S.P., 3 gr (0.19 Gm)—Bottles 25 and 100.

TAKA-DIASTASE, PANCREATIN, NUX VOMICA—Tablets—Chocolate coated containing Taka-Diastase, 0.13 Gm; Pancreatin, U.S.P., 3 gr (0.19 Gm); Extr. Nux Vomica, ½ gr (0.03 Gm)—Bottles 25 and 100.

TAKA-DIASTASE, PEPSIN AND PANCREATIN—Tablets—Chocolate coated containing Taka-Diastase, 2 gr (0.13 Gm); Pepsin 1:3,000, 1 gr (0.06 Gm); Pancreatin, U.S.P., 2 gr (0.13 Gm)—Bottles 25 and 100.

TAKA-DIASTASE, PEPSIN AND PANCREATIN—Capsules, containing Taka-Diastase, 2 gr (0.13 Gm); Pepsin 1:3,000, 1 gr (0.06 Gm); Pancreatin, U.S.P., 2 gr (0.13 Gm)—Bottles of 25, 100 and 500.

TAKA-DIASTASE, PEPSIN AND STRYCHNINE—Tablets—Chocolate coated containing Taka-Diastase, 2 gr (0.13 Gm); Pepsin 1:3,000, 2 gr (0.13 Gm); Strychnine Phosphate, 1/100 gr (0.0006 Gm)—Bottles of 25 and 100.

TAKAZYME TABLETS, containing Taka-Diastase, ½ gr (0.03 Gm); Pepsin 1:3,000, 1 gr (0.06 Gm); Calcium Carbonate, 10 gr (0.6 Gm)—Bottles of 100 and 1,000.

TANNALBIN (Bilhuber-Knoll)

Intestinal Astringent

Chemical Name: Tannin Proteinate.

Description: A light brown odorless, tasteless powder, containing 50% of tannin; insoluble in cold water or alcohol.

Action: A non-irritating intestinal astringent and antidiarrhoeic; is not affected in the stomach, but is broken down in the intestines, liberating tannin which diminishes secretions of the intestinal mucosa.

Uses: In acute and chronic intestinal catarrh, in diarrheas of tuberculosis, dysentery, typhoid and drugs; in summer complaint of children.

Supply: TANNALBIN—Tablets gr 5 (0.324 Gm)—Bottles of 100.

TANNALBIN—Powder—Cartons of ½ oz.

Administration: Adults—½ teaspoonful of powder or 3–6 tablets several times daily.
Infants—5 gr (0.324 Gm) three times a day;
Children—According to age; continued 1–2 days after symptoms subside.
Rectally—Instilled slowly with the addition of opium.

TANNIC ACID SPRAY (Crookes)

Burn Therapy

Composition: A stable 25% non-colloidal solution of Tannic Acid.

Action and Uses: Analgesic and protective; *used* for relief of pain and shock in the treatment of burns.

Supply: TANNIC ACID SPRAY—Ampules 30 cc—Boxes of 3, 6.

TANNIC ACID SPRAY—Adaptor with 1 ampule, cardboard box or metal container.

Administration: Applied by spraying scalded area.

TANNIGEN (Winthrop)

Intestinal Astringent

Chemical Name: Acetic Acid Ester of Tannic Acid. Brand of Acetyltannic Acid.

Formula: $C_{14}H_8(CH_3CO)_2O_9$.

Description: A light gray powder, almost odorless and tasteless; insoluble in cold water and dilute acids, soluble in alcohol.

Action: Passes unchanged through the stomach; in the intestines tannic acid is gradually liberated; exerts an astringent action by contracting the mucous membrane; relieves congestion and checks diarrheal discharges; acts on both the large and small intestines.

Uses: In dysentery, various types of colitis, gastroenteritis, typhoid fever.

Incompatibles: Is decomposed by alkalies which should therefore be avoided after its administration.

Supply: TANNIGEN—Powder (C.A.)—Bottles ½ and 1 oz.

Administration: Adults, 8–15 gr (0.5–1.0 Gm), beginning with the larger dose and reducing to smaller. Children, half dosage.
Is administered in water, milk sugar, or is added to food.

Bibliography: *See Chap. XII.*

TANNISMUT (Heyden)

Intestinal Astringent

Chemical Name: Bismuth Bitannate.

Formula: $BiOH(C_{14}H_9O_9)_2$.

Description: A brownish or yellowish odorless powder of slightly astringent taste; insoluble in water, soluble in dilute acids and alkalies; contains 17–21% bismuth.

Action: An intestinal astringent affecting the entire colon; does not influence the stomach, being but slightly decomposed there; is non-toxic.

Uses: In acute, subacute and chronic intestinal catarrh, summer diarrhea and other intestinal disorders in children.

Supply: TANNISMUT—Powder—Bottles of 25 Gm.
TANNISMUT—Tablets 0.5 Gm—Tubes of 20.

Administration: Adults—1–2 tablets (0.5–1.0 Gm), chewed three to five times daily.
Children under 1 yr.—0.03–0.1 Gm three to five times daily.
Children over 1 yr.—0.1–0.5 Gm, three to five times daily.

Bibliography: *See Chap. XII.*

TARGESIN (Kretschmar)

Gonocide. Astringent

Chemical Name: Diacetyl-silver-tannin-albumen.

Description: A colloidal preparation of silver; occurs in scales of dark color and metallic lustre, readily soluble in water, forming a slightly acid and stable solution; contains 6% metallic silver.

Action and Uses: A gonocide and astringent; a deeply penetrating, non-caustic bactericide; is not precipitated by albumen or salts of urine. *For use* in gonorrheal infections; in ophthalmologic, dermatologic and other disturbances where a silver astringent is desired.

Supply: TARGESIN—Bottles 10, 25, 50, 100 Gm.

Administration: Urology—1–5 % solution for urethral injection and instillation; in 0.2 % solution for bladder irrigation in cystitis; in 5–10 % solution in gonorrheal abortive therapy and female urethritis; as tampon 15–20 % for vaginal use.

Ophthalmology—5 % solution or ointment in conjunctivitis, blepharitis and corneal ulceration.

Rhino-Laryngology—For topical application—2–10 % in chronic rhinitis, pharyngitis; in 2–3 %—for sinus irrigation.

Dermatology—In 2–5 % solution or 5 % ointment in eczema, impetigo, pyodermia, intertrigo.

Surgery—In solution or 5 % ointment—in ulcers and granulating wounds.

Bibliography: *See Chap. XII.*

TETANOL-COLLOSOL (Crookes)

Calcium Therapy

Composition: Calcium Levulinate, containing 13 % Calcium.

Action and Uses: To raise blood calcium, and control spasms in tetany.

Supply: TETANOL-COLLOSOL—Ampules 5 cc, 10 cc and 20 cc, Intravenous—Boxes of 6.

TETANOL-COLLOSOL—Ampules 2 cc, Intramuscular—Boxes of 6.

Administration: *Intramuscular or Intravenous Injection*—1 ampule as necessary.

TETRABROMPHENOLPHTHALEIN SODIUM (Eastman)

X-Ray Contrast Medium

Chemical Name: The Sodium Salt of Dibasic Tetrabromphenolphthalein.

Formula: $NaOOC.\ C_6H_4C{:}\ (C_6H_2Br_2OH)_2Na$.

Description: A bluish odorless powder, freely soluble in water, slightly soluble in alcohol, insoluble in ether; contains about 47 % of bromine.

Action: Is excreted with the bile into the gall bladder in sufficient concentration to produce a dense shadow of the organ and its contents.

Uses: For radiography of the gall bladder.

Caution: Is now rarely used; if employed must be used cautiously; untoward effects such as nausea, dizziness, fall in blood pressure, general pains may occur, and may be relieved by epinephrine, 0.5–1.0 cc, 1:1,000 intramuscularly.

Supply: TETRABROMPHENOLPHTHALEIN SODIUM SALT—Bottles of 100 and 500 Gm.

Administration: 0.1 Gm per kilogram of body weight, or 4.5–5 Gm of the dye for a person of 125 lb.; is dissolved in 35–40 cc of freshly distilled water, filtered and sterilized by heating the container in boiling water for 20 min.; is administered *intravenously* in 2 injections, at half hour intervals, half quantity each time, avoiding extravasation into tissues; x-rays taken at intervals, as with similar preparations.

TETRADOL (National Aniline)

X-Ray Contrast Medium

Composition: A contrast medium for administration in cholecystography; contains Sodium Tetraiodophenolphthalein.

Action and Uses: Assures shadows of good density and is non-irritating to the gastric mucosa; does not deteriorate upon standing if kept in sealed container.

Supply: **TETRADOL EMULSION**—Containing 4 Gm of dye—Individual bottles—1 dose.

TETRADOL POWDER—Intravenous—Vials of 3½ Gm—Packages of 5 vials.

Administration: *Oral Method*—Content of 1 bottle of emulsion is stirred in ½–¾ glass of cold water or fruit juice and taken at 7 P. M.; no food or laxatives are permitted; exposures made at 10 A. M. the next morning.

Intravenous Method—About 50 mg of powder per kilogram of body weight, total not to exceed 3½ Gm; is dissolved in freshly distilled water, filtered, sterilized for 15 min. over water bath, diluted to 200 cc with Ringer's or saline solution and injected slowly for 15 min. by the gravity method. Roentgenograms taken 12 hr. after.

TETRAIODOPHENOLPHTHALEIN SODIUM (Eastman)

Radiopaque Medium

Chemical Name: Sodium Tetraiodophenolphthalein.

Formula: $C_{20}H_8I_4O_4Na_2$.

Description: A bluish, odorless, hygroscopic powder, soluble in water and alcohol.

Action: After absorption by the liver and its elimination with the bile into the gall bladder, the latter may become radiographically opaque and visualized.

Uses: In cholecystography.

Advantages: Is non-poisonous, producing but little gastro-intestinal irritation.

Supply: **TETRAIODOPHENOLPHTHALEIN SODIUM**—Salt (C.A.)—Bottles of 100 and 500 Gm.

TETRAIODOPHENOLPHTHALEIN SODIUM—Capsules 0.5 Gm each—Bottles of 100.

Administration: *Intravenously*—Dosage—For patients 115–160 lb.—3 Gm, over 160 lb.—3.5 Gm, under 115 lb.—reduced accordingly; the dye is dissolved in 30 cc of freshly distilled water, sterilized and injected; radiography 12 hours after; *Orally*—8 capsules 0.5 Gm each or 4 Gm dissolved in 30 cc of distilled water and added to 120–240 cc grape juice are taken during and after evening meal (fat free); examination made the next morning.

TETROPHINE (Riedel-de Haen)

Stimulant

Chemical Name: Dihydro Naphtacridin-carbonic Acid.

Formula: $C_{18}H_{31}NO_2$.

Description: A yellowish fine crystalline powder of weak acid and slightly bitter taste; almost insoluble in water or ordinary organic solvents; soluble in alkalis forming crystalline salts.

Action: Acts as stimulant on both the central and peripheral nervous system, improving muscle tone and reflexes.

Uses: In ataxia and perception disturbances of tabes dorsalis, pseudo-tabes, cerebellar disease; also in multiple sclerosis, polyneuritis, post-poliomyelitis; in paralysis after diphtheria, apoplexy, encephalitis lethargica, Parkinson's disease, amyotrophic lateral sclerosis, syringomyelia and pernicious anemia.

Supply: **TETROPHINE**—Tablets—gr 1½ (0.1 Gm)—Tubes of 20.

TETROPHINE—Ampules—2.2 cc, 5% solution—Boxes of 5.

Administration: *Orally*—½ tablet twice daily, gradually increased to 2 or a maximum of 3 tablets daily.
Intralumbarly—Initial dose 1 cc, after 2 days, 1.5 to 2 cc.

Caution: Treatment to begin with small doses; large doses may produce muscular rigidity.

Bibliography: *See Chap. XII.*

THEAMIN (Lilly)

Diuretic. Vasodilator

Chemical Name: Theophylline Ethanol Amine.

Formula: $C_7H_8N_4O_2$—C_2H_7NO.

Description: A white, crystalline non-hygroscopic, powder; contains 25.32% monoethanolamine and 74.68% anhydrous theophylline.

Action: A diuretic and coronary vasodilator.

Uses: In edema of myocardial insufficiency, chronic passive congestion, chronic hypertension; in angina pectoris, coronary thrombosis, glomerulonephritis, uremia.

Supply: THEAMIN—Pulvules, gr 3 (0.194 Gm)—Bottles of 40, 500.

Administration: 3–5 pulvules daily for 3 or 4 days.

THEELIN (Parke, Davis)

Hormone Therapy

Description: Colorless rhomboid or six-sided tabular crystals; a complex alcohol and thus non-protein in nature; standardized to a potency of at least 3,000 rat units per milligram.

Action and Uses: As ovarian follicular hormone; stimulates estrogenic function in gonadal deficiency and uterine dysfunction; is of particular value in the nervous manifestations of menopause; *also useful* in secondary types of amenorrhea, in oligomenorrhea and dysmenorrhea; good results have lately been observed in hemophilia.

Supply: THEELIN—Ampules, 1 cc, 50 rat units—Boxes of 6 and 100.
THEELIN—Suppositories, Vaginal, 50 rat units each—Boxes of 6.

Administration: 1 or 2 ampules, *subcutaneously* or *intramuscularly;* suppositories—one at night on retiring.

Bibliography: *See Chap. XII.*

THEELOL (Parke, Davis)

Hormone Therapy

Formula: $C_{18}H_{24}O_3$.

Description: A crystalline, colorless, ovarian hormone for oral administration; standardized by Doisy method to a potency of at least 3,000 rat units per milligram.

Action and Uses: Stimulates estrogenic activity in disturbances of the ovarian sexual cycle resulting from gonadal hypofunction; *useful* in menopause, functional oligomenorrhea and amenorrhea; functional sterility, sexual frigidity, uterine atrophy, infantile uterus and hyperemesis gravidarum.

Supply: THEELOL—Kapseals, 50 rat units each—Bottles of 20.

Administration: 1–3 Kapseals daily, administered orally in intervals between Theelin injections.

Bibliography: *See Chap. XII.*

THELESTRIN (G. W. Carnrick)

Hormone Therapy

Composition: A standardized preparation of ovarian follicular, estrus producing hormone; each cubic centimeter represents 25 Allen-Doisy units.

Action and Uses: For intensive therapy in stimulating endometrial proliferation and ovarian function; in functional amenorrhea and menopausal disorders due to uterine atrophy.

Supply: THELESTRIN—Ampules 1 cc—Boxes of 6.

Administration: *Subcutaneously*—1–2 ampules daily.

THEOBROMINE

Cardiac Stimulant. Diuretic

Chemical Name: 3.7 dimethylxanthine; 3.7 dimethyl-2.6 dioxypurine.

Formula: $C_5H_2(CH_3)_2N_4O_2$.

Description: Occurs naturally in the seeds of Theobroma cacao; is also prepared synthetically; a white, bitter crystalline powder, odorless and permanent in air; is slightly soluble in water, alcohol and chloroform; insoluble in petroleum ether, easily soluble in alkalies.

Action and Uses: As for caffeine, but its action is relatively greater on the heart and muscles and less powerful on the central nervous system; is efficient diuretic superior to caffeine but its double salts are preferred in many instances because of greater solubility; *used* in edemas—cardiac, renal or hepatic; also used in aortitis, pleurisy, pericarditis and uremia.

Supply: THEOBROMINE (C.A.)—Bottles 1 oz., ¼ and 1 lb. (Merck)

Administration: 5–8 gr (0.3–0.5 Gm) four times daily.

Combinations: THEOBROMINE AND SODIUM ACETATE (C.A.) (Merck) Bottles of 1 oz, ¼ and 1 lb.

THEOBROMINE AND SODIUM ACETATE (C.A.)—Bottles of 10 Gm and 100 Gm. (Roche)

A mixture of theobromine and sodium acetate, in molecular quantities; a white, almost odorless hygroscopic powder, freely soluble in water, slightly soluble in alcohol; *For use* in the same conditions as theobromine, but often preferable because of greater solubility.

THEOCALCIN (Bilhuber-Knoll)

Diuretic

Chemical Name: Theobromine Calcium Salicylate.

Formula: Calcium Theobromine $(C_7H_7O_2N_4)_2Ca$; Calcium Salicylate $(C_7H_5O_3)_2Ca$.

Description: A double salt comprising calcium theobromine and calcium salicylate and containing 44% theobromine, occurs as a white powder, slightly soluble in water.

Action: Diuretic and chlorides eliminant; is easily absorbed, non-irritating and well tolerated; dilates the coronary blood vessels improving nutrition of the heart muscle and increasing cardiac efficiency; decreases arterial tension and resistance.

Uses: *Used* for relief of angina pectoris, in congestive heart failure of arteriosclerotic origin, in myocarditis, cardiac asthma and cardionephritic edema.

Advantages: Freedom from gastric upset, nausea and renal irritation.

Supply: THEOCALCIN—Tablets (C.A.) gr 7½ (0.5 Gm)—Tubes of 20—Bottles of 100.

THEOCALCIN—Powder (C.A.)—Bottles of 1 oz.

Administration: 1–3 tablets three times daily after meals; reduced when possible; as diuretic, given up to 60 gr daily.

Combinations: POTASSIUM IODIDE-THEOCALCIN—A combination of Theocalcin gr 7½ (0.5 Gm) with Potassium iodide gr 1½ (0.09 Gm) per tablet, for synergistic effect. *Used* in above conditions, 1–2 tablets, crushed and taken with water at meals and bedtime; dosage is reduced as soon as possible—Tubes of 20—Bottles of 100.

Bibliography: *See Chap. XII.*

THEOCIN (Winthrop)

Diuretic

Chemical Name: 1.3 dimethylxanthin. Brand of Theophyllin.

Formula: $C_7H_8N_4O_2$.

Description: A white, odorless, bitter powder; soluble in 180 parts of water at room temperature; soluble with difficulty in alcohol and ether.

Action: Produces prompt and marked diuresis, often when other remedies fail; causes vasodilatation and cardiac stimulation.

Uses: In dropsies of cardiovascular and cardiorenal origin; in chronic myocarditis with decompensation; in arteriosclerosis and angina pectoris.

Supply: THEOCIN—Tablets (C.A.) 1½ gr (0.09 Gm)—Bottles of 25.

THEOCIN—Powder (C.A.)—Bottle of ½ oz.

Combination: THEOCIN—Soluble (C.A.) Theocin-Sodium-Acetate, containing 65% of theocin; a white powder of greater solubility in water—Tablets 2½ gr (0.15 Gm)—Bottles of 25. Powder—Bottles of ½ oz.

Administration: 1 or 2 tablets of either preparation, two or three times daily, on a full stomach or with an abundance of fluid.

Bibliography: *See Chap. XII.*

THEPHYLDINE (Kretschmar)

Diuretic

Chemical Name: Brand of Theophylline-ethylene-diamine.

Formula: $C_{25}H_{40}N_{16}O_6$.

Description: A white or slightly yellow, crystalline powder of ammoniacal odor; is freely soluble in water, readily absorbed and non-irritating; contains 80% Theophylline.

Action and Uses: Cardiac stimulant, vascular dilator, powerful diuretic; *For use* in angina pectoris, coronary sclerosis, cardiac asthma, arteriosclerosis, hypertension, nephritis.

Supply: THEPHYLDINE—Tablets gr 1½ (0.1 Gm), gr 3 (0.2 Gm)—Tubes of 20 and 100.

THEPHYLDINE—Suppositories (0.36 Gm)—Boxes of 12.

THEPHYLDINE—Ampules 2 cc (0.48 Gm), Intramuscular—Boxes of 6.

THEPHYLDINE—Ampules 10 cc (0.24 Gm), Intravenous—Boxes of 5.

THEPHYLDINE—Powder—Bottles of 15 Gm.

Combinations: **THEPHYLDINE WITH BENZYL SUCCINATE**—Tablets—Tubes of 20.

THEPHYLDINE WITH CALCIUM LACTATE—Tablets—Tubes of 20, 100.

THEPHYLDINE WITH CALCIUM LACTATE AND POTASSIUM IODIDE—Tablets—Tubes of 20, 100.

THEPHYLDINE WITH PHENOBARBITAL—Tablets—Tubes of 20, 100.

THEPHYLDINE WITH CALCIUM SALICYLATE AND POTASSIUM IODIDE—Ampules 10 cc—Boxes of 5.

THEPHYLDINE WITH CALCIUM LACTATE—Suppositories—Boxes of 12.

THEPHYLDINE WITH CALCIUM LACTATE AND POTASSIUM IODIDE—Suppositories—Boxes of 12.

Administration: *Oral*—1–2 tablets, three or four times daily, after meals.
Rectal—2–4 suppositories daily.
Intramuscular—1–3 ampules daily.
Intravenous—1–3 ampules daily.

Bibliography: *See Chap. XII.*

THIGENOL (Roche)

Antipruritic. Antiseptic

Composition: A solution of the Sodium salt of synthetic Sulpho-oleic acid; contains 2.85% of Sulphur.

Description: A dark brown liquid of faint sulphurous odor; soluble in one or more parts of water, dilute alcohol, glycerin, chloroform and oily or fatty bases.

Action: Mildly antiseptic, antipruritic and siccative; stimulates granulation and promotes healing.

Uses: In dermatologic and gynecologic conditions.

Advantages: Is devoid of the disagreeable odor of ichthyol, does not stain tissues, is non-irritating, and easily miscible with all ointment bases.

Supply: **THIGENOL** (C.A.)—Bottles of 1 lb., ½ lb., ¼ lb., and 1 oz.

Administration: *Used* pure or diluted with glycerin or alcohol, 5–20%; as ointment—15–25%; on tampons—saturated with 10–50% solution in glycerin or petrolatum; as suppositories—15–25% in cacao butter base.

Caution: Is incompatible with mineral acids and acetic acid; where water is used as vehicle, distilled only should be employed.

THIO-BISMOL (Parke, Davis)

Antiluetic

Chemical Name: Sodium Bismuth Thioglycollate.

Formula: $Bi(SC_2H_2O_2Na)_3$.

Description: A water-soluble compound of bismuth; on injection is not precipitated in the tissue fluids, but is completely absorbed from the site of injection within 2 hr.

Action and Uses: Possesses definite spirocheticidal activity; is of low toxicity and free from local injury to the tissues where injected; is especially useful in neurosyphilis.

Supply: THIO-BISMOL—Ampules (C.A.) 2 cc, containing gr 3 (0.194 Gm) Thio-Bismol—Boxes of 12 and 100, with sufficient distilled water for use of entire contents.

Administration: *Intramuscularly*—Usual dose, 3 gr or 1 ampule twice a week, in 1–2 cc of water for one weighing 150 lb.; increased or decreased in accordance with weight. After 3–4 weeks, may either be substituted by bismuth salicylate or continued for another week or two.

Preparation: Powder to be dissolved in the ampule.

THIOCOL (Roche)

Sedative Expectorant

Chemical Name: The Potassium salt of Orthoguaiacolsulphonic Acid.

Formula: $C_6H_3(OH)(OCH_3)(SO_3K)$.

Description: A colorless crystalline powder of neutral or faintly alkaline reaction; is odorless and practically tasteless; is soluble in water, only partly soluble in alcohol, insoluble in absolute alcohol, ether or oils; contains 52 % of pure guaiacol.

Uses: For coughs, colds or other inflammatory conditions of the respiratory tract and in incipient tuberculosis; as intestinal disinfectant in some types of diarrhea.

Advantages: Over guaiacol in being tasteless and non-toxic; does not disturb digestion and is not constipating.

Supply: THIOCOL—Powder (C.A.)—Bottles of 1 oz.

THIOCOL—Tablets (C.A.), 5 gr (0.324 Gm)—Bottles of 25 and 100.

SYRUP THIOCOL (C.A.)—Containing Thiocol, 6 gr (0.384 Gm) per fluidram is devoid of all sedatives; is well borne and adapted for administration to children —Bottles of 6 oz.

Administration: Syrup 1–2 teaspoonfuls every 2–3 hr.; larger doses where necessary; children—according to age, ½–1 teaspoonful every 2–3 hr.
Powder or tablets 5–10 gr every 2–3 hr.; children—in accordance.

THIOL (Riedel)

Sulphur Therapy

Official Name: Thiol Liquidum; Thiol Siccum.

Description: THIOL LIQUIDUM—Is a thick dark-brown liquid of neutral reaction and pleasant odor; soluble in water, glycerine and alcohol.

THIOL SICCUM—Is a dry brown colored powder of agreeable odor and bitter astringent taste; is hygroscopic and slowly soluble in water and alcohol; both contain sulphurized and sulphonized mineral oil, the sulphur organically combined.

Action and Use: Analgesic, antiphlogistic, vasoconstrictor; *used* in numerous dermatoses where sulphur is active; in acne, dermatitis, eczema, erysipelas, erythema, furunculosis, ulcers, herpes, impetigo, intertrigo, carbuncle, lichen, urticaria, pemphigus, periphlebitis, chilblains, pityriasis, pruritus, prurigo, psoriasis, acne rosacea, sycosis, tinea tonsurans, ulcers, varicosities; also in rhinitis, pharyngitis, angina, otitis; in rheumatism, cervical erosions, mastitis.

Supply: THIOL—Liquid—Tubes 50 Gm.

THIOL—Powder—Bottles of 1 oz.

Administration: On skin—as ointment (10–25 %) or powder 5–10 %.
In nose and throat—as liquid 2 %, painted or sprayed.

In Gynecology—A tampon, diluted with water.
In Arthritis—Rubbed in as ointment.
Internally—1½–3 gr, three times daily after meals.

THOROTRAST (Heyden)

X-Ray Contrast Medium

Description: A solution containing 25% Thorium Dioxide in highly dispersed form; miscible with all body fluids without flocculation; is stable, sterile and of milky appearance in reflected light.

Action and Uses: A radiopaque medium *for use* in intravenous hepato-lienography, arteriography and cystography. In hepato-lienography almost plastic pictures of the liver and spleen are obtainable; in peripheral and cerebral arteriography—sharp visualization, is painless and reactionless; in cystography, it causes no tendency to spasm and offers sharply defined cystograms.

Supply: **THOROTRAST**—Boxes of 3 ampules, each 25 cc.
THOROTRAST—Ampules, each 12 cc—Boxes of 10.
THOROTRAST—Ampules, each 12 cc—Boxes of 2.
THOROTRAST—Bottles of 100 cc.

Technic: **Hepato-lienography**—A total of 50–75 cc of Thorotrast is given in divided daily doses of 20–25 cc; is warmed to body temperature and administered *intravenously*, either daily or every second day. Radiographs are taken 1 or 2 days following the last injection.

Peripheral Arteriography—Upper extremities, 10–12 cc injected into the artery with a 19 gauge needle; lower extremities, 20–25 cc injected into the femoral artery.

Cerebral Arteriography—8–15 cc introduced into the common carotid through a platinum needle 1 mm in diameter.

Cystography—Is introduced into the bladder in the dilution of 1:5; this dilution in no way affects the distinctness of the radiographs.

Bibliography: *See Chap. XII.*

THROMBOPLASTIN

Hemostatic

Description: An extract of brain tissue of cattle containing thromboplastic substances; is physiologically standardized to coagulate one hundred times its quantity of oxalated blood in less than 1 min.; is non-irritating, safe, quickly effective.

Action: A physiological hemostat; checks oozing and bleeding; also believed to stimulate granulation and epithelization and to promote healing.

Uses: *Locally*—After tonsillectomy; in bleeding from umbilical cord, mouth, nose, skin; as dressing after circumcision, in surgical tongue-tie, tooth extraction. *Internally*—In hemophilia, hemophilia neonatorum, hepatic bleeding; in urinary bladder, prostate, bronchoscopic, gastric, intestinal and other internal hemorrhages.

Supply: **THROMBOPLASTIN** (C.A.)—Bottles 25 cc, 16 per box. (Armour)
THROMBOPLASTIN—Local—Bottles 20 cc. (Cutter)
THROMBOPLASTIN—Subcutaneous—Bottles 20 cc. (Cutter)

THROMBOPLASTIN (C.A.)—Vials 20 cc. (Lederle)

THROMBOPLASTIN (C.A.)—Dental—Vials 4 cc—Packages of 6. (Squibb)

THROMBOPLASTIN (C.A.)—Hypodermic—Vials 20 cc, rubber stoppered. (Squibb)

Administration: *Locally*—By direct application with cotton or gauze to bleeding surface, held in contact till firm clot is formed; small clots are previously removed.

Subcutaneously or intramuscularly—never intravenously, 10–20 cc, repeated as necessary in inaccessible hemorrhages.

Oral Surgery—1–2 cc injected into site of bleeding, remainder of vial subcutaneously elsewhere.

Bibliography: *See Chap. XII.*

THYRACOIDS (Reed and Carnrick)

Thyroid Therapy

Composition: An Iodothyroglobulin preparation standardized biologically; represents the entire potency of desiccated thyroid and is of uniform strength.

Description and Action: The iodothyroglobulin contained in the thyroid gland and rich in iodine probably represents thyroxine linked to a protein; in proportion to its iodine content it is apparently more active than thyroxine and represents the entire activity of the thyroid.

Uses: *Used* where thyroid medication is indicated; in congenital athyria (cretinism), cachexia strumipriva (myxedema), athyria acquisita (thyroidectomy); in delayed eruption of deciduous teeth, in general developmental retardation of children; in enuresis nocturna and also in hypothyroidism in adults with cold hands and feet, subnormal temperature, dry skin, sluggish bowels and lack of energy.

Supply: THYRACOIDS—Tablets Plain and Enteric coated gr 1/10 (0.006 Gm), gr 1/4 (0.016 Gm), gr 1 (0.064 Gm) and gr 2 (0.12 Gm)—Bottles of 100.

Administration: 1–3 tablets daily; graded in accordance with age, sex and other conditions.

THYRACTIN (Winthrop)

Hormone Therapy

Chemical Name: Brand of Prothyrin.

Description: An iodine-protein substance isolated from the thyroid gland by a fractionation process; contains 0.4–0.6% of iodine, or about three times that of desiccated thyroid.

Action and Uses: That of biologically standardized thyroid extract; also possesses diuretic action, which is quite pronounced in some cases. *For use* in hypothyroidism, thyrogenous obesity, myxedema, cretinism, retarded mental and physical development, delayed callus formation; in nephrosis.

Supply: THYRACTIN—Tablets, 25 mg, representing 10 guinea pig units—Tubes of 30.

Administration: **In Obesity and Nephrosis**—1–2 tablets daily, gradually increased to 6.

In Hypothyroidism and Allied Conditions—2–3 tablets three times daily.

Children, in accordance with age.

Bibliography: *See Chap. XII.*

THYROXIN (Squibb)

Hormone Therapy

Chemical Name: Triiodo-oxy-indol Beta-propionic Acid.

Formula: $(C_8H_5ONI_3).C_2H_4COOH$.

Description: The active principle of the thyroid gland; is prepared from thyroids of animals in accordance with the Kendall method; occurs as white or slightly yellowish, needle-like, odorless crystals or powder, soluble in alkaline hydroxides, insoluble in water and organic solvents; contains 63 % iodine.

Action: Stimulates general metabolism, raises pulse rate and blood pressure; increases excretion of nitrogenous products and accelerates most of the bodily functions.

Uses: *Useful* in all thyroidal deficiencies: cretinism, myxedema, colloid goitre, thyrogenous obesity; also in nephrosis.

Supply: THYROXIN—Tablets (C.A.)—Oral—1/160 gr (0.4 mg); 1/320 gr (0.2 mg); 1/80 gr (0.8 mg); 1/32 gr (2.0 mg)—Bottles of 100.

THYROXIN—Crystalline—Intravenous—Tubes of 10 mg, or multiples thereof.

Administration:—Dosage guided by basal metabolic rate; **Myxedema**—0.4 mg daily, *intravenously;* 1 mg daily, 1 hr. before meals, *orally.*

In Other Conditions—Administered in accordance with individual requirements.

Bibliography: *See Chap. XII.*

THYROXINE, SYNTHETIC (Roche)

Hormone Therapy

Formula: $HOC_6H_2I_2.OC_6H_2I_2.CH_2CH(NH_2)COOH$.

Composition: A Tetra-iodo para-hydroxyphenyl Ether of Tyrosine, containing not less than 65 % of iodine.

Description: Is identical with natural thyroxine of which it is the dl-form; 1 mg Synthetic Thyroxine is therapeutically equivalent to 3 gr (0.194 Gm) of desiccated thyroid.

Action: *Used* essentially for the same purposes as thyroid, U.S.P., but the dosage may be more accurately determined and controlled and results more quickly obtained.

Uses: Indicated in all forms of hypothyroidism, low basal metabolism, obesity.

Supply: THYROXINE SYNTHETIC—Crystals (C.A.)—Vials of 100 mg or more.

THYROXINE SYNTHETIC—Tablets (C.A.) Oral 1 mg each—Boxes of 30.

THYROXINE SYNTHETIC—Ampules (C.A.), 1.1 cc (1:1,000 solution)—Boxes of 6 and 12.

THYROXINE SYNTHETIC—Liquid (C.A.) (2 mg per cubic centimeter)—Vials of 15 cc.

Administration: 2–4 tablets or 1–2 ampules per day, depending on basal metabolic rate.

TIODINE "COGNET" (Fougera)

Cicatrix Resolvent

Chemical Name: Thiosinamin Ethyliodide.

Formula: $C_6SN_2H_{13}I$.

Description: An organic, iodine sulphur combination.

Action: A powerful vaso-dilator and hypotensor and marked antisclerous agent, promoting absorption of fibrous and scar tissue.

Uses: *For use* in conditions associated with fibrosis—rheumatism, arthritis, tertiary syphilis, leukoplasia, medullary sclerosis; in emphysema, atheroma, arteriosclerosis; in skin disorders, scars, hepatic cirrhosis, otosclerosis.

Supply: TIODINE "COGNET"—Ampules 1 cc, containing gr 0.20 Tiodine—Boxes of 12.

TIODINE "COGNET"—Pills, Gluten coated, each gr 0.05 Tiodine—Boxes of 50.

Administration: 1 ampule *intramuscularly* every other day; 2–5 pills daily, children 1–3 daily.

TISSUE EXTRACT 568 (Sharp and Dohme)

Vasodilator

Description: An extract prepared from pancreas, freed from insulin and of standardized activity; each cubic centimeter contains 10 units and neutralizes the pressor effect of 0.01 mg of epinephrine.

Action and Uses: A vasodilator and epinephrine antagonist; is stated to depress the sensitivity of the sympathetic nervous system, to counteract pain reflexes and other symptoms of the anginal syndrome. *For use* in angina pectoris and similar angiospastic conditions, for its sympathetic relief.

Supply: TISSUE EXTRACT 568—Vials 10 cc, 10 units per cubic centimeter.

Administration: *Hypodermic*—2–5 cc, every 2 or 3 days and gradually reduced during 5–10 weeks course.

Caution: Care is to be exercised in its use during pregnancy and anaphylactic states, as hay fever, asthma.

Bibliography: *See Chap. XII.*

TOLAMINE (Burroughs Wellcome)

Germicide

Chemical Name: Sodium-para-Toluenesulphonchloroamide; referred to as Chloramine-T.

Description: A white stable crystalline substance, soluble in cold and very soluble in hot water; contains 12% active Chlorine.

Action: A powerful germicide; acts by liberation of free chlorine similar to Dakin solution; is more active, less irritating, more continuous in action in the presence of pus and serum than sodium hypochlorite.

Uses: *For irrigation* of wounds, abscesses, pleural cavity; as wet dressings, mouth wash and irrigant.

Supply: "SOLOID" TOLAMINE—Gr 4.6 (0.299 Gm)—Bottles of 100 and 500.

Administration: One soloid in 1 oz. of water makes 1% solution.

Moist Dressings—2%, for bedsores, ulcers, chancroid, burns.

Mouth Wash—1%, in pyorrhea, stomatitis, abrasions, ulcers, jaw injuries.

Nose and Throat—0.2%, as spray in catarrh, ozena, tonsillitis, pharyngitis, Vincent's angina.

Eye Wash—0.1%, pre- and postoperatively, granular lids, purulent ophthalmia.

Irrigations—0.5%, of urethra, bladder and uterus.

TOLYSIN (Calco)

Analgesic. Antipyretic

Chemical Name: The Ethyl Ester of Paramethylcinchophen.

Description: A neutral compound, neither acid nor alkaline; a fine white powder, tasteless and odorless; is insoluble in water but is rapidly disintegrated in the secretions of the mouth or stomach; is absorbed directly from the intestines.

Action: Analgesic, antipyretic and antirheumatic; unlike salicylates does not produce renal irritation and is comparatively non-toxic.

Uses: In arthritis, acute and chronic; in osteo-arthritis, rheumatic fever, neuritis, neuralgia and myositis; also in colds, tonsillitis and facial pain.

Supply: TOLYSIN—Tablets, gr 5 (0.324 Gm)—Packages of 20, 48, 200 and 1,000.
TOLYSIN—Powder, in multiples of 1 oz.

Administration: 1 or 2 tablets every 3 hr., children according to age; frequent rest periods are given during prolonged therapy.

Contraindications: Thyrotoxicosis; active infection of the biliary tract; severe gastroenteritis in infants, idiosyncrasy, extensive surgical operations.

Bibliography: *See Chap. XII.*

TRICHLORETHYLENE

Antineuralgic

Chemical Name: Trichloro-ethylene; Chlorylene; Gemalgine.

Formula: $CHClCCl_2$.

Description: A colorless, volatile fluid, of faintly sweetish odor.

Action and Uses: Is unstable when exposed to air; in therapeutic dosage is practically non-toxic; is apparently a specific in trigeminal neuralgia, giving constant relief.

Supply: TRICHLORETHYLENE (C.A.)—Tubes 1 cc—Packages of 21. (Calco)
TRICHLORETHYLENE—Bottles of 500 Gm. (Eastman)

Administration: Qy *Inhalation*—Crushing 1 cc tube or using 20–25 drops of liquid and inhaling vapor directly from gauze or handerchief, 6–7 breaths, several times a day for 4–6 weeks.

Caution: Must be kept away from open flame or red hot metal; may cause tingling of nasal mucosa, watering of the eyes and other unpleasant symptoms.

Bibliography: *See Chap. XII.*

TRICHOPHYTIN EXTRACT (Metz)

Parasiticide

Composition: A polyvalent extract obtained from various species of trichophyton, comprising T. gypseum (40 %), T. cerebriforme (20 %), T. microides (20 %), and T. rosaceum, T. violaceum and T. crateriforme in equal parts constituting 20 %.

Action and Uses: For diagnosis and therapeusis of trichophyton infections.

Supply: TRICHOPHYTIN EXTRACT—Vials of 1 cc.

Administration: *Diagnostic*—0.1 cc of 1:50 dilution is injected *intradermally*, in the arm; if a wheal is not produced, injection of 0.1 cc of a 1:10 is made in the other arm. Observations are made after 24 hr.: where negative—either no reaction occurs at the site of injection or only a small area of redness appears, without

definite infiltration; if positive—a well defined slightly raised area of redness or a flattened papule ¾–1¼ in. in diameter with slightly depressed center will appear. *Therapeutic:* 1. *Intradermal Method*—0.1 cc, dilution 1:50 is injected in the arm or pectoral region at the first sitting; subsequent treatments of 3 injections at 3 different sites are given at 4 day intervals, using solutions of increasing concentrations, 1:30, 1:10, 1:5 and even higher, 1:2 and 1:1, depending upon the local and systemic reactions.
2. *Subcutaneous Method*—Injections of 0.05 cc, diluted to 1 cc with sterile saline solution; increased at each treatment by 0.1 cc with the same amount of saline until 0.5 cc is reached; injections are given every 4–5 days.

TRILLIN (C. D. Smith)

Hemostatic

Composition: A resinoid extract from the root of Trillium pendulum, 1/10 gr being equivalent to 1 gr powdered Trillium root.

Action and Uses: To control hemorrhage in epistaxis and excessive menstruation; in pre- and postpartum bleeding, in intestinal, pulmonary and dental hemorrhages.

Supply: TRILLIN—Tablets, gr 1/10 (0.006 Gm) and gr ¼ (0.016 Gm)—Bottles of 1,000, 5,000.

Administration: 2–5 tablets, every 3 hr. if required.

TRIONAL (Winthrop)

Hypnotic. Sedative

Chemical Name: Diethylsulfonmethylethylmethane. Brand of Sulphonethylmethane.

Formula: $CH_3.\ C_2H_5:\ C:\ (SO_2)_2.\ (C_2H_5)_2.$

Description: A white, crystalline, odorless powder of bitter taste and neutral reaction; soluble in 300 parts of water of room temperature, more readily in warm water and easily soluble in alcohol and ether.

Action and Uses: Hypnotic, producing restful sleep without depressing the heart or circulation; is not indicated in insomnia with severe pain; is non-narcotic. *Used* in simple insomnia and insomnia of mental disease.

Supply: TRIONAL—Tablets (C.A.), 5 gr (0.324 Gm)—Bottles of 25 and 100.
TRIONAL—Powder (C.A.)—Cartons of 1 oz.

Administration: 10–15 gr (0.6–1.0 Gm), increased if necessary, taken about ½ hr. before retiring, with cupful of warm fluid.

Caution: During prolonged use of Trional, alkalies should be freely administered and constipation prevented by saline laxatives.

TRIPHAL (Metz)

Gold Therapy

Chemical Name: Sodium Aurothiobenzimidazolcarboxylicate. Brand of Aurothiol.

Formula: $C_6H_3N.\ NH.\ CS.\ Au.\ CO_2Na + 2H_2O.$

Description: A light yellow powder, freely soluble in cold water forming slight alkaline reaction; contains approximately 44% gold; solution is stable but readily decomposed by heat.

Action: Affects lesions promptly, affording permanent clinical and good cosmetic results; is of low toxicity.

Uses: In lupus erythematosus.

Supply: TRIPHAL—Ampules (C.A.), 0.025 and 0.1 Gm—Boxes of 1.

Administration: *Intravenously* slowly, twice weekly. Solutions must be freshly prepared; the powder is dusted on 3–5 cc of cool, sterile, distilled water and dissolved without stirring.

Caution: After 12 administrations, 3–6 intravenous injections of Sulfactol should be made; foci of infection in teeth, tonsils and sinuses, should first be eliminated; strong sunlight or actinotherapy should be avoided; if albuminuria or erythema occur treatment must be discontinued.

Contraindications: Pregnancy, renal disease and progressive tuberculosis.

Bibliography: *See Chap. XII.*

TRYPARSAMIDE (Merck)

Antiluetic

Chemical Name: Sodium salt of N-phenylglycineamide-para-arsonic acid.

Formula: $(NH_2COCH_2NH).\ C_6H_4(AsO.\ OH.\ ONa)$.

Description: A white, odorless, crystalline stable powder; freely soluble in water, almost insoluble in alcohol, chloroform, ether, benzene.

Action: Mildly spirocheticidal but highly penetrative to nerve tissue.

Uses: In early paresis and neurosyphilis, particularly in those not responsive to other type of therapy; also in trypanosomiasis (African sleeping sickness).

Supply: TRYPARSAMIDE—Ampules (C.A.) of 1, 2 and 3 Gm.

Administration: Given *intravenously, intramuscularly, subcutaneously;* never orally.
Dosage—Not to exceed 0.04–0.05 Gm per kilo of body weight; administered once weekly, in courses of 8–16 doses.

Bibliography: *See Chap. XII.*

TRYPSIN

Protein Digestant

Description: A light yellow powder, of faint odor and meaty taste; is the proteolytic enzyme of the pancreas, freed as much as possible from other enzymes and gland constituents; is standardized by the Fuld-Gross Method, to digest at least 100 times its weight of casein; has 4–5 times the tryptic power of Pancreatin, U.S.P.

Action and Use: *Used* to assist the digestion of various proteins into soluble, assimilable forms; in duodenal dyspeptic conditions and protein putrefaction; externally—is used as solvent of diphtheritic membranes, in purulent tuberculosis and cancer.

Supply: TRYPSIN (C.A.)—Powder—Bottles of 2 dr. **(Armour)**
TRYPSIN (C.A.)—Bottles ¼ oz. **(Fairchild)**

Administration: *Internally*—8–25 gr (0.5–1.6 Gm) at or after meals, in keratin coated capsules or pills.
Externally—10% solution in 1:1,000 salicylic acid, digested for 4 hr. and made alkaline; or about 6 gr (0.384 Gm) is mixed with 2 Gm of sodium bicarbonate in mortar, triturated and 1 dr. distilled water added, the mixture then warmed

to body temperature and applied to affected area; freshly prepared solutions for every application.

In Purulent Tuberculosis—1–2 cc of 1% solution injected locally into infected tissue.

TUTOCAINE (Winthrop)

Local Anesthetic

Chemical Name: Para-amino-benzoyldimethylaminomethyl-butanol Hydrochloride. Brand of Butamin.

Formula: $(CH_3)_2N.\ CH_2CH(CH_3)CH(CH_3)(O.\ CO.\ C_6H_4NH_2)HCl$.

Description: A whitish, crystalline powder, practically odorless, of faintly bitter taste, and stable in the air; easily soluble in water, forming a neutral solution; soluble in alcohol with difficulty.

Action: A surface anesthetic producing complete and prolonged anesthesia in relatively low concentration.

Uses: In general surgery, gynecology, ophthalmology, rhinolaryngology, otology, urology, wherever anesthetic effect is desired.

Incompatibles: Alkalies.

Supply: TUTOCAIN—Tablets (C.A.)

1. Containing Tutocain 0.03 Gm, Suprarenin 0.00015 Gm—Tubes of 20.
2. Containing Tutocain 0.03 Gm, Suprarenin 0.00006 Gm—Tubes of 20.
3. Containing Tutocain 0.03 Gm—Tubes of 20.
4. Containing Tutocain 0.05 Gm, Suprarenin 0.000125 Gm—Tubes of 10.
5. Containing Tutocain 0.1 Gm—Tubes of 10.
6. Containing Tutocain ¾ gr—Bottles 100.

Administration: Solutions should be freshly prepared; physiologic saline is first heated to the boiling point before the tablet of Tutocain with Suprarenin is added.

Surgery and Gynecology—Infiltration ⅕–¼%; conduction—½–1%, spinal ½–1%.

Rhinolaryngology—Surface application 2–5%; infiltration ⅛%; conduction ½–1%.

Ophthalmology—Surface application 2–5% infiltration ⅕–½%.

Urology—Surface application ½–2%.

Otology—Surface application 2–5%.

Bibliography: *See Chap. XII.*

TYRAMINE

Vasoconstrictor

Chemical Name: Para-hydroxyphenylethylamine Hydrochloride.

Formula: $OH.\ C_6H_4CH_2CH_2NH_2HCl$.

Description: White crystals, soluble in water forming a neutral solution.

Action and Uses: An organic base generally prepared from ergot and its extracts; like epinephrine is a member of the sympathomimetic amines but its action is less powerful and more persistent; raises blood pressure by vaso-constriction but has no local vaso-constrictive effect; *used* in shock, collapse, post-partum hemorrhage, morphine poisoning.

Supply: **TYRAMINE PHOSPHATIS ACIDI**—Tabloid Hypodermic, gr 1/3 (0.02 Gm)—Tubes 12, 50 and 500. **(Burroughs Wellcome)**

TYRAMINE (C.A.)—Bottles of 1, 10 and 100 Gm. **(Roche)**

Administration: 1/3–2/3 gr (0.02–0.04 Gm) dissolved and administered *hypodermically.*

UMBRATHOR (Heyden)

X-Ray Contrast Medium

Description: A 25% non-stabilized Thorium Dioxide solution; is a brownish liquid, of milky appearance in reflected light; forms a sediment upon long standing, which may be redissolved upon shaking.

Action and Uses: The preparation flocculates, forming a surface coating on mucous membranes, affording a relief picture of the intestinal, stomach and bladder walls and showing the finest details of the mucosa with outlines of tumors where present; the mucosal relief picture is claimed to be superior to radiographs obtained by the total filling of the gastro-intestinal canal with solid opaque media; is non-irritating and non-toxic.

Supply: **UMBRATHOR**—Bottles of 200 cc.

Technic: Depiction of intestinal mucosa: On the day preceding the examination, a substantially liquid diet is given and purgative administered. On the day of the examination the intestine is cleaned by an enema. Umbrathor diluted with equal parts of distilled water, in syringe with a thin catheter attached, is then rectally injected, in a thin stream under regulated pressure. Approximately 200–400 cc of the contrast medium are needed; this should be well distributed in the intestines by massaging the abdomen, and drained off after 15–20 min. The intestines are then inflated with air, and the radiograph taken as soon as possible.

Depiction of the stomach mucosa—About 20–30 cc of Umbrathor are given perorally, and the contrast medium well distributed by massaging the upper abdomen for about 10 min. before the radiograph is taken.

Depiction of the bladder mucosa—Umbrathor is injected into bladder, held for 2 min., drained, the bladder inflated with air and radiographed.

Bibliography: *See Chap. XII.*

(UNDILUTED) HALIBUT LIVER OIL (Mead Johnson)

Vitamin Therapy

Description: Pure halibut liver oil free from vegetable oil or other diluents. Each gram contains not less than 32,000 vitamin A units (U.S.P.) and 200 vitamin D units (Steenbock); is biologically assayed for vitamin potency.

Action: Fortifies against infections of the mucous membranes; controls calcium and phosphorus utilization.

Uses: In vitamin A deficiencies; xerophthalmia, xerosis, hemeralopia; as aid in maintaining health in vitamin D deficiencies as rickets, tetany, osteomalacia, non-healing fractures; in allergies, and dental caries.

Supply: **HALIBUT LIVER OIL**—Bottles of 10 and 50 cc.

Administration: Infants—10 drops daily.

In instances of great calcium drain, viosterol may be needed in addition. Special cases may require larger dosage.

Bibliography: *See Chap. XII.*

UREA (Merck)

Diuretic

Chemical Name: Carbonic Acid Diamide; Carbamide.

Formula: $CO(NH_2)_2$.

Description: Colorless, prismatic, transparent, almost odorless crystals, of cooling saline taste; soluble in water and alcohol, insoluble in ether and chloroform.

Action and Uses: Diuretic—*For use* in all cases where diuresis is indicated, especially in ascites.

Supply: **UREA** (C.A.)—Bottles 1 oz., ¼ and 1 lb.

Administration: 10–20 gr (0.6–1.3 Gm); three or four times daily.

Incompatibles: Chloral hydrate; lead acetate.

UROTROPIN (Schering and Glatz)

Urinary Antiseptic

Composition: Prepared by synthesis of Formaldehyde and Ammonia; a brand of Methenamine.

Formula: $(CH_2)_6N_4$.

Description: A white crystalline powder, freely soluble in water, less soluble in alcohol and chloroform, insoluble in ether.

Action: A diuretic and genitourinary antiseptic; liberates formaldehyde which is an active bactericide and antiseptic; is also uricolytic and stimulates detrusor contraction with simultaneous inhibition of vesical sphincter resulting in bladder evacuation; is also effective in systemic infections, intravenously introduced.

Uses: Gall bladder disease, cystitis, pyelitis, urethritis, pyuria, pyelonephritis, post-operative urinary retention; in coryza, colds, bronchitis, tonsillitis, sinusitis, otitis; in meningitis, poliomyelitis, encephalitis, cholangitis, jaundice, eye infections.

Supply: **UROTROPIN**—Tablets, gr 5, (0.324 Gm)—Boxes of 30—Bottles of 50, 100, 500 and 1,000.

UROTROPIN—Tablets, gr 7½ (0.480 Gm)—Boxes of 20—Bottles of 50, 100, 500 and 1,000.

UROTROPIN—Crystals—Bottles 1 oz., ¼, ½ and 1 lb.

UROTROPIN—Ampules 5 cc (gr 31)—Boxes of 6.

Administration: *Intravenously*—In general infections, 5 cc of 40% solution.
Intramuscularly or Subcutaneously—Same dosage.
Orally—Gr 7½ (0.480 Gm) two to four times daily.

VENTRICULIN (Parke, Davis)

Hematopoietic

Description: A desiccated preparation of stomach tissue; palatable, stable, non-hygroscopic, non-nauseating.

Action and Uses: Stimulates reticulocytosis; produces rapid improvement in the blood picture and the general condition of the patient; *is especially indicated* in pernicious anemia.

Supply: VENTRICULIN—Vials 10 Gm (C.A.), each vial equivalent to 120 Gm fresh stomach tissue—Packages of 12 and 25.

VENTRICULIN—Bottles 100 Gm (C.A.) with 10 Gm measuring cap.

Administration: 1 vial daily for each million of red blood cell deficiency below 5,000,000; thus if the red cell count is

	Vials Daily
Less than 2,000,000	4
2,000,000	3
3,000,000	2
4,000,000	1

Is given suspended in fruit juice, tomato juice, or is mixed with cereal or other food.

Bibliography: *See Chap. XII.*

VERODIGEN (Merck)

Cardiac Tonic

Description: An aqueous extract of digitalis leaves known as Gitolin, free from digitalein, digitoxin and inert matter; is an amorphous powder, soluble in 600 parts of water; standardized 1/80 gr (0.0008 Gm) to represent 1½ gr (0.097 Gm) of prime digitalis leaf.

Action and Uses: Heart tonic and diuretic; *For use* in all cases where digitalis is indicated; is promptly absorbed, well tolerated and less cumulative than digitalis.

Supply: VERODIGEN—Tablets, gr 1/80 (0.0008 Gm)—Tubes of 12.

Administration: 1 tablet three times daily, reduced to twice daily or ½ tablet three times daily.

VERONAL

Hypnotic

Official Name: Diethylbarbituric Acid U.S.P.X. Brand of Barbital.

Formula: $(C_2H_5)_2$: C: $(CONH)_2$: CO.

Description: A white, crystalline, sublimable powder, of faintly bitter taste and no odor; soluble in about 130 parts of water, more soluble in boiling water.

Action and Uses: In average dosage is a relatively safe and reliable sedative and hypnotic, inducing calm, refreshing sleep in from ½–1 hr.; is well borne, non-irritating and more prompt than trional and sulfonal. *Useful* in simple agrypnia; in insomnia accompanying hysteria, neurasthenia, hypochondria, alcoholism, melancholia, psychoses and other nervous conditions; also as sedative and soporific in seasickness, vomiting of pregnancy, epilepsy, chorea, morphinism, cocainism, delirium tremens; to lessen tremors in multiple sclerosis, paralysis agitans, hemiplegia; also as preliminary to chloroform anesthesia.

Contraindications: Renal disease, extensive myocarditis, aortic regurgitation; insomnia due to pain.

Supply: VERONAL—Powder—Cartons of 1 oz., ¼ lb., 1 lb. (Merck)

VERONAL—Tablets, gr 5 (0.324 Gm)—Tubes of 10—Bottles of 100, 1,000. (Merck)

VERONAL (C.A.)—Powder—Cartons of 1 oz. (Winthrop)

VERONAL (C.A.)—Tablets gr 5 (0.324 Gm)—Tubes of 10 and 20. (Winthrop)

Administration: *Dosage*—5–15 gr (0.3–1 Gm), best dissolved in hot tea or water; average dose 8 gr (0.5 Gm); in whooping cough ½ gr (0.03 Gm) for young and 1–1½ gr (0.06–0.1 Gm) for older children, three to four times daily; in digestive disturbances and tetanus in children ⅔–1⅙ gr (0.04–0.07 Gm) one to two times daily; preoperatively 15 gr (1 Gm), 1½–2 hr. before anesthesia administration.

Incompatibilities: Calomel, if given at nearly the same time.

Antidote: Stimulation of vasomotor center; camphor, gastric lavage with tannin solution, oxygen, stimulants.

Combination: ELIXIR OF VERONAL (C.A.)—A very agreeable, (Winthrop) stable solution containing gr 2 (0.13 Gm) of veronal to the teaspoonful—Bottles of 12 oz.

Bibliography: *See Chap. XII.*

VERONAL-SODIUM

Hypnotic

Official Name: Monosodium Diethylbarbiturate.

Formula: $(C_2H_5)_2$: C: (CONNa. CONH): CO.

Description: The sodium salt of diethylbarbituric acid; a white, crystalline, powder of somewhat bitter taste; is readily soluble in water (1:5).

Action and Uses: As for Veronal, but being of far greater solubility is especially adapted for hypodermic and rectal uses, as solution and suppository; very effective in seasickness, epilepsy, delirium tremens and convulsive states.

Supply: VERONAL-SODIUM—Powder—Tins of 1 oz., ¼ lb., 1 lb. (Merck)

VERONAL-SODIUM—Tablets gr 5 (0.324 Gm)—Tubes of 10— (Merck) Bottles of 100, 1,000.

VERONAL-SODIUM (C.A.)—Tablets gr 5 (0.324 Gm)—Tubes of (Winthrop) 10—Bottles of 100.

Administration: *Orally*—5–8 gr (0.324–0.512 Gm); *rectally* and *subcutaneously*—8 gr (0.512 Gm) dissolved in 5 cc water.

VIOFORM (Ciba)

Antiseptic. Deodorant

Chemical Name: Iodochloroxyquinoline; a compound where an atom of iodine is introduced into anachlor-ortho-hydroxyquinoline.

Formula: $C_9H_4NOHICl$.

Description: A yellowish gray tasteless powder, of faintly aromatic odor; is insoluble in water, freely soluble in alcohol and hot glacial acetic acid.

Action: Is a non-irritating antiseptic more powerful than iodoform; checks capillary hemorrhage and hastens coagulation; causes no systemic poisoning; dries up wound secretions serving as culture media for pathogenic microorganisms and inhibits bacterial growth; also possesses amebacidal properties.

Uses: *For use* as dusting powder in all conditions where an odorless substitute for iodoform is desirable; in ulcers, septic suppurating wounds, burns, exudative eruptions; orally, in the treatment of amebiasis.

Supply: VIOFORM—Powder (C.A.)—Sprinkler-top cans.

VIOFORM—Powder (C.A.)—Bottles ½ oz. and 1 lb.

Administration: *Locally*—By dusting or sprinkling on lesions.

Internally—8 gr three times daily for 10 days, in amebiasis.

Bibliography: *See Chap. XII.*

VIOSTEROL IN OIL—250 D

Irradiated Ergosterol

Description: A bland neutral vegetable oil containing irradiated Ergosterol, obtained from yeast and other vegetable organisms and plants; is physiologically standardized and of high vitamin D potency, 3,333 units per gram solution or 250 times that of standard cod liver oil; is odorless and tasteless and does not turn rancid.

Action and Uses: That of the antirachitic principle of cod liver oil, but is not a substitute for it since it contains no vitamin A; is easily administered, well tolerated and causes no digestive disturbances; is almost specific in spasmophilia of infants, rachitic tetany and rickets.

Supply: **VIOSTEROL IN OIL—250 D** (C.A.)—Bottles of 5 cc and 50 cc. **(Abbott)**

VIOSTEROL IN OIL—250 D (C.A.)—Bottles of 5 cc and 50 cc anaerobically sealed, with measuring dropper delivering 75 units per drop. **(Squibb)**

VIOSTEROL IN OIL (C.A.)—Bottles of 5 cc and 50 cc, with standard droppers. **(Winthrop)**

Administration: *Prophylactic in Rickets*—8–10 drops daily (600–750 units); 1 drop is equivalent to teaspoonful of Cod Liver Oil.

Curative—Mild rickets and prematures, rapidly growing infants—5 drops, three times daily. Mild and moderate rickets, 15–20 drops daily; severe cases—20 drops and over.

Pregnancy and Lactation—20 drops daily.

Is administered in milk, orange juice and with bottle feedings.

Bibliography: *See Chap. XII.*

VIVARGIN (Kahlenberg)

Germicide

Description: A 1:500 solution of colloidal organic compound containing about 25% Mercury.

Action and Uses: A powerful non-toxic germicide; harmless even if taken internally; *For use* chiefly as a local disinfectant.

Supply: **VIVARGIN**—Bottles of 4 oz.

Administration: *Externally*—in full strength for applications or wet dressings.

Internally—1 teaspoonful to a tablespoonful three times daily.

XEROFORM (Schering and Glatz)

Antiseptic

Chemical Name: Bismuth Tribromphenate.

Formula: $(C_6H_2Br_3O_2)BiOH + Bi_2O_3$.

Description: An amorphous, yellow, tasteless powder, of neutral reaction; is slightly soluble in water, alcohol, chloroform, oils.

Action and Uses: A non-irritating, non-toxic, odorless antiseptic *for use* in weeping eczema, ulcus cruris, gastro-intestinal catarrh, proctitis, dysentery, choleraic diarrheas.

Supply: **XEROFORM**—Powder (C.A.)—Bottles 1 oz., 1 lb.

Administration: Gr 15–45 daily; children 2–5 gr.

Locally—As dusting powder.

YATREN-CASEIN (Winthrop)

Foreign Protein Therapy

Composition: A combination of Yatren with highly purified Casein.

Action: As for non-specific foreign proteins.

Supply: YATREN-CASEIN SOLUTION—Ampules, Strong, 1 cc containing Yatren 0.03 Gm and Casein 0.05 Gm per cubic centimeter—Boxes of 6—Bottles of 25 cc.

YATREN-CASEIN SOLUTION—Ampules, Weak, 1 cc containing Yatren 0.03 Gm and Casein 0.025 Gm per cubic centimeter—Boxes of 6—Bottles 25 cc.

Administration and Uses: Rheumatism—*Intramuscularly*—initial dose 1 cc of Weak solution; increased to 3 cc in regulated dosage, according to type and chronicity of disease; injections given every 2–5 days.

Pulmonary Diseases—1 cc Weak solution, *intravenously;* repeated or increased to 2 cc.

Gynecology—In acute febrile puerperal infections—5 cc. Strong solution. *intramuscularly;* decreased to 3, 2 and 1 cc, at intervals of 2 or 3 days.

In Chronic Affections—1–2 cc Weak solution, *intramuscularly* every 2 days.

Furunculosis and Pustular Eruptions—*Intravenously* 0.5–2 cc Weak solution, up to 2 cc of Strong solution, every 3–5 days.

Eye Affections—Acute—small doses of Strong solution, *intravenously*, repeated several times daily at the start; chronic cases, 0.5–2 cc *intravenously*, gradually increasing to 3 cc at intervals of 2 or 3 days.

Advantages: Free from untoward effects, severe shock or marked rise of temperature.

Bibliography: *See Chap. XII.*

YEAST "FLEISCHMANN'S" (Standard Brands)

Description: A strain of Saccharomyces Cerevisiae, of high enzymatic and vitamin content.

Analysis:

	Dry Substance	Moist
Protein	52.41	14.15
Fat	1.72	0.46
Glycogen	30.25	8.16
Cellulose gum	6.88	1.87
Ash	8.74	2.36
Moisture	.....	73.00

Ash Analysis:

		Percentage
Phosphorus pentoxide	P_2O_5	54.5
Potassium oxide	K_2O	36.5
Magnesium oxide	MgO	5.2
Calcium oxide	CaO	1.4
Silica	S_1O_2	1.2
Sodium oxide	Na_2O	0.7
Sulphur trioxide	SO_3	0.5
Chlorine	Cl	trace
Iron	Fe	trace
Caloric value per lb	625	

Action and Uses: A vitamin A, B, D and G factor; increases bulk and softens intestinal contents stimulating peristalsis. *Used* as adjunct to other therapy in boils, acne, pellagra, constipation, digestive disorders, intestinal intoxication; in vitamin deficiency diseases.

Supply: YEAST "FLEISCHMAN'S" (L.A.)—Boxes of 6 cakes.

Administration: 2–3 cakes daily before meals.

YEASTONE (Merck)

Vitamin Therapy

Description: An extract containing the purified active principles and vitamins of yeast.

Action: Invigorative, growth-promoting, laxative; does not cause fermentation in deficiency diseases.

Uses: In auto-intoxication, furunculosis, boils, acne, carbuncles; in malnutrition, digestive disturbances and for correction of habitual constipation.

Supply: YEASTONE—Pills, Chocolate coated, gr 1½ (0.097 Gm) equivalent to an ordinary yeast cake—Bottles of 100.

Administration: 1–3 pills three times daily.

YOHIMBIN (Cavendish)

Aphrodisiac

Description: An active alkaloid obtained from the bark of Yohimbeh; the hydrochloride ($C_{23}H_{32}H_2O_4HCl$) salts are colorless crystals soluble with difficulty in water.

Action and Uses: Stimulates erection center in the lumbar cord, dilates penile and lower abdominal vessels. *For use* in impotence, deficient libido sexualis, menstrual irregularities; in eye, ear and nose practice—as local anesthetic.

Supply: YOHIMBIN—Tablets, gr 1/12 (0.005 Gm)—Bottles of 10, 40 and 100.

YOHIMBIN—Ampules, 1% solution m 15 (1 cc)—Boxes of 12.

YOHIMBIN—Elixir—Bottles of 8 and 16 oz.

Administration: 1 tablet or teaspoonful of elixir three times daily after meals; ampules—*hypodermatically*.

ZINCOL (Mulford Colloid)

Astringent

Description: A Colloidal Zinc preparation containing 20–25% Zinc.

Action and Uses: In conjunctivitis and other ophthalmic infections; in insect bites and stings.

Supply: Zincol—Vials 10 Gm.

Zincol—Ointment 10%—Tubes ½ oz.—Packages of 12.

Administration: 1–5 gr (0.064–0.324 Gm).

Locally—By instillation into conjunctival sac.

ZINC PERBORATE (Roessler and Hasslacher)

Antiseptic

Formula: $Zn(BO_3)_2$.

Description: A fine white odorless flocculent powder consisting of zinc perborate and zinc hydroxide; is insoluble in water, but decomposes liberating oxygen, boric and zinc oxides; has available active oxygen 7%.

Action and Uses: A soothing antiseptic in minor surgical affections.

Supply: ZINC PERBORATE—Cases 100 lb.

Administration: Applied *locally*, as dusting powder or ointment.

ZINC PERMANGANATE

Astringent

Official Name: Zinci Permanganas.

Formula: $Zn(MnO_4)_2 + 6H_2O$.

Description: Dark brown, lustrous deliquescent crystals, soluble in water (1:3); contains not less than 90% zinc permanganate.

Action and Uses: Oxidizer, astringent, antiseptic; a non-irritating antigonorrheic; *For use* in urethritis, vaginitis, cystitis.

Supply: ZINC PERMANGANATE (C.A.)—Bottles 1 oz., ¼ lb. and 1 lb. **(Merck)**
ZINC PERMANGANATE (C.A.)—Tablets gr 1. **(Sharp and Dohme)**
ZINC PERMANGANATE—Bottles 1 oz. **(Sharp and Dohme)**

Administration: 1:4,000 as injection in gonorrhea; 1:2,000 as eye wash in conjunctivitis.

Incompatible: All easily oxidizable or combustible substances (sugar, glycerin, alcohol, etc.).

ZINC PEROXIDE (Roessler and Hasslacher)

Antiseptic

Formula: ZnO_2.

Composition: Contains Zinc Peroxide 45%, available active Oxygen 7.4%.

Description: A fine yellow-white powder, consisting of zinc peroxide and zinc hydroxide; is insoluble in water, soluble in acid medium; is decomposed by body secretions.

Action and Uses: Non-irritating, odorless germicide, antiseptic and bactericide; *For use* in leg ulcers, burns, wounds, eczema, plant dermatitis, as skin protective.

Supply: ZINC PEROXIDE—In bulk.

Administration: Applied locally as ointment, 2–25% in paraffin or dusting powder, pure or with starch or tartaric acid.

CHAPTER II

EFFECTIVE COMBINATIONS

This chapter presents 492 preparations in 610 forms. Each product contains two or more fully defined ingredients combined for efficient action. The arrangement is alphabetical. Dosages are average and stated in both the metric and U.S. systems, approximately converted.

A. B. D. MALT EXTRACT WITH COD LIVER OIL AND VIOSTEROL 5 D (Abbott)

Nutrient. Vitamin Therapy

Composition: Pure barley Malt Extract, mixed with 30% by volume of standardized Cod Liver Oil and sufficient Viosterol to represent an antirachitic potency of 5 D; contains vitamins A, B, B_2 and D.

Action: Stimulates appetite, assists in bone and tissue building, in nutrition and growth; raises bodily resistance to disease.

Uses: In vitamin deficiencies and malnutrition; as food supplement to mother's milk, when deficient in vitamins A, B and D.

Supply: A. B. D. MALT EXTRACT (C.A.)—Bottles 16 oz.

Administration: Infants—½ teaspoonful three times daily; premature and rapidly growing infants—1 teaspoonful several times daily. Adults—1 teaspoonful four times daily.

ACCESSORONE (Upjohn)

Hematinic. Vitamin Therapy

Composition: Contains per ounce:

Vitamin A concentrate (of liver)	m 24 (1.478 cc)
Glycerinated red bone marrow extract	m 10 (0.616 cc)
Iron and ammonium citrate	gr 4 (0.259 Gm)
Malt extract (non-diastasic) and Citrus concentrate	q.s. 1 oz.

Presents per ounce not less than 15,000 units of vitamin A; contains also vitamins B, C and G.

Action and Uses: Is appetite stimulating and reconstructive in convalescence, debility, anemia, malnutrition and similar affections.

Supply: ACCESSORONE—Bottles 10 oz.

Administration: 1–4 teaspoonfuls three to four times daily before meals.

ACECOLEX (Anglo-French)

Antiseptic

Composition:

Acecoline (acetylcholine hydrochloride)	2%
Fenchone (a terpenic ketone of camphor group)	10%
Ichthyol	1.25%

Oxide of titanium	2%
Butyl para-amino-benzoate	1%
Zinc oxide	15%
Excipient	q.s. ad 100 Gm

Action and Uses: An antiseptic and stimulant for the healing and cicatrization of indolent ulcerations and skin wounds of trophic origin.

Supply: ACECOLEX—Tubes of 1 oz.

Administration: Applied thickly and bandaged without washing or irritating the wound; dressed daily.

ACETIDINE (Sharp and Dohme)

Analgesic

Composition: Each tablet represents:

	Gm	Gr
Acetphenetidin	0.1176	$1\frac{8}{10}$
Acetyl salicylic acid	0.1764	$1\frac{8}{10}$
Caffeine	0.0294	$\frac{45}{100}$

Action and Uses: *For relief* of pain, headache, neuralgia, myalgia and as antipyretic in all febrile conditions.

Supply: ACETIDINE—Capsules gr 5—Packages of 100 and 1,000.

ACETIDINE—Tablets gr 5—In tin box of 12—Packages of 100 and 1,000.

Administration: 1 or 2 tablets, repeated in 2 hr. if necessary.

ACIDONE TABLETS (Battle Creek)

Digestant

Description: A preparation of Hydrochloric Acid in loose combination with Protein.

Action: Liberates hydrochloric acid in stomach slowly and without irritation, and like natural gastric acid activates pepsin and pancreatic secretion, regulates the opening and closing of the pylorus, creates hunger by exciting gastric contractions, disinfects contents of stomach and duodenum.

Uses: *Useful* in achylia gastrica, pernicious anemia, gastrogenic diarrhea, jaundice, cholecystitis and cholelithiasis; postoperatively in gastric operation, in cancer of stomach, typhoid fever, biliousness.

Advantages: Does not injure teeth, is convenient and safe of administration.

Supply: ACIDONE—Tablets, representing 4 drops dilut ehydrochloric acid—Bottles 100.

Administration: Tablets 2–4, half hour before meals, for anorexia.

Tablets 5–10 after meals and 1 hr. later, for digestive purposes.

ACIDO-SODIUM (Westerfield)

Mineralizer

Composition: Contains Sodium Carbonate and Sodium Chloride, in percentage in accordance with Fischer formula, each tablet when dissolved representing 50 cc of Fischer solution.

Uses: As remineralizer in colds, acidosis, nephritis, eclampsia, cardiac decompensation, diarrhea.

Supply: ACIDO-SODIUM—Tablets—Bottles of 100, 500 and 1,000.

Administration: 2 tablets four times daily.

ACTIVIN (Bischoff)

Non-specific Protein Therapy

Description: A purified Casein combined with organic Iodine.

Action: Stimulates increased tissue cell activity in defense against noxious organisms; causes active focal reaction of short duration with but little local irritation.

Uses: In the treatment of numerous infections: arthritis, epididymitis, prostatitis, adnexitis, puerperal pyelitis and sepsis; in purulent sinusitis, iritis, iridocystitis, corneal and indolent ulcers; in gastric and duodenal ulcers and carbuncle.

Supply: ACTIVIN—Ampules 1 cc—Boxes of 6 and 12.
ACTIVIN—Liquid—Bottles of 10 and 25.

Administration: *Intramuscular* injections—beginning with ½ cc, gradually increased in accordance with reaction; in acute conditions—larger doses, generally given daily; in chronic—smaller doses, twice weekly.

Contraindications: Arteriosclerosis, alcoholism, pregnancy, diabetes and myocardial disease.

Bibliography: *See Chap. XII.*

AGO-CHOLAN (Bilhuber-Knoll)

Cholagogue

Chemical Name: Strontium Cholate-salicylate.

Description: Contains, in stable form, the strontium salts of cholic and salicylic acids, 2 gr (0.13 Gm) and phenolphthalein diacetate ⅕ gr (0.012 Gm), per tablet.

Action: A cholagogue, laxative, antiseptic and analgesic; stimulates liver cells to increased bile formation and promotes drainage of biliary tract, thus preventing precipitation of cholesterin and calculus formation; is a physiological aperient by stimulating intestinal peristalsis.

Uses: In cholecystitis, hepatic congestion and insufficiency, cholangitis, habitual constipation.

Advantages: Is well tolerated, quickly effective and but little irritating.

Supply: AGO-CHOLAN—Tablets, sugar coated, gr 2 (0.13 Gm)—Tubes of 20—Bottles 50 and 300.

Administration: 1-3 tablets two or three times daily after meals; reduced where necessary.

Bibliography: *See Chap. XII.*

A.L.A. (Sutliff and Case)

Local Anesthetic

Description: An oily liquid of ethereal odor; not miscible with water or alcohol.

Composition: Contains per fluid ounce:

	Per Cent
Para-aminobenzoic Acid Ethylester	3.0
Phenmethylol	5.0
Ether	10.00
Olive Oil	82.00

Action: Local analgesic and anesthetic effective through nerve endings; causes transient induration, tingling and anesthesia 10 min. after application; non-toxic and non-irritating.

Uses: Surgical—As anesthesic in minor surgery—boils, carbuncles, fistulae, fractures.

Dentistry—For extractions and other painful operations.

Proctology—In hemorrhoids, fissures and various other lesions.

Medical—In neuritis, sciatica and similar conditions.

Supply: A.L.A.—Bottles of 30 cc, 500 cc.

A.L.A.—Ampules, 2 cc—Packages of 6.

Administration: *Intramuscular or subcutaneous injection,* of 0.1–0.5 cc at each of 5–7 points within a 3 in. circle surrounding the painful area, for a total of 1 cc.

Caution: Not to be injected into larger veins.

ALBOMALT (McKesson and Robbins)

Intestinal Lubricant. Nutrient

Description: An emulsion containing:
Malt extract 50% (Vitamin B).
Heavy mineral oil, free from paraffin, 50%.

Action and Uses: Intestinal lubricant in chronic constipation; a nutrient for pregnant women, nursing mothers, undernourished children and the aged.

Supply: ALBOMALT—Bottles of 16 oz.

Administration: 1 level tablespoonful night and morning before breakfast; children—one-half tablespoonful.

ALEPSAL (Fougera)

Hypnotic

Composition: Each tablet represents

	Gm
Gardenal (French Luminal)	0.1
Belladonna	0.02
Trimethylxanthine	0.025

Action and Uses: Hypnotic and antispasmodic in epilepsy, convulsions and nervous excitation.

Supply: ALEPSAL—Tablets—Tubes of 20.

Administration: 1 or 2 tablets as often as required.

ALKARHEIN (Merrell)

Digestive

Composition: Contains per ounce:

Rhubarb	20 gr	(1.296 Gm)
Fluid Hydrastis (alkaline soluble principle)	20 m	(1.232 cc)
Sodium Bicarbonate (free and combined)	18 gr	(1.166 Gm)
Pancreatin Glycerol	8 m	(0.492 cc)
Cinnamon, Peppermint, Aromatics, Elixir, Base	1 oz	

Action and Uses: Indicated in gastrointestinal disorders to decrease acidity and stimulate digestive functions; serves as vehicle for iron, iodides and the salicylates.

Supply: ALKARHEIN—Bottles of 1 pt. and 1 gal.

Administration: In acute gastrointestinal attacks—1–4 teaspoonfuls in hot water at intervals of from ½–2 hr. until relieved; in chronic cases 1–2 teaspoonfuls in water after meals.

Bibliography: *See Chap. XII.*

ALKA-ZANE (Warner)

Alkalizer

Composition: 1 heaping teaspoonful represents:

	Gr	Gm
Calcium glycerophosphate	1.6	0.1
Magnesium phosphate	3.5	0.22
Calcium phosphate	3.5	0.22
Potassium bicarbonate	7.0	0.45
Sodium bicarbonate	17.0	1.1
Sodium citrate	48.0	3.11

Description: An alkaline effervescent compound of the basic salts helpful in maintaining the alkali reserve of the body.

Action and Uses: A systemic alkalizer assisting to maintain alkaline reserve of body; makes a palatable refreshing drink and favorably affects diuresis and acidosis; *For use* in infectious fevers, rheumatism, influenza, pneumonia, nephritis, gout, urticaria and skin diseases.

Supply: ALKA-ZANE—Bottles of 4 oz.

Administration: 1 teaspoonful in a glass of cold water or milk; lemon or orange juice may be added.

ALPHA-NAPHCO (Carel)

Disinfectant. Deodorant

Composition:

	Gm
Alpha naphthol	10.0
Glycerin	32.0
Saponis molle (from cottonseed oil and potassium hydroxide)	23.8
Aqua	q.s. 100.0

Flavored with gluside and essential oils.

Description: Alpha naphthol ($C_{10}H_7OH$), the active component of the preparation, occurs as colorless, glistening crystals or white crystalline powder, of faint phenol odor and pungent taste; is soluble in water, alcohol, ether, chloroform; has phenol coefficient of 1.46 (U.S.H. Lab) and of 3.11 when tested against staphylococcus aureus, in half saline and half blood serum at body heat.

Action and Uses: Is efficient antiseptic and germicide without toxicity; is absorbed from the gastrointestinal tract and excreted through the kidneys; is *used* as general disinfectant, for clinical purposes, for internal and external application in various infections.

Supply: ALPHA-NAPHCO—Liquid—Bottles 1¼, 3, 6½ and 16 oz.
ALPHA-NAPHCO—Ointment—Jars 1, 2, 6½ and 16 oz.

ALPHA-NAPHCO—Rectal Suppositories (C.A.)—Containing 0.1376 Gm in oleum theobromatis and yellow wax—Boxes of 12.

ALPHA-NAPHCO—Vaginal Suppositories—Boxes of 7 and 16.

ALPHA-NAPHCO—Cones (C.A.)—Containing 0.32 Gm in base of boric acid and sodium bicarbonate, equal parts—Boxes of 7 and 16.

ALPHA-NAPHCO MENTHOL—Suppositories (C.A.)—Containing 0.356 Gm and menthol 0.014 Gm in oleum theobromatis and yellow wax—Boxes of 7 and 16.

ALPHA-NAPHCO CAMPHOR—Nasal Ointment (C.A.)—Containing Alphanaphco 2 Gm and Camphor 2 Gm per 100 Gm—Tubes of 2 oz.

ALPHA-NAPHCO—Powder—Cans of 3 oz. and in bulk.

ALPHA-NAPHCO ZINC STEARATE—Powder (C.A.)—Containing 3.65 Gm, Zinc Stearate 8.75 Gm to 100 Gm of talcum, colored and perfumed—Cans of 3 oz.

ALPHA-NAPHCO ZINC STEARATE—Camphor Ointment (C.A.)—Containing 7.5 Gm with Camphor 1½ Gm, Zinc Stearate 10 Gm, starch 10 Gm, petrolatum perfumed—to 100 Gm—Tubes of 2 oz.

ALPHA-NAPHCO JELLY—Capsules—Boxes of 60 and 80.

Administration: For topical use; as gargle, vaginal douche and urethral irrigation—1/10–½%.

ALPHEBIN (Gane-Ingram)

Analgesic. Hypnotic

Chemical Name: Dimethyl-amino-phenyl-dimethyl-pyrazolon; Phenylallyl-barbituric acid.

Composition: Each tablet represents—

	Gr	Gm
Phenyl-allyl-barbituric acid	¼	0.016
Amidopyrine	2½	0.16

Action and Uses: Sedative, analgesic and hypnotic; of minimum toxicity and free from kidney irritation. *For use* where sedation is desired; in nervousness, sleeplessness and headache; in hysteria, chorea, gastric and cardiac neuroses; in vomiting of pregnancy, pre- and postoperatively and in dentistry.

Supply: **ALPHEBIN**—Tablets 2¾ gr (0.18 Gm)—Vials of 20—Bottles of 100.

Administration: *Maximum Daily Dosage*—6 tablets.

In Insomnia—2 tablets on retiring.

In Nervousness—1 tablet twice daily.
As Analgesic—2 tablets, repeated in 1–2 hr.
Preoperatively—1–2 tablets.
Postoperatively—1–2 tablets, repeated in 2–3 hr.

ALQUINCO (McNeil)

Antiseptic

Composition: Each tablet represents—

	Gr	Gm
Powdered Alum, Cryst	12½	0.800
Copper Sulphate U.S.P.	12½	0.800
Quinosol (Oxyquinolin Sulphate "McNeil") and oil rose	q.s.	

Action and Uses: Antiseptic and astringent in vaginal infections, cervicitis, leucorrhea.

Supply: ALQUINCO—Tablets—Bottles of 100 and 1 lb.

Administration: 1 tablet dissolved in 1 pt. of water for use as douche.

ALVESEN (Burroughs Wellcome)

Antacid

Composition:

	Gr	Gm
Sodium Bicarbonate	5	0.324
Calcium Lactophosphate	3	0.194
Potassium Bicarbonate	1	0.065
Magnesium Sulphate Exsicc	1	0.065
Sodium Chloride	1	0.065
Salis Effervescens	q.s.	

In solution produces 29.4 gr soluble citrates.

Action and Uses: An effervescent antacid, *for use* in acidosis of fever, starvation, from vomiting and anorexia; as antacid—in neuritis, gout, diabetes, diarrhea, post anesthesia; as alkaline diuretic—in pyelitis, cystitis, urethritis, gall bladder and liver affections, uric acid calculi.

Supply: ALVESEN—Tablets—Tubes of 25.

Administration: 1–2 tablets dissolved in a glass of water, after meals.

AMERTAN (Lilly)

Burn Therapy

Description: A hygroscopic ointment of Tannic Acid 5% and Merthiolate, 1:5,000, in a water-soluble jelly base; its Tannic Acid precipitates the superficial alkaloids and proteins forming a fixed, unabsorbable protective covering; the Merthiolate exerts antiseptic action.

Action and Uses: Antiseptic and protective; applied on raw surface keeps area dry, prevents fluid depletion and protects from trauma; inhibits bacterial growth and toxic absorption, encourages rapid healing; is *used* for extensive burns and scalds.

Supply: AMERTAN—Ointment—Collapsible tubes, 1 and 5 oz.

AMERTAN—Ointment—Glass jars, 1 and 5 lb.

Administration: Applied liberally, ¼–½ in. thick, with or without dressing, until tanning occurs; tanned area should be left uncovered; oily and greasy substances previously applied should be removed where possible with suitable solvent.

Bibliography: *See Chap. XII.*

AMIFEINE (McNeil)

Analgesic

Description: Combination of Amidopyrine and Caffeine.

Action and Uses: Antipyretic, analgesic and uterine sedative; *For use* in dysmenorrhea and for relief of pain in general.

Composition: **AMIFEINE**—Capsules and Tablets—containing:

	Gr	Gm
Amidopyrine	3½	0.227
Caffeine	1	0.064
Oleoresin Ginger	q.s.	

Combinations: **AMIFEINE COMPOUND 1**—Capsules and Tablets—containing:

	Gr	Gm
Amidopyrine	3¾	0.242
Caffeine	½	0.032
Ext. Hyoscyamus	¼	0.016

AMIFEINE COMPOUND 2—Capsules and Tablets—containing:

	Gr	Gm
Acetphenetidin	1¼	0.081
Amidopyrine	1¼	0.081
Strontium Salicylate	1¼	0.081
Barbital	¼	0.016
Caffeine	⅛	0.008

ELIXIR AMIFEINE (Non-Alcoholic) containing per fluid ounce:

	Gr	Gm
Amidopyrine	21	1.360
Caffeine	6	0.384
Oleoresin Ginger	q.s.	

TABLETS AMIFEINE (Children) containing:

	Gr	Gm
Amidopyrine	7/10	0.044
Caffeine	1/10	0.006
Sodium Bicarbonate	⅕	0.013

Supply: **AMIFEINE AND COMBINATIONS:**
Capsules and Tablets—Bottles of 100, 500, 1,000 and 5,000.
Elixir—Bottles of 2, 3 and 4 oz., ½ and 1 gal.

Administration: Capsules or Tablets—One or two, taken with warm tea or milk, as required.
Elixir—1 teaspoonful, with warm tea or milk as required.
Tablets—Amifeine (Children) 1–3 tablets, according to age.

AMOSAL (McNeil)

Antipyretic

Composition: A light brown powder, containing per tablet or capsule:

	Gr	Gm
Dover's powder	¼	0.016
Acetanilid	1½	0.097
Ammonium Salicylate	2	0.130
Caffeine	¼	0.016
Powdered Camphor	q.s.	

Action and Uses: Antipyretic, diaphoretic and analgesic, *for use* in acute fevers, colds, influenza, tonsillitis, rheumatism.

Supply: **AMOSAL**—Capsules—Bottles of 100, 500, 1,000 and 5,000.

AMOSAL—Tablets, Plain or Enteric coated—Bottles of 100, 500, 1,000, 5,000.

Administration: 1 capsule or tablet with water, as necessary.

AM-PHEN-AL (Stoddard)

Analgesic

Composition: Per tablet:

	Gr	Gm
Amidopyrine	2½	0.150
Phenobarbital	¼	0.016

Action and Uses: Analgesic and hypnotic in headaches, neuritis, neuralgia and for pre- and postoperative use.

Supply: AM-PHEN-AL—Tablets—Bottles of 100, 500 and 1,000.

Administration: 1–2 tablets in water, repeated in 1 hr. if necessary.

AMPOULE "REIPAR" (Fougera)

Antiarthritic

Composition:

	Gm
Salicylic acid C.P.	0.001
Sodium chloride C.P.	0.009
Betula lenta water	0.40
Distilled water	q.s. 1 cc

Action: A hypertonic solution of natural salicylic acid; is non-irritating, analgesic and antirheumatic.

Uses: In articular rheumatism, sciatica, gout, lumbago, myalgia, neuralgia.

Supply: AMPOULE "REIPAR"—1 cc—Boxes of 10.

Administration: *Hypodermically*—At the most painful points of the joint or at nerve exits near involved areas; 1–10 cc as required.

ANALGINE (Sharp and Dohme)

Analgesic

Official Name: Tabella Acetanilidi et Sodii Salicylas Co.

Composition: Each tablet represents—

	Gr	Gm
Acetanilid	2½	0.162
Powd. extr. cannabis	½	0.032
Extr. hyoscyamus	¼	0.016
Sodium bicarbonate	¼	0.016
Sodium salicylate	¼	0.016
Camphor monobromated	¼	0.016
Caffeine	5⁄16	0.020
Aromatic powder	q.s.	

Action and Uses: Analgesic, antipyretic and nerve sedative for conditions where these are indicated.

Supply: ANALGINE—Tablets 5 gr (0.324 Gm)—Bottles of 100 and 1,000.

Administration: 1 or 2 tablets, repeated in 2 hr. if necessary.

ANESTHONE CREAM (IMPROVED) (Parke, Davis)

Analgesic

Composition:

Adrenalin Chloride	1:5,000
Benzocaine	10%
Ephedrine Hydrochloride	10%
Bland Oleaginous Base	q.s.

Description: Benzocaine is a tasteless, odorless powder that dissolves slowly in body secretions and developes a protracted anesthetic effect without, apparently, any habit forming tendency; adrenalin is promptly astringent, which effect is supplemented in this combination by the more lasting astringent action of ephedrine.

Action and Uses: Allays hyperesthesia of nasal mucosa, decreases excessive secretion, relieves pain and itching; is especially useful in hay fever and conjunctivitis, *also used* in urethral caruncle, hemorrhoids, anorectal fissure; in burns, frost bites and varicose ulcers.

Supply: **ANESTHONE CREAM**—Improved—Collapsible tubes ½ oz., with elongated nozzle.

Administration: By local application.

ANTI-ASTHMATIC "HECKEL" (Anglo-French)

Antispasmodic

Composition:

	Per Cent
Suprarenal (total gland)	0.03
Saccharose	2.00
Distilled water	97.97

Action and Uses: An antispasmodic *for use* in asthma, in bronchial spasm, hay fever, urticaria, spastic headache.

Contraindications: Late pregnancy, hypertension, heart failure.

Supply: **ANTI-ASTHMATIC "HECKEL"**—Ampules 5 cc—Boxes of 12.

Administration: *Subcutaneously*—½–1 ampule several times daily.

ANTIFORMIN (American Antiformin)

Germicide

Description: A concentrated stabilized solution of Sodium Hypochlorite and Alkaline Hydrate; contains approximately 7.8 Gm sodium hydroxide, 0.32 Gm sodium carbonate and 5.68 Gm available chlorine, per 100 cc; a clear, yellowish colored liquid of peculiar characteristic odor.

Action and Uses: Solvent, sterilizer, oxidizer, antiseptic, disinfectant and deodorant; is non-poisonous, non-caustic; dissolves organic material and destroys all bacterial organisms except acid fast bacilli; has a phenol coefficient of 3.36; *Used* for disinfection, douching and topical application in infections and surgical conditions; in demonstrating tubercle bacilli in blood and sputum.

Supply: **ANTIFORMIN** (C.A.)—Medicinal—Vials of 4 oz.—Bottles of 1 lb.—Jugs of 1 gal.

Administration: For hand disinfection when caring for individuals with infectious diseases, and for local use—1–2 % watery solution.
For cleansing wounds and ulcerated surfaces—1–2 % watery solution.
For parasitic skin diseases and pruritus—5–10 % solution, applied twice daily.
For vaginal douching and venereal diseases—2 % solution.
For digestion of sputum and demonstration of tubercle bacilli—15 % solution.

Caution: In concentrated solution destroys enamel, lacquer, oil colors and linoleum.

Bibliography: *See Chap. XII.*

ARMERVENOL (Hille)

Alterative

Composition: Contains per cubic centimeter:

	Gr	Gm
Colloidal arsenic	1/24	0.0025
Colloidal mercury	1/12	0.0050
Colloidal copper	1/40	0.0016

Action and Uses: Non-irritant and non-toxic alterative; is readily assimilated and does not disturb gastro-intestinal tract; *For use* in coryza, bronchitis, tonsillitis, influenza and similar infections.

Administration: *Orally*—20 m, three times daily, in water or milk.
Intramuscularly or Intravenously—1–5 cc daily.

Supply: ARMERVENOL—(Oral)—Bottles of 1, 4 and 12 oz.
ARMERVENOL—(Injection)—Vials of 20 and 60 cc.

Bibliography: *See Chap. XII.*

ARMICOL (Mulford Colloid)

Hematinic

Description: A combination of Colloidal Arsenic and Mercuric Iodide; contains 10–12½ % Arsenic and 10–12 % Mercuric Iodide.

Action and Uses: A stable, non-irritating, readily absorbed and assimilated hematinic and alterative; does not cause precipitation of tissue fluids, is slowly eliminated and has prolonged action. *For use* in secondary anemias.

Supply: ARMICOL—Vials, 10 Gm.
ARMICOL—Capsules, Soluble, gr 2½ (0.162 Gm)—Bottles of 100.

Administration: 1–5 gr (0.064–0.324 Gm) three times daily after meals.

ARSCLERO (Irwin, Neisler)

Hypotensive

Composition: Each fluid ounce represents:

Sodium sulphocyanate	gr 20 (1.29 Gm)
Chloroform	m 60 (3.69 cc)
Aromatic vehicle	q.s.

Action and Uses: A light yellow, aromatic elixir of alterative and hypotensive action; *For use* in essential hypertension, in conjunction with other measures.

Supply: ARSCLERO—Bottles 1 gal.

Administration: 1 or 2 teaspoonfuls two to three times daily.

ASPIROFEINE (McNeil)

Analgesic

Description: Combinations of Acetylsalicylic Acid and Caffeine in various dosage and forms.

Action and Uses: Analgesic and antipyretic *for use* in conditions indicated.

Combinations: ASPIROFEINE 1—Capsules and Tablets containing

	Gr	Gm
Acid Acetylsalicylic	4	0.259
Charcoal	½	0.032
Caffeine	⅛	0.008

ASPIROFEINE 2—Capsules and Tablets containing

	Gr	Gm
Acid Acetylsalicylic	4	0.259
Acetphenetidin	1½	0.097
Charcoal	½	0.032
Caffeine	¼	0.016
Ext. Gelsemium	1/10	0.006

ASPIROFEINE 3—Capsules and Tablets containing

	Gr	Gm
Acetphenetidin	2½	0.162
Acid Acetylsalicylic	3¾	0.242
Caffeine Citrated	½	0.032

ASPIROFEINE—Tablets (Children) containing

	Gr	Gm
Acetphenetidin	⅝	0.040
Acid Acetylsalicylic	⅞	0.056
Caffeine	1/16	0.004

Supply: ASPIROFEINE—Capsules and Tablets—Bottles of 100, 500, 1,000 and 5,000.

Administration: 1 or 2 capsules or tablets as necessary.
Tablets Aspirofeine (Children) 1 or 2 tablets, according to age.

ATOMIDINE (Schieffelin)

Iodine Therapy

Description: A stable 1% Iodine compound in saline solution; is stated to liberate nascent iodine on contact with body fluids.

Action: A non-toxic alterative and diuretic; is rapidly absorbed, activating general metabolism.

Uses: Where iodine is indicated in early infections, hypertension, iodine deficiency diseases, asthma.

Administration: 5–10 drops in water; intensive therapy—20 drops.

Supply: ATOMIDINE—Bottles of 2 oz.

ATOMIDINE—Ointment—Tubes of 1 oz.
Bactericidal, hemostatic, non-staining; *For use* in burns, scalds, erosions, enlarged glands; also in gynecologic and rhinolaryngologic practice; *applied* two or three times daily.

ATROBUTIN (Stoddard)

Urinary Antiseptic

Composition: Per tablet:

Arbutin	gr 1/10	(0.006 Gm)
Potassium Citrate	gr 2	(0.130 Gm)
Tr. Belladonna	m 5	(0.308 cc)

Action and Uses: In urinary incontinence and vesical spasm.

Supply: ATROBUTIN—Tablets—Bottles of 100, 500 and 1,000.

Administration: 1 tablet four times daily for a child of 5 yr.

AURALGAN (Doho)

Analgesic

Composition: A solution of 5% pyrazolon phenyl-dimethyl in high specific gravity Glycerin.

Action and Uses: Is helpful in arresting inflammatory processes in acute otitis media before the onset of suppuration, in promoting osmosis through the drum membrane, withdrawing excessive serum from the tympanum and relieving tension and pain.

Supply: AURALGAN—Bottles of 15 Gms.

Administration: Without warming is instilled into external canal, filling it completely, and retained until relief is obtained.

Bibliography: *See Chap. XII.*

BARAMID (McNeil)

Sedative

Description: A combination of Barbital-Sodium and Amidopyrine.

Action and Uses: Antipyretic, analgesic and sedative in conditions indicated.

Combinations:

BARAMID 1—Capsules and Tablets containing	Gr	Gm
Barbital-Sodium	1½	0.097
Amidopyrine	3½	0.227

BARAMID 2—Capsules and Tablets containing	Gr	Gm
Amidopyrine	2½	0.162
Phenobarbital	¼	0.016

BARAMID COMPOUND—Capsules and Tablets containing

Barbital-Sodium	gr ½	(0.032 Gm)
Amidopyrine	gr 1½	(0.097 Gm)
Strontium Salicylate	gr 2½	(0.162 Gm)
Ext. Hyoscyamus	gr ⅛	(0.008 Gm)
Tinct. Gelsemium	m 2	(0.123 cc)

Supply: BARAMID AND COMBINATIONS—Capsules and Tablets—Bottles of 100, 500, 1,000 and 5,000.

Administration: 1 or 2 capsules or tablets as necessary.

BARBENZAL (Searle)

Analgesic

Composition: Each tablet represents—

	Gr	Gm
Sodium monobenzyl succinate	4¾	0.3
Phenobarbital	¼	0.016

Action: Analgesic, antispasmodic and sedative.

Uses: In dysmenorrhea, ovarian neuralgia, periodic headaches, neuritis.

Supply: BARBENZAL—Tablets—Bottles of 100, 1,000.

Administration: 1–2 tablets in warm fluid every 4–6 hr. until relieved.

BARB-ETH-OIL (Abbott)

Rectal Analgesic

Composition: OBSTETRICAL—(Dr. Axelrod's Formula):

n-Butyl Ethyl Barbituric Acid (Neonal)	5 gr (0.324 Gm)
Quinine (alkaloid)	20 gr (1.3 Gm)
Ether	2½ fl. oz.
Mineral oil	1½ fl. oz.
Ethyl (1-methyl-butyl) Barbituric acid (Nembutal)	8 gr (0.324 Gm)

SURGICAL—

Ethyl (1-methyl butyl) Barbituric acid (Nembutal)	10 gr (0.6 Gm)
Ether	2½ fl. oz.
Mineral oil	1½ fl. oz.

Action: Produces analgesia and anesthesia through the rectal route; causes drowsiness within 30 min. and induces deep slumber lasting several hours without excitatory effect during or after administration.

Uses: As preanesthetic in surgical operations and obstetrics; to eliminate fear, produce relaxation and permit the use of high oxygen concentration.

Contraindications: Nephritis, colitis, diabetes, auditory disturbances, pulmonary infections, low metabolism rate and respiratory obstruction.

Caution: Should not be exposed to flame because of its ether content; rectal or vaginal examination is not made for at least 1 hr. after instillation.

Supply: BARB-ETH-OIL—Surgical—Tins of 4 oz.

BARB-ETH-OIL—Obstetrical—Tins of 4 oz.

Administration: Usually 2 plain or soapsud enemas are given until the return flow is clear; in obstetric cases the tube is introduced beyond the pressure point of fetal head or buttocks and about 1 oz. of plain mineral or olive oil is introduced; this is followed by Barb-Eth-Oil in dosage according to body weight: 130 lb. or over—4 fl. oz., 100–130 lb.—3 fl. oz., 100 lb. or less—2 fl. oz.; instillation is made slowly, taking 20–30 min. for its completion.

Bibliography: *See Chap. XII.*

BARBROMID (Columbus Pharmacal)

Hypnotic

Composition: Each tablet represents—

	Gr	Gm
Phenobarbital	½	0.032
Valeryl urea bromide	2	0.130
Amidopyrine	2	0.130

Action and Uses: Analgesic, antispasmodic and sedative; also hypnotic in pre- and post-operative cases.

Supply: BARBROMID—Tablets—Bottles 100, 1,000.

Administration: 1 tablet every 2 hr., for 3–4 doses.

BARBROMIDE (Irwin, Neisler)

Hypnotic

Composition: Each capful represents approximately:

	Gr	Gm
Barbital	1	0.064
Sodium bromide	20	1.296

Description: An effervescent, orange colored and flavored salt.

Uses: In insomnia, nervousness, general excitation.

Supply: BARBROMIDE—Bottles 4 oz., with dose cap—Boxes 12.
BARBROMIDE—Bottles, large size—Boxes 12.

Administration: 1 capful at bedtime.

BARLUPULIN (McNeil)

Sedative

Description: A light brown powder containing—

	Gr	Gm
Barbital-Sodium	1	0.064
Ext. Lupulus (Hops)	1	0.064
Ext. Celery Seed	1	0.064
Ext. Hyoscyamus	¼	0.016
Aromatics	q.s.	

Action and Uses: Nerve sedative in nervous and mental excitation.

Supply: BARLUPULIN—Capsules—Bottles of 100, 500, 1,000 and 5,000.

Administration: 1 or 2 capsules, as necessary.

BARMIPHEN (Fraser)

Antipyretic

Composition: Each capsule represents:

	G	Gm
Cinchophen	2	0.130
Barmidon	½	0.032
Phenacetin	2	0.130
Theobromo-Salicyl-ester	2¼	0.144

Action and Uses: Antipyretic, sedative, analgesic and mildly diuretic; *For use* in colds, grippe and coryza.

Supply: BARMIPHEN—Capsules—Bottles of 100 and 1,000.

Administration: 1–2 Capsules, with sodium bicarbonate in glass of water three times daily.

BELLADENAL (Sandoz)

Antispasmodic. Sedative

Composition: An association of Bellafoline (natural levorotatory alkaloids of belladonna leaves) 1/250 gr (0.00025 Gm) with Phenobarbital 3/4 gr (0.05 Gm), per tablet.

Action: Relieves pain in obstinate spastic conditions; is claimed to be exceptionally effective because of the marked potency of bellafoline on excessive vagus stimulation and the powerful sedative and antispasmodic action of the barbituric acid component.

Uses: As antispasmodic and sedative in epilepsy, Parkinsonism, angina pectoris, cardiac and gastric neuroses, asthma, climacteric disorders; in migraine, hepatic colic, dysmenorrhea, enuresis, infantile convulsions, chorea, seasickness; in nervous erethism, neurasthenia and psychoneuroses.

Supply: BELLADENAL—Tablets—Tubes of 20—Bottles of 100 and 500.

Administration: Adults—Average 2–4 tablets, maximum 6 tablets per day; Fractional dose method, 1/4 tablet every 1/2 hr. or 1/2 tablet every hour, up to 4 tablets a day.
Children—1/4 tablet to four 1/2 tablets daily.

Bibliography: *See Chap. XII.*

B.F.I. POWDER (Sharp and Dohme)

Antiseptic

Official Name: Pulvis Bismuthi, Formici et Iodidi Co.

Composition: Each ounce represents:

	Gr	Gm
Bismuth-formic-iodide	70	4.531
Acetanilid	30	1.944
Zinc sulphocarbolate	10	0.643
Bismuth subgallate	20	1.296
Powdered alum	3	0.194
Boric acid	128	8.294

Action and Uses: A dry surgical dressing for antiseptic and astringent purposes. *Used* as first aid in cuts, scratches, chafing; in minor wounds and skin irritations of various kinds.

Supply: B.F.I.—Powder—Cans, sprinkler-top, small and large size;
Plain, for dispensing, small size—Boxes of 1 lb.

Combinations: B.F.I.—Ointment—containing:

Bismuth-formic iodide comp. powder	42 gr (2.722 Gm)
Balsam peru	7 m (0.431 cc)
Diachylon ointment	60 gr (3.888 Gm)
Petrolatum q.s.	1 oz.

Supply—Collapsible tubes, 1 oz.—Jars 1 and 5 lb.

Uses—Same as for powder.

BENACOL SOLUTION (Marvell)

Analgesic

Description: Contains 5 parts each of Ethacaine and Phenmethylol in 90 parts of pure sweet Almond Oil.

Action and Uses: *For relief* of intense itching and to relax sphincter spasm in anal fissure and pruritus ani.

Supply: **BENACOL SOLUTION**—Ampules 3 cc—Boxes of 6 and 25.

Administration: *Subcutaneously* and *submucously* only; never into skin as it causes sloughing; 1 ampule, injected slowly just below skin of perianal region, and distributed in fan-shaped manner; repeated in 5 days.

BETANAPHTHOL COMPOUND (Stoddard)

Intestinal Antiseptic

Composition: Per tablet:

	Gr	Gm
Betanaphthol	¾	0.048
Bismuth-papaya compound	½	0.032
Strychnine sulphate	1/200	0.0003
Kaskara (Stoddard)	1	0.064
Aromatics	q.s.	

Action and Uses: Stomachic and laxative in flatulence and intestinal infections.

Supply: **BETANAPHTHOL COMPOUND**—Tablets—Bottles 100, 500 and 1,000.

Administration: 1–3 tablets in water as required.

BETULOL (Huxley)

Anodyne. Counterirritant

Composition:

	Per Cent
Methyl Salicylate	84
Menthol	2
Chloral Hydrate	2
Oleic Acid	10
Oils of Lavender and Rosemary	2

Action and Uses: Anodyne, counterirritant for external application in neuritis, arthritis, lumbago, sciatica, muscular aches, sprains, bruises and similar conditions; will not blister.

Supply: **BETULOL**—Bottles 1, 2, 4 and 16 oz.

Administration: Applied locally freely, and covered with hot wet dressing.

BICREOL (Burroughs Wellcome)

Antisyphilitic

Composition: A bismuth cream, containing per cc 0.15 Gm Metallic Bismuth, in Creo-camphor base.

Action and Uses: Antiluetic, *for use* in various syphilitic conditions.

Supply: **BICREOL**—Jars ½ and 2 oz.

Administration: *Intramuscularly*—1–1½ cc weekly for 8 injections; course repeated as necessary.

Bibliography: *See Chap. XII.*

BILE SALTS (Fairchild)

Cholagogue

Description: Comprises the sodium salts of the conjugated cholic acids, the glycocholates and taurocholates, separated from fresh oxgall in proportions in which they exist naturally; is not an artificial mixture of separate salts.

Action and Uses: As cholagogue and stimulant in faulty or deficient bile secretion and in postoperative biliary fistulae.

Supply: BILE SALTS (C.A.)—Bottles of ¼ and 1 oz.

BILE SALTS (C.A.)—Capsules, gr 3—Bottles of 100.

Administration: ½–2 gr (0.03–0.13 Gm) three to four times daily.

Combinations: BILE SALTS WITH SUCCINATE OF SODA AND HOLADIN—Contains per capsule:
Bile salts gr ½, Succinate of Soda, gr 5, Holadin gr 3; *Used*—1 capsule before breakfast and at bedtime, with water; increased if necessary—Bottles of 50 capsules.

BILE SALTS WITH PHENOLPHTHALEIN AND HOLADIN—Contains:
Bile salts gr ½, Phenolphthalein gr 1; Holadin gr 2; *Used*—1 capsule before breakfast and at bedtime, with water—Bottles of 100 capsules.

BILE SALTS WITH SUCCINATE OF SODA AND PHENOLPHTHALEIN—Contains:
Bile Salts gr 1, Succinate of Soda gr 5, Phenolphthalein gr ½; *Used*—1 capsule as indicated—Bottles of 50 capsules.

BILE SALTS WITH SALICYLATE OF SODA AND HOLADIN—Contains:
Bile salts gr 2, Salicylate of Soda gr 2, Holadin gr 2; *Used* when indicated. Bottles of 50 capsules.

BILE SALTS COMPOUND (Boericke and Runyon)

Cholagogue

Composition: Each tablet represents:

	Gr	Gm
Sodium glycocholate and taurocholate comp.	1½	0.097
Phenolphthalein	⅓	0.021
Sodium salicylate	1½	0.097
Sodium oleate	1	0.064
Menthol	1/20	0.003

Action and Uses: Cholagogue and choleretic; promotes flow of bile and stimulates biliary peristalsis; effects intestinal movement; *For use* in hepatic insufficiency, chronic constipation, cholecystitis, cholelithiasis.

Supply: BILE SALTS COMPOUND—Tablets—Bottles of 100, 500, 1,000 and 5,000.

Administration: 2 Tablets night and morning, with hot water; in cholelithiasis, double dosage.

BILOX (McNeil)

Cholagogue

Composition: Contains per tablet

	Gr	Gm
Bile Salts, purified	⅔	0.042
Sodium Salicylate	1	0.064

Phenolphthalein	⅔	0.042
Podophyllin	1/12	0.005

Action and Uses: Cholagogue, anti-fermentative and laxative.

Supply: BILOX—Tablets—Bottles of 100, 500, 1,000 and 5,000.

Administration: 1 or 2 tablets as necessary.

BISALCO (McNeil)

Cholagogue

Composition: Each tablet represents:

	Gr	Gm
Bile salts, purified	1	0.064
Sodium salicylate	1	0.064
Phenolphthalein	½	0.032
Extract cascara sagrada	½	0.032
Menthol	q.s.	

Action and Uses: Cholagogue, antifermentative and laxative; *For use* in hepatic insufficiency, intestinal putrefaction, habitual constipation.

Supply: BISALCO—Tablets—Bottles of 100, 500, 1,000 and 5,000.

Administration: 1–2 tablets, one or two times daily.

BISEMPCO CREAM (Marvell)

Antiluetic

Composition: A 10 % sterile suspension of Bismuth Subsalicylate in hydrogenated oil.

Uses: As antiluetic in syphilis and for topical application in Vincent's angina.

Supply: BISEMPCO CREAM—Ampules, 1 cc—Boxes of 12.

BISEMPCO CREAM—Solution—Bottles of 60 cc.

Administration: 10 m, gradually increased to 40 m, injected intramuscularly twice weekly; topically—by swab, as necessary.

BISMOGEN (Liquid) (Searle)

Intestinal Astringent

Composition: Each fluid ounce represents:

	Gr	Gm
Bismuth subnitrate	41	2.656
Zinc sulphocarbolate	1	0.064
Papain	1	0.064

Action and Uses: Gastro-intestinal astringent and antiseptic; *used* to control diarrhea in dysentery and intestinal fermentation.

Supply: BISMOGEN—Bottles of 1 pt. and 1 gal.

Administration: Adults—1 or 2 dr. every 2 or 3 hr. as required; children—in accordance.

BISMOL (National Drug)

Antiluetic

Composition: Each cubic centimeter represents:

Bismuth subsalicylate	gr 2 (0.130 Gm)
Benzocaine	1%
Guaiacol	½%
Oil sesame q.s.	1 cc

Action and Uses: In all stages of syphilis, especially of the nervous system.

Supply: BISMOL—Ampule-Vial 25 cc and 100 cc.

Administration: 6–15 intramuscular injections at 5 day intervals constituting one course; repeated when necessary after rest period of 1 week.

BISMOLATE (Irwin, Neisler)

Sedative

Composition: Each tablet represents:

	Gr	Gm
Benzocaine	1/12	0.005
Bismuth subnitrate	2	0.130
Cerium oxalate	2	0.130

Action and Uses: Gastric sedative for relief of nausea and gastric irritation.

Supply: BISMOLATE—Tablets—Bottles of 1,000.

Administration: 1 or 2 tablets two to three times daily after meals, or as required.

BISMOSOL (Merck)

Antiluetic

Composition:

Potassium sodium bismuthotartrate	10 Gm (155 gr)
Piperazine	0.3 Gm (4.5 gr)
Glucose solution, aqueous q.s.	100 cc

Description: A pale yellow sterilized glucose-aqueous solution of potassium sodium bismuthotartrate, containing 35% of bismuth (Bi).

Action and Uses: As for bismuth in syphilis.

Supply: BISMOSOL (C.A.)—Ampules 1 cc—Boxes of 10.

Administration: *Intramuscularly*, 1 cc, every 2–7 days for 20 doses; after a rest period of 1 mo. a second course is administered.

BISMUTH AND ANESTHESIN COMPOUND (Searle)

Sedative

Composition: Each tablet or capsule contains—

	Gr	Gm
Bismuth subnitrate	2	0.130
Cerium oxalate	½	0.032
Phenol	1/10	0.0065
Anesthesin	1/10	0.0065
Menthol	q.s.	

Action and Uses: *For use* as gastric sedative in nausea and vomiting due to irritation or excessive mucus secretion.

Supply: BISMUTH AND ANESTHESIN COMPOUND—Tablets—Bottles of 1,000.
BISMUTH AND ANESTHESIN COMPOUND—Capsules—Bottles of 1,000.

Administration: 1–2 tablets or capsules as required.

BISMUTH HYDRATE COMPOUND (Wampole)

Intestinal Astringent

Formula: Each fluid ounce represents:

Chloroform	m 2 (0.12 cc)
Bismuth oxycarbonate	gr 10 (0.643 Gm)
Fluid red gum (Kino Eucalypti)	m 32 (2.16 cc)
Pepsin	gr 4 (0.259 Gm)
Phenyl Salicylate	gr 1 (0.064 Gm)
Alcohol	2%
Oil and Aromatics	q.s.

Action and Uses: Astringent and carminative, *For use* in the treatment of gastro-intestinal irritation and fermentation; and in diarrheas of various origins.

Supply: BISMUTH HYDRATE COMPOUND—Bottles 4 oz., 16 oz., and 1 gal.

Administration: 1–2 teaspoonfuls every half hour for 6 or 8 doses; children 10 drops to half teaspoonful.

BISMUTH THYMOL IODIDE (Strasenburgh)

Antiseptic

Composition: Bismuth Oxyiodide, Thymol Iodide and Boric Acid.

Action and Uses: As surgical dressing in suppurative diseases.

Supply: BISMUTH THYMOL IODIDE—Bottles of 1 lb.
BISMUTH THYMOL IODIDE—Cans, sprinkler top, ½ oz.—Bottles, sprinkler top, 2 oz.

Administration: *Applied freely* as dusting powder.

BLANDINE COMPOUND (Sharp and Dohme)

Emollient

Official Name: Liquid Petrolatum Compound.

Composition: Each fluid ounce contains:

Camphor	gr 1⅓ (0.085 Gm)
Menthol	gr ⅕ (0.013 Gm)
Thymol	gr ⅕ (0.013 Gm)
Eucalyptol	m ⅖ (0.024 cc)
Methyl Salicylate	m 1½ (0.092 cc)
Hydrastine	gr 1/40 (0.0016 Gm)
Liq. Petrolatum	q.s. 1 oz.

Action and Uses: Protective to the mucous membranes of the upper respiratory tract, stimulates the mucosa and its secreting glands. *Used* in colds, catarrhs, nasopharyngeal affections.

Supply: BLANDINE COMPOUND—Bottles of 1 pt. and 1 gal.

Administration: By swabbing or spraying.

BRANDRETH'S PILLS (Allcock)

Cathartic

Composition:

	Gm	Gr
Solid extract sarsaparilla	0.0052	1/12
Curacao and socotrine aloes	0.0547	7/8
Colocynth	0.0132	1/5
Gum gamboge	0.0212	1/3
Gum guaiac	0.0212	1/3
White castile soap	0.0044	1/15
Capsicum	0.0026	1/24

Action and Uses: *For use* as cathartic in more obstinate cases of chronic constipation.

Supply: BRANDRETH'S PILLS (L.A.)—Boxes of 36.

Administration: 1–3 pills at night.

BROMHOSAL (Abbott)

Bromide Therapy

Composition: A combination of 60% Bromine and Hosal (a substitute for table salt) with a small quantity of Sodium but no chlorides; contains Sodium, Calcium Amino-acids and Fatty Acids of low molecular constitution.

Description: A white microcrystalline powder, readily soluble in water.

Action: As for bromides; has the advantage of administering bromides in smaller dosage, because of greater effectiveness in the absence of sodium chloride; makes food palatable, yet salt free.

Uses: Epilepsy and epileptoid states, vasomotor disturbances, menopausal affections.

Supply: BROMHOSAL—Glass shakers with sprinkler tops, 3/4 oz.

BROMHOSAL—Bottles of 8 oz.

Administration: Sprinkled on food as condiment from salt shaker.

Caution: Containers when not in use should be kept closed to prevent caking of contents.

Bibliography: *See Chap. XII.*

BROMIONYL (Upjohn)

Bromide Therapy

Composition: Contains per heaping teaspoonful 60 gr (3.888 Gm)—

	Gr	Gm
Sodium bromide	9.50	0.608
Calcium bromide	3.75	0.240
Potassium bromide	2.50	0.162

on solution citrates and tartrates are formed, with alkilizing effect equal to gr 27 (1.75 Gm) of sodium bicarbonate.

Action and Uses: Indicated where the administration of bromides is desired and where alkilization is also appropriate, as acidosis and gastric irritation accompanying nervousness; in insomnia, seasickness, sexual hyperesthesia, hysteria, exophthalmic goitre, vomiting of pregnancy, delirium tremens, hypertension.

Supply: BROMIONYL—Bottles 2 and 4 oz.

Administration: 60–75 gr daily in 4 or 5 doses; in hypertension—½ teaspoonful six times daily in 6 oz. water.

Combinations: BROMIONYL WITH ACETYL SALICYLIC ACID—Contains in addition gr 5 (0.324 Gm) acetyl salicylic acid per teaspoonful; *Used* in nervous disturbances accompanied by pain; *administered:* 4 teaspoonfuls every ½ hr. *Supply*—Bottles 2 and 4 oz.

BROMIONYL WITH BARBITAL—Contains in addition gr 5 (0.324 Gm) Barbital per teaspoonful, to reinforce hypnotic effect; *Used* in insomnia without pain. *Dosage*—1 or 2–4 teaspoonfuls at bedtime. *Supply*—Bottles 2 oz.

BROMIPHEN ELIXIR (McNeil)

Sedative. Hypnotic

Description: An orange colored elixir containing in each fluid ounce—

		Gr	Gm
Potassium Bromide, Sodium Bromide, Strontium Bromide	aa	60	3.888
Phenobarbital Sodium		2	0.130

Action and Uses: Antispasmodic, sedative and hypnotic—in insomnia, hysteria, nervous depression and similar disturbances.

Supply: BROMIPHEN—Elixir—Bottles of 2, 3, 4 oz., 1 pt., ½ and 1 gal.

Administration: 1–2 teaspoonfuls in water after meals.

BROMOFORM BRONCHIAL ANODYNE COMPOUND

Sedative Expectorant (Nelson, Baker)

Composition: Each ounce represents—

Bromoform	drops
Ammonium Bromide	gr 24 (1.536 Gm)
Ipecac	gr ½ (0.032 Gm)
Benzoin	gr 1 (0.064 Gm)

Action and Uses: Bronchial sedative in acute bronchitis, whooping cough and spasmodic coughs of other origin; is miscible with water and other liquids.

Supply: BROMOFORM BRONCHIAL ANODYNE COMPOUND—Bottles of 1 pt. and 1 gal.

Administration: Children up to 10 yr., 1 dr. every 2 hr; more frequently in severe attacks; adults—1–4 teaspoonfuls three or four times daily.

BROMO-MANGAN "DIETRICH" (Reinschild)

Sedative

Official Name: Liq. Ferro-Mangan Bromopeptone "Dietrich."

Composition: Contains in solution:

	Per Cent
Iron	0.6
Manganese Peptonate	0.1
Bromo-peptone	3.0
Alcohol	10

Action and Uses: A stable, palatable sedative hematinic and digestant, readily assimilated and not injurious to teeth; *For use* in nervous disturbances complicated by anemia.

Supply: **BROMO-MANGAN**—Amber Bottles, 10 oz.

Administration: 1 Tablespoonful as sedative, equivalent to gr 15 Potassium Bromide, three or four times daily.
Children—20 drops to 1 teaspoonful, three or four times daily.

BRONCHOL (Sharp and Dohme)

Expectorant

Official Name: Caps. Terebeni Co.

Composition: Each capsule contains—

Terebene	m 1	(0.061 cc)
Sandalwood Oil	m 1½	(0.091 cc)
Creosote, U.S.P	m ½	(0.030 cc)
Eucalyptol	m ⅕	(0.012 cc)
Strychnine	gr 1/100	(0.00065 Gm)
Olive Oil q.s.	m 5	(0.30 cc)

Action and Uses: Expectorant and restorative in subacute and chronic bronchial affections, chronic emphysema, chronic catarrh, post-influenzal protracted cough.

Supply: **BRONCHOL**—Capsules—Boxes of 24 and 100.

Administration: 1–2 capsules, three to four times daily, after meals.

BUCHUFORM (Strasenburgh)

Urinary Antiseptic

Composition: Each tablet represents:

	Gr	Gm
Ammonoform (hexamethylenamine)	2	0.130
Resorcinol	1	0.064
Barosmin	q.s.	

Action and Uses: A urinary antiseptic *for use* in cystitis, pyelitis.

Supply: **BUCHUFORM**—Tablets—Bottles of 500 and 1,000.

Administration: 1 tablet four times daily, with water.

BY-KEM (Bio Medico)

Cholagogue

Description: A combination of Taurolactic Acid ($CH_2NHCH_2HSO_3.\ C_3H_5O_2$) and Copper Sulphate 1:50,000, as co-ferment for interaction with the natural lipolytic and proteolytic enzymes in the intestines.

Action and Uses: Stimulates gall bladder function, decreases intestinal fermentation and influences physiologic peristalsis; *For use* in acute and chronic cholecystitis, colitis, chronic constipation, intestinal toxicosis, post operative flatulence and hyperemesis gravidarum.

Supply: BY-KEM—Tablets 6.45 gr—Bottles of 50.

Administration: *Medical—Average Dose*—2–6 tablets daily with meals.
Surgical—2 tablets twice daily, 2 days preoperatively, then 1 tablet 4 hr., and 2 tablets 8 hr. after operation, with 2 tablets twice daily for the following 2 days.

Caution: Is not to be combined with other laxatives; vinegar, wine, fats and white bread are best avoided during use of drug.

Bibliography: *See Chap. XII.*

CACTUS COMPOUND (Stoddard)

Cardictonic

Composition:

Tr. Cactus Grandiflora	m 2	(0.123 cc)
Fl. Ext. Digitalis	m 2	(0.123 cc)
Strychnine Sulphate	gr 1/40	(0.001 Gm)
Nitroglycerin	gr 1/200	(0.0003 Gm)

Action and Uses: Cardiac stimulant and tonic for the relief of palpitation in valvular disease, angina pectoris and other cardiac diseases.

Supply: CACTUS COMPOUND—Tablets—Bottles 100, 500 and 1,000.

Administration: 1 tablet three or four times daily.

CAFUMAL (Winthrop)

Sedative

Composition: Formally known as Cafinal. Contains per tablet:

	Gr	Gm
Luminal	3/4	0.048
Caffeine	3/8	0.024

Action and Uses: A combination to counteract the drowsiness induced by luminal if given alone; *For use* as sedative where luminal is indicated; in migraine, dysmenorrhea, hysteria, neurasthenia, vomiting of pregnancy, drug addiction.

Supply: CAFUMAL—Tablets—Tubes of 20—Bottles of 100.

Administration: 1–3 tablets daily.

CAL-BIS-MA (Warner)

Antacid

Composition: One level teaspoonful represents:

	Gr	Gm
Calcium Carbonate	9	0.576
Bismuth Subgallate	1	0.064
Bismuth Subcarbonate	2	0.130
Magnesium Carbonate	5	0.324
Sodium Bicarbonate	10	0.643
Colloidal Kaolin	3	0.194

Action and Uses: Gastric antacid in hyperacidity with heartburn, epigastric pain, flatulence; is also laxative.

Supply: CAL-BIS-MA—Metal Cans of 1¾ and 4 oz. and 1 lb.

CAL-BIS-MA—(Unflavored)—Metal Cans of 1¾ and 4 oz. and 1 lb.

Administration: 1 level teaspoonful several times daily, or as required.

CALCIDIN (Abbott)

Expectorant

Description: A compound of Calcium and Iodine (15%), in assimilable form.

Action: Exerts through its iodine content germicidal properties, affects cellular catabolism, accelerates resorption and elimination, loosens and liquefies secretions from the respiratory tract.

Uses: In respiratory infections, colds, laryngitis, pharyngitis, bronchitis; in simple goiter, bronchial asthma; topically—as dressing for chronic ulcers and septic wounds.

Advantages: Is pleasant to take, well tolerated and gives rise to no gastric distress.

Supply: CALCIDIN—Tablets ⅓ gr (0.02 Gm), 1 gr (0.06 Gm), 2½ gr (0.16 Gm), 5 gr (0.32 Gm)—Bottles of 100, 1,000.

CALCIDIN—Powder—Bottles of 1 oz.

CALCIDIN—Troches—⅓ gr (0.02 Gm)—Bottles 100, 1,000.

Administration: Infants ⅓ gr (0.02 Gm) to 1 gr (0.06 Gm);
Adults 1 gr (0.04 Gm) to 5 gr (0.32 Gm), four or five times daily, followed by copious draughts of water.
Topically—As dusting powder.

Combinations: ANESTHESIN-CALCIDIN—Troches or Lozenges, containing ⅓ gr (0.02 Gm) calcidin, ¼ gr (0.01 Gm) anesthesin (non-toxic)—Packages of 12 boxes containing 24 troches—Bottles of 100, 1,000.

SALICYLIC ACID AND CALCIDIN COMPOUND—Containing calcidin ⅓ gr (0.02 Gm), salicylic acid 1 gr (0.06 Gm), colchicine 1/250 gr (0.0002 Gm), bryonin 1/220 gr (0.0005 Gm), extract of cimicifuga 1/12 gr (0.05 Gm)—Bottles of 100, 1,000.

CAMPHOR AND CALCIDIN COMPOUND—Containing calcidin ⅓ gr (0.02 Gm), camphor ¼ gr (0.01 Gm), hydrastine hydrochloride 1/250 gr (0.0002 Gm), hysocyamine sulphate 1/2,000 gr (0.00003 Gm)—Bottles of 100, 1,000.

CALCILACT (Abbott)

Calcium Therapy

Composition: A palatable effervescent granular combination of approximately 25% Calcium Lactate and 45% Lactose.

Action: Supplies calcium in specific calcium metabolism deficiencies and at the same time, by the slow decomposition of its lactose, provides suitable medium in the intestines for the growth of lactic acid bacteria, inhibiting proteolytic putrefaction with absorption of toxins.

Uses: In systemic calcium deficiencies; in asthma, hay fever, vagotonia, sprue; during growth, pregnancy, lactation and menopause; in decreased blood coagulability, edema and renal disease.

Supply: CALCILACT—Bottles 6 and 14 oz.

Dosage: *Average Dose*—1 capful, containing 60 gr (3.8 Gm) calcium lactate and 95 gr lactose, in a glass of cold water three times daily, 1 hr. before meals; increased or decreased according to requirements; smaller doses to children.

Bibliography: *See Chap. XII.*

CALCIONATES (Upjohn)

Calcium Therapy

Description: A granular, effervescent preparation containing per heaping teaspoonful, calcium phosphate gr 7 (0.384 Gm) in calcium equivalent to gr 20 (1.296 Gm) of calcium lactate; is designed for the administration of calcium as a pleasant, acidulous, supersaturated, effervescent drink.

Action and Uses: As for calcium; *used* where calcium medication is indicated: in rickets, tetany, allergy, dermatitis and to shorten coagulation time of blood.

Supply: CALCIONATES—Bottles of 2, 4 and 8 oz.

Administration: 1 teaspoonful three times daily in 6 oz. of water, between meals.

CALCIUM GRANULAR (Schieffelin)

Calcium Therapy

Official Name: Granular Calcium Lactophosphate Saccharated.

Description: A saccharated soluble granular preparation of calcium lactophosphate; dissolved in water forms a palatable lemonade-tasting drink; is well tolerated by children.

Action: As for calcium; promotes coagulating activity of blood, stimulates heart muscle and nerve tissue, establishes normal irritability of nervous system.

Uses: In conditions of calcium deficiency; in malnutrition, rickets, scrofula; in spasmophilia, tetany, laryngismus stridulus, bronchial asthma, urticaria, angioneurotic edema; in pregnancy and during convalescence from acute diseases.

Supply: CALCIUM GRANULAR—Bottles of 4½ oz.

Administration: 2 teaspoonfuls in glass of water during meals; children according to age.

CALI-CHLORIDES (Westerfield)

Reconstructive

Composition: Each dram represents:

	Gr	Gm
Mercury bichloride	1/128	0.0005
Arsenic chloride	1/280	0.0002
Iron chloride	1/8	0.008
Calisaya	5	0.324
Hydrastis q.s.		

Action and Uses: As general stimulant and reconstructive in infections; is readily absorbed and well tolerated; *For use* in leg ulcers, infected hemorrhoids, abscesses.

Supply: CALI-CHLORIDES—Bottles of 1, 5 pt., 1 gal.

Administration: 1–2 teaspoonfuls four or five times daily in ½ glass water.

CALOMEL CAMPHOR COMPOUND (Stoddard)

Intestinal Astringent

Composition: Each tablet represents:

	Gr	Gm
Ext. stramonium	1/20	0.003
Calomel	1/10	0.006
Camphor	1/10	0.006

Capsicum	1/10	0.006
Ipecac	1/32	0.002
Salcetol (Stoddard)	1/2	0.032

Action and Uses: Astringent in cholera, dysentery and diarrheas.

Supply: CALOMEL CAMPHOR COMPOUND—Tablets—Bottles 100, 500 and 1,000.

Administration: 1 tablet every hour for 4 doses; then 1 every 2 or 3 hr.

CAMPHOGEN (Bischoff)

Stimulant. Antispasmodic

Composition: A water soluble Japanese Camphor in the following combination:

	Per Cent
Camphor	2
Acetdiethylamid	25
Sodium Salicylate	15
Water	58

Action: Is miscible with body fluids, readily absorbed and prompt in action.

Uses: As cardio-respiratory stimulant in syncope, surgical shock, cardiac insufficiency, narcosis; in acute infections, cardio-vascular depression of chronic diseases and toxemia, myocarditis; also for the relief of spasm of unstriped muscle in intestinal colic and pylorospasm.

Advantages: The camphor is water soluble by reason of added substances; is twenty times as efficacious as in oil and two hundred times as in oral administration.

Supply: CAMPHOGEN "INGELHEIM"—Ampules, 1 cc or 2 cc—Boxes of 6.

Administration: Adult—1–2 cc, in extreme cases up to 4 cc, *intramuscularly.* Children 1/2–1 cc; injections repeated as demanded.
Intravenous injections only where instantaneous action is required.

CAMPHOR COMPOUND (Stoddard)

Antipyretic

Composition: Contains per tablet:

	Gr	Gm
Camphor	1/12	0.005
Aconite	1/12	0.005
Ext. stramonium	1/20	0.003
Ext. eucalyptus comp	3	0.194
Salcetol (Stoddard)	2	0.130
Kaskara (Stoddard)	1	0.064

Action and Uses: Antipyretic, diaphoretic; *For use* in colds, grippe, rhinitis, influenza.

Supply: CAMPHOR COMPOUND—Tablets—Bottles of 100, 500 and 1,000.

Administration: 1–2 tablets every half hour for 6 doses; then 1 every 2–4 hr.

CAMPHRO-SALYL AMPULES "FRAISSE" (Fougera)

Analgesic

Composition: Each ampule contains

Benzyl salicylate	gr 0.50	(0.032 Gm)
Camphor	gr 0.10	(0.006 Gm)
Pure olive oil	5 cc	

Action and Uses: Analgesic and sedative; *For use* in cardiac pain, neuritis, sciatica, arthritis, rheumatism.

Supply: **CAMPHRO-SALYL AMPULES "FRAISSÉ"**—Ampules 5 cc each—Boxes of 6.

Administration: *Subcutaneously or intramuscularly* into the painful area; 1 ampule every 2 or 3 days; 5 or 6 injections.

CANNABIN COMPOUND (Stoddard)

Aphrodisiac

Composition: Each tablet represents:

	Gr	Gm
Ext. cannabis	1/6	0.012
Zinc phosphide	1/8	0.008
Strychnine phosphate	1/38	0.001
Ext. quassia	1/32	0.002

Action and Uses: As aphrodisiac in sexual impotence, neurasthenia, alcoholism.

Supply: **CANNABIN COMPOUND**—Tablets—Bottles 100, 500 and 1,000.

Administration: 1 tablet four times daily, increased to 2, four times daily.

CARIPEPTIC LIQUID (Upjohn)

Digestive

Composition: Contains per fluid ounce—

Caripeptic enzymes	14 gr	(0.902 Gm)
Aromatic oils	3/5 m	(0.036 cc)
Ipecac	1/4 gr	(0.016 Gm)
Glycerin and Elixir as vehicles	q.s.	

Description: A palatable, stable solution containing proteolytic, amylolytic and milk curdling enzymes of Carica Papaya, with malt diastase, a vegetable digestant; standardized to uniform digestive capacity of the following strengths: 1.5–2.5 cc will completely convert 2.5 Gm anhydrous starch into sugar, in 30 min.; 3.7 cc will curdle at 50°c 100 cc boiled milk in 10 min.

Action and Uses: A digestant, carminative and stomachic; *For use* in starch indigestion with pyrosis, in gastric subacidity, gastric fermentation of achlorhydria and as a vehicle.

Supply: **CARIPEPTIC LIQUID**—Bottles 1 pt., 1 gal.

CARICA POWDER—Tins 1/4, 1 lb.

Administration: 1–2 teaspoonfuls as indicated; or 2–4 doses during or after meals.

Hypoacidity—1 tablespoonful.

Combinations: **CARICA COMPOUND**—Tablets gr 5 (0.324 Gm)—Bottles of 100, 1,000, 6,000.

CARICA COMPOUND—Tablets gr 7 (0.448 Gm)—Bottles of 100, 1,000, 4,000.

CARICA WITH GLYCEROPHOSPHATE—Tablets gr 7 (0.448 Gm)—Bottles of 100, 1,000, 4,000.

CASCARINE COMPOUND (Stoddard)

Cholagogue

Composition: Contains per tablet:

	Gr	Gm
Cascarine	½	0.032
Aloin	⅙	0.012
Xanthoxylin	¼	0.016
Euonymin	⅕	0.013
Ext. belladonna	1/10	0.006
Ext. nux vomica	1/10	0.006

Action and Uses: Cholagogue and laxative; in constipation and hepatic stasis.

Supply: CASCARINE COMPOUND—Bottles 100, 500 and 1,000.

Administration: 1–2 tablets at night.

CEROGEN (Hance)

Antacid

Composition: Each tablet represents:

	Gr	Gm
Cerium oxalate	2	0.130
Anesthesin	⅕	0.013
Powd. camphor	1/20	0.003
Magnesia carbonate	2	0.130

Action and Uses: Analgesic and antacid; *For use* in vomiting of pregnancy and gastric ulcer.

Supply: CEROGEN—Tablets—Bottles of 100 and 1,000.

Administration: 1–2 tablets as indicated.

CEROSE (Wyeth)

Expectorant

Composition: Each fluid ounce represents:

	Gr	Gm
Codein phosphate	1	0.064
Ipecac	1	0.064
Horehound	2½	0.162
Wild cherry	2½	0.162
Eucalyptus	1	0.064
Lobelia	8	0.512
Aromatic balsamic cordial	q.s.	

Action and Uses: Expectorant and bronchial sedative in respiratory affections.

Supply: CEROSE—Bottles of 8 oz. and 1 gal.

Administration: 1–2 teaspoonfuls three or four times daily.

CHAMOMILLA COMPOUND (Fraser)

Nervine

Composition: Each teaspoonful contains:

Tr. Cinchona	m 11	(0.77cc)
Tr. Chamomille	m 11	(0.77cc)

Tr. Ignatia................................	m 3	(0.18 cc)
Tr. Nux Vomica...........................	m 3	(0.18 cc)
Phosphorus................................	gr 1/250	(0.0002 Gm)

Action and Uses: Nerve stimulant and supportive indicated in asthenia, neurasthenia, convalescence, anemia.

Supply: **CHAMOMILLA COMPOUND**—Bottles of 4, 8 oz., 1 gal.

Administration: 1 teaspoonful in hot water four times daily, before meals and at bedtime.

CHERACOL (Upjohn)

Expectorant

Composition: Contains per ounce:

Potassium Guaiacol Sulphonate..................	gr 8	(0.512 Gm)
Ammonium Chloride...........................	gr 6	(0.512 Gm)
Codeine Phosphate.............................	gr 1	(0.064 Gm)
Antimony and Potassium Tartrate.............	gr 1/12	(0.005 Gm)
Chloroform....................................	m 2	

White Pine and Wild Cherry as vehicle.

Action and Uses: Sedative for cough without checking expectoration; *For use* in bronchial affections and other pulmonary diseases with irritating cough.

Supply: CHERACOL—Bottles of 1 pt. and 1 gal.

Administration: 1–3 teaspoonfuls, repeated every 2–4 hr., as indicated; taken without water.
Children; 1 month, 2–3 drops; 3 months, 4–6 drops; 6 months, 6–10 drops. Over 1 year of age, ½–1 teaspoonful.

CHINOPLASMIN (Winthrop)

Antimalarial

Chemical Name: Brand of Aminoquin with Quinine.

Description: A combination of Plasmochin, a brand of Aminoquine with Quinine, in proportions found most effective in malaria.

Uses: Antimalarial *for use* in tertian, quartan and subtertian types.

Advantages: Affects both the asexual and sexual malarial parasites (schizonts and gametes); promptly controls acute attacks and prevents infection by destroying the gametes which transmit the disease through the mosquito; is well tolerated.

Supply: **CHINOPLASMIN**—Tablets, containing 1/12 gr (0.005 Gm) Plasmochin and 2⅓ gr (0.15 Gm) Quinine Sulphate—Bottles of 100.

Administration: Adults, 2 tablets three or four times daily after meals.
Children 1–5 yr., 1 or 2 tablets, older children 3–4 tablets, daily.

Incompatibles: Contraindications as for Plasmochin.

Caution: Treatment is continued from 10–14 days; in obstinate cases up to 3 weeks. As malarial prophylactic 2 tablets daily or on alternate days.

Bibliography: *See Chap. XII.*

CHIONACEA (Nelson, Baker)

Alterative

Composition: Each fluid ounce represents:

Tinct. Chionanthus	dr.	3
Tinct. Echinacea	dr.	1.5
Euonymus	gr	12 (0.773 Gm)
Lappa	gr	16 (1.027 Gm)
Taraxacum	gr	16 (1.027 Gm)
Syrup Senna	dr.	2
Solution Sodium Phosphate Conc.	m	24 (1.46 cc)

Action and Uses: Stomachic, tonic, hepatic stimulant and depurative; influences digestive secretions; in larger dosage acts as cholagogue-laxative; *used* in conditions where such effect is indicated—in hepatic and biliary disease, fermentation, indigestion, constipation.

Supply: CHIONACEA—Bottles 1 pt., 1 gal.

Administration: 1–2 teaspoonfuls increased to 1 tablespoonful, as demanded.

CHLORHYDRIONIC WITH HEXAMETHYLENE TETRAMINE (Upjohn)

Urinary Antiseptic

Formula: An effervescent salt containing per teaspoonful:

	Gr	Gm
Ammonium Chloride	15	0.972
Hexamethylene Tetramine	15	0.972

Action and Uses: For acidifying urine and as urinary antiseptic in pyelitis and cystitis.

Supply: CHLORHYDRIONIC WITH HEXAMETHYLENE TETRAMINE—Bottles 4 oz.

Administration: 3–5 teaspoonfuls daily. If excessively painful micturition results, this may be counteracted with Citrocarbonate or other alkalies.

CHLORO-CALCIUM (Sharp and Dohme)

Hemostatic

Official Name: Elixir Calcium Chloride.

Description: A palatable elixir, containing Calcium Chloride gr 5 to the fluid dram; alcohol 15%.

Action and Uses: Raises coagulability of blood; is hemostatic and non-astringent. *For use* in hemorrhages due to prolonged blood coagulation time; in conditions where calcium is indicated.

Incompatibles: Carbonates, phosphates, sulphates and tartrates.

Supply: CHLORO-CALCIUM—Bottles of 1 pt. and 1 gal.

Administration: 1–2 dr. in water, as required.

CHOLAPHEN (Stoddard)

Cholagogue

Composition: Each tablet represents:

	Gr	Gm
Sodium Glyco-Taurocholate	1	0.064
Hexamethylenamine	1½	0.09
Sodium Salicylate	1½	0.09
Phenolphthalein	¼	0.016

Action and Uses: Cholagogue and laxative in gall bladder infections, calculus, biliary fistulae and constipation.

Supply: CHOLAPHEN—Tablets, sugar coated—Bottles 100, 500 and 1,000.

Administration: 1–2 tablets with water 2 hr. after meals.

CHOLEOL (C. D. Smith)

Cholagogue

Composition: Contains per ounce:

	Gr	Gm
Ferrum organicum comp	6	0.388
Jateorrhiza miersii	6	0.388
Matricaria	13	0.847
Polygonacia	13	0.847
Sod. glycocholate comp	3	0.194

Action and Uses: Stimulates liver and gall bladder function; is laxative, carminative and astringent in biliary diseases, calculi, flatulence, colic.

Supply: CHOLEOL—Bottles of 1 pt., 1 qt. and 1 gal.

Administration: 1 teaspoonful with water every 3 hr.

CHOLPHENOLATE (Searle)

Cholagogue

Composition: Contains per tablet:

	Gr	Gm
Sodium Glycocholate	¼	0.016
Sodium Taurocholate	⅛	0.008
Sodium Succinate	1	0.06
Dioscorein (Wild Yam)	¼	0.016
Fel Bovis	½	0.03
Phenolphthalein	¼	0.016

Action and Uses: Sodium glycocholate and sodium taurocholate induce cholagogue action, sodium succinate acts as intestinal antiseptic, phenolphthalein as mild laxative; *For use* in chronic constipation, deficient fat digestion, autointoxication, catarrhal jaundice, migraine.

Supply: CHOLPHENOLATE—Tablets—Bottles of 100 and 1,000.

Administration: 1–3 tablets, four times daily.

CIBALGINE (Ciba)

Chemical Name: Dimethyl-amino-phenyl-dimethyl-pyrazolon and Diallyl-malonylurea.

Description: A combination of Amidopyrin and Dial; their synergism enhances the therapeutic action of both and antagonizes any toxicity or either, offering optimum effect in small dosage.

Action: Analgesic, sedative and antipyretic.

Uses: *As analgesic* in various neuralgias—pleurodynia, sciatica, migraine; *as sedative* in general malaise and nervousness accompanying dysmenorrhea; *intramuscularly* in more painful affections, as tabetic crises, biliary and renal colic, angina, labor pains; *as antipyretic* in influenza, arthritis, cephalalgia, coryza, acute rheumatic fever.

Supply: CIBALGINE—Tablets—containing Amidopyrin gr 3½ (0.23 Gm) and Dial gr ½ (0.03 Gm)—Tubes of 12—Bottles of 100 and 1,000.

CIBALGINE—Elixir—each teaspoonful equals 1 tablet—Bottles of 2 and 6 oz. and 1 gal.

CIBALGINE—Ampules—2.3 cc; each cubic centimeter equals 1 tablet—Cartons of 5.

Administration: *Orally*—1 tablet, repeated in 3–4 hr. as indicated; 2 tablets in severe cases, repeated in 4–6 hr. if necessary.
Elixir—1 teaspoonful administered every 3–4 hr. repeated as above; 2 teaspoonfuls in severe instances.
Intramuscularly—1–2 cc, repeated in 4–6 hr.

Bibliography: *See Chap. XII.*

COCI-CODEINE (C. D. Smith)

Expectorant

Composition: Contains per ounce:

Potassium guaiacol sulphonate	gr 12 (0.773 Gm)
Ammonium chloride	gr 16 (1.036 Gm)
Ephedrine HCl	gr ¼ (0.016 Gm)
Fl. extr. coccillana	m 16 (0.976 cc)
Codeine phosphate	gr ¾ (0.048 Gm)
Chloroform	m 2 (0.12 cc)
Syrup wild cherry and tolu	q.s.

Action and Uses: Expectorant and sedative in respiratory affections.

Supply: COCI-CODEINE—Bottles of 4, 8, 16 oz., and 1 gal.

Administration: 2 Teaspoonfuls every 3–4 hr.

COCIPHEN SYRUP (McNeil)

Sedative

Composition: A syrup containing per fluid ounce:

Phenobarbital-Sodium	gr 1½	(0.097 Gm)
Tinct. Euphorbia Pil	m 120	(2 dr.)
Syr. Wild Lettuce	m 120	(2 dr.)
Tinct. Cocillana	m 40	(⅔ dr.)
Syr. Squill Comp	m 24	(⅖ dr.)
Cascarin, Menthol, Aromatics and Syrup	q.s.	

Action and Uses: Cough sedative, analgesic and antispasmodic *for use* in respiratory affections.

Supply: COCIPHEN SYRUP—Bottles of 2, 3, 4 and 16 oz., ½ and 1 gal.

Administration: 1–2 teaspoonfuls, as necessary.

COCO-QUININE (Lilly)

Antimalarial

Description: Each teaspoonful contains gr 2 (0.13 Gm) of Quinine Sulfate crystals suspended in a bland, chocolate flavored medium which disguises its taste, but does not alter the action.

Action and Uses: Analgesic, tonic, stomachic and specific against malaria; quickly assimilable, palatable and especially useful for children.

Supply: COCO-QUININE (C.A.)—In 3 oz., pint and gallon bottles.

Administration: 1 teaspoonful several times daily.

COCO-VITAMIN (Lilly)

Nutrient

Composition:

	Per Cent
Cod liver oil	40
Vitamin extracts	40
Malt extract	10
Potassium hypophosphite	1.7
Chocolate and aromatics.	

Standardized for vitamin content:	Units per Ounce	Units per 100 Cc
Vitamin A	5,500	18,400
Vitamin B	16	54

Each ounce equivalent in vitamin strength to 10 oz. milk or 1½ lb. spinach.

Action and Uses: Rickets; and as food tonic.

Supply: COCO-VITAMIN—Bottles of 1 pt.

Administration: Infants—¼-½ teaspoonful in each feeding.
Children—1-3 teaspoonfuls } three times daily after meals.
Adults—1-2 tablespoonfuls }

COD LIVER OIL EMULSION (Crookes)

Nutrient. Vitamin Therapy

Composition: A 50% emulsion, prepared from fresh cod livers; is finely subdivided, easily absorbed and digested; is palatable, miscible with other liquids and of standardized iodine content.

Action and Uses: As for cod liver oil.

Supply: EMULSION WITH CALCIUM—Containing gr 4 (0.259 Gm) calcium gluconate per ounce—Bottles, 6, 12 and 80 oz.

EMULSION WITH COLLOSOL IODINE—Containing collosol iodine equivalent to 1 m Tr. Iodine U.S.P. per teaspoonful of emulsion—Bottles, 6, 12 and 80 oz.

EMULSION WITH COLLOSOL CALCIUM LECITHIN—Bottles, 6, 12 and 80 oz.

EMULSION WITH YEAST—Containing vitamins A, B and D—Bottles 6, 12 and 80 oz.

Administration: 1 teaspoonful to 1 tablespoonful in milk, water, wine, three times daily.

COD LIVER OIL WITH VIOSTEROL 10 D

Nutrient. Vitamin Therapy

Composition: Cod Liver Oil with Viosterol added to make a vitamin A potency of not less than 500 units per gram and a vitamin D potency of cod liver oil with viosterol 10D.

Action and Uses: As preventive against Vitamin A and D deficiencies in the treatment of infants and young children with disturbances in normal growth, decreased resistance, or early symptoms of rickets.

Supply: **COD LIVER OIL WITH VIOSTEROL 10 D** (C.A.)—Bottles of 3 and 16 oz. **(Abbott)**

COD LIVER OIL WITH VIOSTEROL 10 D (C.A.)—Bottles of 3 and 16 oz. **(Parke, Davis)**

Administration: Prophylactic, infants and young children, 35–40 drops daily; mild or moderate rickets—½–⅔ teaspoonful three times daily.

Bibliography: *See Chap. XII.*

COD LIVER OIL WITH VIOSTEROL 10D

(Mead Johnson)

Vitamin Therapy

Description: Cod Liver Oil, increased to "10D" vitamin potency by the addition of Viosterol; biologically assayed.

Action: Fortifies against infections of the mucous membranes; aids in the utilization of calcium and phosphorus.

Uses: Wherever vitamins A and D are useful; in ophthalmias as xerosis, hemeralopia, xerophthalmia; in rickets, tetany, osteomalacia, allergies, tuberculosis and dental caries.

Supply: **COD LIVER OIL WITH VIOSTEROL 10D** (C.A.)—Bottles 3 and 16 oz.

Administration: *Prophylactic Dosage*—For infants and young children—1½ teaspoonfuls (6 cc) daily.

Curative Dosage—For infants and young children—3 teaspoonfuls (12 cc) daily.

Bibliography: *See Chap. XII.*

CODAMINES **(Stearns)**

Vitamin Therapy

Description: A palatable chocolate flavored Emulsion of Cod Liver Oil of standardized vitamin content with Malt Extract.

Composition: Each fluid ounce represents—Cod Liver Oil 25%, containing vitamin A, 7,500 units and Vitamin D, 1,900 units with Malt Extract 55 gr containing Vitamin B complex.

Supply: **CODAMINES**—Bottles of 12 oz.

CODAMINES—Tablets—Each representing 250 Vitamin A and 100 Vitamin D units—Bottles of 100.

Action and Uses: As for cod liver oil and malt; is easily retained and assimilated; *Used* in all conditions where vitamin therapy and nutritive aid is desired.

Administration: *Dosage*—Adults, 1 tablespoonful.
Children, 1 dessertspoonful.
Infants, 1 teaspoonful.
Pregnant and nursing mothers, 1 tablespoonful.

COLCHICUM COMPOUND (Stoddard)

Analgesic

Composition: Each tablet represents:

Tr. aconite } Tr. belladonna } Tr. bryonia comp. (Stoddard) } aa	m ¾ (0.054 cc)
Tr. cimicifuga } Tr. colchicum } aa	m ¾ (0.054 cc)
Salcetol (Stoddard)	gr 2 (0.130 Gm)
Sodium comp. (Stoddard)	gr 3 (0.194 Gm)

Action and Uses: Antipyretic and diaphoretic; *For use* in colds, grippe, influenza, rheumatism, neuralgia.

Supply: COLCHICUM COMPOUND—Tablets—Bottles 100, 500 and 1,000.

Administration: 1 tablet in water every ½ hr. for 6 doses; followed by 1 every 2–4 hr.

COLLOSOL "F.C.V.D." (Crookes)

Hematinic

Composition: Contains per teaspoonful:

	Mg
Colloidal iron	1
Colloidal copper	1/20
Irradiated ergosterol 250 D.	
Malt extract including Vitamin B.	
Orange juice containing Vitamin C.	

Action and Uses: Hematinic and tonic *for use* in metabolism deficiency diseases and as nutritional restorative.

Supply: COLLOSOL "F.C.V.D."—Bottles of 4, 40 and 80 oz.

Administration: ½–2 teaspoonfuls three times daily after meals.

COLLOSOL FERRO-ARSENICUM (Crookes)

Hematinic

Composition: Contains Colloidal Iron Hydroxide 0.05 %, Colloidal Arsenic Sulphide 0.033 %.

Action and Uses: Hematinic in simple anemia, chlorosis, nervous debility, neurasthenia, convalescence and splenic anemia of infancy.

Supply: COLLOSOL FERRO-ARSENICUM—Ampules 1, 2 cc—Boxes of 6.
COLLOSOL FERRO-ARSENICUM—Injection—Bottles, 30 cc.
COLLOSOL FERRO-ARSENICUM—Oral—Bottles, 4, 8, 16 oz.

Administration: *Hypodermically*—2 cc once or twice weekly for 6 doses; repeated after rest period of 1 week.
Orally—1 teaspoonful, well diluted, three times daily after meals.

Combination: COLLOSOL FERRO-ARSENICUM AND STRYCHNINE 0.1%—Contains in addition strychnine, 0.1%; Supply and dosage as above.

Bibliography: *See Chap. XII.*

COLLOSOL FERRO-MANGANESE (Crookes)

Hematinic

Description: A slightly alkaline colloidal mixture containing Manganese Hydroxide 0.5% and Iron Hydroxide 0.05%; is of similar action to Collosol Manganese with the additional hematinic property of iron.

Composition: Contains in colloidal solution:

For Oral Use—

Colloidal iron hydroxide	1:1,200
Colloidal manganese hydroxide	1:1,000

For Injection—

Colloidal iron	1:1,200
Colloidal manganese	1:1,000

Action and Uses: Hematinic in chlorosis and anemias accompanying dysmenorrhea, amenorrhea, suppurative processes, impetigo contagiosa, follicular impetigo, seborrhoeic eczema, gonorrhea, staphylococcus and streptococcus infections.

Supply: COLLOSOL FERRO-MANGANESE—Ampules 1, 5 cc—Boxes of 6.

COLLOSOL FERRO-MANGANESE—Bottles, Injection 30 cc.

COLLOSOL FERRO-MANGANESE—Bottles, Oral 4, 8, 16, 80 oz.

Administration: *Intramuscularly*—0.5–1.5 cc one or two times weekly.
Orally—1 teaspoonful, diluted, three times daily after meals.

Bibliography: *See Chap. XII.*

COLLOSOL FERRO-MANGANESE-ARSENIC (Crookes)

Hematinic

Composition: Contains in colloidal solution:

For Oral Use—

Colloidal iron	1:5,000
Colloidal manganese	1:800
Colloidal arsenic	1:8,000

For Injection—

Colloidal iron as hydroxide and arsenite	1:4,000
Colloidal manganese arsenite	1:1,000
Colloidal arsenic	1:2,000

Action and Uses: Hematinic *for use* in chlorosis, anemias and in chronic skin diseases, where arsenic is useful.

Supply: COLLOSOL FERRO-MANGANESE-ARSENIC—Ampules ½, 1, 2 cc—Boxes of 6.

COLLOSOL FERRO-MANGANESE-ARSENIC—Bottles (injection) 30 cc.

COLLOSOL FERRO-MANGANESE-ARSENIC—Bottles (oral) 4, 8, 16, 80 oz.

Administration: *Injection*—1–2 cc twice weekly.
Oral—1 teaspoonful in water two or three times daily after meals.

COLLOSOL SILICA WITH DROSERA ROTUNDIFOLIA

Vasodilator (Crookes)

Composition: Contains per teaspoonful—

Extr. Drosera rotundifolia (whole plant)	gr 6 (0.39 Gm)
Organic iodine	gr ⅝ (0.04 Gm)
Silica	0.1%

Action and Uses: A vasodilator in arterial hypertension with gastrointestinal disorders and for relief of stenocardia.

Supply: COLLOSOL SILICA WITH DROSERA ROTUNDIFOLIA—Bottles of 4, 10, 20 oz.

Administration: 1–2 teaspoonfuls in water three times daily after meals for 6 weeks.

COLLOSOL SULPHUR PARAFFIN EMULSION (Crookes)

Laxative

Composition: Contains Colloidal Sulphur 0.2%; Liquid Paraffin B.P. 50%.

Action and Uses: An intestinal lubricant and disinfectant; *For use* in diverticulitis and other bowel affections.

Supply: COLLOSOL SULPHUR PARAFFIN EMULSION—Bottles of 6, 12, 80 oz.

Administration: 1–2 tablespoonfuls night and morning.

COMBINAL (Morgenstern)

Analgesic. Hypnotic

Composition: Contains per tablet—

	Gr	Gm
Dimethylaminoantipyrine	2½	0.16
Dimethylmalonylurea	1	0.06
Phenylethylmalonylurea	¼	0.016
Theobromine-sodium-salicylate	¼	0.016

Action and Uses: Sedative, analgesic and hypnotic; is devoid of irritant and depressive effect; quickly induces sound sleep without after effects. *For use* in nervous insomnia with pain, neuralgia, wound pains, acute rheumatism and various other painful affections.

Supply: COMBINAL—Tablets—Boxes of 20.

Administration: As sedative—1 tablet three times daily.
As analgesic—1 or 2 tablets.
As hypnotic—2 or 3 tablets at bedtime.

COMPRAL (Winthrop)

Analgesic. Antispasmodic

Chemical Name: A molecular compound of Pyramidon and Voluntal. Brand of Cyrinal.

Formula: Pyramidon: $C_6H_5N.\ (CO.\ CH)N(CH_3)C(CH_3).\ N.\ (CH_3)$ + Voluntal: $NH_2.\ CO.\ NH.\ CO.\ OCH_2C.\ Cl_3$.

Description: A bitter, white crystalline powder, insoluble in water, readily soluble in alcohol.

Action: The trichlorethanolurethane or voluntal affects the nervous system and establishes sedation; the pyramidon is the analgesic, antispasmodic and moderately antipyretic factor and gives prompt relief from pain for many hours; is free from gastric disturbances, cardiac depression and drowsiness; is non-toxic, non-narcotic.

Uses: Dysmenorrhea, climacteric disorders, postpartum and postoperative pains; influenza, neuralgia, headache, migraine, pleurisy, rheumatic pains.

Supply: COMPRAL—Tablets gr 5 (0.3 Gm)—Tubes of 10—Bottles of 100.

Administration: 1 or 2 tablets, repeated if necessary three or four times daily.

Bibliography: *See Chap. XII.*

COPRAL (Brewer)

Hematinic

Composition: Each fluid ounce represents:

	Gr
Colloidal Copper	1/40
Iron Citrate Soluble	iv
Manganese Citrate Soluble	iii

Action and Uses: An assimilable, palatable, non-irritating hematinic and general tonic, increasing the hemoglobin and red cell content of blood; *For use* in all types of secondary and nutritional anemias.

Supply: COPRAL—Bottles 1 pt.

Administration: 1 Dessertspoonful three times daily after meals in milk or water; children 1 teaspoonful.

CREMO CARBONATES (Sharp and Dohme)

Antacid

Composition: Contains per ounce:

Magnesium Carbonate	gr 20 (1.296 Gm)
Bismuth Subnitrate	gr 20 (1.296 Gm)
Calcium Carbonate	gr 10 (0.643 Gm)
Chloroform	m 1 (0.06 cc)

Description: A creamy even colloidal suspension of great surface tension and high acid neutralizing power; insoluble in water and thus not absorbed in the intestinal tract; is palatable, soothing and neither constipating nor laxative.

Action and Uses: As antacid in gastric and duodenal ulcer, acid dyspepsia, pyrosis.

Supply: CREMO CARBONATES—Bottles of 12 oz.

Administration: ½–2 fl. dr. in water; increased if necessary; three to seven times daily.

CREOSOTIDE (Nelson, Baker)

Phthisis Therapy

Chemical Name: Creosote Iodide.

Composition: A compound containing about 25% of Iodine in combination with Phenols, Guaiacol, Cresol and other constituents of beechwood creosote.

Description: A brownish powder of mild creosote odor and taste.

Action and Uses: Upon decomposition in the gastrointestinal tract the iodine is liberated, absorbed and excreted through the urinary tract, while the creosote component is eliminated through the respiratory mucosa. *For use* as disinfectant, antiseptic and iodine therapy in chronic pulmonary disease, tuberculosis, tubercular adenitis; in hypertrophic goitre and intestinal fermentation.

Supply: CREOSOTIDE—Tablets, Chocolate coated, gr ¼ (0.016 Gm)—Bottles of 100, 500 and 1,000 gr ½ (0.032 Gm)—Bottles of 100, 500 and 1,000.

Combinations: **CREOSOTIDE AND BISMUTH COMPOUND**—Tablets containing

	Gr	Gm
Creosotide	¼	0.016
Bismuth Subnitrate	2	0.130
Pepsin 1:3,000	1	0.064

Chocolate coated—Bottles of 100, 500 and 1,000.

CREOSOTIDE AND PEPSIN COMPOUND—Tablets containing

	Gr	Gm
Creosotide	¼	0.016
Ext. Nux Vomica	⅛	0.008
Pepsin 1:3,000	1	0.064

Chocolate coated—Bottles of 100, 500 and 1,000.

CREOSOTIDE AND STRYCHNINE—Tablets containing

	Gr	Gm
Creosotide	¼	0.016
Strychnine Sulphate	1/80	0.0008

Chocolate coated—Bottles of 100, 500 and 1,000.

CREOSOTIDE, IRON AND ARSENIC—Tablets containing

	Gr	Gm
Creosotide	¼	0.016
Reduced Iron	1	0.064
Arsenic Trioxide	1/60	0.001

Chocolate coated (s-c)—Bottles of 100, 500 and 1,000.

CREOSOTIDE BRONCHIAL SEDATIVE—containing per ounce:

Creosotide	gr 2 (0.130 Gm)
Guaiacol	gr 2 (0.130 Gm)
Syrup Wild Cherry	dr. 1
Aromatics, etc.	q.s.

Supply—Bottles of 1 pt., 1 gal.

Administered: 1 tablet or 1 teaspoonful every 4 hr., or in accordance with requirements.

CREO-TERPIN (Wampole)

Expectorant

Composition: Contains per fluid ounce:

Chloroform	m 1 (0.06 cc)
Creosote	m 2 (0.12 cc)
Terpin Hydrate	gr 2 (0.130 Gm)
Calcium Glycerophosphate	gr 4 (0.259 Gm)
Sodium Glycerophosphate	gr 4 (0.259 Gm)
Alcohol	25%

Action and Uses: A stimulating expectorant for coughs and colds, to allay bronchial irritation; *Used* in chronic bronchitis and various other respiratory affections.

Supply: CREO-TERPIN—Bottles 3, 10 oz. and 1 gal.

Administration: ½ teaspoonful every 20–30 min.; children 10–15 drops.

CUPRIFERRUM (Squibb)

Hematinic

Description: A mixture of copper and iron in suitable vehicle.

Composition:

		Mg	
Tablets	Copper	0.5	per tablet
	Iron	30	
Syrup	Copper	0.5	per teaspoonful
	Iron	12.5	
Elixir	Copper	0.5	per teaspoonful
	Iron	12.5	

Action and Uses: As hematinic in secondary anemias, nutritional anemias in children and idiopathic hematopoietic disturbances.

Supply: CUPRIFERRUM—Tablets—Chocolate coated—Bottles 100, 1,000 for adults and older children only.

CUPRIFERRUM—Syrup—Bottles of 16 fl. oz.; intended primarily for children.

CUPRIFERRUM—Elixir—Bottles 16 fl. oz., for adults.

Administration: SYRUP OF CUPRIFERRUM—½–1 teaspoonful, one to three times daily after meals.

ELIXIR, CUPRIFERRUM—1–2 teaspoonfuls, one to three times daily after meals.

TABLETS, CUPRIFERRUM—1 or 2 tablets, one to three times daily after meals.

Bibliography: *See Chap. XII.*

DERMOCAINE (Walker Pharmacal)

Antiseptic

Composition:

	Parts
Bismuth subnitrate	12.5
Benzocaine	3.0
Zinc oxide	12.5
Acid salicylic	1.0
Liq. potassii arsenitis	0.2
Thuja occidentalis	1.0
Amylum	12.5
Petrolatum	q.s. 100.0

Action and Uses: Antiseptic and antipruritic for the relief of itching and dermatitis of athlete's foot (epidermophytosis); also used as local analgesic and soothing agent in eczema, impetigo, parasitic lesions, pruritus.

Supply: DERMOCAINE—Jars 2 oz.

Administration: Applied locally three times daily or as required.

DEXTRETTES "ESKAY"

(Smith, Kline and French)

Reduction Therapy

Composition: Tablets containing Dextrose gr 30 (1.94 Gm) and Magnesium Oxide gr ½ (0.32 Gm).

Action and Uses: To overcome material craving for carbohydrates and thus to facilitate reduction therapy. *Used* in obesity, also in circulatory and digestive disturbances in addition to dietary regime.

Supply: DEXTRETTES "ESKAY"—Tablets—Packages of 100.

Administration: 1 Tablet every half hour between meals, beginning 1 hr. after a meal and stopping 1 hr. before the next; a special diet schedule with "Eskay's Dextrettes" is recommended.

Bibliography: *See Chap. XII.*

DIALKALOS

(Sharp and Dohme)

Uric Acid Eliminant

Official Name: Lithium and Formamine Co.

Composition: Contains:

	Gr	Gm
Caffeine	½	0.032
Potassium Bicarbonate	5	0.324
Lithium Carbonate	2½	0.162
Potassium Phosphate	5	0.324
Formamine	2½	0.162

Action and Uses: As uric acid eliminant in gout, rheumatism and urinary affections; in prophylaxis against kidney infection in scarlet fever, typhoid and other bacterial diseases.

Supply: DIALKALOS—Bottles of 4 oz. and 1 lb.

Administration: 1 tablespoonful in water, two or three times daily after meals.

DIASYSTOL

(Rorer)

Hypotensor

Composition: Each fluid dram represents:

	M	Cc
Tr. passiflora	2.8	0.17
Tr. aconite	2.8	0.17
Tr. veratrum	2.8	0.17

Action and Uses: As hypotensor *for use* in hypertension, irritable heart, valvular disorders, arteriosclerosis.

Supply: DIASYSTOL—Bottles 14 oz., 5 pt., 1 gal.

Administration: 1 teaspoonful, three to four times daily.

DI-EFRIN

(Buffington)

Expectorant

Official Name: Syrupus Ephedra Vulgaris Co.

Composition: Each ounce represents

Ephedra vulgaris	gr 30	(1.944 Gm)
Wild cherry	gr 10	(0.643 Gm)
Squill	gr 1	(0.064 Gm)
Horehound	gr 1	(0.064 Gm)
Ammon. chloride	gr 1	(0.064 Gm)
Ethylmorphine HCl	gr ¼	(0.016 Gm)
Potassium guaiacol sulphonate	gr 8	(0.512 Gm)
Alcohol	3%	

Action and Uses: As bronchial sedative and expectorant in asthma, bronchitis and upper respiratory catarrh.

Supply: **DI-EFRIN**—Bottles of 3 oz., 1 pt., 1 gal.

Administration: 1–2 teaspoonfuls as required.

DINITRENAL CAPSULES (Drug Products)

Reduction Therapy

Composition: Each capsule represents:

	Gr	Gm
Dinitrophenol sodium	1½	0.096
Suprarenal, desiccated	⅛	0.008
Carbo vegetalis	q.s.	

Action and Uses: To stimulate metabolism in the reduction treatment of the obese.

Supply: **DINITRENAL**—Capsules—Bottles of 20 in packages of 20 bottles; Bottles of 100 in packages of 20 bottles.

Administration: 1 or 2 capsules daily with meals, with water; increased cautiously to 3–4 capsules a day.

DIOVIBURNIA (Dios Chemical)

Antispasmodic

Composition: Contains per ounce.

Viburnum Prunifolium	¾ dr.
Viburnum Opulus	¾ dr.
Dioscorea Villosa	¾ dr.
Aletris Farinosa	¾ dr.
Helonias Dioica	¾ dr.
Mitchella Repens	¾ dr.
Caulophyllum Thalictroides	¾ dr.
Scutellaria Lateriflora	¾ dr.
Alcohol	18%
Aromatic Elixirs	q.s.

Action and Uses: Antispasmodic, uterine tonic and alterative in dysmenorrhea, menorrhagia, uterine subinvolution, menopause and threatened abortion.

Supply: **DIOVIBURNIA**—Bottles of 10 oz.

Administration: 1 dessertspoonful in water three times daily after meals.

DISKETS ALKALINE (Lilly)

Alkalizer

Composition: Per disket:

	Gr	Gm
Sodium bicarbonate	15	0.972
Potassium bicarbonate	15	0.972
Calcium glycerophosphate	5	0.324
Magnesium sulphate	2½	0.162
Sodium chloride	4	0.259
Effervescent base	q.s.	

Action: Antacid; is more acceptable to some because of effervescence.

Uses: For oral alkalization in acidosis of acute infectious diseases, cyclic vomiting in children; also in gastric acid fermentation and urine hyperacidity.

Supply: DISKETS ALKALINE—Vials of 25, hermetically sealed.

Administration: 1 disket in glass of water, repeated as necessary.

DISKETS BROMIDES (Lilly)

Sedative

Composition: Contains per disket:

	Gr	Gm
Potassium bromide	6	0.384
Sodium bromide	6	0.384
Ammonium bromide	3	0.194
Effervescent base	q.s.	

Action and Uses: Effervescent hypnotic and sedative; *For use* in cases where bromides are indicated: insomnia, restlessness, hysteria, seasickness, functional hypertension, nervous palpitation, epilepsy.

Supply: DISKETS BROMIDES—Vials of 25, hermetically sealed.

Administration: 1 disket dissolved in water.

DISKETS SODIUM BROMIDE COMPOUND (Lilly)

Sedative

Composition: Contains per disket:

	Gr	Gm
Sodium bromide	15½	1.0
Sodium bicarbonate	15½	1.0
Sodium phosphate (dibasic)	15½	1.0
Effervescent base	q.s.	

Action and Uses: An effervescent, palatable, hypnotic, sedative and mild laxative; *useful* in milder cases of nausea of pregnancy; in migraine; in nervous cases with gastric distress without demonstrable organic lesions; in vasomotor instability; also in hyperthyroidism, menopause, dysmenorrhea and hypertension.

Supply: DISKETS SODIUM BROMIDE COMPOUND—Tablets—Vials of 25, hermetically sealed.

Administration: 1 disket in ½ glass of water on empty stomach; repeated in 1 hr.

Bibliography: *See Chap. XII.*

DISKETS SODIUM SALICYLATE COMPOUND (Lilly)

Antiarthritic

Composition: Contains per disket:

	Gr	Gm
Sodium salicylate	10	0.643
Sodium bicarbonate	20	1.296
Effervescent base	q.s.	

Action and Uses: Antipyretic, analgesic, antirheumatic; *For use* in tonsillitis, rheumatic affections and as cholagogue in various biliary disturbances.

Contraindications: Nephritis; salicylate idiosyncrasy.

Supply: **DISKETS SODIUM SALICYLATE COMPOUND**—Vials of 25, hermetically sealed.

Administration: 1–2 diskets in glass of warm water every 2 or 3 hr., repeated as necessary.

DIUROL (Sharp and Dohme)

Diuretic

Composition: Contains per fluid ounce:

	Gr	Gm
Buchu	16	1.024
Triticum	16	1.024
Saw palmetto	16	1.024
Hydrangea	16	1.024
Pichi	16	1.024
Hyoscyamus	2	0.130
Potassium bicarbonate	8	0.512
Lithium benzoate	4	0.259

Action and Uses: A soothing alkaline diuretic for the relief of vesical and renal disturbances and conditions where diuresis is desired.

Supply: **DIUROL**—Bottles of 1 pt., 1 gal.

Administration: 2–4 fl. dr.—three or four times daily.

DYSCO (Abbott)

Antispasmodic

Composition: Each tablet contains:

	Gr	Gm
Ephedrine hydrochloride	1/8	0.008
Amidopyrine	1½	0.09
Aromatics	q.s.	

Action and Uses: Analgesic, antispasmodic, sympathetic stimulant; *For use* in conditions where relaxation of smooth musculature is desired, and to relieve pain in dysmenorrhea.

Supply: **DYSCO**—Tablets—Tins of 12—Bottles of 100, 1,000.

Administration: Initial dose 2 tablets, continued with 1 tablet every 4–6 hr.

Bibliography: *See Chap. XII.*

DYSMENATONE (Norwich)

Uterine Sedative

Composition: Contains per tablet:

	Gr	Gm
Ovarian Substance	1	0.064
Thyroid	1/4	0.016
Calcium Glycerophosphate	1	0.064
Blaud's mass	1	0.064
Strychnine Sulphate	1/120	0.0005
Arsenous Acid	1/80	0.008

Action and Uses: As uterine sedative in amenorrhea, dysmenorrhea, menopause and ovarian dysfunction.

Supply: DYSMENATONE—Tablets—Bottles 100, 1,000 and 5,000.

Administration: 1 or 2 tablets three times daily.

ELIXIR ARSYLENE COMPOSITUM (Roche)

Reconstructive. Tonic

Composition: Contains per fluid ounce:

Ext. Kolae, glycerinat. sacch., equiv. to Sem. Kolae	gr 90	(5.731 Gm)
Arsylene (Natrium-allyl-arsonat.)	gr 1/4	(0.016 Gm)
Ext. Nucis Vomicae	gr 1/7	(0.009 Gm)
Natrium Biphosphoricum	gr 18	(1.166 Gm)
Manganese	gr 1/10	(0.006 Gm)
Alcohol	3.5%	
Elix. Aromat. (Roche)	q.s.	

Description: Arsylene, the chief constituent, is an organic arsenical compound, containing an unsaturated allyl radicle and is adapted in arsenical therapeusis over an extended period.

Action and Uses: Improves general tone and resistance; restores appetite in impaired digestion; *For use* in anemia and low bodily resistance; for hastening convalescence after operation; restoring strength after colds, grippe and influenza; for debility in chronic diseases, physical and mental depression.

Advantages: Is devoid of the garlic like odor of cacodylates objectionable to many; is readily oxidized and of low toxicity.

Supply: ELIXIR ARSYLENE COMPOSITUM—Bottles of 6 oz.

Administration: 1–2 teaspoonfuls, three times daily, before meals.

ELIXIR BARMIVAL (Fraser)

Sedative

Composition: Each dram represents Brom isolvaleryl hydroxybenzylmalonylurea gr 1 (0.064 Gm), in stable, palatable liquid form.

Action and Uses: Sedative and hypnotic; *For use* in hysteria, neurasthenia, neuroses, insomnia and menopausal excitation.

Supply: ELIXIR BARMIVAL—Bottles of 1 pt. and 1 gal.

Administration: 1 teaspoonful one or two times daily.

ELIXIR BROMO VALERIANATE (Anglo-French)

Sedative

Description: An odorless, tasteless valerian preparation.

Composition: Contains per tablespoonful:

	Gr	Gm
Extract valerian	4	0.259
Valerianic acid	1	0.064
Strontium bromide	4	0.259

Action and Uses: Nerve tonic and sedative *for use* in functional nervous disorders as hysteria, neurasthenia, nervous irritability and insomnia.

Supply: ELIXIR BROMO VALERIANATE—Bottles of 17.5 cc.

Administration: 1 teaspoonful three times daily in water.

ELIXIR DIGITALIN COMPOUND (Nelson, Baker)

Stimulant

Composition: Each fluid ounce represents:

	Gr	Gm
Digitalin	8/100	0.005
Strychnine sulphate	8/50	0.010
Nitroglycerin	8/100	0.005

Action and Uses: As stimulant in shock, cardiac depression, acute heart failure.

Supply: ELIXIR DIGITALIN COMPOUND—Bottles 1 pt., 1 gal.

Administration: *Average Dose*—1 dr. orally.

ELIXIR I.A.S. (Fougera)

Hematinic

Composition:

	Gr	Gm
Iron	5	0.324
Arsenic	1/100	0.00065
Strychnine	1/65	0.001
Copper (catalyst)	Traces	

Action and Uses: Palatable tonic *for use* in anorexia, debility, convalescence, asthenia; as hematinic—in secondary anemias, chronic malaria, arthritis, osteitis deformans.

Supply: ELIXIR I.A.S.—Bottles of 6 oz.

Administration: 1 teaspoonful, four times daily after meals.

ELIXIR MA HUANG (McNeil)

Antispasmodic

Composition: Each ounce represents:
Ma Huang (Ephedra vulgaris) 240 gr (15.5 Gm), standardized to contain 0.25 Gm ephedrine per 100 cc.

Action and Uses: Antispasmodic and decongestive in hay fever, dysmenorrhea, spasmodic coughs.

Supply: **ELIXIR MA HUANG**—Bottles of 2, 3, 4 oz., 1 pt., ½ and 1 gal.

Administration: 1–2 teaspoonfuls, as often as required.

EMMENAGOGUE (Medicone)

Uterine Stimulant

Composition: Each pill represents—

	Gr	Gm
Yohimbin	1/16	0.004
Aloes	1½	0.09
Reduced iron	3/5	0.036
Asafetida	2	0.13

Action and Uses: Indicated in amenorrhea and dysmenorrhea.

Supply: **EMMENAGOGUE**—Pills—Boxes of 24.

Administration: 3 or 4 pills after meals for 1 day only.

EMULSION OF COD LIVER OIL

Nutritive Tonic

Description: Emulsion of Cod Liver Oil standardized for vitamin content of not less than 140 U.S.P. vitamin A units and 70 A.D.M.A. vitamin D units per gram.

Action and Uses: As for cod liver oil; is pleasant tasting, easily digested and *most useful* for children and adults who cannot take plain cod liver oil.

Supply: **EMULSION COD LIVER OIL**—Containing (McKesson and Robbins) Norwegian cod liver oil with Sodium and Calcium Hypophosphites, 4 gr (0.259 Gm) of each per ounce—Bottles of 8 and 16 oz.

SCOTT'S EMULSION OF COD LIVER OIL (C.A.)— (Scott and Bowne) Containing Scott's cod liver oil, of potencies, vitamin A 140 units (U.S.A.), vitamin D 70 units (A.D.MA.), per Gm.

Administration: 3 Tablespoonfuls per day, equivalent to at least 6,300 U.S.P. vitamin A units and 3,450 A.D.M.A. vitamin D units.

ENDOMIN TABLETS (Reed and Carnrick)

Hematinic

Composition: Each tablet represents in lipoid soluble form:

	Mg
Iron	8.0
Copper	0.6
Manganese	0.4
Zinc	0.3
Nickel	0.03
Cobalt	0.03
Sodium Germanate	0.05

Action and Uses: Stimulates red blood cell formation; is non-irritating and readily assimilable; *For use* in various types of secondary anemia, especially those with gastric symptoms.

Supply: **ENDOMIN**—Tablets—Bottles of 100, 500 and 1,000.

Administration: 1–3 tablets, three times daily.

Bibliography: *See Chap. XII.*

ENTACARB (Reed and Carnrick)

Alkalizer

Composition: Each tablet represents:

	Gr	Gm
Sodium bicarbonate	5	0.31
Calcium carbonate	½	0.03
Potassium carbonate	¼	0.016
Magnesium carbonate	¼	0.016

Action and Uses: An alkalizer; each tablet is protected by a coating resistant to the gastric secretion, passes through the stomach unchanged without causing local disturbances, disintegrating only in the duodenum and other parts of the intestine; is absorbed there and produces general systemic alkalization. *For use* in prophylaxis and treatment of acidosis, of colds, various infections, pregnancy; also in cystitis, nephritis, diabetes, rheumatic conditions and urticaria.

Supply: ENTACARB—Tablets, Enteric coated—Boxes of 75, 500, 1,000.

Administration: 2 or more tablets every 2–3 hr. as required.

ENTERI-DRASTIS (Westerfield)

Astringent

Description: An enteric coated tablet of Hydrastis, each gr 2 (0.13 Gm).

Action and Uses: Soothing, tonic and astringent in colitis and entero-colitis.

Administration: 2 tablets, three times daily, as long as necessary.

Supply: ENTERI-DRASTIS—Tablets—Bottles of 100, 500 and 1,000.

ENZYMATASE (Schieffelin)

Digestive

Description: An agreeable, palatable elixir containing per dram:

	Gr	Gm
Pepsin	1	0.06
Diastase	1	0.06
Aromatics		

Action and Uses: As digestive in gastrointestinal disorders, in protein and starch indigestion; as vehicle for iodides, bromides, salicylates.

Supply: ENZYMATASE—Bottles of 1 pt., 1 gal.

Administration: 1–2 teaspoonfuls after meals.

EUPHORBIA COMPOUND SYRUP (Sharp and Dohme)

Sedative Expectorant

Official Name: Syrupus Euphorbia Co.

Composition: Each fluid ounce contains:

Tr. euphorbia	m 120	(7.776 cc)
Syrup squills	m 180	(11.664 cc)
Wine ipecac	m 30	(1.944 cc)
Jamaica dogwood	gr 16	(1.00 cc)

Menthol	gr	⅛	(0.008 Gm)
Chloroform	m	2	(0.130 cc)
Syrup tolu	q.s.		

Action and Uses: A palatable sedative and expectorant; relieves cough, dyspnea, spasm; *useful* in spasmodic asthma, asthmatic bronchitis and other respiratory affections with spasmodic cough and irritation.

Supply: EUPHORBIA COMPOUND SYRUP—Bottles 1 pt. and 1 gal.

Administration: 1–2 teaspoonfuls, repeated in 2 hr. if needed.

EPHCABEN (Kretchmar)

Antiasthmatic

Composition: Each tablet represents

	Gm	Gr
Ephedrine	0.025	⅜
Calcium lactate	0.050	¾
Benzyl succinate	0.100	1½
Amidopyrine	0.100	1½
Theophylline	0.050	¾

Action and Uses: In bronchial asthma as prophylactic.

Supply: EPHCABEN—Tablets, 0.3 Gm—Vials of 20.

Administration: To prevent an attack, 1 or 2 tablets are given daily or every second day; in nocturnal types—is administered at bedtime; where attack is not aborted dosage is repeated in ½ hr. and continued with 1 tablet at longer intervals until relief is obtained.

EPHEDRINE AND AMYTAL (Lilly)

Sedative

Composition: Each pulvule contains:

	Gr	Gm
Ephedrine sulphate	⅜	0.025
Amytal	¾	0.048

Action and Uses: As sedative and antispasmodic for bronchial spasm and congestion in asthma and hay fever; also as sedative and hypnotic in nervous conditions indicated.

Supply: EPHEDRINE AND AMYTAL—Pulvules—Bottles of 40, 500.

Administration: 1 pulvule three times daily before meals.
To abort attack of asthma—1–2 pulvules before retiring.

EPHETAL TABLETS (Abbott)

Antispasmodic

Composition: Each tablet contains

	Gr	Gm
Ephedrine hydrochloride	⅜	0.024
Phenobarbital	¼	0.016

Action and Uses: Combines the physiologic effect of ephedrine with the mild sedative action of a small dose of phenobarbital. *For use* in asthma, hay fever and various allergies.

Supply: EPHETAL—Tablets—Bottles of 40, 100, 500.

Administration: 1–2 tablets every 2–4 hr. as needed.

ETHYL MORPHINE AND EPHEDRINE COMPOUND

(Abbott)

Expectorant

Composition: Each fluid ounce represents:

Ephedrine Hydrochloride	gr 1/16	(0.004 Gm)
Fl. Extr. Ipecac	m 1	(0.064 cc)
Ethyl Morphine Hydrochloride	gr 1/32	(0.002 Gm)
Chloroform	gr 1/8	(0.008 Gm)
Thyme and menthol	q.s.	

Action and Uses: *Used* as sedative expectorant in spasmodic coughs and colds.

Supply: ETHYL MORPHINE AND EPHEDRINE COMPOUND—Bottles 4 and 16 oz.

Administration: 1 teaspoonful four to eight times daily; children 1/4–1/2 teaspoonful four to eight times daily.

EUPHILLANA

(Norwich)

Expectorant

Composition: Each fluid ounce represents:

Tincture Euphorbia Pilulifera	120 m	(7.776 cc)
Tincture Cocillana	40 m	(2.592 cc)
Syrup Wild Lettuce	120 m	(7.776 cc)
Cascarin "Norwich"	8 gr	(0.52 cc)
Syrup Squill compound	24 m	(1.60 cc)
Menthol and Aromatics	q.s.	
Alcohol	5%	

Action and Uses: Expectorant in bronchial affections.

Supply: EUPHILLANA—Bottles 1 pt.

EUPHILLANA WITH DIONIN—(Gr 1/4 to 1 oz.)—Bottles 1 pt.

Administration: 1–2 teaspoonfuls every 4 hr.

EUPHYDIGTAL

(Hurst)

Diuretic. Vasodilator

Composition: A combination of Metaphyllin (Aminophyllin) with Digitalis.

Action and Uses: Powerful diuretic and cardiac stimulant without the constrictive effect on coronary vessels of digitalis when administered alone; stimulates excretion of urinary chlorides and nitrogenous products. *For use* in coronary disease, arteriosclerosis, hypertension, cardiorenal edema.

Supply: EUPHYDIGTAL—Tablets, containing 0.1 Gm Metaphyllin and 0.1 Gm (150 frog doses) fol. Digitalis—Tubes of 20.

EUPHYDIGTAL—Suppositories, containing 0.2 Gm Metaphyllin and 0.15 Gm (225 frog doses) fol. Digitalis—Cartons of 6 and 12.

Administration: 1–2 tablets three to four times daily.
2–3 suppositories daily.

EVACUANT (Medicone)

Biliary Laxative

Composition: Each pill represents—

	Gr	Gm
Aloin	¼	0.016
Podophyllin	⅙	0.012
Sodium benzyl succinate (Mobenate)	½	0.032
Bile salts compound	4	0.259

Action and Uses: Cholagogue and choleretic, inhibiting putrefaction; *For use* in spastic constipation, in habitual constipation with biliary insufficiency.

Supply: EVACUANT—Pills—Boxes of 50.

Administration: 1 or 2 pills at bedtime.

EXTRALIN (Lilly)

Liver-Stomach Concentrate

Description: A preparation of liver or its extracts with ground fresh hog stomach tissue or extract; is suitably treated for oral administration; is standardized, tasteless and easily administered.

Action and Uses: As hematopoietic in specific oral therapy of pernicious anemia.

Advantages: Three times as potent as Cohn Fraction G (Liver Extract 343) and other liver extracts; permits the use of smaller dosage.

Supply: EXTRALIN (C.A.)—Pulvules 0.5 Gm—Bottles of 84 and 500.

Administration: In Relapse—4 pulvules three times a day; maintenance dose—3 pulvules three times a day.

Bibliography: *See Chap. XII.*

FELAMINE (Sandoz)

Cholagogue

Description: A molecular association of crystalline Cholic Acid and Methenamine.

Action: Cholagogue, biliary and urinary antiseptic; favors fat digestion and intestinal peristalsis; its laxative effect is due to the cholic acid.

Uses: *Used* in hepatic dysfunction and bile tract infections; in catarrhal jaundice and chronic constipation; as biliary disinfectant after abdominal operations and in typhoid fever; during and after pregnancy to stimulate liver function.

Supply: FELAMINE—Tablets, Sugar coated, 5 gr (0.3 Gm)—Bottles 50 and 250.

Administration: Biliary Disease—Acute, 2–3 tablets, three times daily.

Chronic, 1–2 tablets, three times daily for several weeks, repeated several times a year.

Constipation—2 tablets, three times daily, reduced to 4 a day; given for 2 weeks each month.

Enterocolitis—2 tablets, three times daily.

Bibliography: *See Chap. XII.*

FELSOL (American Felsol)

Antispasmodic

Composition: Each powder contains:

	Gm
Metozin	0.9
Phenazone	0.25
Anilipyrine	0.4
Iodopyrin	0.25
Caffeine	0.1
Digitalis and Strophanthus glucosides	0.0015
Lobelia Inflata Alkaloid	0.005

Description: A colorless crystalline powder of acid reaction and somewhat bitter but not unpleasant taste; is especially soluble in warm water.

Action and Uses: Stimulates the respiratory center by action of its lobelia; tones the heart with its caffeine, digitalis and strophanthus; is analgesic, antipyretic and sedative to the nervous system through the medium of its anilipyrine. Is not cumulative and may be taken for long periods without after effect. *For use* in bronchial and cardiac asthma, as prophylactic or for treatment; in hay fever, chronic bronchitis, spasmodic or convulsive cough; in angina pectoris and neuralgic headache.

Supply: FELSOL—Powders 15 gr (1 Gm)—Boxes of 15 and 90.

Administration: Adults—1 powder 1–3 times daily in water or followed by drink; if attack is very severe, first dosage is followed by a second in ½ hr.
Children—¼–½ the full dose, given in sweetened lukewarm water.

Bibliography: *See Chap. XII.*

FER-IODINE (C. D. Smith)

Oral Diabetic Therapy

Composition: Per tablet:

Iron arsenate	gr 1/200 (0.0003 Gm)
Phosphoric acid	gr 1/200 (0.0003 Gm)
Syzygium powder (Jambul)	gr 2 (0.130 Gm)
Tr. iodine carbolized	m 1

Action and Uses: Has inhibitory effect on diastatic fermentation, affecting excess sugar formation and excretion; tonic, stomachic and hematinic; *For use* in diabetes, flatulent diarrhea and certain skin diseases, connected with carbohydrate metabolism.

Supply: FER-IODINE—Tablets—Bottles of 500.

Administration: 1–2 tablets every 2 hr.

FERRI-QUIN (McNeil)

Hematinic

Description: An apple-green, odorless, astringent and bitter tasting powder containing

	Gr	Gm
Iron Phosphate	1	0.064
Quinine Phosphate	½	0.032
Strychnine Phosphate	1/64	0.001

Action and Uses: A tonic, nervine and hematinic in secondary anemia and convalescence.

Supply: FERRI-QUIN—Capsules—Bottles of 100, 500, 1,000 and 5,000.

Administration: 1 or 2 capsules two or three times daily after meals.

FERRO-CU-MANG (Drug Products)

Hematinic

Description: A combination of Colloidal Iron, Colloidal Copper and Colloidal Manganese in palatable form; is non-astringent, non-toxic.

Action and Uses: Increases red cell count and hemoglobin; *For use* in secondary anemia.

Supply: FERRO-CU-MANG—Solution, containing per fluid ounce:

	Mg
Iron colloidal	112.5
Copper colloidal	1.125
Manganese colloidal	37.5
Beef peptone, glycerine and aromatics	

Bottles of 8 oz., 1 pt., 1 gal.

FERRO-CU-MANG—Pulvoids, Sugar coated, each containing:

	Mg
Iron colloidal	14
Copper colloidal	0.14
Manganese colloidal	4.70

Bottles of 100 and 1,000.

FECUMN—Hyposols, 5 cc containing:

	Mg
Iron colloidal	4
Copper colloidal	1
Manganese colloidal	1.5
Isotonic solution	q.s. 5 cc

Boxes of 12, 25 and 100.

Administration: *Solution*—1–2 fl. dr. after meals, in milk or water.
Pulvoids—2–4 three times daily after meals.
Hyposols—*Intravenously* or *intragluteally*, twice weekly.

FERRO-COP (Strasenburgh)

Hematinic

Composition: Each tablet represents:

	Gr	Gm
Copper	1/200	0.0003
Iron (ferrous)	1/4	0.016

Action and Uses: A carbohydrate free hematinic; *For use* in secondary, nutritional and other anemias.

Supply: FERRO-COP—Tablets—Bottles of 500, 1,000.

Administration: 1–3 tablets three times daily; children in accordance with age.

FERRO-MANGAN PEPTONIZED (Reinschild)

Hematinic

Official Name: Liquor Ferro-Mangan Peptonatis "Dieterich"

Composition:

	Per Cent
Iron	0.6
Manganese peptonate	0.1
Alcohol	10

Action and Uses: Stable, palatable, hematinic and digestant; non-injurious to teeth; *For use* in various types of anemia.

Supply: FERRO-MANGAN PEPTONIZED—Bottles 10 oz.

Administration: 1 tablespoonful three to four times daily, in water or milk. Children 1 teaspoonful, three times daily.

FERRO-MANGANESE PEPTONATED (Sharp and Dohme)

Tonic

Composition: A liquid preparation of peptonized Albuminates of Iron and Manganese; contains Metallic Iron 1¾ gr (0.112 Gm), Manganese gr ¾ per fluid ounce (0.048 Gm); Alcohol 17%; palatable, readily assimilable and of neutral reaction.

Uses: As hematinic and tonic in anemia, chlorosis, general debility and convalescence.

Supply: FERRO MANGANESE PEPTONATED—Bottles 12 ounces and 1 gal.

FERRO MANGANESE PEPTONATED WITH ARSENIC—Containing 1/30 gr (0.00216 Gm) arsenic per ounce—Bottles 14 oz. and 1 gal.

Administration: 1 or 2 fl. dr. three times daily before or after meals.

FERRUGINOUS COMPOUND "FRAISSE" (Fougera)

Hematinic

Composition: Each ampule contains:

	Gr	Gm
Iron cacodylate	1/6	0.011
Sodium glycerophosphate	1½	0.10
Strychnine cacodylate	1/120	0.0005

Description: Stable, sterile, easily absorbed and non-irritating solution.

Action: Reconstructive and hematinic; stimulates blood generation.

Uses: Anemias of convalescence, pregnancy and rickets.

Supply: FERRUGINOUS COMPOUND "FRAISSE"—Ampules 1cc—Boxes of 12 and 50.

FERRUGINOUS COMPOUND "FRAISSE"—Solution—Oral—Bottles of 25 Gm.

Administration: *Subcutaneously or Intramuscularly*—1 ampule daily for 12 days; repeated after 5-day interval.

Orally—25 drops in sweetened water, daily, for 12 days; repeated after 5-day interval.

FIBROGEN LOCAL (Merrel)

Hemostatic

Description: A sterile suspension of tissue Fibrinogen prepared from lung tissue extract; contains 1.5% tissue fibrinogen (globulin phospholipin) and 0.5% cephalin preserved, in saline solution; is a gray yellow fluid, sterile, free from albuminous matter and physiologically standardized.

Action and Uses: Controls bleeding by promoting the formation of tough contractile clots; *Used* in surgical, traumatic, dental and other surface hemorrhages.

Supply: FIBROGEN LOCAL (C.A.)—Vials of 7 cc.

Administration: Undiluted, by tampon, gauze or is poured into wound and gentle pressure applied; in *dentistry*—saturated cotton pledget packed into tooth sockets.

Caution: Must be thoroughly agitated before use; must be kept in cool place, below 70°F.

FIBROGEN ORAL and SUBCUTANEOUS (Merrell)

Hemostatic

Description: A sterile suspension of purified tissue Fibrinogen and Cephalin, free from albumin or extraneous protein matter.

Action and Uses: A hemostatic *for use* in concealed hemorrhages, where topical application to site of hemorrhage cannot be made, as in pulmonary, gastric, intestinal and similar bleeding.

Supply: FIBROGEN—Oral—Vials 3 cc—Boxes of 4.

FIBROGEN—Subcutaneous—Ampules 2 cc—Packages of 4; Ampules 1 cc—Boxes of 6.

Administration: *Oral*—3–6 cc in 6–8 oz. of ice water on empty stomach.

Subcutaneous—2–4 cc into non-fatty tissue, repeated if necessary; *never intravenously.*

Contraindications: Not to be administered within 6 hr. before or after blood transfusion, or the injection of sera or vaccines.

Bibliography: *See Chap. XII.*

FIROLYPTOL (Tilden)

Tonic

Composition: Contains:

Eucalyptol	m 10	(0.643 cc)
Ol. gossypium purificat	oz. ½	(15.55 cc)
Firwein	oz. 1	(31.103 cc)

Action and Uses: Easily assimilated nutrient and roborant *for use* in respiratory diseases and tuberculosis.

Supply: FIROLYPTOL—Plain—Bottles of 16 oz. and 1 gal.

FIROLYPTOL WITH KRESOTE "TILDEN"— (Morson's White Label) Bottles of 16 oz. and 1 gal.

Administration: 1–2 teaspoonfuls three to four times daily after meals.

FORMOHYDRION (Upjohn)

Urinary Antiseptic

Composition: A granular effervescent salt containing per teaspoonful (gr 60):

	Gr	Gm
Acid Sodium Phosphate	20	1.296
Methenamine	5	0.324

Action and Uses: Urinary acidifier and antiseptic; a pleasant means of administering simultaneously hexamethylene tetramine with an acidifier; *For use* in urethritis, cystitis, pyelitis.

Supply: FORMOHYDRION—Bottles of 4 and 8 oz.

FORMOHYDRION—Tablets, gr 10 (Methenamine gr 5 and Acid Sodium Phosphate gr 5)—Bottles 100 and 1,000.

Administration: Dosage necessary to acidify urine, 1 heaping teaspoonful (60 gr) in 6 oz. water, five to eight times daily between meals; tablets—accordingly.

GALLO-BISMUTH COMPOUND (Nelson, Baker

Intestinal Astringent

Official Name: Mist. Bismuthi Subgallatis Comp.

Composition: Each fluid ounce represents:

	Gr	Gm
Bismuth Subgallate, superhydrated	8	0.518
Salol	1.6	1.036
Aromatics	q.s.	

Action and Uses: Intestinal sedative and astringent in diarrhea, intestinal fermentation, ulceration; may be used in combination with other similar preparations.

Supply: GALLO-BISMUTH COMPOUND—Bottles of 3 oz., 1 pt. and 1 gal.

Administration: Adults—1 tablespoonful; children—1 teaspoonful; infants—5–15 m per dose.

GALLO-GOGUE (Westerfield)

Cholagogue

Composition: Each tablet represents:

	Gr	Gm
Purified Oxgall	1	0.064
Acid Sodium Oleate	1	0.064
Phenolphthalein	1/3	0.021
Menthol	1/10	0.006
Sodium Salicylate	1½	0.097

Action and Uses: Cholagogue and biliary antiseptic in cholelithiasis, gall-bladder colic, hepatic congestion and constipation.

Supply: GALLO-GOGUE—Tablets—Bottles of 100, 500 and 1,000.

Administration: 1 or 2 tablets, four or five times daily.

GASTRON (Fairchild)

Digestant

Description: An aqueous 0.25% Hydrochloric Acid-Glycerin extract containing entire soluble contents of the fresh gastric mucosa, including: the pyloric portion, with amino-acids, colloidal proteins, activated enzymes, nitrogenous extractives, organic and inorganic cell principles; is alcohol and sugar free.

Action and Uses: An agreeable stomachic; standardized, 1 cc to digest 200 Gm coagulated egg-albumin; is *useful* in disorders of gastric function.

Supply: GASTRON—Bottles of 6 oz.

Dosage: 2–4 dr. after meals.

Combinations: GASTRON WITH IRON—Contains in addition ferric ammonium citrate gr 5 per tablespoonful; *For use* in anemias with lowered digestive function. *Dosage*—1 or 2 teaspoonfuls after meals.

GENITONE (Merrell)

Uterine Sedative

Composition:

Viburnum Prunifolium	64 gr	(4.00 Gm)
Senecio Aureus	40 gr	(2.592 Gm)
Passiflora Incarnata	80 gr	(5.184 Gm)
Pulsatilla	16 gr	(1.00 Gm)
Colorless Hydrastis	16 m	(1.00 cc)
Aromatic Cordial	q.s. ad. 1 fl. oz.	

Action and Uses: To restore normal uterine tone, relieve congestion, muscular spasm and nerve irritability; to check excessive bleeding in threatened abortion, in functional menorrhagia; to quiet abnormal uterine contractions.

Supply: GENITONE—Bottles of 16 oz.

Administration: 1–2 teaspoonfuls, three times daily.

GERMICIDAL DISCS (Parke, Davis)

Antiseptic

Description: Mercuric Iodide in disc form for the preparation of germicidal solutions; the discs are readily soluble in water.

Composition: *Small size:* to make 4 oz. of a 1:5,000 mercuric iodide solution:

	Gr	Gm
Mercuric Iodide	3/8	0.025
Potassium Iodide	3/8	0.025
Sodium Bicarbonate	q.s.	

Large size: to make 1 pt. of a 1:5,000 solution:

	Gr	Gm
Mercuric Iodide	1½	0.097
Potassium Iodide	1½	0.097
Sodium Bicarbonate	q.s.	

Action and Uses: Antiseptic and germicidal for topical use in various surgical conditions; for vaginal irrigation in dilution 1:20,000.

Supply: GERMICIDAL DISCS (C.A.)—Small size—Screw-cap vials of 25—Bottles of 100 and 500.

GERMICIDAL DISCS (C.A.)—Large size—Bottles of 25, 100 and 500.

Caution: To be used only for the preparation of antiseptic, germicidal solutions, which must be kept in closed vessels to prevent evaporation and alteration in concentration.

Advantages: The 1:5,000 solution does not coagulate tissue albumin or corrode steel or nickeled instruments.

GLYCANA (Schieffelin)

Tonic

Composition: Contains per ounce:

	Gr	Gm
Sodium Glycerophosphate	8	0.52
Calcium Glycerophosphate	8	0.52
Strychnine Glycerophosphate	1/15	0.004
Phosphoric Acid, sugar wine	q.s.	

Action and Uses: Appetizer and nerve tonic, in neuroses, debility, convalescence.

Supply: GLYCANA—Bottles 16 oz.

Administration: 1 dessertspoonful three times daily.

GLYCEROPHAN (Balmogen)

Tonic

Composition: Each fluid ounce represents:

	Gr	Gm
Calcium Glycerophosphate	10	0.64
Sodium Glycerophosphate	16	1.06
Iron Glycerophosphate	1½	0.09
Manganese Glycerophosphate	1	0.06
Quinine Glycerophosphate	½	0.03
Strychnine Glycerophosphate	1/16	0.004
Sherry Wine	q.s.	

Action and Uses: Nerve tonic and alterative in debility, convalescence, neuroses.

Supply: GLYCEROPHAN—Bottles 12 oz.

Administration: 1–2 teaspoonfuls three times daily, after meals. Children, in proportion to age.

GLYCO-CYPRESS (Irwin, Neisler)

Antispasmodic

Composition: Each fluid ounce represents:

	Gr	Gm
Menthol	⅕	0.013
Sodium Mono-benzyl-succinate	2½	0.162
Gelsemium	6	0.384
Cypress	q.s.	

Description: An opalescent, yellow-green fluid, of pleasant odor and flavor.

Action and Uses: Sedative and antispasmodic, *For relief* of spasm in whooping cough and bronchial asthma.

Supply: GLYCO-CYPRESS—Bottles of 1 gal.

Administration: 1–2 teaspoonfuls every 4–6 hr.

GLYKERON (Smith)

Sedative Expectorant

Composition: Contains per teaspoonful:

	Gr	Gm
Codeine phosphate	1/8	0.008
Hyoscyamus	1	0.064
Ammonium hypophosphite	3	0.193
Balsam tolu	1/4	0.016
White pine bark	3 1/2	0.224
Glycerine	q.s.	

Action and Uses: *For relief* of cough and pectoral pain, to promote bronchial secretion and allay irritation; as antispasmodic in asthma, pertussis, asthmatic bronchitis, laryngitis.

Supply: GLYKERON—Bottles 4 oz. and 16 oz.

Administration: Adults—1–2 teaspoonfuls every 2 or 3 hr, or as required. Children—10 drops to 1 teaspoonful.

GLYPECTUS (Schieffelin)

Expectorant

Composition: Contains per fluid ounce:

Syrup squill	160 m (7.776 Gm)
Syrup senega	8 m (0.490 Gm)
Syrup ipecac	20 m (1.296 Gm)
Syrup sanguinaria	10 m (0.648 Gm)
Syrup white pine	60 m (3.888 Gm)
Syrup wild cherry	90 m (5.832 Gm)
Chloroform (pure)	1 gr (0.064 Gm)
Honey and eucalyptol	q.s.

Description: A combination of expectorants in palatable form.

Action and Uses: Exerts soothing action on respiratory mucous membrane, liquefying thick tenacious mucus and promoting expectoration with relief of cough; *For use* in bronchial and laryngeal catarrh with irritating and painful coughs.

Supply: GLYPECTUS—Plain—Bottles of 1 pt.

GLYPECTUS WITH CODEIN—1 gr (0.06 Gm) per fluid ounce—Bottles of 1 pt.

Administration: 1–2 teaspoonfuls as required; children in proportion.

GRAVOCAIN (Metz)

Obstetric Spinal Anesthetic

Description: A 40% solution of Novocain with small amount of Strychnine; is specially prepared to have a higher specific gravity than spinal fluid and to be non-diffusible.

Action: Injected into spinal canal anesthetizes the pudendal and sacral plexuses and induces anesthesia of pelvic organs. Its viscosity prevents rapid diffusion in the spinal fluid, thus regulating the intensity and duration of anesthesia and diminishing the possibility of a rapid fall in blood pressure with resulting nausea, vomiting and other untoward symptoms.

Uses: Principally in obstetrics, for spinal anesthesia lasting about 3 1/2 hr.

Caution: To be used in primiparae *only* after cervix is fully dilated; in multiparae when cervix has opened 5–6 cm; must be injected while patient is in sitting position; if this is not feasible, the head and shoulders must be raised 15–20 deg.

Supply: GRAVOCAIN—Ampules, 0.75 cc, each containing 300 mg Novocain and 2.2 mg of Strychnin Sulphate—Packages of 5 ampules, with 5 ampules of Ephedrin-Novocain solution, the latter for controlling blood pressure and anesthetizing site of puncture.

GUAIACOSE (Winthrop)

Expectorant

Description: A combination of 7% Calcium Guaiacolsulphonate with Somatose; a dark brown liquid of agreeable taste and aromatic odor, freely miscible with water in all proportions.

Action: Its calcium guaiacolsulphonate component endows it with antiseptic and expectorant properties, but unlike creosote and guaiacol, is not toxic, does not irritate the gastrointestinal tract and is palatable; it reduces and liquefies secretions, deodorizes offensive sputum and controls putrefactive and fermentative processes; the somatose component adds nutrient, tonic and appetizing qualities to the preparation.

Uses: In all pulmonary affections—chronic bronchitis, tuberculosis, emphysema, whooping cough, measles, influenza.

Supply: GUAIACOSE—Bottles of 4 oz.

Administration: Adults—1 teaspoonful three or four times daily.
Children—½ teaspoonful in milk, cocoa and other fluids.

GUAIAPHEDRA SYRUP (McNeil)

Expectorant

Composition:

Potassium Guaiacol Sulphonate	gr 20	(1.29 Gm)
Ma Huang (Ephedra)	gr 120	(7.77 Gm)
Aromatics, Syrup	q.s.	1 oz.

Action and Uses: Expectorant, cough sedative and stimulant in bronchial affections, especially with spasmodic cough.

Supply: GUAIAPHEDRA SYRUP—Bottles of 2, 3, 4 and 16 oz., ½ and 1 gal.

Administration: 1–2 teaspoonfuls, as required.

GUAIAPHON (McNeil)

Expectorant

Description: Combinations containing Potassium Guaiacol Sulphonate.

Action and Uses: Cough sedative and expectorant in various pulmonary affections.

Combinations: SYRUP GUAIAPHON—Containing per fluid ounce:

	Gr	Gm
Potassium Guaiacol Sulphonate	40	2.592
Aromatics and Syrup	q.s.	

SYRUP GUAIAPHON WITH CODEINE SULPHATE—Gr ½ (0.032 Gm), per ounce.

SYRUP GUAIAPHON COMPOUND—(Non-narcotic) each fluid ounce represents:

Potassium Guaiacol Sulphonate	gr 8 (0.512 Gm)
Sodium Benzoate	gr 4 (0.259 Gm)
Syrup Squill	48 m (3.200 Gm)
Tincture Sanguinaria	48 m (3.200 Gm)
Chloroform	1 m (0.064 Gm)
Aromatics and syrup	q.s.

SYRUP GUAIAPHON COMPOUND 1—Same as above with Morphine Acetate 3/16 gr (0.012 Gm) per fluid ounce.

SYRUP GUAIAPHON COMPOUND 2—Same as Syrup Guaiaphon Compound with ½ gr (0.032 Gm) Codeine Sulphate per fluid ounce.

SYRUP GUAIAPHON COMPOUND 3—Same as Syrup Guaiaphon Compound with Codeine Sulphate gr 1 (0.064 Gm) per fluid ounce.

Supply: **SYRUP GUAIAPHON AND COMBINATIONS**—Bottles of 2, 3, 4, oz., 1 pt., ½ and 1 gal.

Administration: Adults, 1–2 teaspoonfuls; Children ½–1 teaspoonful, according to age; the Syrup Guaiaphon Compound—(Non-narcotic) Adults, 2–4 teaspoonfuls, Children ½–2 teaspoonfuls, according to age.

GUAIATONIC (Warner)

Tonic. Expectorant

Composition: Each fluid ounce represents:

Guaiacol Sulphonate	4 m	(0.259 cc)
Creosote Sulphonate	4 m	(0.259 cc)
Quinine Sulphate	½ gr	(0.032 Gm)
Strychnin Hypophosphite	1/32 gr	(0.002 Gm)
Hypophosphites of Iron, Calcium, Manganese, Potassium and Aromatics	q.s.	

Action and Uses: Tonic, alterative and expectorant *for use* in various bronchial, laryngeal and pulmonary disturbances.

Supply: GUAIATONIC—Bottles of 8 and 16 oz. and 1 gal.

Administration: 1 teaspoonful, three to four times daily.

HAIMASED (Tilden)

Vasodilator

Composition: Aromatic solution of Sodium Sulphocyanate, gr 2½ (0.162 Gm) to the dram.

Action and Uses: *For use* in reducing blood pressure and alleviating symptoms, as headache, nervousness, insomnia in hypertension; also as sedative and hypnotic.

Supply: HAIMASED—Bottles 8 and 16 oz.

Administration: 1 teaspoonful two to three times daily for 1 week, then on alternate days.

HALEY'S M-O (MAGNESIA-OIL) (Haley)

Laxative

Composition: Each tablespoonful contains:

Magma magnesia	3 dr
Petrolatum liquidum	1 dr

Description: An emulsion of milk of magnesia and pure mineral oil.

Action and Uses: Lubricates intestinal mucosa, allays irritation and inflammation, absorbs toxins, checks putrefaction, softens fecal material; *For use* in gastric hyperacidity, constipation, flatulence, enteritis, colitis, hemorrhoids, ulceration, fistula, fissure in ano and in pregnancy.

Supply: HALEY'S M-O—Bottles of 4, 8 oz.

Administration: 1–2 tablespoonfuls before breakfast and at bedtime.

HEMABOLOIDS (Arlington)

Hematinic

Description: An Organic Iron preparation in stable combination with Nucleoprotein; each tablespoonful, in addition to other ingredients, contains:

Iron	gr 0.92 (0.05 Gm)
Nucleoproteins	gr 9.6 (0.6 Gm)
Alcohol	17%

Action and Uses: Hematinic, increasing red cell count and hemoglobin; is readily assimilable, non-constipating, non-irritating. *For use* in anemia, chlorosis and other forms of blood impoverishment.

Supply: HEMABOLOIDS—Liquid—Bottles of 12 fl. oz.

HEMABOLOIDS—Tablets—Bottles of 50, 100.

Administration: 1 Tablespoonful or 2 tablets three to four times daily, increased if desired.

Combinations: HEMABOLOIDS ARSENIATED WITH STRYCHNIA—Contains Hemaboloids with gr 1/40 (0.0016 Gm) arsenious acid and strychnine gr 1/80 (0.0008 Gm) to the tablespoonful; *For use* in severer types of anemia. Dosage as for Hemaboloids.

HEMEC TABLETS (Schieffelin)

Hematinic

Composition: Contains per tablet:

	Gr	Gm
Hematin	1/2	0.032
Extr. nux vomica	1/20	0.003
Acid arsenous	1/36	0.0018
Oleoresin capsicum	1/720	0.00009
Extr. cascara sagrada	1/7	0.009
Aloin	1/45	0.0014

Action and Uses: Hematinic *for use* in anemia, chlorosis.

Supply: **HEMEC**—Tablets—Bottles of 100.

Administration: 1 or 2 tablets, three times daily after meals.

HEMOGLOBIN COMPOUND (Stoddard)

Hematinic

Composition: Contains per tablet:

	Gr	Gm
Hemoglobin	1	0.064
Iron peptonized	1	0.064
Ext. nux vomica	1/12	0.005
Kaskara (Stoddard)	1/4	0.016

Action and Uses: Non-astringent slightly laxative tonic; *For use* in anemia, chlorosis, amenorrhea, convalescence.

Supply: **HEMOGLOBIN COMPOUND**—Tablets—Bottles 100, 500 and 1,000.

Administration: 1–3 tablets at meals with water.

HEMO-NUCLEO-SPLEEN COMPOUND (Marvell)

Hematinic

Composition: Each capsule contains:

	Gr	Gm
Hemoglobin	4	0.259
Nucleinic acid	1/4	0.016
Spleen	1/8	0.008
Peptonized iron	1/4	0.016
Calcium glycerophosphate	1/4	0.016
Sodium glycerophosphate	1/4	0.016

Action: Hematinic, nervine tonic.

Uses: Secondary anemias of various origins and in convalescence.

Supply: **HEMO-NUCLEO-SPLEEN COMPOUND**—Capsules—Bottles of 50.

Administration: 3–6 capsules daily after meals.

HEMO-S (Chappel)

Hematinic

Description: A concentrate of all the water soluble secondary fractions of 450 Gm of fresh liver with its contained copper and of 520 mg of elementary iron in the form of a neutral semi-colloidal glycerol compound, in 8 oz. of defibrinated blood; alcohol 14½% as preservative.

Action and Uses: As hematopoietic to stimulate especially hemoglobin production in secondary anemias only: in infectious, toxic, hemorrhagic, hemolytic and other secondary anemias; as pre- and post-operative hematinic to favorably affect convalescence.

Supply: **HEMO-S**—Bottles of 8 oz.

Administration: 1 tablespoonful after meals, two to four times daily, taken plain, or in milk or fruit juices.

HEMO-VITOL (C. D. Smith)

Tonic

Composition: Contains per tablet—

	Gr	Gm
Calcium glycerophosphate	½	0.032
Hemoglobin	2	0.130
Iron albuminized	½	0.032
Nucleinic acid	1/20	0.003
Strychnine arsenate	1/200	0.0003

Action and Uses: Reconstructive, nerve and cell stimulant and hematinic in chlorosis, debility, neurasthenia and similar disturbances.

Supply: HEMO-VITOL—Tablets—Bottles of 1,000, 5,000.

HEMO-VITOL—Capsules, (double strength of tablets)—Bottles of 100, 500 and 1,000.

Administration: 2 Tablets or 1 capsule three times daily.

HEPATICON (United Laboratories)

Hematopoietic

Composition: Prepared from desiccated fetal calves' liver; 1 Gm is equivalent to 6 Gm of fresh liver substance.

Action and Uses: *For use* in pernicious anemia.

Supply: HEPATICON—Vials 4.5 Gm—Boxes of 12.

Administration: 1 vial twice daily.

HEPATONE (Sharp and Dohme)

Laxative

Official Name: Sodii Phosphas Effervescens Co.

Composition: Contains about 50% Sodium Phosphate, 3 gr (0.194 Gm) Phenolphthalein, 2 gr (0.130 Gm) Lithium Citrate to the ounce.

Action and Uses: A cholagogue-laxative devoid of objectionable taste; is effective eliminant in biliousness, jaundice and constipation, especially in children.

Administration: ½–1 tablespoonful well diluted in glassful of water ½ hr. before breakfast.

Supply: HEPATONE—Bottles of 5 oz.

HEPVISC (Anglo-French)

Hypotensive

Description: A combination of Mistletoe with Glandular Extracts each tablet containing—

	Gr	Gm
Viscum album extract	1¼	0.075
Hepatic extract	1¾	0.10
Pancreatic extract	⅞	0.05

Action and Uses: A symptomatic remedy for hypotensive, diuretic and antispasmodic uses in arteriosclerosis, arterial hypertension, albuminuria, congestion of heart, kidneys and of other abdominal organs.

Supply: HEPVISC—Bottles of 50.

Administration: 3–6 tablets daily, increased or decreased as necessary; given ½ hr. before meals, for 15–20 weeks; after interval of rest, course may be repeated.

Bibliography: *See Chap. XII.*

HEX-ARBUTIN (Searle)

Antiseptic

Composition: Contains per tablet—

	Gr	Gm
Methenamine	3	0.194
Arbutin	½	0.032
Ammonium benzoate	3	0.194

Action and Uses: Urinary antiseptic in various genito-urinary affections.

Supply: HEX-ARBUTIN—Tablets—Bottles of 1,000.

Administration: 1 tablet three times daily with water.

HOLADIN (Fairchild)

Digestant

Description: An extract of the entire pancreas with all its enzyme constituents.

Action and Use: Contains trypsin, amylopsin and lipase and is highly potent in its enzymatic action upon proteins, starches and fats, its diastasic action predominating. *For use* in assisting digestion in the feeble and convalescent.

Supply: HOLADIN—Capsules, gr 3—Bottles of 25 and 100.

Administration: One or more capsules after each meal and at bedtime.

Combination: HOLADIN AND BILE SALTS—Contains Holadin gr 2½, Bile salts gr ½. *Supply*—Capsules, Enteric coated—Bottles of 25 and 100. *Administration:* 1 or 2 capsules at bedtime and mornings before breakfast, with glass of water; *For use* where an additional laxative effect is desired.

HOMIODIN (American Bio-Chem.)

Iodine Therapy

Composition: 5% Sodium Iodide solution, containing traces of free iodine.

Action and Uses: Stimulates respiratory mucosa and affords relief in catarrhal and vasomotor rhinitis, catarrhal otitis media, bronchial catarrh, coryza.

Supply: HOMIODIN—Ampules, 1 cc—Boxes of 10 and 50.

Administration: *Subcutaneously*—1 cc. Infants—½ cc, given twice weekly, for 2–6 injections.

HYCLORITE (Bethlehem)

Antiseptic

Chemical Name: Sodium Hypochlorite Concentrated.

Description: A non-irritating, concentrated solution of chlorinated soda, of special alkalinity; contains over 3.85% available chlorine.

Composition:

	Per Cent
Sodium hypochlorite (NaOCl)	4.05
Sodium chloride	2.00
Calcium hydrate	0.14
Inert salts	1.30

Action: An antiseptic, deodorant and disinfectant; disintegrates necrosed tissue and promotes healthy granulation; does not precipitate proteins.

Uses: **Surgery**—Where Dakin solution is indicated: in bone suppurations, chronic ulcers, empyema, abdominal infections; in skin grafting and burns.

Laryngology—As spray, snuff or gargle—in suppurative nasal, throat and ear conditions; in purulent sinus disease and tonsillar infection.

Ophthalmology—In purulent conjunctivitis.

Urology—In acute and chronic gonorrhea; vaginitis and cystitis, chancroids and ulcers.

Dentistry—As oral cleanser after extraction; in the treatment of putrescent pulps, fistulae and pyorrhea alveolaris.

Supply: **HYCLORITE** (C.A.)—Bottles 2, 5, 10, 32 oz. and 1 gal.

Administration: As Dakin solution (0.45–0.50% of NaOCl)—by dilution with 7 parts of water.
As Wet Dressing—In 1:200 solution.
For Irrigation—1:2,000 to 1:200 solution.
For Topical Use and Swabs—Half or full strength.

Caution: In preparing solutions of definite chlorine concentration, allowance is to be made for a yearly decrease of 12% of available chlorine content of the drug used.

Advantages: Has more available active chlorine than U.S.P. chlorinated soda.

Bibliography: *See Chap. XII.*

HYDRAGOGIN (Bischoff)

Diuretic

Composition:

	Parts
Oxysaponin	0.5
Tr. Digitalis	1.5
Tr. Strophanthus with Scillipicrin and Scillitoxin	2.5
Alcohol	q.s. 15

Action: Is a powerful vegetable diuretic; the digitalis and strophanthus are aided by the oxysaponin, a glucoside-like substance obtained from Herniaria Glaba.

Uses: In cardiorenal edema, hepatic cirrhosis and other affections where powerful diuresis is indicated.

Supply: **HYDRAGOGIN**—Bottles of 15 cc.

Administration: From 3–15 drops every 3–4 hr. in water; in severe cases—15 drops every hour for 24–36 hr.

HYGEM (Bloomfield)

Laxative

Composition: An emulsion of milk whey and mineral oil, suspended in a medium of agar-agar, gelatine and malt extract and inoculated with culture of lactobacillus. Contains per ounce:

Mineral oil	3 dr. (11.664 Gm)
Gelatine and Agar	4 dr. (15.552 Gm)
Milk whey	1 dr. (3.888 Gm)
Saccharin	1/12 gr
Lactose and malt extract bacterial medium	27 gr
Peppermint	trace

Action and Uses: Intestinal detoxicant and antiseptic in putrefaction, flatulence, colitis; in eczema, dermatitis, rheumatism, arthritis.

Supply: **HYGEM**—Bottles of 16 oz.

Administration: 1–2 tablespoonfuls increased or decreased as demanded, once or twice daily.

HYOS-ZEA (Noyes)

Urinary Sedative

Composition: Each fluid ounce represents:

Liquid potassium hydroxide	40 m (2.592 cc)
Methenamine	40 gr (2.592 cc)
Tincture hyoscyamus	80 m (5.184 cc)
Fluid extract zea	80 m (5.184 cc)
Aromatics	q.s.

Action and Uses: *For relief* of vesical spasm, to correct acidity in dysuria, cystitis or urethral irritation.

Supply: **HYOS-ZEA**—Bottles of 1 pt., 1 gal.

Administration: 2 teaspoonfuls in water every 3 hr.

HYOTOLE (Sharp and Dohme)

Expectorant

Composition: Contains per 100 cc:

	Gm
Tolu	31.2
Sanguinaria	0.65
Squill	2.2
Wild cherry bark	6.6
Balm of gilead buds	0.82
Hyoscyamus	0.04
Alcohol, glycerin and syrup	q.s.

Uses: *For use* as expectorant and sedative in bronchial affections, especially of children.

Supply: **HYOTOLE**—Bottles of 4 and 16 oz. and 1 gal.

Administration: 1 or 2 fl. dr., repeated if necessary.
Children—1–3 mo., 10 drops
4–12 mo., 20 drops
1–3 yr. 30 drops
4–8 yr. ½–1 teaspoonful.

HYPNO-BROMIC COMPOUND (Wampole)

Hypnotic

Formula: Contains per fluid ounce:

	Gr	Gm
Cannabis extract	1	0.064
Chloral hydrate	96	6.218
Potassium bromide	48	3.109
Hyoscyamus extract	1	0.064

Action and Uses: Hypnotic in insomnia, nervousness, hysteria.

Supply: HYPNO-BROMIC COMPOUND—Bottles of 16 oz.

Administration: ½–1 teaspoonful in water.

HYPOTAN (Anglo-French)

Hypotensive

Composition: Each tablet contains:

α-Methylacetylcholine bromide	gr 1/12 (5 mg)
Bromocholine bromide	gr 1/12 (5 mg)
Chloral hydrate	gr ¾ (5 cg)

Action and Uses: Dilates blood vessels and relieves arterial spasm; is non-depressant to cardiac, respiratory and nervous systems. *For use* in hypertension, Raynaud's disease, endarteritis obliterans, senile or diabetic gangrene and impending cerebral apoplexy.

Supply: HYPOTAN—Tablets—Boxes of 44.

Administration: 4–6 Tablets daily.

Bibliography: *See Chap. XII.*

ICHTHOLDINE (Sharp and Dohme)

Local Antiseptic

Official Name: Glyceritum Ichthyoli Co.

Composition: Contains per ounce:

Ichthyol	gr 4	(0.259 Gm)
Iodine (free and combined)	gr 1	(0.064 Gm)
Liquefied phenol	m 4	(0.259 Gm)
Hydrastine hydrochloride	gr 1/32	(0.002 Gm)
Boroglyceride	gr 9	(0.582 Gm)
Eucalyptol	m 1/20	(0.003 cc)

Action and Uses: Local antiseptic for topical application, for the relief of inflammation, especially of the female genitalia.

Supply: ICHTHOLDINE—Bottles of 4, 8 oz., 1 pt., 1 gal.

Administration: Applied locally with fine brush or cotton applicator, or on wool tampons.

IDOZAN (Sterling and Jensen)

Hematinic

Description: A neutral colloidal preparation containing 5% Iron; does not discolor teeth, is very palatable and non-constipating.

Composition:

	Per Cent
Solution colloidal iron	83
Alcohol	6
Sugar	10
Flavoring	1

Action and Uses: As hematinic in chlorosis, anemia and hemoglobin deficiencies in general.

Supply: IDOZAN—Bottles of 8 oz.

Administration: 1 teaspoonful three times daily after meals.

Bibliography: *See Chap. XII.*

INOTON "DEBAT" (Fougera)

Antiphlogistic

Composition: An ointment containing—

	Gm
Lithol, a hypersulphonated oil of schiste	0.50
Ammonium-ichthyol sulphonate	0.25
Extract witchhazel	0.50
Titanium oxide	2.50
Hydroxide orthotitanique colloidal	0.50
Zinc oxide	7.50
Sodium borate	0.05
Non-oxidizable base	39.00

Action: Soothing, mild antiseptic, antiphlogistic and antipruritic; accelerates healing by stimulating proliferation of epithelium.

Uses: *For use* in acne, burns, cuts, chapped skin, eczema, fissures, intertrigo, pityriasis, pruritus, ulcers, herpes zoster.

Administration: Applied liberally to lesions, and covered with 2 thicknesses of gauze.

Supply: INOTON "DEBAT"—Tubes of 50 Gm—Tins of 500 Gm.

INOTON POWDER—Cartons of 125 Gm with shaker top.

Contains:

	Gm
Sulfo-schistol	0.010
Lithol	0.030
Extract of hamamelis	0.200
Sodium borate	0.080
Zinc oxide	0.400
Calcium carbonate	1.600
Magnesium silicate	36.000

For use as dusting powder and supplementary dressing for sensitive skins and dermatologic affections; as continuation treatment to Inoton ointment.

IOCAMFEN (Schering and Glatz)

Parasiticide

Composition:

	Per Cent
Iodine	10
Camphor	70
Phenol	20
Free iodine	7½

Description: A dark, reddish-brown liquid of camphoraceous odor; insoluble in water, soluble in alcohol, benzine, petrolatum; when mixed with fats or wax its free iodine forms combinations.

Action and Uses: Analgesic and antipruritic; relieves irritation, promotes healing; is antiseptic, fungicidal, keratolytic, deodorant; *For use* in ringworm infections of the feet, body, scalp and nails; also on wounds and denuded surfaces.

Supply: **IOCAMFEN** (C.A.)—Liquid—Bottles 1 oz., ¼ and ½ lb.

Administration: *Locally*—By swab or brush after cleaning parts; to be applied to dried surfaces only.

IOCOL (McNeil)

Expectorant

Description: Contains approximately 4% Iodine and 40% Guaiacol.

Action and Uses: Expectorant, respiratory disinfectant and alterative. *For use* in pulmonary disturbances.

Combinations: Capsules and Tablets, Enteric coated:

IOCOL COMPOUND 1:

	Gr	Gm
Iocol	2	0.130
Terpin Hydrate	2	0.130
Strychnine Sulphate	1/120	0.0005
Oil Eucalyptus	q.s.	

CAPSULES IOCOL COMPOUND 2:

Iocol	gr 2	(0.130 Gm)
Blaud's Mass	gr 3	(0.194 Gm)
Calcium Glycerophosphate	gr 1	(0.064 Gm)
Ext. Nux Vomica	gr 1/20	(0.003 Gm)
Arsenic Trioxide	gr 1/250	(0.2 mg)

CAPSULES IOCOL COMPOUND 3:

	Gr	Gm
Iocol	2	0.130
Bismuth Subnitrate	2½	0.162
Cerium Oxalate	2½	0.162
Orthesin (Anesthesin "McNeil")	1/5	0.013

CAPSULES IOCOL COMPOUND 4:

Iocol	gr 2	(0.130 Gm)
Atropine Sulphate	gr 1/600	(0.1 mg)
Aloin	gr 1/20	(0.003 Gm)
Tinct. Gelsemium	m 1	
Tinct. Aconite	m 1	

SYRUP IOCOL—Containing in each fluid ounce:

Iocol.. gr 12 (0.768 Gm)

Supply: IOCOL AND COMBINATIONS:

Capsules and Tablets, each gr 2—Bottles of 100, 500, 1,000 and 5,000.
Syrup—Bottles of 2, 3, 4 oz. by the dozen; 1 pt., ½ and 1 gal.

Administration: Capsules or Tablets, 1 or 2 when necessary.
Capsules Iocol Compound 4—1 capsule every hour for 4 hr., then 1 every 3 or 4 hr.
Syrup Iocol—1–2 teaspoonfuls.

IODALBIN (Parke, Davis)

Iodine Therapy

Description: A compound of Iodine and Albumin; a brown almost tasteless powder, containing approximately 21.5% iodine; insoluble in water, alcohol, acids and other ordinary solvents; soluble in alkaline liquids.

Action and Uses: Being insoluble in acids, it passes through the stomach unchanged causing no gastric disturbance; is broken up in the alkaline secretions of the small intestine and there absorbed. Acts like other soluble iodides, but owing to its protein character is believed to be less rapidly eliminated. *For use* in all conditions where iodine therapy is indicated.

Supply: IODALBIN—Capsules (C.A.), gr 5 (0.324 Gm)—Bottles of 100, 500, 1,000.
IODALBIN—Bottles (C.A.) 1 oz. and ¼ lb.

Combination: IODALBIN AND MERCUROL (C.A.)—Tablets, containing Iodalbin gr 5 (0.324 Gm) and Mercurol gr 1 (0.064 Gm)—Bottles of 100.

Administration: *Dosage*—Gr 5 (0.324 Gm) after meals.

Advantages: Freedom from gastric disturbances; prolonged effect of small dosage, minimizing risk of iodism.

IODEIKON EMULSION (Abbott)

Radiopaque Medium

Description: A brownish powder containing Iodeikon (tetraiodophenolphthalein sodium) and an organic acid, in chocolate malted milk; when mixed with cool water it forms a flocculent palatable mixture, easily administered.

Action and Uses: *Used* as cholecystographic medium in x-ray diagnosis of gall bladder.

Supply: IODEIKON EMULSION—Vials ½ oz.—Packages of 1 and 6.

Administration: Contents of 1 vial in a glass of cool water, taken the evening before radiographic examination; radiography 12, 15 or 18 hours after.

IODICALCIUM TABLETS (Searle)

Iodine-Calcium Therapy

Description: Calcium, combined with Iodine 15%, in palatable and assimilable form.

Action and Uses: Alterative and antispasmodic; *For use* to relieve bronchial spasms in children and affections of upper respiratory tract; also in prophylaxis and treatment of simple goitre.

Supply: IODICALCIUM—Tablets, gr ⅓, gr 1, gr 2, gr 5 (0.03, 0.064, 0.130, 0.324 Gm)—Bottles of 1,000.

Administration: Tablets gr 1–2 crushed in water, every 10–15 min.; 6–10 doses, until relieved; or one gr 2 tablet every 3 hr.; or one gr 5 tablet three times daily.

IODOBESIN (Anglo-French)

Reduction Therapy

Formula: Each opocrin represents:

	Gm
Liver extract	0.050
Pituitary extract	0.004
Testicular extract	0.040
Ovarian extract	0.050
Thyroid (lipoid free)	0.005
Suprarenal extract	0.001
Iodalbumin (colloidal)	0.050

Description: A pluriglandular preparation for the control of carbohydrate and fat metabolism.

Action and Uses: *For use* in obesity of endocrine origin, with headache, faintness, amenorrhea and edematous lower extremities.

Supply: IODOBESIN—Dragees—Bottles of 60.

Administration: 2 Opocrins daily for 10 days, followed by 3 or 4 opocrins daily for another 10 days; then rest period of 10 days.

Bibliography: *See Chap. XII.*

IODOBISMITOL (Squibb)

Antiluetic

Description: A solution of Sodium Iodobismuthite and Sodium Iodide in Ethylene Glycol, with total iodine content of 0.32–0.34 gr per ampule. Sodium Iodobismuthite is a red, crystalline, inorganic powder, containing 21.5% bismuth; is odorless, hygroscopic and astringent to taste; Ethylene Glycol is a penetrating and antiseptic solvent of sodium iodide, added in excess.

Action and Use: Antisyphilitic; presents bismuth in a form with marked penetrating power for the central nervous system. *Recommended* in syphilis of cerebrospinal system; also in visceral syphilis, in aortitis, hepatitis and parasyphilis (general paralysis), tabes; is administered *intramuscularly*.

Supply: IODOBISMITOL—Ampules (C.A.)—2 cc—Containing, Sodium Iodobismuthite, gr 2 (0.130 Gm), Sodium iodide, gr 4 (0.260 Gm), Ethylene glycol with 0.1% Acetic acid, q.s. 2 cc—Boxes of 10 and 100—Vials 50 cc.

Administration: 1 ampule every 3 days, 10 injections constituting a course; rest periods of 2–4 weeks between courses.

Bibliography: *See Chap. XII.*

IODO-CASEIN (Sharp and Dohme)

Iodine Therapy

Description: A compound of Iodine with milk Casein organically combined; a yellowish-brown powder, odorless and tasteless; insoluble in water and acid solutions, partly soluble with decomposition in alcohol; iodine content 18%.

Action and Uses: As for iodine therapy in goitre prophylaxis.

Supply: IODO-CASEIN (C.A.)—Tablets gr 5 (0.3 Gm) Chocolated—Bottles of 50 and 100.

IODO-CASEIN (C.A.)—Tablets gr 5 (0.3 Gm) Plain—Bottles of 50.

Administration: 1–4 tablets as often as required.

IODO-MANGAN (Reinschild)

Hematinic

Official Name: Liq. Ferro-Mangan Iodopeptone "Dieterich"

Composition:

	Per Cent
Iron	0.1
Manganese peptonate	0.1
Iodo-peptone	1
Alcohol	10

Each tablespoonful contains 1¼ gr Iodo-peptone, equivalent to 1/12 gr elemental iodine.

Action and Uses: A palatable hematinic and digestant, *for use* in anemia and various conditions where iodine therapy is indicated.

Supply: IODO-MANGAN—Bottles, 10 oz.

Administration: 1 Tablespoonful three or four times daily. Children—20 drops to 1 teaspoonful, three or four times daily.

IODOTONE (Eimer and Amend)

Iodine Therapy

Composition: A standardized Glycerole of Hydrogen Iodide, each dram containing Iodine gr 1, in solution; palatable, readily assimilable and non-irritating.

Action and Uses: Indicated where iodine medication is used; in hypothyroidism, obesity, cretinism, myxedema; in bronchial irritation, bronchitis, influenza, pneumonia, tuberculosis; in syphilis, asthma, arteriosclerosis, hypertension, angina pectoris, aneurysm, myocardial sclerosis, and rheumatism.

Supply: IODOTONE—Bottles 10 oz.—Boxes of 12 bottles.

Administration: 1–2 teaspoonfuls three or four times daily before meals. Children—½ teaspoonful three times daily.

Bibliography: *See Chap. XII.*

IODOXYL (Argy)

Antiarthritic

Composition: Magno-iodo-cinchophen; a compound of Cinchophen with Iodine and Magnesium Oxide; each capsule represents:

	Gr	Gm
Cinchophen	3.75	0.25
Iodine	1.50	0.10
Magnesium Oxide	1.50	0.10

Action and Uses: Analgesic, antipyretic, alkalizer and uric acid eliminant; is well tolerated causing minimum gastric disturbances. *For use* in arthritis, rheumatism, gout, neuralgia, neuritis, myositis.

Contraindications: Liver, kidney and gastro-intestinal diseases.

Supply: IODOXYL—Capsules—Boxes of 48 and 500.

Administration: 2 capsules three times daily, after meals, with water; in long-standing cases—larger dosage is indicated.

Bibliography: *See Chap. XII.*

IRRADOL-A (Parke, Davis)

Vitamin Therapy

Composition: Contains per fluid ounce—

Liver Oil (100 A)	5 m (0.324 Gm)
Viosterol (250 D)	10 m (0.643 Gm)
Vitamin B Extract	25 gr (1.600 Gm)
Iron and Ammonium Citrate	4 gr (0.259 Gm)
Malt Extract	Base

Action and Uses: A hematinic and palatable tonic, especially rich in vitamins A, B and D: *useful* as dietary supplement in infant feeding and for growing children.

Supply: IRRADOL-A—Jars 1 lb.

Administration: Infants—½–1 dr., Children—2 dr., Adults—1 tablespoonful; administered three times daily, after meals.

Bibliography: *See Chap. XII.*

I-X BARIUM MEAL (Dick X-Ray)

Radiopaque Medium

Description: A mixture of 85% of fine natural amorphous Barium Sulfate, U.S.P. with 10% of native Silicate as suspension agent, which coats each grain of barium with a gelatinous, film-like lubricant; also contains 5% Malted Milk and Saccharin for palatability.

Action: Is radiopaque; non-gritty, non-irritating, non-constipating and stays in suspension; *used* in X-ray study of gastro-intestinal tract.

Supply: I-X BARIUM MEAL—Cans of 8 oz. 5, 10, 25 and 100 lb. with 4 oz. measuring cup.

Administration: 1 measureful, 4 oz. in 8 oz. water thoroughly mixed before use.

Combinations: I-X BARIUM—Unflavored—containing 90% barium sulphate; *For use* as X-ray enema; 4 oz. in 8 oz. water, mixed and injected; may be used for oral administration and flavored if desired.

Supply: Cans of 8 oz. 5, 10, 25 and 100 lb. with 4 oz. measuring cup.

JECULIN (Upjohn)

Hematinic

Official Name: Extr. Jecoris Comp.

Composition: Contains per ounce

Whole liver extract, equivalent to	2.66 oz. fresh liver
Orange juice concentrate, representing	1.35 oz. orange juice

Glycerinated extract of red bone marrow.......	10 m (0.616 cc)
Iron and ammonium citrate..................	8 gr (0.518 Gm)
Malt extract, non-diastasic.................q.s.	

Action and Uses: Contains both hematinic fractions of liver which are effective in primary and secondary anemias; *For use* in pernicious and various other anemias, primary and secondary.

Supply: JECULIN—Bottles of 12 oz.

Administration: 2–4 teaspoonfuls three times a day after meals.

KACYAN (McNeil)

Hypotensive

Description: A preparation of chemically pure Potassium Sulphocyanate.

Action and Uses: Vasodilator in arterial hypertension.

Supply: KACYAN—Capsules and Tablets—Containing Potassium Sulphocyanate C.P. gr 1 (0.064 Gm)—Bottles of 100, 500 and 1,000.

ELIXIR KACYAN—(Sugarless and non-alcoholic), pleasantly flavored, aromatic solution of Potassium Sulphocyanate C.P. gr 8 (0.512 Gm) in each fluid ounce—Bottles of 2, 3 and 4 oz. 1 pt., ½ and 1 gal.

Administration: Elixir—1 teaspoonful three times daily.
Capsules and Tablets—1 or 2 capsules or tablets two or three times daily.

KALMERID GERMICIDAL TABLETS (Davis and Geck)

Germicide

Chemical Name: Potassium Mercuric Iodide.

Composition: Contains per tablet—

	Gr	Gm
Potassium mercuric iodide..........................	7.72	0.5
Potassium iodide....................................	5.7	0.37
Ammonium chloride..................................	1.8	0.125
Eosin "Y"..	0.077	0.005

Description: Rectangular shaped red-colored tablets; very hygroscopic, but nevertheless stable; readily soluble in water, 70% alcohol and 85% acetone.

Action: Has high bactericidal potency and is free from irritant action; is of comparatively low toxicity, forming no insoluble combinations with proteins.

Uses: External only; for disinfection of skin, sterilization of instruments and suture tubes; for hand disinfection, wet dressing, irrigation of nasal and other sinuses and of the genito-urinary tract.

Supply: KALMERID GERMICIDAL—Tablets (C.A.)—Bottles of 100.

Administration: *Skin Disinfection*—operation sites, abrasions, cuts and infected areas: 1:100 alcoholic solution (1 tablet in 50 cc of 70% alcohol).
Sterilization of Instruments—1:2,000 aqueous solution (1 tablet in 1,000 cc of water with 100 Gm sodium carbonate or bicarbonate).
Sterilization of suture tubes—1:2,000 alcoholic solution. (1 tablet in 1,000 cc of 70% alcohol.)
Hand disinfection—1:5,000. (1 tablet in 2½ liters of water.)

Solutions: Solutions are prepared by first dissolving tablet in small quantity of water; then water, or 70% alcohol, or 85% acetone is added to desired dilution.

Wet dressings—1:1,000 to 1:5,000.
Sinus irrigation—1:5,000 to 1:20,000. (1 tablet in 2½–10 liters of water.)
Irrigation of genito-urinary tract—1:20,000. (1 tablet in 10 liters of water.)

Antidotes: Gastric lavage, emetics, castor oil.

Bibliography: *See Chap. XII.*

KAOMIN (Lilly)

Sedative

Composition:

	Parts
Bismuth subcarbonate	100
Kaolin	280
Magnesium hydroxide	60
Sucrose	180
Vegetable mucilage	20
Vanillin	0.60

Action: Forms a protective dressing on wall of the intestines decreasing secretion, absorbing gases, deodorizing stools and favoring the healing of ulcerated areas; is non-irritating and sedative.

Uses: In intestinal fermentation and ulceration, diarrhea, flatulence; in colon dysfunction with distention and constipation.

Supply: KAOMIN—Jars 4 oz. and 1 lb.

Administration: 1 level tablespoonful every morning in a half glass of water.

Bibliography: *See Chap. XII.*

KASAGRA (Stearns)

Laxative

Description: A concentrated aromatic Cascara Sagrada, treated in a special manner to remove its bitter taste and griping tendency; is palatable and thus adapted for use in children.

Action and Uses: As tonic laxative in ordinary constipation.

Supply: KASAGRA—Bottles 2 and 16 oz.

Dosage: *Laxative*—½ dr. (2.0 Gm) diluted with water, ½ hr. before meals and at bedtime.
Cathartic—½–1 dr. (2.0–4.0 Gm) twice daily, diluted with water.

KATOLOX (Eimer and Amend)

Iodine Therapy

Composition: A stable, aqueous solution of Organic Iodine, gr ⅛ (0.008 Gm) to 10 drops; is almost neutral in reaction and does not precipitate albumen.

Action and Uses: Is indicated where iodine is *used;* in bronchitis, bronchial asthma, pleurisy; in arthritis, goitre prophylaxis, scrofula, malnutrition, syphilis, tuberculosis, sinusitis, tonsillitis.

Supply: KATOLOX—Bottles, 2 oz.

Administration: *Internally*—10–20 drops before meals, 2 or 3 doses; children—5–10 drops before meals.
Intramuscularly—5 cc with 0.3 Gm sodium bicarbonate.

Externally—Diluted in 3 parts of water, as surface antiseptic; also for douching and vaginal tampons.
Topically—Full strength on gums, dental sockets and other tissues.

KIDNOIDS (Noyes)

Diuretic

Composition: Each tablet represents:

	Gr	Gm
Ext. asparagus	1/4	0.016
Pulv. digitalis	1/5	0.013
Pulv. squill	1/2	0.032
Ext. epigea repens	1/2	0.032
Potassium nitrate	1	0.064
Ext. chimaphila umbeliforme	1/2	0.032

Action and Uses: A stimulating diuretic in cardiac and renal edema, chronic nephritis.

Supply: KIDNOIDS—Tablets, Sugar coated—Bottles of 100 and 1,000.

Administration: 1–3 tablets three or four times daily.

KOLA "ASTIER" (Gallia)

Stimulant. Tonic

Description: A granulated preparation of agreeable flavor; contains the active principles of Kola nut, Sterculia Acuminata, in their natural proportions.

Composition:

	Parts	
Caffeine	2.346	in 100 parts
Theobromine	0.023	
Fatty bodies	0.585	
Tannin	1.620	
Kola red	1.290	
Sugar	2.875	

Action: Stimulant and diuretic like coffee, but three times as powerful; assists in resisting fatigue, regulates heart action, toning up its muscles and checking profuse perspiration associated with muscular activity; is sustaining in mental strain and senility.

Uses: Functional nervous disorders, neurasthenia, mental disturbances; its tannin is helpful in persistent diarrhea; *also used* as stimulant tonic in infectious diseases; influenza, measles, small pox, scarlatina, typhoid.

Supply: KOLA "ASTIER"—Bottles of 100 Gm.

Administration: 2 Teaspoonfuls daily taken either pure or in water or other liquid.

KOLAGOG (Sutliff and Case)

Cholagogue

Composition: Contains per fluid ounce:

Cascara sagrada	gr 160 (10.4 Gm)
Lappa	gr 48 (3.11 Gm)
Taraxacum	gr 64 (4.15 Gm)
Euonymus	gr 32 (2.07 Gm)
Leptandra	gr 32 (2.07 Gm)

Fringe tree bark	gr	48	(3.11 Gm)
Sodium phosphate	gr	40	(2.59 Gm)
Citric acid	gr	12	(0.77 Gm)
Alcohol		18%	

Action and Uses: Hepatic stimulant and alterative with cholagogue effects; *For use* in hepatic congestion, catarrhal jaundice, intestinal fermentation, constipation.

Supply: KOLAGOG—Bottles of 1 pt., 1 gal.

Administration: ½–2 teaspoonfuls after meals.

KONDREMUL (Patch)

Laxative

Composition: Prepared from Irish moss (Chondrus Crispus) with 55% Mineral oil, held in very fine suspension.

Action: Mixes intimately in intestines with feces, forming a soft moist bulky mass and preventing hardening and drying of intestinal contents without causing leakage of the mineral oil.

Uses: In regulating bowel action in constipation.

Supply: KONDREMUL—Plain—Bottles of 16 fl. oz.

KONDREMUL WITH PHENOLPHTHALEIN—Gr 2.2 per tablespoonful—for more obstinate cases—Bottles of 16 fl. oz.

KONDREMUL WITH CASCARA—Bottles of 14 oz.

Administration: 1 Tablespoonful night and morning. Children 1 teaspoonful at night; may be taken with hot fluid.

Bibliography: *See Chap XII.*

LAC BISMO (Hart)

Antacid

Official Name: Mistura Bismuthi-Hart.

Description: A suspension in finely divided state of Bismuth Hydroxide and Bismuth Subcarbonate, 2½ gr (0.15 Gm) per dram of mixture.

Action and Uses: A gastric antacid and sedative *for use* in hyperacidity, gastritis and peptic ulcer.

SUPPLY: LAC BISMO (C.A.)—Bottles of 4 and 16 oz.

Administration: 1–4 teaspoonfuls every 2–3 hr.

LACTOBACILLUS (Towt-Nolan)

Acidophilus Milk

Description: An Acidophilus Milk, containing protein, 3.5%; fat, 0.5%; carbohydrate, 4%; lactic acid, 0.8%.

Action and Uses: Effective in supplanting intestinal putrefactive organisms, maintaining intestinal digestion and thus promoting bodily health. *For use* in constipation, chronic colitis, diarrhea, gastroenteritis, infantile digestive disorders.

Supply: LACTOBACILLUS ACIDOPHILUS MILK (C.A.)—Cases of 6 pt.

Administration: 1 pt. to 1 qt. daily, in 4 portions, at meal time and on retiring; continued for 6–12 weeks; in obstinate cases 6–10 teaspoonfuls of lactose are added per glass.

Bibliography: *See Chap. XII.*

LAPACTIC PILLS (Sharp and Dohme)

Laxative

Official Name: Pil. Lapacticae.

Composition: Each pill represents—

	Gr	Gm
Aloin	$\frac{1}{4}$	0.016
Strychnine	$\frac{1}{60}$	0.001
Ext. Belladonna	$\frac{1}{8}$	0.008
Powdered Ipecac	$\frac{1}{16}$	0.004

Action and Uses: Tonic laxative in chronic constipation, intestinal atony and dyspepsia; pills are small, readily soluble and seldom gripe.

Supply: LAPACTIC—Pills—Bottles of 100.

Administration: 1 or 2 pills at bedtime.

LECITHIN GLYCEROLE (Fairchild)

Nervine

Description: Contains per dram:
Pure Lecithin gr 1 (0.064 Gm), equivalent to gr 1.25 (0.0007) phosphorus, in chemically pure Glycerine.

Action and Uses: Tonic in neurasthenia, debility, various psychoses.

Supply: LECITHIN GLYCEROLE—Bottles of 8 oz.

Administration: Teaspoonful in ice water or on cracked ice.

LINCTUS COMPOUND (Sharp and Dohme)

Expectorant

Composition: Each fluid ounce contains—

Codeine sulphate	gr $\frac{1}{2}$ (0.032 Gm)
Chloroform	m 2 (0.130 cc)
Wine of ipecac	m 20 (1.30 cc)
Dilute phosphoric acid	m 16 (1.00 cc)
Tinct. 'squillis	m 20 (1.30 cc)
Alcohol	3–4%

Action and Uses: A palatable sedative and expectorant *for use* in coughs, colds and similar respiratory affections.

Supply: LINCTUS COMPOUND—Bottles of 4 oz., 1 pt., 1 gal.

Administration: 1 or 2 fl. dr. repeated if necessary.

LIQUID PEPTONOIDS (Arlington)

Nutritive, Tonic

Description: A clear, palatable liquid of pleasant odor and after taste; has a solid content of 28%, or more than twice that of milk including fat with only 12% solids; prepared from beef, wheat and predigested milk.

Composition:

	Per Cent
Proteins (peptones and propeptones)	5.25
Lactose and dextrose	11.3
Cane sugar	2.5
Alcohol	17.95

Food Value 10 calories per cubic centimeter.

Action and Uses: Stimulates appetite and food tolerance, assists nutrition saving waste of tissues; causes no gastric irritation; is *used* in numerous nutritional disturbances, also as vehicle.

Supply: LIQUID PEPTONOIDS—Bottles of 12 oz.

Administration: ½–1 tablespoonful several times daily.

Combinations: 1. LIQUID PEPTONOIDS WITH CREOSOTE—Containing per tablespoonful

Pure beechwood creosote	m 2
Guaiacol	m 1
Proteins (peptones and propeptones)	5.25%
Lactose and dextrose	11.3%
Cane sugar	2.5%
Minerals	0.95%
Alcohol	12%

A palatable sedative, expectorant and intestinal antiseptic; checks cough and intestinal fermentation. Useful in influenza, tonsillitis, laryngitis, bronchitis, bronchopneumonia. *Supply*—Bottles of 12 oz. *Dosage*—2–4 teaspoonfuls three to four times daily.

2. CASCARA PEPTONOIDS—Containing per tablespoonful

Fluid extract cascara sagrada	m 30 (1.944 cc)
Tr. nux vomica	m 1 (0.064 cc)
Liquid peptonoids	q.s.

Useful as tonic and laxative. *Supply*—Bottles of 6 and 12 oz. *Dosage*—1–2 tablespoonfuls two or three times daily.

3. IODO-PEPTONOIDS—Containing per tablespoonful

Assimilable iodine gr 1 (0.06 Gm) in organic combination with peptones. *Supply*—Bottles of 12 oz. *Dosage*—1 tablespoonful four times daily.

LIQUID PETROLATUM WITH AGAR (Squibb)

Laxative

Composition:

Liquid petrolatum (heavy)	50 cc
Agar	1.5 Gm
Benzyl benzoate	0.1 Gm
Acacia, glycerine and water	q.s. 100 cc

Description: A palatable emulsion of mineral oil, of milk white color and creamy consistency, with 30% by volume of agar content in minute particles; does not separate on standing or freezing.

Action and Uses: Intestinal lubricant; mixes readily with colon content, softens and increases its bulk, thus aiding normal evacuation; does not gripe and is not habit forming.

Supply: LIQUID PETROLATUM (C.A.)—Plain—Bottles of 16 fl. oz.

LIQUID PETROLATUM WITH AGAR (C.A.)—Bottles of 16 fl. oz.

LIQUID PETROLATUM WITH AGAR AND PHENOLPHTHALEIN (C.A.)—Gr 1½ per fluid ounce—Bottles of 16 oz.

Administration: Adults—1–2 tablespoonfuls in ½ glass water, between meals or at bedtime.
Children—1–2 teaspoonfuls in water.

LIQUOR DIASTOS (Sharp and Dohme)

Digestant

Composition: Each fluid ounce contains:

Pepsin (1:3000)	gr 8	(0.518 Gm)
Papain	gr 1⅓	(0.087 Gm)
Rennin	gr ¾	(0.048 Gm)
Dil. nitrohydrochloric acid	m 5	(0.324 Gm)
Lactic acid	m ½	(0.032 Gm)
Nux vomica	gr 9/10	(0.058 Gm)
Alcohol	18%	

Action and Uses: Helpful digestant in achylia gastrica, gastric atony, subacidity and biliousness.

Supply: LIQUOR DIASTOS—Bottles 1 pt. and 1 gal.

Administration: 1 or 2 teaspoonfuls after meals.

LIQUOR SANTAIVA (Sharp and Dohme)

Genitourinary Sedative

Official Name: Liquor Santali et Copaibae Compositum.

Composition: Contains per fluid dram Santal oil 5 m (0.324 cc), Copaiba 10 m (0.648 cc) with Flavoring and Alcohol 52%.

Description: A clear yellow, aromatic, palatable liquid, miscible with water in all proportions; forms a permanent emulsion.

Uses: Recommended in all genitourinary diseases where the administration of above drugs in liquid form is desired.

Supply: LIQUOR SANTAIVA—Bottles 4 oz. and 1 pt.

Administration: 1 fl. dr. in wine-glassful of milk (also water), two to three times after meals.

LITHIUM SALICYLATE 30% WITH TUTOCAINE 1% (Crookes)

Sclerosing Agent

Action and Uses: Sclerosing solution *for use* in obliteration of varicose veins.

Supply: LITHIUM SALICYLATE 30% WITH TUTOCAINE 1%—Ampules 2, 5 cc—Boxes of 6—Bottles 30 cc.

Administration: 1–4 cc per injection.

Bibliography: *See Chap. XII.*

LIVER EXTRACT WITH IRON 55 (Lilly)

Hematopoietic

Description: A combination of the hemoglobin-forming fraction of liver and soluble iron; standardized so that each level teaspoonful will produce at least 75 % of the hemoglobin stimulated by 100 Gm fresh liver.

Action and Uses: As hematopoietic for increasing erythrocytosis and hemoglobin in secondary anemia.

Advantages: Is more effective than either component alone.

Supply: LIVER EXTRACT WITH IRON 55—Powdered Extract—Bottles of 125 Gm.

Administration: 2–4 level teaspoonfuls, taken with orange juice, grape juice, lemonade, ginger ale, soup, water, milk, cereal.

Bibliography: *See Chap. XII.*

LIVER MEAL (Liver Meal)

Hematopoietic

Description: Whole liver substance in concentrated form.

Composition:

	Per Cent
Fresh beef liver, desiccated	81
Malted milk	18
Cinnamon flavor	1

Action and Uses: As hematinic in all anemias where fresh liver is indicated.

Supply: LIVER MEAL (C.A.)—Glass jars 8 and 16 oz., net—5½ and 11 oz.

Administration: 2 heaping teaspoonfuls three times daily; best given in soups, milk, cereal, gravy, stewed fruit, fruit juices, cocoa and chocolate.

Caution: Should not be cooked or boiled, but added to soups or stews when ready to serve.

Bibliography: *See Chap. XII.*

LUMALGIN (Winthrop)

Hypnotic

Composition: Each tablet represents

	Gr	Gm
Luminal	¼	0.016
Acetyl salicylic acid	5	0.32

Action: Prompt, safe and efficient hypnotic in painful affections, combining the sedative effect of Luminal and analgesic action of Acetylsalicylic acid; produces prolonged analgesia with relief of nervous tension.

Uses: Nervousness, cardiac and gastrointestinal neuroses, climacteric disorders, hyperthyroidism, hysteria, insomnia, migraine; in dental practice and pre- and postoperatively.

Supply: LUMALGIN—Tablets—Tubes of 10—Bottles of 25.

Administration: *Dosage*—1-3 tablets, according to severity of condition.

Bibliography: *See Chap. XII.*

LUMODRIN (Winthrop)

Antispasmodic

Composition: Each tablet represents—

	Gr	Gm
Luminal	¼	0.016
Ephedrine Hydrochloride	⅜	0.024
Pyramidon	2	0.12

Action: Sedative, decongestive, antispasmodic and analgesic; relaxes smooth musculature.

Uses: In colds, influenza, bronchitis, laryngitis, pertussis, asthma.

Supply: LUMODRIN—Tablets—Bottles of 25.

Administration: Adults—1 or 2 tablets, three to four times daily, children above 5 yr.—½-1 tablet.

MACARBO (McNeil)

Antacid

Composition:

	Per Cent
Magnesium Carbonate	50
Calcium Carbonate	50
Carminatives and Aromatics	q.s.

Action and Uses: Antacid, stomachic, sedative and carminative; *For use* in acid dyspepsia, epigastric distress, flatulence.

Combinations: TABLETS MACARBO—Containing Calcium Carbonate gr 2 (0.130 Gm). Magnesium Carbonate gr 2 (0.130 Gm).

TABLETS MACARBO WITH BISMUTH SUBCARBONATE—Gr ½ (0.032 Gm).

POWDER MACARBO WITH BISMUTH SUBCARBONATE—14%.

POWDER MACARBO WITH ORTHESIN—1¼ gr per dram.

TABLETS MACARBO WITH ORTHESIN—Gr ⅒ (0.006 Gm).

TABLETS MACARBO WITH PAPAIN—Gr ½ (0.032 Gm).

TABLETS MACARBO WITH PHENOLPHTHALEIN—Gr ⅛ (0.008 Gm).

LOZENGES MACARBO WITH BISMUTH—Containing: Magnesium Carbonate, 2½ gr (0.162 Gm), Calcium Carbonate, 5 gr (0.324 Gm), Bismuth Subcarbonate, 2½ gr (0.162 Gm), Carminatives and Aromatics, q.s.

Supply: MACARBO AND COMBINATIONS—Tablets—Bottles of 100, 500, 1,000 and 5,000.

Lozenges—Bottles of 1 and 5 lb.

Powder—In large jars.

Administration: Tablets—1 or 2 with water.

Lozenges—1 or 2 dissolved on the tongue.

Powder—1 teaspoonful with water.

MAGNESPIRIN (Calco)

Analgesic. Antipyretic

Composition: Contains Acetylsalicylic Acid potentiated by Magnesium, making 3⅓ gr (0.215 Gm) of the former equivalent in potency to 5 gr.

Description: A white or slightly colored powder of sour taste; insoluble in water or ordinary solvents.

Action: Antipyretic, analgesic, diaphoretic and antirheumatic.

Uses: Common colds, headaches, minor surgical pain; in prophylaxis of rheumatic fever in children, in painful infections of the eye, ear, nose and throat.

Incompatibilities: Strong alkalies, iron salts, tannates.

Supply: MAGNESPIRIN—Tablets, 5 gr (0.324 Gm)—Packages 12, 100 and 1,000.

Dosage: 2 tablets three or four times daily with water.

Bibliography: *See Chap. XII.*

MALT EXTRACT "KEPLER" (Burroughs Wellcome)

Nutrient

Composition: Contains Maltose, Dextrins, assimilable sugars useful as food, with Vitamin B and Diastase.

Action and Uses: As nutrient, tonic, hematinic in disturbed nutrition of children; also as vehicle.

Supply: MALT EXTRACT "KEPLER"—Bottles of 8 and 16 oz.

Administration: 1–4 teaspoonfuls whenever necessary.

Combinations: MALT EXTRACT WITH CASCARA SAGRADA—gr 6 (0.389 Gm) per oz.—Bottles of 8 oz.

MALT EXTRACT WITH GLYCEROPHOSPHATES—Contains per ounce Calcium Glycerophosphates gr 4 (0.13 Gm), Potassium Glycerophosphate gr 2 (0.13 Gm), Sodium Glycerophosphate gr 2 (0.13 Gm), Magnesium Glycerophosphate gr 2 (0.13 Gm)—Bottles of 8 oz.

MALT EXTRACT WITH HAEMOGLOBIN—Gr 8¾, (0.567 Gm) per ounce—Bottles of 8 oz.

MALT EXTRACT WITH HYPOPHOSPHITES—Calcium—Gr 8 (0.518 Gm), Potassium gr 4 (0.259 Gm) and Sodium gr 4 (0.259 Gm) per ounce—Bottles of 8 and 16 oz.

MALT EXTRACT WITH IRON IODIDE—Gr 2 (0.13 Gm) per ounce—Bottles of 8 oz.

MALT EXTRACT WITH IRON-PYROPHOSPHAS—Gr 4 (0.259 Gm) per ounce—Bottles of 8 oz.

MALT EXTRACT WITH IRON, QUININE AND STRYCHNINE PHOSPHATE—Containing Iron Phosphate gr ½ (0.032 Gm) Quinine Phosphate gr ⅜ (0.024 Gm), Strychnine Phosphate gr 1/64 (0.001 Gm) per ounce—Bottles of 8 oz.

MALT EXTRACT WITH PHOSPHORUS—Gr 1/64 (0.001 Gm)—Bottles of 8 oz.

MALT EXTRACT PLAIN (Borcherdt)

Nutrient

Description: Prepared from malted winter barley; contains the whole crushed grain, including germ and bran portions of the kernel.

Composition:

	Per Cent
Maltose	52.45
Dextrins	9.15
Protein	4.40
Mineral salts, including potassium, calcium, sodium, magnesium, iron, sulphur, phosphorus	1.06
Lactic acid	0.65
Moisture	22.29
Glycerine	10

Food Value: 58 calories per tablespoonful.
Vitamin Content: B (antineuritic), B_2 (G) antipellagric.
1 Gm is equivalent to 0.8 Gm dried brewers' yeast or 3.2 Gm moist yeast.

Action and Uses: An easily assimilable nutrient food, carbohydrate digestant and vehicle *for use* in numerous instances where these are helpful.

Supply: MALT EXTRACT, PLAIN—Bottles of 8 and 16 oz.

Administration: 1–4 teaspoonfuls three times daily after meals.

Combinations: MALT WITH IRON IODIDE—Contains Malt Extract with gr 4 (0.259 Gm) Ferrous Iodide per ounce; 1 teaspoonful equals 10 m of Syrup Ferrous Iodide; *For use* as hematinic and alterative.

Dosage—1–4 teaspoonfuls three to four times daily. *Supply*—Bottles 8 and 16 oz.

MALT EXTRACT WITH CASCARA SAGRADA (C.A.)—Contains Malt Extract with Extract Cascara Sagrada gr 60 (3.888 Gm), per ounce; *For use* as tonic laxative in constipation.

Dosage—1–2 teaspoonfuls as often as required. *Supply*—Bottles 8 and 16 oz.

MALT EXTRACT WITH YERBA SANTA COMPOUND—Contains Malt Extract with Ammonium Chloride gr 8 (0.518 Gm) and Yerba Santa Extract 32 m (1.92 cc) per ounce; *For use* in irritating cough.

Dosage—1 teaspoonful every 15–30 min. until relieved; then every 2 or 3 hr. *Supply*—Bottles 8 and 16 oz.

MALT EXTRACT WITH COD LIVER OIL (C.A.)—Contains Malt Extract plain 75% and Cod Liver Oil 25% with Vitamins A, B_1, B_2 (G) and D; *For use* as tonic food and nutrient in rickets.

Dosage—1–4 teaspoonfuls three to four times daily. *Supply*—Bottles 8 and 16 oz.

MALT EXTRACT, AND COD LIVER OIL WITH IRON IODIDE (C.A.)—Contains per ounce: Malt Extract Plain 75%, Cod Liver Oil 25%, Iron Iodide gr 2 (0.130 Gm); *For use* as alterative and hematinic in goitre, malnutrition and numerous other instances.

Dosage—1–4 teaspoonfuls three times daily. *Supply*—Bottles 8 and 16 oz.

MALT COD LIVER OIL WITH SPLEEN MARROW—Contains per ounce: Malt Extract plain 75%, Cod Liver Oil 25%, Spleenmarrow gr 10 (0.643); *For use* as hematinic, nutrient and food tonic in anemia, malnutrition.

Dosage—1–4 teaspoonfuls three times daily after meals. *Supply*—Bottles of 8 and 16 oz.

MALT EXTRACT WITH CREOSOTE (C.A.)—Contains Malt Extract Plain with Creosote U.S.P. 4 m (0.83 cc) per 100 cc; *For use* in respiratory diseases and tubercular affections.

Dosage—1–4 teaspoonfuls three times daily after meals. *Supply*—Bottles of 8 and 16 oz.

MALT EXTRACT WITH COD LIVER OIL

(Parke, Davis)

Nutrient

Description: Contains 25% Cod Liver Oil of standardized potency of vitamin A not less than 500 units per gram (U.S.P. method) and vitamin D of not less than 112 units (McCollum, *et al.*); also 75% of unmedicated Malt Extract, flavored with chocolate and vanilla extract.

Supply: MALT EXTRACT WITH COD LIVER OIL—Capsules, Soluble gelatin, 10 and 20 m—Boxes of 12 and 100. Capsules, 2½ and 5 Gm—Boxes of 6 and 50.

Administration: 1-3 capsules three to four times daily, in accordance with requirements.

MANAKALI (Tilden)

Antirheumatic

Composition: Each fluid ounce represents—

	Gr	Gm
Manaca	20	1.296
Sodium salicylate	40	2.592
Potassium iodide	8	0.512
Gelsemium	8	0.512
Colchicum root	8	0.512

Action and Uses: Analgesic and antirheumatic; *For use* in rheumatic affections.

Supply: MANAKALI—Bottles 16 oz. and 1 gal.

Administration: ½–1 teaspoonful three times daily with water.

MANCUHEMIN (Searle)

Hematinic

Description: A palatable Iron compound containing also small quantities of Manganese and Copper especially adapted for use in women and children.

Composition: Contains per tablet—

	Gr	Gm
Iron glycerophosphate	1	0.064
Copper glycine	1/100	0.00065
Manganese hypophosphite	1/100	0.00065
Calcium gluconate	1	0.064

Action and Uses: A readily absorbed, hematinic and tonic; stimulates blood forming organs in chlorosis and in anemias following hemorrhage, malnutrition, pregnancy and other causes.

Supply: MANCUHEMIN—Tablets—Bottles of 100 and 1,000.

MANCUHEMIN—Elixir—Each teaspoonful being equivalent to 1 tablet—Bottles of 2, 3 and 4 oz.

Administration: Tablets, 1 or 2 three or four times daily.
Elixir—1–2 teaspoonfuls three to four times daily, taken with milk or fruit juices. Children in proportion.

Bibliography: *See Chap. XII.*

MANOLA (Manola)

Tonic

Composition: Contains in each dessertspoonful:
4 m (0.2566 cc) of concentrated solution of combined salts of Iron, Calcium, Magnesium, Sodium and Potassium, 0.5 m (0.032 cc) each of Tincture Cinchona and Diluted Phosphoric Acid, ¼ m (0.016 cc) Fowler's solution, 1/240 gr (0.0005 Gm) Strychnine Phosphate and aromatics.

Action and Uses: Reconstructive, tonic and hematinic in anemia, debility, convalescence and neurasthenia.

Supply: MANOLA—Bottles of 16 oz.

Administration: 1–2 teaspoonfuls four times daily.
Children—½–1 teaspoonful after meals.

MARADOL (Smith-Dorsey)

Tonic. Vitamin Therapy

Composition: Each ounce represents—

Cod Liver Oil	120 m (7.776 cc)
Glycerinated Ext. Red Bone Marrow	10 m (0.643 cc)
Calcium Hypophosphite	4 gr (0.259 Gm)
Potassium Hypophosphite	2 gr (0.130 Gm)
Sodium Hypophosphite	2 gr (0.130 Gm)
Malt Extract	q.s.

Action and Uses: Its cod liver oil content presents Vitamin A—500 units, Vitamin B—250 units per gram; its malt extract—vitamines B and G. *For use* in malnutrition, anemia, rachitis, convalescence, debility and dental caries.

Supply: MARADOL—Jars 16 oz.

Administration: 2–4 teaspoonfuls three times daily.

MEBLUCO (McNeil)

Antiseptic

Composition: Each tablet represents—

	Gr	Gm
Methylene Blue	1	0.064
Ext. Kava Kava	1	0.064
Powdered Cubeb	½	0.032
Massa Copaiba	½	0.032
Oil Nutmeg	q.s.	

Action and Uses: An emollient and antiseptic *for use* in infections of the genito-urinary tract.

Supply: MEBLUCO—Tablets—Bottles of 100, 500, 1,000, 5,000.

Administration: 1 tablet three times daily after meals.

MENTHOLIC COMPOUND (Stoddard)

Antispasmodic

Composition: Contains per tablet:

Tr. opii camphoratae (equiv.)	m 5	(0.324)
Salcetol (Stoddard)	gr 1	(0.064 Gm)
Menthol	gr 1/20	(0.003 Gm)
Acid benzoic	gr 1/20	(0.003 Gm)
Eucalyptol compound	gr 1/20	(0.003 Gm)

Action and Uses: Bronchial sedative and antispasmodic for upper respiratory irritations and infections.

Supply: MENTHOLIC COMPOUND—Tablets—Bottles 100, 500 and 1,000.

Administration: 1 tablet dissolved on tongue as required.

MERGAL (Riedel)

Antiluetic

Chemical Name: Oxide of Mercury Cholate.

Formula: $(C_{24}H_{39}O_5)_2Hg$.

Composition: A combination of Mercuric Cholate and Tannalbin or Albumin Tannate.

Description: A cream colored or light brown, fine powder of metallic taste; sparingly soluble in water, soluble in saline; contains 6.5 % mercury.

Action and Uses: Antiluetic and cholagogue; causes no renal irritation. *Used* in syphilis and parasyphilis, tabes and general paralysis.

Supply: MERGAL—Capsules, containing gr 2½ (0.162 Gm) Cholate of Mercury Oxide and 1½ gr (0.097 Gm) Tannalbin—Boxes of 50.

Administration: 1 Capsule three times daily after meals; increased to 2 capsules five or six times daily.

Caution: Warm baths should be taken frequently, dental and oral hygiene observed.

MERVENOL (Hille)

Non-specific Therapy

Description: A colloidal solution, containing 0.58 % Mercury Sulphide and 0.1856 % Copper Sulphide.

Action: A non-specific therapy agent stimulating leucocytosis; is non-toxic, non-irritant and non-corrosive.

Uses: In affections of respiratory organs—cold, grippe, influenza, pneumonia.

Administration: 20 m every 3 hr. in water, between meals; in severe cases—*Intramuscularly and Intravenously*—3 cc daily.

Supply: MERVENOL—For Oral Use—Bottles of 1, 4 and 12 oz.

MERVENOL—For Injection—Vials 20 and 60 cc.

Bibliography: *See Chap. XII.*

METATONE (Parke, Davis)

Alterative. Tonic

Description: A palatable vitamin-containing combination of alterative and tonic ingredients.

Composition: Each fluid ounce contains:

	Gr	Gm
Vitamin B extract	10	0.643
Nucleic acid	2	0.130
Calcium glycerophosphate	4	0.259
Potassium glycerophosphate	4	0.259
Sodium glycerophosphate	2	0.130
Manganese glycerophosphate	½	0.032
Strychnine glycerophosphate	8/200	0.0026

Action: The vitamin B extract is antineuritic and growth promoting; the glycerophosphates supplement the phosphorus of nucleic acid which stimulates phagocytosis; the combined minerals are native to the human organism, and strychnine exerts tonic action.

Uses: In malnutrition, anemia, neurasthenia, convalescence from acute diseases; after surgical operation and as an appetizer for the utilization of food.

Supply: METATONE—Bottles of 12 fl. oz.

Administration: 1–4 teaspoonfuls three to four times daily, after meals; children—½–1 teaspoonful.

METHENOS (Sharp and Dohme)

Analgesic

Official Name: Elixir Methenamine Compound.

Composition: Each fluid ounce represents:

Methenamine, U.S.P.	gr 10	(0.643 Gm)
Potassium citrate	gr 8	(0.512 Gm)
Ammonium salicylate	gr 4	(0.259 Gm)
Cascara sagrada	gr 24	(1.536 Gm)
Ipecac	gr 1	(0.064 Gm)
Caffeine citrate	gr 1	(0.064 Gm)
Podophylin	gr ¼	(0.016 Gm)
Camphor	gr ¼	(0.016 Gm)
Alcohol	9%	

Action and Uses: Antipyretic, analgesic and laxative in colds, grippe, malaise, headaches and similar disturbances.

Supply: METHENOS—Bottles of 1 pt. and 1 gal.

Administration: 1 or 2 teaspoonfuls every 3–4 hr. in water.

METHYLETS (Sharp and Dohme)

Gonocide

Composition: Each pearl contains—

Methylene blue	gr 1	(0.064)
Santal oil	m 1½	(0.097)
Copaiba	m 1½	(0.097)
Cinnamon oil	m ½	(0.032)

Action and Uses: Antiseptic and sedative in genito-urinary affections.

Supply: METHYLETS—Bottles of 40.

Administration: 1 or 2 pearls three or four times daily.

MINERAL MIXTURE TABLETS 85

(Mead, Johnson)

Mineralizer

Description: A mixture of mineral salts, principally Calcium, Phosphorus, Iron and Copper.

Composition:

	Per Cent
Alfalfa ash	4.0
Dicalcium phosphate	32.0
Edible bone meal	64.0

Analysis: Each tablet 7.5 gr (0.486 Gm) supplies:

	Mg
Calcium	140.0
Phosphorus	83.0
Iron	1.0
Copper	0.05
Magnesium	2.8
Sodium	5.0
Potassium	5.0

Uses: A mineral supplement to all diets in cases demanding remineralization.

Supply: MINERAL MIXTURE TABLETS 85 (C.A.)—Bottles of 100 and 500.

Administration: 6 tablets daily.

Bibliography: *See Chap. XII.*

MINERAL OIL EMULSION

(Abbott)

Laxative

Composition: Contains Liquid Petrolatum 40 cc with Agar, Tragacanth and Gelatine 2 Gm, sugar and flavoring 2 Gm, water in sufficient quantity to make 100 cc.

Action and Uses: Laxative; *For use* in constipation, and other intestinal disorders.

Supply: MINERAL OIL EMULSION (C.A.)—Bottles of 12 oz.

Administration: 1 tablespoonful one or two times daily.

MINERAL OIL EMULSION

(Drug Products)

Intestinal Lubricant

Composition: A palatable emulsion containing—

	Per Cent
Russian mineral oil, heavy	70
Glycerine	5
Gelatin	0.07
French psyllium seed	0.30
Agar agar	0.10
Sodium benzoate.	

Action and Uses: A mechanical lubricant, readily miscible with intestinal contents and softening fecal masses; *For use* in intestinal stasis and similar disorders.

Supply: MINERAL OIL EMULSION—Bottles of 16 fl. oz.

MINERAL OIL EMULSION WITH PHENOLPHTHALEIN—Containing in addition 3 gr (0.194 Gm) of phenolphthalein per ounce—Bottles of 16 oz.

Administration: 1–2 tablespoonfuls at night; children in proportion.

MISCIDINE (Rorer)

Iodine Therapy

Composition: A soluble Iodine, each fluid dram containing gr 1 (0.064 Gm) elemental iodine; is not precipitated in watery dilution; Alcohol 17 %.

Action and Uses: *For use* where iodine is indicated; goitre, pleurisy, chronic bronchitis, rheumatism, lues.

Supply: MISCIDINE—Bottles of 1 oz.

Administration: 5–20 drops, as required.

MYCOZOL (Parke, Davis)

Fungicide

Composition:

		Per Cent
Chloretone (chlorbutanol)		5
Salicylic acid		4
Mercury salicylate		4
Aromatics and ointment base	q.s.	100

Action and Uses: Exfoliative and fungicidal in epidermomycosis, athlete's foot, swimmer's itch, fungus infections in interdigital spaces, thighs, axillae; also for soft corns.

Supply: MYCOZOL—Collapsible tubes of 1 oz.—Packages of 12.

Administration: Affected area is scrubbed with antiseptic soap on a soft brush, washed with alcohol and dried; the ointment is then rubbed in freely and covered with bandage; the process is repeated next night. Between ointment applications Boro-Chloretone is dusted on and protected by a light bandage.

Caution: Contact of Mycozol with sound skin is to be avoided.

MYELADOL (Upjohn)

Tonic. Vitamin Therapy

Composition: Contains per ounce:

Super D Cod Liver Oil	120 m (7.392 cc)
Ext. Red Bone Marrow Glycerinated	10 m (0.616 cc)
Iron and Ammonium Citrate	4 gr (0.259 Gm)
Malt Extract	q.s.

Action and Uses: A nutritive, reconstructive and easily absorbed tonic, presenting per ounce not less than 2,500 (A. D.M.A.) units Vitamin D, 6,250 (U.S.A.) units Vitamin A and a food value of 150 calories. *For use* in all conditions where vitamin D therapy is indicated.

Supply: MYELADOL—Bottles of 12 and 32 oz.

Administration: 1–2 dessertspoonfuls after meals.
Children, 1–2 teaspoonfuls three times daily.

NARKOGEN (Tilden)

Hypnotic

Composition: Each fluid dram contains:

	Gr	Gm
Chloral hydrate	10	0.643
Potassium bromide	10	0.643
Hyoscine hydrobromate	1/200	0.00032
Narkine (Tilden)	1/2	0.032

Action and Uses: *For use* as hypnotic, anodyne and antispasmodic in nervous irritability and mania; also in tenesmus of cystitis, in erethism, priapism, chordee and nymphomania.

Supply: NARKOGEN—4, 8 and 16 oz. and 1 gal.

Administration: 1 or more teaspoonfuls as demanded.

NATIBAINE "NATIVELLE" (Fougera)

Cardiotonic

Composition: A preparation containing 1 part Digitaline "Nativelle" and 2 parts Ouabaine "Arnaud" in 1 Gm of the 2 glucosides per 1,000 cc of a glycero-alcoholic solution.

Action: A powerful cardiac stimulant, offering the combined effects of both constituents; its action is rapid, prolonged and non-cumulative.

Uses: Recommended in ventricular diiatation, auricular fibrillation, myocardial insufficiency and hypertensive heart disease.

Supply: NATIBAINE "NATIVELLE"—Solution 10 cc.

Administration: 10–25 drops daily; in emergencies 30–60 drops a day.

NEOBOVININE-20 (Bovinine)

Hematinic

Description: A palatable compound of liver extract and defibrinated beef blood; contains hematopoietic elements, organic iron, minerals, protein and complements; each tablespoonful is equivalent to 0.83 oz. fresh whole liver.

Composition:

	Per Cent
Beef Blood	53.3
Liver Extract	26.6
Alcohol (by volume)	15.0
Glycerin	2.7
Salt and Water	2.4

Analysis: Mineral Content per 100 cc:

Chlorine	816 mg	Calcium	8.8 mg
Iron	34 mg	Magnesium	2.9 mg
Copper	0.76 mg	Potassium	238 mg
Zinc	5.0 Gm	Sodium	537 mg
Phosphorus	121 mg	Sulphur	170 mg
Manganese	trace		

Action and Uses: Improves appetite, stimulates metabolism and supplies elements for blood regeneration; *Used* in secondary anemias, malnutrition and debility.

Supply: **NEOBOVININE-20**—Bottles of 12 fl. oz.

NEOBOVININE WITH MALT AND IRON—Containing Liver Extract concentrate 26%, Iron 10.6%, Malt Extract 30%, Alcohol 9.5%, Glycerine 3.6%, Water 20.3%; *Supply*—Bottles of 8 oz.

Administration: 1 Tablespoonful, four times daily.
Children—½-1 teaspoonful according to weight.

NEOFERRUM (Maltine)

Hematinic

Composition: Contains per fluid ounce:
Elemental Iron 1.4 gr (0.08 Gm), Manganese 0.33 gr (0.02 Gm), Arsenious Acid, 0.00353 gr; Maltine and Sherry wine; Alcohol 18%.

Description: A palatable iron preparation of neutral reaction.

Action and Uses: Easily assimilable and non-constipating; does not stain nor injure teeth. *Useful* in debility from blood impoverishment.

Supply: **NEOFERRUM**—Bottles 12 oz. and 5 pt.

Administration: 1 tablespoonful three times daily; children—teaspoonful or less.

NEOGESTIN (Morgenstern)

Antacid

Composition: Each powder represents—

	Gr	Gm
Colloidal Aluminum Silicate	15	0.97
Magnesium Peroxide	5	0.32
Pancreatin Concentrated	2	0.13
Extract Papaya	½	0.03
Oil Peppermint, Saccharin	q.s.	

Action and Uses: Gastric antacid, sedative and digestant; allays irritation, catarrh; mechanically protects mucosa and assists in digestion; *For use* in gastric hyperacidity and ulceration, intestinal insufficiency, fermentation and flatulence.

Supply: **NEOGESTIN**—Powders 24 gr each—Boxes of 40.

Administration: 1 powder before meals or when necessary; in water or milk.

NEOMAGNEPHEN (Calco)

Analgesic. Antiarthritic

Composition: Per tablet 3 grains of the Ethyl Ester of Paramethylcinchophen potentiated by Magnesium.

Description: A white powder, almost tasteless and odorless; insoluble in water and ordinary solvents.

Action: As for neocinchophen; has a selective sedative effect upon bone, joints and periarticular tissues; is comparatively non-toxic and non-irritating to gastric mucosa.

Uses: Acute and chronic rheumatic fever, osteo-arthritis, synovitis, neuritis, neuralgia; also in mild types of tabes dorsalis.

Supply: NEOMAGNEPHEN—Tablets gr 5 (0.32 Gm)—Packages of 24, 100 and 1,000.

Incompatibilities: Acids, alkalies in strong solution, tannates, iron salts.

Contraindications: Thyrotoxicosis, active infection of the biliary tract; major surgical operations with protein absorption.

Administration: 2–3 tablets three times daily and at bedtime.

Bibliography: *See Chap. XII.*

NERVINAL (Morgenstern)

Nerve Sedative

Composition: Contains per tablet:

	Gr	Gm
Bromural	2	0.13
Phenobarbital	¼	0.016
Ephedrine Hydrochloride	⅛	0.008
Benzyl Succinate	½	0.03
Calcium Glycerophosphate	2	0.13

Action and Uses: Sedative and antispasmodic; *For use* in dysmenorrhea and menopausal disturbances, in neurasthenia, insomnia, hysteria, neuritis, sciatica, neuralgia, migraine and bronchial asthma.

Supply: NERVINAL—Tablets—Box of 30.

Administration: 1–2 tablets, three times daily; reduced when relief is obtained.

NEUREMPCO (Marvell)

Tonic

Composition: NEUREMPCO 3, Ampule 1 cc containing—

	Gm
Iron citrate	0.03
Sodium glycerophosphate	0.10
Sodium cacodylate	0.06
Strychnine sulphate	0.001

NEUREMPCO 4, Ampule 1 cc, containing—

	Gm
Iron cacodylate	0.02
Strychnine cacodylate	0.0005
Sodium arsenate	0.001
Sodium glycerophosphate	0.03

NEUREMPCO 8, Ampule 1 cc, containing—

	Gm
Iron cacodylate	0.01
Sodium glycerophosphate	0.065
Strychnine cacodylate	0.0005
Chlorbutanol less than ½ %	

Action and Uses: Hematinic and tonic in various anemias and in neurasthenia.

Supply: Boxes of 12.

Administration: *Intramuscular* injections, two to three times weekly.

NEURO-CALM (Westerfield)

Sedative

Composition: Each tablet represents:

	Gr	Gm
Ext. Passiflora	1½	0.097
Ext. Valerian	1½	0.097
Ext. Henbane	⅛	0.008
Barbital	1	0.064

Action and Uses: Sedative in nervous instability, insomnia and restlessness.

Supply: NEURO-CALM—Tablets—Bottles of 100, 500 and 1,000.

Administration: 1 or 2 tablets, three or four times daily.

NEURONIDIA (Schieffelin)

Sedative. Hypnotic

Chemical Name: Elixir Diethylmalonylurea.

Description: Contains 16 gr (1.0 Gm) of Barbital to the ounce, in stable palatable form; Alcohol 35%.

Action: Induces restful sleep without after effects; does not depress heart and respiration; acts promptly and is readily eliminated.

Uses: In insomnia of mild psychoses, neuroses, acute febrile diseases, chronic organic diseases; as sedative in hysteria, neurasthenia, seasickness.

Supply: NEURONIDIA—Bottles of 8 oz., 1 gal.

Administration: *As Hypnotic*—2 teaspoonfuls.
As Sedative—1 teaspoonful, two or three times daily.

NEUROPHOSPHATES "ESKAY" (Smith, Kline and French)

Tonic

Composition: Contains in each 2 teaspoonfuls:

Sodium glycerophosphate	2 gr	(0.13 Gm)
Calcium glycerophosphate	2 gr	(0.13 Gm)
Strychnine glycerophosphate	1/64 gr	(0.001 Gm)
Alcohol	20 m	(1.296 cc)

Action: Nerve tonic and roborant.

Uses: Nervous depression, neurasthenia; as tonic in convalescence and debility; as vehicle for administration of other medicaments.

Incompatibles: Sodium bicarbonate, sodium salicylate and all similar salts.

Advantages: Agreeable taste; bitterness of strychnine is "masked."

Supply: NEUROPHOSPHATES "ESKAY"—Bottles of 8 and 16 oz.

Administration: 2 teaspoonfuls three or four times daily.

Bibliography: *See Chap. XII.*

NEUROSINE (Dios Chemical)

Hypnotic

Composition: Contains per fluid ounce:

Potassium Bromide	gr 40	(2.59 Gm)
Ammonium Bromide	gr 40	(2.59 Gm)
Sodium Bromide	gr 40	(2.59 Gm)
Zinc Bromide	gr 1	(0.06 Gm)
Extract Lupulin	gr 32	(2.07 Gm)
Extract Cannabis Indica	gr 0.60	(0.036 Gm)
Extract Belladonna	gr 0.075	(0.0016 Gm)
Extract Henbane	gr 0.075	(0.0016 Gm)
Extract Cascara Sagrada	m 40	(2.46 cc)
Alcohol and aromatic elixirs	5%	

Action and Uses: Sedative, antispasmodic and hypnotic; *For use* in epilepsy, delirium tremens, hysteria, neurasthenia, insomnia; in migraine, neuralgia, chorea; in whooping cough and asthma.

Supply: NEUROSINE—Bottles of 2, 4 and 8 oz.

Administration: 1 dessertspoonful in water three or more times daily.

Bibliography: *See Chap. XII.*

NEUSTHENIC "FRAISSE" (Fougera)

Stimulant

Composition: Contains Sodium Glycerophosphate gr 1½ (0.09 Gm), and Strychnine Cacodylate gr 1/120 (0.0005 Gm).

Action: A stimulant and nerve tonic in atony of nerve tissue.

Uses: Nervous debility and exhaustion, especially after prolonged illness; in drug habitués and in exhausting lactation.

Supply: NEUSTHENIC—Ampules 1 cc—Boxes of 12 and 50.

NEUSTHENIC—Bottles of 25 Gm, for oral use.

Administration: *Subcutaneously or Intramuscularly*—1 ampule daily for 12 days; after 5 days' interval a second series is recommended.

Orally—25 drops in sweetened water, daily for 12 days; after 5 days' interval, a similar series is repeated.

NEUROTROPHOL "BYLA" (Fougera)

Tonic

Composition:

Sodium glycerophosphate 50%	1	Gm
Nucleinic acid	0.5	Gm
Tr. bitter orange peel	1	cc
Tr. ceylon cinnamon	1	cc
Fl. extr. condurango	1	cc
Quinine sulphate	0.5	Gm
Sodium methylarsenate	0.5	Gm
Alcohol 95%	16	cc
Simple syrup	52	Gm
Orchitic juice	11.5	Gm
Aqua	q.s. ad 100	Gm

Action and Uses: A palatable elixir *for use* in neurasthenia, neurocirculatory asthenia, exhaustion, convalescence; improves appetite in anorexia and stimulates general metabolism.

Supply: NEUROTROPHOL "BYLA"—Bottles, 300 Gm.

Administration: Adults, 1 tablespoonful twice daily after meals.
Children, 1 teaspoonful two times daily after meals.

NITROBAR (McNeil)

Hypotensive

Chemical Name: Bismuth Subnitrate-Phenobarbital Compound.

Composition: Each tablet represents

	Gr	Gm
Bismuth subnitrate	5	0.032
Phenobarbital	1/8	0.008
Extr. passiflora and Extr. lupulus	q.s.	

Action and Uses: Antispasmodic, arteriolar sedative and vasodilator; acts by slowly liberating nitrite ions in the intestinal tract; *For use* in hypertension and angina pectoris.

Supply: NITROBAR—Tablets, Enteric coated—Bottles of 100, 500, 1,000.

Administration: 1–2 tablets three times daily, administered for a long period.

NITROCON (McNeil)

Hypotensive

Description: A light brown, bitter powder containing

Sodium Nitrite	gr 1/2	(0.032 Gm)
Nitroglycerin	gr 1/200	(0.0003 Gm)
Tinct. Aconite Root	m 1 1/2	(0.097 cc)
Podophyllin	gr 1/40	(0.001 Gm)
Sodium Bicarbonate	q.s.	

Action and Uses: Vasodilator in arterial hypertension.

Supply: NITROCON—Tablets and Capsules—Bottles of 100, 500, 1,000 and 5,000.

Administration: 1 or 2 capsules or tablets three times daily.

NITROSCLERAN (Tosse)

Vasodilator

Description: Sodium Nitrite in saline solution, potentiated with Phosphates of Sodium and Potassium; occurs as dry white crystals of saline taste and soluble in water.

Action and Uses: Is claimed to be more effective than ordinary nitrites; relaxes blood vessels, lowers blood pressure and improves general circulation; *For use* in hypertension for relief of symptoms; headache, vertigo, dyspnea, palpitation; in arteriosclerosis, coronary sclerosis, angina pectoris, nephrosclerosis and degenerative myocarditis; in toxic amblyopia and preceding ocular operation.

Supply: Nitroscleran—Ampules 1 cc—Containing 0.1 and 0.04 Gm of sodium nitrite—Boxes of 6 and 30.

Nitroscleran Salts—Oral—Containing 0.75 Gm of sodium nitrite per bottle—Bottles of 100 Gm, with measuring caps.

Administration: *Subcutaneous Injection*—Beginning with 0.04 and slowly increasing to 0.1 Gm, for 8–15 injections; course repeated at 4–6 week intervals in intensive treatment.
Intravenous Injection—Where more rapid action is desired.
Orally—1 measureful of salts dissolved in 1 cup of water, taken ½ hr. before breakfast in prophylaxis or continuation treatment after course of injections.

Bibliography: *See Chap. XII.*

NOVATONE (Brooklyn Scientific)

Tonic

Composition: Each tablet contains:

	Gr	Gm
Vitamin B Concentrate	1	0.064
Nucleinic Acid	⅙	0.012
Calcium Glycerophosphate	1½	0.09
Strychnine Glycerophosphate	1/100	0.0006
Reduced Iron	1	0.064

Action and Uses: Tonic and hematinic; stimulates appetite and leucocytosis; *For use* in anorexia, debility, convalescence and in prophylaxis and treatment of polyneuritis.

Supply: NOVATONE—Tablets—Bottles of 50.

Administration: 1–2 tablets, three times daily, after meals.

Bibliography: *See Chap. XII.*

NUCHOL TABLETS (Maltbie)

Cholagogue

Composition: Each tablet represents:

	Gr	Gm
Sodium salicylate	1½	0.097
Sodium oleate	1½	0.097
Sodium choleate	1	0.064
Phenolphthalein	⅓	0.021
Menthol	1/10	0.006

Action and Uses: As cholagogue in liver and gall bladder disorders.

Supply: NUCHOL TABLETS—Bottles of 100, 500 and 1,000.
NUCHOL "B" TABLETS—Containing Cascara sagrada gr 1 (0.064 Gm) in place of phenolphthalein—Bottles of 100, 500 and 1,000.

Administration: 2 tablets night and morning.

NUCLEIN (Burroughs Wellcome)

Leucocyte Stimulant

Description: A compound of Nucleinic Acid with Albuminates and Carbohydrates.

Action and Uses: Stimulates leukocytosis in pneumonia, influenza, tuberculosis and typhoid.

Supply: **HYPOLOID NUCLEIN**—1 cc, gr ½ (0.032 Gm)—Boxes of 10.
TABLOID—Nucleo-Lecithin Compound—Sugar coated, containing:

	Gr	Gm
Nuclein	¼	0.016
Lecithin	½	0.032
Potassium Glycerophosphate	1	0.065
Calcium Glycerophosphate	1	0.065

Bottles of 25 and 100.

Administration: 1 Ampule *subcutaneously*, daily.
Tabloids—1 or more twice daily after meals.

NUMOTIZINE (Numotizine)

Antiphlogistic

Composition: Contains in 1,000 parts:

	Parts
Guaiacol U.S.P.	2.6
Beechwood creosote	13.02
Methyl salicylate	2.6
Formalin	2.6
Quinine sulphate	2.6

Glycerine C.P., Colloidal aluminum silicate, Kaolin as base.

Action and Uses: An endermic plaster aiding in diminishing local congestion and relieving pain; *for use* externally in bronchitis, pleurisy, colds, tonsillitis, adenitis, mastitis, orchitis, epididymitis, ovaritis, abscesses, felons, boils, carbuncles, sprains, bruises.

Supply: **NUMOTIZINE**—Jars of 3½, 7¼, 14½, 27 oz.

Administration: Applied externally over affected area, at body temperature, ⅛ in. thick on thin cloth, for a period until the fever falls or until dried; repeated when desired after skin cleansing.

Bibliography: *See Chap. XII.*

NUROBROMYDS (Rorer)

Sedative. Antispasmodic

Composition: Contains in elixir form, per fluid ounce:

Sodium Bromide	gr 20 (1.296 Gm)
Strontium Bromide	gr 20 (1.296 Gm)
Ammonium Bromide	gr 20 (1.296 Gm)
Tinct. Valerian	m 60 (3.888 Gm)
Tinct. Hyoscyamus	m 60 (3.888 Gm)
Alcohol	25%

Action and Uses: As sedative in nervous conditions, where bromides and valerianates are indicated.

Supply: **NUROBROMYDS**—Bottles 14 oz., 5 pt.—Jugs 1 gal.

Administration: 1 or 2 teaspoonfuls, in water, every 3 hr.; increased as indicated.

OMNADIN (Metz)

Non-specific Lipo-Protein Therapy

Chemical Name: Brand of Prolipin.

Description: A sterile solution containing non-pathogenic bacterial proteins (sarcinae and B. mycoides), various animal fats and lipoids derived from bile.

Action: When injected causes prompt and favorable reaction, resulting in rapid fall of temperature, increased leucocytosis and phagocytosis, improving the general condition and shortening the disease; the animal fats and lipoids stimulate the defensive powers of the body, producing more complete non-specific immunization than foreign proteins alone.

Uses: In all acute infectious diseases with high temperature: influenza, colds, pneumonia, erysipelas, scarlatina, measles, puerperal sepsis, surgical sepsis, gonorrhea, furunculosis, arthritis, tonsillitis, otitis media.

Advantages: Injections are practically painless and free from disagreeable reactions.

Supply: OMNADIN—Ampules 2 cc—Boxes of 5.

Administration: Adults, 1 ampule *intramuscularly*, once daily; double dosage and repeated, several times if necessary, where no symptoms of intolerance or of local irritation appear.
Children, 1–2 cc.

Bibliography: *See Chap. XII.*

OPTALIDON (Sandoz)

Anodyne. Sedative

Composition: A combination of Sandoptal (isobutylallylmalonylurea) gr ¾ (0.05 Gm) with Amidopyrine, 2 gr (0.125 Gm) and Caffeine ⅜ gr (0.025 Gm) to each tablet.

Action: Relieves pain without causing depression, drowsiness or other by-effects; dilates cerebral blood vessels, thus favoring quicker analgesia; has a mild stimulating effect upon the kidneys.

Uses: In painful states associated with nervous excitability and restlessness; headache, toothache, neuralgia, insomnia due to pain; also in colds, influenza, dysmenorrhea, post-operative pain.

Supply: OPTALIDON—Tablets—Tubes of 10—Bottles of 100, 250—Tins of 1.000.

Administration: 1–2 tablets as required; average daily dose 6 tablets.
Children 1–3 tablets per day.

Bibliography: *See Chap. XII.*

OPTARSON (Winthrop)

Tonic. Alterative

Composition: Ammonium Heptenchlorarsonate and Strychnine Nitrate; Brand of Chlorarsenol with Strychnine.

Description: A sterile solution, each cubic centimeter containing ⅙ gr (0.01 Gm) of ammonium heptenchlorarsonate with 1/64 gr (0.001 Gm) of strychnine nitrate.

Action and Uses: Stimulates metabolism, improves nutrition and anemia; the arsenic (equal to 1/16 gr of arsenious acid) is uniformly and adequately liberated and eliminated and without toxicity; injections are painless and non-irritating. *For use* in malaria, tuberculosis, skin diseases, neuralgias; in convalescence from exhausting illness.

Supply: OPTARSON—Ampules, 1.2 cc—Boxes of 12.

Administration: *Subcutaneously or Intramuscularly*—1 ampule every other day; in hypersensitive cases twice weekly.

Bibliography: *See Chap. XII.*

ORARGOL (Anglo-French)

Non-specific Therapy. Antiseptic

Description: A colloidal suspension of Gold and Silver, electrically prepared from an alloy of 10% gold and 90% silver; stabilized and sterilized by tyndallization.

Action: Is stated to be bactericidal, to raise resistance against infection and favor leukocytosis.

Uses: In severe infectious fevers; influenza, pneumonia, bronchopneumonia, sepsis, typhoid fever, epidemic encephalitis; also in minor affections as ordinary colds, tonsillitis, nasopharyngeal disease, conjunctivitis.

Supply: ORARGOL—Injectable—Ampules 5 and 10 cc *for intravenous and intramuscular use.*
Ampules 5 cc—Package of 2 and 6,
Ampule 10 cc—Package of 1.

ORARGOL—Non-injectable—Bottles of 4 oz.

ORARGOL—O.R.L. with nasal instillator and eye dropper—Bottles of 20 cc.

Administration: *Intravenously or Intramuscularly*—5–20 cc, injectable, daily or every other day.
Children—1 cc for each year of age.
Oral—Non-injectable, 20–100 drops daily, or 1 teaspoonful morning and evening; used as continuation to parenteral therapy. O.R.L.—4–5 drops applied through instillator; also as collyrium.

ORCHATON (Norwich)

Aphrodisiac

Composition: Each tablet represents:

	Gr	Gm
Strychnine Phosphate	1/120	0.0005
Zinc Phosphide	1/10	0.006
Yohimbine Hydrochloride	1/12	0.005
Orchic substance	1	0.064
Muirapauma	1	0.064

Action and Uses: Nerve tonic and aphrodisiac in sexual impotence, asthenia, sexual neuroses.

Supply: ORCHATON—Bottles of 100.

Administration: 1 tablet three times daily.

ORGANIDIN (Wampole)

Iodine Therapy

Composition: An organic iodine preparation, containing 2½ Gm combined Iodine per 100 cc.

Description: Is stable, tasteless, non-irritating, freely miscible with water, non-alcoholic.

Action and Uses: In all conditions where iodine is indicated, as in goitre, arterial hypertension, arteriosclerosis, syphilis, asthma, gout, scrofula.

Supply: ORGANIDIN—Bottles of 1 oz.

Administration: 5–20 drops, diluted, three times daily, before meals.

Bibliography: *See Chap. XII.*

ORTHOBEN (Stoddard)

Expectorant

Composition: Contains per ounce:

Potassium guaiacol sulphonate	gr 16	(1.024 Gm)
Mono-sodium benzyl succinate	gr 8	(0.512 Gm)
Syrup wild cherry	dr. 1	(3.888 Gm)
Infusion senna	dr. 1½	(5.832 Gm)
Syrup ipecac	m 12	(0.777 Gm)
Sugar, glycerin, aromatics	q.s.	

Action and Use: As sedative and expectorant in spasmodic coughs, whooping cough and bronchial affections.

Supply: ORTHOBEN—Bottles 16 oz. and gallons.

Administration: 1–2 teaspoonfuls every 2 or 3 hr.

OVARITONE (Sharp and Dohme)

Uterine Tonic

Composition: Contains per fluid ounce:

Black haw	gr 64 (4.147 Gm)
Pulsatilla	gr 16 (1.036 Gm)
Golden seal	gr 16 (1.036 Gm)
Passion flower	gr 32 (2.072 Gm)
Life root	gr 40 (2.592 Gm)
Aromatic cordial	q.s.
Alcohol	18%

Action: Anodyne and antispasmodic, suitable for administration in functional disorders of female generative organs.

Uses: In menorrhagia of ovarian origin, in puberty and menopausal neuroses, in uterine irritability.

Supply: OVARITONE—Bottles of 1 pt. and 1 gal.

Administration: *As Anodyne or Antispasmodic*—1 or 2 fl. dr., repeated four or five times daily if necessary, beginning several days prior to onset of menstruation. *As Uterine Tonic*—2 fl. dr., three times daily.

OXACHOL (Columbus Pharmacal)

Cholagogue

Official Name: Elixir Oxgall Comp.

Composition: Each ounce contains:

Oxgall	gr 8	(0.512 Gm)
Cascara	gr 40	(2.592 Gm)
Pepsin	gr 4	(0.259 Gm)
Papain	gr 4	(0.259 Gm)
Taraxacum	gr 20	(1.296 Gm)
Podophyllin	gr ½	(0.032 Gm)
Tr. nux vomica	m 16	(1 cc)
Aromatics	q.s.	

Action and Uses: Cholagogue and laxative; *For use* in liver stasis, constipation and intestinal autointoxication.

Supply: OXACHOL—Bottles 1 pt. and 1 gal.

Administration: 1 or 2 teaspoonfuls three times daily after meals.

OXIPHEN (Pitman-Moore)

Cholagogue

Composition: Each tablet represents:

	Gr	Gm
Sodium glycocholate	¼	0.016
Sodium taurocholate	¼	0.016
Phenolphthalein	½	0.032
Extr. cascara	½	0.032
Aloin	⅛	0.008

Action and Uses: A cholagogue cathartic *for use* in habitual constipation, producing gentle stimulation of the secretory and muscular functions of the intestinal tract; in biliary stasis, catarrhal jaundice, hepatitis.

Supply: OXIPHEN—Tablets—Bottles of 100.

Administration: 1 tablet after evening meal or on retiring, increasing to 1 tablet after meals and at bedtime, when required.

OXYCAINE (Strasenburgh)

Antacid. Sedative

Composition: Each tablet represents:

	Gr	Gm
Cerium oxalate	1	0.064
Bismuth subcarbonate	2	0.130
Light magnesia	4	0.259
Benzocaine	¼	0.016

Action and Uses: Gastric sedative and antacid in gastralgia, nausea, vomiting and hyperacidity.

Supply: OXYCAINE—Tablets—Bottles of 500 and 1,000.

Administration: 1–2 tablets after meals.

PABUTOLE (Sharp and Dohme)

Nutrient. Tonic

Description: Each fluid ounce contains—

Calcium Hypophosphite	gr ⅜	(0.024 Gm)
Calcium Iodide	gr ⅛	(0.008 Gm)

Iron Hypophosphite	gr 1/4	(0.016 Gm)
Manganese Hypophosphite	gr 1/8	(0.008 Gm)
Potassium Hypophosphite	gr 1/4	(0.016 Gm)
Sodium Salicylate	gr 3/4	(0.048 Gm)
Sodium Hypophosphite	gr 1/8	(0.008 Gm)
Alcohol	17%	
Flavor	q.s.	

In addition, Carbohydrates, 18½%; Proteins, 5%; Fats, 2% and vitamins A B D and E, with traces of C.

Action and Uses: A palatable nutrient and tonic for impaired digestion, disordered nutrition, in convalescence and other conditions where easily digested food is indicated.

Supply: PABUTOLE—Bottles of 14 oz.

Administration: 1–2 tablespoonfuls four times daily in water or milk.

PALPEBRINE (Dios Chemical)

Antiseptic

Composition: Contains per ounce

	Gr	Gm
Zinc Sulphate	1/7	0.009
Mercury Bichloride	1/11	0.0058
Salicylic Acid	3/4	0.0486
Boric Acid	5 3/8	0.348

Action and Uses: As antiseptic and astringent in conjunctivitis, blepharitis and other external eye affections.

Supply: PALPEBRINE—Bottles of 3 oz.

Administration: By dropper, three or four times daily.

PANACOIDS (Reed and Carnrick)

Digestant

Composition: Each tablet contains 2 gr (0.130 Gm) of desiccated Pancreas and 1 gr (0.064 Gm) of desiccated Duodenal substance.

Action and Uses: Stimulates the production of pancreatic enzymes and hormones and is of importance in activating proenzymes; *For use* in intestinal indigestion and functional disorders of the pancreas.

Supply: PANACOIDS—Bottles of 100, 500 and 1,000.

Administration: 1–4 tablets, several times daily.

PANALGYN (Sharp and Dohme)

Analgesic. Antiarthritic

Composition: Contains per fluid ounce:

Strontium salicylate	gr 20	(1.296 Gm)
Strontium iodide	gr 8	(0.520 Gm)
Colchicine	gr 1/50	(0.0013 Gm)
Pilocarpine	gr 1/8	(0.008 Gm)
Gelsemium	gr 1	(0.065 Gm)
Alcohol	8%	

Action and Uses: Analgesic and alterative; the unpleasant taste of the ingredients is favorably disguised; *For use* in diseases benefited by iodides and salicylates—rheumatism, gout, lumbago and similar affections.

Supply: PANALGYN—Bottles of 1 pt. and 1 gal.

Administration: 1–2 Teaspoonfuls increased to 1 tablespoonful every 3–4 hr., followed by glass of water or milk.

PAN-BIS-CAL (Noyes)

Digestant

Composition: Each fluid ounce represents:

	Gr	Gm
Pancreatin	8	0.52
Malt diastase	4	0.26
Bismuth subcarbonate	20	1.29
Calcium phenolsulphonate	4	0.26
Calcium carbonate, pure	40	2.59
Aromatics	q.s.	

Action and Uses: Digestant of starchy foods, gastric sedative and antacid; *For use* in gastric dyspepsia, pyrosis, intestinal fermentation and diarrhea.

Supply: PAN-BIS-CAL—Bottles of 1 pt., 1 gal..

Administration: 2–4 teaspoonfuls, repeated as necessary; children in proportion.

PANOPEPTON (Fairchild)

Nutrient

Description: A sterile, readily assimilable solution of all the soluble substances in prime lean beef and whole wheat.

Composition: Contains approximately 24% of nutritive constituents; Protein 6.5%, Carbohydrates 16.5%, Inorganic Salts 1%, Alcohol by weight 15%.

Action and Uses: An easily digestible, revivifying and restorative nutrient; *For use* in acute diseases, fevers, pre- and post-operative surgical cases, convalescence, weakness, fatigue, defective assimilation, seasickness, insomnia.

Administration:

Adults—1 dessertspoonful or 1 tablespoonful several times daily and at bedtime.
Infants—from a few drops to ½ teaspoonful.
May be taken as *hot drink*—1 tablespoonful in ⅔ cup of boiling water and 1 teaspoonful lemon juice, sugar to taste; as *hot bouillon*—1 tablespoonful in cup of boiling water, a pinch of salt, pepper, celery salt; *as whey*—1 tablespoonful in cup of whey with cracked ice; *iced*—placed in cup half full of cracked ice.

Supply: PANOPEPTON—Plain—Bottles of 6 and 12 oz.

Combinations: PANOPEPTON FERRUGINOUS—Each tablespoonful contains metallic iron equivalent to ¼ gr of official ferric salt; *dosage* same as Panopepton.

PAN-PEPTIC ELIXIR (Sharp and Dohme)

Digestant

Composition: Each fluid ounce contains—

Pepsin	gr 6	(0.39 Gm)
Pancreatin saccharated	gr 4	(0.26 Gm)

Lactic acid	m	17–20	(0.12 Gm)
Caffeine	gr	1	(0.065 Gm)
Celery seed	gr	1⅕	(0.078 Gm)
Aromatics and Alcohol		20%	

Action and Uses: A digestive and palatable tonic in gastrointestinal diseases, as gastric atony and nervous dyspepsia; also useful as menstruum for the administration of iodides, bromides and salicylates.

Supply: PAN-PEPTIC—Elixir—Bottles of 1 pt. and 1 gal.

PAN-PEPTIC—Powder—Bottles of 1 oz.

PAN-PEPTIC—Tablets—equivalent to 1 dessertspoonful of the elixir—Bottles of 25, 50 and 100.

Administration: 1 or 2 Dessertspoonfuls after meals.

PARAFFIN COMPOUND (Sharp and Dohme)

Dressing for Burns

Composition:

	Per Cent
Beta-naphthol	0.25
Oil eucalyptus	2
Olive oil	5
Paraffin ointment	25
Paraffin	67¾

Action and Uses: A paraffin compound *for use* in extensive burns; serves to apply compression to affected tissues, fulfilling the function of a constant pressure bandage; hastens cicatrization, excludes air; is pliable, ductile and easily removable.

Supply: PARAFFIN COMPOUND—Packages of 2 half pounds each.

Administration: Applied after cleansing and drying burned area; is melted, sprayed with nebulizer or painted with fine camel's hair brush; preceded, if desired, by spray of plain liquid paraffin, with or without antiseptics; dressed, bandages saturated with paraffin compound and covered with ordinary bandage; if necessary, treatment renewed when cicatrization slackens.

Bibliography: *See Chap. XII.*

PARA-PSYLLIUM (Abbott)

Laxative

Composition: An emulsion containing 80% Liquid Petrolatum with Psyllium Seed Jelly, a gelatinous substance obtained by soaking European psyllium seed in water.

Action: A mild creamy laxative, mucilaginous, non-absorbable, non-irritating, non-toxic and palatable.

Uses: Chronic obstipation in hemorrhoids, pregnancy, diabetes; also for infants and children.

Advantages: No leakage of oil; thorough mixing with intestinal contents; pleasant flavor; free from sugar.

Supply: PARA-PSYLLIUM—Plain—Bottles of 16 fl. oz.

PARA-PSYLLIUM WITH PHENOLPHTHALEIN—Bottles of 16 oz.

Administration: 1 teaspoonful to 1 tablespoonful one or two times daily after meals.

PARATHYROID WITH CALCIUM

Calcium Therapy

Description: Preparations containing Parathyroid and Calcium.

Action and Uses: Controls blood calcium level influencing function of muscular and nerve tissues; *For use* in tetany, nursing mothers, rickets; in congenital syphilis, gastroenteritis and bronchial pneumonia.

Supply: **PARATHYROID WITH CALCIUM LACTATE**—Tablets containing: (Armour)

	Gr	Gm
Parathyroid	1/20	0.003
Calcium Lactate	2½	0.15

Bottles of 100, 500 and 1,000.

PARATHYROID WITH CALCIUM LACTATE—Powder—Bottles 1 dr. (Armour)

PARATHYROID WITH CALCIUM LACTATE—Tablets containing: (Reed and Carnrick)

	Gr	Gm
Desiccated Parathyroid	1/20	0.003
Calcium Lactate	5	0.324

Bottles of 100, 500 and 1,000.

PARATHYROID AND CALCIUM CITRATE COMPOUND— (Searle) Capsules containing Parathyroid, desiccated gr 1/20 (0.003 Gm) equivalent to 2 gr fresh gland, Calcium Citrate gr 5 (0.324 Gm)—Bottles of 100 and 500.

Administration: 1 or 2 tablets or capsules three times daily, or as directed.

PARRESINE (Abbott)

Emollient. Dressing

Composition:

	Per Cent
Paraffin	94–96
Gum elemi	0.2 –0.25
Japan wax	0.4 –0.5
Asphalt	0.2 –0.25
Eucalyptol	2.0
Alkannin	0.5 –1
Gentian violet	q.s.

Action and Uses: Splints wounded surfaces, maintains uniform tension and offers an air tight dressing in the treatment of burns and skin abrasions.

Supply: PARRESINE (C.A.)—Cakes ½ lb.

Administration: Applied in thin layer by spray, covered lightly with cotton, resprayed and bandaged.

PASANOL (Tilden)

Cardiac Stimulant

Composition: Each fluid dram represents:

	Gr	Gm
Cactus grandiflora	1/16	0.004
Digitalin	1/100	0.0006

Nitroglycerin	1/100	0.0006
Strychnine sulphate	1/100	0.0006
Strophanthin	1/200	0.0003

Action and Uses: Cardiovascular stimulant; *For use* in functional disorders of the heart with palpitation, weakness, precordial distress.

Supply: PASANOL—Bottles 1 pt.

Administration: 1 teaspoonful two to three times daily.

PASSIFLORA COMPOUND (C. D. Smith

Sedative

Composition: Contains in each tablet:

Tr. Passiflora	m 1	(0.0616 cc)
Tr. Chamomilla	m 1	(0.0616 cc)
Tr. Ignatia	m 1	(0.0616 cc)
Tr. Hyoscyamus	m 2	(0.1232 cc)
T. Pulsatilla	m 2	(0.1232 cc)
Lupulin	gr 1/10	(0.006 Gm)

Action and Uses: Sedative in insomnia, nervous and mental irritability, hysteria.

Supply: PASSIFLORA COMPOUND—Bottles of 1,000 and 5,000.

Administration: 1–2 tablets, two or three times daily after meals.

PASSIPHEN (McNeil)

Sedative

Composition: Each tablet represents:

	Gr	Gm
Extract of Passiflora	1	0.064
Extract of Valerian	1	0.064
Extract of Hyoscyamus	1/8	0.008
Phenobarbital	1/4	0.016

Action and Uses: Sedative and antispasmodic in insomnia, restlessness, nervous depression.

Supply: PASSIPHEN (C.A.)—Tablets—Bottles of 100, 500, 1,000, 5,000.

Administration: 1 or 2 tablets when required.

PEPANA (Burroughs Wellcome)

Digestant

Composition: A combination of digestive ferments; each tablet contains:

	Gr	Gm
Pepsin	1	0.064
Pancreatin	1	0.064
Calcium Lactophosphate	1	0.064

Action and Uses: A gastrointestinal digestive; after the sugar coating is dissolved in the stomach, the tablet liberates pepsin which functions there locally; the pancreatin, enclosed in an inner coating of keratin is freed only in the alkaline medium of the intestines and becomes effective there; *For use* in gastric and intestinal digestive disorders.

Supply: PEPANA—Bottles of 25, 100 and 500.

Administration: 1–3 tablets in water, two to three times daily after meals.

PERTUSSIN (Seeck and Kade)

Expectorant. Antispasmodic

Description: Extractum Thymi Saccharatum "Taeschner"; a saccharated, syrupy extract of the active principles of Thymus Vulgaris, prepared by the Taeschner process.

Action and Uses: Aids in liquefying mucus, relieving spasmodic attacks of whooping cough, in colds, bronchial affections and in asthma; helpful in coughs of the aged.

Supply: PERTUSSIN—Bottles of 4 and 11 oz.

Administration: 1 tablespoonful every hour; children ½–1 teaspoonful.

Bibliography: *See Chap. XII.*

PETROBRAN (Sargent)

Laxative

Composition:

	Per Cent
Petrolatum	74
Bran	22
Powdered licorice with ethyl butyrate	4

Action and Uses: As for petrolatum; *useful* as laxative in spastic constipation with small, dry and hard stools.

Supply: PETROBRAN (C.A.)—Jars 4 oz.

Administration: 1–2 tablespoonfuls at bedtime.

PETROLAGAR (Petrolagar)

Laxative

Composition: An emulsion of Liquid Petrolatum, 65% by volume, with Agar Agar; contains in addition Sugar and Sodium Benzoate 0.1%; is readily miscible with water and completely homogenized; flavored for palatability.

Action and Uses: Induces normal physiologic motor function of intestines; protects the mucosa mechanically like natural mucus; is not absorbed, but mixes freely with the intestinal contents, providing for normal fecal consistency and producing a laxative effect.

Supply: PETROLAGAR—Plain (C.A.)—Bottles of 16 oz.

PETROLAGAR WITH CASCARA (NON-BITTER) (C.A.)—Containing 13.2 cc fluid extract of Cascara Sagrada per 100 cc; for constipation.—Bottles of 8 and 16 oz.

PETROLAGAR WITH PHENOLPHTHALEIN (C.A.)—Gr ⅔ (0.32 Gm) per tablespoonful—for more obstinate constipation—Bottles of 16 oz.

PETROLAGAR WITH MILK OF MAGNESIA (C.A.)—8%, for constipation with hyperacidity—Bottles of 16 oz.

PETROLAGAR—Unsweetened (C.A.) (without sugar), for diabetics—Bottles of 16 oz.

Administration: *Orally*—1 tablespoonful night and morning.

Rectally—2–4 oz. in pint of warm water.

Infants—1 teaspoonful plain with feeding formula.

Obstetrics—In nausea of pregnancy—1 tablespoonful of Petrolagar with Milk of Magnesia, in ½ glass grape juice, mornings and at bedtime.

Proctology—2 oz. introduced into rectum to protect wound after injection treatment for hemorrhoids.

Surgery—As post operative prophylactic to prevent distention, meteorism; in usual dosage.

Ophthalmology—To prevent straining at stool after cataract extraction; usual dosage.

Bibliography: *See Chap. XII.*

PHEDROS (Sharp and Dohme)

Sedative

Official Name: Syrupus Ephedra Co.

Composition:

Fl. ex. ephedra vulgaris	m 40
Chloroform	m 2
Syrup squill	m 180
Syrup ipecac	m 40
Ammonium chloride	gr 8
Syrup tolu	q.s.
Alcohol	6%

Action and Uses: An active sedative and expectorant; is especially effective in spasmodic and irritating coughs.

Supply: PHEDROS—Bottles of 1 pt. and 1 gal.

Administration: 1 or 2 teaspoonfuls, repeated in 2 hr. if necessary.

PHENOBILIN (Norwich)

Cholagogue. Laxative

Composition: Each tablet represents:

	Gr	Gm
Phenolphthalein	½	0.032
Sodium Salicylate	1	0.064
Sodium Glyco-Taurocholate	1	0.064
Extract Cascara Sagrada	½	0.032
Menthol	Trace	

Action and Uses: Cholagogue, liver stimulant, biliary antiseptic and laxative in toxemia of intestinal origin.

Supply: PHENOBILIN—Tablets—Bottles of 100 and 1,000.

Administration: 1 or 2 tablets, before meals, with water.

PHENO-SAGRA (McNeil)

Laxative

Description: Combinations of Phenolphthalein and Cascara.

Action and Uses: Laxative and carminative *for use* in all types of constipation, flatulence and intestinal toxemia.

Combinations: PHENO-SAGRA 1—Each tablet represents:

	Gr	Gm
Phenolphthalein	1	0.064
Ext. Cascara Sagrada	⅔	0.042
Podophyllin	1/16	0.004
Powdered Ipecac	1/16	0.004
Ext. Belladonna	1/16	0.004
Ext. Nux Vomica	⅛	0.008

PHENO-SAGRA 2—Each tablet represents:

	Gr	Gm
Phenolphthalein	½	0.032
Cascarin	¼	0.016
Aloin	¼	0.016
Podophyllin	¼	0.016
Ext. Belladonna Leaves	⅛	0.008
Carminatives	q.s.	

Supply: PHENO-SAGRA—Tablets—Bottles of 100, 500, 1,000 and 5,000.

Administration: 1 or 2 tablets as necessary.

PHENOBARBOID "LOWENTHAL" (American Organotherapy)

Sedative

Composition: Contains per tablet—

	Gr	Gm
Phenobarbital	1½	0.09
Sodium bromide	1/10	0.006
Excipient	1	0.06

Action and Uses: As sedative in insomnia, chorea, epilepsy and other nervous disorders.

Supply: PHENOBARBOID "LOWENTHAL"—Tablets—Bottles of 60.

Administration: In epilepsy, 1½ gr mornings and evenings; insomnia, 1½ gr at bedtime, repeated in 4 hr.; chorea, 1 gr twice daily.

PHENOCO (West Disinfecting)

Antiseptic

Composition: A mixture of coal tar Creosote, 27 %, obtained by destructive distillation of coal, with 43 % of higher Phenol homologues, or Phenol containing 2 or more methyl groups, in a solution of Vegetable Soap (30 %).

Description: A dark brown liquid of tar odor, miscible with water in all proportions and forming a white emulsion; is soluble in alcohol, ether, acetone and fixed oils; is miscible with normal saline solution; has a phenol coefficient of 15–16, but is less than half as toxic as phenol.

Action: Strong germicide, antiseptic and disinfectant.

Uses: In surgery, obstetrics, eye, ear, nose and throat diseases and dermatologic infections.

Supply: PHENOCO (C.A.)—Bottles of 16 oz. and Tin cans 1 gal.

Administration: May be used in dilutions of 1–5% or higher, in accordance with requirements.
Solutions of 1–300 parts of water are equal in antiseptic potency to 5% carbolic acid.

Incompatibles: Strong acids and alkaloids.

PHOS-HEPATIC EXTRACT (Liver Meal)

Tonic

Composition: A combination, in palatable form, of stimulating ingredients; contains per fluid ounce:

	Gr	Gm
Extract beef liver	5	0.324
Sodium glycerophosphate	5	0.324
Manganese glycerophosphate	½	0.032
Iron and ammonium citrate	1½	0.097
Alcohol	14%	
Copper, carminatives, digestants		

Action and Uses: A general tonic and hematinic in simple and secondary anemia, nutritional anemias, debility, impaired nutrition, convalescence.

Supply: PHOS-HEPATIC EXTRACT—Bottles 12 oz.

Administration: 1 tablespoonful three times daily after meals; children ½ tablespoonful.

PHOSPHO-LECITHIN (Wampole)

Tonic

Composition: Each fluid ounce contains:

	Gr	Gm
Sodium Glycerophosphate	8	0.512
Calcium Glycerophosphate	4	0.259
Potassium Glycerophosphate	4	0.259
Strychnine Glycerophosphate	1/60	0.001
Lecithin	1/16	0.004
Avenin	1/30	0.002
Alcohol	14%	

Action and Uses: A general tonic, particularly in cases of disordered nervous system; also an appetizer; *For use* in convalescence, debility, neurasthenia, malnutrition.

Supply: PHOSPHO-LECITHIN—Bottles of 16 oz.

Administration: 2 teaspoonfuls, four times daily, before meals.
Children ½–1 teaspoonful.

PHOSPHORCIN (Eimer and Amend)

Tonic

Composition: Contains per ounce:

	Gr	Gm
Phosphoric acid (U.S.P.)	8	0.512
Calcium glycerophosphate	6	0.384
Sodium glycerophosphate	10	0.643
Lactated pepsin	2	0.130
Powder extract nux vomica, (U.S.P.)	⅕	0.013
Glycerin C.P.	50%	

Action and Uses: Supplies phosphorus in assimilable form; is a reconstructive and nerve tonic in anemia, chlorosis, debility, exhaustion; also in general paralysis, impotence, rickets, osteomalacia.

Supply: **PHOSPHORCIN**—Bottles 10 oz.

Administration: 1–2 teaspoonfuls three times daily.
Children 1 teaspoonful.

PHOSTONE ELIXIR (McNeil)

Nerve Tonic

Description: A palatable elixir. Each fluid ounce represents:

Calcium Glycerophosphate Sodium Glycerophosphate Potassium Glycerophosphate	gr 16 (1.024 Gm)
Strychnine Glycerophosphate	gr 1/30 (0.002 Gm)
Lecithin Albuminate	gr ¼ (0.016 Gm)
Papain	gr 2 (0.130 Gm)
Alcohol	18%

Action and Uses: Nerve stimulant, tonic and reconstructive in anemia, convalescence and similar conditions.

Supply: **PHOSTONE ELIXIR**—Bottles of 2, 3, 4 oz.—Cartons of 12; also 1 pt., ½ and 1 gal.

Administration: 2–4 teaspoonfuls, two or three times daily.

PHYTOLACCA COMPOUND (Drug Products)

Reduction Therapy

Composition: Each pulvoid represents:

	Gr	Gm
Phytolacca fructus powdered extract	2	0.130
Powdered Apocynum	1	0.064
Thyroid, fresh gland	1	0.064
Pituitary, whole gland	½	0.032

Action and Uses: Is stated to affect fat and water metabolism. For use in reduction therapy of obesity.

Supply: **PHYTOLACCA COMPOUND**—Pulvoids—Bottles of 100, 500, 1,000.

Administration: 1 pulvoid 3 times daily, increased to 2 pulvoids after third week.

PHYTOSALICYL (Sutliff and Case)

Antiarthritic

Composition: Contains per fluid ounce:

	Gr	Gm
Sodium Salicylate	80	5.18
Phytolaccin	8	0.52
Colchicine	8/300	0.00173
Macrotine	2	0.13
Pilocarpine	8/200	0.0026
Alcohol	13.2%	

Action and Uses: Antiarthritic *for use* in rheumatic fever, acute articular rheumatism, gout and other arthritic disorders.

Supply: PHYTOSALICYL—Bottles of 1 pt., 1 gal.

Administration: 1–2 teaspoonfuls diluted with water, five or six times daily.

PICRATOL (Wyeth)

Antiseptic

Chemical Name: Silver Picrate; contains 30% silver as the trinitrophenolate.

Action and Uses: Mildly germicidal, antiseptic, styptic, analgesic; non-caustic, non-irritating; *For use* in hemorrhoids, burns, infections.

Supply: PICRATOL—Ointment 2%—Collapsible tubes of 1 oz.

PICRATOL—Rectal Suppositories, gr ¼ and gr ½, in boroglyceride base, for fissures, hemorrhoids—Boxes of 20.

PICRATOL—Urethral Suppositories, gr ½ and gr 1—Boxes of 20.

PICRATOL—Vaginal Suppositories, gr 1, gr 2, in boroglyceride and gelatin—Boxes of 20.

Administration: *Externally*, applied as required.

PINE AND SOMNOS CORDIAL (Sharp and Dohme)

Expectorant

Composition: Contains per fluid ounce:

		Gm
Somnos (Sharpe and Dohme)	m 120	7.392
Syrup white pine	m 30	1.848
Syrup wild cherry	m 60	3.696
Syrup tolu	m 48	2.956
Syrup squill	m 60	3.696
Syrup ipecac	m 24	1.478
Syrup sanguinaria	m 30	1.848
Chloroform	m 3	0.184
Elixir glycerophosphate	m 48	2.956
Alcohol	9%	

Action and Uses: A sedative expectorant and tonic; allays cough and promotes expectoration in chronic bronchitis, emphysema and similar pulmonary affections.

Supply: PINE AND SOMNOS CORDIAL—Bottles of 1 pt. and 1 gal.

Administration: 1 or 2 teaspoonfuls; repeated when necessary.

POTASSIUM IODIDE-THEOCALCIN (Bilhuber-Knoll)

Vasodilator

Composition: Contains Theocalcin gr 7½ (0.5 Gm) with Potassium iodide gr 1½ (0.09 Gm) per tablet.

Action and Uses: A myocardial stimulant and diuretic *for use* in stenocardia, hypertensive cardiovasculo-renal disease, arteriosclerosis, luetic aortitis.

Supply: POTASSIUM IODIDE-THEOCALCIN—Tablets—Tubes of 20—Bottles of 100.

Administration: 1–2 tablets, crushed and taken with water, at meals and at bedtime; dosage reduced as soon as possible.

Bibliography: *See Chap. XII.*

PROKLIMAN (Ciba)

Sedative

Composition: Each tablet represents:

Sistomensin	gr ⅛	(20 mg)
Nitroglycerine	gr 1/320	(0.2 mg)
Amidopyrine	gr 1½	(0.01 Gm)
Caffeine sodio-salicylate	gr ¾	(50 mg)
Peristaltine	gr ¼	(15 mg)

Action and Uses: Combines the effects of its constituents; is *used* for the relief of disturbances associated with climacterium: nervous and mental manifestations, hypertension, hot flushes, sweating, cardiac disturbances, headaches, irregular bleeding.

Supply: PROKLIMAN—Tablets—Bottles of 40 and 100.

Administration: 2 tablets two to three times daily after meals.

Bibliography: *See Chapter XII.*

PROTEOLAC (Searle)

Non-Specific Protein Therapy

Description: A clear solution of Peptones and Proteoses derived from milk.

Action: Stimulates leukocytosis, increases resistance to infection.

Uses: In acute infections: influenza, arthritis, furunculosis; in allergic conditions—asthma, hay fever; dermatologic lesions—acne, eczema; genito-urinary-gonorrhea and its complications; in eye infections; purulent disease—mastitis, lymphangitis, abscesses; in sepsis, septicemia, puerperal fever; in thrombophlebitis, peptic ulcer and adenitis.

Supply: PROTEOLAC—Ampules 1 and 2 cc—Boxes of 12, 25, 100.
PROTEOLAC—Ampules 5 and 10 cc—Boxes of 6, 25, 100.

Administration: *Intradermal*—In diseases of skin, mucous membranes, joints; 3 m to raise wheal.
Intramuscularly—In systemic diseases—initial test dose 1–2 cc, rapidly increased to 5 and 10 cc, given at intervals of 2–5 days, using 5 and 10 cc ampules.
Intravenously—Beginning with smallest dose and increased slowly; given where strong and rapid action is desired, every 2–5 days.

PROTONUCLEIN (Reed and Carnrick)

Endocrine Stimulant

Composition: Each tablet represents:

	Gr	Gm
Thyroid	1/14	0.004
Suprarenal	1/14	0.004
Lymphatic substance	1/6	0.012
Brain	1/6	0.012
Spleen	1/3	0.018
Pancreas	1/3	0.018
Thymus	1/9	0.006

Pepsin, Salivary gland, Excipients.

Action and Uses: Represents hormones of the principal endocrine glands, in physiological association, for the promotion of metabolism and improvement of nutrition; actuates defensive forces of the organism and stimulates the glands of internal secretion; *For use* in various types of malnutrition, debility, neurasthenia and convalescence; externally—to stimulate granulation of wounds.

Supply and Dosage: PROTONUCLEIN—Tablets, gr 3 (0.19 Gm)—Bottles of 100, 500 and 1,000.

Dosage—2–4 tablets after meals and at bedtime.

PROTONUCLEIN—Powder—Bottles of 1 and 8 oz.

Dosage—3–9 gr (0.19–0.57 Gm) after meals and at bedtime.

PROTONUCLEIN—Special Tablets, gr 2 (0.130 Gm)—Bottles of 80, 500 and 1,000, containing extracts of Spleen and Pancreas 50%; *For use* especially in diabetes.

Dosage—2–4 tablets, three or four times daily.

PROTONUCLEIN—Beta Cubes—containing 50% Spleen with Protonuclein; *For use* in tuberculosis, hypertension.

Dosage—2–4 cubes after meals, chewed thoroughly—Bottles of 60, 300 and 600.

PROTONUCLEIN—Special Dusting Powder—containing also Boric Acid; *For use* to stimulate granulation; applied externally; Supply—1/8, 1 oz.

PROTONUCLEIN—Ointment—containing 19% Protonuclein Special Powder and 12% Balsam of Peru; *For use* as stimulating ointment—Jars 1 oz.

PTHALOX (Sutliff and Case)

Cholagogue. Laxative

Composition: Contains per tablet:

	Gr	Gm
Ricinoleic acid	1	0.06
Phenolphthalein	1/2	0.03
Sodium glycocholate	1/4	0.016
Sodium taurocholate	1/4	0.016
Ext. cascara	1/2	0.03
Aloin	1/8	0.008

Action and Uses: Hepatic, stimulant laxative and intestinal detoxicant; *For use* in constipation, catarrhal jaundice, intestinal fermentation.

Supply: PTHALOX—Tablets—Bottles of 500, 1,000.

Administration: 1–2 tablets at night.

PULVULES LEXTRON 55 (Lilly)

Hematinic. Hematopoietic

Composition: Each pulvule contains:

	Gm
Liver-Stomach concentrate	0.433
Iron ammonium citrate (green)	0.2
Vitamin B complex (adsorbed on Lloyd's reagent)	0.016

Description: Contains both of the antianemic liver potencies, the Cohn-Minot Fraction G and the Whipple fraction.

Action and Uses: Stimulates formation of hemoglobin and erythrocytes, increases appetite, weight and strength. *For use* in pernicious anemia and in anemias of secondary character as after hemorrhage; also in undernutrition.

Supply: PULVULES LEXTRON 55—Bottles of 84 and 500.

Administration: 3 pulvules three times daily immediately before meals; children 3–6 pulvules daily.

PYRAMINAL (Metz)

Sedative. Analgesic

Composition: A combination of Pyramidon 2½ gr (0.162 Gm) and Luminal ⅛ gr (0.008 Gm) per tablet.

Action and Uses: The action of each constituent is intensified by the other, making their combined effect more prolonged and giving greater tranquility and mental composure without languor during the day. Valuable as analgesic and sedative in headache, migraine, neuralgia, dysmenorrhea, climacteric disorders.

Supply: PYRAMINAL—Tablets—Tubes of 10—Bottles of 100.

ELIXIR PYRAMINAL—Bottles of 4 and 12 oz.

A palatable preparation especially adapted for children; 1 teaspoonful of elixir is equal to 1 tablet; is best prescribed alone without admixture of other drugs to avoid precipitation.

Administration: Adults--1–2 Tablets, as required. Children—¼–1 teaspoonful of elixir. The doses of both may be repeated in ½–1 hr., if necessary; in cases of intense pain may be doubled.

QUICAMPHOL (Spicer)

Quinine Therapy

Description: A solution of insoluble basic Quinine with Camphor and Aromatic Terpenes; prepared for injection therapy.

Composition: Ampules 1 cc containing:

	Gm
Anhydrous basic quinine	0.03
Camphor	0.025
Eucalyptol	0.18
Menthol	0.08

Action: These components accumulate in the lung tissues, where they act as pneumococcicides and counteract inflammatory processes.

Use: In pulmonary infections; bronchial disease, chronic purulent bronchitis, broncho-, croupous, and postoperative pneumonia; also for prevention of postoperative pneumonia.

Supply: QUICAMPHOL—Ampules 1.2 cc—Boxes of 6.
QUICAMPHOL—Bottles of 25 cc.

Administration: 1–2 cc *intramuscularly* daily for 7–14 days; in chronic affections with purulent expectoration, every 2–3 days.

Bibliography: *See Chap. XII.*

QUINARSIN (Sharp and Dohme)

Antimalarial

Composition: Contains per fluid ounce:

Quinine	gr 4	(0.259 Gm)
Cinchonine	gr 8	(0.512 Gm)
Sodium arsenate	gr 1/16	(0.004 Gm)
Tinct. nux vomica	m 16	(0.985 cc)
Potassium iodide	gr 5	(0.324 Gm)
Iron, other synergists and alcohol	12½%	

Action and Uses: An antimalarial; is used in malarial fevers; particularly valuable as tonic in malarial anemia.

Supply: QUINARSIN—Bottles of 1 pt. and 1 gal.

Administration: 1–2 teaspoonfuls three to four times daily.

QUININE HYDROCHLORIDE AND URETHANE (Parke, Davis)

Sclerosing Agent

Description: An aqueous solution of Quinine Hydrochloride 4 gr (0.266 Gm) and Urethane 2 gr (0.133 Gm) in 2 cc of distilled water.

Action and Uses: Injected into varicose veins acts as a sclerosing agent, gradually obliterating the lumen of the vein, thus directing the return blood flood to the deeper veins of the leg.

Supply: QUININE HYDROCHLORIDE AND URETHANE—Ampules 2 cc—20% solution; Boxes of 12.

Administration: *Intravenously*—In serial injections to cover the entire varicosed area, beginning at the lowest point;
Dosage—Depends upon the condition of the veins.

Contraindications: Pregnancy, menstruation, uterine fibroids, phlebitis, severe kidney disease, myocardial degeneration, extreme old age.

Caution: Deposition of any part of the solution in the subcutaneous tissues is to be avoided.

Bibliography: *See Chap. XII.*

QUININE AND URETHANE (Burroughs Wellcome)

Sclerosing Agent

Composition: Each hypoloid represents—

	Gm
Quinine Bihydrochloride	0.26
Urethane	0.13

Action and Uses: As sclerosing agent for the injection of varicose veins and hydrocele.

Supply: HYPOLOID QUININE AND URETHANE—2 cc—Boxes of 5.

Administration: ½–1 cc injected into each varicosity.

QUININE CAMPHOR COMPOUND (Stoddard)

Antipyretic

Composition: Each tablet represents:

	Gr	Gm
Salcetol (Stoddard)	¼	0.016
Atropine sulphate	1/600	0.0001
Quinine sulphate	⅛	0.008
Strychnin sulphate	1/200	0.0003
Potassium bromide	⅙	0.012
Camphor	¼	0.016

Action and Uses: Antipyretic and analgesic in colds and respiratory affections.

Supply: QUININE CAMPHOR COMPOUND—Tablets—Bottles 100, 500 and 1,000.

QUININE CAMPHOR COMPOUND WITH MORPHINE SULPHATE—Tablets containing gr 1/80 (0.0008 Gm) of morphine sulphate—Bottles 100, 500 and 1,000.

Administration: 1 tablet every hour; then every 2 or 3 hr, as required.

QUINOTHESIN (McNeil)

Antiseptic

Description: Combinations of Quinosol (Oxyquinolin Sulphate "McNeil") and Orthesin (Anesthesin "McNeil").

Action and Uses: Antiseptic and analgesic; *For use* in infections of the throat, nose, and intestinal mucous membranes; externally in burns, scalds, psoriasis and ringworm of the feet (athlete's foot).

Combinations: LOZENGES QUINOTHESIN—containing:

	Gr	Gm
Orthesin	¼	0.016
Quinosol	1/100	0.0006
Aromatics	q.s.	

OINTMENT QUINOTHESIN 1—(Skin) containing:

	Per Cent
Orthesin	1
Quinosol	1/10
Sodium Bicarbonate and White Petrolatum	q.s.

OINTMENT QUINOTHESIN 2—(Nasal) containing:

	Per Cent
Ephedrine Hydrochloride	1
Orthesin, Quinosol, Aromatics and Petrolatum	q.s.

OINTMENT QUINOTHESIN 3—(Rectal) containing per ounce:

Orthesin	gr 10 (0.643 Gm)
Sol. Epinephrine Hydrochloride	m 45 (2.772 cc)
Quinosol, Zinc Oxide, Aromatics, Lanum and Petrolatum	q.s.

POWDER QUINOTHESIN—Containing:

	Per Cent
Orthesin	5
Quinosol Salicylate	1/10
Sodium Hyposulphite and Acid Boric	q.s.

TABLETS QUINOTHESIN, chocolate coated—Containing:

	Gr	Gm
Orthesin	1/2	0.032
Quinosol	1/2	0.032
Lead Acetate	1/6	0.012
Powd. Ipecac	1/8	0.008
Camphor	q.s.	

Supply: QUINOTHESIN AND COMBINATIONS—Lozenges and Tablets—Bottles of 100, 500, 1,000 and 5,000.
Ointment 1—Tubes of 1 and 12—Jars 1 and 5 lb.
Ointment 2—Tubes (nasal tip) 12.
Ointment 3—Tubes (rectal tip) 12—Jars 1 lb.
Powder—sprinkler top—Cartons 1 and 12.

Administration: Lozenges—whenever required as throat anodyne.
Tablets—1 or 2, as intestinal astringent and anodyne.
Ointment 1—applied freely as emergency relief in burns and scalds, and for treatment of psoriasis.
Ointment 2—applied freely to nasal mucous membrane.
Ointment 3—in the treatment of hemorrhoids, fissures, pruritus.
Powder—dusted freely on affected area in athlete's foot; as prophylactic, dusted into shoes and stockings.

QUINOXYL (Burroughs Wellcome)

Amebacide

Description: A mixture of Iodohydroxyquinoline Sulphonic Acid, 80%, with Sodium Bicarbonate 20%.

Action and Uses: An amebacide; causes little nausea and toxicity and no iodism; in milder cases demands no diet restriction or confinement; safe for children; *For use* in amebic dysentery.

Supply: TABLOID QUINOXYL—Gr 4 (0.25 Gm), Oral—Bottles 25.
SOLOID QUINOXYL—Gr 77 (5 Gm), For Enema—Bottles of 10 Gm.

Administration: *Internally*—1–4 tabloids three times daily.
Rectal—daily retention enemas of 200 cc of 2½% solution prepared from soloids.

Bibliography: *See Chap. XII.*

RECTAL ANALGESIA (Gwathmey) (Lilly)

Description: A preparation especially devised for rectal anesthesia; is represented in 2 strengths and contains—

Formula 1	Ether		2½	oz.
	Alcohol		45	m
	Quinine alkaloid		20	gr
	Mineral oil	q.s. ad	4	oz.
Formula 2	Ether		2½	oz.
	Alcohol		45	m
	Quinine alkaloid		10	gr
	Mineral oil	q.s. ad	4	oz.

Action and Uses: Rectal anesthetic and analgesic; *For use* in relieving pain in childbirth.

Supply: **RECTAL ANALGESIA 1**—Tin contains Formula 1 and 1 ampule mineral oil sufficient for primary rectal instillation.

RECTAL ANALGESIA 2—Tin contains Formula 2 and 1 ampule mineral oil sufficient for secondary rectal instillation.

Administration: After rectal cleansing is administered as retention enema, by means of a rectal analgesia set which contains—

1 rubber pressure bulb, 1 catheter, 1 tube clamp, 2 special rubber connecting tubes.

RESTOPHEN (Noyes)

Sedative

Composition: Each tablespoonful represents:

	Gr	Gm
Extract Hyoscyamus	½	0.032
Powdered Valerian	½	0.032
Extract Sumbul	½	0.032
Phenobarbital	½	0.032
Camphor	q.s.	

Action and Uses: In nervous disorders where a sedative is indicated.

Supply: **RESTOPHEN**—Bottles of 100 and 1,000.

Administration: 1 tablespoonful; repeated when necessary.

ROBOLINE (Reed and Carnrick)

Tonic

Composition: Each ounce represents:

Strychnine sulphate	gr 1/100	(0.00065 Gm)
Quinine sulphate	gr 1/10	(0.006 Gm)
Phosphoric acid, dilute	m 6	

Action: Stimulates appetite, improves tone of nervous system and general circulation.

Uses: In "nervousness" of the aged and convalescents.

Supply: **ROBOLINE**—Bottles of 16 oz. and 1 gal.

Administration: 1–2 tablespoonfuls before meals.

SALADIN (Strasenburgh)

Antipyretic

Composition: Each tablet represents:

	Gr	Gm
Phenacetin	2	0.130
Acetyl salicylic acid	2	0.130
Salol	2	0.130

Action and Uses: Analgesic and antipyretic, in colds, influenza, grippe, malaise.

Supply: **SALADIN**—Tablets—Bottles of 500, 1,000.

SALADIN, JR.—Containing half dosage—Bottles of 500 and 1,000.

SALADIN IMPROVED—Bottles of 500 and 1,000. Containing per tablet:

	Gr	Gm
Phenacetin	2	0.130
Acetyl salicylic acid	2	0.130
Salol	1	0.064
Caffeine	½	0.032

Administration: 1 tablet every 3 hr. or 2 at night as required.

SALICIONYL (Upjohn)

Analgesic. Antacid

Description: A granular effervescent salt containing per heaping teaspoonful (60 gr), when dissolved, 10 gr Sodium Salicylate and 20 gr free Alkaline Bicarbonate, with Citrates and Tartrates to assure systemic alkalinization.

Action and Uses: Antipyretic and antirheumatic causing little unpleasantness from intestinal and gastric irritation, nausea or vomiting; *For use* to combat acidosis and foster general alkalinization in rheumatic fever, tonsillitis and other conditions where salicylates are employed.

Supply: SALICIONYL—Bottles 4 and 8 oz.

Administration: 1 dr. in 6 oz. of water every 1 or 2 hr. until relief is obtained, or until point of tolerance is reached; then at longer intervals.

SANGUINARIA COMPOUND (Stoddard)

Expectorant

Composition: Contains per tablet—

Morphine Sulphate	gr 1/60	(0.001 Gm)
Sanguinarin (conc.)	gr 1/60	(0.001 Gm)
Tartar Emetic	gr 1/60	(0.001 Gm)
Ext. Piscidia	gr ¼	(0.016 Gm)
Ipecac	gr ⅛	(0.008 Gm)
Fl. Ex. Wild Cherry	m 1	(0.064 Gm)
Ammonium Chloride	gr 1	(0.064 Gm)
Ext. Licorice	q.s.	

Action and Uses: As expectorant in bronchitis, pharyngitis, laryngitis, throat irritations and cough.

Supply: SANGUINARIA COMPOUND—Tablets—Bottles of 100, 500 and 1,000 tablets.

Administration: 1–2 tablets, every 2–3 hr., dissolved on tongue.

SANPAIBA (McNeil)

Urinary Antiseptic

Description: A soft elastic globule-capsule containing:

	M
Oil Sandalwood	1¾
Copaiba	1¾
Haarlem Oil (equivalent)	1½
Oil Cassia	q.s.

Action and Uses: Urinary anticatarrhal and astringent, *For use* in urinary disorders.

Supply: SANPAIBA—Capsules soft elastic—Bottles of 100 and 500.

Administration: 2 capsules several times daily.

SARAKA (Schering)

Laxative

Composition: Granules of a species of Bassorit sap and Cortex frangula.

Action and Uses: Increases bulk of intestinal contents, stimulates peristalsis, induces evacuation without griping; *useful* in habitual constipation as a stimulating intestinal lubricant.

Supply: SARAKA—Boxes of 10 oz.

Administration: 1 teaspoonful ½ hr. after meals.

Bibliography: *See Chap. XII.*

SEDACO (Strasenburgh)

Expectorant

Composition: Each ounce represents

Ethyl morphine hydrochloride	gr ⅛	(0.008 Gm)
Chloroform	gr 2	(0.130 Gm)
Sanguinaria nitrate	gr 1/16	(0.004 Gm)
Ammonium chloride	gr 4	(0.259 Gm)
Terpene hydrate, Syrup tolu, Syrup of wild cherry aa	q.s.	
Alcohol	5%	

Action and Uses: Bronchial sedative in respiratory affections.

Supply: SEDACO—Bottles of 4 oz., 1 pt. and 1 gal.

Administration: 1–2 teaspoonfuls, as required.

SEDOBROL (Roche)

Bromide Therapy

Composition: Each Sedobrol cube contains 17 gr of Sodium Bromide, U.S.P., combined with pure vegetable extractives and flavoring matter; 1 or 2 cubes dissolved in a cupful of hot water furnishes a palatable broth in which the taste of the bromides is completely disguised; the hot broth enhances and quickens the absorption and action of the medication.

Uses: As sedative in all conditions in which bromides are indicated: restlessness, neurasthenia, nervous dyspepsia, hyperemesis gravidarum, epilepsy.

Supply: SEDOBROL—Tins of 10, 30 and 100 cubes.

Administration: 2–4 cubes a day; in insomnia—2 cubes dissolved in very hot water, taken with crackers late in the afternoon, or in the evening in lieu of the last meal.

Advantages: Especially useful in the administration of bromides to neurotics and other sensitive patients, the hot bouillon being without a suspicion of medicinal taste or odor.

SELENIUM "OEFELE" (Marvell)

Cancer Prophylactic

Composition: Each tablet contains:

	Gr	Mg
Colloidal selenium	1/64	1
Less soluble selenium	1/40	1½

Normal saline mixture, of 5 cc normal serum content.

Action and Uses: Is claimed to be of value as palliative in the treatment of carcinoma; also to be of use in faulty sulphur metabolism disorders.

Supply: SELENIUM "OEFELE"—Tablets, 1 mg—Bottles of 40.

Administration: 4 Tablets daily.

SILVER NITRATE-ANESTHESIN COMPOUND (Searle)

Sedative

Composition: Each tablet contains:

	Gr	Gm
Silver nitrate	¼	0.016
Anesthesin	⅛	0.008
Ext. nux vomica	¼	0.016
Ext. belladonna	⅛	0.008
Potassium nitrate	½	0.032

Action and Uses: Sedative in acute gastric irritation and pain.

Supply: SILVER NITRATE-ANESTHESIN COMPOUND—Tablets—Bottles of 1,000.

Administration: 1–2 tablets three times daily with water.

SKIABARYT (Merck)

Radiopaque Medium

Composition: A mixture of Barium Sulphate U.S.P., 75–85%, with Sugar, Tragacanth, Vanillin, Cinnamon and Cacao.

Description: A prepared X-ray meal; a fine brown powder of pleasant odor, palatable and easily administered.

Action and Uses: For radiography of esophagus, stomach and intestines; affords dense, compact, continuous and plastic skiagrams; causes no impairment of secretory and kinetic gastrointestinal properties; is smoothly and painlessly excreted with no annoying retention of excreta.

Supply: SKIABARYT—Oral (C.A.)—Tins of 1, 5 and 25 lb.

SKIABARYT—Rectal (C.A.)—Tins of 1, 5 and 25 lb.

Administration: *Oral*—5–6½ oz. (150–200 Gm) or 4–6 heaping tablespoonfuls is made into thin paste with cold water; then enough hot or cold water is added to make the total quantity 1 pt. (0.5 l), ready for administration; the mixture may be taken in 1 or 2 portions.

Rectal—6½ oz. (200 Gm) of Skiabaryt Rectal is mixed with cold water and stirred into a paste; is then diluted with warm water to make a fine suspension of about 2 qt., ready for use.

SODINCO (Irwin, Neisler)

Antacid

Composition: Contains per teaspoonful:

	Gr	Gm
Sodium phosphate	8	0.512
Citric acid	9	0.576
Sodium bicarbonate	15	0.972

Description and Uses: An effervescent yellow-colored, flavored salt. *For use* as alkalizer in acidosis, acute infections, childrens' intestinal disorders.

Supply: SODINCO—Bottles, with dose cap, small and large size.

Administration: 1 teaspoonful between meals.

SODIUM GLYCOCHOLATE COMPOUND (Wampole)

Cholagogue

Composition: Each tablet contains:

	Gr	Gm
Sodium Glyco- and Taurocholate	1½	0.097
Sodium Salicylate	1½	0.097
Sodium Succinate	1½	0.097

Action and Uses: Cholagogue and biliary stimulant; *For use* in hepatitis, jaundice and cholelithiasis.

Marketed: SODIUM GLYCOCHOLATE COMPOUND—Tablets—Bottles of 100.

Administration: 2–3 tablets, 2–3 hr. after meals.

Bibliography: *See Chap. XII.*

SODIUM MORRHUATE 5% WITH BENZYL ALCOHOL (Searle)

Sclerosing Agent

Description: A stable solution of Sodium Salts of the Fatty Acids of cod liver oil and Benzyl Alcohol; is of amber color and soapy consistency.

Action and Uses: For the obliteration treatment of varicose veins, internal hemorrhoids, varicocele, hydrocele, bursae and nevae.

Advantages: Does not produce sloughing on extravasation; causes no pain, no cramps.

Supply: SODIUM MORRHUATE 5 % WITH BENZYL ALCOHOL (C. A.)—Ampules 5 cc—Boxes of 6, 25 and 100.

Administration: ½–2 cc injected into one vein; multiple injections may be given at one sitting, but total not to exceed 5 cc; is administered at 2–7 day intervals.

Bibliography: *See Chap. XII.*

SOLMIDES (Sharp and Dohme)

Bromide Therapy

Composition:	Large Tablet, Gr	Small Tablet, Gr
Ammonium bromide	5	2½
Sodium bromide	5	2½
Potassium bromide	5	2½

Action and Uses: An effervescent preparation *for use* where bromides are indicated.

Supply: SOLMIDES—Tablets, large 15 gr—Tubes of 25.

SOLMIDES—Tablets, small 7½ gr—Tubes of 25.

Administration: As for all bromides.

SOLUREA (McNeil)

Diuretic

Composition: Hexamethylenamine "McNeil."

Action and Uses: Uricolytic, urinary prophylactic and diuretic; *For use* in cystitis and infections of the urethral tract.

Combinations: **CAPSULES AND TABLETS SOLUREA**—Containing Hexamethylenamine, 5 gr (0.324 Gm).

TABLETS SOLUREA—Containing Hexamethylenamine, 7½ gr (0.580 Gm).

CAPSULES SOLUREA COMPOUND—Containing Solurea, 3 gr (0.194 Gm); Ext. Saw Palmetto, 1 gr (0.064 Gm), Ext. Pichi, 1 gr (0.064 Gm), Ext. Corn Silk, ½ gr (0.032 Gm), Ext. Hydrangea, ½ gr (0.032 Gm), Atropine Sulphate, 1/600 (0.1 mg).

TABLET SOLUREA COMPOUND 2—Containing Solurea, 2 gr (0.130 Gm), Acid Boric, 2 gr (0.130 Gm), Potassium Nitrate, 1 gr (0.064 Gm), Ext. Saw Palmetto, ½ (0.032 Gm), Ext. Corn Silk, ½ gr (0.032 Gm), Aromatics, q.s.

TABLETS SOLUREA COMPOUND 3—Chocolate coated—Containing Solurea, 1½ gr (0.097 Gm), Lithium Salicylate, ½ gr (0.032 Gm), Lithium Benzoate, ¾ gr (0.048 Gm), Ext. Corn Silk, ½ gr (0.032 Gm).

TABLETS SOLUREA COMPOUND 4—Plain and flavored—Containing Solurea, 5 gr (0.324 Gm), Acid Sodium Phosphate, 5 gr (0.324 Gm).

TABLETS SOLUREA COMPOUND 5—Containing Solurea, 2½ gr (0.162 Gm), Potassium Citrate, 1½ gr (0.097 Gm), Lithium Carbonate, 1 gr (0.064 Gm).

TABLETS SOLUREA COMPOUND 6—Containing Solurea, 2½ gr (0.162 Gm), Calcium Lactate, 2½ gr (0.162 Gm).

Supply: **SOLUREA AND COMBINATIONS:**
Capsules—Bottles of 100, 500, 1,000 and 5,000.
Tablets—Bottles of 100, 500, 1,000 and 5,000.
Tablets Solurea gr 7½—Bottles of 500, 1,000 and 5,000.

Administration: All capsules or tablets are administered 1 or 2, with water, several times daily.

SOMNOS (Sharp and Dohme)

Sedative. Soporific

Official Name. Elixir Chloral Glycerolate.

Description: A solution of Chloral Glycerolate, 25 gr per fluid ounce, in palatable and sugar-free elixir form.

Action: Hypnotic, producing drowsiness, soon passing into natural sleep; pulse, respiration and blood pressure are slightly lowered; heart is not depressed, nor is circulation or respiration affected as commonly ascribed to ordinary chloral hydrate.

Uses: Recommended as sedative and hypnotic in insomnia from various causes; also in hysteria, delirium, mania, nocturnal epilepsy; as antispasmodic in whooping cough, spasmodic croup, colic and convulsions in children.

Supply: SOMNOS—Bottles of 16 oz.

Administration: *Oral*—As sedative 1 teaspoonful every ½–1 hr.; as hypnotic 1–2 tablespoonfuls at bedtime.
Rectal—In tetanus and strychnine poisoning, in emergencies, in spasmophilia and postoperatively—2 oz. in 5 % sodium bicarbonate solution, as retention enema.

SPINOCAIN (Metz)

Spinal Anesthetic

Description: A solution of Novocain, 10 %, in a solvent of a specific gravity lower than that of spinal fluid with Strychnine Sulphate 1.1 mg per cubic centimeter.

Action and Uses: For spinal anesthesia.

Advantages: Is stated to be safer than ordinary Novocaine, and to eliminate shock almost entirely; rarely causes nausea, vomiting, headache or other complications affecting convalescence after spinal anesthesia.

Supply: SPINOCAIN—Ampules 2 cc—Boxes of 10.
Ephedrine Novocaine Solution, containing 5 % Ephedrine Hydrochloride and 1 % Novocaine to anesthetize site of puncture and maintain blood pressure; Ampules 1 cc—Boxes of 10.
Combination Packages containing 5 ampules each of above products.

Administration: The procedure demands attention to technical details which are fully described in a special pamphlet issued by the manufacturer.

STANNO-YEAST (Stoddard)

Corrective

Composition: Contains per tablet—

	Gr	Gm
Tin proteinate	1	0.064
Yeast desiccated	4	0.259
Aromatics	q.s.	

Action and Uses: *For use* in acne, furunculosis and intestinal infections.

Supply: STANNO-YEAST—Tablets—Bottles of 100, 500 and 1,000 tablets.

Administration: 1–3 tablets, every 3 hr.

STOMACHON (United Laboratories)

Hematopoietic

Composition: Contains desiccated entire hog stomach; each gram is equivalent to 6 Gm of fresh organ substance.

Action and Uses: Hematopoietic *for use* in pernicious anemia.

Supply: STOMACHON—Vials of 10 Gm—Boxes of 12 and 24.

Administration: 1 or 2 vials per diem.

SULPHODINE (Strasenburgh)

Astringent

Composition: Each tablet represents:

	Gr	Gm
Bismuth subgallate	2	0.130
Calcium sulphocarbolate	1	0.064
Sodium sulphocarbolate	2	0.130
Copper sulphocarbolate	1/25	0.0006
Caloxidine (Oxidized calcium)	½	0.032
Menthol and eucalyptol	q.s.	

Action and Uses: Astringent in diarrheal diseases.

Supply: SULPHODINE—Bottles of 500 and 1,000 tablets.

Administration: Two (2) tablets later followed by 1, every 3 hr.

SURGODINE (Sharp and Dohme)

Iodine Therapy

Composition: A miscible solution of Iodine in 92 % Alcohol; contains 2.25 % available iodine, and no glycerin or potassium iodide.

Action and Uses: As for iodine; especially adapted to surgical use.

Supply: SURGODINE—Bottles of 4 oz. and 1 pt.

Administration: 2–10 ♏ well diluted, several times daily;
Externally—Applied in pure form.

SUSTO (Stearns)

Hematinic

Composition: Each teaspoonful represents:

Predigested hog stomach	gr 7½	(0.5 Gm)
Ferrous carbonate	gr 10	(0.6 Gm)
Copper sulphate	gr 1/50	(0.0013 Gm)

Action and Uses: Stimulates hematogenesis in simple and secondary anemias; in anemia of chronic nephritis, cardiorenal disease and following radiotherapy; in the treatment of myelogenous leukemia.

Supply: SUSTO—Powder 5 oz. jars
SUSTO—Capsules—Bottles of 60.

Administration: Usual dosage—1 dr. (3.8 Gm) or 2 capsules with meals, in soup, bouillon, milk or tomato juice. Dosage governed in accordance with conditions presented.

SUXIPHEN "ESKAY" (Smith, Kline and French)

Expectorant. Antispasmodic

Composition: Each dose (2 teaspoonfuls) represents:

Sodium Phenobarbital	1/6 gr (0.012 Gm)
Squill	¾ gr (0.048 Gm)
Sanguinaria	1 gr (0.064 Gm)

Phenolphthalein	1/8 gr	(0.008 Gm)
Alcohol	6 m	(0.369 cc)
Mentholated Syrup of Tolu	q.s.	

Action: Antispasmodic; allays irritation, stimulates expectoration, promotes elimination.

Uses: Bronchitis and bronchial affections with spasm; also in respiratory diseases of children and as general sedative.

Supply: SUXIPHEN—Bottles of 12 oz.

Administration: 2 teaspoonfuls after meals three to four times daily.

SYNDROME TABLETS (Noyes)

Cardiac Stimulant

Composition: Each tablet represents:

Tincture Digitalis	m 4	
Tincture Nux Vomica	m 1	
Caffein Alkaloid	gr 1/2	(0.032 Gm)
Extract Hyoscyamus	gr 1/4	(0.016 Gm)
Nitroglycerin	gr 1/100	(0.00065 Gm)

Action and Uses: As cardiac stimulant, vasodilator and tonic in cardiac arrhythmia with dyspnea, precordial distress or lack of compensation.

Supply: SYNDROME TABLETS—Bottles of 100, 1,000.

Administration: 1 tablet every 4 hr.

SYNODAL (Metz)

Non-specific Therapy

Composition: Brand of Emetabol; is a combination of Lipoproteins with Emetine.

Action and Uses: That of non-specific protein; *For use* in gastric ulcer to allay pain, gastric tonus and hunger contractions; to diminish pylorospasm and increase vascularity and thus improve the circulation around the ulcer.

Supply: SYNODAL—Ampules, 6 cc—Boxes of 5.

Administration: *Intravenously*—1 ampule twice weekly, with 1 week interval after sixth dose; in severe cases administered more frequently; maximum number of injections during 1 course, 10; intervals between courses 6–8 weeks. May be used intramuscularly, but with slight discomfort.

Caution: To be administered on empty stomach; in acidosis and dehydration, a dram of bicarbonate of soda is given 5–10 min. before administration.

Bibliography: *See Chap. XII.*

SYRUP GUAIACOL AMMONIUM COMPOUND (Stoddard)

Expectorant

Composition: Represents per ounce—

	Gr	Gm
Potassium Guaiacol Sulphonate	16	1.024
Ammonium Chloride	16	1.024
Ammonium Bromide	8	0.512
Compound Syrup Thyme	q.s.	

Action and Uses: A light amber syrupy liquid, *for use* as a stimulating expectorant in non-productive coughs and for bronchial sedation in various respiratory affections.

Supply: SYR. GUAIACOL AMMONIUM COMPOUND—Bottles 1 pint and 1 gallon.

Administration: 1–2 teaspoonfuls every 2–4 hr.

SYRUP OF AMMONIUM HYPOPHOSPHITE (Gardner)

Expectorant

Chemical Name: Ammonium Hypophosphite.

Formula: $NH_4PH_2O_2$.

Descriptions: Contains gr 16 Ammonium Hypophosphite C.P. per fluid ounce; is a colorless, odorless liquid of slight acid reaction and agreeable taste.

Action and Uses: Stimulating expectorant, resolvent, alterative and eliminant; is non-narcotic and palatable; *For use* in coughs of colds and influenza; in laryngitis, pharyngitis, bronchitis, pertussis and bronchopneumonia.

Supply: SYRUP OF AMMONIUM HYPOPHOSPHITE—Bottles 4 and 8 oz.

Administration: 1–2 teaspoonfuls, with or without water, as frequently as necessary. Children in proportion.

Caution: Not to be used in tuberculosis.

SYRUP OF HYDRIODIC ACID (Gardner)

Iodine Therapy

Description: Contains 6.66 gr (0.426 Gm) of resublimed Iodine or 6.72 gr (0.430 Gm) gaseous Hydrogen Iodide (HI) per fluid ounce; is clear, colorless, odorless, of acid taste and reaction.

Action and Uses: That of active iodine; is antiseptic, alterative, eliminative; stimulates metabolism and glandular action; is non-irritant to gastric mucosa; *For use* in acute or chronic infections of the respiratory tract, resolution stage of pneumonia; in bronchial asthma, influenza, arthritis, arteriosclerosis; in syphilis and endocrinopathies.

Supply: SYRUP OF HYDRIODIC ACID—Bottles 4 and 8 oz.

Administration: Dosage regulated by existing conditions; usually ½–3 teaspoonfuls is taken with plenty of water on starch-free stomach.

SYRUP HYPOPHOSPHITE OF CALCIUM (Gardner)

Calcium Therapy

Composition: Contains per fluid ounce gr 20 (1.296 Gm) of Calcium Hypophosphite.

Action and Uses: A preparation supplying 2 important elements in the treatment of rickets, delayed dentition and non-union of fractures; also in anemia, scrofula, cachexia, during pregnancy and lactation, and in incipient tuberculosis.

Supply: SYRUP HYPOPHOSPHITE OF CALCIUM—Bottles 4 and 8 oz.

Administration: 1–2 teaspoonfuls after meals; in tuberculosis ½–1 teaspoonful, guided by the character of expectoration.

SYRUP HYPOPHOSPHITES OF IRON AND QUININE (Gardner)

Hematinic

Composition: Contains per fluid ounce:

	Gr	Gm
Ferrous Hypophosphite C.P.	4	0.259
Quinine Hypophosphite C.P.	1	0.064

Action and Uses: Hematinic; *For use* in anemia, chlorosis, anorexia, convalescence and malarial prophylaxis.

Supply: SYRUP HYPOPHOSPHITES OF IRON AND QUININE—Bottles of 4 and 8 oz.

Administration: 1 dessertspoonful after meals.

SYRUP HYPOPHOSPHITE OF SODIUM (Gardner)

Alterative

Composition: Contains per fluid ounce gr 20 (1.296 Gm) of pure Hypophosphite of Sodium.

Action and Uses: A preparation for use in the treatment of neurasthenia, insomnia, convalescence, anemia and incipient tuberculosis.

Supply: SYRUP HYPOPHOSPHITE OF SODIUM—Bottles 4 and 8 oz.

Administration: 1–2 teaspoonfuls after meals; in tuberculosis ½–1 teaspoonful, guided by the quantity of expectoration.

TABLET THEOBUTIN COMPOUND (Stoddard)

Diuretic

Composition: Each tablet contains—

	Gr	Gm
Powdered Digitalis	¼	0.016
Theobromine Sodium Salicylate	2	0.130
Potassium Nitrate	½	0.032
Arbutin	1/10	0.006
Aromatics	q.s.	

Action and Uses: Diuretic *for use* in nephritis with edema.

Supply: Bottles of 100, 500 and 1,000 tablets.

Administration: 1–3 tablets, three to four times daily.

TARTRO-QUINIOBINE (Spicer)

Antiluetic

Composition: A combination of Quiniobine 0.072 Gm with water soluble Sodium Potassium Bismuth Tartrate 0.032 Gm, finely suspended in oil, with Camphor 0.003 Gm; Each cubic centimeter represents—

	Gm
Metallic Bismuth	0.030
Iodine	0.037
Quinine	0.022

Action and Uses: An active spirocheticide; effective in all stages of syphilis and its various manifestations; being absorbed slowly, its action is prolonged. *Used also* in iritis, neuritis, and neuroretinitis.

Supplied: TARTRO-QUINIOBINE—Ampules (C.A.) 2 cc—Boxes of 6.

TARTRO-QUINIOBINE—Liquid—Bottles of 25 cc.

Administration: *Intragluteally:*

Week	Cc	Injections	
1	1–2	3	followed by 2 weeks' rest
2	2	2	
3	2	2	
4	2	2	followed by 3 weeks' rest and continued
5	1–2	2	

Visceral, Neurosyphilis—7 weeks' course.

Infants—Initial dose 0.1 cc; total dosage 2.5 cc.

Bibliography: *See Chap. XII.*

TENAMIN (Winthrop)

Uterine Hemostatic

Chemical Name: Hydrochlorides of Paraoxyphenylethylamin (Tyramine) and Betaimidazolethylamin (Histamine). Brand of Amergine.

Formulae: $(CH)_2NH.\ N.\ C.\ (CH_2)_2.\ NH_2.\ HCl$ and $OH.\ C_6H_4(CH_2)_2NH_2.\ HCl$.

Description: Contains two active principles of ergot in the form of hydrochlorides in proportion of 1:50 and free from ergotoxin or inert matter; is a clear, colorless, tasteless, stable solution.

Action: Offers the combined action of the two components, one closely allied to epinephrine with its qualifications, the other to histamine with some synergistic and other antagonistic effects; is a powerful uterine hemostatic.

Uses: *For use* in postpartum hemorrhage, metrorrhagia and other pelvic conditions where ergot is indicated.

Supply: TENAMIN—Liquor—Bottles of ½ oz.

TENAMIN—Ampules, 1.2 cc each—Boxes of 10.

Administration: *Orally*—15–20 drops, three to four times daily;

Subcutaneously and Intramuscularly—1 ampule, repeated if necessary.

Caution: Should never be injected intravenously.

Bibliography: *See Chap. XII.*

TEROGON "SCHUFTAN" (Cavendish)

Urinary Antiseptic

Formula: Each tablet represents—

	Per Cent
Extract Pichi-Pichi	75.0
Extract Kava-Kava	14.5
Lecithin	5.5
Chamomile Oil, Ethereal	0.01

Action and Uses: *For relief* of pain and strangury in gonorrhea.

Supply: TEROGON "SCHUFTAN"—Tablets—Boxes of 60.

Administration: 3 or 4 Tablets, three times daily.

Bibliography: *See Chap. XII.*

TERPAL (Lederle)

Common Cold Therapy

Composition:

Oil of Melaleuca Alternifolia	0.5
Glycol Stearate	0.1
Glycerine	1.5
Borax	1.5
Water	q.s. 100.0

Description: An emulsion *for use* as prophylactic and in the treatment of common colds; is non-irritating to the mucous membrane.

Supply: TERPAL—Bottles of 2 and 6 oz.

Administration: *Used* as gargle, nasal instillation by dropper, douche and spray; also by swallowing small amount to reach epiglottis, larynx. Applied every ½ hr. for at least 3 treatments; if required may be used for several days.

TERPAZONE (Strasenburgh)

Expectorant

Composition: Each tablet represents:

	Gr	Gm
Sanguinarin nitrate	1/100	0.00065
Caloxidine (iodized calcium)	1/6	0.012
Ammonium muriate	½	0.032
Cubebs	¼	0.016
Terpin hydrate	1	0.064
Extract licorice		
Sugar and aromatics	aa q.s.	

Action and Uses: Bronchial sedative in coughs and respiratory affections.

Supply: TERPAZONE—Tablets—Bottles of 500 and 1,000.

Administration: 1 tablet every 2 hr., dissolved on tongue.

TERPICHIN (Beisner)

Non-specific Therapy

Composition: A sterile solution of purified Turpentine Oil 15 %, Quinine ½ %, Anesthesin ½ %, Olive oil 84 %.

Action and Uses: Is similar in action to non-specific agents; stimulates favorable reaction in various infections—gonorrhea, adnexitis, arthritis, skin suppurations, sinusitis, mastoiditis, eye infections, sepsis; also in phlebitis, bronchopneumonia, bronchiectasis.

Supply: **TERPICHIN**—Ampules 1 cc—Boxes of 10.

Administration: *Intragluteal Injections*—1 cc twice weekly or every 2 days; may be increased to 2 cc.

Caution: Needles for injection should not be sterilized with alcohol.

Bibliography: *See Chap. XII.*

THANTIS LOZENGES

(Hynson, Westcott and Dunning)

Antiseptic. Anesthetic

Chemical Name: Merodicein (Sodium salt of Monohydroxy Mercuridiiodoresorcin-sulphonphthalein) and Saligenin (Orthodroxybenzyl alcohol).

Formula: $NaO_3S.\ C_6H_4C{:}\ C_6H_2IO.\ OC_6HI(ONa)(HgOH)$.

Action and Uses: Antiseptic and anesthetic to the mucous membrane of the mouth and throat; affords continuous medication of a local area; *For use* in all oral irritations and inflammations.

Supply: **THANTIS LOZENGES**—Tablets, containing Merodicein gr ⅛ (0.008 Gm), Saligenin gr 1 (0.064 Gm)—Boxes of 2 tubes, each 12 lozenges.

Administration: *Orally*—Dissolved in the mouth, as often as desired.

THEOMINAL

(Winthrop)

Antispasmodic. Vasodilator

Composition: Contains Theobromine 10 parts and Luminal 1 part, a proportion found effective in various circulatory conditions in which these drugs are employed.

Action and Uses: Combines the vasodilator action of theobromin with the antispasmodic effect of luminal offering greater efficiency in cardiovascular disorders than either alone; *Used* in angina pectoris, arterial hypertension, arteriosclerosis, climacteric disorders.

Supply: **THEOMINAL**—Tablets, containing Theobromin, 5 gr (0.32 Gm) and Luminal ½ gr (0.03 Gm)—Vials of 20.

Administration: 1 tablet two or three times daily, according to indications.

Bibliography: *See Chap. XII.*

THIATE

(Merrell)

Sedative. Expectorant

Composition: Represents per fluid ounce:

	Gr	Gm
Potassium Guaiacol Sulphonate	6	0.384
Benzocaine Benzoate	¼	0.016
Sodium Monobenzyl Succinate	5	0.324
Sodium Salicylate	14	0.907

Action and Uses: Sedative and expectorant; local analgesic and antispasmodic; *Used* for asthma, incipient tuberculosis, tonsillitis, bronchitis, dysphagia.

Supply: **THIATE**—Bottles of 16 oz. and 1 gal.

Administration: 1 teaspoonful swallowed slowly; repeated when necessary.

Combination: **THIATE AND CODEINE**—Represents per fluid ounce: Potassium Guaiacol Sulphonate, 40 gr (2.592 Gm); Codeine Phosphate, 1 gr (0.064 Gm)—*For use* where quicker relief of cough is desired. *Supply*—Bottles of 12 oz. and 1 gal. *Administration*—½ Teaspoonful as required.

THIOCYAN-ELIX (Sutliff and Case)

Hypotensive

Composition: Contains Potassium Thiocyanate gr 1½ (0.09 Gm), Aromatic Fluid Extract Cascara m 5, per teaspoonful; Alcohol 8.1 %.

Action and Uses: To reduce blood pressure in hypertension.

Supply: **THIOCYAN-ELIX**—Bottles of 1 pt. and 1 gal.

Administration: 1 teaspoonful three times daily after meals for first week, reduced to twice daily and once daily during second and third weeks.

Bibliography: *See Chap. XII.*

THYMEPHEN SYRUP (McNeil)

Sedative

Description: A dark brown syrup containing in each fluid ounce—

	Gr	Gm
Phenobarbital-Sodium	⅜	0.024
Wild Thyme	25	1.600
Thyme	25	1.600
Potassium and Sodium Bromide	8	0.512
Atropine Sulphate	1/100	0.00065
Aromatics and Syrup	q.s.	

Action and Uses: Antispasmodic and cough sedative, *for use* in pertussis and other spasmodic respiratory disorders.

Supply: **THYMEPHEN SYRUP**—Bottles of 2, 3, 4 and 16 oz., ½ and 1 gal.

Administration: Adults, 4 teaspoonfuls; Children 1–4 teaspoonfuls according to age.

THYROCALX (Sharp and Dohme)

Calcium Therapy

Composition: Tablet 1 contains:

	Gr
Calcium lactate	5
Desiccated parathyroid	1/20
Desiccated thyroid	¼

Tablet 2 contains above ingredients except thyroid.

Action and Uses: Is indicated in calcium deficiencies; chronic ulceration, tetany, chronic sepsis, spasmophilia, sprue.

Supply: **THYROCALX 1**—Bottles of 100.

THYROCALX 2—Bottles of 100.

Administration: 3 Tablets daily, gradually reduced to 1 tablet.

Bibliography: *See Chap. XII.*

TIN OXIDE (Smith-Dorsey)

Staphylocide

Composition: Contains per capsule:

	Gr	Gm
Tin	1.7	0.108
Tin oxide	0.3	0.019

Action and Uses: Effective against staphylococcus infections; *For use* in boils and furuncles.

Supply: TIN OXIDE—Capsules—Bottles of 100.

Administration: 1 capsule every 3 hr.

TINPRONATE (Searle)

Non-specific Therapy

Description: An organic combination of Tin, (Stannum) with an insoluble protein base.

Action: The tin in ionizable form is gradually absorbed in the intestine; stimulates body defense mechanism and leukocytosis; is non-toxic.

Uses: Recommended for the relief of pain and inflammation in staphylococcus infections: furunculosis, acne, styes, sinusitis, abscesses and suppurating wounds.

Supply: TINPRONATE—Tablets gr 2 (0.13 Gm)—Bottles of 100.

Administration: 2 tablets every 3 hr. first day.
2 tablets every 4 hr. second day.
1 tablet every 3 hr. thereafter.

TOLUPHEN (McNeil)

Expectorant

Description: A dark, green colored syrup containing per fluid ounce:

Chloroform	m 2	
Cannabis	gr 7½	(0.480 Gm)
Lobelia	gr 7½	(0.480 Gm)
Phenobarbital-Sodium	gr 1½	(0.097 Gm)
Tartar Emetic	gr ⅛	(0.008 Gm)
Syr. Tolu and Aromatics	q.s.	

Action and Uses: Expectorant and cough sedative in various respiratory affections.

Supply: TOLUPHEN—Bottles of 2, 3, 4 oz.
Bottles of 1 pt., ½ and 1 gal.

Administration: Adults, 2–4 teaspoonfuls.
Children, ½–2 teaspoonfuls according to age.

TONICINE (Reed and Carnrick)

Endocrine Tonic

Tonicine—Male: Contains per fluid dram:

	Gr	Gm
Hormones, representing fresh testicle	25	1.6
Strychnin sulphate	1/200	0.0003
Sodium glycerophosphate	1	0.064

Tonicine—Female: Contains per fluid dram:

	Gr	Gm
Hormones representing fresh ovary	5	0.3
Strychnin sulphate	1/200	0.0003
Sodium glycerophosphate	1	0.06

Description: A general tonic and reconstructive; improves appetite and digestion, stimulates nerve centers, raises metabolism.

Uses: Asthenia, anorexia, convalescence, neurasthenia and hypogonadism.

Supply: TONICINE—Bottles 8 oz. and 1 gal.

Administration: 2 teaspoonfuls before meals.

TRITUSSIS (Noyes)

Expectorant

Composition: Each fluid ounce represents:

Prunus Virginiana	gr 7½ (0.480 Gm)
Scilla	gr 3 (0.194 Gm)
Sanguinaria	gr 3 (0.194 Gm)
Ipecac	gr 2 (0.130 Gm)
Antimony Potassium Tartrate	gr 3/40 (0.004 Gm)
Dil. Hydriodic acid	m 20.6 (1.262 cc)
Dil. Hydrobromic acid	m 31.9 (1.971 cc)

Action and Uses: Astringent, sedative, expectorant; indicated in bronchitis, bronchial coughs, croup, laryngitis.

Supply: TRITUSSIS—Bottles 1 pt., 1 gal.

Administration: ½–1 teaspoonful diluted or plain.

TYLOID "LOWENTHAL" (American Organotherapy)

Cholagogue

Composition: Each tablet contains—

	Gr	Gm
Thiocol	½	0.03
Holadin	¼	0.016
Sodium choleate	½	0.03
Ext. colocynth compound	¼	0.016
Eserine salicylate	1/200	0.00032
Extr. cascara sagrada	⅛	0.008
Oil betula	⅛	0.008

Action and Uses: Cholagogue, *for use* in indigestion, constipation, colitis, jaundice, diabetes, nephritis.

Supply: TYLOID "LOWENTHAL"—Tablets—Bottles of 100.

Administration: 1 tablet after meals.

URIFORM (Schieffelin)

Urinary Antiseptic

Composition: Each ounce represents—

	Gr	Gm
Sandalwood	10	0.64
Saw-palmetto	20	1.29
Methenamine	30	1.94

Action: Antiblenorrhagic, antiseptic, sedative; liberates formaldehyde, preventing ammoniacal decomposition of the urine; reduces congestion, bacteriuria, discharge, tenesmus.

Uses: Cystitis, urethritis, prostatitis, vesiculitis, pyelitis.

Supply: URIFORM—Bottles of 8 oz.

Administration: 1–2 teaspoonfuls three times daily, with liberal use of water.

UROCEDROL (Anglo-French)

Urinary Antiseptic

Composition: Each capsule represents—

	Gm
Cedrus Allantica essential oil	0.25
Urotropine camphorate	0.05

Action and Uses: Non-irritating antiblenorrhoeic; relieves backache, burning, strangury; diminishes discharge and shreds; *For use* in cystitis, orchitis, gonorrheal, prostatitis, vesiculitis, epididymitis.

Supply: UROCEDROL—Capsules—Bottles of 50, 500.

Administration: Acute Gonorrhea—10 capsules daily, 5 before midday and 5 before evening meal.

Chronic Gonorrhea, Cystitis, Pyelitis—6 capsules daily, before meals.

Bibliography: *See Chap. XII.*

UTROS (Sharp and Dohme)

Uterine Sedative

Composition: Contains per fluid ounce:

Viburnum prunifolium	gr 20
Viburnum opulus	gr 30
Hydrastis	gr 10
Aletris	gr 15
Mitchella repens	gr 15
Caulophylum	gr 15
Cascara sagrada	gr 15
Somnos	m 160
Alcohol	23%

Action and Uses: A sedative for uterine disorders; *For use* in dysmenorrhea, menorrhagia, metrorrhagia.

Supply: UTROS—Bottles 1 pt. and 1 gal.

Administration: 1–2 teaspoonfuls every 3–4 hr.

VALITAL (Leeming)

Analgesic

Composition: Each tablet contains:

	Gr	Gm
Ephedrine Hydrochloride	1/8	0.008
Bromisovalerylurea	1¼	0.016
Amidopyrine	1¼	0.016
Aromatics	q.s.	

Action and Uses: Antispasmodic and analgesic; relaxes smooth muscle fibre; *For use* in relieving pain in functional dysmenorrhea; in headache, irritating coughs and in bronchitis.

Supply: VALITAL—Tablets—Boxes of 12.

Administration: 1–2 tablets every 4 hr.; in more severe cases 2 tablets repeated in 1 hr. if necessary.

VAPOROLE CHLOROFORM WITH ETHYL IODIDE COMPOUND (Burroughs Wellcome)

Antispasmodic

Composition: Contains—

Chloroform	m 10 (0.6 cc)
Ethyl Iodide	m 5 (0.3 cc)
Menthol	gr 1/8 (0.008 Gm)

Description: An inhalant in thin glass, surrounded by absorbent cotton in silken netting.

Action and Uses: *For inhalation* to lessen severity of asthmatic attacks, prevent epileptic fits and as aid in whooping cough, bronchitis, laryngitis and angina pectoris.

Supply: VAPOROLE CHLOROFORM WITH ETHYL IODIDE COMPOUND—Boxes of 6.

Administration: Is crushed and contents inhaled.

VARITOSE (Ulmer)

Sclerosing Agent

Composition: Contains Invert Sugar 7.5 Gm per 10 cc with 5% Cane Sugar, by weight.

Action and Uses: A mild sclerosing agent in the treatment of smaller varicose veins.

Supply: VARITOSE—Ampules 10 cc—Boxes of 12, 25 and 100.
VARITOSE—Vials 20 cc—Boxes of 12, 25 and 100.

Administration: In varicose vein therapy by the injection method.

VIBURNO (Viburno)

Uterine Tonic

Composition: Represents per 2 dr.:

Viburnum prunifolium	gr 8 (0.52 Gm)
Piscidia erythrina	gr 3 (0.19 Gm)
California port wine	q.s. dr. 2

Action and Uses: Nervine and uterine tonic *for use* in functional amenorrhea, dysmenorrhea, menopausal and puerperal disturbances.

Supply: VIBURNO—Bottles 11 oz.

Administration: 2 Teaspoonfuls three or four times daily before meals.

VIOSTEROL IN HALIBUT LIVER OIL 250 D (Mead Johnson)

Vitamin Therapy

Description: A preparation rich in vitamin A and equivalent in its vitamin D content to viosterol 250D. Each gram contains not less than 100,000 vitamin A units (U.S.P.) and 3,333 vitamin D units (Steenbock); biologically essayed.

Action: Fortifies organism against infections of mucous membranes and aids in maintaining health; controls calcium and phosphorus utilization.

Use: Is especially indicated where greater quantities of vitamins A and D are needed and cod liver oil of equivalent potency would not be tolerated; *For use* in xerophthalmia, hemeralopia, xerosis; as specific in rickets, tetany and osteomalacia; helpful in calcium-phosphorus deficiencies, as in tuberculosis, dental caries, fractures, tetanoid syndrome of pregnancy, allergies.

Supply: VIOSTEROL IN HALIBUT LIVER OIL 250 D (C.A.)—Bottles of 5 and 50 cc; Capsules m 3—Boxes of 25 and 100.

Administration: Infants—10 drops daily; prematures and rapidly growing children, 15 drops.
Pregnant and nursing women—25 drops or more.
Special cases may require larger dosage.

Bibliography: *See Chap. XII.*

VIOSTEROL IN OIL 250 D (Mead Johnson)

Vitamin Therapy

Description: A tasteless, odorless oil, high in vitamin D potency; biologically standardized by Steenbock assay.

Action: Controls calcium and phosphorus utilization.

Uses: A specific in rickets, tetany and osteomalacia; a helpful agent in other calcium-phosphorus deficiencies, as in tuberculosis, dental caries, fractures, tetanoid syndrome of pregnancy, allergies. Especially indicated where large amounts of Vitamin D are needed and cod liver oil of equivalent potency would not be tolerated.

Supply: VIOSTEROL IN OIL 250D (C.A.)—Bottles of 5 and 50 cc.

Administration: *Prophylactic Dosage*—Infants growing at normal rate—10 drops daily. Premature and rapidly growing infants—15 drops daily.
Nursing and expectant mothers—25 drops or more daily.
Curative Dosage—Mild and moderate rickets—15–20 drops daily.
Severe rickets—20–60 drops daily.

Bibliography: *See Chap. XII.*

VITAFOOD (Vitamin Food)

Vitamin B Therapy

Composition: Dried brewers' yeast containing the vitamin B complex; is practically salt, starch and sugar free; contains Protein 54%, Minerals, including Iron, 10%. Food value—83 calories per ounce.

Action: Stimulates appetite, aids normal digestion and promotes growth.

Uses: In nutritional disorders of mother and child; in pellagra, beri-beri, liver diseases, endocrine deficiencies, malnutrition and nervous affections.

Supply: VITAFOOD—Packages of ½, 1, 2 and 5 lb.

Administration: 1–3 teaspoonfuls in milk, meats, cooked vegetables or prepared dishes.

VITAMINS "A" AND "D" (S.M.A.)

Vitamin Therapy

Description: A potent combination of Primary Vitamin A (carotene) and Natural Vitamin D; 10 drops are equivalent to 3 teaspoonfuls of standard, potent cod liver oil; is free from fishy taste.

Action and Uses: Suitable for individuals who object to taste or bulk of cod liver oil.

Supply: VITAMINS "A" AND "D"—Bottles, dropper top, 5 cc and 50 cc.

Administration: 10 drops or more to meet individual requirements, taken *orally* daily.

VITO-LECITHIN (National Drug)

Tonic

Formula: Each fluid ounce represents—

Iron Glycerophosphate	gr 4	(0.259 Gm)
Calcium Glycerophosphate	gr 4	(0.259 Gm)
Manganese Glycerophosphate	gr 3	(0.194 Gm)
Sodium Glycerophosphate	gr 8	(0.512 Gm)
Strychnine Sulphate	gr 1/60	(0.0010 Gm)
Cerebrin Lecithin	m 4½	(0.259 cc)
Tr. Hyoscyamus	m 6¼	(0.369 cc)

Action and Uses: Nerve stimulating hematinic and tonic. *Used* in functional nervous disorders, neurasthenia, nervousness, melancholia, insomnia; as hematinic in anemia and nursing mothers.

Supply: VITO-LECITHIN—Bottles of 1 pt.

Administration: 1 Dessertspoonful, increased gradually to 1 tablespoonful, before meals and on retiring. Children ½–1 teaspoonful.

YEAST BOUILLON CUBES (Harris)

Vitamin Therapy

Composition: A concentrated powdered extract from fresh cultures of Brewer's Yeast; palatable and rich in Vitamin B complex.

Action and Uses: Stimulates appetite and is growth promoting; is a convenient means of administering Vitamin B in deficiency diets to expectant and nursing mothers; in anemias, diabetes, pellagra; as intestinal detoxicant in constipation.

Supply: YEAST BOUILLON CUBES—4 Gm—Boxes 12, 48, 500 and 1,000.

YEAST VITAMIN—Tablets, 200 mg Vitamin B Concentrate—Bottles of 50. 500, 1,000.

YEAST VITAMIN—Powder—Bottles of 1, 4, 8 oz., 1 lb.

Administration: 2 tablets three times daily; children in proportion; minimum—2 tablets a day for smallest infant.

As broth—1 cube dissolved in boiling water, or placed as flavoring agent in soups, gravies.

YERSANCO (McNeil)

Expectorant

Composition: Each fluid ounce represents:

Yerba Santa	gr 56	(3.624 Gm)
Ammonium Chloride	gr 16	(1.036 Gm)
Grindelia	gr 40	(2.592 Gm)
Senega	gr 12	(0.773 Gm)
Sanguinaria	gr 4	(0.259 Gm)
Chloroform	m 2	(0.123 cc)
Mentholated Syrup	q.s.	

Action and Uses: Expectorant in bronchial affections.

Combinations: SYRUP YERSANCO WITH CODEINE SULPHATE—Gr ½ (0.032 Gm) per fluid ounce.

SYRUP YERSANCO WITH PHENOBARBITAL-SODIUM—Gr 1½ (0.097 Gm) per fluid ounce.

Supply: YERSANCO AND COMBINATIONS—Bottles of 2, 3, 4 and 16 oz.; ½ and 1 gal.

Administration: 1–4 teaspoonfuls as required.

YOHIMBOID "LOWENTHAL" (American Organotherapy)

Stimulant

Composition: Contains per tablet:

		Gr	Gm
Yohimboid hydrochloride		1/12	0.005
Excipient	q.s.	2	0.13

Action and Uses: *For use* in impotence, sexual neurasthenia, senility, debility.

Supply: YOHIMBOID "LOWENTHAL"—Tablets—Bottles of 100.

Administration: 1 tablet after meals and at bedtime.

ZILATONE (Drew Pharmacal)

Cholagogue

Formula: Each tablet contains:

	Gr	Gm
Pepsin / Pancreatin } U.S.P. equivalent	2	0.130
Bile salts compound	1⅛	0.072
Ext. cascara sagrada	⅝	0.040
Ext. nux vomica U.S.P.	1/16	0.004
Phenolphthalein (white)	½	0.032
Oleoresin capsicum	1/64	0.001

Action and Uses: Choleretic and cholagogue; stimulates active peristalsis and digestive processes; *used* in biliary disease and cholelithiasis, as stomachic tonic in atonic dyspepsia, constipation, especially in the aged, diabetic and pregnant; in intestinal stasis and toxemia; in hypertension, hepatic insufficiency and other disorders of intestinal origin.

Supply: ZILATONE—Tablets—Packages of 40, 80

Administration: 2 tablets with 2 glasses of water 2 hr. after breakfast and at bedtime; in resistant cases—2 tablets after each meal; dosage reduced when desired results are obtained.

ZONITE (Zonite)

Antiseptic

Description: A stabilized solution of Sodium Hypochlorite, presenting 1% of available Chlorine, or twice the concentration of Dakin's solution; is mildly alkaline and thus aids liquefaction of pus and necrotic tissue; contains approximately 10% Sodium Chloride, to render the usual dilutions slightly hypertonic and more effective upon living tissue.

Action and Uses: A general antiseptic, bactericide and deodorant; a powerful bleaching agent; non-toxic, if taken internally.

Supply: ZONITE—Bottles of 2½, 6 and 14 oz.

Administration: *For Oral Uses*—1 teaspoonful to ⅓ glass of water.

As Local Antiseptic—3 teaspoonfuls to ¼ glass of water; vaginal douching, 2 tablespoonfuls to quart of warm water.

Dentistry—Used as mouth wash and bactericide in oral infections, pyorrhea, trench mouth, antrum disease; in the disinfection of cavities before filling, after extraction; in oral surgery in general.

Surgery—As general antiseptic in abrasions, ulcers, purulent wounds; as gargle in the treatment of sore throat; as cleanser, moist dressing and as vaginal douche.

Caution: Should not be permitted to come in contact with dyed fabrics because of its bleaching tendency.

Combinations: ZONITE—Ointment—A greaseless cream, containing the equivalent of 2% chloramine-T in a mixture of stearates as base; *useful* for scratches, abrasions, burns, chafing, sunburn, insect bites, cold sores, cracked lips, chapped hands, and after shaving; *supplied* in tubes.

ZONITE—Suppositories—Contains chlorine compounds in a mixture of stearates, softening and melting at body temperature; *used* for feminine hygiene and as substitute for the vaginal spray or douche in the treatment of local inflammatory conditions; *supplied* in small glass vials—Boxes of 12.

CHAPTER III

PREPARATIONS OF UNDECLARED COMPOSITION

This chapter presents 346 preparations in 441 forms. Their full composition is not stated, exact data not having been made available. The arrangement is alphabetical; the dosages are average and stated in both the metric and U.S. systems, approximately converted.

ACETONYL (Upjohn)

Analgesic

Composition: Granular, effervescent, alkaline acetyl-salicylates with bicarbonates, citrates and tartrates of sodium, potassium, calcium and magnesium; contains when dissolved gr 7½ (0.480 Gm) of acetyl salicylic acid per heaping teaspoonful (gr 60).

Action and Uses: An analgesic and antipyretic in carbonated palatable form, *for use* in neuralgia, headache, colds, influenza, fevers.

Supply: ACETONYL—Bottles 2 and 4 oz.

Administration: 1 teaspoonful dissolved in 6 oz. cold water; repeated as necessary.

ACRIVIOLET "NATIONAL" (National Aniline)

Germicide

Description: A combination of neutral acriflavine, gentian violet and a mixture of triphenyl methane dyes.

Action and Uses: Germicide and antiseptic; equally effective against gram positive and gram negative organisms; penetrates deeply into tissues; is non-toxic, non-irritating and stimulates cell regeneration. *For use* in otolaryngological and dental practice; in grippe, colds, tonsillitis, Vincent's infection; in leukoplakia, tracheobronchitis, furunculosis of nose and ear, otitis media, sinusitis.

Supply: ACRIVIOLET "NATIONAL"—1% Aqueous solution—Vials 1 oz.

ACRIVIOLET "NATIONAL"—Powder—Bottles 5, 10, 25 and 50 Gm.

ACRIVIOLET "NATIONAL"—Tablets 2.4 gr, (0.156 Gm)—Bottles of 50.

Administration: In Nose and Throat Affections—As spray and gargle every 3 hr., 1% solution.

In Ear Furunculosis—For pencilling, 1% solution two times daily, drying lesions first.

In Otitis Media—Canal is filled with 1% solution and patient is instructed to swallow.

In Sinusitis—4–6 cc of 1% solution injected into sinuses, 4–6 times.

Dentistry—In trench mouth, pyorrhea, gingivitis, ulceration, stomatitis, pus pockets, 1% solution by direct application.

Bibliography: *See Chap. XII.*

ADEX TABLETS—10 D (Squibb)

Vitamin Therapy

Description: A concentrate of cod liver and halibut liver oil vitamins and viosterol; is stable, potent, palatable, readily assimilable and physiologically standardized.

Composition: Each tablet represents

Vitamin A	1,500 U.S.P. Units
Vitamin D	2,450 A.D.M.A. Units

Action: Antirachitic and growth promoting; heightens immunity against infections; assists in the maintenance of normal calcium-phosphorus metabolism.

Uses: Recommended for pregnant and nursing mothers; as adjunct in infant feeding and as dietary supplement for older individuals.

Supply: ADEX—Tablets 10 D (L.A.). Chocolate coated—Bottles of 80.

Administration: 1–3 tablets daily at meals, with water, milk or orange juice; invalids and convalescents 3–6 tablets daily; children 2–4 tablets daily.

Bibliography: *See Chap. XII.*

ADGENE (Adgene)

Nutrient

Composition: Contains in concentrated form barley, cocoa, sugar and vanilla flavoring, comprising carbohydrates, proteins, calcium, phosphates and a vitamin-carrying organic catalyst.

Action and Uses: An easily digested, readily tolerated food-beverage, of high nutritive value; *For use* at all ages as reconstructive—in malnutrition, states of exhaustion, convalescence, pregnancy, anorexia, nervous irritability.

Supply: ADGENE—Cans of 14 oz., 5 lb.

Administration: 1 level tablespoonful per cup, or 6 level tablespoonfuls per quart of milk; boiled before serving.

ADSORGAN (Heyden)

Adsorbent

Description: A powder containing charcoal, colloidal silica gel, cocoa 50%, sugar, aromatics and silver chloride.

Action: An adsorbing agent, combining with bacteria and their toxins and rendering these innocuous; does not affect gastric or intestinal enzymes and is not constipating.

Uses: *For use* in infections of gastrointestinal tract, acute and recurrent enteritis; in summer diarrhea, intestinal flatulence and fermentation; in dysentery and typhlitis; also in chronic arthritides with intestinal disturbances.

Supply: ADSORGAN—Powder—Tins of 25 and 50 Gm.

Administration: 1–2 teaspoonfuls two or three times daily, plain as powder or mixed with water.

Bibliography: *See Chap. XII.*

AEROPHAGYL "BEYTOUT" (Fougera)

Gastric Sedative

Composition: A combination of hexamethylene tetramine, sodium citrate, bromine and calcium.

Action and Uses: Is stated to be antispasmodic, antiseptic and sedative in conditions accompanied by eructations; *For use* in aerophagia, cholecystitis, cholelithiasis, gastro-duodenal ulceration; also in neurasthenics.

Supply: AEROPHAGYL "BEYTOUT"—Tablets—Boxes of 45.

Administration: 1 or 2 tablets in a half glass of water, during meals or belching attacks; children—half dosage.

AGAROL (Warner)

Laxative

Composition: An emulsion of mineral oil with agar-agar and phenolphthalein.

Description: A palatable efficient laxative.

Action and Uses: Stimulates intestinal peristalsis and regulates bowel action without griping; *useful* in constipation and intestinal flatulence.

Supply: AGAROL,—Bottles of 6 and 14 oz.

Administration: 1 tablespoonful night and morning; children—½–1 tablespoonful.

ALAXA (Burroughs Wellcome)

Laxative

Composition: Presents in palatable form the laxative properties of cascara sagrada, combined with other stomachic and carminative principles; each dram is equivalent to m 24 fl. extract cascara sagrada.

Action and Uses: As laxative in various types of obstipation.

Supply: ALAXA—Bottles of 4 oz.

Administration: 1–2 fl. dr. as necessary.

ALBAGAR (McKesson and Robbins)

Laxative

Description: A palatable emulsion of agar-agar and albolene, a Russian mineral oil.

Action and Uses: Laxative in chronic constipation.

Administration: 1 tablespoonful mornings and evenings.

Supply: ALBAGAR—Plain—Bottles of 8 and 16 oz.

ALBAGAR COMPOUND—Contains, in addition, phenolphthalein—Bottles 8 and 16 oz.

ALCAROID (American Ferment)

Antacid. Digestant

Description: An antacid and digestant containing the vegetable ferment caroid, with calcium carbonate, bismuth subcarbonate, calcined magnesia, sodium bicarbonate, aromatics.

Action and Uses: As antacid and sedative in gastric distress, hyperacidity and intestinal flatulence; also as systemic alkalizer.

Supply: ALCAROID—Cans 2 and 4 oz.

Administration: In Gastric Disturbances—1 teaspoonful well mixed in glass of water, after meals or when indicated; repeated if necessary every 2–4 hr.

In Acidosis—As systemic alkalizer, 1 teaspoonful every 4–6 hr. until the urine is alkaline.

ALKA CARB (Searle)

Antacid

Composition: A mixture of acid sodium and potassium carbonates, magnesium phosphate, calcium lactate, iodine, manganese and tartrates, together with peptic and pancreatic digestive enzymes.

Description: A yellowish-white, granular, effervescent powder.

Action and Uses: Indicated in the treatment of hyperacidity and its sequelae.

Administration: 1 teaspoonful dissolved in glass of water after meals; given only where necessary to relieve attack.

Supply: ALKA CARB—Bottles 4 oz., 1 lb. and 10 lb. containers.

ALKA-SAL (Maltbie)

Alkalizer

Composition: A mixture containing potassium, sodium, calcium and magnesium salts.

Action and Uses: *For use* as systemic alkalizer in uric acid diathesis, gout and vesical irritation; as local antacid in gastric hyperacidity.

Supply: ALKA-SAL—Bottles of 2 and 4 oz.

Administration: *Initial Dosage*—1–3 teaspoonfuls daily; continued until urine is alkaline, then reduced in accordance.

ALKANITE (Sharp and Dohme)

Antiphlogistic

Composition: An aluminum potassium nitrate compound.

Description: Occurs as fine, white, odorless crystals.

Action and Uses: For sterilization of rolled-oats poultices for application in the treatment of pyogenic infections of bone tissues, felons and carbuncles.

Supply: ALKANITE—Bottles of ½ and 1 lb.

Administration: 5–10 gr (average strength 13 gr) per ounce of rolled oats, boiled in water to plastic consistency and spread thickly on gauze; applied while hot; repeated as frequently as desired.

ALLISATIN (Sandoz)

Antispasmodic

Description: Presents the therapeutically active principles of garlic (Allium sativum) in a form in which the adsorptive power of vegetable charcoal is utilized to render the garlic odorless and tasteless.

Action: On contact with stomach juices the combined garlic is gradually liberated from the charcoal and becomes therapeutically active; is sedative, stomachic and corrective; is non-narcotic; is antiputrefactive in the alimentary tract, modifying the intestinal flora.

Uses: As sedative antispasmodic in intestinal hyperperistalsis, colic, enterocolitis, spasm, flatulence, diarrhea; effective in the relief of general symptoms in arteriosclerosis.

Supply: ALLISATIN—Tablets, each 0.55 Gm equivalent to 16 gr (1 Gm) fresh garlic—Bottles of 30, 100 and 250.

Administration: Adults—2 tablets three times a day after meals, to be taken with small quantity of water; in special cases dose may be raised to 10 or 12 tablets per day; in anorexia—taken ½–1 hr. before meals.
Children—1 or 2 tablets three times a day.

Bibliography: *See Chap. XII.*

ALTERATIVE COMPOUND (Burnham)

Alterative

Description: A preparation of iodine and vegetable alteratives.

Action and Uses: *For use* as tonic and alterative in muscular rheumatism, anemia, hepatic and skin affections.

Supply: ALTERATIVE COMPOUND—Bottles of 8 oz.

Administration: 1–3 teaspoonfuls three times daily.

ALYCIN (Merrell)

Antiarthritic

Composition: A balanced combination containing ⅓ of natural sodium, calcium and magnesium salicylates and ⅔ of an alkaline base consisting of sodium bicarbonate, calcium and magnesium carbonates.

Action and Uses: Analgesic, antipyretic and antiarthritic; *For use* in colds, tonsillitis, influenza, neuralgia, rheumatism, arthritis.

Supply: ALYCIN—Bottles of 1, 4 and 16 oz.

Administration: 1 level teaspoonful 30 gr (1.94 Gm) every hour for 4 doses, then every 2–3 hr.; in severe cases, gr 3 (0.194 Gm) per pound of body weight, daily; 60 gr (3.888 Gm) daily to maintain salicylization.

Bibliography: *See Chap. XII.*

AMMOFORM COMPOUND (Strasenburgh)

Urinary Antiseptic

Composition: An effervescent powder each ounce containing—
Ammoform (hexamethylenamine) gr 8 (0.52 Gm) with sodium phosphate, sodium sulphate, lithium carbonate, sodium tartrate and aromatics.

Action and Uses: Urinary antiseptic and diuretic in infections of genitourinary tract.

Supply: AMMOFORM COMPOUND—Bottles 4 oz.

Administration: 1–2 teaspoonfuls in water, three to four times daily, before meals.

AMYLGESTIN (McNeil)

Digestant

Description: A compressed tablet containing the equivalent of pancreatin, U.S.P., gr 15.

Action and Uses: Digestant in amylaceous dyspepsia, fermentative colitis.

Supply: AMYLGESTIN—Tablets Enteric coated—Bottles of 100, 500, 1,000 and 5,000.

AMYLGESTIN COMPOUND—Enteric coated; contains Amylgestin with Bile salts purified, gr 1 (0.064 Gm) Podophyllin, gr 1/24 (0.002 Gm); *For use* where gentle laxative effect is desired—Bottles of 100, 500, 1,000 and 5,000.

Administration: 1–2 tablets as necessary.

ANACIN (Anacin)

Analgesic

Composition: A combination of acetylsalicylic acid, caffein, quinine sulphate with para-acetphenetidin gr 3 per tablet.

Action and Uses: A non-narcotic, non-habit forming analgesic; *For use* in dental surgery for relief of pain in operative manipulation; also for colds, headache, neuralgia, neuritis and dysmenorrhea.

Supply: ANACIN—Tablets—Tins of 12—Bottles 50, 100, 250 and 500.

Administration: 1–2 tablets in water; repeated in 1 hr.

ANALAX (McKesson and Robbins)

Laxative

Composition: A combination of agar-agar and phenolphthalein, flavored with fruit juices.

Action and Uses: A mild laxative in ordinary constipation.

Supply: ANALAX—Tablets—Tins of 6 and 25.

Administration: 1 or 2 tablets at night.

ANALEPTINE (Reed and Carnrick)

Antiarthritic

Composition: Contains sodium iodide, lithium salicylate, potassium acetate, extracts of black cohosh and of cascara.

Action and Uses: Assists in alleviating symptoms, eliminating excess of uric acid and stimulating diuresis; *For use* in rheumatism, gout and uric acid diathesis.

Supply: ANALEPTINE—Bottles 14 oz. and 1 gal.

Administration: ½–1 tablespoonful after meals, three to four times daily.

ANGIER'S EMULSION (Angier)

Expectorant

Composition: An emulsion of petroleum, with calcium and sodium hypophosphites.

Action and Uses: Soothing, antiphlogistic and laxative; is stated to promote bronchial secretion, to facilitate expulsion of viscid adherent mucus and allay cough; to assist normal bowel action and reduce intestinal intoxication; *For use* in tubercular infections, grippe, influenza and convalescence.

Supply: ANGIER'S EMULSION—Bottles of 6 and 12 oz.

Administration: 1 tablespoonful four times daily; children in proportion.

Combination: ANGIER'S—Throat Tablets—Contains purified petroleum, pure elm bark and excipients; palatable, non-narcotic. *For use* to allay faucial irritation with hoarseness and dryness in singers, clergymen and speakers. *Supply*—Angier's Throat Tablets—Boxes of 50.

Bibliography: *See Chap. XII.*

ANTIPHLOGISTINE (Denver Chemical)

Antiphlogistic

Composition: Contains dehydrated silicate of aluminum, compounds of iodine, boric and salicylic acids, oils of peppermint, gaultheria, eucalyptus and glycerine.

Description: A plastic, non-toxic, soothing poultice and dressing, possessing hygroscopic, osmotic, bacteriostatic, relaxant and analgesic properties.

Action: Induces active hyperemia, stimulates cutaneous reflexes, aids local phagocytosis and tissue resistance.

Uses: Inflammations and congestions, both superficial and deep-seated; in pneumonia, pleurisy, bronchitis and other affections of the respiratory tract; in tonsillitis and laryngitis; in rheumatism, arthritis, lumbago and gout; in orchitis, epididymitis, buboes; in sprains and bruises; as tampon in cervicitis and endocervicitis.

Administration: By direct application, ¼ in. thick, as hot as possible and covered with absorbent cotton and bandage.

Supply: ANTIPHLOGISTINE—Tins 34½, 17½, 10½ and 5½ oz.—Tins 5 lb. (Hospital size).

Bibliography: *See Chap. XII.*

APHRODIN TABLETS (Fraser)

Aphrodisiac

Composition: Is stated to contain the active principles of Pansinystalia, Yohimbe and Turnera aphrodisiaca with the addition of phosphorus, gold and sodium chloride.

Action and Uses: *For use* as nerve stimulant in neurasthenia, functional impotence, spermatorrhea and reflex nervous disorders.

Supply: APHRODIN—Tablets—Bottles of 100, 500 and 1,000.

Administration: 1 Tablet after meals, three times daily.

AQUADINE (Govett)

Iodine Therapy

Composition: A combination of colloidal iodine with sodium, containing 0.25% iodine; is practically tasteless, easily absorbed, of little or no toxicity or irritation.

Action and Uses: That of iodine; *For use* in hypertension, arthritis, rheumatic and systemic infections, in prophylaxis of goitre and in luetic conditions.

Supply: AQUADINE—Solution, 0.2% (2 mg per cubic centimeter)—Bottles 8 oz.

AQUADINE—Tablets, ½ gr (0.032 Gm)—Bottles of 45.

Administration: 1–3 tablets or 2–4 teaspoonfuls three times daily, with half glassful of water.

Combinations: **AQUADINE**—Ointment—containing 0.15% iodine; is non-staining, non-irritating; for local application in arthritis, inflammatory conditions, to promote absorption of indurations; also in ringworm and other skin diseases. *Supply*—Jars of 2 oz., 1 lb.

AQUAPHOR (Duke)

Ointment Base

Description: Contains complex high molecular hydroxyl animal fat compounds, readily binding water incorporated in indifferent aliphatic hydrocarbons; an odorless and non-irritating ointment base which readily absorbs at least three times its own weight of water or aqueous solution of medicaments to form a stable homogeneous mixture; is colorless, neutral and bland.

Action and Uses: *For use* as ointment base and soothing emollient cleanser in acne rosacea, chapped skin.

Supply: AQUAPHOR—Tins of 1 and 5 lb.

Administration: May be mixed with other medicaments in any desired proportion.

ASCARIDOLE (Burroughs Wellcome)

Anthelminthic

Composition: Contains the vermicidal principle of oil of chenopodium, free from inert matter; is of constant and definite composition.

Action and Uses: *For use* as anthelminthic in hook worm disease; also against other nematodes and cestodes.

Supply: ASCARIDOLE—Bottles of 25 and 100 cc.

Administration: **Hookworm**—Adults 12–20 m (maximum 30 m) in 3 divided doses, taken in 3 consecutive hours; dropped on sugar or in other vehicle. Children ½–¾ m for 2 yr. child, increased by ½ m per year up to 12 yr. Castor oil or magnesium sulphate is given after last dose.

ASPARAGUS COMPOUND (Boericke and Runyon)

Diuretic

Composition: Is stated to contain the aqueous extracts of asparagus, kava kava, zea and triticum with potassium acetate and sodium salicylate; alcohol 8%.

Description and Uses: A concentrated aqueous extract with diuretic, eliminant and sedative properties for conditions where diuresis is desired.

Supply: ASPARAGUS COMPOUND—Bottles 1 gal.

Administration: 1–2 teaspoonfuls in glass of water.

ASPIRO-LITHINE (McKesson and Robbins)

Analgesic

Composition: A combination of aspirin with lithium citrate and lithium bitartrate.

Action and Uses: *For use* as analgesic in muscular pain, rheumatic disturbances, gout.

Supply: ASPIRO-LITHINE—Tablets—Bottles of 50.

Administration: 1 tablet in half glass of water three to four times daily.

ASTHMOLYSIN (Beisner)

Antispasmodic

Description: Contains the active principles of posterior pituitary and of suprarenal gland, combined for synergistic effect; is a clear sterile solution, non-toxic, non-narcotic.

Action and Uses: Relaxes unstriped bronchial musculature, affects sensitization and cardiovascular system; *used* for relief of attacks of bronchial asthma, hay fever, urticaria, angina pectoris.

Supply: ASTHMOLYSIN—Ampules 1 cc—Boxes of 10.

Administration: Asthma—During attack 1–3 ampules *subcutaneously* or *intramuscularly*, never intravenously; for prevention of attack in chronic asthma—1 ampule at night, in nocturnal type, mornings where necessary, for 20–30 injections; in impending attack an extra injection is given.

Children: 3 mo.–3 yr.—¼ ampule. 3 yr.–8 yr.—½ ampule. 8 yr.–14 yr.—¾ ampule.

Angina Pectoris and Hypertension—½ ampule only.

Bibliography: *See Chap. XII.*

BAGA (Townes and James)

Laxative

Description: A hygroscopic vegetable mucilage, insoluble in water; is prepared from the powdered sap or dried juice derived from the tree of the astragalus species indigenous to Persia, Syria and Kurdistan; fortified with a small amount of phenolphthalein.

Action and Uses: Absorbs water, forming a soft jelly; *used* as laxative in chronic and habitual constipation, producing a smooth, easily gliding stool without griping or other intestinal disturbance; does not affect digestion; useful also in children, in postoperative and hemorrhoidal conditions, in pregnancy and lactation.

Supply: BAGA—Capsules gr 7½ (0.486 Gm)—Packages of 36.

Administration: 1–2 capsules night and morning, followed by a full glass of water.

BARMIDON TABLETS (Fraser)

Analgesic

Composition: A combination of dimethylaminoantipyrine with diethylmalonylurea.

Action and Uses: *For use* as analgesic in migraine, headache, irritating cough; in neuritis, sciatica, dysmenorrhea, tabetic crises and cancer pain.

Supply: BARMIDON—Tablets—gr 2½ (0.160 Gm)—Bottles 100, 250, 500 and 1,000.

Administration: *As Analgesic*—1–2 tablets daily.
As Sedative—Double dosage.

BEMAX (Schieffelin)

Vitamin Therapy

Description: A preparation in the form of shredded wheat, containing 1,400 Sherman-Spohn units of Vitamin B, per ounce.

Action and Uses: Supplies Vitamin B in dietary deficiencies; stimulates the appetite; assists gastrointestinal function, increases resistance to disease; is protective against beri-beri and polyneuritis.

Supply: **BEMAX**—Tins of 12 oz.

Administration: 1 heaping tablespoonful (15 Gm) daily, equivalent to 700 units of Vitamin B; may be used uncooked.

BENZO-ACETATE (Westerfield)

Urinary Sedative

Composition: Each dram represents:
Potassium acetate, gr 5 (0.324 Gm), strontium bromide, gr 5 (0.324 Gm) with hyoscyamus, sodium benzoate and tincture belladonna.

Action and Uses: *For the relief* of urinary discomfort and strangury in prostatic hypertrophy and cystitis.

Supply: **BENZO-ACETATE**—Bottles 1 and 5 pt., 1 gal.

Administration: 1–2 teaspoonfuls, four times daily.

BENZOINOL (Benzoinol)

Local Anesthetic

Description: A refined and purified petroleum product incorporated with gum benzoin in definite proportions; a colorless, tasteless, limpid liquid of agreeable odor; stable at all temperatures.

Action and Uses: A bland, soothing, mild anesthetic and antiseptic for topical use in catarrhal affections of mucous membrane; allays irritation, diminishes discharges and prevents crust formation; also as solvent and vehicle for surface medicament. *For use* by speakers, singers and travelers in preventing throat irritation; in rhinitis, tonsillitis, laryngitis, bronchitis; in whooping cough, hay fever, sinusitis, otitis; in vaginitis, urethritis, cervicitis, cystitis, proctitis, hemorrhoids.

Supply: **BENZOINOL AND COMBINATIONS**—Bottles of 4, 16 oz., 5 pt.

Administration: Topically by brush, cotton wrapped applicator, or by atomizer and Benzoinol Inhaler.

Combinations: **DR. DOUGLAS' FORMULA**—Contains benzoinol with eucalyptol, oil of cubebs, menthol, oil of rose; *For use* in chronic nasal and pharyngeal catarrhs.

BENZOINOL AND RESORCIN COMP.—Contains benzoinol, resorcin, eucalyptol, menthol; *For use* in subacute nasopharyngeal cases.

BENZOINOL WITH CAMPHOR—Indicated in profuse and purulent discharge.

BENZOINOL WITH MENTHOL—For engorged turbinates with scanty viscid secretion.

BENZOINOL CAMPHOR-MENTHOL—As decongestant.

BENZOINOL WITH EUCALYPTOL—For prophylaxis of colds.

BENZOINOL WITH CARBOLIC ACID—As deodorant in otitis, sinusitis, ozena, vaginitis, cervicitis.

BENZOINOL WITH IODINE—For hypertrophy of turbinates, post-operatively; also in gynecological affections.

BENZOINOL WITH IODINE AND CARBOLIC ACID—*For use* in proctological affections.

BENZYL AROMATIC (Stoddard)

Antispasmodic

Composition: Is stated to contain benzyl benzoate m 2½ per capsule, with willow charcoal in alkaline aromatic base.

Action and Uses: As antispasmodic in dysmenorrhea, biliary and renal colic; in singultus and pertussis.

Supply: BENZYL AROMATIC—Capsules—Bottles 100, 500 and 1,000.

Administration: 2 or 3 capsules in hot water or milk three or four times daily.

BETA LACTOSE "NATIONAL" (National Milk)

Milk Sugar

Description: A palatable and soluble milk sugar; 1 oz. by weight yields 120 calories.

Action: Encourages the growth and predominance of Bac. Acidophilus in the intestinal tract; reduces putrefaction of bowel content and autointoxication.

Uses: As a carbohydrate in routine infant feeding; in the feeding of infants with gastrointestinal disturbances, prolonged diarrhea, vomiting, constipation; in malnutrition as supplementary food; in adults—for similar disorders and intestinal autointoxication.

Advantages: Has all therapeutic and nutritional values of old type milk sugar, but is more palatable and six times as soluble.

Supply: BETA LACTOSE—Packages of 1, 5 and 25 lb. tins.

Administration:
Dosage—3–9 oz. daily, alone or during acidophilus therapy; in infant feeding—3–12% of formula, in accordance with development and dentition; in constipation—2 tablespoonfuls in ½ glass cold water ½ hr. before breakfast, in the afternoon and on retiring; may be used as substitute for ordinary sugar on fruit, cereals and in beverages—coffee, tea, lemonade, orangeade.

Bibliography: *See Chap. XII.*

BETAPHOS (Alphaden)

Cholagogue

Description: A combination of sodium acid phosphate with an effervescent alkaline buffer salt base.

Action and Uses: A pleasant cholagogue cathartic, causing no griping. *For use* in gall bladder stasis, dyspepsia, constipation, eructations.

Supply: BETAPHOS—Powder—Bottles of ½, 1 lb.

Administration: 1 teaspoonful of powder in ¾ glass of hot water, taken ½ hr. before meals, one to three times daily, as required.

BILINA (Carnrick)

Cholagogue

Composition: Contains the peristaltic principle extracted from the mucosa of the pylorus and duodenum, with bile salts and cascara sagrada gr 1 (0.064 Gm) per tablet.

Action and Uses: Cholagogue cathartic in biliary stasis and constipation.

Supply: BILINA—Tablets—Bottles 40, 100, 500 and 1,000.

Administration: 1–3 tablets at night.

BISMODIDE (Central Pharmacal)

Antiluetic

Description: A complex organic compound containing approximately 25% of metallic bismuth and 60% of metallic iodide; is insoluble in water and gastric acid secretions.

Action: A spirocheticide; is gradually hydrolyzed and slowly eliminated from the system; is readily penetrating to the central nervous apparatus and non irritating to the renal organs.

Uses: In all stages of syphilis, particularly in neurosyphilis, Wassermann-fast cases, and where arsenic and mercury are not well tolerated.

Supply: BISMODIDE—Capsules 3.85 gr (0.25 Gm)—Bottles of 60.

Administration: Average dosage—1 capsule per kilo of body weight; in primary syphilis 4–6 capsules daily, reduced to 2–4 capsules daily, graded by improvement; rest periods of 4–6 weeks after each course; in tertiary syphilis 2–3 capsules daily for 6 to 8 weeks, with rest period following.

Caution: As for metallic poisoning; if stomatitis, fetor ex ore, salivation or pigmented mucosa appear, treatment must be suspended.

BISODOL (Bisodol)

Antacid. Digestant

Composition: A combination of sodium bicarbonate, magnesium carbonate, bismuth subnitrate, carica papaya, malt diastase, mentha piperita.

Action and Uses: Systemic and gastric antacid and digestant. *For use* in gastric hyperacidity, gastritis, peptic ulcer, nausea and vomiting, diarrhea and flatulence; in systemic acidosis of nephritis, rheumatism, influenza, colds, pneumonia and pregnancy.

Supply: BISODOL—Boxes of 2, 5 and 16 oz.

Administration: 1 teaspoonful in water after meals, or as needed.

Bibliography: *See Chap. XII.*

BISURATED MAGNESIA (Bisurated)

Antacid

Composition: A combination of magnesium carbonate (light), sodium bicarbonate, calcium carbonate prec. (light), bismuth subcarbonate, papaya comp. and malt diastase.

Action and Uses: Antacid, alkalizer and digestant in gastric hyperacidity and for systemic alkalization.

Supply: BISURATED MAGNESIA—Cans 2 and 5 oz.

Administration: 1 teaspoonful in water after meals, and as required.

BLENOL (Merrell)

Gastric Sedative

Description: A clear, palatable, stable solution of bismuth and hydrastine.

Action and Uses: In the gastrointestinal tract is split into its components, acts as emollient and astringent on the mucosa of the stomach and intestines and increases muscular tone; is stated to be *useful* in gastric hyperacidity, gastric ulcer and enteritis.

Supply: BLENOL—Bottles of 16 oz.

Administration: 1 teaspoonful in water three to four times daily.

BOERENZYME (Boericke and Runyon)

Digestant

Composition: Is stated to contain digestive enzymes in pineapple juice; alcohol 10%.

Description: A palatable preparation *for use* as substitute for natural digestive ferments where deficient or absent.

Uses: Indicated in dyspepsia, hypoacidity, intestinal fermentation; as vehicle for the administration of bitter drugs.

Supply: BOERENZYME—1 and 5 gal.

Administration: 1–3 teaspoonfuls after meals.

BONE MEDULLA (Burroughs Wellcome)

Hematinic

Composition: Extract of Bone Marrow.

Action and Uses: Hematinic in anemias.

Supply: TABLOID BONE MEDULLA—Gr 5 (0.324 Gm)—Boxes of 50.

Administration: 1 or more tabloids after meals with water.

BREWER'S YEAST (Mead, Johnson)

Vitamin Therapy

Description: Dried yeast; a fine yellowish gray powder of characteristic odor and taste, miscible with cold or hot water, milk and other food; has a vitamin B and G potency sixteen times that of the commercial wet cake yeast with tapioca and twice that of dried cake yeast without tapioca; contains no diluent or excipient;

Uses: In anorexia; partial vitamin B deficiency with spasticity, fretfulness and malnutrition in infants; for lactating mothers—to increase the vitamin B content of breast milk; in beriberi, pellagra, intestinal stasis.

Supply: BREWERS' YEAST (C.A.)—Powder (3 level tablespoonfuls weigh 1 oz.)—Bottles 6 oz.

BREWERS' YEAST—Tablets, gr 6 (70 tablets weigh 1 oz.)—Bottles 250 and 1,000.

Administration: Nursing mothers—20–30 tablets or up to 3 tablespoonfuls of powder, daily. Infants—1–3 teaspoonfuls or 6–10 tablets per day mixed with the feedings.

Pellagra—½–1 oz. daily; or 35–70 tablets.

Bibliography: *See Chap. XII.*

BROMIDIA (Battle)

Hypnotic. Sedative

Composition: A combination of potassium bromide 91 gr, chloral hydrate 91 gr with hyoscyamus 1 gr and cannabis indica 1 gr in each fluid ounce.

Action and Uses: *For use* in nervousness, irritability, insomnia, neuralgia, headache; in acute alcoholism, delirium of fever, mania, epilepsy and drug addiction.

Supply: BROMIDIA—Bottles 4 and 16 oz.

Administration: ½–1 teaspoonful in water every hour until sleep is produced; maximum dose 3 teaspoonfuls in 24 hr.

BROMIDONNA ELIXIR (McNeil)

Sedative

Description: A dark, reddish brown, pleasantly flavored preparation containing per fluid ounce—

Ammonium Bromide, Potassium Bromide, Sodium Bromide } gr 108 (6.192 Gm)
Cannabis Indica, Belladonna, Hyoscyamus, Cascara } small quantities
Alcohol 1½ %

Action and Uses: Antispasmodic and nerve sedative in various nervous manifestations, melancholia and hysteria.

Incompatibles: Barbital sodium.

Supply: BROMIDONNA ELIXIR—Bottles of 2, 3 and 4 oz., pint, ½ and 1 gal.

Administration: 1 or 2 teaspoonfuls in water.

BROMO-ADONIS (Tucker Pharmacal)

Sedative

Composition: Is stated to contain: Bromo-Adonis 1—adonidin, potassium and sodium bromide, gr 17 (1.1 Gm) per dram; Bromo-Adonis 2—potassium, sodium and ammonium bromide gr 17 (1.1 Gm) per dram with extract of Cypripedium pubescens.

Action and Uses: A sedative *for use* in epilepsy, hysteria, insomnia, spasmodic neuroses, nervous indigestion; for more lasting sedation as in chronic idiopathic epilepsy Bromo-Adonis 2 is indicated.

Supply: BROMO-ADONIS 1 and 2—Bottles of 8 oz., 1 gal.

Administration: Epilepsy—1 teaspoonful four times daily with water after meals; may be increased to 1½ teaspoonfuls; in nocturnal type a larger dose at bedtime may be required.
Children under 12—half dosage.
In Other Conditions—Dosage in accordance.

BROMSALIZOL (Hynson, Westcott and Dunning)

Antispasmodic

Chemical Name: Monobromo-salicyl-alcohol.

Description: Very slightly soluble in water and in normal saline.

Action and Uses: Antispasmodic and marked local anesthetic; relaxes smooth muscle and inhibits peristaltic contractions; does not depress the heart, respiratory center nor impair renal function. *Indicated* in hypertension due to angiospasm; in gastrointestinal hyperperistalsis, gastralgia, enteralgia; in spasmodic dysmenorrhea, spasm of ureter or bladder, renal calculus.

Supply: BROMSALIZOL—Tablets gr 5—Vials of 10—Boxes of 2 vials.

Administration: 1-3 tablets daily.

BROSEDAN (Beisner)

Sedative

Description: A liquid preparation of pleasant meat-soup flavor, containing 28% bromides and vegetable yeast; 1 dr. is equivalent to 1 Gm sodium bromide.

Action and Uses: Sedative and hypnotic; *For use* in menopausal disorders, cardiac and gastric neuroses, insomnia, hysteria; in intoxications of alcohol and narcotics; also in neuralgia, neurasthenia, vomiting of pregnancy.

Supply: BROSEDAN—Bottles of 5⅓ oz.

Administration: 1-3 teaspoonfuls two or three times daily, in hot fluid.

Bibliography: *See Chap. XII.*

BULBOCAPNINE PHOSPHATE (Burroughs Wellcome)

Psychic Sedative

Composition: An alkaloidal extract from Corydalis cava.

Action and Uses: Is stated to ameliorate behavior disorders in children with chronic epidemic encephalitis; also to be useful in milder types of ambulatory mental disorders with lack of moral control, impulses and behavior.

Supply: TABLOID BULBOCAPNINE PHOSPHATE—Hypodermic, gr 1½ (0.097 Gm)—Tubes of 12.

Administration: 1 tabloid hypodermically or orally, three times daily.

Bibliography: *See Chap. XII.*

CACTINA PILLETS (Od Peacock)

Cardiac Stimulant

Composition: Prepared from Cactus Grandiflorus (Mexicana).

Action and Uses: An antispasmodic *for use* in functional heart disturbances.

Supply: CACTINA PILLETS—Bottles of 100.

Administration: 1–4 pillets, three times daily.

Bibliography: *See Chap. XII.*

CAGESTOL ELIXIR (McNeil)

Digestant

Description: A dark brownish, pleasantly flavored solution, containing per fluid ounce:

Cascara Sagrada	gr 60 (3.888 Gm)
Sodium Salicylate	gr 32 (2.074 Gm)
Sodium Benzoate	gr 8 (0.512 Gm)
Diastase, Pancreatin, Aromatics	q.s.
Alcohol	10%

Action and Uses: Laxative, digestant, intestinal antifermentative; *For use* in intestinal putrefaction and habitual constipation.

Incompatibles: Acidulous solutions.

Supply: CAGESTOL ELIXIR—Bottles of 2, 3, 4 oz., pint, ½ gal. and gallon.

Administration: 1 teaspoonful as often as required.

CALCIPHOS (Bilhuber-Knoll)

Calcium Therapy

Description: A compound of calcium and phosphoric acid, comprising hexa-calcium and tetra-ferri hexa-phosphate of inosite, with approximately calcium 17%, phosphorus 15% and iron 2%; is a grayish powder but sparingly soluble in water and dilute mineral acids.

Action: That of organic calcium; is not affected by gastric juices but is split into its components by the alkaline intestinal secretions and is readily assimilated; is not constipating.

Uses: In calcium-phosphorus deficiencies: rickets, marasmus, osteomalacia; in pregnancy and lactation; in malnutrition, dental decay.

Supply: CALCIPHOS—Tablets gr 6—Boxes of 180.
CALCIPHOS—Powder—Boxes of 3 oz.

Administration: 12 gr three times daily with meals; in water, milk or fruit juices; children, same dosage.

CALCIUM BISMUTH COMPOUND (Boericke and Runyon)

Antacid

Composition: Is stated to contain calcium carbonate, magnesium carbonate, bismuth subcarbonate, bismuth subgallate, sodium bicarbonate.

Description: A gastric antacid producing neutralization in part immediate and partly after prolonged action.

Action and Uses: *For use* in gastric hyperacidity, gastric and duodenal ulcer, pyrosis, flatulence.

Supply: CALCIUM BISMUTH COMPOUND—Boxes of 2 and 3 oz.

Administration: 1 teaspoonful in glass cold water, stirred and taken while in suspension: repeated every 2–4 hr.

CALCIUM LACTOPHOSPHATE (Schieffelin)

Calcium Therapy

Description: Granular, saccharated calcium salt of slight acidulous taste.

Action and Uses: Reconstructive tonic *for use* in tuberculosis, rickets, spasmophilia and convalescence.

Supply: CALCIUM LACTOPHOSPHATE—Bottles of 4½ oz.

Administration: 2 teaspoonfuls in water three times daily.

CALCULI-SOL (Westerfield)

Uricolytic

Composition: Contains columbo, lobelia, nux vomica, epigaea, cascara.

Action and Uses: Antispasmodic, analgesic and uricolytic in renal, vesical and biliary colic due to calculi.

Supply: CALCULI-SOL.—Bottles 8 oz.

Administration: 1–2 teaspoonfuls, three or four times daily, with water.

CALMITOL (Leeming)

Antipruritic

Description: A solution of chlorocamphoric aldehyde, organically combined iodine (0.5 %), menthol and laevo-hyoscine oleinate in ether-alcohol-chloroform base; a transparent, greenish liquid, drying quickly on application and leaving a cooling sensation.

Action and Uses: Non-irritating, non-toxic, germicidal and antipruritic; *For use* in acne, tinea trichophyton, eczema, pruritus ani et vulvae, prurigo senilis; in varicose ulcer, neurodermatitis and hemorrhoids.

Supply: CALMITOL—Liquid—Bottles of 2 oz.
CALMITOL—Ointment—Collapsible tubes.
CALMITOL—Suppositories—Boxes of 12.

Administration: Applied daily without rubbing; washing parts is to be avoided; scabs where present should first be raised with oil, liquid calmitol then applied and covered with ointment; on mucous surfaces only ointment is to be used.

Bibliography: *See Chap. XII.*

CALMOXIDE (Drug Products)

Alkalizer

Composition: Is stated to contain in balanced ratio:
magnesium phosphate tribasic, calcium phosphate tribasic, aluminum hydroxide colloidal, magnesium peroxide, effervescent powder and aromatics.

Description: Small effervescent granules, palatable.

Action and Uses: Antacid and alkalizer with no effect upon alkali tissue reserve; *For use* in gastric hyperacidity, gastrosuccorrhea, peptic ulcer, gastrointestinal irritation.

Supply: CALMOXIDE—Bottles of 6 oz.

Administration: 1 level teaspoonful in ½ glass hot water after meals.

CALOXIDINE (Strasenburgh)

Expectorant

Composition: Contains iodine in loose chemical combination with calcium and starch; yields 15% free available iodine.

Action and Uses: Antiphlogistic *for use* in frequently occurring colds, laryngitis bronchitis; also in iodine therapy of goitre.

Supply: CALOXIDINE—Tablets, gr ⅓—Bottles of 1,000

CALOXIDINE—Tablets gr 1—Bottles of 500.

Administration: ⅓ gr or more according to conditions.

Combination: CALOXIDINE COMPOUND THROAT TABLETS: Contains—

	Gr
Caloxidine	⅓
Belladonna powder	3/200
Benzoic acid	1/12

For use in tonsillitis, pharyngitis. *Supply*—Tablets—Bottles of 500 and 1,000. *Dosage*—1 tablet every hour dissolved on tongue.

CALSOMA (Abbott)

Gastric Antacid

Composition: An effervescent mixture of buffer salts: tribasic phosphates of calcium and magnesium, sodium biphosphate and magnesium citrate.

Action: The sodium biphosphate maintains a slightly acid condition with buffer effect, preventing an alkaline reaction of gastric contents or alkalosis of general system; excess thus does not produce gastric alkalinity; is non-toxic, practically inert and is excreted by the intestines.

Uses: *For use* as corrective in gastric hyperacidity, acid indigestion, heartburn, gastrosuccorrhea.

Supply: CALSOMA—Bottles 2, 4 and 16 oz.

CALSOMA—Mint Tablets—Boxes 24—Bottles 1,000.

Administration: 1 teaspoonful to a glass of cool water, ¼–2 hr. after meals; in acid diarrhea, 1 teaspoonful hourly till relief is secured.

Bibliography: *See Chap. XII.*

CAL-SO-MAG (Smith-Dorsey)

Antacid

Composition: Is stated to contain calcium carbonate, magnesium carbonate, sodium bicarbonate, bismuth subgallate, papain and colloidal kaolin.

Action and Uses: Sedative, antacid and neutralizer in gastric hyperacidity.

Supply: CAL-SO-MAG—Cans 4 oz.

Administration: 1 Teaspoonful in water, every 2–4 hr.

CAMPHENOL (Johnson and Johnson)

Antiseptic

Description: A liquid disinfectant and antiseptic, prepared as emulsion of cresols; non-poisonous, non-corrosive, non-staining.

Action: Germicidal.

Use: As disinfectant in home and hospital; as surgical and dental antiseptic.

Supplied: CAMPHENOL—Bottles of 1, 3 and 8 oz.

Administration: Applied diluted with large quantities of water.

CANNABINE TANNATE (Burroughs Wellcome)

Sedative

Composition: A compound prepared by precipitating the glucoside cannabin with tannic acid.

Action and Uses: *For use* as sedative in dysmenorrhea and menorrhagia in combination with hydrastine and ergot.

Supply: TABLOID HYDRASTINE COMP.—Sugar coated, containing:

	Gr	Gm
Hydrastine Hydrochloride	1/4	0.016
Ergot	1/2	0.032
Cannabine Tannate	1/2	0.032

Bottles of 25 and 100.

Administration: 1–3 taken with little water; repeated if necessary.

CARBOVESCENT (Columbus Pharmacal)

Alkalizer

Composition: Contains citrates, tartrates, phosphates, sulphates, carbonates and bicarbonates of magnesium, potassium, sodium with calcium gluconate, in effervescent, palatable form.

Action and Uses: A non-injurious, non-toxic systemic alkalizer *for use* in rheumatism, gout, lumbago, uric acid diathesis, skin affections.

Supply: CARBOVESCENT—Bottles 4 oz. or 1 lb.

Administration: 1/2–2 teaspoonfuls two to four times daily, in water.

CARMINZYM (Fairchild)

Digestant

Description: Composed of pancreatic diastase of standardized potency, alkaline carbonates, soda, creta preparata, minute amounts of ipecac, vegetable aromatic antiseptics and gastric stimulants.

Action and Uses: Digestive, antacid and carminative, *For use* in gastric and intestinal indigestion, flatulence, nausea, hyperacidity, pyrosis and vomiting of pregnancy.

Supply: CARMINZYM—Bottles of 30 and 100 tablets.

Administration: 1 or 2 tablets several times a day.

CAROID POWDER (American Ferment)

Digestant

Description: A highly concentrated digestive prepared from the juices of specially grown and selected ferment-yielding plants.

Action and Uses: An efficient proteid digestant active throughout the gastrointestinal tract, in all media—acid, alkaline or neutral; is not inhibited by antiseptics, even where simultaneously administered; dissolves effete material covering alimentary walls and stimulates flow of natural digestive juices. *Indicated* internally in peptic ulcer, cholera infantum and for duodenal drainage; externally—as solvent of dead, diseased and sloughing tissues; in indolent ulcers, abscess cavities, carbuncles, ischio-rectal fistulae, sloughing cancer; also used in chronic cystitis, leucorrhea and tonsillitis.

Supply: **CAROID POWDER**—Bottles 1 oz.

CAROID ESSENCE—Each fluid dram represents 1½ gr (0.09 Gm) Caroid.
Dosage—Adults, 1–4 teaspoonfuls. Children, ½–1 teaspoonful.

CAROID TABLETS—Plain, gr 1½ (0.09 Gm)—Bottles 45, 150 and 500.
Dosage—1–3 tablets.

Administration: *Externally*—As dusting powder, applied daily and area covered with wet antiseptic dressing.
As 5% Solution—½–1 oz. for irrigation.
As Paste—Prepared with glycerine and eucalyptol or as powder for direct application on diphtheritic membrane, every 2 hr.

In Suppurative Otitis Media—10–20% solution.
Internally—In Cholera—Gr 1–3 (0.064–0.194 Gm), the essence—1–2 teaspoonfuls, three to four times daily.

Infantile Diarrhea—Given with calomel or lactic acid.
Infants—dr. 1 of essence or gr 1 (0.064 Gm) to gr 2 (0.130 Gm) of powder in sweetened water during feeding.

Combinations: **CAROID AND SODA**—Each tablet contains: Caroid, 1½ gr (0.09 Gm); Soda Bicarbonate, 3 gr (0.194 Gm); Sacch. Lactis, Mentha Piperita, Aromatics, q.s. *For use* in hyperacidity, pain, and nausea.
Dose—2–4 tablets, crushed and taken with hot water; repeated as necessary.
Supply—Bottles of 45, 150 and 500.

CAROID AND CHARCOAL—Each tablet contains: Caroid, 1½ gr (0.09 Gm); Charcoal, Acid Boric, aa, 1½ gr (0.09 Gm); Aromatics, q.s. *For use* in flatulence.
Dose—2–4 tablets, crushed and taken with hot water.
Supply—Bottles of 45, 150 and 500.

CAROID AND BILE SALTS—Each tablet contains: Pulv. Caroid, 2 gr (0.130 Gm); Bile Salts Comp. (Sod. Glycocholate and Taurocholate), 1 gr (0.064 Gm); Ext. Cascara Sagrada, ½ gr (0.032 Gm); Phenolphthalein, ½ gr (0.032 Gm); Ext. Nux Vomica, 1/16 gr (0.004 Gm); Oleoresin Capsicum, 1/40 gr (0.001 Gm); *For use* in cholecystitis, cholangitis, cholelithiasis, constipation.
Supply—Bottles of 50, 100, 500 and 1,000.
Administration—2 tablets night and morning, best taken with 2 glasses water and 8–10 glasses of water during the day.

CAROID LAXATIVE—Each tablet contains: Caroid, 1½ gr (0.09 Gm); Ext. Cascara Sag., 2 gr (0.130 Gm); Podophyllin Resin, ⅛ gr (0.008 Gm); Ext. Belladonna, 1/16 gr (0.004 Gm); Gingerine and Aromatics, q.s.
For use in chronic constipation.
Supply—Bottles of 20, 150 and 500.
Administration—1–2 tablets, as required.

CAROID AND BANA DIASTASE—Each tablet contains: Caroid, 1½ gr (0.09 Gm); Bana Diastase, 2 gr (0.130 Gm); Soda Bicarbonate, Sacch. Lactis, Aromatics, aa. q.s.

For use in indigestion accompanied by distension, pain and flatulence; in constipation and diarrhea.
Supply—Bottles of 45, 150 and 500.
Administration—In commencing treatment, 4 tablets immediately after each meal, crushed and swallowed with warm or hot water; as symptoms improve, dosage is gradually decreased.

CAROID AND NUX VOMICA—Each tablet contains: Pulv. Caroid, 1½ gr (0.09 Gm); Ext. Nux Vomica, ⅕ gr (0.013 Gm); Pulv. Rhubarb, ½ gr (0.032 Gm); Pulv. Ipecac, $\frac{1}{20}$ gr (0.003 Gm); Pulv. Capsicum, ¼ gr (0.016 Gm); Sacch. Lactis, Pulv. Arom., aa. q.s.
For use in gastric atony.
Supply—Bottles 45, 150 and 500.
Administration—1–2 tablets three times daily—½ hr. before meals.

C. C. C. TONIC (Boericke and Runyon)

Stimulant

Composition: Contains cinchona, calisaya, hydrastis canadensis with hypophosphites of calcium, potassium and sodium; alcohol 10%.

Action and Uses: A stimulant for use as tonic in states of exhaustion, debility, nervousness with anorexia, insomnia and anemia.

Supply: C.C.C. TONIC—Bottles of 16 oz.

Administration: 1 tablespoonful 3–4 times daily; children in proportion.

CEANOTHYN (Flint, Eaton)

Hemostatic

Composition: A hydro-alcoholic extract of the alkaloids from the bark of the root of Ceanothus Americanus, in liquid form.

Action and Uses: Accelerates blood coagulation; is rapidly absorbed and effective in increasing blood coagulability; *For use* in operative cases, surgical and dental to prevent and check hemorrhage.

Supply: CEANOTHYN—Bottles of 1 pt.

Administration: *Orally*—In active hemorrhage—4 teaspoonfuls every ½ hr. or every 15 min.
Rectally—Double dosage.
As Prophylactic—4 teaspoonfuls 45 min. before operation.

Bibliography: *See Chap. XII.*

CHIQUENIA (Buffington)

Expectorant

Composition: Is stated to contain euphorbia, horehound, coccillana with ¼ gr ethylmorphine per ounce, in mucilaginous base.

Action and Uses: *For use* as cough sedative and expectorant in various bronchial affections.

Supply: CHIQUENIA—Bottles of 1 pt.

Administration: 1 teaspoonful every 3 hr.

CHLOMIN (Columbus Pharmacal)

Antiseptic

Official Name: Chlorbutanol and Borate Compound.

Composition: Is stated to contain chlorbutanol, boric acid, sodium borate, thiosulphate and aromatics; soluble in water.

Action and Uses: Alkaline, antiseptic, fungicide and deodorant; non-corrosive and non-staining; *For use* in ringworm, trichophytosis, scabies, sycosis, infected ulcers, pelvic diseases; also in minor surgery affections.

Supply: CHLOMIN—Cans 4 oz.

Administration: *Wet Dressing*—2–3 teaspoonfuls per pint.
Dusting Powder—Pure or mixed with bland powder; used freely.

CHYMOGEN (Armour)

Digestant

Description: Prepared from cleaned gastric mucosa of suckling calves and mixed with milk sugar.

Action and Uses: To curdle cow's milk in preparation for infant feeding.

Supply: CHYMOGEN—Powder—Bottles 4 oz.

Administration: ½ teaspoonful to 1 pt. of sterilized warm (104°F) milk, stirred for 15 sec., cooled on ice.

CITRICO "ESKAY" (Smith, Kline and French)

Alkalizer

Composition: A granular effervescent compound containing 120 gr of potassium, sodium and magnesium citrates and tartrates, citric and tartaric acids, calcium lactate 7 gr, citrated caffeine 1.25 gr per dessertspoonful, with lactose and flavoring matter; forms with water an acidulous, carbonated, hypertonic solution.

Action: Supplies essential salts for normalizing body alkalinity; promotes elimination of acid waste products and is diuretic.

Uses: *For use* as systemic alkalizer in acidosis of febrile states, in rheumatic and gouty conditions; as gastric antacid in acid dyspepsia and similar disorders.

Supply: CITRICO "ESKAY"—Bottles of 4 oz.

Administration: 2 teaspoonfuls in water before breakfast; in systemic acidosis is repeated as often as necessary until urine is alkaline.

CITROCARBONATE (Upjohn)

Alkalizer

Composition: Each teaspoonful (about 60 gr, 4 Gm) when dissolved presents approximately 12½ gr (0.8 Gm) free sodium bicarbonate, 28 gr (1.8 Gm) sodium and potassium bicarbonates, as citrates and tartrates, 2½ gr (0.162 Gm) calcium lactate, with correct proportions of phosphates, sulphates, and magnesium, and about 2% sodium chloride.

Description: A palatable systemic alkalizer, supplying buffer salts and alkaline bases in percentage relationship of the blood and designed to replenish or maintain alkali reserve; is also an agreeable and effective gastric antacid.

Action and Uses: As antacid, as diuretic and systemic alkalizer in cases where blood alkalinization is desirable as in fevers, rheumatism, gout, diabetes, acidosis.

Supply: Bottles of 4 and 8 oz.

Administration: 1 or 2 teaspoonfuls, three to four times daily with water, slowly poured over powder; continued until alkalization is obtained.

CITROSALVEN (Medicinal Products)

Non-specific Therapy

Composition: Is stated to contain sodium citrate, sodium chloride and buffer salts.

Action and Uses: Anticoagulant, antitoxemic and stimulant to healing; *For use* in peptic ulcer.

Supply: CITROSALVEN—Ampules 50 and 100 cc.

Administration: *Intravenously*—Initial dose—50 cc, succeeding doses—100 cc, slowly injected; at first given two to three times weekly, then once weekly for 1 yr., or until improvement is noted; food is withheld for 1–2 hr. after each injection.

CITRO-SODA (Abbott)

Alkalizer

Composition: An effervescent combination of sodium citrate, sodium bicarbonate and citric acid.

Action: Dissolved in water forms a solution of sodium citrate with citric acid slightly in excess; in the body—the latter is decomposed and the base functions as alkali, inducing diuresis, diaphoresis, increased blood alkali reserve and decrease of acidosis; also increases and liquefies bronchial secretions.

Uses: *For use* in dry coughs; in acidosis of fever, rheumatism, toxemia, influenza, gout, hepatic sclerosis, inanition.

Supply: CITRO-SODA—Bottles of 4 oz. and 1 lb.

Administration: 1–2 teaspoonfuls in water, taken between meals.

CITROSODINE "LONGUET" (Fougera)

Gastric Sedative

Description: Pure trisodium citrate, which decomposes in the stomach with formation of sodium chloride and citric acid.

Action and Uses: Gastric alkalizer and sedative; diuretic, diaphoretic and anticoagulant; *For use* to neutralize gastric hyperacidity in gastric ulcer and gastritis; in vomiting of infants, alcoholics and that due to gastric dilatation; as anticoagulant in phlebitis, thrombosis, embolism, pneumonia.

Supply: CITROSODINE "LONGUET"—Tablets, gr 4 (0.25 Gm)—Boxes of 100.

Administration: Adults—4–8 tablets, two or three times a day.
Children—3–4 tablets, two or three times a day.
Infants—1 tablet dissolved in water and added to feeding bottles.

In Pneumonia—4 tablets every hour in ½ glass of water, day and night until third day after crisis

COFRON (Abbott)

Hematopoietic

Composition: Each capsule represents approximately—

Fresh liver	1/3 oz. (10.0 Gm)
Iron	1/10 gr (0.007 Gm)
Copper	1/250 gr (0.0027 Gm)

Description: Contains a standardized extract prepared from fresh mammalian liver and elements required for the production of hemoglobin.

Action: Is stated to have at least four times the Vitamin B potency of compressed yeast and approximately forty times its Vitamin G content.

Uses: For treatment of anemia—primary, pernicious and secondary.

Supply: COFRON CAPSULES—Bottles of 100 and 1,000.

Administration: Adults—3-5 capsules three times daily.
Children—1-2 capsules three times daily.

Bibliography: *See Chap. XII.*

COFRON ELIXIR (Abbott)

Hematopoietic

Composition: Prepared from concentrated liver extract obtained from fresh mammalian livers, inorganic copper and iron; 3 tablespoonfuls are stated to represent—

Fresh liver	2 oz.
Iron	1½ gr (0.09 Gm)
Copper	1/16 gr (0.004 Gm)

Action and Uses: A palatable, tonic and hematinic; *For use* in secondary and nutritional anemias, in infectious and pernicious types.

Supply: COFRON ELIXIR—Bottles 12 oz.

Administration: Adults—1 tablespoonful three times daily.
Children—1 teaspoonful three times daily.

Bibliography: *See Chap. XII.*

COLACTIN (Spicer)

Laxative

Description: An emulsion of petroleum and lactose.

Action and Uses: An intestinal lubricant, accelerating peristalsis. The mineral oil coating of lactose prevents its absorption until it reaches the colon, where it supplies sustenance to the bacillus acidophilus, encouraging the growth and multiplication of the antiputrefactive organisms. *For use* in intestinal stasis, chronic constipation and colitis.

Supply: COLACTIN—Plain—Bottles of 12 oz.

COLACTIN WITH PHENOLPHTHALEIN gr 4 (0.256 Gm) per ounce—Bottles of 12 oz.

Administration: 1 tablespoonful ½ hr. before meals, or in the morning and at bedtime.

COLALIN (Schieffelin)

Cholagogue. Laxative

Description: A mixture of hyoglycocholic and hyotaurocholic acids obtained from bile and magnesium carbonate.

Action: That of the component acids; stimulates hepatic cell function, increases bile formation keeping cholesterol in solution; enhances pancreatic digestion of fats; assists bowel movement.

Uses: *For use* in diseases of liver and gall bladder, intestinal autotoxemia, constipation.

Supply: COLALIN—Powder—Vials of ⅛ and 1 oz.

COLALIN—Tablets, gr ½ (0.032 Gm) gr ¼ (0.016 Gm) gr ⅛ (0.008 Gm)—Bottles of 100.

COLALIN AND PHENOLPHTHALEIN—Tablets:

Colalin	gr ⅙ (0.012 Gm)	Bottles of 100.
Phenolphthalein	gr 1 (0.064 Gm)	

Dosage—1–2 tablets at night.

COLALIN—Laxative Tablets, containing Colalin, cascara and podophyllin—Bottles of 100; *Dosage*—1–3 tablets at night.

Administration: Colalin—Adults, gr ¼ (0.016 Gm) to gr 1 (0.064 Gm), three or four times daily.

Children, gr ⅛ (0.008 Gm) to gr ¼ (0.016 Gm)

In Cholelithiasis—2 tablets gr ½ (0.032 Gm) three times daily after meals for 1 week; 1 tablet gr ½ (0.032 Gm) three times daily during second week; 1 tablet gr ¼ (0.016 Gm) three times daily in the third week; reduced when necessary.

Bibliography: *See Chap. XII.*

COLCHI-SAL (Huxley)

Antirheumatic

Composition: Is stated to contain colchicine and methyl salicylate.

Action and Uses: As antiarthritic in rheumatism, arthritis, gout and uratic manifestations.

Supply: COLCHI-SAL—Bottles 50 and 100 capsules.

Administration: 1 capsule every hour for 16 doses the first day; every hour and half for 10–12 doses the second day; subsequently continued in reduced dosage.

COLLODAURUM (Kahlenberg)

Gold Therapy

Description: A colloidal gold preparation containing metallic gold dispersed in distilled water.

Action and Uses: In inoperable carcinoma is stated to be hematinic, improve appetite, increase weight and relieve pain; is *used* as prophylactic following cancer surgery.

COLLODAURUM—Bottles of 4 oz.

Administration: *Intravenously*—2–5 cc two to three times weekly.
Orally—30 drops, increased by 1 drop to 60, in water three times daily for 3 mo.; reduced to 15 drops three times daily for the following 2 yr.

Bibliography: *See Chap. XII.*

COLLOSOL BROMOFORM COMPOUND (Crookes)

Sedative Expectorant

Composition: A colloidal preparation containing ½ m of bromoform and ⅛ gr (0.008 Gm) codein hydrochloride per dram; with senega, wild cherry and krameria, in a demulcent base.

Advantages and Uses: A stable, effective expectorant and pulmonary sedative; is palatable and safe for administration to children; constituent elements do not separate on standing. *For use* in whooping cough, post-influenzal infections, dry bronchitis, and tubercular disease.

Supply: **COLLOSOL BROMOFORM COMPOUND**—Bottles of 2, 4, 8, 16 and 80 oz.

Administration: 1 dr. in wineglassful of water at bedtime.
Children under 10 years—5–10 drops.
Children 10–15 years—10–30 drops.

Bibliography: *See Chap. XII.*

COLLOSOL FERROMALT (Crookes)

Nutritive

Composition: Contains colloidal iron and extract of malted barley, standardized for content of protein, diastase, mineral salts.

Action and Uses: Nutritive and tonic in anemias, asthenia, digestive disorders and debility.

Supply: **COLLOSOL FERROMALT**—Bottles of 4, 8, 16, 80 oz.

Administration: 1 teaspoon to 1 tablespoonful three times daily after meals.

Combinations: **COLLOSOL FERROMALT AND HYPOPHOSPHITES**—Contains Ferromalt and gr 2 each of potassium, sodium and calcium hypophosphites per ounce; *For use* in tuberculosis, to promote bone formation and as tonic. *Dose*—1–3 teaspoonfuls three times daily after meals. *Supply*—Bottles 8, 16, 80 oz.

COLLOSOL FERROMALT AND GLYCEROPHOSPHATES—Contains Ferromalt and gr 2 each of sodium, calcium and potassium glycerophosphates per ounce; especially useful in nervous debility, to stimulate growth and metabolism and as general tonic. *Dose*—1–3 teaspoonfuls three times daily after meals. *Supply*—Bottles 8, 16, 80 oz.

COLLOSOL FERROMALT AND CASCARA—Contains Ferromalt and gr 2 extr. cascara sagrada siccum U.S.P. per ounce; *For use* in constipation, in bowel irregularity in anemias. *Dose*—1–3 teaspoonfuls three times daily after meals. *Supply*—Bottles 8, 16, 80 oz.

COLLOSOL FERROMALT AND HEMOGLOBIN—Contains Ferromalt and gr 2 defibrinated hemoglobin per ounce; is indicated in the more severe anemias. *Dose*—1–3 teaspoonfuls three times daily after meals. *Supply*—Bottles 8, 16, 80 oz.

COLLOSOL FERROMALT AND MANGANESE—Contains Ferromalt and gr ½ (0.1 %) colloidal manganese hydroxide per ounce; is indicated in anemia and debility from coccogenic infections. *Dose*—1–3 teaspoonfuls three times daily. *Supply*—Bottles 8, 16, 80 oz.

COLLOSOL LACTO-CALAMINE (Crookes)

Astringent

Composition: Contains pure, finely divided zinc carbonate (calamine) combined with milk of almonds and witch-hazel.

Action and Uses: Emollient, soothing and antiseptic; *For use* in various skin affections where calamine is helpful.

Supply: COLLOSOL LACTO-CALAMINE—Bottles of 4, 80 oz.

Administration: Applied with sponge or cotton pad and massaged gently.

COLLOSOL LEAD M.A. (Crookes)

Lead Therapy

Composition: A colloidal suspension of lead and mercury, combined in organic form and adapted for intravenous use.

Action and Uses: Is claimed to be palliative in malignant disease; to be helpful in cancer.

Supply: COLLOSOL LEAD M.A.—Ampules, 5 cc, 10 cc, 20 cc—Boxes of 3.
COLLOSOL LEAD M.A.—Bottles of 10 cc, 20 cc.

Administration: *Intravenously*—For directions and technic see "References's accompanying package.

Combination: COLLOSOL PLUMBUM—Also known as "Choriotrope"—Ampule" 10, 20 cc.

Bibliography: *See Chap. XII.*

COLLOSOL TRIMINE (Crookes

Gonocide

Composition: Contains colloidal iron, colloidal manganese hydroxide and colloidal zinc hydroxide.

Action and Uses: *For use* in subacute recurrent urethritis and its complications; also in gonorrheal ophthalmia.

Supply: COLLOSOL TRIMINE—Ampules 1 cc—Boxes of 6.
COLLOSOL TRIMINE—Oral—Bottles 1, 4 oz.

Administration: 0.5–1.5 cc injected *intramuscularly;* repeated in 3 days and continued till 6 cc have been given.

COMBINED CARBONATES COMPOUND (Rorer)

Antacid

Composition: Is stated to contain bismuth subcarbonate, magnesium carbonate and cerium oxalate.

Description: A white fluffy powder, odorless and tasetless; is insoluble in water but stays temporarily in suspension.

Action and Uses: A combination of alkalies; for use as local antacid in gastric ulcer, gastritis; as a systemic alkalizer in acidosis; as sedative in nausea and inflammatory irritative intestinal conditions.

Supply: COMBINED CARBONATES COMPOUND—Dispensing boxes.

Administration: 1 teaspoonful, diffused in ½ glass of water, 3–4 times daily; in pernicious nausea, is given with menthol in olive oil.

COPFERTABS (Fraser)

Hematinic

Composition: Is stated to contain in each tablet reduced iron, gr 5 (0.324 Gm) and a copper compound equivalent to 0.0063 gr of metallic copper.

Action and Uses: Hematinic in secondary anemias.

Supply: COPFERTABS—Tablets—Adult—gr 5 (0.324 Gm)—Bottles 100, 500, 1,000.
COPFERTABS—Tablets—Children (containing reduced iron gr 1½ (0.09 Gm) metallic copper 0.0020 gr)—Bottles 100, 500, 1,000.

Administration: Adults, 2 tablets three times daily with meals.
Children, in proportion to age.

COPPER-IRON COMPOUND (McKesson and Robbins)

Hematinic

Composition: Is stated to contain organic proteid salts of copper and iron.

Description: A palatable, clear, brown solution, practically free from astringency.

Action and Uses: For regeneration of hemoglobin in various forms of anemia.

Supply: COPPER-IRON COMPOUND—Liquid—Bottles 8 oz., 1 qt. and 1 gal.
COPPER-IRON COMPOUND—Tablets—Boxes of 40.

Administration: 1–2 teaspoonfuls or 1–2 tablets after meals in water or milk.

COTEREMUL (McNeil)

Urinary Antiseptic

Description: A brownish colored powder containing emulsified copaiba and terebenthene, combined with cubebs, potassium nitrate, iron sulphate and alum; flavored with wintergreen.

Action and Uses: A prophylactic and genito-urinary antiseptic, in infections of the urethral tract.

Supply: COTEREMUL—Capsules—Bottles of 100, 500, 1,000, 5,000.

Administration: 2 capsules several times daily.

CREOLIN-PEARSON (Merck)

Antiseptic

Description: A mixture of coal tar oils and phenols rendered emulsifiable with water by a special process; a dark brown liquid of tar odor.

Action and Uses: Deodórizer, disinfectant and antiseptic, of phenol coefficient 8; *useful* in minor wounds, cuts, bites, burns, ulcers and surgical operations; also in cervical catarrh, leukorrhea, gonorrhea; as deodorizer and disinfectant in the sick room, bathroom and general household.

Supply: **CREOLIN-PEARSON**—Bottles 3 oz., ½ and 1 lb.

Administration: *As Disinfectant and Deodorant*—2–4 tablespoonfuls to the gallon of water.
For Antisepsis—1 dr. per pint.
As Douche—1 dr. per liter.
As Compress—0.5% solution.
For Scalp Treatment—½ dr. per quart.
For Disinfection of Hands—1.0% solution.

Bibliography: *See Chap. XII.*

CREOSOTE CARBONATE (Schering and Glatz)

Phthisis Therapy

Composition: A mixture containing guaiacol and creosote carbonate.

Description: A clear, colorless or slightly yellow viscid oily liquid, soluble in alcohol and oils, insoluble in water.

Action and Uses: As for creosote, in pulmonary and intestinal affections.

Supply: **CREOSOTE CARBONATE**—Bottles 1 oz., ¼, ½ and 1 lb.

Administration: M 5–20, increased slowly to m 80, several times daily; average dose 15 m.

CREOTHYOL (Strasenburgh)

Expectorant

Composition: Contains creosote and ichthyol with dilute hydrocyanic acid 1 m per dram; alcohol 27%.

Action and Uses: A sugar free bronchial sedative and antispasmodic *for use* in persistent cough, particularly of tubercular origin and in pulmonary complications of diabetes.

Supply: **CREOTHYOL**—Bottles, 1 pt. and 1 gal.

Administration: 1–2 teaspoonfuls four times daily, or as required.

CUPRAMIN (Buffington)

Hematinic

Composition: Each ounce represents
Copper (organic) gr 0.032; iron glycerophosphate gr 7 with manganese glycerophosphate and red bone marrow in equal parts.

Action and Uses: *For use* as reconstructive tonic in secondary anemia and neurasthenia.

Supply: **CUPRAMIN**—Bottles of 12 oz.

Administration: 1–2 teaspoonfuls three or four times daily.

CUPROGLOBIN (Bates)

Hematinic

Composition: A combination of pure hemoglobin with copper, glycerine and aromatics; contains approximately ½% of iron.

Action and Uses: A clear, stable, palatable solution *for use* in secondary anemias of various origin particularly anemias of children; in malnutrition and debility.

Supply: CUPROGLOBIN—Bottles of 8 oz. and 1 gal.

Administration: Adults 1–2 tablespoonfuls; Children 1 teaspoonful twice daily. Infants 20–30 drops, twice daily.

Bibliography: *See Chap. XII.*

DAROL (McKesson and Robbins)

Antipyretic

Composition: Is stated to contain phenacetin, aspirin and other antipyretics.

Action and Uses: Analgesic, antipyretic in colds, grippe, fevers.

Supply: DAROL—Tablets—Tins of 12 and 36.

Administration: 2 Tablets every 3 hr., with water for 5 doses; then 1 tablet every 3 hr. till relieved.

DELBIASE (Fougera)

Biologic Stimulant

Composition: Is stated to contain halogen salts of magnesium in certain fixed proportions, of dehydrated chloride, bromide, iodide and fluoride of magnesium.

Action and Uses: Is claimed to be a general biologic and metabolic stimulant of cytophylactic character, and to be useful in cancerous and precancerous states; also in asthenia, debility, intestinal toxemia, ulcers, cholecystitis, biliary insufficiency and Parkinsonism.

Supply: DELBIASE—Tablets gr 10 (0.6 Gm)—Vials of 10—Boxes of 4 vials.

DELBIASE—Ampules (Gelodelbiase) 5 cc, for intramuscular use—Boxes of 6.

DELBIASE—Ampules Isotonic Solution—100, 250 and 500 cc, for hypodermoclysis and topical application.

Administration: Tablets—2 daily, dissolved in water before breakfast; in severe cases increased to 4 tablets.

Ampules—1 ampule *intramuscularly* every other day.

DERMALGEN (National Drug)

Antiseptic

Description: A fine powder of light yellow color and pleasant odor, containing alum, bismuth, iodine, acetanilid, phenol, boric acid and antiseptic oils.

Action and Uses: Absorbent, deodorant, bactericide and analgesic; promotes healthy granulations. *Used* as dusting powder and stimulating dressing for abrasions, wounds, indolent ulcers, moist skin diseases; in syphilitic and tubercular ulcers; as styptic in continued bleeding.

Supply: DERMALGEN—Bottles with sprinkler top, 2 oz.

Administration: Is dusted freely, after cleansing surface with hydrogen peroxide.

DIATUSSIN (Bischoff)

Antispasmodic

Description: An alcoholic extract of the active principles of Thymus Vulgaris and Pinguicula Alpine.

Action: Is stated to be antiseptic and anesthetic to the respiratory mucous membrane and to liquify accumulated mucus.

Uses: In spasmodic coughs; in whooping cough, night cough of the aged and bronchial asthma; in coughs of influenza, measles, bronchitis and laryngitis.

Supply: DIATUSSIN—Bottles of 6 cc.

DIATUSSIN—Syrup—containing 2 drops Diatussin per dram—Bottles ot 6 oz.

Administration: Children—1–3 drops, two to three times daily in ½ oz. of water. Adults—up to 5 drops at bedtime or when required; in severe cases as often as every 2 hr.

DIAZYME GLYCEROLE (Fairchild)

Carbohydrate Digestant

Description: A glycerin extract of fresh pancreas gland, containing amylopsin without appreciable quantities of trypsin or lipase; is palatable and alcohol-free.

Action and Uses: *For use* as supplementary starch digestant in carbohydrate fermentation.

Supply: DIAZYME GLYCEROLE—Bottles, 8 oz.

Administration: 1–2 dr. diluted with several volumes of water; or is added directly to farinaceous foods, of temperature below 100°F.

DIGESTONE ELIXIR (McNeil)

Digestant

Description: A pleasantly flavored elixir containing per fluid ounce:

Tinct. Nux Vomica	6 m
Pepsin, Papain, Rennin	gr 12 (0.768 Gm)
Lactic Acid, Nitrohydrochloric acid, dilute	q.s.
Alcohol	15%

Action and Uses: Digestant and stomachic in chronic gastritis and dyspeptic states; also used as vehicle.

Incompatibles: Alkaline solutions.

Supply: DIGESTONE ELIXIR—Bottles of 2, 3, 4 oz., pt., ½ and 1 gal.

Administration: Adults—2–4 teaspoonfuls.
Children—½–1 teaspoonful.

DI-PHEN (Squibb)

Antiseptic

Description: A soapy solution of a diphenyl compound, a phenol derivative; is non-corrosive, non-poisonous and of pleasant odor.

Action and Uses: Antiseptic, germicide, detergent and cleanser; *useful* in sterilization of surgical instruments, sick room utensils and as hand wash; as antiseptic in cuts, bites, abrasions and as douche.

Supply: DI-PHEN—Bottles of 3 and 12 oz.

Administration: *Disinfection of instruments*—1 tablespoonful (½ oz.) in 1 qt. water, boiled for 5 min.
Hand and Foot Wash, Cuts, Abrasions and other skin affections—1 teaspoonful in 1 qt. water.
Douche—1 teaspoonful in 2 qt. water.

DRY PEPTONOIDS (Arlington)

Nutrient

Description: Prepared from milk, wheat and beef in proper proportions, thoroughly digested, concentrated, assayed and brought to uniform composition by the addition of lactose; is a light brown, granular powder of pleasant taste and odor, soluble in water.

Action and Uses: *For use* in conditions of low digestive capacity and for rectal alimentation; *Food Value* per 100 Gm, 375 calories, comprising proteins 164 calories, carbohydrates 211 calories.

Supply: DRY PEPTONOIDS—Bottles 2½, 5 and 28 oz.

Administration: Adults—2–4 teaspoonfuls in milk, broth, soup, water or other fluids.

DUODENIN (Armour)

Digestant

Description: Prepared from the glandular layer of hog duodenum containing secretin and enterokinase.

Action and Uses: Digestant; stimulates flow of pancreatic, hepatic and intestinal secretions. *For use* in intestinal disorders, duodenal insufficiency; in impaired protein digestion.

Supply: DUODENIN—Tablets, gr 1 (0.064 Gm)—Bottles of 100.
DUODENIN—Powder—Bottles of 1 oz., 1 lb.

Administration: 1 or more tablets (or 1–3 gr) three times daily after meals.

ECTHOL (Battle)

Alterative

Description: Contains the active principles of Echinacea and Thuja.

Action and Uses: Is claimed to stimulate leucocytosis and raise body resistance in infections: *For use* in sepsis, typhoid, small pox, erysipelas; in boils, carbuncles, gangrenous wounds, ulcers, abscesses.

Supply: ECTHOL—Bottles 8 oz.

Administration: 1 teaspoonful every 2 or 3 hr.
Locally—As wet dressing full strength or diluted with 2–10 parts of water.

ECZEMOL (Frasér)

Antipruritic

Composition: Is stated to consist of antiseptic oils, hydrocyanic acid, mercury nitrochloride and glycerin.

Action and Uses: Antipruritic and antiseptic; *For use* in eczema.

Supply: ECZEMOL—Bottles of 4 and 12 oz. and 1 gal.

Administration: Applied freely and allowed to dry or used as a wet dressing.

EKZEBROL (Tosse)

Antipruritic

Composition: Combines for synergistic effect bromine and strontium in isotonic sodium chloride solution.

Action and Uses: As antipruritic in prurigo, eczema, urticaria, psoriasis; sedative and analgesic in acute arthritis, neuralgia, migraine and allergic disturbances.

Supply: EKZEBROL—Ampules 10 cc—Boxes of 6 and 25.

Administration: 1 ampule, previously warmed to body temperature, *intravenously*, slowly injected, daily or every other day; 3–4 injections in acute cases, more in chronic cases.

Bibliography: *See Chap. XII.*

ELDOFORM (Winthrop)

Intestinal Astringent

Chemical Name: Tannin-Yeast Combination. Brand of Cervitan.

Description: A light gray, tasteless, odorless powder, slightly soluble in water, organic solvents and dilute acids, readily soluble in dilute alkalies; is unaffected by atmospheric heat and moisture, therefore well adapted for use in warm climates.

Action and Advantages: An effective astringent in both upper and lower intestinal tract; is without irritating effect upon the stomach and therefore well tolerated; is of agreeable taste, hence easily administered to children; constricts intestinal mucosa, reduces congestion and arrests discharges; the yeast content inhibits putrefactive and fermentative processes.

Uses: In various types of enterocolitis, dysentery, intestinal tuberculosis, typhoid fever.

Supply: ELDOFORM—Tablets 5 gr (0.3 Gm)—Bottles of 25.

Administration: Adults, 2 or 3 tablets, three or four times daily, thoroughly chewed before swallowed.

Children, 1 or 2 tablets several times daily, crushed and stirred in some fluid.

Bibliography: *See Chap. XII.*

ELIXIR ASPIRAL (Eastern Pharmacal)

Antipyretic

Composition: A palatable preparation of acetyl salicylic acid, blended with glycerin, aromatics and other media; 1 dr. represents 5 gr (0.324 Gm) of the sodium salt of aspirin.

Action: Analgesic and antipyretic; sweet, fragrant, miscible with water.

Uses: Acute infections—colds, influenza, tonsillitis, headaches, neuralgia, rheumatism, lumbago; also as gargle and as vehicle.

Supply: ELIXIR ASPIRAL—Bottles of 6 oz., 5 pt.

Administration: 1 dr. every 3 or 4 hr.; children—½–1 teaspoonful diluted in water; as gargle—full strength.

ELIXIR CARICANS (Fraser)

Digestant

Composition: A combination of the enzyme principles of Papaya, tropical melon, with pepsin and pancreatin.

Action and Uses: A protein and carbohydrate digestant, stimulating secretions and aiding nutrition; *For use* in various types of indigestion with eructation and flatulence; in gastralgia and duodenal catarrh, in vomiting of pregnancy; also as vehicle and solvent in the administration of other remedies.

Supply: ELIXIR CARICANS—Bottles of 16 oz. and 1 gal.

Administration:. 1–2 teaspoonfuls after meals.

ELIXIR IODO-BROMIDE OF CALCIUM COMPOUND (Tilden)

Alterative

Composition: Is stated to contain salts of iodine, bromine, potassium, sodium, calcium and magnesium with stillingia, rumex, dulcamara, lappa, taraxacum and menispermum.

Action and Uses: Alterative; *For use* in scrofula, syphilis and leprosy.

Supply: ELIXIR IODO-BROMIDE OF CALCIUM COMPOUND—Containing per dram gr 1½ (0.097 Gm) combined iodides—Bottles 12 and 16 oz.

ELIXIR IODO-BROMIDE OF CALCIUM COMPOUND WITH MERCURY BICHLORIDE—Containing per dram gr 1½ (0.097 Gm) combined iodides and gr 1/100 (0.0006 Gm) mercury bichloride—Bottles 12 and 16 oz.

Administration: 1–2 teaspoonfuls three to four times daily, in ½ glass water, ½ hr. before meals and at bedtime; increased if necessary.

ELIXIR MALTOPEPSINE (Tilden)

Digestant

Composition: Contains malt diastase, dioscorein, nitromuriatic, phosphoric and lactic acids with pepsin gr 1 (0.064 Gm) per dram.

Action and Uses: Digestive, tonic and vehicle; *For use* in cholera infantum, children's summer diarrhea and other intestinal disturbances.

Supply: ELIXIR MALTOPEPSINE—Bottles of 16 oz.

Combinations: ELIXIR MALTOPEPSINE WITH GLYCEROPHOSPHATES, containing Sodium gr 2 (0.130 Gm), Calcium gr 1 (0.064 Gm), Magnesium gr ⅛ (0.008 Gm), Strychnine gr 1/64 (0.001 Gm), Iron gr 3/16 (0.0121 Gm)—Bottles of 16 oz.

ELIXIR MALTOPEPSINE WITH IRON, ARSENIC, QUININE AND STRYCHNINE—Bottles 16 oz.

ELIXIR MALTOPEPSINE WITH SALICYLATES COMPOUND—Bottles of 16 oz.

LIQUOR MALTOPEPSINE—Sugar free—Bottles of 16 oz.

Administration: 1 or 2 teaspoonfuls three to four times daily, after meals.

ELIXIR NEUROGENIC (Cavendish)

Tonic

Description: Is stated to contain glycerophosphates of calcium, sodium, and strychnine, in addition to other constituents.

Action and Uses: Tonic and reconstructive; improves appetite and gastrointestinal function; relieves depressed states and thus used in neurasthenia, nervous exhaustion and postfebrile convalescence.

Supply: **ELIXIR NEUROGENIC**—Bottles of 6 and 16 oz.

Administration: 1 teaspoonful in water one to three times daily before meals.

ELIXIR OF ENZYMES (Armour)

Digestant. Vehicle

Description: A palatable preparation of proteolytic and milk curdling ferments active in acid medium.

Action and Uses: Gastric stimulant, digestant and mild carminative; *For use* in faulty protein digestion and proteolytic intoxication; as vehicle in the administration of iodides, salicylates and other drugs, and for preparation of junket, curds and whey.

Supply: **ELIXIR OF ENZYMES**—Bottles 1 pt.—Jugs 1 or 5 gal.

Administration: 1–2 dr. after meals.

For making junket—1 teaspoonful in ½ pt. of lukewarm milk, stirred and cooled.

EMULSION METAGEN AND COD LIVER OIL (Parke, Davis)

Nutrient. Vitamin Therapy

Description: An emulsion of cod liver oil 40% with Metagen, an extract containing Vitamins A and B, and fresh eggs as the emulsifying agent; a small amount of phosphoric acid is added. The bulk of the fat-soluble vitamin is supplied by the cod liver oil.

Action and Uses: Alterative and reconstructive tonic *for use* in nutritional disorders of infants and young children; fortifies resistance to disease in persons of all ages.

Supply: **EMULSION METAGEN AND COD LIVER OIL**—Bottles of 16 oz.

Administration: *Dose*—½–2 teaspoonfuls three times daily.

ENDO-MANGALAC (Endo)

Non-specific Therapy

Composition: A combination of manganese butyrate with a standardized, concentrated, non-specific protein.

Action and Uses: *For use* as non-specific protein agent in the therapy of infectious processes, as epididymitis, prostatitis, gonorrhea, colitis and pelvic infections in women; in eye, nose and throat diseases; in acne vulgaris, furunculosis, carbunculosis.

Supply: **ENDO-MANGALAC**—Ampules 1 cc—Packages of 12, 25, 100.

Administration: *Intramuscularly*, 1 cc daily for 3 days, then 2–3 doses weekly, in accordance with reaction.

ENEMOSE (Fairchild)

Colon Alimentation

Composition: Is stated to contain the entire soluble, digestible content of lean beef and whole wheat with organic and inorganic extractives as natively associated; is a converted, concentrated and diffusible nutrient.

Action and Uses: For colon alimentation; prepared by simple dilution; contains no fat, cane sugar or alcohol.

Supply: ENEMOSE—Vials 1 oz.—Boxes of 6.

Administration: 1 oz. dissolved in 4 oz. of water administered rectally; offers protein 2.4%, maltose and dextrins 9%, ash 0.9%; caloric value—about 15.

ENZYMES SOLUTION (Noyes)

Digestive

Composition: Is stated to contain pepsin, pancreatin, diastase, malt, hydrochloric acid and aromatics.

Action and Uses: *For use* in digestive disorders of the aged, in convalescence and dyspepsia.

Supply: ENZYMES SOLUTION—Bottles of 1 pt., 1 gal.

Administration: 1 dessertspoonful after meals.

ENZYMOL (Fairchild)

Surgical Solvent

Description: A light, straw colored, liquid extract prepared from fresh mucous membranes of animal stomachs; contains all the enzymes and the soluble organic and inorganic substances derived from gastric cells; has glycerine 25%, a trace of thymol, no alcohol; acidity equivalent to 0.26–0.3% hydrochloric acid; is assayed for its proteolytic power.

Action and Use: A physiological surgical solvent and proliferant; eliminates offensive odor, dissolves necrotic and sloughing tissues and stimulates healing of indolent wounds; *For use* in ulcers, old sores, slow healing wounds.

Supply: ENZYMOL (C.A.)—Bottles 4 oz., with vial of HCl and pipette.

Administration: Applied topically in 1 or 2 parts of water; for irrigation of abscess cavities, bone sinuses, in 0.2% HCl solution.

ERGOAPIOL (Smith)

Emmenogogue

Composition: Composed of specially extracted apiol, ergot, savin and aloin.

Action and Uses: Produces congestion and hyperemia of pelvic organs, increases menstrual activity and is employed in menstrual disorders, amenorrhea, dysmenorrhea, and menorrhagia.

Supply: ERGOAPIOL—Packages of 20 capsules.

Administration: 1 or 2 capsules three to four times daily.

ERNUTIN (Burroughs Wellcome)

Uterine Stimulant

Composition: A clear solution stated to contain ergotoxin 0.033% with chemically pure ergamine and tyramine in definite proportions.

Action and Uses: Induces uterine contraction of long continued spasm, tetanic in character, beginning 20–30 min. after hypodermic injection; effects are more durable on oral administration, lasting from 7–12 hr. *Uses*—as for ergot, in post partum and in uterine hemorrhages, after curettage.

Supply: ERNUTIN—Oral—Bottles of 30 cc, 4 and 16 oz.

ERNUTIN—Hypoloids 0.6 cc, containing 0.1% ergotoxin salt—Boxes of 6 and 100.

Administration: *Orally*—30–60 m.
Subcutaneously or Intramuscularly—0.3–0.6 cc, or ½–1 hypoloid.

Caution: Preparation should be protected from light.

ESTIVIN (Schieffelin)

Astringent

Description: A liquid preparation of Rosa Gallica.

Action: Relieves congestion of the conjunctivae and nasal mucosa, abating ocular discomfort, nasal irritation and discharge.

Uses: Principally in hay fever; also in conjunctivitis, blepharitis, episcleritis, trachoma, vernal catarrh, rhinitis.

Supply: ESTIVIN—Vials 2 dr., with dropper.

Administration: Moderate cases—1 drop instilled into inner canthus of each eye, three or four times daily.
Severe cases—1 drop applied at half-hour intervals three or four times in the morning, repeated during the day when necessary.

Bibliography: *See Chap. XII.*

EUPEPTIC HYPOPHOSPHITES (Nelson, Baker)

Tonic

Composition: Is stated to contain the hypophosphites of potassium, calcium, iron and manganese with quinine, strychnine, pancreatic ferments and wine.

Action and Uses: Reconstructive tonic; *For use* in mental and nervous exhaustion, debility, wasting diseases, tuberculosis.

Supply: EUPEPTIC HYPOPHOSPHITES—Bottles 1 pt. and 1 gal.

Administration: 1 teaspoonful three or four times daily.

EUPINOL (Tilden)

Antiseptic

Composition: A specially prepared distillate from the resinous wood of Pinus Palustris; is mostly laevo-menthone, a product superior to terebenthine antiseptics; phenol coefficient 1.7 (Rideal-Walker).

Action and Uses: Antiseptic and anodyne, non-toxic and non-escharotic; *For use* in minor surgery, trauma, burns, contusions, insect bites.

Supply: **EUPINOL**—Bottles 3 and 8 oz. and 1 pt.

EUPINOL—Ointment—Contains eupinol, ichthyol, camphor, resorcin, dried alum in petrolatum—Jars 2 and 16 oz.

Administration: *Locally*—5–10 %, as wet dressing and spray, in nose and throat affections.

Internally—5–10 drops every 3–4 hr., as emulsion, in bronchitis and intestinal fermentation.

EXICOL (Brooklyn Scientific)

Cholagogue

Composition: A combination of oleic acid and biliary salts.

Action: Stimulates liver cell activity, promotes bile secretion and gall bladder evacuation; aids in overcoming biliary stasis.

Uses: In functional hepatic insufficiency, postoperative biliary and intestinal stasis, cholecystitis, cholangitis; also applicable in cholecystography to empty gall bladder in place of the Boyden meal (fat meal).

Supply: **EXICOL**—Capsules, Soluble elastic—Boxes of 36 and 100.

EXICOL WITH PHENOLPHTHALEIN—Capsules soluble elastic—Boxes 36 and 100.

Administration: Average Dose—2 capsules, two to three times daily before meals given for 6–8 weeks, continued where necessary; in persistent intestinal stasis Exicol with Phenolphthalein is preferable.

Bibliography: *See Chap. XII.*

EXTRACT OF RED BONE MARROW (Armour)

Hematinic

Description: A medullary glyceride prepared from short-rib fresh marrow of growing cattle; is stated to contain in stable form the erythropoietic principles of marrow cells and hemoglobin.

Action and Uses: As hematinic in anemias following hemorrhage and tuberculosis; in chlorosis, marasmus, leukemia, Bright's disease; in anemias of bone necrosis, syphilis, malaria, rickets.

Supply: **EXTRACT OF RED BONE MARROW**—Bottles of 16 oz.

Administration: Adults—2 teaspoonfuls with water or milk three times daily; children in proportion.

Rickets—4–5 teaspoonfuls daily.

FERRODINE (Govett)

Hematinic

Description: Colloidal iodine and iron; contains 0.1 % of ferrous iodide; is nearly tasteless, of little toxicity, non-constipating, non-staining.

Action and Uses: That of iron and iodine; *For use* in anemias, especially those accompanying arthritis, infections, thyroidal disease and lues.

Supply: **FERRODINE**—Bottles of 8 oz.

Administration: ½–4 teaspoonfuls in half glass of water half hour before meals.

FLA-MIN-OL (Schieffelin)

Laxative

Description: Extra heavy, colorless Russian mineral oil, flavored.

Action and Uses: Palatable intestinal lubricant and mechanical laxative. *For use* in all types of chronic obstipation.

Supply: FLA-MIN-OL—Bottles of 1 pt.

Administration: 1 teaspoonful to 1 tablespoonful two or three times daily or 1–2 tablespoonfuls at night.

FOMOS (Fomos)

Antiseptic

Composition: A combination of quinone oxyquinolin sulphate, boric acid, tartaric acid and sodium bicarbonate.

Action and Uses: A potent non-irritating antiseptic and deodorant; on contact with vaginal secretions it disintegrates with formation of carbon dioxide which diffuses the antiseptic ingredients throughout the vaginal canal, distended by the gas. *For use* as prophylactic, in leukorrhea, cervicitis, vaginitis; in catarrhal infection and contraception.

Supply: FOMOS—Tablets 1¼ Gm—Tubes of 10.

Administration: 1 tablet inserted vaginally twice daily, or before exposure.

FOOD FERRIN (Battle Creek)

Hematinic

Description: A compound of iron, copper and chlorophyll of green plants; is of agreeable taste and does not affect the teeth.

Action and Uses: Hematinic and food tonic; *For use* in nervousness, anemia, convalescence.

Supply: FOOD FERRIN—Sweetened—for children—Bottles of 18 oz.

FOOD FERRIN—Unsweetened—for normal adults and the diabetic—Bottles of 1 pt.

Administration: 1 teaspoonful four times daily; children half dosage.

Bibliography: *See Chap. XII.*

FORTO-TESTIN (Remogland)

Aphrodisiac

Composition: Contains per tablet—
orchic substance, suprarenal substance, anterior pituitary, nux vomica ⅛ gr and dicalcium phosphate ½ gr.

Action and Uses: Aphrodisiac in sex gland deficiency; in disturbed metabolism and asthenia.

Supply: FORTO-TESTIN—Bottles of 100 tablets.

Administration: 1 Tablet three times daily after meals.

GADUOL CORDIAL (Noyes)

Tonic

Description: Contains Gaduol, an extract of cod liver oil, with malt, wild cherry bark and strychnine sulphate gr 1/32 per ounce; palatable and nutritive.

Action and Uses: Nutrient tonic in convalescence, anemia, undernutrition and for children of lowered vitality.

Supply: GADUOL CORDIAL—Bottles of 1 pt., 1 gal.

Combination: GADUOL WITH HYPOPHOSPHITES COMPOUND—Containing Gaduol 2.4 gr and hypophosphites of calcium, sodium, potassium, magnesium—4 gr with strychnine sulphate gr 1/32 per ounce—Bottles 1 pt., 1 gal.

Administration: 1 dessertspoonful three to four times daily after meals. Children ½ teaspoonful.

GASTRO-GALLATE (Westerfield)

Antacid

Composition: Is stated to consist of heavy calcium carbonate, magnesium carbonate ponderosa, bismuth subgallate, bismuth subcarbonate, sodium bicarbonate, hydrastis.

Action and Uses: Antacid and gastric sedative in gastritis, hyperacidity with nausea, in peptic ulcer, intestinal infections.

Supply: GASTRO-GALLATE—Bottles of 1 pt.

Administration: 1 teaspoonful in ½ glass of water, four or five times daily.

GASTROGEN TABLETS (Bristol-Myers)

Antacid

Composition: Is stated to contain calcium carbonate, magnesium carbonate, calcium phosphate and aromatics.

Action and Uses: As antacid in acid dyspepsia, hyperacidity and flatulence.

Supply: GASTROGEN—Tablets—Tins of 20—Bottles of 60 tablets.

Administration: 2 or 3 tablets chewed and swallowed with water; repeated in 15 min. if necessary.

GINGAMENT (Burroughs Wellcome)

Antacid

Composition: Is stated to contain sodium bicarbonate gr 5 (0.324 Gm) and equal parts of ammonium bicarbonate, gingament, saccharin and peppermint oil.

Action and Uses: Antacid and carminative *for use* in symptomatic flatulence, nausea and pyrosis.

Supply: TABLOID GINGAMENT—Bottles of 25, 100 and 500.

Administration: 1 or more tabloids taken with water or dissolved slowly in mouth, as often as necessary.

GLUCAL (McNeil)

Calcium Therapy

Description: A light yellow, pleasantly flavored, creamy emulsion containing 100 gr calcium gluconate in each fluid ounce.

Action and Uses: Alterative and tonic *for use* in calcium deficiency diseases.

Supply: GLUCAL—Emulsion—Bottles of 2, 3, 4 oz., pint, ½ gal., 1 gal.

GLUCAL—Lozenges—(containing 15 gr Calcium Gluconate)—Bottles of 1 and 5 lb.

Administration: Adults—2–4 teaspoonfuls, three or four times daily.
1–4 lozenges three or four times daily.
Children—½–2 teaspoonfuls three or four times daily.

GLUCO-CALCIUM (Lilly)

Calcium Therapy

Description: A solution of the calcium salts of various glucose acids, including gluconic acid.

Action and Uses: Raises blood calcium content; is easily dissociated and ionized in the blood and tissues; is non-irritating, readily absorbed and well tolerated. Recommended in calcium deficiencies; in bone, joint or peritoneal tuberculosis; in delayed calcification, rickets, osteomalacia, infantile tetany, eclamptic conditions; in delayed blood coagulability and allergic states.

Supply: GLUCO-CALCIUM—Vials, rubber-capped, 30 cc.

Administration: *Intramuscularly*—2–5 cc. *Intravenously*—5–20 cc.
May be repeated several times per day if necessary.

Bibliography: *See Chap. XII.*

GLYCO-HYDRASTIN (Stoddard)

Digestive

Composition: Is stated to contain hydrastis, pepsin, nux vomica, chamomile and aromatics in a non-alcoholic acidulated base, containing nitromuriatic acid.

Action and Uses: Stomachic, digestant and tonic in indigestion, gastrointestinal catarrh, intestinal stasis.

Supply: GLYCO-HYDRASTIN—Bottles 4 oz., 1 pt. and 1 gal.

Administration: 1–2 teaspoonfuls in water.

GLYCONDA (Lloyd Brothers)

Vehicle

Description: A concentrated sugarless cordial containing rhubarb, bicarbonate of potassium, golden seal, cinnamon, glycerin and peppermint; a dark, wine colored, pleasant aromatic liquid.

Action and Uses: Carminative, antacid, antifermentative and palatable vehicle. *For use* in cholera, diarrhea, dysentery, children's summer diarrhea, as tonic and stomachic and for masking bitter unpleasant substances.

Supply: GLYCONDA—Bottles of ½, 1 and 5 pt.

Administration: 1–2 teaspoonfuls every ½–2 hr.; Children—quarter of adult dose.

GLYCOSURETICS (Rorer)

Oral Diabetotherapy

Composition: A concentrated extract from the splenic portion of pancreas.

Action and Uses: *For oral therapy,* especially in early cases, of glycosuria and diabetes mellitus.

Supply: GLYCOSURETICS—Capsules, gr 2½ (0.162 Gm) Plain and Enteric coated—Bottles of 100.

Administration: 2 capsules after meals and at bedtime.

GONOSAN (Riedel)

Urinary Sedative. Antiseptic

Description: A combination of East Indian sandal wood oil and kava-kava resins.

Action: Exercises a bland, emollient effect upon inflamed urethral membrane; reduces dysuria and tenesmus; modifies inflammatory symptoms and shortens gonorrheal attack; is non-irritating and well tolerated.

Uses: Gonorrheal urethritis, cystitis, prostatitis, epididymitis, chordee; in gonorrheal diseases of women.

Supply: GONOSAN—Capsules, 5 m—Boxes of 40.

Administration: 2 capsules three times daily, after meals.

Bibliography: *See Chap. XII.*

GRAY'S GLYCERINE TONIC COMP.

(Purdue Frederick)

Alterative

Composition: Contains gentian, taraxacum, phosphoric acid, glycerine, sherry wine and carminatives.

Action and Uses: Is stated to stimulate digestion and enzyme activity; to increase appetite and produce general improvement; *For use* in anemia, convalescence, debility, coughs, colds, influenza; in cardiovascular and gastrointestinal disorders; *also* as vehicle for other drugs.

Supply: GRAY'S GLYCERINE TONIC COMP.—Bottles of 6 and 16 oz.

Administration: 2–4 teaspoonfuls before meals, three or four times daily; children ½–1 teaspoonful before meals.

GUAIACOL COMPOUND (Boericke and Runyon)

Expectorant

Composition: Is stated to contain guaiacol, 12 m per ounce, hypophosphites of calcium, sodium and potassium; alcohol 6%.

Description: A palatable expectorant with guaiacol in soluble form; is better tolerated than creosote U.S.P.

Action: Antiseptic, expectorant and sedative.

Uses: Colds, bronchitis, chronic pulmonary tuberculosis, emphysema.

Supply: GUAIACOL COMPOUND—In 1 and 5 gal.

Administration: 1–2 teaspoonfuls in milk or water, three to four times daily.

GYNALGOS. ALGOS (Wyeth)

Analgesic

Official Name: Elixir Amidopyrine and Potassium Bromide Comp.; now known as Algos.

Action and Uses: A palatable, analgesic, antipyretic and sedative; *For use* in dysmenorrhea, headache, colds, neuralgia and rheumatism.

Supply: ALGOS—Bottles of 1 pt., 1 gal.

Administration: 1–2 teaspoonfuls repeated every 3–4 hr.

HAEMOBUMINATE (Strasenburgh)

Hematinic

Composition: Each ounce represents:

	Gr	Gm
Hemoglobin	4	0.26
Ferric Albuminate	4	0.26
with other ingredients.		

Action and Uses: Hematinic in secondary anemia.

Supply: HAEMOBUMINATE—Bottles of 1 pt., 1 gal.

Administration: 1–2 teaspoonfuls three times daily.

HAEMOGLOBIN (Burroughs Wellcome)

Hematinic

Composition: Organic iron.

Action and Uses: A non-irritating, readily absorbed hematinic.

Supply: TABLOID HAEMOGLOBIN—Gr 5 (0.324 Gm)—Bottles of 100 and 500.

Administration: 1 or more tabloids three times daily.

Combinations: KEPLER MALT EXTRACT WITH HAEMOGLOBIN—Contains 9.2 gr (0.58 Gm) hemoglobin to the ounce; administered—1–2 dr., two to three times daily, after meals. *Supply*—Bottles of 9 oz.

HAGEE'S ORIGINAL CORDIAL COMPOUND (Katharmon)

Tonic

Composition: Is stated to contain calcium glycerophosphate, sodium glycerophosphate, salicylic acid, sherry wine, ext. cod liver oil and aromatics.

Action and Uses: Palatable reconstructive nutrient; *For use* in calcium deficiency diseases—rickets, osteomalacia, hay fever, asthma; in debility, anorexia and neurasthenia.

Supply: HAGEE'S ORIGINAL CORDIAL COMPOUND—Bottles of 16 oz.

Administration: Tablespoonful at meal times.

HAYDEN'S VIBURNUM COMPOUND

(N. Y. Pharmaceutical)

Uterine Antispasmodic

Description: Is stated to contain: Viburnum opulus, Dioscorea villosa, with aromatics; alcohol 50%.

Action and Uses: An antispasmodic and uterine sedative; non-narcotic, non-depressive, palatable. *For use* in threatened or habitual abortion, menorrhagia, metrorrhagia, menopause and following labor.

Supply: **HAYDEN'S VIBURNUM COMPOUND**—Bottles of 4 and 16 oz.

Administration: 1–2 teaspoonfuls in 3–6 teaspoonfuls of boiling water, taken hot; repeated when necessary; in severe dysmenorrhea—twice daily for 7 days prior to menstruation.

HAZELINE

(Burroughs Wellcome)

Astringent

Description: A preparation of the volatile principles of the bark of fresh young twigs of Hamamelis Virginiana.

Action and Uses: Styptic for small cuts, superficial bleeding and epistaxis; as dressing in skin irritations and slight burns; as mouth wash and spray in coryza, sore throat; in suppositories for hemorrhoids; as cream for hands, feet and axillae in hyperhidrosis, chafing and skin affections.

Supply: **HAZELINE**—Bottles 4 and 16 oz.

HAZELINE—Cream—Glass pots and Jars of 1 lb.—Large and small collapsible tubes—Tube with nozzle for hemorrhoids.

HAZELINE—Soap—soothing, non-greasy, super-fatted—Boxes of 3 tablets.

HAZELINE—Snow—non-greasy, vanishing preparation for skin—Glass pots and Jars of 1 lb.

HAZELINE—Suppositories—Boxes of 12.

Administration: *For External Use*—In conditions above enumerated.

HEMA-GLYCON

(Boericke and Runyon)

Tonic

Composition: Each tablet represents peptonate of iron with manganese, calcium glycerophosphate, nux vomica, berberine, hypophosphites of calcium, potassium and sodium and tissue phosphate salts.

Action and Uses: A general tonic to increase appetite, nutrition and energy production in asthenia, anemia, neurasthenia and convalescence.

Supply: **HEMA-GLYCON**—Tablets—Bottles of 100, 500, 1000, 5000.

Administration: 1 or 2 tablets three times daily before meals.

HEMAGULEN

(Lilly)

Hemostatic

Description: Prepared from fresh brain substance; contains some of the hemostatic elements most essential in clot production.

Action and Uses: Physiological hemostatic for topical application in capillary bleeding from nose, throat, gums and in other superficial hemorrhages.

Supply: HEMAGULEN—Bottles 1 oz.

Administration: Topical application to bleeding surface.

HEMO-GENIN (Stearns)

Hematinic

Description: Is stated to contain chlorophyll, ferric oxide and bone marrow.

Action and Uses: Supplies in readily assimilable form material for bone marrow and hemoglobin production; stimulates appetite, is hematinic and general tonic; *For use* in chlorosis, anemias of inanition, infections, pregnancy and from hemorrhage.

Supply: HEMO-GENIN—Capsules gr 6—Bottles of 100, 500 and 1,000.

Administration: 1 capsule three times daily with meals.

HEMOL (Irwin, Neisler)

Tonic. Nutrient

Composition: Contains gaduol, malt, wild cherry, hypophosphite compounds and aromatics.

Description: A brown liquid of wild cherry flavor.

Action and Uses: As for cod liver oil.

Supply: HEMOL—Bottles of 1 gal.

Administration: 1 teaspoonful to a tablespoonful two to three times daily, after meals.

HEMOPROTEIN "BROOKS" (Parke, Davis)

Non-specific Therapy

Description: A definite mixture of protein fractions, prepared from ox-blood fibrin by acid digestion, precipitation and fractionation.

Action and Uses: Stimulates antigenic function without causing protein reactions; promptly induces leukocytosis. *For use* as non-specific therapy agent in various conditions as arthritis, influenza, allergic disorders, infections, peptic ulcer, colitis, septic diseases, endocarditis, rheumatism, pleurisy and others.

Supply: HEMOPROTEIN "BROOKS"—10% sterile solution—Vials 10 cc.

Administration: 0.1 cc increased by 0.1 cc till 0.5 cc is reached; administered first daily then every second day; may be given *intravenously*, *intramuscularly* or *subcutaneously*. In urgent, especially acute cases, larger doses are given; in chronic, smaller doses.

HEMOQUININE (Schieffelin)

Hematinic

Composition: Is stated to contain the peptonates of iron, manganese, and sodium arsenate.

Action and Uses: Tonic, alterative and hematinic; *For use* in anemia, chlorosis, chronic malaria; to hasten convalescence after exhausting diseases.

Supply: HEMOQUININE—Bottles of 1 pt. and 1 gal.

Administration: 1 dessertspoonful in water, milk or wine, three times daily after meals.

HEPATIC SALINE (Schieffelin)

Laxative

Composition: Contains sodium phosphate, sodium sulphate and lithia.

Action and Uses: Cholagogue, laxative, uric acid eliminant; *For use* in constipation, gastrointestinal catarrh, gout and rheumatism.

Supply: HEPATIC SALINE—Bottles of 3, 6 oz.

Administration: ½–1 teaspoonful.

HYDROSAL (Hydrosal)

Astringent

Description: A colloidal suspension of aluminum acetate; stable, uniform and non-toxic.

Action: Astringent and antiseptic; is relatively non-irritating to tissue cells.

Supply: HYDROSAL—Liquid—Bottles of 4, 8 and 16 oz.

HYDROSAL—Ointment—Jars of ½ and 2 oz.

Combinations: HYDROSAL—Compound Ointment—Contains in addition belladonna, tannic acid in lanolin-petrolatum base—Tubes of 1 oz.

Uses and Administration: Liquid—As wet dressing for cuts, wounds, burns, skin affections, leg ulcers, eye and ear inflammations.

Ointment—Applied ⅛ in. thick directly to affected part and covered with waxed paper, in infant skin affections, furunculosis, burns.

Bibliography: *See Chap. XII.*

HYPEROL (Purdue Frederick)

Uterine Tonic

Composition: Contains ergotin, hydrastine, apiol, aloin, iron and quinine.

Action and Uses: Is stated to affect utero-ovarian circulation, reducing congestion and relieving painful spasm in amenorrhea, dysmenorrhea, menorrhagia, metrorrhagia; also effective in subinvolution, incomplete abortion and menopause.

Supply: HYPEROL—Capsules—Bottles of 28—Boxes of 12.

Administration: Acute conditions—1 capsule every 4 hr., followed by hot drink; chronic—3 capsules daily, one week preceding and after menstrual period. In acute menstrual suppression—2 capsules three times daily; in hemorrhage—1 capsule every 4 hr.

HYPOTENS "FRAISSE" (Fougera)

Hypotensive

Composition: A combination of Viscum album and sodium nitrite.

Action and Uses: Hypotensive and cardiac tonic in arterial hypertension, arteriosclerosis, Bright's disease, angina pectoris.

Supply: HYPOTENS—Hypodermic, Ampules, 2 cc—Boxes of 12.

HYPOTENS—Oral—Bottles of 25 Gm.

Administration: *Subcutaneously or Intramuscularly*—1 ampule daily for 12 days; after a 5 days' interval series is repeated.
Orally—25 drops in sweetened water, daily for 12 days.

ICHTHAMOL (Burroughs Wellcome)

Analgesic

Description: An ichthyol derivative.

Action and Uses: Is stated to be *useful* in fibrositis and rheumatic arthritis; also to relieve menopausal distress.

Supply: TABLOID ICHTHAMOL—Gr 2½ (0.162 Gm)—Bottles 25, 100 and 500.

Administration: 1–4 tabloids, three times daily after meals.

IODEX (Menley and James)

Iodine Therapy

Description: Contains elemental iodine combined with absorbent mixed fatty acids; is non-irritating, non-corrosive.

Action and Uses: For ready surface absorption in arthritis, rheumatism, glandular enlargements, goitre; in hemorrhoids, leukorrhea, pruritus, skin diseases; in strains and sprains, ulcers, wounds, burns and scalds.

Supply: IODEX—Ointment—Tubes ½ oz.—Jars 1 oz.
IODEX—Liquid—Bottles 2 oz.
IODEX—Soap—Individual cakes—Packages of 3.
IODEX WITH METHYL SALICYLATE—Tubes ½ oz.—Jars 1 oz.

Administration: Applied locally to affected area, freely, by inunction.

IODIA (Battle)

Alterative

Description: A combination of vegetable alteratives of active potentiality; each fluid dram represents 2½ gr (0.162 Gm) of potassium iodide and 1½ gr (0.097 Gm) of phosphated iron.

Action and Uses: *For use* in syphilis, scrofula, glandular disturbances, gout, rheumatism, skin affections.

Supply: IODIA—Bottles 8 oz.

Administration: 1 or 2 teaspoonfuls three times daily before meals.

IODO-ALBOID "LOWENTHAL" (American Organotherapy)

Antiluetic

Composition: Is stated to be an organic combination of iodine and protein, the iodine constituting 21%.

Action and Uses: *For use* in syphilis.

Supply: IODO-ALBOID "LOWENTHAL"—Tablets gr 5—Bottles of 100.

Administration: 1–2 tablets after meals, with water.

KAOSYL (Columbus Pharmacal)

Laxative

Official Name: Colloidal Kaolin Compound.

Composition: Contains colloidal kaolin, psyllium, bismuth subcarbonate, magnesium oxide, precipitated calcium carbonate and aromatics.

Action and Uses: Carminative, sedative, laxative, antacid; *For use* in gastric hyperacidity, intestinal stasis and toxicosis.

Supply: KAOSYL—Packages 4 oz. and Bulk.

Administration: 1–2 teaspoonfuls twice daily.

KATHESINA "HEISLER" (Kretschmar)

Hypotensive

Composition: A synthetic, stable derivative of cholin.

Action and Uses: Is stated to dilate the blood vessels of the general circulation, to reduce arterial tension and thus favorably affect the organism; recommended in the prophylaxis of cardiac weakness and failure, in vascular fibrosis with spasm, in arterial hypertension; also tends to raise pressure in hypotension.

Supply: KATHESINA "HEISLER"—Pills, 0.01 Gm—Vials of 20.

KATHESINA "HEISLER"—Ampules, 1 cc—Boxes of 10.

Administration: 1 pill two to three times daily for 1–4 weeks; then 1 pill daily. *Subcutaneously*—1 ampule daily or every second day.

KAVALACTOL (Tosse)

Urinary Sedative

Composition: Contains the ester of santalol and lactic acid, combined with extract of Kava-Kava, hexamethylenamine, resin guaiaci and radix rhei.

Action and Uses: Urinary antiseptic and sedative; relieves dysuria, chordee, deodorizes urine; *For use* in gonorrheal urethritis, cystitis.

Supply: KAVALACTOL—Pills, Keratin coated, equivalent to 4 m sandal wood oil—Bottles of 100, 1,000.

KAVALACTOL—Tubules of 30 pills—Boxes of 5 tubules.

Administration: 2 pills with water three times daily after meals.

KELPAMALT (Seedol)

Laxative

Composition: A combination of dehydrated Pacific marine algae (Macrocystis pyrifera) with dried malt extract, the former containing: iodine 0.17 %, phosphorus 0.36 %, calcium 1.88 %, magnesium 0.69 %, iron 0.02 %, sulphur 0.91 %, sodium 3.35 %, potassium 6.40 %; manganese 1 part and copper 18 parts per million.

Description: A hygroscopic substance capable of absorbing large quantities of water and forming a soft jelly-like mass.

Action and Uses: A laxative *for use* in intestinal functional deficiencies.

Supply: KELPAMALT—Tablets—Packages of 200, 600.

Administration: 2–4 tablets daily; in obstinate constipation—larger doses.

LACTIN PREPARATIONS (Hurst)

Antiseptics

Composition: Prepared from lactinium, a combination of aluminum and lactic acid, aluminum lactate, in aqueous solution and as basic lactate; pH-3.8.

Action and Uses: Astringent and antiseptic; in vaginal infections, gonorrheal disease, pelvic inflammation.

Supply: GLOBULACTIN—Pellets, contain lactinium with gelatine and glycerine; for vaginal use—Boxes of 12.

BOLOLACTIN—Powder, contains làctinium, bole and talcum; for dry treatment—Boxes of 100 Gm.

STYLOLACTIN—Rods, contains lactinium, gelatine; for urethral introduction —Boxes of 6.

TAMPOLACTIN—Liquid, contains lactinium dissolved in glycerine; for tampon treatment—Bottles 100 Gm.

Administration: *Vaginal*—Globulactin pellets.
Dry Application—Bololactin powder.
Urethral—Stylolactin rods.
Tampon—Tampolactin liquid.

Combinations: TAMPOLACTIN COMP.—Containing also iodine and potassium iodide; indicated in pelvic inflammation and adnexitis.
Supply—Bottles 100 Gm.

GLOBULACTIN COMP.—Containing also iodine and potassium iodide; indicated in pelvic inflammation and adnexitis.
Supply—Boxes of 12.

TAMPOLACTIN WITH ARGENTUM PROTEINICUM—Contains also argentum proteinicum; indicated in gonorrheal cases.
Supply—Bottles 100 Gm.

GLOBULACTIN WITH ARGENTUM PROTEINICUM—Contains also argentum proteinicum; indicated in gonorrheal cases.
Supply—Boxes of 6.

STYLOLACTIN WITH ARGENTUM PROTEINICUM—Contains also argentum proteinicum; indicated in gonorrheal cases.
Supply—Boxes of 12.

LACTOPEPTINE (Arlington)

Digestant

Composition: A combination of digestive and enzymogenic agents—pepsin, pancreatin, diastase, hydrochloric and lactic acids.

Action: Digestive; is proteolytically active in acid or alkaline medium.

Uses: *For use* in conditions of lowered digestive function; also as vehicle.

Supply: LACTOPEPTINE—Powder—Bottles of 1 oz.

LACTOPEPTINE—Tablets—Bottles of 40.

ELIXIR LACTOPEPTINE—Containing lactopeptine gr 38 per ounce, alcohol 16%; a clear, pink-colored, pleasant liquid—Bottles of 15½ oz.

Administration: Elixir—1–2 dr. after meals.
Powder—20 gr (1.3 Gm) after meals.
Tablets—2–4 tablets after meals.

LACTO-PROTEIN (Rorer)

Non-specific Therapy

Description: A sterile preparation of milk proteins with fat content largely removed and controlled hydrogen ion concentration.

Action and Uses: Increases leucocytosis and tissue resistance to pathogenic microorganisms and improves circulation through infected area. *For use* in chronic gonorrhea, chronic pelvic inflammatory disease, infectious arthritis, bronchopneumonia and suppurative diseases, and in gastric ulcer. Produces a minimum of pain and discomfort and a maximum of protein reaction.

Supply: LACTO-PROTEIN—Ampules 1, 5, 10 cc—Packages of 6, 12 and 100.

Administration: Initial dose 1–1.5 cc *intramuscularly* (gluteal) every 3–4 days in accordance with the reaction; dose is cautiously increased to 5–10 cc; course of 10–20 injections.

LAXAMEL (Burroughs Wellcome)

Laxative

Description: A palatable jelly-like preparation of paroleine, a liquid paraffin; contains 80% paroleine.

Action and Uses: Laxative for constipation.

Supply: LAXAMEL—Glass jars 4 oz.

Administration: 1 teaspoonful to 2 dessertspoonfuls before meals.

LECIBRIN (Fairchild)

Nervine

Description: A complex phosphorized-fat constituent of the brain combined with nucleo-proteins; standardized to contain 33⅓% by weight of brain lecithin.

Action and Uses: Nerve tonic *for use* in various nervous disorders.

Supply: LECIBRIN—Capsule, each representing gr $\frac{1}{25}$ elementary phosphorus—Bottles of 50.

Administration: 1–3 capsules daily, increased if indicated.

LECITHOL (Armour)

Nutritive. Hematinic

Description: An emulsion of lecithin obtained from fresh brain and spinal cord substance; is mixed with kephalin in normal proportions; is superior to lecithol of egg.

Action and Uses: Nerve tonic and hematinic in defective nutrition and impairment of nervous system; *used* in early paralysis of central origin; in neurasthenia, sexual debility, malnutrition, rickets, scrofula and secondary anemia.

Supply: LECITHOL—Bottles 8 oz.

Administration: 1 or 2 teaspoonfuls in cold water, immediately before or after meals.

LEUCOCYTE EXTRACT

Systemic Roborant

Description: Prepared from fresh, normal blood.

Action and Uses: For acute infections.

Supply: LEUCOCYTE EXTRACT—Syringes 10 cc—Vials 20 cc. *Administration*—10 cc every 4–6 hr. until 40–60 cc are administered in each 24 hr. (Squibb)

LEUCOCYTIC EXTRACT—Ampules 2 cc, 5 cc—Boxes of 6, 12 and 24; 2–5 cc per diem, *intramuscularly*. (United Laboratories)

LIBRADOL (Lloyd)

Counterirritant

Description: A plastic, homogenous, medicated plasma containing dracontium, sanguinaria cephaelis, melaleuca, lobelia, laurus, capsicum, tobacco; a green colored, fragrant, non-irritating substance of ointment-like consistency, easily spread and completely removable by washing with water.

Action and Uses: *For external use* as counterirritant and antiphlogistic in colds, croup, bronchitis, pleuritis, and other inflammatory conditions.

Supply: LIBRADOL—Jars of ¼, ½ and 1 lb.

LIBRADOL—Mild—Jars of ¼ and ½ lb.

Administration: Is spread freely over affected area.

LIPOLYSIN (Cavendish)

Reduction Therapy

Composition: Two varieties: Masculine—contains testicular extract, pancreatic hormone, ferments, enzymes and pituitary gland. Feminine—contains extract of ovaries, pancreatic hormone, ferments, enzymes and pituitary gland.

Action and Uses: In obesity to affect sugar metabolism and fat combustion.

Supply: LIPOLYSIN—Ampules—Packages of 12 and 100.

LIPOLYSIN—Tablets—Packages of 100, 250 and 500.

Administration: 1 ampule two to three times weekly, *intramuscularly*, accompanying oral tablet therapy.

Oral—1–3 tablets twice daily, ½ hr. before meals.

Bibliography: *See Chap. XII.*

LIQUENZYME (Wyeth)

Digestant

Composition: An elixir of digestive ferments; contains pepsin and rennin with aromatics; standardized by U.S.P. method, 1 dr. to digest 3,000 gr coagulated egg albumen.

Action and Uses: Assists digestion in gastro-intestinal disturbances; in children, convalescence, gastric hypoacidity and secondary anemia; as vehicle used for administration of unpalatable drugs; for preparation of junket.

Supply: LIQUENZYME—Bottles 8 oz., 1 gal.

Administration: 1–2 teaspoonfuls after meals, children ½ dose; junket—1 teaspoonful to quart of warm milk.

LITHIATED SORGHUM COMPOUND

(Sharp and Dohme)

Diuretic

Composition: Is stated to contain per fluid ounce 120 gr of broom corn seed, corn silk, saw palmetto and hydrangea, with 16 gr of benzoate and citrate of lithium.

Action and Uses: Diuretic, uric acid eliminant, genito-urinary demulcent and sedative in vesical atony and bladder irritability, in nocturnal incontinence of children.

Supply: LITHIATED SORGHUM COMPOUND—Bottles of 14 oz., 1 gal.

Administration: 1–2 fl. dr., three or four times daily.

LIVER EXTRACT

(United Laboratories)

Hypotensive

Description: A preparation from fresh bovine liver.

Action and Uses: Hypotensive *for use* in essential hypertension.

Supply: LIVER EXTRACT—Ampules 2 cc—Boxes 6, 12 and 24.

Administration: 2 cc injected daily.

LOINGIA

(Columbus Pharmacal)

Expectorant

Official Name: Lobelia et Stillingia Compound.

Composition: Contains lobelia, stillingia, oils of cajuput, lavender and cinnamon in syrupy base.

Action and Uses: Antispasmodic expectorant, sedative and abortive in croup, coughs, colds, asthma.

Supply: LOINGIA—Bottles of 1 pt. and in Bulk.

Administration: 20–30 m, repeated as indicated.

LUIZYM

(Kretschmar)

Amylolytic

Description: Contains carbohydrate digesting enzymes, including cellulase and hemicellulase; is hygroscopic, palatable and of seasoned-broth taste.

Action and Uses: Assists in the complete digestion of carbohydrates and in the enzymatic, hydrolytic decomposition of cellulose into its simplest non-fermenting components; *For use* in flatulence, colic, fermentation due to carbohydrate indigestion; in abdominal radiography to eliminate undesirable gas in the intestines.

Supply: LUIZYM—Tablets—Tubes of 20—Bottles of 50 and 200.

Administration: 2 tablets three times daily chewed after meals; later 1 tablet three times daily, as long as necessary. In radiography—2–3 tablets three times daily after meals; in achlorhydria simultaneously with dilute HCl, for 2 days preceding the examination; alcohol, large meals and cathartics should be avoided.

Bibliography: *See Chap. XII.*

LYSOL (Lehn and Fink)

Germicide and Antiseptic

Description: A 60% cresylic acid compound, free from naphthalene, pyridin, oily and tarry matter; is uniform in composition, active in high dilution, clearly soluble in water with neutral reaction; phenol coefficient 5 (F.D.A.)

Uses and Dosage: *For use* as irrigation, douche and local application—in 0.5–1.0% dilutions; for wounds, burns, scalds, 1–2%; for disinfection of hands, instruments, rubber gloves—2%; for disinfecting discharges (sputum, feces, urine, utensils, bacterial cultures, etc.) 5%.

Supply: LYSOL (L.A.)—Bottles of 3, 7, 16 oz. and 1 gal.—Drums 5, 10, 30 and 50 gal.

MARINOL (Fairchild)

Nutritive

Description: A vitamin-standardized cod liver oil, 40%, in combination with sea water and sea plants, the oil is homogenized, held in colloidal suspension, highly diffusible, digestible and palatable.

Action and Use: A supplementary food and antirachitic in rickets, malnutrition.

Supply: MARINOL—Bottles of 2 and 12 oz.

Administration: Adults—Tablespoonful doses several times daily.
Children—Dram dosage; Infants in drop doses, as above.

MAR-PHEDACO (Strasenburgh)

Expectorant

Composition: Contains per ounce—

	Gr	Gm
Codein sulphate	½	0.032
Ephedra	30	1.944
Calcium guaiacol sulphonate	5	0.324

with marrubium, menthol and aromatics.

Action and Uses: Bronchial sedative of sustained action in bronchitis, laryngitis, colds.

Supply: MAR-PHEDACO—Bottles of 1 pt. and 1 gal.

Administration: 1 teaspoonful as required.

MARROW MALT COMPOUND (C. D. Smith)

Nutritive. Reconstructive

Composition: Is stated to contain red bone marrow extract, glycerophosphates of calcium, iron, manganese and sodium, alfalfa, soluble copper, diastatic malt, nuclein and vitamin D in its cod liver oil; alcohol 15%.

Action and Uses: Reconstructive, tonic, hematinic and nutritive; *For use* in convalescence after acute infections, in chronic disease, anemia, neurasthenia.

Supply: MARROW MALT COMPOUND—Bottles of 4, 8, 16 oz. and 1 gal.

Administration: Dessertspoonful followed by wineglassful of water, three or four times daily, before meals.

MERRILLIZED YEAST (MacDowell)

Detoxicant

Description: A concentrated dehydrated, vitamin B_1 and B_2 product prepared from brewers' yeast; palatable and non-fermenting.

Action and Uses: An antiseptic and detoxicant in dysentery, colitis, arthritis, boils, anorexia, obesity and malnutrition.

Supply: MERRILLIZED YEAST—Tins of 6 oz.

Administration: 1 tablespoonful, equivalent to about 8 bakers' yeast cakes, taken twice daily.

METABOL (McNeil)

Intestinal Antiseptic

Composition: A combination of benzoated ricinoleates and other glyceryl esters of the higher fatty acids.

Action and Uses: Assists the liver in its detoxifying function; in the intestinal tract is laxative and reestablishes normal peristalsis. *For use* in detoxication treatment of arthritis, rheumatism, myalgia, neuritis, sciatica, dysentery; in cholecystitis, spastic colon, colitis, urticaria.

Supply: METABOL—Bottles of 4, 6 oz., 1 pt., ½, 1 gal.

Administration: 1 teaspoonful before meals; later 1 teaspoonful daily.

METALLIC BISMUTH (COLLOSOL BRAND) (Crookes)

Antiluetic

Composition: A non-colloidal suspension of metallic bismuth.

Action and Uses: Antiluetic; is readily and continuously absorbed.

Supply: METALLIC BISMUTH—Bottles 5, 10, 20% in 5, 10, 30 cc each.

Administration: 1–2 gr once weekly by *intramuscular* injection.

MILK OF MAGNESIA "PHILLIPS" (Phillips)

Antacid

Composition: A concentrated liquid magnesia, odorless and almost tasteless.

Action and Uses: Antacid, laxative and gastric sedative in hyperacidity, pyrosis, peptic ulcer; in intestinal flatulence, constipation, seasickness and nausea of pregnancy.

Supply: MILK OF MAGNESIA "PHILLIPS"—Bottles, 4 and 12 oz. and 3 pt.
MILK OF MAGNESIA "PHILLIPS"—Tablets, Mint flavored, each equal to 1 teaspoonful of fluid—Boxes of 30—Bottles of 75.

Administration: *Internally* as Antacid—1 teaspoonful in water 2 hr. after meals.
As Laxative—2–4 tablespoonfuls in water 1 hr. after breakfast.
Children—under 1 yr.—5–10 drops, 1–3 yr.—10–20 drops, 3–7 yr.—½ teaspoonful, under 14 yr.—1 teaspoonful.
Externally—In burns, as wet dressing, full strength or mixed with oil.

MINERALIZATION TABLETS (Manola)

Remineralizer

Composition: Is stated to contain silica, manganese, phosphates of iron and magnesium, and salts of sodium, potassium and calcium.

Action and Uses: For remineralization in various conditions associated with mineral salt deficiencies.

Supply: MINERALIZATION TABLETS—Boxes of 100.

Administration: 2 tablets dissolved in the mouth four or five times a day.

MINERASAL (Searle)

Remineralizer

Description: A combination of aluminum, calcium, chlorine, fluorine, magnesium, iodine, iron, manganese, phosphorus, potassium, sodium, silicon and sulphur, in granulated effervescent powder form.

Action and Uses: To supply the mineral elements in the growing child, in pregnancy and lactation; in peptic ulcer, diabetes mellitus, arterial hypertension, respiratory affections.

Supply: MINERASAL—Bottles of 4 oz., with measuring cap.

Administration: 1 measuring cap three or four times daily; children—half dosage.

MOBÉ (Norwich)

Expectorant

Composition: Is stated to contain mobenate, potassium guaiacol sulphonate, sodium benzoate, sodium citrate, aromatics; alcohol 10%.

Action and Uses: A palatable syrupy expectorant in coughs, colds and bronchitis and sedative to allay throat irritation.

Supply: MOBÉ—Bottles of 4 oz.

Administration: 1–2 teaspoonfuls every 3–4 hr.

MOROTOL (Morotol)

Nutrient

Composition: Extract of malt with 50% cod liver oil, aromatic cascara sagrada, glycerine, chocolate, aromatics; alcohol (as solvent) 4%.

Description: A chocolate flavored cod liver oil with extract of malt; freed from disagreeable odor and taste.

Action and Uses: That of cod liver oil, with slightly laxative properties added.

Supply: MOROTOL—Bottles of 12 oz.

Administration: 1 tablespoonful three times daily.
Children—according to age.

MORRHUOL "CHAPOTEAUT" (Fougera)

Vitamin Therapy

Description: An alcoholic extract of cod liver oil available in capsule form.

Action and Uses: Has a high vitamin content, exerting a stimulating effect upon metabolism; improves appetite, increases digestive and assimilative powers; *uses* as for cod liver oil.

Supply: MORRHUOL "CHAPOTEAUT"—Capsules, each of vitamin content of 1 teaspoonful of fat free oil—Bottles of 100.

Administration: Children—2–4 capsules daily, after meals.
Adults—4–8 capsules daily, after meals.

Combinations: MORRHUOL CREOSOTE—Contains Morrhuol 3 m with creosote U.S.P. 1 m per capsule; combines the effects of cod liver oil with the soothing expectorant action of creosote. *Supply*—Capsules—Bottles of 80. *Administration*—4–10 capsules daily after meals.

MUCIN (Burroughs Wellcome)

Gastric Sedative

Composition: The principle constituent of mucus.

Action and Uses: Soothes mucous membranes locally, neutralizes gastric acidity. *Used* largely in the treatment of peptic ulcer.

Supply: MUCIN—Scales—Bottles of 1 oz.

Administration: 1 dr. to 1 oz. three times daily after meals.

Bibliography: *See Chap. XII.*

MUSKOLA (Strasenburgh)

Nerve Sedative

Composition:

	Gr	Gm
Kola nuts (caffeine)	½	0.032
Ammonium bromide	15	0.972
Hyoscyamine hydrobromide	1/128	0.0005
Muskroot, iron citro-chloride, aromatics ... q.s.		

Action and Uses: Nerve sedative, in hysteria, neurasthenia, anemia.

Supply: MUSKOLA—Bottles of 1 pt. and 1 gal.

Administration: 1 teaspoonful three to four times daily.

MYORGAL (Winthrop)

Cardiac Stimulant

Description: A preparation of nucleosides, derivatives of nucleic acid; is free from choline, histamine and epinephrine, and contains no potassium or calcium ions of pharmacologic significance; is biologically standardized.

Action: Chiefly on the coronary arteries, causing dilation and increased rate of blood flow; slightly accelerates pulse, causing flushing of face and sensation of warmth; also stimulates respiration with decrease of residual air.

Uses: In angina pectoris; in precordial distress due to excessive use of alcohol, tobacco, tea or coffee; in chronic myocarditis, syphilitic aortitis and some cases of glomerular nephritis; combined with digitalis is also helpful in cardiac dilatation and decompensation.

Supply: MYORGAL—Tablets—Bottles of 25.

Administration: 1 tablet two or three times daily, either alone or in association with other therapy.

Bibliography: *See Chap. XII*

MYOSTON (Cavendish)

Cardiac Stimulant

Description: An extract obtained from calf muscle.

Action and Use: Is stated to relax spasm of cardiac vessels and thus relieve precordial distress and dyspnoea; is *used* in angina pectoris, in sclerosis of the aorta and coronaries; also in asthenia, nervous exhaustion and convalescence from acute infections.

Supply: MYOSTON—Bottles of 20 cc.
MYOSTON—Ampules—Boxes of 12.

Administration: *Subcutaneously*—1 ampule, repeated in acute attacks; then as required.

Bibliography: *See Chap. XII.*

NACITRA (McNeil)

Diuretic

Description: An effervescent, compressed tablet containing sodium citrate, with or without flavoring of lemon.

Action and Uses: Diuretic, diaphoretic and antacid; *For use* as diuretic and milk modifier in feeding of children and in the early stages of bronchial infection.

Supply: NACITRA—Tablets, gr 5, 10, 15—Bottles of 100, 500, 1,000 and 5,000.

Administration: 1–3 tablets dissolved in water or milk.

NEODYNE (National Drug)

Expectorant

Composition: Is stated to contain creosote carbonate, guaiacol, terpene hydrate, ammonium chloride, tartar emetic, sodium glycerophosphate, calcium glycerophosphate, glycerin, with tr. hyoscyamus m 4 per fluid ounce; alcohol 22%.

Action and Uses: A non-irritating expectorant, liquifying mucus and relieving congestion; *indicated* in coughs, colds, throat irritation, bronchitis, whooping cough, grippe, pneumonia; also as stomachic to increase flow of gastric juice and improve digestion.

Supply: NEODYNE—Bottles of 1 pt.

Administration: 1–3 teaspoonfuls every 2–3 hr.
Children—10 drops to ½ teaspoonful.

NEO-REARGON (Akatos)

Antiseptic. Gonocide

Composition: Is a chemical compound of silver nitrate and anthrachinonglucosides; contains about 15% of silver.

Action and Uses: A penetrating gonocide and antiseptic, free from irritation and pain, and forming a stable solution; *For use* in anterior and posterior gonorrheal urethritis and in gonorrheal infections in the female; also in nose, throat and ear affections.

Supply: NEO-REARGON—Vials 10, 25 and 100 Gm.

Administration: *For Hand Injection*—5 cc of 5% solution, two to three times daily and at bedtime; continued later with 2½% solutions.
As Irrigation—250 cc of ¼% solution.
As Abortive Therapy—5–6 injections daily for several days.
For Vaginal Irrigation—30 cc of 1–2% solution.
For Tampons—5% solution.

In Nose and Throat Affections—5% solution in glycerin, applied directly, two to three times daily, or by tampons; as irrigation, 0.5% aqueous solution twice daily.

In Ear Diseases—Several drops of 5% solution instilled two to three times daily; as irrigation, 0.5% solution.

In Eye Disorders—As irrigation, 1% aqueous solution every hour; 1 drop of 5% solution for instillation.

Caution: Solutions must be freshly prepared, using distilled water only. Stains may be removed by washing and 10% bichloride of mercury solution.

NEO-SEVETOL (Wyeth)

Nutrient

Official Name: Emulsio Sevi Comp.

Composition: An emulsion of 40% mixed fats, proteins and carbohydrates; each tablespoonful is equivalent in vitamin A and D content to 1 dr. of standard cod liver oil.

Action and Uses: As nutrient and vitamin stimulant in malnutrition, emaciation, marasmus of infancy and childhood and in convalescence.

Supply: NEO-SEVETOL—Bottles of 12 oz.

Administration: 2–4 teaspoonfuls two to three times daily, taken plain or diluted. Children 1–2 teaspoonfuls.

NEPENTHÉ (Tilden)

Intestinal Astringent

Composition: Contains blackberry root, nut gall, cinnamon, ginger, sodium bicarbonate, prickly ash bark and aromatics.

Action and Uses: Carminative, antispasmodic and sedative; *For use* in diarrhea, cholera infantum and cholera morbus; in dysentery, intestinal fermentation, flatulence and autointoxication.

Supply: NEPENTHÉ—Bottles 16 oz. and 1 gal.

Administration: ½ teaspoonful every hour until relieved. Children 10–30 drops, as required.

NEPHROSON (Merrell)

Diuretic

Composition: A combination of active extractives of the following plants: Oxydendron arboreum, Eupatoreum purp., Eryngium yuccaefol, Hydrangea arborescens, Polytrichum juniper, Stigmata maydis together with Tr. apis mellifica, lithium benzoate and spirit juniper, a sourwood compound.

Action and Uses: Diuretic and uricolytic; *For use* in Bright's disease, cystitis, urine retention and incontinence, anasarca, gout, calculus.

Supply: NEPHROSON—Bottles of 12 oz.

Administration: 1 teaspoonful every 1–6 hr. in accordance with symptoms.

NEURILLA (Od Peacock)

Sedative

Composition: Prepared from Scutellaria passiflora, calamus, lavender; alcohol 20.3%.

Action and Uses: Sedative *for use* in insomnia, nerve exhaustion, depression; also as nervine, antispasmodic and tonic.

Supply: NEURILLA—Bottles of 8 oz.

Administration: 1–2 teaspoonfuls as required.

NEURINASE (Fougera)

Sedative

Composition: Is stated to contain per teaspoonful 0.15 Gm sodium diethylmalonylurea dissolved in fluid extract of valerian.

Action and Uses: Sedative and hypnotic in nervous excitability, insomnia, melancholia.

Supply: NEURINASE—Bottles of 90 Gm.

NEURINASE—Tablets, each containing 0.2 Gm sodium diethylmalonylurea with 0.5 Gm extract valerian—Tubes of 20.

Administration: 1 teaspoonful or 1 tablet, three or four times daily after meals.

NEUTRALIZING CORDIAL (Columbus Pharmacal

Antacid

Official Name: Rhei et Potassii Comp.

Composition: Each ounce represents

	Gr	Gm
Rhubarb	17	1.091
Potassium carbonate	6⅔	0.428
Berberis aquifolium	10	0.643
Cinnamon	10	0.643
Aromatics	q.s.	
Special menstruum without sugar	q.s.	

Action and Uses: Antacid, carminative, laxative; *For use* in gastric hyperacidity, chronic dyspepsia, chronic constipation.

Supply: NEUTRALIZING CORDIAL—Bottles 1 pt. and 1 gal.

Administration: 1–4 teaspoonfuls three or four times daily after meals.

NITROPHEN (McNeil)

Hypotensive

Composition: Each tablet contains—

	Gr	Gm
Bismuth subnitrate..	5	0.324
Phenobarbital..	⅛	0.008

With ext. passiflora and ext. lupulus (Hops).

Action and Uses: Is stated to be a vaso-dilator and to reduce diastolic blood pressure; *For use* in acute nephritis and renal insufficiency.

Supply: NITROPHEN—Tablets—Bottles of 100, 500, 1,000 and 5,000.

Administration: 1 or 2 tablets three times daily, continued for a considerable time.

NOPIRINE "VICARIO" (Fougera)

Antiarthritic

Composition: Is stated to contain aspirin (acetylsalicyl radicle) with acetphenetidin and caffeine.

Action and Uses: As analgesic in arthritis, neuralgia, headache, toothache, influenza, acute bronchitis.

Supply: NOPIRINE "VICARIO"—Boxes of 12 tablets.

Administration: 1 tablet when necessary.

OBTUNDIA (Otis Clapp)

Antiseptic

Description: A limpid, red-brown liquid of pungent odor; insoluble in water, soluble in alcohol and ether; volatilizes slowly and is of low surface tension; phenol coefficient 6.9.

Action and Uses: Non-corrosive, non-irritating germicide; antipruritic and local anesthetic; *For use* in minor surgical affections, burns, boils, toothache.

Supply: OBTUNDIA—Bottles 1 and 4 oz., 1 pt. and 1 qt.

Administration: Local application.

Combinations: OBTUNDIA CREAM—Contains obtundia, calendula in creamy base; *For use* as anesthetic antiseptic in burns. *Supply*—Tubes of 1½ oz. *Administration*—Local application.

OBTUNDIA INHALANT—Contains obtundia in light mineral oil; *For use* as decongestive in nasal affections. *Supply*—Bottles 1 and 4 oz., 1 pt. and 1 qt.; *Administration*—By inhalation.

OBTUNDIA NASAL CREAM—Tubes of ¼ and ½ oz.; for local application.

OBTUNDIA EPHEDRINE INHALANT—Contains obtundia and ephedrine 1% in light mineral oil; *For use* in sinus and nasal affections as decongestive; *Supply*—Bottles 1 and 4 oz., 1 pt. and 1 qt; *Administration*—By spray to nose and throat.

OBTUNDIA EPHEDRINE NASAL CREAM—Tubes of ¼ and ½ oz.

OBTUNDIA VAGIOBULBS—Contains obtundia in glyco-boron or cocoa butter base; *For use* in vaginal affections. *Supply*—Boxes of 12 suppositories. 323A—cocoa butter base. *Administration*—Locally applied.

OBTUNDORRHOID—Contains obtundia with hamamelis and aesculus, *For use* in rectal irritations, for astringent effect. *Supply*—Tubes of 1 oz. *Administration*—Locally applied.

OBTUNDOBULBS—Contains obtundia with hamamelis and aesculus; *For use* in bleeding, irritated rectal conditions. *Supply*—Suppositories—Boxes of 12. *Administration*—Locally applied.

OCCY-CRYSTINE (Occy-Crystine)

Laxative. Detoxicant

Composition: A neutral hypertonic solution of the sulphates of sodium, potassium, calcium and magnesium.

Action: Causes precipitation of a colloidal sulphur on contact with gastric hydrochloric acid; in small doses is laxative and detoxicant, in larger doses acts as hydragogue cathartic.

Uses: In gastric indigestion with gaseous distention and hyperacidity; in constipation and intestinal auto-intoxication; for detoxication purposes in dermatologic and systemic conditions: acne, neuritis, lumbago, sciatica, headache; as hydragogue cathartic in general anasarca and ascites.

Supply: OCCY-CRYSTINE—Bottles of ½, 1, 2, 4 and 8 oz.

Administration: *Laxative*—½–2 teaspoonfuls in cold water before meals.
Cathartic—2–6 teaspoonfuls.
Children—up to 12 years of age—10–30 drops, in prune juice.
In Gall-Bladder drainage, through duodenal tube—2 oz., warmed.
As Mineral Table Water—2 teaspoonfuls to quart of water.

OLEOTHESIN (Oleothesin)

Local Anesthetic

Composition: A solution of procaine base in colloidal state, in an oily solvent.

Action and Uses: Produces prompt local anesthesia by direct action on nerve tissue; is non-irritating to mucous membranes, denuded areas or open wounds. *For use* in dentistry—for needle puncture, in scaling of teeth, in gingivitis and plate discomfort; in minor surgery—in lancing abscesses, in cysts, fractures, burns, cuts; also in nose and throat work.

Supply: OLEOTHESIN—Solution—Bottles of ½ and 1 oz.
OLEOTHESIN—Packing—Jars of ½ in. selvage edged gauze.
OLEOTHESIN—Spray—in De Vilbiss Atomizer.
OLEOTHESIN—Socket Paste.
OANDA—Ointment, containing Oleothesin in ointment base.

Administration: By swab, spray or dropper directly to affected area; for deeper or prolonged effect, repeated applications.

OCTOZONE "ROYER" (Octozone)

Oxidizing Agent

Chemical Name: Octozone.

Composition: Is thought to be a condensation product of 3, 4 or 8 atoms of oxygen, O_3 or O_4 or O_8, with characteristics not observed in other oxygen basic gases.

Description: A concentrated, pungent form of ozone prepared by passing oxygen under 5 lb. pressure through a "electroniseur," an apparatus which subjects the gas to silent electrical discharges, forming an unstable, concentrated, non-explosive gas; decomposes in 30 min. if exposed to light and cannot be preserved or transferred.

Action: Strong oxidizer, disinfectant, deodorizer and bleaching agent; favors oxidation of waste products deposited in subcutaneous tissues, muscles and fasciae with liberation of lactic acid.

Uses and Administration: For general external application patient is enclosed, up to the neck, in fabric suit filled with the gas and is exposed to its action and absorption by the skin for ½–1 hr. For local external application, is put in arm and leg bags, for treatment of varicose ulcers, wounds, skin diseases; *Subcutaneously:* 10–50 cc, for boils, furuncles. *Intramuscularly* 10–50 cc for infection of joints. Also applied by spraying wounds and abscesses, rectal injection—250–1,000 cc; and orally by drinking Octozonised water. Is claimed to be *useful* in rheumatism, sciatica, neuritis, fibrositis, osteomyelitis and infections: carbuncle, sinusitis, hemorrhoids.

Supply: By an octozone producing apparatus, the "electroniseur" only.

Caution: In severe cough from inhalation, tincture benzoin compound, or spiritus ammonium aromaticus, or 10 m spirits of chloroform are helpful.

Bibliography: *See Chap. XII.*

ORALSULIN (Lafayette Pharmacal)

Oral Diabeto-Therapy

Description: Prepared from desiccated pancreas of young cattle and from other interdependent endocrines; is of uniform composition and protected against gastric action by Enterocap preparation.

Action and Uses: *For use* as supplement to dietotherapy, to reduce glycosuria and hyperglycemia in diabetes mellitus.

Supply: ORALSULIN—In 4 types of doubled strength capsules, Enteric-salol coated —A, B, C, D; 2 capsules of A are equivalent to 1 of B; 2 capsules of B to 1 of C; 2 capsules of C to 1 of D—Packages of 100.

ORALSULIN WITH DUODENAL EXTRACT—Containing Oralsulin A—with duodenal extract gr 2.
Capsules, Enteric coated—Packages of 100.

ORALSULIN MIXTURE—Containing Oralsulin A with

	Gr	Gm
Thyroid	1/16	0.004
Pituitary	⅛	0.008
Duodenal	1	0.065

Capsules, Packages of 100.

Administration: First week—Oralsulin A, 1 capsule three or four times daily ½–1 hr. before meals and on retiring; increased slowly to dosage B for 1 week; subsequent dosage is controlled by urinary and blood sugar findings, with diet regulated in accordance.

OVOFERRIN (Barnes)

Hematinic

Composition: An easily assimilable colloidal iron solution; contains per fluid ounce 2 gr of elementary iron, held in suspension by means of a protective colloid, protein in nature; alcohol 9 %, as preservative.

Action and Uses: General tonic and hematinic in anemia associated with anorexia and gastrointestinal sensitiveness; increases hemoglobin and red blood cell count without disturbing digestion, causing constipation or affecting the teeth.

Supply: OVOFERRIN—Bottles 11 oz.

Administration: ½ to 1 tablespoonful in wine-glass full of water or milk, before or after meals and at bedtime; children, 1 or 2 teaspoonfuls in water or milk.

OXINOL (Oxinol)

Antacid

Composition: Is stated to contain magnesium peroxide, calcium peroxide, magnesium carbonate, bismuth subcarbonate, sodium bicarbonate, malt diastase, fennel oil, caraway seed oil, peppermint.

Action and Uses: Antacid and digestant; forms in gastrointestinal tract nascent oxygen which affects toxins, ptomains and bacteria; *For use* in gastric hyperacidity, pyrosis, peptic ulcer; in flatulence, intestinal toxicosis and vomiting of pregnancy.

Supply: OXINOL—Boxes of 2 and 5 oz.

Administration: 1 teaspoonful in water or milk after meals; as alkalizer—½-1 teaspoonful every 2 hr.

Bibliography: *See Chap. XII.*

PADUTIN (Winthrop)

Vasodilator

Description: A complex substance prepared from the pancreas; dialyzes with great difficulty and is extremely labile, being easily destroyed by increased temperature, acids, bases, alcohol; is insoluble in ordinary solvents.

Action: A powerful dilator of the smallest peripheral blood vessels of the heart, lungs, brain, musculature and skin; increases cardiac output, accelerates the circulation and reduces blood pressure.

Uses: In angina pectoris, vascular diseases with trophic changes, as Buerger's disease, Raynaud's disease, intermittent claudication; in essential and thyrotoxic hypertension; in varicose ulcers.

Supply: PADUTIN—Ampules, 1 cc (2 biologic units)—Boxes of 5.

Administration: *Intramuscularly* (never intravenously), beginning with ½ ampule daily for 2 days and continued with full ampule from third day, twice daily for a period of 10–14 days; in obstinate cases 4 ampules daily, in 2 injections.

Bibliography: *See Chap. XII.*

PANCRASIN (Smith-Dorsey)

Oral Diabetotherapy

Composition: A desiccation product of pancreas.

Action and Uses: *For use* in oral therapy of diabetes mellitus.

Supply: PANCRASIN—Capsules—Enteric coated—Bottles of 100 (each capsule stated to be equivalent to ½ rabbit unit of insulin).

Administration: 1 capsule, ½ hr. before meals and at bedtime; dosage increased as necessary.

PANCREO-BISMUTH AND PEPSIN (Frye)

Digestant

Composition: Is stated to contain pancreatin, pepsin, taka-diastase, bismuth subnitrate, sodium bicarbonate, powdered ginger.

Action and Uses: Affords symptomatic relief and is indicated in deficient protein digestion, flatulence and gastric hyperacidity, dyspepsia and functional neuroses.

Supply: **PANCREO-BISMUTH AND PEPSIN**—Powder—Bottles of 2 oz.

Administration: ½–1 teaspoonful in water, preferably lukewarm, three times daily, after meals.

PANCREPATINE (Anglo-French)

Oral Diabeto-Therapy

Description: Prepared from pancreas and liver substance; each globule contains 0.25 Gm of active principle and is protected by gluten coating.

Action and Uses: As substitution therapy in glycosuria and hyperglycemia for relief of symptoms in diabetes mellitus; of use especially in those averse to insulin hypodermics, and where the injections are avoidable.

Supply: **PANCREPATINE**—Globules—Gluten coated—Boxes of 100.

Administration: Adults—2–4 globules, three times daily after meals, increased by 2 globules daily till 12 are taken; dosage maintained till urine is sugar free, then diminished to 3 globules daily and continued for 1 mo.; course repeated three to four times a year.

Bibliography: *See Chap. XII.*

PANCRESAL (Pancresal Sales)

Oral Diabeto-Therapy

Composition: A preparation from fresh pancreatic gland and activated by an electrolyte mineral-vitamin assisting in the catalytic action of the hormone.

Action and Uses: For the reduction of glycosuria and hyperglycemia in diabetes mellitus.

Supply: **PANCRESAL**—Tablets, Enteric-coated, each stated to correspond to 15 insulin units—Tubes of 15—Bottles of 50 and 100.

Administration: 1–3 tablets 10 min. after meals three times daily; reduced after a 10-day course.

Bibliography: *See Chap. XII.*

PANCROBILIN (Reed and Carnrick)

Cholagogue. Laxative

Composition: Contains pancreatic enzymes and pure bile salts.

Action and Uses: The association of the two components affords a natural means of restoring intestinal harmony and aids in the re-establishment of normal function of the intestinal tract. *For use* in habitual constipation, intestinal indigestion, auto-intoxication, jaundice, abdominal post-operative procedures.

Supply and Dosage: PANCROBILIN PILLS—Plain—Containing pancreatic enzymes with 4 gr (0.26 Gm) of dehydrated bile; *dosage* 1–3 after each meal—Bottles of 100, 500, 1,000.

PANCROBILIN PILLS COMPOUND—Containing in addition to above, aloin 1/5 gr (0.012 Gm), strychnia gr 1/200 (0.00032 Gm) and belladonna gr 1/40 (0.0016 Gm); *dosage* 1–3 after each meal—Bottles of 100, 500, 1000.

PANCROBILIN PILLS WITH PODOPHYLLIN—Gr 1/10 (0.0064 Gm); *dosage* 1 three times daily and at bedtime—Bottles of 100, 500 and 1,000.

PANCROBILIN LIQUID—Used frequently for women and children; *dosage* 1–3 tablespoonfuls after meals—Bottles 14 oz. and 1 gal.

PANCROBILIN PILLS WITH CASCARA—Gr 1 (0.064 Gm); *dosage* 1 three times daily and at bedtime—Bottles 100, 500 and 1,000.

PANCROBILIN PILLS WITH PHENOLPHTHALEIN—Gr 1/2 (0.032 Gm); *dosage* 1 three times daily and at bedtime—Bottles of 100, 500 and 1,000.

PANKREON "RHENANIA" (Kretschmar)

Digestant

Description: Prepared from fresh pancreas; is not a synthetic product.

Action and Uses: As auxiliary in low grade digestive function; effective in gastro intestinal disorders, debility and in diarrheas of children.

Supply: PANKREON—Tablets, gr 4—Bottles of 25, 50 and 100.

PANKREON—Powder—Bottles of 25 and 50 Gm.

Administration: 3–4 tablets, crushed, or its equivalent 1 teaspoonful of powder taken with meals; in severe cases 4–6 tablets or 2 teaspoonfuls of powder with each meal.
Infants 1/4 teaspoonful with each feeding.
Where dilute hydrochloric acid is prescribed in conjunction with Pankreon, the acid should be given 1/2–1 hr. after the meal.

Bibliography: *See Chap. XII.*

PANSULINE "FORNET" (Kretschmar)

Oral Diabetotherapy

Description: Prepared from pancreas of healthy cattle in a manner to assure stability and complete absorption.

Action and Uses: Influences carbohydrate metabolism causing after preliminary rise a fall in glycosuria; standardized—30 pills Concentration 1 to represent 30 units of Insulin; 30 pills Concentration 2—60 units; 30 pills Concentration 3—120 units insulin.

Supply: PANSULINE "FORNET"—Pills, Concentration 1, 2 and 3, each in boxes of 35 and 100.

Administration: Initial dose 2 pills 1/2 hr. before meals, three times daily; the dosage is then regulated in accordance with the extent of glycosuria.

PAPINE (Battle)

Anodyne

Description: Contains, in addition to other ingredients 1/8 gr (0.008 Gm) of morphine per fluid dram.

Action and Uses: As for morphine or opium for all forms of pain; also *for use* in cough mixtures; is claimed not to interfere with normal secretions.

Supply: PAPINE—Bottles of 12 oz.

Administration: 1 teaspoonful for adults, 2–10 m for children under 1 yr.

PARALAX (Battle Creek)

Laxative

Description: An emulsion of pure, tasteless, highly refined mineral oil.

Action and Uses: Is non-irritating, not absorbed and causes no leakage. *Used* as mechanical lubricant and laxative in constipation, colitis, intestinal intoxication, chronic appendicitis, catarrhal proctitis.

Supply: PARALAX—Bottles of 1 pt.

Combinations: PARALAX WITH AGAR—Contains also Agar to add bulk to its laxative properties—Bottles of 1 pt.

Administration: 2 tablespoonfuls in water with meals.
Children: 1–2 teaspoonfuls.

PASCARNATA (Merrell)

Sedative

Composition: An alcoholic extract of fresh leaves of Passiflora incarnata.

Action and Uses: Sedative; is non-depressant, non-toxic and does not impair digestion. *For use* in allaying nervous symptoms accompanying menopause, menstrual cycle; in neuralgia, epileptic seizures and asthma.

Supply: PASCARNATA—Bottles of 12 oz.

Administration: 5–60 m according to age and conditions.

PEACOCK'S BROMIDES (Od Peacock)

Sedative

Composition: Each fluid dram is stated to contain 15 gr of the combined bromides of potassium, sodium, ammonium, calcium and lithium; alcohol 6 %.

Action and Uses: Sedative in epilepsy, nervousness, insomnia and headache.

Supply: PEACOCK'S BROMIDES—Bottles of 8 oz.

Administration: 1–4 teaspoonfuls, as indicated.

PENTABROMIDES (Merrell)

Sedative

Composition: Is stated to contain bromides of calcium, sodium, potassium, lithium and ammonium; each fluid dram represents 15 gr of the combined salts in palatable vehicle.

Action and Uses: Nervous sedative; *For use* in insomnia, hysteria, mild types of epilepsy, convulsions of children, laryngeal crises.

Supply: PENTABROMIDES—Bottles of 1 pt. and 1 gal.

Administration: 1–2 teaspoonfuls in water, three to four times daily.

PEPETAL (Sharp and Dohme)

Digestant

Description: An elixir containing proteolytic enzymes, with a digestive capacity, according to U.S.P. assay process, of 3,000 gr of freshly coagulated and disintegrated egg albumin to the ounce; alcohol 20%.

Action and Uses: *For use* in gastrointestinal disturbances due to lowered digestive functions.

Supply: PEPETAL—Bottles of 1 pt. and 1 gal.

Administration: 1 or 2 fl. dr., as often as required.

PEPSENCIA (Fairchild)

Digestant

Description: Also known as Essence of Pepsine. Obtained by direct extraction from the gastric mucous membrane of the fresh animal stomach; contains the proteolytic and milk curdling enzymes with the entire soluble constituents of the gastric glands in an aromatized sterile medium; alcohol by weight 15%.

Action and Uses: *Used* as digestant; also as vehicle in the administration of drugs of disagreeable taste; in making of junket and whey, and as vehicle.

Supply: PEPSENCIA—4, 8, 16, 32 oz., and 5 pt. bottles.

Administration: As digestant, 1 teaspoonful or more after meals; for making junket and whey directions are enclosed with preparation.

PEPTENZYME (Reed and Carnrick)

Digestant

Composition: Contains the enzymes and secretions active in the process of digestion, of the salivary, peptic and intestinal glands, with pancreas and spleen.

Description: Performs every phase of enzymatic function; assists the digestion of protein, converts starches into soluble carbohydrates, splits and emulsifies fats; is easily administered and agreeable to taste.

Uses: Indicated in gastrointestinal dysfunction; in various types of indigestion; in acute, chronic and alcoholic gastritis, nervous dyspepsia, vomiting of pregnancy; in anorexia, gastralgia, duodenal catarrh.

Supply and Administration: PEPTENZYME—Tablets—gr 5 (0.3 Gm)—Bottles of 25, 100, 500 and 1,000; *Dosage*—2 tablets before and after each meal.

PEPTENZYME—Powder—Bottles of 1 and 8 oz.; *Dosage*—10–20 gr (0.6–1.2 Gm) before or after meals.

PEPTENZYME—Elixir—Bottles of 8 and 16 oz., 5 pt. and 1 gal.; a very palatable vehicle for administration of nauseant drugs; is compatible with all therapeutic drugs; is of neutral reaction and free from sugar or acids; *Dosage*—1–2 teaspoonfuls.

PEPTENZYME—Effervescent Granules—Bottles, large and small sizes; Contains Peptenzyme combined with effervescent substances to assist gastric function and decrease gas fermentation; *Dosage*—1 heaping teaspoonful in ½ glass water, repeated if necessary.

Bibliography: *See Chap. XII.*

PEPTOGENIC POWDER (Fairchild)

Milk Modifier

Description: A powder for the modification of cow's milk to resemble closely in chemical, physical and physiological properties average normal mother's milk.

Use: For infant feeding, partial breast feeding.

Supply: PEPTOGENIC POWDER—Cartons—large and small.

Administration: Proportions of milk, water, cream and peptogenic powder used in accordance with requirements in each case, as per accompanying directions.

PEPTO-MANGAN "GUDE" (Breitenbach)

Hematinic

Description: A neutral organic solution of the peptonates of manganese and iron in the presence of copper; is readily and completely absorbed in gastrointestinal tract.

Action and Uses: Hematinic and reconstructive; is non-irritating, non-astringent and palatable; does not stain the teeth, disturb digestion or cause constipation; *For use* in secondary anemia, chlorosis and nutritional anemias; as reconstructive tonic and nutrient in many disturbances with malnutrition and debility.

Supply: GUDE'S PEPTO-MANGAN (L.A.)—Tablets—Packages of 60.
GUDE'S PEPTO-MANGNAN (L.A.)—Bottles of 11 oz.

Administration: Liquid—1 Tablespoonful after meals, plain or in milk or water; Children—1-2 teaspoonfuls, according to age.
Tablets—2 tablets followed by water, three times daily, after meals.

PEPTONAL (Armour)

Nutrient

Description: Is stated to contain predigested lean beef and malt extract, in a palatable and stable medium.

Action and Uses: Nutrient and tonic in malnutrition, especially for those unable to digest solid food.

Supply: PEPTONAL—Bottles of 16 oz.—Jugs of 1 and 5 gal.

Administration: 1-3 teaspoonfuls three or four times daily, or as demanded.

PEPTONISING TUBES (Fairchild)

Digestant

Description: A peptonizing powder in small glass tubes.

Action and Uses: Contents of 1 tube will peptonize 1 pt. of milk; a most convenient means of utilizing the proteolytic principle of the pancreas for the preparation of peptonized milk, and other foods for the sick.

Supply: PEPTONISING TUBES—Boxes of 12 tubes.

Administration: Directions for peptonization accompany each box.

"WAMPOLE'S" PREPARATION (Wampole)

Tonic

Composition: Contains a solution of an extract of fresh cod livers combined with malt extract, fluid extract of wild cherry, calcium, sodium, potassium, iron, manganese, quinine and strychnine.

Action and Uses: Stimulating tonic, hematinic and growth promoting; *For use* in convalescence, debility and nutritional anemia.

Supply: "WAMPOLE'S" PREPARATION—Bottles of 16 oz.

Administration: 1 tablespoonful before meals and on retiring. Children under 10 yr., 1–2 teaspoonfuls.

PHEDROCAINE (Colwell)

Local Anesthetic

Composition: A combination of ephedrine with ethyl aminobenzoate and para-amino-benzoyl-diethylaminoethanol.

Action: An anesthetic of localized, prolonged and intensified action; is non-toxic, non-irritating, non-habit forming and without systemic effect.

Uses: As for cocaine; *For use* in tonsillectomy and tonsil electro-coagulation; in sore throat, quinsy, tubercular laryngitis, acute rhinolaryngeal and sinus infections.

Supply: PHEDROCAINE—Tablets—Vials of 15—Bottles of 50.

PHEDROCAINE—Oil, 10% Solution—Bottles 2 oz.

PHEDROCAINE—Suppositories, gr ½ (0.032 Gm) in cocoa butter base—Boxes of 12.

Administration: Tablets—1 tablet dissolved in mouth 5 min. before operation or for other purposes.

Oil—for sponging, swabbing and shrinking mucosa in rhinitis, sinusitis and similar affections.

Suppositories—for anal fissure, inflamed hemorrhoids, ulceration.

Incompatibles: To be kept water free.

Bibliography: *See Chap. XII.*

PETRO-MUL (Irwin, Neisler)

Laxative

Composition: Contains Russian mineral oil, phenolphthalein gr 6 (0.384 Gm) per ounce and agar-agar q.s.

Action and Uses: Laxative; *For use* in constipation, hemorrhoids.

Supply: PETRO-MUL—Bottles 1 pt., 1 gal.

Administration: ½–1 tablespoonful at bedtime.

PHENO-BROMATE (Foster)

Analgesic

Description: A combination of phenetidin and bromine derivatives; a white powder of saline taste, slightly soluble in water.

Action and Uses: Sedative, antipyretic and analgesic; *For use* in dysmenorrhea, nervous irritability, hysteria, insomnia; in infectious fevers, rheumatic affections, sciatica, lumbago, neuralgia, headache.

Supply: PHENO-BROMATE—Powder—Packages of 1 oz.

PHENO-BROMATE—Tablets gr 5 (0.324 Gm)—Tubes of 12—Boxes of 100.

Administration: *As Antipyretic*—5–10 gr every 1–4 hr.
As Analgesic—15–25 gr every hour for 2–3 doses.
As Antispasmodic and Hypnotic—20–25 gr.

PHENOL-PROCAINE "D.F." (C. D. Smith)

Anesthetic

Composition: Is stated to contain phenol, procaine, benzocaine and other antiseptics.

Action and Uses: A bland, colorless fluid for surface sterilization and desensitization in dental, nasolaryngeal and genitourinary work; also as local anesthetic in treatment of boils, pustules, ulcers; in plant poisoning, skin eruptions, burns, hemorrhoids.

Supply: PHENOL-PROCAINE "D.F."—Bottles 1, 4 oz., 1 pt.

Administration: Applied locally on swab.

PHOSPHO-SODA (Fleet)

Laxative

Description: A clear, yellow, concentrated solution of monobasic sodium phosphate in palatable form; is not precipitated in cold water.

Action and Uses: Cholagogue, hepatic stimulant and laxative; *For use* in constipation, gastrointestinal disorders, catarrhal jaundice, vomiting of pregnancy; in acute infections and in genitourinary diseases.

Supply: PHOSPHO-SODA—Bottles of 2½, 6 and 16 oz.

Administration: *As Aperient*—1 teaspoonful before meals, well diluted.
As Laxative 2–4 teaspoonfuls before meals, well diluted.

PHOSPHO-VITAMIN B (McKesson and Robbins)

Nervine

Description: Is stated to contain glycerophosphates of sodium, calcium, manganese, iron and strychnine, with a vitamin B concentrate.

Action and Uses: A palatable liquid preparation; *For use* as tonic in neurasthenia, asthenia, anorexia, nervous irritability and susceptibility to fatigue.

Supply: PHOSPHO-VITAMIN B—Bottles of 8 oz.

Administration: 2 teaspoonfuls in water after meals; children in proportion.

PHYSILIN (McNeil)

Detergent

Description: A clear, pale yellow, slightly acid solution containing dilute hydrochloric acid, pepsin, menthol, eucalyptol, glycerin, alcohol and water.

Action and Uses: Detergent, *for external use* in cleansing of wounds, ulcers.

Supply: **PHYSILIN**—Bottles of 100 cc.

Administration: Applied freely.

PINUS-CODEIA (Stoddard)

Expectorant

Composition: Is stated to contain white pine bark, wild cherry bark, ipecac, belladonna, eucalyptus, terpene hydrate, glycerine, cane sugar and codein acetate gr ⅛ (0.008 Gm) per teaspoonful.

Action and Uses: A palatable syrupy liquid *for use* in cough of bronchitis, laryngitis, tonsillitis; especially adapted for children.

Supply: **PINUS-CODEIA**—Bottles 4 oz., 1 pt. and 1 gal.

Administration: 1–2 teaspoonfuls as required. Children 10 drops to 1 teaspoonful, by age.

PMC (Protein Mineral)

Mineralizer

Composition: A palatable powder derived from the serum or whey fraction of milk, and fortified with a protein mineral fraction of milk; contains lactose, non-casein soluble protein, potassium, calcium, sodium and magnesium, combined as phosphates, chlorides and citrates. Average dose furnishes 1 Gm of calcium daily.

Action and Uses: A source of readily assimilable calcium *for use* in growing children, malnutrition, convalescence from infectious and respiratory disorders and tuberculosis; in calcium deficiencies as rickets, osteomyelacia, delayed union of fractures, faulty dentition; in pregnancy and lactation, urticaria, neuromuscular irritability (tetany).

Supply: **PMC (C.A.)**—Glass jars of 12 oz.

Administration: 1 tablespoonful three times daily; children—2 teaspoonfuls three times daily; stirred in milk, water, cocoa, or sprinkled over soup, or as milk shake, or with fruit drinks.

POLYGALYSATE (Bischoff)

Expectorant

Composition: Is stated to contain the active principles of Radix Polygalae Senegae in stable, concentrated form; is well tolerated.

Action and Uses: Alleviates bronchial irritation, and stimulates secretion; *used* as expectorant in catarrhs and bronchial affections of influenza, measles, whooping cough.

Supply: **POLYGALYSATE**—Bottles of 15 cc.

Administration: 10–20 drops three to six times a day.

Bibliography: *See Chap. XII.*

PROTENZAMYL (Strasenburgh)

Digestant

Composition: Is stated to contain papain 16 gr to 1 oz. combined with diastase, malt extract and aromatics.

Action and Uses: A protein and starch digestant in chronic dyspeptic conditions, intestinal fermentation, chronic gastritis.

Supply: **PROTENZAMYL**—Bottles of 1 pt., 1 gal.

Administration: 1–2 teaspoonfuls after meals.
Infants 3–5 drops with each feeding.

PROVIDIN TABLETS (Fraser)

Iodine Therapy

Composition: An organic iodine for internal administration.

Action and Uses: Is slowly absorbed and excreted, providing for prolonged action of iodine; *used* in simple goitre.

Supply: **PROVIDIN TABLETS**—Bottles of 100, 500 and 1,000 tablets.

Administration: 2 tablets, three times daily, increased to 16 daily.

Contraindications: Exophthalmic goitre.

PSYLLA

Laxative

Description: Indian Plantago seeds, sterilized, clear and of attractive appearance; gives bulk when soaked in water and promotes elimination; *For use* as laxative in chronic constipation.

Supply: **PSYLLA WHITE**—Packages 16 oz. and 5 lb. **(Battle Creek)**
PSYLLIUM SEED—Tins of 1 lb. **(Chicago Dietetic)**
PSYLLIUM—Cans 12 oz. also 5 lb. **(MacDowell)**

Administration: Adults: 2–3 teaspoonfuls with meals, soaked in hot water before use. Children—1 teaspoonful with meals.

Combination: **PSYLLA WAFERS**—Contains psyllium seed, 1 teaspoonful per wafer, with agar, lacto-dextrin, whole wheat flour, milk, fig and bran cereal and vegetable shortening; a laxative food. *Dosage*—1–2 wafers three times daily. *Supply*—Boxes 16 oz., 5 lb. **(Battle Creek)**

PULVIS ALKANTIS (Lafayette Pharmacal)

Antacid

Composition: Is stated to contain bismuth subcarbonate, magnesium carbonate, calcium carbonate, aromatics and cerium oxalate gr 4 (0.259 Gm) to the dram.

Action and Uses: A palatable, stable powder forming a fine mixture upon addition of water; *For use* in gastric hyperacidity, ulcer, nausea, reflex vomiting.

Supply: **PULVIS ALKANTIS**—Powder—Boxes of 1 oz.

Administration: 1 teaspoonful three times daily on empty stomach; is prepared by making first a thick paste of the powder with a small quantity of water, triturating thoroughly and then adding more water.

PULVOIDS NATRICO (Drug Products)

Hypotensive

Description: A combination of potassium nitrate, sodium nitrite, nitroglycerine and Crataegus Oxyacantha for synergistic action.

Action and Uses: A vasodilator, minimizing tendency to rise in blood pressure and reducing existing hypertension; relieves headache, vertigo, flushes and other symptoms of high blood pressure; is readily absorbed, non-irritating.

Supply: **PULVOIDS NATRICO**—Enteric sugar coated—Bottles of 100, 1,000.

Administration: 1–3 Pulvoids four times daily; reduced as soon as permitted; may be given with alkaline waters or saline laxatives.

QUINBOLIN (Huxley)

Antiseptic

Composition: Contains oxyquinoline sulfate with salol and thymol, in soothing absorbent base.

Action and Use: An antiseptic, bacteriostatic dressing in minor surgery, skin affections, burns and ulcers.

Supply: **QUINBOLIN**—Tin boxes, approximately ¾ oz.

Administration: *As dusting powder*—in pruritus ani and pruritus vulvae.
As dry dressing—in minor surgery, dermatitis and venereal eruptions.

RADOLATUM (Squibb)

Irradiated Mineral Oil

Description: An ultraviolet-irradiated mixture of specially selected mineral oils and petrolatum-like products known to be susceptible to activation under irradiation; a bland non-irritating and non-toxic oil, retaining its therapeutic properties for prolonged period.

Action and Uses: Is bactericidal; diminishes discharges, stimulates granulation and healing. *For use* in suppurating wounds, cellulitis, infections of tendon sheaths, persisting sinuses; in fistula in ano, chronic bone disease; in varicose, decubital and diabetic ulcers; in cutaneous infections as echthyma.

Supply: **RADOLATUM**—Jelly—Bottles of ¼ and 1 lb.
LIQUID RADOLATUM—Bottles of ¼ and 1 lb.

Administration: Is applied freely, at 110°F, to the wound or diseased surface, or is flooded from large syringe over infected area; bandaged lightly. In bone affections the liquid is preferred, drainage being provided for.
Rectally—From 4–6 oz. is injected to be retained overnight.

REARGON (Akatos)

Gonocide

Composition: A mixture of silver gelatose and anthrachinonglucosides; contains about 6% silver.

Action and Uses: A penetrating gonocide and antiseptic, free from irritation and pain; *For use* in anterior and posterior gonorrheal urethritis and gonorrheal disease in the female; also used in nose, throat and ear affections.

Supply: **REARGON**—Vials 10, 25 and 100 Gm.

Administration: *As Abortive Therapy*—5–6 injections daily for several days.
Hand Injection—5 cc of 5% solution two to three times daily and at bedtime; continued later with 2½% solutions.
As Irrigation—250 cc of ¼% solution.
For Vaginal Irrigation—30 cc of 1–2% solution.
For Tampons—5% solution.

In Nose and Throat Affections—5 % solution for topical application.

Caution: Solutions must be freshly prepared, with distilled water only. Stains may be removed by washing and with 10 % bichloride of mercury solution.

RECVALYSATE (Bischoff)

Sedative. Soporific

Description: A dialysate of fresh valerian root, containing all its active principles with inactive constituents eliminated.

Action: Sedative and soporific.

Uses: Nervous disturbances, climacterium, neurasthenia, hypertension, cardiac neuroses.

Supply: RECVALYSATE—Bottles of 15 and 60 cc.

Administration: As sedative 20–30 drops; as soporific 40–50 drops at bedtime.

Bibliography: *See Chap. XII.*

REGULIN (Reinschild)

Laxative

Composition: A combination of agar-agar with an aqueous extract of cascara sagrada.

Action and Uses: Lubricates bowel, softens and adds bulk to contents and stimulates intestinal peristalsis; *For use* in constipation and intestinal toxicosis.

Supply: REGULIN—Bottles 10 oz.

Administration: 1–2 tablespoonfuls night and morning, mixed with fluids; larger quantities in obstinate cases; children in accordance.

Bibliography: *See Chap. XII.*

REMOGLAND (Remogland)

Aphrodisiac

Composition: A combination of extracts of the gonads, adrenals, anterior pituitary with thyroid extract gr 1/10 (0.006 Gm), calcium glycerophosphate gr 1/8 (0.008 Gm) and nux vomica gr 1/8 (0.008 Gm) per tablet.

Action and Uses: Aphrodisiac *for use* in sexual impotence and defective testicular secretion.

Supply: REMOGLAND—Tablets—Box of 40 and 100.

REMOGLAND—Ampules—Boxes of 12.

Administration: 1–2 tablets, three times daily, before meals.

1 Ampule every 2 days, *intramuscularly*, restricting tobacco and alcohol.

Bibliography: *See Chap. XII.*

REMOLYSIN (Remogland)

Reduction Therapy

Composition: Is stated to contain extracts of thyroid, pituitary, pancreas and of the female generative glands.

Action and Uses: Is said to reduce obesity by stimulating metabolism and tissue oxidation and to decrease the weight gradually without causing systemic disturbances.

Supply: REMOLYSIN—Tablets—Vials 50, 100.

Administration: 1–3 tablets after meals, as addition to regulated diet.

RENNET (Armour)

Digestant

Description: Gastric enzyme prepared from the fourth stomach of suckling calves; curdles 30,000 times its own weight of pasteurized milk in 12–15 min.

Action and Uses: To curdle cheese, to prepare ice cream; to curdle milk in the preparation of junket and whey; in diets to convert glucose of food into lactic acid.

Supply: RENNET—Bottles of 1, 4, 8 and 16 oz.

Administration: 10–30 gr (0.6–2.0 Gm).

ROBINOL (Wyeth)

Tonic

Composition: Is stated to contain glycerophosphates of lithium, calcium, sodium, iron, manganese and quinine, with strychnine glycerophosphate gr 1/16 to the fluidounce.

Action and Uses: A readily absorbed nervine, tonic and reconstructive causing no gastro-intestinal disturbances; indicated in anemia, chlorosis, neurasthenia, convalescence.

Supply: ROBINOL—Bottles of 10 oz., 1 gal.

Administration: 1–2 teaspoonfuls in water three to four times daily. Children in proportion.

RYTHMIN (Carnrick, G. W.)

Cathartic

Composition: Contains peristaltic principles extracted from duodenal and pyloric mucosa with spleen, bile salts and phenolphthalein gr ½ (0.032 Gm) per tablet.

Action and Uses: Cholagogue and cathartic *for use* in constipation, fat indigestion, intestinal toxemia, bile stasis.

Supply: RYTHMIN—Tablets—Bottles of 50.

Administration: 1–3 tablets at night.

SALCETOL (Stoddard)

Analgesic

Composition: A mixture of equal parts of acetanilid and salicylates.

Action and Uses: Antipyretic, antirheumatic, analgesic; *For use* in rheumatism, neuralgia, grippe, tonsillitis, dysmenorrhea.

Supply: SALCETOL—Powder—Bottles 1 oz., 1 lb.

SALCETOL—Tablets (gr 5)—Bottles 100, 500 and 1,000.

Administration: Gr 5–15 (0.324–0.972 Gm), repeated in 1 hr. if necessary, *As gargle*—Gr 10 (0.643 Gm) in ½ glass hot water.

Combinations: **SALCETOL CAFFEINE COMPOUND**—Containing: Salcetol, gr 3 (0.194 Gm); Caffeine, gr ¼ (0.016 Gm); Tr. zingiber, m 5.
Dosage—1–2 tablets every 1–4 hr. or 2 every hour for 3 doses.
Supply—Tablets—Bottles of 100, 500 and 1,000.

SALCETOL CALOMEL COMPOUND—Containing: Salcetol, gr 1 (0.064 Gm); Calomel, gr ⅙ (0.012 Gm); Podophyllin, gr 1/16 (0.004 Gm).
Dosage—1 every 15 min. for 6 doses, followed by saline cathartic.
Supply—Tablets—Bottles of 100, 500 and 1,000.

SALCETOL CODEIA—Containing: Codein sulphate, gr ¼ (0.016 Gm); Salcetol, gr 5 (0.324 Gm).
Dosage—1–3 at once, in 1 hr.—1 tablet.
Supply—Tablets—Bottles 100, 500 and 1,000.

SALCETOL COMPOUND 1—Containing: Morphine sulphate, gr 1/20 (0.003 Gm); Capsicum, gr 1/20 (0.003 Gm); Salcetol, gr 5 (0.324 Gm).
Dosage—1–2 tablets every hour till relieved; then 1–2 as required.
Supply—Bottles of 100, 500 and 1,000.

SALCETOL COMPOUND 2—Containing: Capsicum, gr 1/20 (0.003 Gm); Salcetol, gr 5 (0.324 Gm)—Tablets Ext. Piscidia gr 1 (0.064 Gm)—Bottles of 100, 500 and 1,000.

SALCETOL CORRECTIVE—Containing: Salcetol, 1/16 gr (0.004 Gm); Ipecac, gr 1/100 (Gm 0.0006); Calomel, gr 1/30 (Gm 0.002); Bismuth-papaya comp. with zinc sulphocarbolate gr 3/10 (Gm 0.018).
Dosage—1 tablet crushed, on tongue, every 10 min. for 3 doses; then 1 every hour for 3 doses.
Supply—Bottles 100, 500 and 1,000.

SALCETOL SALOL—Containing Salcetol, gr 3 (0.194 Gm); Salol gr 2 (0.130 Gm).
Supply—Bottles 100, 500 and 1,000.

SALINE LAXATIVE (Abbott)

Laxative

Composition: Magnesium sulphate, U.S.P., 60%, in effervescent combination.

Action and Uses: Diuretic and eliminant; *For use* in constipation and intestinal toxemia.

Supply: SALINE LAXATIVE—Bottles of 2½, 5 and 12½ oz.

Administration: 1 capful in water, lemonade or sweetened liquid, on retiring or every 2–4 hr.

SALITHIA (Abbott)

Uricolytic

Composition: An effervescent combination of magnesium sulphate, lithium carbonate and colchicine.

Action and Uses: To remove toxic waste, uric acid deposits and as diuretic.

Supply: SALITHIA—Bottles of 2½, 5 and 12½ oz.

Administration: 1–2 heaping teaspoonfuls in water, repeated at intervals of several hours.

SALUSOL (Schieffelin)

Antiseptic

Composition: A soluble aromatic distillate of alkyl acetates and strongly antiseptic volatile oils, forming a compound spirit of acetic ether; in 10% dilution destroys typhoid bacilli, in 20% most pyogenic organisms.

Action and Uses: Antiseptic, analgesic, astringent in typhoid, dysentery, cholera morbus; externally is used in rheumatism, cellulitis, lymphangitis, indolent ulcers; as spray in catarrh of nose and throat.

Supply: SALUSOL—Bottles of 8 oz., 1 gal.

Administration: *Internal*—1–4 teaspoonfuls in wineglassful of water three or four times daily, half hour before or after meals; children ¼–1 teaspoonful.
External—As wet dressing, 1 part to 2–5 parts of water; changed twice daily.
Spray or Gargle—With 5 parts of water.
Enema or Douche—With 5–10 parts of water.

SALVYSATE (Bischoff)

Anhidrotic

Description: A dialysate of Folia Salviae, containing in concentrated form the active principles of the fresh leaves without inert material.

Action and Uses: Anhidrotic and astringent; is stable, well tolerated and non-irritating; *For use* in night sweats of tuberculosis and climacterium; also topically in inflammation of naso-pharyngeal membranes.

Supply: SALVYSATE—Bottles of 15 cc.

Administration: 20–30 drops three times daily.

Bibliography: *See Chap. XII.*

SANMETTO (Od Peacock)

Urinary Sedative

Composition: A combination of saw palmetto, sandalwood and zea in palatable form; alcohol 20%.

Action and Uses: Sedative, antiseptic and demulcent *for use* in cystitis, urethritis and gonorrheal infections.

Supply: SANMETTO—Bottles 8 oz.

Administration: 1 teaspoonful four times daily.

SAVITA (Battle Creek)

Vitamin Therapy

Description: A brewers' yeast and vegetable extract, seasoned with salt; is rich in minerals, vitamin B complex and available iron; has a meat-like flavor but contains no proteins.

Action and Uses: As food seasoning and nutritive agent *for use* in anemia, convalescence and similar conditions.

Analysis: Moisture 26.0, estimated nitrogen protein substance 31.9, fat—trace, crude fiber—none, ash—27.8, NaCl—15.2, phosphate—(P_2O_5)5.1, iron—0.03, copper—0.0028.

Supply: SAVITA (C.A.)—Cans of 3½ and 6½ oz.
SAVITA—Bouillon Cubes—Boxes of 10.

Combination: SAVITA—Yeast Tablets (C.A.)—*for use* in infections with pus forming organisms, beriberi, pellagra, vitamin B deficiencies and intestinal sluggishness; dosage 4–6 tablets daily.
Supply—SAVITA—Yeast Tablets—Bottles of 90.

Bibliography: *See Chap. XII.*

SECRETOGEN (Carnrick, G. W.)

Digestant Laxative

Composition: Is stated to contain homostimulating extracts from the stomach and duodenum, prosecretin, enterokinase, pancreatic proferments and hydrochloric acid 0.1 %.

Action and Uses: Digestant with laxative properties in chronic gastric catarrh, intestinal indigestion, fermentative diarrhea, flatulence, marasmus, inanition and constipation.

Supply: SECRETOGEN—Tablets—Bottles of 100, 500 and 1,000.
SECRETOGEN—Elixir—Bottles of ½, 1 and 5 pt. and 1 gal.

Administration: 1–3 tablets or 1–3 teaspoonfuls of elixir, three times daily.

SEDATOLE (Sharp and Dohme)

Expectorant

Description: Is stated to contain tolu, sanguinaria, squill, wild cherry, balsam, balm of gilead buds and codeine sulphate, 1/16 gr to the fluid dram; alcohol 6 %.

Action and Uses: Sedative, anodyne and palatable expectorant, *for relief* of cough, colds, influenza and other respiratory affections.

Supply: SEDATOLE—Bottles of 4 oz., 1 pt. and 1 gal.

Administration: Children 1 yr.—10–15 drops; 1–4 yr.—15–30 drops; 5–12 yr.—½–1 teaspoonful.
Adults—1–3 teaspoonfuls three times daily.

SENG (Od Peacock)

Stomachic

Composition: A preparation of Panax quinquifolium and pleasant aromatics.

Action and Uses: A bitter stomachic, tonic and secernent; stimulates secretory glands and assists digestion. *For use* especially in achlorhydria, nervous indigestion, chronic gastritis, subacidity.

Supply: SENG—Bottles of 10 oz.

Administration: 1–2 teaspoonfuls before meals.

SENNETAL (Sharp and Dohme)

Laxative

Official Name: Syrupus Senna et Cascara Co.

Composition: Comprises senna leaves, cascara bark, Rochelle salts, fruit acids and aromatics; alcohol 10 %.

Action and Uses: A palatable laxative *for use* in constipation.

Supply: SENNETAL—Bottles of 4 oz., 1 pt. and 1 gal.

Administration: 1 or 2 Teaspoonfuls once or twice daily.

SIDEROL (Wyeth)

Tonic

Official Name: Liquor Ferruginous.

Composition: Is stated to contain saccharated iron peptonate, glycerophosphate of soda, fl. ex. ignatia amara; fl. ext. taraxacum, beef extract and aromatics.

Action and Uses: A palatable hematinic, nutrient tonic in anemia, chlorosis, convalescence, malnutrition and postoperative conditions.

Supply: SIDEROL—Bottles of 12 oz.

Administration: 2 teaspoonfuls four times daily before meals, with or without water. Children to 1 yr.—10–15 drops; 5–10 yr.—1 teaspoonful.

SILARGEL (Heyden)

Adsorbent

Description: A white powder of silver chloride-silicic acid gel; odorless and tasteless.

Action: Has adsorbing power, attracting pathogenic bacteria, toxins and metabolic products without affecting ferments normally present in gastrointestinal tract; is harmless and causes neither irritation nor toxicity.

Uses: Autointoxication, intestinal fermentation, flatulence, dysentery, paratyphoid; externally—in burns, infected wounds, weeping eczema, fluor albus, nasopharyngitis.

Supply: SILARGEL—Tins of 25 Gm.

SILARGETTEN—Gum pastilles of 10 % Silargel—Boxes of 60.

Administration: *Internal*—1–2 Gm, several times daily.

External—As antiseptic dusting powder for dry treatment.

Bibliography: *See Chap. XII.*

SILIFORM (Heilkraft)

Non-specific Therapy. Analgesic

Description: A preparation of silicic and formic acids, in clear sterile colloidal solution.

Action and Uses: Employed in non-specific therapy; injections are painless and reactions very mild; *For use* in articular and muscular rheumatism, arthritis, spondylitis, chronic recurrent sciatica, neuralgia, gout.

Supply: SILIFORM—Ampules, 1 cc—Boxes of 5 and 100.

Administration: In Sciatica—3 deep injections in the region of nerve pressure points, at intervals of 4–5 days; then 2 injections at intervals of 6–8 days; in severe cases, it is advisable to give a second course after an interval of 3–6 mo., but the full beneficial effect should be awaited before repeating treatment.

Other Conditions—***Intragluteally*** **or** ***subcutaneously*** **in region of affected parts.**

SILVER SAL (Smith-Dorsey)

Antiseptic

Official Name: Argento-Proteinum Mite.

Action and Uses: A colloidal silver preparation of penetrating, non-irritating action; *For use* in gonorrheal disease as prophylaxis, irrigation and injection; in conjunctivitis—simple, purulent, gonorrheal; in gynecologic affections—as tampon, ointment, suppository.

Supply: SILVER SAL—Crystals—Bottles 1 and 4 oz.,—Bottles dropper 1 oz. to make 1 pt. 5% solution.

SILVER SAL—Suppositories—5% in glycero-gelatin base—Box of 12.

Administration: In 5–10% solution in conditions above enumerated.

SODA MINT TABLETS (McKesson and Robbins)

Antacid

Composition: A combination of bicarbonate of soda with peppermint.

Action and Uses: *For use* as antacid in hyperacid conditions of the stomach.

Supply: SODA MINT TABLETS—Bottles of 45.

SODA MINT AND PEPSIN—Tablets—Bottles of 45.

Administration: 1–2 tablets when necessary.

SODIUM MORRHUATE 7% SOLUTION (Ulmer)

Sclerosing Agent

Composition: Aqueous solution of sodium morrhuate.

Action and Uses: *Used* to sclerose varicose veins; does not produce cramps, and has no toxic effect in proper dosage; in accidental injection into tissues surrounding the vein, causes sloughing but rarely.

Supply: SODIUM MORRHUATE 7% SOLUTION—Packages of 6—Vials 5 cc.

Administration: Usual technique under strict asepsis.

SOLUBLE IODINE (Burnham)

Alterative

Description: A solution of active iodine, free from alkaline and other metallic iodides or complex organic molecules; is freely soluble without precipitation in all dilutions of water and gastric juices.

Action: Is stated to often be many times as effective (weight for weight of iodine) as metallic or complex organic iodine products and less injurious to eliminating channels; in therapeutic dosage is non-irritating to gastro-intestinal tract; is antiseptic, bactericidal, alterative and endocrine stimulator.

Uses and Administration: Indicated in all conditions where iodine is useful.

Orally—In arterio-sclerosis, asthma, emphysema, chronic bronchitis, glandular enlargement, syphilis, goitre, arthritis and auto-intoxication.

Locally—In tonsillitis, adenitis, in nasal, rectal and vaginal infection.

Dental uses—In root canal infection, periapical disease, Vincent's infection, gingivitis and for ionization.

Supply: SOLUBLE IODINE—Bottles of ½, 1, 2 and 4 oz.

Dosage: 3–60 m (average dose 8 m) three times daily, on empty stomach, well diluted in water, milk, fruit juices. In syphilis *orally* for quick saturation—larger dosage; *intravenously*—same dosage, diluted in 20 parts distilled water. In mixed infections—broncho-pneumonia, influenzal pneumonia, in septicemia and staphylococcus diseases—10 m three timesdaily in water, increased to 60 and 80 m every 2 hr. in severe toxemias.
Intramuscularly—Same dosage, undiluted.
Topically—Full strength for painting, injection, ionization and in dental therapy.
For Vaginal, Rectal and Bladder Uses—1–2 teaspoonfuls in 1 pt. of water, as irrigation.

Bibliography: *See Chap. XII.*

SOLUTION OF INVERT SUGAR (Lilly)

Sclerosing Agent

Description: A mixture of dextrose and levulose, prepared by inverting cane sugar with tartaric acid and adjusted with sodium hydroxide to pH 6.8; a clear pale yellow, sweet watery solution.

Action and Uses: As sclerosing agent in the treatment of varicose veins; causes no irritability, pain or sloughing.

Supply: SOLUTION OF INVERT SUGAR (C.A.)—5 Gm in 10 cc.
SOLUTION OF INVERT SUGAR (C.A.)—6 Gm in 10 cc.
SOLUTION OF INVERT SUGAR (C.A.)—7.5 Gm in 10 cc.

Administration: *Intravenously*—5–20 cc in the concentration of 50–60% in the young and in early cases; in old and protracted varicosities concentrations of the 75% is used.

SPASMOLYSIN (Beisner)

Antispasmodic

Description: A combination of asthmolysin, a preparation of posterior pituitary and suprarenal gland, and parathyroid extract; a sterile colorless solution.

Action and Uses: Is claimed to depress sympathetic tonus and to act as antispasmodic in spasmophilia, rickets, gastric and intestinal colic, transitory spasms, bronchial asthma; also to relieve attacks of epilepsy.

Supply: SPASMOLYSIN—Ampules 1 cc—Boxes of 10.

Administration: Epilepsy, Attack—1 ampule *subcutaneously* or *intramuscularly*, never intravenously; repeated in 10 min. if necessary; may be given preliminary to an expected seizure to prevent its occurrence.

Epilepsy, Treatment—1–2 injections daily, more if necessary; continued for several weeks, or until relief is obtained.
Children up to 8 yr.—¼–½ ampule. 8–14 years—¾ ampule, each injection.

Other Diseases—Beginning with 1 ampule, *subcutaneously* or *intramuscularly* in accordance with conditions.

Bibliography: *See Chap. XII.*

SPLEEN LIQUID (Armour)

Non-specific Therapy

Description: A sterile isotonic solution extracted from the spleen.

Action and Uses: Is recommended in eczema, urticaria, angioneurotic edema.

Supply: SPLEEN LIQUID—Ampules 2 cc—Boxes of 12 and 50.
Ampules 5 cc—Boxes of 12.
Solutions, 40 and 150%.

Administration: *Subcutaneously*, in doses of 1–20 cc every 2 days, for 4 injections, at different sites.

Bibliography: *See Chap. XII.*

STANPROTEIN (McNeil)

Staphylocide

Description: A yellowish white tablet of casein-like odor, containing stannous proteinate.

Action and Uses: Alterative; *used* in the treatment of boils, carbuncles and other staphylococcus infections.

Supply: STANPROTEIN—Tablets, Compressed, gr 1½, gr 3—Bottles of 100, 500 and 1,000.

Administration: 6 gr every 3 hr. for 24 hr., then every 4 hr. for another 24 hr.; thereafter 3 gr every 3 hr.
Children—half dosage in same order.

STYPTYSATE (Bischoff)

Hemostatic

Description: Prepared from Capsella Bursa Pastoria, a medicinal plant.

Action: Reduces bleeding time, hastens clotting, does not coagulate albumin; is non-escharotic, non-narcotic and non-depressant.

Uses: In controlling hemorrhage from the respiratory, digestive and genitourinary tracts; in bleeding from operation and injury; in preventing probable secondary hemorrhage.

Supply: STYPTYSATE—Liquid—Bottles of 10 cc, for oral and topical use.

STYPTYSATE—Tablets—Each equivalent to 15 drops of liquid—Bottles of 25 and 100.

Administration: *Preoperative*—1–2 tablets or 15–30 drops, for 3 doses on day preceding, and 1 dose just before operation.

In Hemophilia—5–10 drops, three times daily.

In Uterine Bleeding—3 tablets daily, several days before onset of menses.

In Internal Hemorrhage—25 drops, three times daily.

Locally—Applied by tampon or on gauze.

Bibliography: *See Chap. XII.*

SULBUMIN (Thiophene)

Hematinic

Description: An organic sulphur-albumin complex; formerly known as Thio-Albin. Is a brown powder of characteristic odor and taste.

Action and Uses: Is stated to be hematinic and roborant; *For use* in various types of secondary anemia.

Supply: SULBUMIN—Tablets gr 5 (0.3 Gm)—Bottles of 60 and 500.

Administration: 2–3 tablets before meals and before retiring.

SYL-AG-OL (Schieffelin)

Laxative

Composition: Is stated to contain psyllium seed, agar-agar, heavy mineral oil, in emulsion.

Action and Uses: As laxative in habitual constipation, and intestinal stasis.

Supply: SYL-AG-OL—Bottles of 16 oz.

Administration: 1 Tablespoonful one or two times daily.
Children 1–2 teaspoonfuls daily.

SYRUP HISTOSAN (Bischoff)

Sedative. Expectorant

Chemical Name: Triguaiacol Albuminate.

Composition: Pure guaiacol in combination with egg albumin.

Description: Occurs as light brown powder of aromatic odor and taste; is dispensed as a clear amber colored syrup (5% strength) of pleasant taste; is non-narcotic, does not upset digestion and is acceptable to children.

Action: An expectorant and sedative; anhidrotic, alterative and antipyretic.

Uses: *For use* in acute and chronic coughs, associated with various respiratory infections.

Incompatibles: Acids.

Supply: SYRUP HISTOSAN—Bottles of 6 oz.
HISTOSAN—Powder—Cartons 1 oz.

Administration: Adults, 1 teaspoonful of syrup or 1–3 gr of powder three or four times daily. Children in proportion.

SYRUP HYPOPHOSPHITE OF IRON (Gardner)

Hematinic

Description: Is stated to contain per fluid ounce, gr 4 (0.259 Gm) of pure ferrous hypophosphite.

Action and Uses: Is indicated in chlorosis, anemia, asthenia, nervous disturbances, convalescence.

Supply: SYRUP HYPOPHOSPHITE OF IRON—Bottles of 4 and 8 oz.

Administration: ½–2 teaspoonfuls, preferably after meals.

SYRUP HYPOPHOSPHITES OF LIME AND SODA (Gardner)

Calcium Therapy

Description: A combination of the individual syrups of calcium and of sodium, containing per fluid ounce gr 20 (1.296 Gm) of the combined chemically pure salts.

Action and Uses: *For use* where these elements are indicated, as in nervous disturbances, convalescence, blood calcium deficiency.

Supply: SYRUP HYPOPHOSPHITES OF LIME AND SODA—Bottles of 4 and 8 oz.

Administration: ½–1 teaspoonful, preferably after meals.

SYRUP HYPOPHOSPHITE OF MANGANESE (Gardner)

Hematinic

Composition: Contains per fluid ounce, gr 4 (0.259 Gm) of chemically pure manganese hypophosphite.

Action and Uses: Indicated in cases where iron compounds are not well tolerated; in anemia, chlorosis and for excitation of biliary secretion.

Supply: SYRUP HYPOPHOSPHITE OF MANGANESE—Bottles of 4 and 8 oz.

Administration: ½–2 teaspoonfuls, preferably after meals.

TARTARLITHINE (McKesson and Robbins)

Antiarthritic

Composition: A combination of lithium salts with tartaric acid.

Action and Uses: For the relief of pain in gout, rheumatism and in muscular aches.

Supply: TARTARLITHINE—Tablets—Bottles of 100.

Administration: 1–2 tablets with water, four to five times daily.

TASTELESS CASTOR OIL "KELLOGG'S" (Janvier)

Laxative

Description: A brand of U.S.P. Castor Oil of absolute purity; refined by an exclusive process which removes the free fatty acids and renders the oil tasteless, odorless and free from after-nausea.

Action and Uses: Those of castor oil.

Supply: TASTELESS CASTOR OIL—Bottles 1, 3 and 7 oz.

Administration: 1 teaspoonful to 2 tablespoonfuls, warmed, whenever required.

TAUROCOL (Plessner)

Cholagogue. Laxative

Composition: Sodium glycocholate and taurocholate with cascara sagrada, phenolphthalein and aromatics.

Action and Uses: A cholagogue, stimulating bile secretion and intestinal peristalsis; *For use* in catarrhal jaundice, cholelithiasis, early hepatic cirrhosis and insufficiency, intestinal intoxication and constipation.

Supply: TAUROCOL—Bottles of 100, 500.

Administration: 1–2 tablets before meals.

Combination: TAUROCOL COMPOUND—each tablet contains:

	Gr	Gm
Taurocol	2	0.1296
Pepsin 1:3,000	½	0.0324
Pancreatin	½	0.0324
Extract nux vomica	⅛	0.0081
Aromatics	q.s.	

For use in gastric and intestinal insufficiency with autointoxication.

Supply—Taurocol Compound—Tablets—Bottles of 100, 500.

Administration—1–2 tablets 1 hr. before or 2 hr. after meals.

Bibliography: *See Chap. XII.*

TAUROPHEN (Drug Products)

Cholagogue

Composition: Contains sodium succinate, natural sodium salicylate, sodium glycocholate, sodium taurocholate, extract of cascara, phenolphthalein, menthol.

Action and Uses: A cholagogue *for use* in hepatic insufficiency, constipation, intestinal toxemia.

Supply: TAUROPHEN—Pulvoids—Bottles of 100 and 1,000.

Administration: 1–2 pulvoids two times daily with cup of hot water.

TETRA-CITRATES, EFFERVESCENT (National Drug)

Alkalizer

Description: A palatable, effervescent alkalizing salt, containing sodium, potassium, magnesium and calcium as citrates and tartrates.

Action and Uses: *For use* as antacid in maintaining body alkali reserve, favoring oxidation processes, and enhancing blood gas absorption; also as diuretic in conditions indicated.

Supply: TETRA-CITRATES—Bottles of 4 oz.

Administration: 1–2 heaping teaspoonfuls in a glass of cold water, three to four times daily; as table water—½ teaspoonful to glassful of water.

THALEOCOLATES (Tailby-Nason)

Cholagogue

Composition: Is stated to contain sodium glycocholate, sodium taurocholate, cascara sagrada and phenolphthalein.

Action and Uses: As cholagogue and laxative in gall bladder disorders, hepatic and biliary stasis and constipation.

Supply: THALEOCOLATES—Tablets—Bottles 40, 100.

Administration: 1–3 tablets at night, or 1 tablet three times daily before meals.

THIALION (Vass Chemical)

Antacid. Laxative

Composition: A combination of sodium sulphate, sodium citrate, sodium chloride and lithium citrate, in correct proportions for synergistic action.

Action and Uses: A general antacid, alkaline diuretic and uricolytic; also cholagogue laxative. *For use* in acute colds, various fevers, rheumatism, gout, urticaria; as laxative in constipation, jaundice and intestinal stasis in general.

Supply: THIALION—Bottles of 4 oz.

Administration: 1 dr. in hot water taken 1 hr. before meals, three times daily.

THYMO PITSIN (Searle)

Oxytocic

Description: A solution of the oxytocic principle of the posterior pituitary with thymus gland hormone substance.

Action and Uses: Stimulates strong and rhythmic uterine contractions; useful in second and third stages of labor, in controlling post-partum hemorrhage and in non-operative induction of labor by the castor oil and quinine method.

Supply: THYMO PITSIN—Ampules 0.5 cc—Boxes of 10, 25 and 100.

Administration: *Intragluteally*—1 ampule; where necessary repeated every hour for 3 doses.

Contraindications: Marked contracted pelvis, malpositions, malformation of fetus or of maternal organs; cardiorenal disease.

TIN-OX (Sutliff and Case)

Staphylocide

Chemical Name: A tin oxide compound.

Action and Uses: An abortive and therapeutic agent in furunculosis, styes, carbuncles and other staphylococcus infections.

Supply: TIN-OX—Capsules, Soluble—Bottles of 100, 500 and 1,000.

Administration: 1–2 capsules, three to four times daily.
Children—1 capsule, three times daily.

TONGALINE (Mellier Drug)

Analgesic

Composition: Is stated to contain sodium salicylate, cimicifuga racemosa, pilocarpine, colchicum, tonga; alcohol 20%.

Action: Antiseptic, antipyretic, sedative and mildly laxative; stimulates gastric and respiratory processes; dilates peripheral vessels, lowers arterial tension and increases diaphoresis; relieves pain, congestion and inflammation.

Uses: Rheumatism, gout, arthritis, myalgia, myositis, torticollis, lumbago, pleurodynia; in bronchial congestion, colds, coryza, tonsillitis, grippe; in headache, migraine, neuralgia and neuritis.

Supply: TONGALINE—Liquid—containing with other agents per dram—Sodium salicylate gr 2.7 (0.162 Gm), Colchicum gr 1.2 (0.076 Gm)—Bottles 4, 8 oz., 5 pt.

TONGALINE—Tablets—containing—Sodium salicylate gr 2 (0.130 Gm), Colchicum gr 0.13 (0.008 Gm), with other agents—Boxes of 50, 100.

Administration: 1 dr. or 1 tablet as often as required.

Combinations: TONGALINE WITH QUININE—Each tablet contains Tongaline with Quinine Sulphate gr 2 (0.130 Gm) *for use* in colds, grippe, malaria—Boxes of 50 and 100.

TONGALINE WITH LITHIA—Each tablet contains Tongaline with Lithia gr 0.7 (0.042 Gm) *for use* in uric acid diathesis—Boxes of 50 and 100.

TRIGLUCON (McNeil)

Hematinic

Description: A preparation containing iron 32 mg, copper 0.64 mg per capsule, with calcium in the form of gluconates.

Action and Uses: Alterative, tonic and hematinic in secondary anemias.

Supply: TRIGLUCON—Capsules—Bottles of 100, 500, 1,000 and 5,000.

Administration: Infants and small children—the contents of 1 capsule given in food or drink.

Older children—2 capsules, three times a day.

Adults—2 capsules three times a day, increased with safety.

TROPHONINE (Reed and Carnrick)

Nutrient

Description: A concentrated palatable, liquid preparation from beef, malt, barley, milk and cocoa, with their proteins and carbohydrates in partially predigested and easily assimilable form; alcohol 19.5% by volume.

Action and Uses: Is an efficacious and nourishing liquid food of pleasant taste; *For use* in supplementary feeding after surgical operation; in intestinal disorders, laryngeal and esophageal stenosis; after tonsillectomy; in dyspepsia, neurasthenia and tubercular cases.

Supply: TROPHONINE—Bottles of 12 oz. and 1 gal.

Administration: 1 or 2 tablespoonfuls every 2 or 3 hr., taken over crushed or shaved ice, in charged water, milk, egg nog, jello, ice cream.

For babies—1 oz. in 15 oz. warm distilled water.

TRYPSOGEN (Carnrick, G. W.)

Oral Diabetotherapy

Composition: Contains pancreas principles concerned with sugar metabolism; also includes proteolytic, lipolytic and other digestive ferments.

Action and Uses: *For use* in diabetes mellitus, glycosuria.

Supply: TRYPSOGEN—Tablets, Plain and Enterosol coated—Bottles of 100, 500 and 1,000 each.

TRYPSOGEN—Capsules—Bottles of 100.

Administration: 2–7 tablets or capsules, after meals.

URASAL (Horner)

Urinary Antiseptic. Uricolytic

Composition: Each 2 dr. represent in granular effervescent form—hexamethylenamine gr 7½, combined for synergistic effect with benzoic acid, piperazine and lithium carbonate.

Action and Uses: Urinary antiseptic and uric acid eliminant; indicated in genitourinary infections; also in rheumatism, gout, respiratory affections, hypertension, pyorrhea alveolaris and in gall bladder disease.

Supply: URASAL—Bottles 3½ and 10½ oz.

Administration: 2–3 teaspoonfuls, three to four times daily, before meals; children, dosage in proportion.

URASEPTINE "ROGIER" (Fougera)

Urinary Antiseptic

Composition: Is stated to contain hexamethylene-tetramine, hexamine methylene citrate, sodium benzoate, lithium benzoate, diethylene-diamine.

Action: Is claimed to be effective as urinary antiseptic and acidifier, diuretic, and uric acid eliminant; non-toxic in therapeutic dosage.

Uses: In pyelitis, pyelonephritis, cystitis, urethritis, vesiculitis, prostatitis; renal and vesical calculosis.

Supply: URASEPTINE "ROGIER"—Bottles of 80 Gm.

Administration: 1–2 dr. in a half glass of non-alkaline water, three times daily before meals.

UVALYSATE (Bischoff)

Urinary Antiseptic

Composition: A dialysate prepared from fresh leaves of Uvae Ursi; is pure, concentrated and of constant composition.

Action: A urinary antiseptic of rapid, dependable action and agreeable taste; the contained tannin results in the formation of pyrogallol, its arbutin—in hydroquinone, both inducing astringent, palliative and secretion checking effects.

Uses: *For use* in cystitis, pyelitis, urethritis, gonorrheal disease.

Supply: UVALYSATE—Bottles of 15 cc.

Administration: 20–40 drops three times daily.

Bibliography: *See Chap. XII.*

UVURSIN (Uvursin)

Oral Diabetotherapy

Composition: A combination of chimaphila, eupatorium, pareira, taraxacum, uva ursi, juglans, lappa, inula, eriodictyon, zea mais, senna; also potassium nitrate, sodium borate, 1 gr of each per dose.

Action and Uses: Is claimed to reduce glycosuria because of a particular action on renal cells, affecting their tonus and permeability: *For use* in the oral treatment of diabetes mellitus and glycosuria.

Supply: UVURSIN—Capsules—Boxes of 56.

Administration: 2 capsules three times daily, after meals.

VARI-CHLOR-OSE (Ulmer)

Sclerosing Agent

Composition: Contains invert sugar, cane sugar, sodium chloride, phenylcarbinol.

Action and Uses: Harmless, non-toxic, relatively painless, and with comparatively little danger of sloughing in paravenous injection; *For use* in obliteration of varicose veins.

Supply: VARI-CHLOR-OSE—Ampules 10 cc—Boxes of 12, 25 and 100.

VARI-CHLOR-OSE—Vials 20 cc (serum capped)—Boxes of 12, 25 and 100.

Administration: Usual technique under strict asepsis.

Bibliography: *See Chap. XII.*

VEGEX (Vitamin Food)

Vitamin B Therapy

Description: A water-soluble extract of brewers' yeast, condensed in vacuum to a paste; contains proteins, potassium phosphate, iron, iodine and vitamin B complex; is of vegetable origin and meat-like flavor.

Analysis:

	Per Cent
Protein	45
Minerals	11
Salt	11
Starch	0
Sugar	0

Food Value: 40 calories per ounce.

Action: Stimulates appetite, aids normal digestion and promotes growth.

Uses: In nutritional disorders of mother and child, pellagra, beri-beri, liver dysfunction, endocrine deficiencies, malnutrition and nervous disorders.

Supply: VEGEX—1, 3¼, 6½ oz., 1 and 2 lb. Hospital size 7 and 56 lb.

Administration: ½–1 teaspoonful in milk, meats, cooked vegetables or prepared dishes.

VERACOLATE (Marcy)

Cholagogue. Laxative

Composition: Is stated to contain sodium glycocholate, sodium taurocholate, cascara sagrada, phenolphthalein and capsicum.

Action and Uses: Cholagogue and laxative; stimulates hepatic function and bile production; *useful* in gall bladder and liver affections and in constipation.

Supply: VERACOLATE—Tablets—Bottles of 50, 100 and 500.

Administration: 3 tablets at night or 1 after meals.

Combinations: 1. VERACOLATE WITH PANCREATIN AND PEPSIN—Contains, Veracolate gr 1½, Pancreatin gr 1, Pepsin (aseptic) 1:3,000 gr ½, Oil Peppermint m ¹⁄₁₀, per tablet; combines action of veracolate with digestive function of pepsin and pancreatin; *supply*—Bottles of 50, 100 and 500 tablets; *administered*, 2 tablets, 2 hr. after meals.

2. VERACOLATE WITH IRON, QUININE AND STRYCHNINE—Contains, Veracolate gr ¾, Reduced Iron gr 1, Quinine Sulfate gr ¾, Strychnine Sulphate gr ¹⁄₁₀₀, per tablet; *For use* as tonic and cholagogue in anemia, chlorosis, neuroses,

in gastric atony, anorexia, debility and convalescence associated with constipation; *supply*—Bottles of 100 and 500 tablets; *administered* 2 tablets three times daily.

VERA PERLES (Plessner)

Urinary Antiseptic

Composition: Contains santal oil, haarlem oil and oil of copaiba.

Action and Uses: A stimulant to the genitourinary and respiratory mucous membranes and a diuretic; *For use* in urethritis, cystitis, pyelitis; also in chronic bronchitis.

Supply: **VERA PERLES**—Bottles of 50 and 500.

Administration: 2 Perles three to four times daily.

VISCYSATE (Bischoff)

Vasodilator

Composition: A dialyzation product of the fresh leaves and stems of Viscum album or apple tree mistletoe; is non-toxic, of constant composition and stable.

Action: Vasodilator and sedative; may be given for prolonged periods without affecting heart and producing arrhythmia or disturbing digestion.

Uses: *For use* in hypertension and vasomotor disturbances; to relieve cephalalgia, tinnitus aurium, vertigo in climacterium and arteriosclerosis.

Supply: VISCYSATE—Liquid—Bottles of 30 cc.
VISCYSATE—Tablets—Bottles 25 and 50.

Administration: 20 drops of liquid or 1–2 tablets three times daily, after meals.

Bibliography: *See Chap. XII.*

VITAMEXOL (Strasenburgh)

Vitamin Therapy

Composition: Contains vitamins B (F and G) and D, proteins, carbohydrates and minerals.

Action and Uses: A food accessory and reconstructive *for use* in malnutrition, anemia, convalescence, in expectant and lactating mothers.

Supply: VITAMEXOL—Bottles of 8 oz., 1 pt.

Administration: ½–1 tablespoonful before meals and at bedtime; Children—in accordance with age.

WATERBURY'S COMPOUND (Waterbury)

Hematinic

Composition: Is stated to contain predigested liver, pancreas and spleen, unfermented malt extract, hypophosphites, iron and manganese peptonates, wild cherry extract, nux vomica and aromatics.

Action and Uses: Tonic, hematinic and respiratory sedative, *for use* in respiratory infections, anorexia, anemia, convalescence.

Supply: WATERBURY'S COMPOUND—Plain—Bottles of 1 pt., 1 gal.
WATERBURY'S COMPOUND WITH CREOSOTE AND GUAIACOL—Bottles 1 pt., 1 gal.

Administration: 1 Tablespoonful four to six times daily.
Children—1-2 teaspoonfuls daily.

YEAST CAPSULES (Westerfield)

Alterative

Composition: Is stated to contain yeast gr 3 (0.194 Gm) with extracts of chionanthus, echinacea and alfalfa.

Action and Uses: Alterative *for use* in acne, boils, intestinal disorders; laxative and digestant.

Supply: YEAST CAPSULES—Bottles 100, 500 and 1,000.

Administration: 2 capsules, three to four times daily.

YEASTAMINE (Norwich)

Vitamin Therapy

Composition: Contains vitamin B; 2 tablets are equivalent in active water-soluble vitamin B to one cake of fresh yeast.

Action and Uses: In malnutrition, convalescence and lowered vitality.

Supply: YEASTAMINE—Tablets, gr 1¼—Bottles of 1,000.

Administration: 1-4 tablets, three times daily.

YERBA SANTA-CREO COMPOUND (Boericke and Runyon)

Expectorant

Composition: Is stated to contain yerba santa, eucalyptus, ipecac, menthol with creosote m 4 and chloroform m 2 per ounce; alcohol 6 %.

Action: Sedative, antiseptic, expectorant; a palatable, well tolerated creosote expectorant.

Uses: Coughs, colds, bronchitis.

Supply: YERBA SANTA-CREO COMPOUND—1 and 5 gal.

Administration: 1-2 teaspoonfuls every 2-3 hr.; dosage if desired may gradually be increased without fear of gastro-intestinal disturbances.
Children 15-60 m.

YOHIMBIN (Lehn and Fink)

Aphrodisiac

Composition and Action: An alkaloid said to be of specific effect upon the lower spinal cord and erection center; induces hyperemia of pelvic organs and stimulates aphrodisiac function.

Uses: *For use* in frigidity, impotence, sexual exhaustion; also in amenorrhea, dysmenorrhea, vaginismus, infantile genitalism.

Supply: **YOHIMBIN**—Tablets, gr 1/12 (0.006 Gm)—Vials of 20.

Administration: 1 tablet three times daily, increased after 1 week.

Caution: If vertigo, palpitation, insomnia, headache, nervousness appear, treatment must be reduced or discontinued.

ZYMOCIDE (Reed and Carnrick)

Antiseptic

Composition: A solution of eucalyptol, thymol, menthol, methyl salicylate, boric and benzoic acids and aromatics.

Uses and Administration: *As Antiseptic*—In 10%–50% warm saline—as spray, gargle or mouth wash in pharyngitis, tonsillitis, acute rhinitis; as cleanser of wounds, cuts, burns, ulcers.

As Douche—Mixed with 1–2 parts of warm saline, is used in middle ear disease to control discharge, foul odor and promote healing.

As Wash—In 2–4 teaspoonfuls to a pint of hot water, hot or cold—in conjunctivitis, blepharitis, lachrymal catarrh; as compresses in prickly heat, insect bites, acne, pruritus.

In Ice Cold Solution—For sunburn, ivy poisoning and some forms of pruritus.

Supply: **ZYMOCIDE**—Bottles of 2½, 6, 14 oz., 1 gal.

Pharmaceutical Drug *and* Drugs Products

(With their description, medicinal preparations, administrations and therapeutic uses)

Pharmaceutical Drug *and* Drugs Products

(With their description, medicinal preparations, administrations and therapeutic uses)

A presentation of 8160 modern, non-pharmacopeal, medicinal preparations, comprising: 1878 drugs and chemicals, 535 biologicals, 860 endocrines, 1563 ampule medicaments, 209 medicinal foods, 129 mineral waters, 2344 individual and group allergens and 642 miscellaneous products.

By :

JACOB GUTMAN, M.D., Phar.D., F.A.C.P.

WILLIAM E. FITCH

Consulting Physician, Manhattan General Hospital, New York; the Riverdale, Shore Road, Williamsburg Maternity and Borough Park General Hospitals of Brooklyn; Director, Brooklyn Diagnostic Institute. Formerly Professor of Materia Medica College of Dentistry, University of State of New Jersey; Professor Clinical Chemistry Jersey City College of Pharmacy; Instructor of Medicine, New York Post Graduate Medical School and Hospital; Attending Physician Wyckoff Heights and Unity Hospitals.

Volume 2

SHREE PUBLISHERS & DISTRIBUTORS

NEW DELHI-110 002

Edition : 2008

Published by :
SHREE PUBLISHERS AND DISTRIBUTORS
20, Ansari Road, Daryaganj
New Delhi-110 002

3 Volumes Set

ISBN : 978-81-8329-255-9

Printed by :
Ruchika Printers
Delhi-110032

PREFACE

This treatise is designed to meet the demand of the progressive physician for information concerning the most modern therapeutic agencies placed at his command by Research Laboratories. It presents without bias or comment all the popular non-pharmacopeal preparations and other remedies found useful in the treatment of disease.

The pharmaceutical concerns of America spend millions of dollars yearly for the discovery and preparation of medicinal agents of high merit. Medicine is indeed indebted to these organizations for the many epoch-making discoveries and invaluable additions to modern therapeusis made during the past few decades; most of the curative sera, vaccines, allergens, potent drugs and endocrines are the result of their researches. The physician, however, has at present no adequate means of keeping informed on all the newer additions to his armamentarium; commercial descriptions of these reach him at inopportune times and usually find their way into the waste basket, thus seldom being on hand when wanted; and except for the official publication of only Council-Accepted products, there are no authoritative sources of information embracing all the modern preparations. To provide such source is the purpose of this work.

An endeavor is here made to present without favoritism or discrimination all the non-official products-proprietary, patented, Council Accepted and others, that are popular with the medical profession. Descriptions, statements, analyses and all other data are offered without change or comment, but as found available in the numerous standard works and references consulted, or as obtained from the producers and distributors of the respective products. Every effort has been made to present the information accurately yet concisely, excluding elaborate discussions, quotations, theories and other time consuming topics of but little practical value to the clinician. The embodiment in three volumes of such a mass of material necessitated the use of phraseology as brief as was found consistent with the complete description of every important feature.

To insure ease in locating a desired preparation and to afford equal consideration to all products and producers, the arrangement throughout the book is alphabetical, by drug or distributor. Separate chapters are devoted to preparations of similar character; in each chapter like products are grouped, and preceded in each instance by a brief description with suggestions for their practical application; for each drug its various methods of administration, with dosages in the metric and U. S. systems, are presented. Incompatibilities, contraindications, strengths of solutions and methods of their preparation are given where deemed serviceable; where emphasis is desirable, italics or capitals are employed; verbiage is avoided throughout the book.

The Therapeutic Guide is intended to provide for the clinician, whether general practitioner or specialist, a wide choice of preparations of use in the numerous pathologic conditions encountered in his daily service to the sick; also to assist him in the selection of a remedy for a particular purpose. The comprehensive Index is arranged into three sections-Distributors', Drug and Therapeutic, this to assure convenience and rapidity in locating a desired drug, disease or other topic.

GLOSSARY

Definitions of the Newer Trade Terms

Alkpule: A specially treated glass vial containing chemically pure, normal 4% sodium hydroxide solution, in the exact quantity necessary to alkalize the corresponding dose of the accompanying drug.

Ambot: An ampule-bottle containing a solution for hypodermic use.

Ampacoid: A sterile, isotonic solution containing a physiologically standardized hormone of high concentration and purity.

Ampule-vial: A vial containing a sterile solution for hypodermic injection.

Aspirol: A trade name for Ampule-vial.

Bacterin: A bacterial vaccine; a suspension of killed bacteria for use in immunization.

Billet: A small tablet.

C.A.: Council or Committee Accepted (accepted by the Council on Pharmacy and Chemistry or Committee on Foods of the A.M.A., 1933).

Carpule: A glass cartridge-ampule containing in sterile solution a medicament, in definite dosage and strength.

Collosol: A suspensoid colloid with the active ingredient in the disperse phase; non-dialysable, slowly diffusible and disintegrating; is electrically charged and affected by electrolytes.

Crinogen: A preparation of glandular substance, protein and alcohol-free, in concentrated solution.

Dragee: A sugar coated pill or medicated confection.

Elixoid: A fluid preparation favorably flavored.

Emplet: An endocrine product with a protective, inert, salol-free enteric coating, insoluble in stomach but soluble in duodenal and intestinal secretions.

Enteric Coated: Specially coated to traverse the stomach intact without causing irritation, and disintegrating only in the intestines.

Enterocap: A capsule devised to protect its contents against gastric action.

Enterosol Coated: So coated as to be insoluble in gastric secretion.

Enule: A rectal suppository wrapped individually in tin foil.

Glaseptic Ampule: An ampule made of an alkali-free, non-soluble glass, assuring stability of contents.

Hypoloid: An ampule containing a solution for hypodermic injection.

Immunogen: Extraction from living bacterial culture, principally ectoplasm, free from toxic autolysates, bacterial substances, with only 1/10% of the protein content of ordinary vaccines.

Isopule: An ampule containing a measured dose of a medicament.

Kapseal: A special gelatine capsule with joints hermetically sealed to keep contents airtight and prevent deterioration.

Kerakote: A keratin-composition acid resisting, coating, for carrying into the intestines medicinal products which may be impaired or destroyed in the stomach.

Keratin Coated: Coated with acid-resistant keratin, enabling contained medication to pass through the stomach unimpaired.

L.A.: Laity Advertised; popular preparations advertised to the public.

Phylacogen: A bacterial culture filtrate free from organisms.

Pulvule: A dry powdered preparation enclosed in thin walled, quickly soluble capsule of a special gelatin, assuring stability of medication.

Sanitablet: A tablet mechanically packed in cellophane to prevent contamination from handling.

Serobacterin: A bacterin or vaccine sensitized with its corresponding immune serum and of use in smaller dosage.

Soloid: A tablet of soluble ingredients for the making of solutions.

Sucret: A preparation with sucrose.

Swab-Seal: An Ampule-vial mechanically sealed for preservation of contents in sterile state.

Tabloid: A form of medicinal tablet or lozenge.

TABLE OF CONTENTS

CHAPTER V

HYPODERMIC MEDICAMENTS

CHAPTER VI

BIOLOGICALS

CHAPTER VII

ALLERGENS

CHAPTER VIII

FOODS AND BEVERAGES

CHAPTER IX

BOTTLED MINERAL WATERS

CHAPTER X

MISCELLANEOUS PRODUCTS

CHAPTER XI

THERAPEUTIC GUIDE

CHAPTER XII

CHAPTER XIII

CHAPTER XIV

CHAPTER XV

CHAPTER IV

ENDOCRINE PREPARATIONS

In this chapter are presented 860 endocrine products, in 1523 forms, Uniglandular (Part I) and Pluriglandular (Part II).

Description: Endocrine products are prepared from the fresh organs of normal, healthy animals. After careful selection, dissection and separation from inert matter, the glandular tissues are subjected to various processes—defattening, fractionation, solvent action, vacuum drying, etc., precaution being taken that the potency of hormonal factors of cells is not disturbed. The products thus obtained are concentrated and standardized in units, each unit to represent a definite quantity of fresh glandular substance; they are made available as powdered extracts, expressed juices, glandular solutions and as definite crystalline bodies; some endocrine agents are prepared synthetically.

Uses: Glandular preparations are used quite extensively; because of demonstrated clinical value, their demand is very considerable. Opotherapy is employed: (1) for substitutional purposes, in prenatal or postoperative total absence of a gland, or its complete atrophy and inactivity; (2) for homostimulating effects where a gland is physiologically inactive yet still responsive to stimulation; (3) for symptomatic relief and pharmacodynamic effect, and (4) empirically in many instances, where experience has shown glandular therapy to be of benefit.

Most of the available endocrine preparations are for oral administration; the claim that all except thyroidal products, if orally administered, are destroyed by the gastric juices is debatable. Hypodermically, as in all parenteral therapy, endocrines are often more potent and more dependable, and should thus be employed wherever advisable, especially where rapid pharmacologic effect is desired.

PART I

UNIGLANDULAR PRODUCTS

The 614 uniglandular preparations here to follow are arranged in sections, by gland; each section is alphabetical by producer of preparations and is preceded by a brief summary of the best known actions and uses of the gland represented, with dosages stated for each preparation

---

ADRENAL PRODUCTS

Adrenal glandular products are prepared from the Cortex, the Medulla and the Whole Gland.

CORTICAL PRODUCTS: The cortex is endowed with important functions and is essential to life. It has a controlling influence over bodily growth and the development of male sexual organs; over hair distribution, pigmentation and masculinity; it regulates lipoid metabolism, cerebral development, muscular activity with increased heat production. Cortin, Eschatin and Interrennin are the available cortical hormones. *Used* in all hypoadrenal manifestations, in Addison's disease, in Graves' disease; also in paralysis agitans, Parkinsonism, gastric neuroses, myositis.

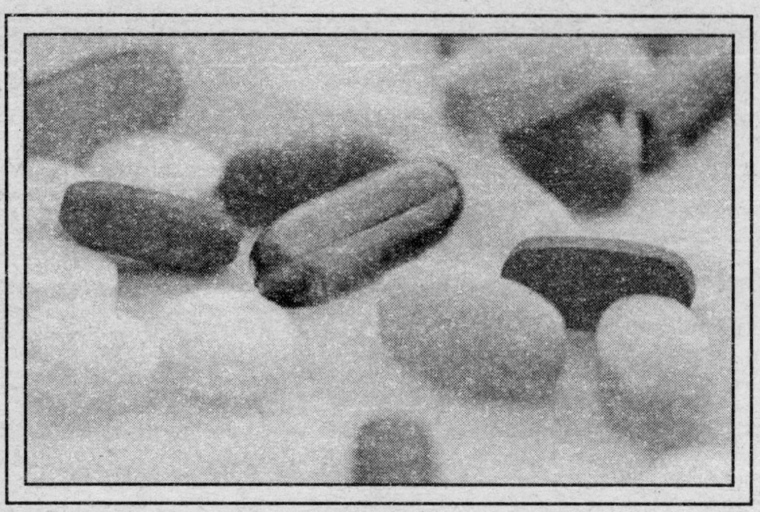

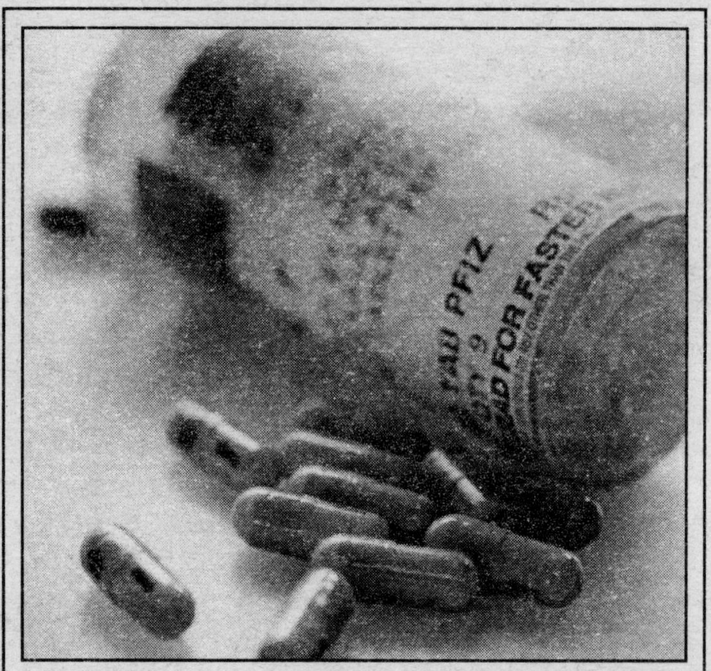

Pharmaceutical Drugs Products

MEDULLARY PRODUCTS: The active principle of the medulla affects arterial tone and blood pressure, is a marked vasoconstrictor, hemostatic and stimulator of most non-striated musculature. The medullary preparations are available as powdered extracts or as the isolated hormone, known as Epinephrin, Suprarenalin, Suprarenin, Adrenalin. *Used* in collapse, shock, cardiac weakness, myasthenia; in asthma, hay fever and other allergies; in numerous conditions for local effect.

WHOLE GLAND PRODUCTS: These are prepared from the total gland and embody the functions of the cortex and medulla. The active principles assist in sexual development, especially in early life; maintain muscular tone and arterial pressure; exert protective influence against systemic infections. *Used* in various hypoadrenal disorders.

---

1. Suprarenal Cortex Preparations

Adrenal Cortex Liquid (Armour)
Ampules 1 cc.......................... Boxes of 12, 50

Dosage: 1 ampule *subcutaneously*, daily.

Suprarenal Cortex Substance (Armour)
Powder.............................. Bottles of 1, 4, 16 oz.
Tablets gr 3......................... Bottles of 100, 500, 1,000

Dosage: 3–6 gr two to three times daily.

Suprarenal Cortex (Carnrick)
Capsules gr 3......................... Bottles of 40
Powder.............................. Bottles of ⅛, 1 oz.
Tablets gr 1......................... Bottles of 50, 100, 500
Tablets gr 2......................... Bottles of 50, 100

Dosage: 3–6 gr two to three times daily.

Adrenal Cortex (Colwell)
Solution............................. Bottles of 1 oz.
5 m representing gr 1 desiccated gland.

Dosage: 3–5 gr, *subcutaneously*, daily.

Adrenal Cortex (Glandular Laboratories)
Capsules gr 1........................ Bottles of 25
in physiologic salt solution.

Dosage: 1 capsule, increased slowly to 4–5 capsules daily.

Adreno-Cortin (Harrower)
Capsules............................. Boxes of 40
containing gr 5 of concentrate, representing gr 30 fresh tissue.

Dosage: 1–2 capsules two to three times daily, preferably with 1 ampule Adreno-Cortin solution daily, *parenterally*.

Adreno-Cortin Solution (Harrower)
Ampules 1 cc......................... Boxes of 5
representing 5 Gm fresh cortex tissue.

Dosage: 1 ampule daily, *subcutaneously*.

Suprarenal Cortex (Lafayette Pharmacal)
Enterocaps, gr 1..................... Bottles of 100
representing gr 6 fresh gland.

Dosage: 3–4 capsules daily.

Suprarenal Cortex Extract **(Lang)**
Glycerol extract........................ Bottles of ½, 1, 2 oz.
each cc representing 1 Gm fresh gland.

Dosage: 15–30 drops three to four times daily.

Adrenal Cortex **(Marvell)**
Powdered extract..................... Bottles of ⅛, 1 oz.
Capsules gr 1......................... Bottles of 100
each capsule representing gr 1 desiccated substance.

Dosage: 1 capsule three times daily, increasing slowly.

Interrenin **(Marvell)**
Ampules 1 cc.......................... Boxes of 6, 12
representing 5 Gm fresh gland.

Dosage: 1–3 ampules three times daily, *intramuscularly.*

Suprarenal Cortex **(Miller)**
Capsules gr 1, gr 2, gr 5................ Bottles of 100, 1,000
Powder.............................. Bottles of 1 oz., ¼, 1 lb.

Dosage: 1–2 gr two to three times weekly.

Eschatin **(Parke, Davis)**
Vials 10 cc
each cc representing 30 Gm fresh beef cortex.

Dosage: 1–5 cc as required. *See Chap. I.*

Suprarenal Cortex **(Reed and Carnrick)**
Powder.............................. Bottles of 1 oz., ¼, 1 lb.
Tablets, Plain, Enteric coated, gr 2...... Bottles of 100, 500, 1,000

Dosage: 2–4 gr three times daily.

Glycortal (Schieffelin)
Pills................................. Bottles of 50
Glycerine extract of suprarenal cortex.

Dosage: 1 pill three times daily, before meals.

Suprarenal Cortex Extract **(Miller)**
Ampules 1 cc, 2 cc.................... Boxes of 12, 100
Ampule-vials 30 cc.................... Packages of 1

Dosage: 1–2 cc two to three times weekly.

---

2. Suprarenal Medulla Preparations

Epinephrine Hydrochloride **(Abbott)**
Ampules 1 cc......................... Boxes of 12, 100
containing epinephrine hydrochloride 1:1,000, chlorbutanol 0.5%.

Dosage: ⅓–1 cc as necessary, *subcutaneously.*

Suprarenal Medulla **(Armour)**
Powder.............................. Bottles of 1 oz.
Tablets gr 1.......................... Bottles of 100
physiologically standardized, containing not less than 2% epinephrine.

Dosage: 1–3 gr two to three times daily.

Suprarenalin **(Armour)**
Crystals............................. Vials 1 gr.
Solution 1:1000....................... Bottles 1 oz.
Ampules—1 cc, 1:1,000 and 1:10,000
solution............................ Boxes of 6, 50 and 100

Dosage: 5–30 m every 2–3 hours, if necessary; *hypodermically*—10–15 m; topically 1:1,000–1:15,000 sol. *See Chap. I.*

Epinephrine Solution (1:1,000) (Burroughs Wellcome)
Hypoloids 1 cc........................ Boxes of 10, 100
Solution........................... Bottles of 1 oz.

Dosage: (Hypoloids) *Intravenously*—1 cc in 500 cc normal saline. *Hypodermically* 5–15 m. (Solution) 10–30 m two to three times daily. *See Chap. I.*

Epinine (Burroughs Wellcome)
Bottles of 25 cc...................... Cartons of 1
a 1:100 solution of synthetic epinephrine.

Dosage: 5–15 m as required. *See Chap. I.*

Epinephrine Hydrochloride (Berwyn)
Ampules 1 cc, solution 1:1,000.......... Boxes of 12, 100, 500
Ampules 1 cc, solution 1:10,000......... Boxes of 12, 100, 500

Dosage: ½–1 ampule, *subcutaneously*, daily. *See Chap. I.*

Epinephrin Solution (Breon)
Ampules 1 cc......................... Boxes of 12, 100
solution 1:1,000.

Dosage: For relief of asthmatic attacks, 5–10 m, *intramuscularly;* for lung hemorrhage, 7–10 m every 20–30 min. *See Chap. I.*

Epinephrine (Carnrick, G. W.)
Powder.............................. Bottles of 1 gr

Dosage: 1–3 gr three times daily.

Epinephrine Chloride Solution 1:1,000 (Carnrick, G. W.)
Solution............................ Bottles of 1 oz.

Dosage: ½–1 cc *intramuscularly*, as required. *See Chap. I.*

Epinephrine 1:10,000 (Carnrick, G. W.)
Ampules 1 cc........................ Boxes of 6

Dosage: ½–1 cc *intramuscularly*, as required. *See Chap. I.*

Suprarenal Medulla (Carnrick, G. W.)
Tablets gr 2......................... Bottles of 100

Dosage: 1–3 gr three times daily.

Epinephrin 1:1,000 (Colwell)
Ampules 1 cc........................ Boxes of 12

Dosage: Used intramuscularly, ½–1 ampule, as required. *See Chap. I.*

Epinephrin Chloride Solution 1:1,000 (Colwell)
Solution............................ Bottles of 1 oz.
containing epinephrin gr ⅖, chlorbutanol gr 2¼.

Dosage: ½–1 ampule, *intramuscularly. See Chap. I.*

Adrenapit (Epinephrin Chloride 1:1,000) (Harvey-Pittenger)
Solution, Hypodermic................... Bottles "Swab Seal" 15 cc

Dosage: ½–1 cc *intramuscularly*, as required.

Adrenapit (Epinephrin Chloride 1:1,000) (Harvey-Pittenger)
Solution, Local and Oral............... Bottles "Swab Seal" 1 oz.

Dosage: Small dose, increased as necessary, *intramuscularly.*

Endo-Suprarenalin, Solution 1:1,000 (Intravenous Products)
Ampules 1 cc......................... Boxes of 12, 100

Dosage: ½–1 cc, *intramuscularly.*

Suprarenal Medulla Extract **(Lang)**
Glycerol extract........................ Bottles of ½, 1, 2 oz.
each cc representing 1 Gm fresh gland.

Dosage: 30–45 drops three times daily.

Epinephrine Hydrochloride **(Lederle)**
Vials 5 cc............................ Boxes of 12
Ampules 1 cc, 1:1,000 solution.

Dosage: 3–10 m as required. *See Chap. I.*

Epinephrine Hydrochloride U.S.P. **(McNeil)**
Solution 1:1,000...................... Bottles of 1 oz.

Dosage: Hypodermically—1–15 m, as required. Locally—full strength. Orally—5–30 m every 2 hr. *See Chap. I.*

Suprarenin **(Metz)**
Ampules 1 cc.......................... Boxes of 20
Liquid................................ Bottles of 1 oz.
a 1:1,000 solution of synthetic epinephrin.

Dosage: 8–15 m as required. *See Chap. I.*

Suprarenal Medulla (Epinephrine or Adrenalin) (Solution 1:1,000) **(Miller)**
Ampules 1 cc.......................... Boxes of 12, 100
Solution.............................. Bottles of 1 oz.

Dosage: ½–1 ampule, *hypodermically*, as required.

Suprarenal Medulla **(Miller)**
Capsules gr 1, gr 2, gr 3................ Bottles of 100, 1,000
Powder................................ Bottles of 1 oz., ¼, 1 lb.

Dosage: 1–3 gr three times daily.

Epinephrine U.S.P. 1:1,000 Solution **(National Drug)**
Ampules 1 cc.......................... Boxes of 12, 25, 100
Ampule-vials 25 cc.................... Boxes of 1

Dosage: ½–1 cc *subcutaneously*. *See Chap. I.*

Adrenalin **(Parke, Davis)**
Ampules 1 cc.......................... Boxes of 5
Liquid................................ Bottles of 1 oz.
a 1:1,000 solution of epinephrine hydrochloride.

Dosage: 8–15 m as required. *See Chap. I.*

Suprarenal Medulla **(Reed and Carnrick)**
Powder................................ Bottles of 1 oz., ¼, 1 lb.
Tablets, Plain, Enteric coated, gr 1...... Bottles of 100, 500, 1,000

Dosage: 1–2 gr three times daily.

Adrenal Residue **(Schieffelin)**
Fluid................................. Bottles of ½ oz.
Pills 5 m............................. Bottles of 50
containing 4 mg epinephrine per cc.

Dosage: 3–5 gr or 10 m two to three times daily.

Epinephrin 1:1,000 **(Searle)**
Ampules 1 cc.......................... Boxes of 12, 25, 100

Dosage: Subcutaneously or *intramuscularly*, ½–1 cc as required. *See Chap. I.*

Adrin Solution **(Sharp and Dohme)**
Liquid................................ Bottles of 1 oz.
a 1:1,000 solution of epinephrine hydrochloride.

Dosage: 8–15 m as required. *See Chap. I.*

Epinephrin Chloride 1:1,000 (Sherman)
Ampules 1 cc........................ Boxes of 12, 100
Solution........................ Vials of 1 oz.

Dosage: ½–1 ampule *intramuscularly*, according to the occasion. *See Chap. I.*

Epinephrine Chloride (Solution 1:1,000) (Zemmer)
Ampules 1 cc........................ Boxes of 12, 100

Dosage: 1 cc *intramuscularly*, as indicated. *See Chap. I.*

---

3. Suprarenal Whole Gland Preparations

Suprarenal Substance (Armour)
Powder........................ Bottles of 1, 4, 8, 16 oz.
Tablets gr 1, gr 2........................ Bottles of 100, 500, 1,000

Dosage: 1–2 gr several times daily.

Suprarenal (Boericke and Tafel)
Capsules gr 5........................ Bottles of 60
containing gr ⅕ suprarenal gland.

Dosage: 1 capsule three times daily.

Suprarenal (Burroughs Wellcome)
Tabloids gr 1, gr 5........................ Bottles of 100, 500

Dosage: 1–5 gr several times daily.

Suprarenal (Carnrick)
Powder........................ Bottles of 1 oz.
Tablets gr 1........................ Bottles of 100, 500, 1,000

Dosage: 1–5 gr as required.

Suprarenal Whole (U.S.P.) (Colwell)
Solution........................ Bottles of 1 oz.
5 m representing gr 1 desiccated gland.

Dosage: 1–3 gr two to three times daily.

Suprarenal Substance (Glandular Laboratories)
Capsules gr 1........................ Bottles of 25
in physiologic saline.

Dosage: 1 capsule three times daily.

Suprarenal (Harvey-Pittenger)
Capsules gr 2........................ Bottles of 50, 100, 500, 1,000
Powder........................ Bottles of 1, 4, 8 oz., 1 lb.
1 gr desiccated substance representing gr 6 fresh gland.

Dosage: 3–5 gr as required.

Suprarenal (Lafayette Pharmacal)
Enterocaps, gr 1, gr 2
each grain desiccated substance representing gr 5 fresh gland.

Dosage: 1–2 capsules two to three times daily.

Suprarenal Extract (Whole) (Lang)
Glycerol extract........................ Bottles of ½, 1, 2 oz.
each cc representing 1 Gm fresh gland.

Dosage: 15–30 drops three to four times daily.

Suprarenal **(Lilly)**

Powder.............................. Bottles of 1, 4 oz.
Pulvules gr 2.......................... Bottles of 100, 500
Tablets, Plain, Enteric coated, gr 2..... Bottles of 100, 500
Tablets, gr 5.......................... Bottles of 100
each grain desiccated substance representing gr 5 fresh gland.

Dosage: Gr 2–5 two to three times daily.

Suprarenal Substance **(Marvell)**

Tablets gr 1........................... Bottles of 100

Dosage: 1–2 tablets several times daily.

Suprarenal (Whole Gland) **(Miller)**

Capsules gr 1, gr 2, gr 5............... Bottles of 100, 1,000
Powder.............................. Bottles of 1 oz., ¼, 1 lb.
Tablets, Enteric coated, gr 1, gr 2....... Bottles of 100, 1,000

Dosage: 1–5 gr three times daily.

Suprarenal Extract (Whole Gland) **(Miller)**

Ampules 1 cc, 2 cc..................... Boxes of 12, 100
Ampule-vials 30 cc..................... Packages of 1

Dosage: 1–2 cc two to three times weekly, *subcutaneously*.

Suprarenal Gland **(McNeil)**

Capsules, Enteric coated, gr 2........... Bottles of 100, 500
Tablets, Enteric coated, gr 2............ Bottles of 100, 500

Dosage: 1–2 capsules or tablets, three times daily.

Suprarenal **(National Drug)**

Tablets gr 1........................... Bottles of 100, 500, 1,000
representing gr 6 fresh gland.

Dosage: 1–2 tablets three times daily.

Suprarenal **(Parke, Davis)**

Capsules gr 2.......................... Bottles of 100, 500
Powder.............................. Vials 1 oz.—Bottles ¼ lb.
Emplets, Enteric coated, gr 2........... Bottles of 100, 500
Tablets gr 2........................... Bottles of 100, 500
each grain desiccated substance representing gr 5 fresh gland.

Dosage: 2–4 gr three times daily.

Suprarenal Whole Gland **(Reed and Carnrick)**

Powder.............................. Bottles of 1 oz., ¼, 1 lb.
Tablets, Plain, Enteric coated, gr 2..... Bottles of 100, 500, 1,000

Dosage: 2–4 gr three times daily.

Adrenal Substance **(Rorer)**

Powder.............................. Bottles of 1 oz.

Dosage: Gr 1–5 three times daily.

Adrenal Extract **(Schieffelin)**

Tablets gr 1........................... Bottles of 100
representing gr 10 dried extract.

Dosage: 1–2 tablets daily.

Adrenal Nucleoprotein **(Schieffelin)**

Powder.............................. Bottles of ½ oz.
Tablets gr 1........................... Bottles of 100
each tablet containing gr $\frac{1}{10}$ nucleoproteins, and traces of epinephrine.

Dosage: 1–2 tablets three to four times daily.

Glyadrenal (Schieffelin)
Pills gr 2.............................. Bottles of 50
A glycerin extract.

Dosage: 1 pill three to four times daily.

Suprarenal Substance (U.S.P.) (Searle)
Tablets, Enteric coated, gr 2............ Bottles of 100, 500
each grain representing gr 6 fresh gland.

Dosage: 1–2 tablets three times daily.

Suprarenal Gland (Wyeth)
Powder.............................. Vials of 1 oz.; Bottles of ¼, 1 lb.
Tablets gr 2......................... Bottles of 100, 1,000
each grain representing gr 5 fresh gland.

Dosage: 1 tablet several times daily.

Suprarenal (U.S.P.) (Zemmer)
Tablets, Plain, Keratin coated, gr 2...... Bottles of 100, 1,000
each grain representing gr 6 fresh gland.

Dosage: 1–2 tablets as required.

LIVER PRODUCTS

Description: Liver products are prepared from fresh liver substance, some to contain the hypotensive element, others—the hematopoietic principles of the organ; most preparations are standardized to represent a definite quantity of fresh liver; are available in powder form, as liquids and as two active principles.

Action and Uses: The action is represented by two hormonal substances: 1 Hemopoietin which stimulates bone marrow and red cell regeneration with reticulocytosis; and 2 Anabolin, a detoxicator and hypotensor. *For use*—the antianemic principle substance in specific therapy of pernicious anemia, also in severe secondary anemia; the hypotensor product—in arterial hypertension not due to sclerotic kidney or marked arteriosclerosis.

Dosage: In accordance with preparation.

Preparations

Hepasol (Abbott)
Ampules 1 cc........................ Boxes of 12, 100
representing gr 25 fresh liver tissue; as hypotensor.

Dosage: 1 cc *subcutaneously*, daily till blood pressure is reduced, then at longer intervals.

Liver Liquid (Armour)
Ampules 1 cc........................ Boxes of 6
contains anti-pressor principles of liver.

Dosage: 1 cc daily, *subcutaneously*.

Liver Substance (Armour)
Powder.............................. Bottles of 1, 4, 8, 16 oz.
Tablets gr 2......................... Bottles of 100, 500, 1,000
1 part desiccated substance representing 5 parts fresh gland.

Dosage: 2–3 gr. two to three times daily in pernicious anemia.

Concentrated Liver Extract (Armour)
Liquid.............................. Bottles of 16 oz.
each tablespoonful representing soluble extractives of ¼ lb. fresh liver.

Dosage: In pernicious anemia—1 tablespoonful three times daily in milk or orange juice.

Liver Substance (Carnrick, G. W.)
Capsules gr 5........................ Bottles of 100
Powder.............................. Bottles of 1 oz.
Tablets gr 3......................... Bottles of 100, 500

Dosage: 2–3 gr. two to three times daily in pernicious anemia.

Liver Extract (Erythgen Brand) (Carnrick, G. W.)
Ampules 2½ cc....................... Boxes of 6
representing 50 Gm fresh liver.
Capsules............................ Bottles of 100
Glycerin solution (Liquid).............. Bottles of 8 oz.
1 part representing 40 parts fresh liver substance.

Dosage: 1–4 teaspoonfuls or 6 capsules three times daily. *Subcutaneously,* 1 ampule daily. *See Chap. I.*

Hemo-S (Chappel)
Liquid.............................. Bottles of 8 oz.
a hemic solution of liver, iron and liver copper.

Dosage: 1 tablespoonful two to four times daily. *See Chap. II.*

Liver Extract, Oral (Chappel)
Liquid.............................. Bottles of 8, 16 oz.
contains per oz. the extract from 600 Gm liver.

Dosage: 1 oz. three times daily; maintenance dose ½ oz. daily. *See Chap. I.*

Liver Extract, Subcutaneous (Chappel)
Ampules 2.5 cc....................... Boxes of 12
representing 25 Gm liver.

Dosage: 1 ampule daily; maintenance dose 1 ampule weekly. *See Chap. I.*

Hepati-Cole (Cole)
Ampules 5 cc........................ Boxes of 6
each cc representing 20 Gm fresh liver.

Dosage: 1–2 cc daily in relapse; maintenance dose 1–2 cc weekly. *See Chap. I.*

Liver Extract (Fairchild)
Vials................................ Boxes of 20; Packages of 4 oz.
each representing 100 Gm fresh liver.

Dosage: 3–4 vials daily, in fluid. *See Chap. I.*

Anabolin (Harrower)
Tablets............................. Vials 15; Bottles of 50
1 gr reducing arterial tension 12 millimeters in a 10 kilogram dog.

Dosage: 1 tablet three times daily. *See Chap. I.*

Heparhemin (Harrower)
Ampules 5 cc........................ Boxes of 5
representing 100 Gm fresh liver.

Dosage: 1 ampule *intramuscularly* daily, then 1–2 injections weekly.

Endo-Liver Extract (Intravenous)
Ampules 1 cc........................ Boxes of 12, 25, 100
containing 50 Gm refined and concentrated liver.

Dosage: 1 ampule daily, *intramuscularly.*

Hepatrat (Kretschmar)

Ampules 2 cc........................ Boxes of 3 and 10
representing 500 Gm liver.

Dosage: 3–6 cc daily for 6–8 weeks. *See Chap. I.*

Liver (Lafayette Pharmacal)

Enterocaps, gr 1, gr 2, gr 5... Bottles of 100
each grain desiccated substance representing 6 gr fresh gland.

Liver Concentrate (Lafayette Pharmacal)

Enterocaps, gr 5.
each grain desiccated substance representing 20 gr fresh gland.

Lamb Liver Extract (Lang)

Glycerol extract...................... Bottles of 4 oz., 1 pt.
each cc representing 1 Gm fresh gland.

Dosage: Adults—1 tablespoonful three to four times daily. Children—1 teaspoonful three to four times daily.

Liver Extract (Lederle)

Vials.............................. Packages of 24
representing 100 Gm liver.

Dosage: 3–4 vials daily; maintenance dose 2–3 vials daily. *See Chap. I.*

Liver Extract 343 (Lilly)

Vials 3½ oz......................... Boxes of 24
representing 100 Gm fresh raw liver.

Dosage: 3 vials daily, or 2 cc *intramuscularly. See Chap. I.*

Liver Extract with Iron 55 (Lilly)

Bottles............................ Cartons of 1
representing extract from 6½ lb. fresh liver with 231 gr ferrous ammonium citrate; each level teaspoonful contains 3.75 Gm, representing 125 Gm fresh liver and 0.65 Gm ferrous ammonium citrate.

Dosage: 2–4 teaspoonfuls in fluid. *See Chap. II.*

Liver Extract (Maltbie)

Capsules gr 7½...................... Bottles of 100, 1,000
representing 10 Gm fresh liver.

Dosage: 10–15 capsules daily, reduced in accordance with blood picture. *See Chap. I.*

Liver Extract (McNeil)

Capsules........................... Bottles of 100, 500
45 capsules representing 1 lb. fresh liver.
Powder, Vials—small, large............. Cartons of 12
8 small or 4½ large vials representing 1 lb. fresh liver.

Dosage: 3–5 capsules, or 1 small or ½ large vial, two to three times daily. *See Chap. I.*

Liver Extract (Concentrated) (McNeil)

Ampule-vials 5 cc..................... Cartons of 1

Dosage: 5 cc *intramuscularly*, weekly. *See Chap. I.*

Liver Solution (McNeil)

Ampules 1 cc........................ Boxes of 6, 100

Dosage: ½–1 cc *intramuscularly*, one to two times daily.

Liver Substance (McNeil)

Capsules gr 5........................ Bottles of 100, 500

Dosage: 3–6 capsules three to four times daily, before meals.

Liver Extract (Hematopoietic) **(Miller)**
Capsules 5 gr........................ Bottles of 100, 500, 1,000
Desiccated water soluble extract from fresh veal livers.

Dosage: 3 capsules three times daily. *See Chap. I.*

Liver Extract (Hypotensive) **(Miller)**
Ampules 1 cc........................ Boxes of 12, 100
Ampules 5 cc........................ Boxes of 6, 50
Ampule-vials 30 cc.................... Packages of 1.

Dosage: 1–5 cc daily, *intramuscularly.* *See Chap. I.*

Liver Extract **(National Drug)**
Capsules............................ Bottles of 100
representing 10 Gm fresh liver.

Dosage: 30–40 capsules during relapse; maintenance dose 20–30 capsules daily. *See Chap. I.*

Liver Extract **(Parke, Davis)**
Ampules 2 cc........................ Packages of 6
representing 10 Gm of liver.
Vials, 3–3½ Gm...................... Packages of 24
representing approximately 100 Gm of liver.

Dosage: 300–400 Gm liver equivalent in relapse; 200–300 Gm—for maintenance. *See Chap. I.*

Liver Substance (1:20) **(Rorer)**
Capsules gr 5........................ Bottles of 100

Liver Substance **(Searle)**
Capsules gr 5........................ Bottles of 100, 500
each grain representing 5 gr fresh gland.

Liver Extract (Fraction A5) **(Sharp and Dohme)**
Vials............................... Packages of 24
representing 100 Gm liver.
Capsules ½ Gm....................... Boxes of 100, 1,000
representing 10 Gm fresh liver.

Dosage: 1 vial three times daily, or 8–15 capsules in any palatable fluid. *See Chap. I.*

Liver Extract **(Smith-Dorsey)**
Capsules gr 7½...................... Bottles of 100, 500, 1,000
representing ⅓ oz. fresh liver.

Dosage: 12–15 capsules daily. *See Chap. I.*

Liver Extract, Plain **(Stearns)**
Capsules............................ Bottles of 100
45 capsules containing the extract from 1 lb. of liver.

Dosage: As required. *See Chap. I.*

Liver Extract 100 X (Concentrated) **(Stearns)**
Capsules............................ Bottles of 40, 500
5 capsules representing the extract of ½ lb. liver.

Dosage: As required. *See Chap. I.*

Liver Extract **(Stoddard)**
Vials............................... Packages of 24
representing 100 Gm fresh mammalian liver.

Dosage: 3–6 vials daily with fluid. *See Chap. I.*

Liver Extract (United Laboratories)
Ampules 2 cc........................ Boxes of 6, 12, 24
for reducing hypertension.

Dosage: 2 cc daily. *See Chap. III.*

Liver Extract (Upjohn)
Capsules............................ Boxes of 100, 1,000
representing 10 Gm fresh whole liver.

Dosage: 15 capsules three times daily. *See Chap. I.*

Liver X (Liver Extract) (Zemmer)
Capsules gr 5....................... Boxes of 100, 1,000
each grain representing 20 gr fresh gland.

Dosage: 3–6 capsules three or four times daily, reduced.

Liver Substance (Zemmer)
Capsules gr 5....................... Boxes of 100, 1,000
Tablets, Keratin coated, gr 5........... Bottles of 100, 1,000
each grain representing 5 gr fresh gland.

Dosage: 1–3 capsules or tablets four times daily, before meals and at bedtime.

Liver Substance Solution (Zemmer)
Ampules 1 cc........................ Boxes of 12, 100
representing 25 gr fresh liver.

Dosage: 1 cc daily.

MAMMARY PRODUCTS

Description: Although no active hormones have been isolated from the mammary gland, clinically the organ is, nevertheless, known to antagonize ovarian hyperactivity, to represent during puerperium the functions of placenta and corpus luteum of checking menstruation and ovulation with consequent conception, to favor uterine involution during nursing period, and to exert a galactogogue action. Mammary products are prepared from mammary glands usually of lactating cattle, one part to represent 8–10 parts of fresh glandular substance. *Used* in deficient lactation and mastitis; to check, especially in young girls, profuse or too frequent menstruation, and in functional bleeding from hyperovarism.

Dosage: In accordance with preparation.

Preparations

Mammary Substance (Armour)
Powder............................ Bottles of 1, 4, 8, 16 oz.
Tablets gr 2........................ Bottles of 100, 500, 1,000

Dosage: Gr 2 three times daily.

Mammary Substance (Boericke and Tafel)
Capsules gr 5.

Dosage: 1 capsule three times daily.

Mammary Gland (Burroughs Wellcome)
Tabloid "Mamos" gr 5............... Bottles of 100, 500

Dosage: 1 tablet three times daily.

Mammary Substance (Carnrick, G. W.)

Capsules gr 5 .... Bottles of 100
Powder .... Bottles of 1 oz.
Tablets gr 1 .... Bottles of 100
Tablets gr 3 .... Bottles of 100, 500

Dosage: Gr 1–5, three times daily.

Mammary (Colwell)

Crinogen .... Bottles of 1 oz.
5 m representing gr 1 desiccated gland.

Dosage: 3–4 gr, three times daily.

Mammary (Drug Products)

Capsules gr 1 .... Bottles or 100
representing gr 8 fresh substance.

Dosage: 1 capsule after meals; increased as necessary.

Mammary Substance (Glandular Laboratories)

Capsules gr 2 .... Bottles of 25
in physiological salt solution.

Dosage: 1 capsule three times daily.

Mammary Substance (Harvey-Pittenger)

Capsules gr 5 .... Bottles of 50, 500, 1,000
Powder .... Bottles of 1, 4, 8 oz., 1 lb.
1 part desiccated substance representing 10 parts fresh gland.

Dosage: 2–10 gr, three times daily.

Mammary (Lafayette Pharmacal)

Enterocaps, gr 2, gr 5.
each grain desiccated substance representing gr 10 fresh gland.

Dosage: Gr 2–5 three times daily.

Mammary Extract (Lang)

Glycerol extract .... Bottles of ½, 1, 2 oz.
each cc representing 1 Gm fresh gland.

Dosage: 15–60 drops three to four times daily.

Mammary Substance (Lilly)

Powder .... Bottles of 1, 4 oz.
Pulvules gr 5 .... Bottles of 50
Tablets, plain, Enteric coated, gr 5 .... Bottles of 100, 500
each grain representing gr 8 fresh gland.

Dosage: 2–10 gr, three times daily.

Mammary Substance (Marvell)

Powdered extract .... Bottles of 1 oz., ¼, ½, 1 lb.
Tablets gr 2 .... Bottles of 100

Dosage: Gr 2 three times daily.

Mammary Gland (McNeil)

Capsules, Enteric coated, gr 5 .... Bottles of 100, 500
Tablets, Enteric coated, gr 5 .... Bottles of 100, 500

Dosage: 1–2 capsules or tablets three times daily.

Mammary Substance (Miller)

Capsules gr 2, gr 5 .... Bottles of 100, 500, 1,000
Powder .... Bottles of 1 oz., ¼, 1 lb.
Tablets, Compressed, gr 5 .... Bottles of 100, 500, 1,000
Tablets, Enteric coated, gr 5 .... Bottles of 100, 500, 1,000
1 part desiccated powder representing 8 parts fresh tissue.

Dosage: 1–2 capsules or tablets three times daily.

Mammary (National Drug)

Capsules gr 1........................ Bottles of 100, 500, 1,000
Tablets gr 1........................ Bottles of 100, 500, 1,000
each grain representing gr 10 fresh gland.

Dosage: 1 capsule or tablet three times daily, for 1 week before menses.

Mammary Substance (Parke, Davis)

Emplets, Enteric coated, gr 5........... Bottles of 100, 500
Powder............................ Bottles of 1 oz., ¼ lb.
Tablets, Compressed, gr 5.............. Bottles of 100, 500
each grain representing gr 8 fresh substance.

Dosage: 5–10 gr three times daily.

Mammary Gland (Reed and Carnrick)

Powder............................ Bottles of 1 oz., ¼, 1 lb.
Tablets, Plain and Enteric coated, gr 2, gr 5 Bottles of 100, 500, 1,000

Dosage: 2–10 gr three times daily.

Mammary Substance (Rorer)

Capsules gr 2, gr 5.................... Bottles of 100
Powder............................ Bottles of 1, 4 oz.
Tablets gr 2, gr 5.................... Bottles of 100

Dosage: gr 2–5 three times daily.

Mammary Substance (Zemmer)

Tablets, plain, gr 2.................... Bottles of 100, 1,000
Tablets, Keratin coated, gr 5........... Bottles of 100, 1,000

Dosage: 1–3 tablets three to four times daily.

OVARIAN PRODUCTS

Ovarian preparations are available as products of the Whole Gland, Ovarian Residue with Corpus Luteum, and Follicular Fluid.

Whole Ovary Products: Represent the functions of all hormones of ovary and are prepared in powdered and liquid form. *For use* in general ovarian dysfunction; as substitution therapy in hypo-ovarism, amenorrhea, dysmenorrhea; in natural and surgical menopause.

Ovarian Residue Products: Are prepared from whole ovary and stroma after removal of corpus luteum and concentrated, each part of residue to represent about 6 parts of fresh glandular substance, retaining all the elements of the interstitial tissue and follicular estrus-inducing hormone. *Action*—stimulates ovary without increasing the activity of corpus luteum; stimulates interstitial elements and thus the secondary characteristics: mammae, body contour, voice, psyche and uterine functions of ovulation and menstruation; also relieves discomfort of over-stimulated breasts. *For use* in hypo-ovarism to stimulate delayed puberty, in oligo- and dysmenorrhea with asthenia; in allaying nervous disorders in natural and surgical menopause; in functional sterility, female genital infantilism, frigidity and scanty menstrual flow.

Corpus Luteum Products: Are available as dried powdered extracts, prepared from corpus luteum and follicular fluid, representing 1 to 3 to 5 parts of fresh substance, as standardized solutions and as two active principles, Progestin and Lutin.

Progestin—A physiological antithesis of ovarian hormone; assists in inducing estrus changes, rupture of ripe follicle and extrusion of ovum (ovulation); causes progestational proliferation of endometrium and decidual growth.

Lutin—is estrus inhibiting, nidatory; prevents maturation of other graafian follicles; sensitizes uterine mucosa for nesting of fertilized ovum, enabling its development.

Uses: To inhibit ovarian activity and menstruation during pregnancy, in ovarian irritability, in habitual abortion, in nausea and vomiting of pregnancy, and other endocrine upsets.

---

1. Corpus Luteum Preparations

Corpus Luteum (Abbott)

Ampules 1 cc........................ Boxes of 6, 100
containing 1/3 gr soluble corpora lutea, representing 0.2 Gm desiccated gland, chlorbutanol 1/12 gr.
Capsules Kerakote gr 5................ Bottles of 100, 500

Dosage: 2–3 ampules weekly, *subcutaneously* or *intramuscularly;* in severe cases, daily or on alternate days. Orally: gr 5 three times daily.

Corpus Luteum (Armour)

Capsules gr 2, gr 5..................... Bottles of 50, 100, 500, 1,000
Powder............................ Bottles of 1, 4, 8, 16 oz.
Tablets gr, 2 gr 5.................... Bottles of 50, 100, 500, 1,000
Liquid—Ampules 1 cc................. Boxes of 6

Dosage: 1 ampule *intramuscularly,* two to three times weekly. Orally—gr 2–5, three times daily.

Corpus Luteum Extract (Berwyn)

Ampules 1 cc........................ Boxes of 6, 100, 500
representing 3 gr corpus luteum.

Dosage: 1 ampule *intramuscularly,* two to three times weekly.

Corpus Luteum (Boericke and Tafel)

Capsules gr 5......................... Bottles of 60
containing gr 1 corpus luteum.

Dosage: 1 capsule three times daily.

Corpus Luteum Solution (Breon)

Ampules 1 cc........................ Boxes of 12, 100
containing 1/3 gr soluble extract of corpus luteum with 1/12 gr chlorbutanol.

Dosage: 1–2 ampules daily as indicated, for 12 injections.

Agomensin (Ciba)

Ampules gr 3/4....................... Cartons of 5, 20
Tablets sugar coated gr 1/3............. Bottles of 20, 100
Represents an aqueous solution corpus luteum.

Dosage: *Oral*—1–3 tablets three times daily, supplemented by 1 ampule hypodermically every other day. *Subcutaneous* and *intramuscular*—1–4 ampules every 2–3 days, with 6 tablets daily on intervening days. *See Chap. I.*

Corpus Luteum (G. W. Carnrick)

Ampules 1 cc 20% solution............ Boxes of 6
Capsules gr 5......................... Bottles of 50, 100
Tablets gr 2.......................... Bottles of 50, 100, 500
Tablets gr 5.......................... Bottles of 50, 100
Powder............................ Bottles of 1/8, 1 oz.

Dosage: 1 ampule *intramuscularly,* two to three times weekly. *Orally,* gr 2–5, three times daily.

Corpus Luteum (Colwell)
Ampules 1 cc........................ Boxes of 12
representing gr 3 water soluble content of desiccated gland.
Crinogen 5 m....................... Bottles of 1 oz.
representing gr 1 desiccated gland.

Dosage: 1–2 gr three times daily; Ampules *intramuscularly*, 2 to 3 times weekly.

Corpus Luteum (Drug Products)
Capsules gr 1....................... Bottles of 100
representing gr 6 fresh gland.

Dosage: 1 capsule after meals, increased as indicated.

Corpus Luteum (Glandular Laboratories)
Capsules gr 1½..................... Bottles of 25
in physiologic salt solution.

Dosage: 3 capsules daily.

Corpus Luteum Extract (Harvey-Pittenger)
Capsules gr 2, gr 5.................... Bottles of 50, 100, 500, 1,000
Powder.............................. Bottles of 1, 4, 8 oz., 1 lb.
1 gr desiccated substance representing 6 gr fresh gland.
Solution............................ Bottles "Swab Seal" of 6, 15 cc
each cc representing gr 3 dried substance.

Dosage: 2–10 gr or 1 cc daily.

Lutein (Hynson, Westcott and Dunning)
Powder.............................. Bottles of 1 oz.
Tablets gr 2......................... Tubes of 100
Tablets gr 5......................... Tubes of 45

Dosage: 1–3 tablets three times daily.

Lutein Solution (Hynson, Westcott and Dunning)
Ampules 1 cc........................ Boxes of 6
representing 0.2 Gm water soluble extract of dry substance.

Dosage: 1 cc *intramuscularly* every 2 days.

Endo-Corpus Luteum (Intravenous Products)
Ampules 1 cc........................ Boxes of 12, 100
containing gr 3 fresh gland.

Dosage: 1 cc *intramuscularly*, two to three times weekly.

Corpus Luteum (Lafayette Pharmacal)
Enterocaps, gr 2, gr 5.................. Bottles of 100
each grain desiccated substance representing 6 gr fresh gland.

Dosage: gr 2–5, three times daily.

Corpus Luteum Extract (Lang)
Glycerol extract of fresh gland.......... Bottles ½, 1, 2 oz.
each cc representing 1 Gm fresh substance.

Dosage: 1 cc *intramuscularly*, two to three times weekly.

Corpus Luteum (Lederle)
Tablets gr 2......................... Bottles of 100
representing 10 gr fresh substance.

Dosage: 1 or more tablets daily.

Corpus Luteum Extract (Lederle)
Ampules 1 cc........................ Boxes of 6
Vials 5 cc........................... Boxes of 1
each cc containing 0.02 Gm.

Dosage: 1 cc *intramuscularly* every other day; in severe cases, daily.

Corpus Luteum **(Lilly)**

Ampules 1 cc........................ Boxes of 6
representing gr 3 desiccated gland.
Pulvules gr 2, gr 5.................... Bottles of 50, 100, 500
Powder.............................. Bottles of 1, 4 oz.
Tablets, Plain, gr 2, gr 5............... Bottles of 50, 100, 500
Tablets, Enteric coated, gr 2............ Bottles of 100, 500
Tablets, Enteric coated, gr 5............ Bottles of 100
each grain representing gr 5 fresh gland.

Dosage: 2–5 gr *orally;* or 1 ampule daily or twice weekly, *hypodermically.*

Corpus Luteum Substance **(Marvell)**

Powdered extract..................... Bottles ½, 1 oz., ¼, ½ lb.
Tablets gr 2.......................... Bottles of 100
Tablets gr 5.......................... Bottles of 50

Dosage: Gr 2–5 three times daily.

Corpus Luteum Solution **(Marvell)**

Ampules 1 cc........................ Boxes of 12
representing water soluble extract from 3 gr desiccated corpus luteum; chlorbutanol less than 0.5%.

Dosage: 1 ampule daily, *intramuscularly.*

Corpus Luteum **(McNeil)**

Ampules 1 cc........................ Boxes of 6, 100
representing gr 3 desiccated substance.
Capsules, Enteric coated, gr 2, gr 5...... Bottles of 100, 500
Tablets, Enteric coated, gr 2, gr 5....... Bottles of 100, 500

Dosage: 2–10 gr *orally* three times daily; or 1 cc *hypodermically* every 2 days.

Corpus Luteum Extract **(Miller)**

Ampules 1 cc........................ Boxes of 12, 100
Ampule-vials 30 cc.................... Packages of 1
each cc representing gr 25 fresh substance; chlorbutanol 0.5%.
Capsules gr 2, gr 5................... Bottles of 100, 500, 1,000
Powder.............................. Bottles of 1 oz., ¼, 1 lb.
Tablets compressed, Chocolate and
Enteric coated, gr 5................ Bottles of 100, 500, 1,000
1 gr desiccated substance representing 6 gr fresh gland.

Dosage: 1 capsule or tablet three times daily. 1 ampule *intramuscularly,* three times weekly.

Corpus Luteum **(National Drug)**

Ampules 1 cc........................ Boxes of 6, 12, 25, 100
Ampule-vials 15 cc, 25 cc.............. Packages of 1
each cc representing 18 gr fresh or 3 gr desiccated substance.
Tablets gr 1.......................... Bottles of 100, 500, 1,000
representing gr 6 fresh gland.

Dosage: 1–2 tablets three times daily; or 4–8 m *intramuscularly* every 2–3 hr.

Corpora Lutea **(Parke, Davis)**

Ampules 1 cc........................ Boxes of 6, 100
containing soluble extract gr $3/10$ with chlorbutanol 0.5%.
Emplets, Enteric coated, gr 2½, gr 5..... Bottles of 100, 500
Capsules gr 5......................... Bottles of 50, 100, 500
Powder.............................. Bottles of 1 oz., ¼ lb.
Tablets gr 2, plain.................... Bottles of 50, 100, 500
Tablets, Chocolate coated, gr 5.......... Bottles of 50, 500
each grain representing gr 5 fresh gland.

Dosage: gr 2½–5, repeated as necessary; or 1 ampule two to three times weekly.

Lipo-Lutin (Parke, Davis)
Ampules 1 cc........................ Boxes of 6.
containing lipoidal extract corpus luteum.

Dosage: 1–2 cc daily for 6 or 8 days, *subcutaneously* or *intramuscularly*.

Corpus Luteum (Reed and Carnrick)
Powder............................. Bottles of 1 oz., ¼, 1 lb.
Tablets, Plain and Enteric coated, gr 2, gr 5 Bottles of 100, 500, 1,000

Dosage: gr 2–5 three times daily.

Corpora Lutea (Rorer)
Ampules 1 cc........................ Boxes of 6, 12, 100
Capsules gr 2, gr 5................... Bottles of 100
Powder............................. Bottles of 1, 4 oz.
Tablets gr 2......................... Bottles of 100

Dosage: 1 ampule two times weekly. Orally—gr 2–5, three times daily.

Corpus Luteum Substance (Searle)
Ampules 1 cc........................ Boxes of 12, 25, 100
containing gr 3.
Tablets, enteric coated, gr 2............ Bottles of 100, 500
each grain representing about 6 gr fresh gland.

Dosage: 1–2 tablets two to three times daily. 1 ampule *intramuscularly*, three times weekly.

Corpus Luteum Extract (Sharp and Dohme)
Ampules 1 cc........................ Boxes of 6
representing gr 3 desiccated substance.
Capsules gr 5....................... Bottles of 50, 100
Tablets, Plain, gr 2, gr 5............... Bottles of 50, 100
Tablets, Chocolate coated, gr 2.......... Bottles of 50, 100
each grain representing 6 gr fresh substance.

Dosage: 1 ampule *intramuscularly*, three times weekly. *Orally*, gr 2–5, three times daily.

Corpus Luteum (Sherman)
Ampules 1 cc........................ Boxes of 6, 100
containing soluble extractives from gr 3 desiccated substance.

Dosage: 1 ampule *intramuscularly*, three times weekly.

Corpus Luteum Solution (Stoddard)
Ampules 1 cc........................ Boxes of 6, 100
representing gr 3 water soluble extract of desiccated gland; chlorbutanol 0.5%.
Tablets gr 1......................... Bottles of 100, 500, 1,000

Dosage: 1 tablet three times daily; or 1 ampule two to three times weekly, *intramuscularly* or *subcutaneously*.

Ovestrumon (United Laboratory)
Ampules 2 cc........................ Boxes of 6, 12, 24

Dosage: 1 ampule three to four times weekly.

Luthorm (Upjohn)
Ampules 1 cc........................ Boxes of 12
0.02 Gm extract representing gr 5–7 fresh corpora lutea.

Dosage: 1 cc *intramuscularly*, daily, for 5–10 doses.

Corpus Luteum (Upjohn)
Tablets gr 2......................... Bottles of 100, 1,000
representing gr 10 fresh gland.

Dosage: 1–3 tablets daily.

Corpus Luteum (Westerfield)

Tablets, Enteric coated, gr 2½.......... Bottles of 100, 500
each grain representing gr 5 fresh gland.

Dosage: 1–2 tablets two to three times daily.

Corpus Luteum Gland (Wyeth)

Ampules 1 cc.......................... Boxes of 6
representing gr 3.
Powder.............................. Bottles of 1, 4 oz.
Tablets gr 2.......................... Bottles of 50, 100

Dosage: Ampule given *intramuscularly* or *subcutaneously*. *Orally:* gr 2–5 three times daily.

Corpus Luteum (Zemmer)

Ampules 1 cc containing gr 3........... Boxes of 6, 25, 100
Capsules gr 2, gr 5.................... Boxes of 100, 1,000
Tablets, Plain or Keratin coated, gr 2, gr 5 Bottles of 100, 1,000
gr 1 representing gr 5 fresh gland.

Dosage: 1–2 capsules or tablets three to four times daily; ampule given *intramuscularly*, as indicated.

---

2. Whole Ovary Preparations

Ovarian Substance (Abbott)

Ampules 1 cc.......................... Boxes of 12, 100
containing soluble constituents of gr 22½ fresh ovary.
Capsules Kerakote gr 5................ Bottles of 100, 500
Tablets Kerakote gr 2½, gr 5.......... Bottles of 100, 500
each 2½ gr representing gr 18¾ fresh ovarian substance.

Dosage: 1 cc intramuscularly every 2 or 3 days. Oral gr 2–5 three times daily.

Ovarian Substance (Armour)

Capsules gr 2.......................... Bottles of 50, 100, 500, 1,000
Capsules gr 5.......................... Bottles of 50, 100, 500
Liquid—Ampules 1 cc................... Boxes of 6, 50, 100
Powder................................ Bottles of 1, 4, 8, 16 oz.
Tablets gr 2.......................... Bottles of 100, 500, 1,000
Tablets gr 5.......................... Bottles of 50, 100, 500

Dosage: 2–5 gr three times daily before period. 1 ampule *intramuscularly* two to three times weekly.

Ovarian Extract (Berwyn)

Ampules 1 cc.......................... Boxes of 12, 100, 500
representing gr 10.
Ampules 1 cc.......................... Boxes of 12, 100, 500
representing gr 31.

Dosage: ½–1 ampule daily, *intramuscularly*.

Ovarian Extract Solution (Breon)

Ampules 1 cc.......................... Boxes of 12, 100
containing gr 40 fresh gland substance with chlorbutanol gr $\frac{1}{12}$.

Dosage: 1 ampule *intramuscularly* every 2–3 days.

Ovarian Substance (Boericke and Tafel)

Capsules gr 5.......................... Bottles of 60
containing gr 2½ ovarian substance.

Dosage: 2 capsules three times daily.

Ovarian Substance (Burroughs Wellcome)
Tabloid Varium gr 5.................. Bottles of 100, 500

Dosage: 1–2 tabloids, increased to 4–5 two to three times daily.

Ovarian Substance (Carnrick, G. W.)
Capsules gr 5........................ Bottles of 50, 100
Powder............................... Bottles of 1 oz.
Tablets gr 1......................... Bottles of 100
Tablets gr 2......................... Bottles of 100, 500
Tablets gr 5......................... Bottles of 50, 100, 500

Dosage: Gr 1–5 three times daily.

Thelygan (Cavendish)
Ampules 1.1 cc....................... Boxes of 12
2.1 cc representing 2 Gm ovary and containing 1 mg yohimbin.
Tablets.............................. Boxes of 40, 100

Dosage: 1 ampule three times weekly. *Orally*, 1 tablet three times daily.

Ovarian Substance (Cheplin)
Ampules 1 cc......................... Boxes of 12
containing soluble substance from gr 40 fresh gland.

Dosage: 1 ampule *intramuscularly*, three times weekly.

Sistomensin (Ciba)
Ampules 1.1 cc }
Tablets gr 1/5 } .... Boxes of 5, 20
representing a lipoidal solution of ovarian hormone.

Dosage: 1–3 tablets three times daily, with 1 ampule three times weekly. *See Chap. I.*

Ovarian Whole (Colwell)
Ampules 1 cc......................... Boxes of 12
representing gr 40 soluble ingredients of fresh gland.
Crinogen............................. Bottles of 1 oz.
5 m representing gr 1 desiccated gland.

Dosage: 1–5 gr (Crinogen); ampules used intramuscularly, three times weekly.

Ovarian (Drug Products)
Capsules gr 1........................ Bottles of 100
representing gr 7½ fresh substance.

Dosage: 1–2 capsules after meals, increased, in accordance.

Ovarian Solution (Drug Products)
Ampuls (Hyposols) 1 cc.............. Boxes of 12, 100
representing gr 40 fresh substance.

Dosage: 1 ampule three to four times weekly, *intramuscularly*.

Ovarian Substance (Glandular Laboratories)
Capsules gr 2........................ Bottles of 25
in physiological salt solution.

Dosage: 1 capsule three times daily.

Endovarin (Harrower)
Ampules 1 cc......................... Boxes of 5
representing gr 23 fresh active ovarian substance.
Tablets gr 2......................... Bottles of 50
representing gr 2 whole ovary with follicular fluid.

Dosage: *Oral*—1–2 tablets three times daily. *Intramuscular*—10 days before menstruation, 1 cc every other day for 3 injections, then 1 cc daily until menstruation.

Ovarian Extract (Harvey-Pittenge

Solution .... "Swab-Seal" Bottles of 6 cc, 15 cc

each cc representing gr 3 dry substance.

Dosage: 1 cc three times weekly.

Ovarian Substance (Harvey Pittenge

Capsules gr 5 .... Bottles of 50, 100, 500, 1,000

Powder .... Bottles of 1, 4, 8 oz., 1 lb.

1 part desiccated substance representing 7 parts fresh gland.

Dosage: 1–10 gr three times daily.

Ovary (Whole) (Hynson, Westcott and Dunning

Ampules 1 cc .... Boxes of 6

representing 0.2 Gm water soluble extract of dry substance.

Powder .... Bottles of 1 oz.

Tablets gr 5 .... Bottles of 50

Dosage: 1 ampule three times weekly, *intramuscularly. Orally,* gr 5 three time daily.

Endo-Ovarian Liquid (Intravenous Products

Ampules 1 cc .... Boxes of 12, 100

representing gr 30 fresh substance.

Dosage: 1 ampule on alternate days, *intramuscularly.*

Ovarian (Lafayette Pharmacal)

Capsules, Enterocap, gr 2, gr 5.

each grain desiccated substance representing 7½ gr fresh gland.

Dosage: Gr 2–5 three times daily.

Ovarian Extract (Lang)

Glycerol extract .... Bottles of ½, 1, 2 oz.

each cc representing 1 Gm fresh gland.

Dosage: 12–30 drops three to four times daily.

Ovary (Whole) (Lederle)

Tablets gr 2½ .... Bottles of 100, 500

Tablets gr 5 .... Bottles of 50, 500

each grain desiccated substance representing gr 6 fresh gland.

Dosage: 1 or more tablets daily.

Ovarian Extract (Lilly)

Ampules 1 cc .... Boxes of 6, 12

representing gr 10 fresh gland.

Ampules 1 cc .... Boxes of 12

representing gr 31 fresh gland.

Dosage: ½–1 ampule three times weekly, *intramuscularly.*

Ovarian Substance (Lilly)

Powder .... Bottles of 1, 4 oz.

Pulvules gr 5 .... Bottles of 100, 500

Tablets gr 2, Plain and Enteric coated ... Bottles of 100

Tablets gr 5, Plain and Chocolate coated Bottles of 100, 500

Tablets gr 5, Enteric coated .... Bottles of 100

each grain desiccated substance representing gr 6 fresh gland.

Dosage: Gr 2–5 three times daily.

(Marvell)

Ovamone (Ovarial Hormone Solution)
Ampules 1 cc.......................... Boxes of 6, 12
representing 25 rat units.
Capsules.......................... Bottles of 50
containing Ovamone 0.06 (desiccated ovarian hormone, 1 Gm standardized to 16½ rat units), ovarian desiccated 0.12.

Dosage: 1 ampule *intramuscularly,* three times weekly. *Orally*—1 capsule three times daily.

(Marvell)

Ovarian Substance
Powdered extract.......................... Bottles of 1 oz., ¼, ½, 1 lb.
Tablets gr 2, gr 5.......................... Bottles of 100

Dosage: Gr 2–5 three times daily.

(Marvell)

Ovowop (Standardized)
Tablets.......................... Boxes of 50
containing 0.15 Gm desiccated ovarian substance and 5 units Ovarialhormon Folliculin Menformon.

Dosage: 1 tablet three times daily.

(Marvell)

Ovarian Solution
Ampules 1 cc.......................... Boxes of 12

Dosage: 1 ampule *intramuscularly,* three times weekly.

(McNeil)

Ovarian Substance Whole
Ampules 1 cc.......................... Boxes of 6, 100
representing gr 23 fresh substance.
Capsules gr 2, gr 5.......................... Bottles of 100, 500
Tablets gr 2.......................... Bottles of 100, 500

Dosage: 2–10 gr three times daily; or 1 cc *intramuscularly* every 2–3 days.

(McNeil)

Ovaracon (Ovarian Solution Concentrated)
Ampules 1 cc.
representing 20 Allen-Doisy rat units.
Ampule-vials 5 cc.
each cc representing 50 Allen-Doisy rat units.

Dosage: 1 cc *intramuscularly,* three times weekly.

(Miller)

Ovarian (Whole)
Capsules gr 2, gr 5.......................... Bottles of 100, 500, 1,000
Powder.......................... Bottles of 1 oz., ¼ lb., 1 lb.
Tablets, Compressed, Chocolate coated or
Enteric coated, gr 5.......................... Bottles of 100, 500, 1,000
1 part desiccated substance representing 6 parts fresh gland.

Dosage: 1 capsule or tablet three times daily.

(Miller)

Ovarian Extract (Whole)
Ampules 1 cc, 2 cc.......................... Boxes of 12, 100
Ampul-vials 30 cc.......................... Packages of 1
each cc representing 25 Allen-Doisy rat units.

Dosage: 1–5 cc *intramuscularly* two to three times weekly.

(National Drug)

Ovarian Extract
Ampules 1 cc.......................... Boxes of 12, 25, 100
Ampule-vials 15 cc, 25 cc.......................... Boxes of 1
each cc representing gr 31 fresh substance.

Dosage: 1 cc *intramuscularly,* daily for 1 week, then on alternate days as indicated.

Ovarian Substance (McNeil)

Capsules gr 1, gr 5.................... Bottles of 100, 500, 1,000
Tablets gr 1, gr 5.................... Bottles of 100, 500, 1,000
each grain desiccated substance representing gr 7 fresh gland.

Dosage: 1–5 capsules or tablets three times daily after meals.

Ovarian Substance (Parke, Davis)

Ampules 1 cc........................ Boxes of 12, 100
representing 0.04 Gm (gr 3/5) entire substance.
Emplets, Enteric coated, gr 5.......... Bottles of 100, 500
Capsules gr 5........................ Bottles of 50, 500
Powder.............................. Bottles of 1 oz., 1/4 lb.
Tablets, Chocolate coated, gr 5.......... Bottles of 100, 500
each grain desiccated substance representing gr 6 fresh gland.

Dosage: Gr 5 daily; or 1 cc *intramuscularly.*

Whole Ovary (Reed and Carnrick)

Powder.............................. Bottles of 1 oz., 1/4 lb., 1 lb.
Tablets, Plain and Enteric coated, gr 2, gr 5. Bottles of 100, 500, 1,000

Dosage: 2–10 gr three times daily.

Ampacoids Ovary (Reed and Carnrick)

Ampacoids 25 Rat Units............... Boxes of 6
representing gr 77 fresh gland.

Dosage: 1 cc three to six times weekly, *subcutaneously* or *intramuscularly.* *See Chap. I.*

Ovarian Substance (Rorer)

Capsules gr 2, gr 5.................... Bottles of 100
Powder.............................. Bottles of 1, 4 oz., 1 lb.
Tablets gr 2......................... Bottles of 100

Dosage: Gr 2–5 three times daily.

Glovarian (Schieffelin)

Pills................................ Bottles of 36
glycerine extract of fresh whole ovaries, each representing gr 2 fresh gland.

Dosage: 1 pill two to three times daily.

Ovarian Nucleoprotein (Schieffelin)

Powder.............................. Bottles of 1/2 oz.
Tablets gr 1......................... Bottles of 100
representing 10% nucleoprotein of entire ovary.

Dosage: 1–2 gr every 3 hr.

Ovarian Substance (Searle)

Tablets, Enteric coated, gr 2, gr 5....... Bottles of 100, 500
each grain desiccated substance representing gr 7½ fresh gland.

Dosage: 1–2 tablets three times daily.

Ovarian Extract (Sharp and Dohme)

Ampules 1 cc........................ Boxes of 12
representing gr 10.
Ampules 1 cc........................ Boxes of 12
representing gr 31.

Dosage: ½–1 ampule *intramuscularly,* three times weekly.

Ovarian Substance Desiccated **(Sharp and Dohme)**
Capsules gr 5 .... Bottles of 100
Powder .... Jars of 1 oz.
Tablets, Plain, Chocolate coated, gr 5.

Dosage: Gr 5, three times daily.

Ovarian Substance **(Smith-Dorsey)**
Tablets, Salol coated, gr 5 .... Bottles of 100

Dosage: 1–2 tablets three times daily.

Ovarian **(Stoddard)**
Tablets gr 2 .... Bottles of 100, 500, 1,000

Dosage: 1 to 3 tablets three times daily.

Ovarian Solution **(Stoddard)**
Ampules 1 cc .... Boxes of 6, 100
representing water soluble ingredients from gr 23 fresh substance; chlorbutanol 0.5 %.

Dosage: 1 cc two to three times weekly, *subcutaneously* or *intramuscularly.*

Ovarian Extract **(United Laboratories)**
Ampules 1 cc .... Boxes of 100

Dosage: 1 cc, *intramuscularly,* three times weekly.

Ovarian Extract **(Upjohn)**
Ampules 1 cc .... Boxes of 12
representing 2 Gm water soluble extract.

Dosage: 1 cc *intramuscularly* every 2 days.

Ovarian Substance **(Upjohn)**
Tablets gr 5 .... Bottles of 100
representing gr 30 fresh substance.

Dosage: 1 tablet three or more times daily.

Ovarian Substance **(Wyeth)**
Ampules 1 cc .... Boxes of 12
representing gr 15 fresh substance.
Powder .... Bottles of 1, 4 oz.
Tablets gr 5 .... Bottles of 100
each grain desiccated substance representing gr 6 fresh gland.

Dosage: 1 ampule *intramuscularly,* three times weekly. Orally, gr 5.

Ovarian **(Westerfield)**
Tablets, Enteric coated, gr 2 .... Bottles of 100, 500

Dosage: 1 tablet three times daily.

Ovarian Substance **(Zemmer)**
Tablets, plain, Keratin coated, gr 2, gr 5 .. Bottles of 100, 1,000
each grain desiccated substance representing gr 8½ fresh gland.

Dosage: 1–3 tablets four times daily.

---

3. Ovarian Residue Preparations

Ovarian Residue **(Armour)**
Capsules gr 2 .... Bottles of 100, 500, 1,000
Capsules gr 5 .... Bottles of 50, 100, 500
Powder .... Bottles of 1, 4, 8, 16 oz.
Tablets gr 2 .... Bottles of 100, 500, 1,000
Tablets gr 5 .... Bottles of 50, 100, 500

Dosage: 5 gr three times daily, beginning 15 days before menstrual period, stopping with onset; additional 5 gr daily may be required.

Ovarian Residue Extract **(Berwyn)**
Ampules 1 cc........................ Boxes of 12, 100, 500
representing gr 31.

Dosage: 1 ampule three times weekly.

Ovarian Residue **(Colwell)**
Ampules 1 cc........................ Boxes of 12
representing soluble ingredients from gr 40 fresh gland.
Crinogen........................ Bottles of 1 oz.
5 m representing gr 1 desiccated gland.

Dosage: 2 to 6 gr (Crinogen); one ampule *intramuscularly*, three times weekly.

Ovarian Residue **(Harvey-Pittenger)**
Capsules gr 5........................ Bottles of 50, 500, 1,000
Powder........................ Bottles of 1, 4, 8 oz., 1 lb.
1 part desiccated substance representing 4 parts fresh gland.

Dosage: 5–10 gr, three times daily.

Ovarian Residue Extract **(Harvey-Pittenger)**
Solution........................ Bottles "Swab-Seal" 6 cc
15 cc
each cc representing gr 3 dried substance.

Dosage: 1 cc *intramuscularly*, three times weekly.

Ovarian Residue **(Hynson, Westcott and Dunning)**
Ampules 1 cc........................ Boxes of 6
representing 0.2 Gm water soluble extract of dry substance.
Powder........................ Bottles of 1 oz.
Tablets, uncoated, gr 5........................ Tubes of 50

Dosage: 1 cc every 2 days for 5–6 doses. *Oral*—gr 5 three times daily.

Ovarian Residue **(Lang)**
Glycerol extract........................ Bottles of ½, 1, 2 oz.
each cc representing 1 Gm fresh gland.

Dosage: 12–30 drops three to four times daily after meals.

Ovarian Residue **(Lederle)**
Tablets gr 3........................ Bottles of 100
representing approximately 15 gr fresh substance.

Dosage: 1 or more tablets daily.

Ovarian Residue **(Lilly)**
Powder........................ Bottles of 1, 4 oz.
Pulvules gr 5........................ Boxes of 50, 500
Tablets, Plain, gr 5........................ Bottles of 50, 500
Tablets, Enteric coated, gr 5........................ Bottles of 100, 500
each gr representing gr 6 fresh gland.

Dosage: Gr 5 three times daily.

Ovarian Residue Extract **(Lilly)**
Ampules 1 cc........................ Boxes of 12
representing gr 31 fresh gland.

Dosage: 1 ampule *intramuscularly*, three times weekly.

Ovarian Residue **(McNeil)**
Ampules 1 cc........................ Boxes of 6, 100
representing 40 gr fresh residue.
Capsules gr 2, gr 5........................ Bottles of 100, 500

Dosage: 2–6 gr three times daily; or 1 cc *intramuscularly*, daily.

Ovarian Residue Extract (Miller)
Ampules 1 cc, 2 cc.................... Boxes of 12, 100
Ampules 5 cc.......................... Boxes of 6, 50
Ampule-vials 30 cc.................... Packages of 1
each cc representing 25 rat units (Allen-Doisy).

Dosage: 1–5 cc two to three times weekly.

Ovarian Residue (Miller)
Capsules gr 5......................... Bottles of 100, 500, 1,000
Powder................................ Bottles of 1 oz., ¼, 1 lb.
Tablets gr 5, Compressed, Chocolate coated, or Enteric coated............ Bottles of 100, 500, 1,000
1 part desiccated substance representing 6 parts fresh gland.

Dosage: 5 gr three times daily.

Ovarian Residue (Parke, Davis)
Ampules 1 cc.......................... Boxes of 12, 100
representing gr ¾ soluble extract ovarian residue; chloretone 0.5%.
Capsules gr 5......................... Bottles of 50, 500
Emplets, Enteric coated, gr 5........... Bottles of 100, 500
Powder................................ Bottles of 1 oz., ¼ lb.
Tablets, Compressed, gr 5.............. Bottles of 50, 500
containing follicular hormone, each grain representing gr 6 fresh ovarian residue.

Dosage: 5–20 gr; or 1 cc *intramuscularly* daily.

Ovarian Residue (Reed and Carnrick)
Powder................................ Bottles of 1 oz., ¼, 1 lb.
Tablets, Plain and Enteric coated, gr 5... Bottles of 100, 500, 1,000

Dosage: Gr 2–10 three times daily.

Ovarian Residue (Schieffelin)
Solution.............................. Bottles of ½ oz.
slightly hydrolized extract of standard N content.

Dosage: 10–15 drops three times daily.

Glystitial (Schieffelin)
Pills................................. Bottles of 36
glycerine extract of interstitial cells, representing gr 2 fresh substance.

Dosage: 1 pill two to three times daily.

Ovarian Residue Extract (Sharp and Dohme)
Ampules 1 cc.......................... Boxes of 12
representing gr 31.

Dosage: 1 ampule *intramuscularly*, three times weekly.

---

4. Follicular Preparations

Thelestrin (Carnrick, G. W.)
Ampules 1 cc.......................... Boxes of 6
each cc represents 25 Allen-Doisy units, ovarian follicular hormone.

Dosage: 1–2 ampules daily. *See Chap. I.*

Ovarialhormon Folliculin Menformon (Colwell)
Crinogen Ampules 1 cc.................. Boxes of 12
representing per cc 40 mouse units.

Dosage: ½–2 ampules, daily for 30 injections. *See Chap. I.*

Ovarialhormon Folliculin Menformon **(Kretschmar)**
Dragees 100 units.................... Packages of 10, 25
Ampules 1 cc........................ Boxes of 3
each cc containing 40 mouse units of ovarian follicular hormone.

Dosage: 1–2 ampules daily for 30 doses. *See Chap. I.*

Ovarialhormon Folliculin Menformon **(Marvell)**
Ampules 1 cc........................ Boxes of 3
Representing 100 mouse units.

Dosage: ½–2 ampules. *See Chap. I.*

Estrogen **(Parke, Davis)**
Ampules 1 cc........................ Boxes of 6
representing 25 rat units of follicular hormone, in colloidal suspension.

Dosage: 1–2 cc *intramuscularly*, daily for 6–8 days.

Theelin **(Parke, Davis)**
Ampules 1 cc........................ Boxes of 6, 100
Suppositories........................ Boxes of 6
each representing 50 rat units ovarian follicular hormone.

Dosage: 1–2 ampules and 1 suppository daily. *See Chap. I.*

Theelol **(Parke, Davis)**
Kapseals............................ Bottles of 20
representing 50 rat units of ovarian follicular hormone.

Dosage: 1–3 kapseals daily, in intervals between Theelin therapy. *See Chap. I.*

Amniotin **(Squibb)**
Vials 5 cc (oral)
representing 2,000 rat units.
Vials 10 cc (hypodermic)
representing 500 rat units.
Pessaries........................... Packages of 6 and 12
representing 75 rat units of ovarian follicular hormone.

Dosage: 1 cc two or three times weekly, or 10 drops (oral) twice daily, or 3 pessaries weekly. *See Chap. I.*

PANCREAS PRODUCTS

Description: Pancreas preparations are available as powdered extracts, as liquids and as 2 hormone products, Padutin and Panocrin. Those prepared from the whole organ contain mostly excretory glandular elements with their enzymes, trypsin, amylopsin and steapsin, and less of the incretory part; those from the splenic portion contain more of the Langerhans antidiabetic principle, Insulin, Iletin.

Action and Uses: Pancreas products assist the digestive function of the gastro-intestinal tract and are helpful as supplement in insulin therapy of diabetics; *For use* in carbohydrate indigestion, pancreatic insufficiency, in digestive disturbances of diabetes; in hyperthyroidism and diabetes mellitus. Insulin products are used in the treatment of diabetes mellitus and its complications.

Dosage: In accordance with preparation.

Preparations

Islands of Langerhans **(Abbott)**
Capsules, Kerakote, gr 5................ Bottles of 100, 500

Dosage: 1–3 capsules before meals.

Pancreas Substance **(Abbott)**
Powder.............................. Bottles of 1, 4, 8, 16 oz.
Tablets gr 2.......................... Bottles of 100, 500, 1,000

Dosage: Gr 2, three times daily.

Islands of Langerhans **(Boericke and Tafel)**
Capsules gr 5......................... Bottles of 60
containing gr 2½ pancreas tail.

Dosage: 1 capsule three times daily before meals, gradually increased to 10 or 15 gr.

Pancreatin **(Boericke and Tafel)**
Capsules gr 5......................... Bottles of 60

Dosage: 1 capsule three times daily, gradually increased to 2 capsules three times daily.

Pancreas Substance **(Carnrick, G. W.)**
Capsules gr 5......................... Bottles of 100
Powder.............................. Bottles of 1 oz.
Tablets gr 2.......................... Bottles of 100, 500
Tablets gr 5.......................... Bottles of 50

Dosage: 2–5 gr three times daily.

Pancreatin (U.S.P.) **(Carnrick, G. W.)**
Powder.............................. Bottles of 1 oz.

Dosage: Gr 2–5 three times daily.

Pancreatin and Soda **(Carnrick, G. W.)**
Tablets.............................. Bottles of 100, 500, 1,000

Dosage: 1 tablet three times daily.

Pancreas Substance **(Glandular Laboratories)**
Capsules gr 1......................... Bottles of 25
in physiological salt.

Dosage: 1 capsule three times daily.

Pancreas **(Lafayette Pharmacal)**
Enterocaps, gr 2, gr 5.................. Bottles of 100
each grain desiccated substance representing gr 5 fresh gland.

Dosage: Gr 2–5 three times daily.

Pancreatin (U.S.P.) **(Lafayette Pharmacal)**
Enterocaps, gr 2, gr 5.................. Bottles of 100

Dosage: Gr 2–5 three times daily.

Pancreas Extract **(Lang)**
Glycerol extract .... Bottles of 2, 8 oz., 1 pt.
each cc representing 1 Gm fresh gland.

Dosage: 15–60 drops three to four times daily.

Iletin **(Lilly)**
Vials 5 cc
containing 10, 20, 40 units per cc.
Vials 10 cc
containing 10, 20, 40, 80 units per cc.

Dosage: *Subcutaneously,* as required. *See Chap. I.*

Islands of Langerhans **(Maltbie)**
Tablets, Enteric coated, gr 5........... Bottles of 100, 1,000

Dosage: 5 gr before meals, gradually increased to 10 or 15 gr.

Islands of Langerhans **(Marvell)**
Powdered extract...................... Bottles of 1 oz., ¼ lb.

Pancreas Substance (Marvell)
Powdered extract.................... Bottles of 1 oz., ¼, ½, 1 lb.
Dosage: Gr 2–5 three times daily.

I-lan-glans (McNeil)
Capsules gr 5........................ Bottles of 100, 500
Dosage: 1 capsule three times daily before meals, for 2 weeks.

Pancreas Substance (Miller)
Powder............................. Bottles of 1 oz., ¼, 1 lb.
1 part representing 5 parts fresh gland.
Dosage: Gr 2–5 three times daily.

Pancreatic Extract (Miller)
Ampules 1 cc.......................... Boxes of 12, 100
representing gr 30 fresh tissue.
Dosage: 1 cc *intramuscularly* two to three times weekly.

Pancreatin (U.S.P.) (Miller)
Powder............................. Bottles of 1 oz., ¼, 1 lb.
Tablets gr 5........................ Bottles of 100, 500, 1,000
Dosage: Gr 5 three times daily.

Pancreas (Reed and Carnrick)
Powder............................. Bottles of 1 oz., ¼, 1 lb.
Tablets, Enteric coated without sugar or starch........................... Bottles of 100, 500, 1,000
Dosage: Gr 2 and upward, three times daily.

Panacoids (Reed and Carnrick)
Tablets gr 2......................... Bottles of 100, 500, 1,000
Dosage: 1 tablet three times daily.

Islands of Langerhans (Searle)
Capsules gr 5........................ Bottles of 100, 500
Tablets, Enteric coated, gr 5............ Bottles of 100, 500
Intesti-sols, Enteric coated.............. Bottles of 100, 500
Dosage: 1 capsule or tablet or 2 pills (Intesti-sols) three times daily before meals.

Insulin (Sharp and Dohme)
Vials 5 cc
containing 10, 20 and 40 units per cc.
Dosage: *See Chap. I.*

Pancreatin (U.S.P.) (Sharp and Dohme)
Powder............................. Bottles of 1 oz., 1 lb.
Dosage: Gr 2–5 three times daily.

Pancrasin (Smith-Dorsey)
Capsules............................ Boxes of 100
representing ½ rabbit unit Insulin.
Dosage: 1–3 capsules before meals.

Insulin (Squibb)
Vials 5 cc
containing 10, 20, 40 units per cc.
Vials 10 cc
containing 10, 20, 40, 80, 100 units per cc.
Dosage: *See Chap. I.*

Insulin **(Stearns)**
Vials 5 cc
containing 10, 20, 40 units per cc.
Vials 10 cc
containing 100 units per cc.

Dosage: *See Chap. I.*

Pancreo Cauda **(Stoddard)**
Tablets gr 4........................ Bottles of 100, 500, 1,000

Dosage: 1–3 tablets three to four times daily.

Pancreatin **(Stoddard)**
Tablets gr 5........................ Bottles of 100

Dosage: 1 tablet three times daily.

Pancreatin, Pure (U.S.P.) **(Wyeth)**
Powder............................ Vials of 1 oz., Bottles of 4 oz., 1 lb.

Dosage: Gr 2–5 three times daily.

PARATHYROID PRODUCTS

Description: These preparations are made from parathyroid gland; each grain of the desiccated product represents from 8–10 gr of fresh glandular substance; they are available in solid form, in solution and as pure principles: Parathyrin, Paroidin and Parathormone, all physiologically standardized.

Action and Uses: The parathyroid gland is the principal regulator of calcium metabolism; it also assists in the coagulation of blood and prevents accumulation in the organism of toxic products of the amino acid type (methylguanidin) affecting the central and myoneural nervous systems. *Used* in hypocalcemia, tetany, paralysis agitans, puerperal convulsions, epilepsy, muscle irritability and spasticity; also in pulmonary and other hemorrhages, in varicose and skin ulceration; in dermatologic affections and allergic states.

Dosage: In accordance with preparation.

Preparations

Parathyrin **(Abbott)**
Ampules 1 cc........................ Boxes of 6, 100
representing gr $\frac{1}{10}$ desiccated substance.

Dosage: 1 ampule twice daily, *intramuscularly.*

Parathyroid Substance **(Armour)**
Powder............................ Vials of 1 dr.
Tablets gr $\frac{1}{20}$, gr $\frac{1}{10}$.................. Bottles of 100, 500, 1,000

Dosage: Gr $\frac{1}{20}$–$\frac{1}{10}$ three times daily.

Parathyroid Substance and Calcium Lactate **(Armour)**
Tablets............................ Bottles of 100, 1,000
containing parathyroid gr $\frac{1}{20}$, calcium lactate gr $2\frac{1}{2}$.

Dosage: 1 tablet three times daily.

Parathyroid **(Boericke and Tafel)**
Capsules gr 5........................ Bottles of 60

Dosage: 1 capsule two times daily.

Parathyroid (Burroughs Wellcome)
Tabloids gr 2/3........................ Bottles of 25, 100
containing gr 1/10 parathyroid, desiccated.

Dosage: 1–2 tabloids two to three times daily ½ hr. before meals.

Parathyroid Substance (Carnrick, G. W.)
Powder............................ Bottles of 1/8 oz.
Tablets gr 1/20...................... Bottles of 100, 500, 1,000
Tablets gr 1/10...................... Bottles of 100

Dosage: Gr 1/20–1/10 three times daily.

Parathyroid (Colwell)
Crinogen.......................... Bottles of 1 oz.
5 m representing gr 1/20 desiccated gland.

Dosage: 5 m, *intramuscularly*, daily.

Parathyroid Solution (Colwell)
Ampules 1 cc....................... Boxes of 12
representing gr 2 fresh gland.

Dosage: *Used intramuscularly* 1 cc three to four times weekly.

Parathyroid (Drug Products)
Capsules gr 1/10..................... Bottles of 100
representing gr 4/5 fresh gland.

Dosage: 1 capsule one to two times daily.

Parathyroid Substance (Glandular Laboratories)
Capsules gr 1/10..................... Bottles of 25
in physiological salt.

Dosage: 1 capsule three times daily.

Paracalcin (Harrower)
Tablets............................ Bottles of 50
representing gr 1 parathyroid, or 1 unit.

Dosage: 1 tablet three times daily.

Paracalcin Solution (Harrower)
Ampules 1 cc....................... Boxes of 5
representing 10 units.

Dosage: 1 cc *intramuscularly* every 2 days.

Endo-Paradin (Intravenous Products)
Ampules 1 cc....................... Boxes of 12, 100
representing gr 0.6 fresh substance.

Dosage: 1 ampule twice weekly, *subcutaneously*.

Parathyroid (Lafayette Pharmacal)
Enterocaps, gr 1/20, gr 1/10............. Bottles of 100
each grain desiccated substance representing gr 10 fresh gland.

Parathyroid Extract (Lang)
Glycerol extract...................... Bottles of ½, 1, 2 oz.
each cc representing 1 Gm fresh gland.

Dosage: 6–10 drops three to four times daily.

Parathyroid (Lilly)
Powder............................ Bottles of 1/8 oz.
Tablets gr 1/10, 1/20.................. Bottles of 100
Tablets, plain, Enteric coated, gr 1/10.... Bottles of 100, 500
each grain representing gr 10 fresh gland.

Dosage: 1/40–1/10 gr, three times daily.

Para-thor-mone (Lilly)
Ampules 1 cc........................ Boxes of 6
Vials 5 cc.
each cc representing 20 units.

Dosage: 20–60 units daily, as required. *See Chap. I.*

Parathyroid Solution (Marvell)
Ampules 1 cc........................ Boxes of 12
representing equivalent of gr 2 fresh gland.

Dosage: 1 ampule *intramuscularly,* three to four times weekly.

Parathyroid Substance (Marvell)
Powdered extract..................... Bottles of 1/8, 1 oz.
Tablets gr 1/20, 1/10..................... Bottles of 100

Dosage: Gr 1/20–1/10 three times daily.

Parathyroid Gland (McNeil)
Capsules, Enteric coated, gr 1/10........ Bottles of 100, 500
Tablets, Enteric coated, gr 1/10.......... Bottles of 100, 500

Dosage: 1 capsule or tablet one to two times daily.

Parathyroid (Miller)
Powder............................. Vials 1/8 oz., 1 oz.
Tablets gr 1/20, 1/10..................... Bottles of 100, 1,000
1 part desiccated substance representing 10 parts fresh gland.

Dosage: Children—gr 1/20 three times daily; Adults—gr 1/10 three times daily.

Parathyroid (National Drug)
Tablets gr 1/20, gr 1/10.................. Bottles of 100, 500, 1,000
each grain representing gr 6 fresh gland.

Dosage: 1 tablet three times daily.

Parathyroidin Solution (National Drug)
Ampules 1 cc........................ Boxes of 6, 12, 25, 100
representing 0.2 Gm fresh gland.

Dosage: 1 ampule *intramuscularly,* three times weekly.

Parathyroid (Parke, Davis)
Emplets, Enteric coated, gr 1/10........ Bottles of 100, 500
Tablets, compressed, gr 1/10............ Bottles of 100, 500
representing gr 1 fresh substance.

Dosage: 1 emplet or tablet one to two times daily.

Paroidin (Parke, Davis)
Bottles 5 cc......................... Cartons of 1
each cc representing 150 Hanson units.

Dosage: 30–60 units every 12 hr. for 5–6 days. *See Chap. I.*

Parathyroid (Reed and Carnrick)
Powder............................. Bottles of 1/8, 1 oz., 1/4, 1 lb.
Tablets, plain, Enteric coated, gr 1/10.... Bottles of 100, 500, 1,000

Dosage: 1 tablet three times daily.

Parathyroid with Calcium Lactate (Reed and Carnrick)
Tablets............................. Bottles of 100, 500, 1,000

Dosage: 1 tablet three times daily.

Parathyroid (Rorer)
Capsules gr 1/10...................... Bottles of 100
Powder............................. Bottles of 1/8 oz.
Tablets gr 1/10....................... Bottles of 100

Dosage: Gr 1/10 three times daily.

Paraglythoid **(Schieffelin)**
Pills.................................. Bottles of 25
each containing 5 m glycerine extract, representing gr 1 fresh gland.
Dosage: 1–2 pills every 4 hr.

Parathyroid Nucleoprotein **(Schieffelin)**
Tablets gr 1.......................... Bottles of 25
containing 5% dry nucleoprotein.
Dosage: 1 tablet every 2–4 hr.

Parathyroid **(Sharp and Dohme)**
Tablets gr 1/10........................ Bottles of 100
representing gr 3/5 fresh gland.
Dosage: Gr 1/10 three times daily.

Parathyroid Hormone **(Squibb)**
Vials 5 cc, 100 units
each cc contains 20 units.
Dosage: 10–30 units daily, as required.

Parathyroid **(Zemmer)**
Tablets, Plain, Keratin coated, gr 1/10.... Bottles of 100, 1,000
each grain representing gr 8 fresh gland.
Dosage: 1 tablet twice daily.

PINEAL PRODUCTS

Description: Are prepared from pineal glands of young cattle and believed to affect the somatic sexual development, and to exercise an auxiliary control over bodily and mental progress.

Action and Uses: Helpful in cases of mental retardation and sexual disturbances in children, in infantilism; also used experimentally in behavior disorders in infancy.

Dosage: 1/10 gr.

Preparations

Pineal Substance **(Armour)**
Powder.................................. Vials of 1 dr.
Tablets gr 1/20........................ Bottles of 100, 500, 1,000
Dosage: Gr 1/20, three times daily.

Pineal Gland **(Boericke and Tafel)**
Capsules gr 5.......................... Bottles of 60
containing gr 1/20 pineal gland.
Dosage: 1 capsule three times daily.

Pineal Substance **(Carnrick, G. W.)**
Powder.................................. Bottles of 1/8 oz.
Tablets gr 1/10........................ Bottles of 100, 500, 1,000
Dosage: gr 1/10 three times daily.

Pineal Substance **(Glandular Laboratories)**
Capsules gr 1/10....................... Bottles of 25
in physiological salt.
Dosage: 1 capsule three times daily.

Pineal **(Lafayette Pharmacal)**
Capsules, Enteric coated, gr ½, gr 1..... Bottles of 100
each grain desiccated substance representing gr 10 fresh gland.
Dosage: Gr ½–1 three times daily.

Pineal Extract **(Lang)**
Glycerol extract...................... Bottles of ½, 1, 2 oz.
1 cc representing 1 Gm fresh gland.
Dosage: 6–10 drops three to four times daily.

Pineal **(Lilly)**
Tablets gr ½ .... Bottles of 100
Tablets, enteric coated, gr 1/10.......... Bottles of 100, 500
each grain desiccated substance representing gr 6 fresh gland.
Dosage: ½ gr three times daily.

Pineal **(National Drug)**
Tablets gr 1/10....................... Bottles of 100, 500, 1,000
representing gr ⅗ fresh gland.
Dosage: 1 tablet three times daily.

Pineal Gland **(Parke, Davis)**
Emplets, Enteric coated, gr 1/10......... Bottles of 100, 500
Tablets, triturate, gr 1/10............... Bottles of 100
representing gr ⅗ fresh gland.
Dosage: 1 emplet or tablet three times daily.

Pineal **(Reed and Carnrick)**
Powder.............................. Bottles of ⅛, 1 oz., ¼, 1 lb.
Tablets, plain, Enteric coated, gr 1/10.... Bottles of 100, 500, 1,000
Dosage: gr 1/10–⅕ three times daily.

Pineal Substance **(Zemmer)**
Tablets gr ½........................ Bottles of 100, 1,000
each grain representing gr 5 fresh tissue.
Dosage: 1 tablet three times daily.

PITUITARY GLAND PRODUCTS

1. Anterior Pituitary

Description: The products of the anterior portion of the pituitary gland are available in powdered form and as active principles, Prolan and Tethelin.

Action and Uses: Contains a growth promoting hormone, affecting skeletal and male sexual development; a gonadotrope hormone, supplying a female sex principle with luteinizing and estrogenic, follicle stimulating properties; and a calorigenic hormone, influencing the thyroid. Is *used* in retarded physical growth and dwarfism; in sexual underdevelopment and infantilism; in dystrophia adiposogenitalis; in pituitary epilepsy, mental defects, late stages of acromegaly; in delayed puberty, amenorrhea and other forms of menstrual disturbances of pituitary origin.

Dosage: In accordance with preparation.

Preparations

Pituitary (Anterior) **(Abbott)**
Capsules, Kerakote, gr 2½............ Bottles of 100, 500
representing gr 15 fresh gland.
Dosage: 1 or more capsules after each meal.

Pituitary Substance (Anterior) **(Armour)**
Liquid—Ampules 1 cc.................. Boxes of 6, 50, 100
Powder.............................. Bottles of 1, 4, 8, 16 oz.
Tablets gr 2, gr 5.................... Bottles of 50, 100, 500, 1,000

Dosage: gr 2–5 three times daily. 1 ampule *intramuscularly,* three times weekly.

Pituitary Anterior Lobe **(Berwyn)**
Ampules 1 cc.......................... Boxes of 6, 100, 500

Dosage: 1 ampule *intramuscularly,* three times weekly.

Pituitary Solution Anterior **(Breon)**
Ampules 1 cc.......................... Boxes of 6, 100
representing gr 18.5 of gland with chlorbutanol gr 1/12.

Dosage: 1 cc every 1–2 days, *intramuscularly* and *intravenously.*

Pituitary Gland (Anterior) **(Burroughs Wellcome)**
Tabloid gr 2.......................... Bottles of 100, 500

Dosage: 1–2 tabloids three to four times daily after meals, increased as required.

Pituitary (Anterior) **(Carnrick, G. W.)**
Powder.............................. Bottles of 1/8, 1 oz.
Tablets gr 1/2, gr 1, gr 2............... Bottles of 50, 100, 500, 1,000

Dosage: gr 1/2–2 three times daily.

Anteri-Cole **(Cole)**
Ampules 5 cc, 15 cc................... Boxes of 6
each cc representing 100 mouse units.

Dosage: 1 cc once or twice daily for 8–10 days following menses. *See Chap. I.*

Pituitary (Anterior) **(Colwell)**
Ampules 1 cc.......................... Boxes of 12
representing gr 18.5 fresh gland.
Solution............................. Bottles of 1 oz.
5 m representing gr 1 desiccated gland.

Dosage: 1–3 gr (solution) 1 ampule used *intramuscularly,* daily.

Pituitary (Anterior) **(Glandular Laboratories)**
Capsules gr 1......................... Bottles of 25
in physiological salt.

Dosage: 1 capsule three times daily.

Apestrin Solution **(Harrower)**
Ampules 1 cc.......................... Boxes of 5
anterior pituitary estrin.

Dosage: 1 cc daily or every other day.

Pituitary (Anterior) **(Harvey-Pittenger)**
Capsules gr 5......................... Bottles of 50, 500, 1,000
Powder.............................. Bottles of 1, 4, 8, 16 oz.
1 part desiccated substance representing 5 parts fresh gland.

Dosage: 1–10 gr three times daily.

Endo-Pituitary Liquid (Anterior) **(Intravenous Products)**
Ampules 1 cc.......................... Boxes of 12, 100.

Dosage: 1 ampule *intramuscularly,* three to four times weekly.

Pituitary Anterior **(Lafayette Pharmacal)**
Enterocaps, gr 2, gr 5................. Bottles of 100
each grain desiccated substance representing gr 6 fresh gland.

Dosage: Gr 2–5 three times daily.

Pituitary Extract (Anterior) (Lang)
Glycerol extract..................... Bottles of ½, 1, 2 oz.
each cc representing 1 Gm fresh gland.

Dosage: 6–8 drops three to four times daily.

Pituitary Anterior (Lederle)
Tablets gr 2, gr 5.................... Bottles of 100

Dosage: 15–30 gr daily.

Pituitary (Anterior) (Lilly)
Powder............................. Bottles of 1, 4 oz.
Tablets, Plain, Enteric coated, gr 2½... Bottles of 50, 100, 500
Tablets, gr 5......................... Bottles of 50, 100, 500
each grain desiccated substance representing gr 5 fresh gland.

Dosage: 2–5 gr three times daily.

Anterior Pituitary Sex Hormone Solution (Marvell)
Vials 5 cc (sterile)................... Cartons of 1
each cc representing 60 mouse units (Aschheim-Zondek).

Dosage: Two 1 cc injections daily for 4–5 days.

Pituitary Substance (Anterior Lobe) (Marvell)
Powdered extract...................... Bottles of 1 oz.
Tablets gr 2.......................... Bottles of 100

Dosage: gr 2 three times daily.

Pituitary Solution (Anterior) (Marvell)
Ampules 1 cc.......................... Boxes of 12
representing extraction from 18.5 gr fresh gland.

Dosage: 1 ampule *intramuscularly,* three to four times weekly.

Pituitary Anterior (McNeil)
Capsules, Enteric coated, gr 2........... Bottles of 100, 500
Tablets, Enteric coated, gr 2............ Bottles of 100, 500

Dosage: 1–2 capsules or tablets three to four times daily.

Pituitary Sex Hormone Solution (McNeil)
Ampule-vials 5 cc.................... Cartons of 1
each cc representing 100 Aschheim-Zondek mouse units.

Dosage: 1 cc *intramuscularly,* three to four times weekly.

Pituitary Extract (Anterior) (Miller)
Ampules 1 cc.......................... Boxes of 12, 100
Ampule-vials 30 cc.................. Cartons of 1
each cc representing gr 45 fresh gland.

Dosage: 1 cc *intramuscularly* two to three times weekly.

Pituitary (Anterior) (Miller)
Capsules gr 3, gr 5.................... Bottles of 100, 1,000
Powder............................... Bottles of 1 oz., ¼, 1 lb.
Tablets gr 2½......................... Bottles of 100, 1,000
Tablets, compressed, Chocolate coated or
Enteric coated, gr 5.................. Bottles of 100, 1,000
1 part desiccated powder representing 5 parts fresh gland.

Dosage: 1 capsule or tablet three times daily.

Pituitary (Anterior) (National Drug)
Tablets gr 1.......................... Bottles of 100, 500, 1,000
representing gr 5 fresh gland.

Dosage: 1–4 tablets three to four times daily between meals.

Pituitary Extract (Anterior) **(National Drug)**
Ampules 1 cc........................ Boxes of 6, 12, 25, 100
representing 1.2 Gm fresh gland.

Dosage: 1 cc *intramuscularly*, three to four times weekly.

Pituitary (Anterior) **(Parke, Davis)**
Powder.............................. Bottles of 1 oz., ¼ lb.
Emplets, Enteric coated, gr 2½, gr 5.... Bottles of 100, 500
Tablets gr 2½, gr 5.................. Bottles of 50, 100, 500
each grain desiccated substance representing gr 5 fresh gland.

Dosage: 5–10 gr daily.

Antuitrin-S **(Parke, Davis)**
Vials 10 cc.......................... Packages of 1
each cc representing 100 rat units.

Dosage: 50–200 units daily. *See Chap. I.*

Pituitary (Anterior) **(Reed and Carnrick)**
Powder.............................. Bottles of 1 oz., ¼, 1 lb.
Tablets, plain, Enteric coated, gr 2, gr 5.. Bottles of 100, 500, 1,000

Dosage: 2–10 gr three times daily.

Pituitary Substance (Anterior) **(Rorer)**
Capsules gr 2......................... Bottles of 100
Powder.............................. Bottles of 1 oz.
Tablets gr 2......................... Bottles of 100

Dosage: gr 2 three times daily.

Follutein **(Squibb)**
Vials of 1,250 rat units.
each cc containing 250 rat units.

Dosage: 750–1,250 units daily. *See Chap. I.*

Pituitary Sex Hormone Solution (Anterior Lobe) **(Stoddard)**
Ampules 5 cc........................ Boxes of 1
each cc representing 100 mouse units (maturing and luteinizing hormones).

Dosage: 1 cc, *intramuscularly* three to four times weekly.

Antophysin **(Winthrop)**
Ampules............................. Boxes of 5
representing 100 rat units.

Dosage: 100–300 units daily. *See Chap. I.*

Pituitary (Anterior) **(Wyeth)**
Powder.............................. Bottles of 1, 4 oz.
each grain desiccated substance representing gr 5 fresh gland.

Dosage: gr 2, three times daily.

Pituitary Substance (Anterior) **(Zemmer)**
Tablets, Plain, Keratin coated, gr 2...... Bottles of 100, 1,000
each grain representing gr 5 fresh gland.

Dosage: 1–3 tablets three times daily.

---

2. Posterior Pituitary

Description: Most preparations are in liquid form for hypodermic use; few are powdered for oral use. Also available as hormones: Pituitrin, Infundin, Pitocin, Pitressin, Pituitary liquid.

Action and Uses: Contains pressor, oxytocic and diuretic principles; stimulates non-striated musculature of various organs; controls sexual development in the female and regulates menstrual function; affects carbohydrate metabolism; is galactogogue and most reliable oxytocic. *Used* pharmacologically in numerous instances: in shock to raise arterial blood pressure, in infections, sudden heart failure; in inertia uteri and hemorrhage; in enuresis, polyuria, anuria, diabetes insipidus; in tympanites, intestinal atony and paresis.

Dosage: In accordance with preparation.

Preparations

Pituitary Solution (U.S.P. Obstetrical) **(Abbott)**
Ampules ½ cc, 1 cc.................... Boxes of 6, 100

Dosage: ⅕–2 cc, repeated cautiously as necessary, *subcutaneously*. *See Chap. I.*

Pituitary Solution (Surgical, Double U.S.P. Strength) **(Abbott)**
Ampules 1 cc........................ Boxes of 6, 100

Dosage: ½–1 cc *intramuscularly* immediately after operation; repeated as required. *See Chap. I.*

Pituitary Liquid **(Armour)**
Ampules 0.5, 1 cc (Obstetrical)......... Boxes of 6, 50 and 100
Ampules 1 cc (Surgical)............... Boxes of 6, 50 and 100
Ampules 1 cc (Surgical and Obstetrical). Boxes of 6, 50 and 100

Dosage: 0.5–2 cc as necessary. *See Chap. I.*

Pituitary Substance (Posterior) **(Armour)**
Powder............................ Bottles of 1 dr.
Tablets gr 1/10....................... Bottles of 100, 500, 1,000

Dosage: Gr 1/10 three times daily.

Pituitary Extract U.S.P. Obstetrical **(Berwyn)**
Ampules ½ cc, 1 cc.................... Boxes of 6, 100, 500

Pituitary Extract Surgical (Double U.S.P. Strength) **(Berwyn)**
Ampules 1 cc........................ Boxes of 6, 100, 500

Dosage: ¼–1 cc according to the occasion, *intramuscularly*. *See Chap. I.*

Pituitary Extract (Obstetrical) **(Breon)**
Ampules ½ cc, 1 cc.................... Boxes of 6, 100
with chlorbutanol gr 1/12.

Dosage: ⅕–2 cc, *intramuscularly*, according to the occasion. *See Chap. I.*

Pituitary Extract (Surgical, Double Strength) **(Breon)**
Ampules 1 cc........................ Boxes of 6, 100

Dosage: ½–1 cc immediately after or 4 hr. after operation as indicated, *intramuscularly*. *See Chap. I.*

Pituitary Gland **(Burroughs Wellcome)**
Tabloid gr ½........................ Bottles of 100, 500

Dosage: 1–2 tabloids, increased, three to four times daily after meals.

Infundin **(Burroughs Wellcome)**
Hypoloids ½ cc, 1 cc.................. Boxes of 6, 100
5 I.U. per cc.
Hypoloids ½ cc, 1 cc.................. Boxes of 6, 100
10 I.U. per cc.

Dosage: ½–1 cc *intramuscularly*, according to the occasion.

Pituitary Posterior (U.S.P.) **(Carnrick, G. W.)**
Powder........ Bottles of 1/8 oz.
Tablets gr 1/10, gr 1/2........ Bottles of 100, 500, 1,000
Dosage: Gr 1/10–1/2 three times daily.

Pituitary Posterior (Obstetrical) **(Carnrick, G. W.)**
Ampules 1/2 cc, 1 cc........ Boxes of 6
Dosage: 1/2–1 cc *intramuscularly*, according to the occasion.

Pituitary Posterior (Surgical) **(Carnrick, G. W.)**
Ampules 1 cc........ Boxes of 6
Dosage: 1/2–1 cc *intramuscularly*, according to the occasion.

Pituitary Solution Obstetrical (U.S.P.X.) **(Colwell)**
Ampules 1 cc........ Boxes of 12
Dosage: *Use intramuscularly*, 1 cc according to the occasion. *See Chap. I.*

Pituitary Solution Surgical (Double U.S.P. Strength) **(Colwell)**
Ampules 1 cc........ Boxes of 12
Dosage: *Use intramuscularly*, 1 cc according to the occasion. *See Chap. I.*

Pituitary Solution U.S.P. (Surgical and Obstetrical) **(Drug Products)**
Ampuls (Hyposols) 1/2 cc, 1 cc........ Boxes of 12, 100
10 units per cc.
Dosage: 1/2–1 cc *intramuscularly*, according to the occasion. *See Chap. I.*

Pituitary Solution (Surgical) **(Drug Products)**
Ampuls 1 cc........ Boxes of 12, 100
20 units.
Dosage: 1/2–1 cc *intramuscularly*, according to the occasion. *See Chap. I.*

Liquor Pituitary U.S.P. (Obstetrical) **(Harrower)**
Ampules 1 cc........ Boxes of 5
10 I.U.
Dosage: 1/2–1 cc *intramuscularly*, according to the occasion. *See Chap. I.*

Pituitary Extract (Posterior) **(Harvey-Pittenger)**
Solution........ Bottles "Swab-Seal" 6 cc, 15 cc
Dosage: 1 cc *intramuscularly*, according to the occasion. *See Chap. I.*

Endo-Pituitary Liquid (Obstetrical) **(Intravenous Products)**
Ampules 1/2 cc, 1 cc........ Boxes of 12, 100
Dosage: 1/5–2 cc, repeated cautiously as necessary, *intramuscularly.*

Endo-Pituitary Liquid (Surgical, Double Strength) **(Intravenous Products)**
Ampules 1 cc........ Boxes of 12, 100
Dosage: 1/2–1 cc as required, *intramuscularly.*

Pituitary Posterior **(Lafayette Pharmacal)**
Enterocaps, gr 1/10, gr 1/5.
each grain desiccated substance representing gr 6 fresh gland.
Dosage: Gr 1/10–1/5 three times daily.

Pituitary Extract (Posterior) **(Lang)**
Glycerol extract........ Bottles of 1/2, 1, 2 oz.
each cc representing 1 Gm fresh gland.
Dosage: 6–8 drops three to four times daily. *See Chap. I.*

Pituitary Extract (Lederle)
Ampules 1 cc........................ Boxes of 6, 100
representing 5, 10 or 20 units.

Dosage: 20 units every 4–6 hr. *See Chap. I.*

Pituitary Posterior (Lederle)
Tablets gr 1/10........................ Bottles of 100

Dosage: 1/10–1/2 gr three times daily.

Pituitary Posterior (Lilly)
Powder........................ Vials 1 dr.
Tablets, Plain, Enteric coated, gr 1/10.... Bottles of 100, 500
each grain representing 6 gr fresh gland.

Dosage: Gr 1/10 three times daily.

Pituitary Extract U.S.P. (Obstetrical) (Lilly)
Ampules 1/2 cc, 1 cc.................. Boxes of 6

Dosage: 1/2–1 cc; repeated in 1/2–1 hr. if necessary, *intramuscularly.*

Pituitary Extract (Surgical, Double U.S.P. Strength) (Lilly)
Ampules 1/2 cc, 1 cc.................. Boxes of 6

Dosage: 1/2–1 cc; repeated in 1/2–1 hr. if necessary, *intramuscularly.* *See Chap. I.*

Pituitary Posterior (McNeil)
Ampules 1/2 cc, 1 cc, 10 cc.............. Boxes of 6

Dosage: 1/2–1 cc *intramuscularly*, as required.

Pituitary Extract Obstetrical (U.S.P.X.) (Miller)
Ampules 1 cc........................ Boxes of 12, 100
Ampule-vials 30 cc.................... Packages of 1
each cc representing 10 I.U.

Dosage: 1/2–1 cc *intramuscularly*, according to the occasion.

Pituitary Extract Surgical (Double U.S.P. Strength) (Miller)
Ampules 1 cc........................ Boxes of 12, 100
Ampule-vials 30 cc.................... Packages of 1
each cc representing 20 I.U.

Dosage: 1/2–1 cc *intramuscularly*, according to the occasion.

Pituitary Posterior (Miller)
Powder........................ Vials of 1/8 oz.—Bottles of 1 oz.
1 part desiccated substance representing 6 parts fresh gland.

Dosage: Gr 1/10–1/2 three times daily.

Pituitary Extract (U.S.P.) (National Drug)
Ampule-vials 15 cc, 25 cc.............. Packages of 1
each cc representing 10 I.U.

Dosage: 1/4–1 cc according to the occasion, *intramuscularly.*

Pituitary Liquor U.S.P. (Obstetrical) (National Drug)
Ampules 1/2 cc, 1 cc.................. Boxes of 6, 12, 25, 100
each cc representing 10 I.U.

Dosage: 1/4–1 cc according to the occasion, *intramuscularly.*

Pituitary Posterior (National Drug)
Tablets gr 1/10........................ Bottles of 100, 500, 1,000
each grain desiccated substance representing gr 5 fresh gland.

Dosage: Gr 1/10 three times daily.

Pituitary Posterior (Parke, Davis)
Emplets, gr 1/10 .... Bottles of 100, 500
Tablets, Compressed, gr 1/10 .... Bottles of 100, 500
representing gr 3/5 fresh substance.
Dosage: 4–8 emplets or tablets daily.

Pitocin (Parke, Davis)
Ampules 0.5 cc, 1 cc .... Boxes of 6 and 100
Dosage: 3–8 m every 30 min. *See Chap. I.*

Pitressin (Parke, Davis)
Ampules 1 cc .... Boxes of 6, 100
Nasal Jelly .... Tubes of 3 Gm, Boxes of 6 tubes
Dosage: 3–5 m as necessary. *See Chap. I.*

Pituitrin (Parke, Davis)
Ampules 0.5 cc, 1 cc (obstetrical) .... Boxes of 6, 100
Ampules 1 cc (surgical) .... Boxes of 6, 100
Dosage: 8–15 m as required. *See Chap. I.*

Pituitary Posterior (Reed and Carnrick)
Powder .... Bottles of 1/8, 1 oz., 1/4, 1 lb.
Tablets, plain, Enteric coated, gr 1 .... Bottles of 100, 500, 1,000
Dosage: gr 1/10–1/2 three times daily.

Pituitary Extract Obstetrical (Rorer)
Ampules 1/2 cc, 1 cc .... Boxes of 6, 12, 100
Dosage: 1/5–2 cc as indicated. *See Chap. I.*

Pituitary Substance (Rorer)
Powder .... Bottles of 1/8 oz.
Dosage: Gr 1/10 three times daily.

Pituitary Solution (Posterior and Middle Lobe) (Searle)
Ampules 1/2 cc, 1 cc .... Boxes of 12, 25, 100
Dosage: *Use subcutaneously* or *intramuscularly* 1/2–1 cc, according to the occasion.

Pituitary Extract (Obstetrical) (Sharp and Dohme)
Ampules 1/2 cc, 1 cc .... Boxes of 6
Dosage: 1/2–1 cc *intramuscularly*, according to the occasion. *See Chap. I.*

Pituitary Extract (Surgical, Double Strength) (Sharp and Dohme)
Ampules 1 cc .... Boxes of 6
Dosage: 1/2–1 cc *intramuscularly*, according to the occasion.

Pituitary Extract (Obstetrical) (Sherman)
Ampules 1/2 cc, 1 cc .... Boxes of 6, 100
Dosage: 1/2–1 cc *intramuscularly*, according to the occasion. *See Chap I.*

Pituitary Extract (Surgical) (Sherman)
Ampules 1 cc .... Boxes of 6, 100
Dosage: 1/2–1 cc *intramuscularly*, according to the occasion.

Pituitary Solution (Squibb)
Ampules 1 cc .... Boxes of 6, 100
containing 5, 10 or 20 units.
Dosage: 3–30 units every 1/2–1 hr. *See Chap. I.*

Pituitary Solution U.S.P. **(Stoddard)**
Ampules ½ cc, 1 cc.................... Boxes of 6, 100
water soluble ingredients, with chlorbutanol 0.5%.

Dosage: ½–1 cc *subcutaneously* or *intramuscularly*, according to the occasion. *See Chap. I.*

Pitamin (Obstetrical) Pituitary Extract **(Upjohn)**
Ampules ½ cc, 1 cc.................... Boxes of 6

Dosage: ½–1 cc according to the occasion, *intramuscularly*.

Pitamin (Surgical, Double Strength) **(Upjohn)**
Ampules 1 cc.......................... Boxes of 6

Dosage: ½–1 cc *intramuscularly*, according to the occasion.

Pituitary Extract (Obstetrical) **(Wyeth)**
Ampules ½ cc, 1 cc.................... Boxes of 6

Dosage: In labor—¼–1 cc; in surgery—1–2 cc postoperatively, *intramuscularly*. *See Chap. I.*

Pituitary Extract (Infundibular) **(Zemmer)**
Ampules ½ cc, 1 cc.................... Boxes of 6, 25, 100

Dosage: 1 cc *intramuscularly*, in severe shock intravenously.

Pituitary Substance **(Zemmer)**
Tablets, Plain, Keratin coated, gr 1/10.... Bottles of 100, 1,000
each grain desiccated substance representing gr 5 fresh gland.

Dosage: 1 tablet three times daily.

---

3. Whole Pituitary

Description: Pituitary whole gland preparations are obtained from both lobes and are available mostly as desiccated extracts, representing about 1 part of the extract to 5 parts of fresh gland; also obtainable in liquid form for oral and hypodermic administration.

Action and Uses: Those of the anterior and posterior parts combined; also influences libido and hair growth; *used* in hypopituitarism, adiposogenitalism, infantilism, pituitary obesity and in some cases of Graves' disease; also in enuresis, lethargy, somnolence, stupor and dullness of hypopituitary origin.

Dosage: In accordance with preparation.

Preparations

Pituitary (Whole) **(Abbott)**
Capsules Kerakote, gr 2½.............. Bottles of 100, 500
representing gr 12½ fresh pituitary substance.

Dosage: 1–2 capsules after each meal.

Pituitary Liquid **(Armour)**
Ampules 1 cc.......................... Boxes of 6, 50, 100

Dosage: 1 ampule *intramuscularly*, three to four times weekly.

Pituitary Substance **(Armour)**
Powder................................ Bottles of 1, 4, 8, 16 oz.
Tablets gr 1, gr 2.................... Bottles of 100, 500, 1,000

Dosage: Gr 1–2 three times daily.

Pituitary (Whole) **(Boericke and Tafel)**
Capsules gr 5........................ Bottles of 60
containing gr 2½ pituitary gland.

Dosage: 1 capsule two times daily.

Pituitary (Whole) **(Burroughs Wellcome)**
Hypoloids 1 cc, representing gr ⅙........ Bottles of 100, 500
Hupoloids 1 cc, representing gr ⅓....... Bottles of 100, 500
Tabloids gr ½, 1, 2.................... Bottles of 100, 500

Dosage: ½–1 cc *intramuscularly,* three to four times weekly. Orally: gr ½–2 three times daily.

Pituitary (Whole) **(Carnrick, G. W.)**
Powder............................. Bottles of ⅛, 1 oz.
Tablets gr ½, 1, 2.................... Bottles of 50, 100, 500

Dosage: Gr ½–2 three times daily.

Pituitary (Whole) **(Colwell)**
Ampules 1 cc........................ Boxes of 12
representing gr 15.43 whole gland.
Crinogen........................... Bottles of 1 oz.
5 m representing gr 1 desiccated gland.

Dosage: 1–2 gr (Crinogen) three times daily; ampules used *intramuscularly* 1 cc three times weekly.

Pituitary (Whole) **(Glandular Laboratories)**
Capsules gr ¼........................ Bottles of 25
in physiological salt.

Dosage: 1 capsule three to six times daily.

Pituitary Substance (Whole) **(Harvey-Pittenger)**
Capsules gr 1........................ Bottles of 100, 500, 1,000
Powder............................. Bottles of 1, 4, 8, 16 oz.
1 part desiccated substance representing 5 parts fresh gland.

Dosage: 1–2 gr three times daily.

Pituitary (Whole) **(Lafayette Pharmacal)**
Enterocaps, gr ½, gr 1 .... Bottles of 100
each grain desiccated substance representing gr 5 fresh gland.

Dosage: Gr ½–1 three times daily.

Pituitary Extract (Whole) **(Lang)**
Glycerol extract of fresh gland.......... Bottles of ½, 1, 2 oz.
each cc representing 1 Gm fresh gland.

Dosage: 6–8 drops three to four times daily.

Pituitary Whole **(Lederle)**
Tablets gr 1, gr 3.................... Bottles of 100

Dosage: 2–6 gr daily.

Pituitary Whole **(Lilly)**
Powder............................. Bottles of 1, 4 oz.
Tablets, plain, Enteric coated, gr 1...... Bottles of 100, 500
each grain desiccated substance representing gr 5 fresh gland.

Dosage: Gr 1 three times daily.

Pituitary Solution **(Marvell)**
Ampules 1 cc........................ Boxes of 12
representing extraction from 15.43 gr fresh gland.

Dosage: 1 cc intramuscularly, three times weekly.

Pituitary Substance (Marvell)
Powdered extract...................... Bottles of 1 oz.
Tablets gr 1.......................... Bottles of 100

Dosage: Gr 1 three times daily.

Pituitary Whole (McNeil)
Capsules, Enteric coated, gr ½......... Bottles of 100, 500
Tablets, Enteric coated, gr ½.......... Bottles of 100, 500

Dosage: 1–4 capsules or tablets three to four times daily.

Pituitary (Whole) (Miller)
Capsules gr 2½, gr 5.................. Bottles of 100, 1,000
Powder............................. Bottles of 1 oz., ¼, 1 lb.
Tablets gr 1, gr 2½.................. Bottles of 100, 1,000
Tablets, Compressed, Chocolate coated or
Enteric coated, gr 5.................. Bottles of 100, 1,000
1 part desiccated substance representing 5 parts fresh gland.

Dosage: 1 capsule or tablet three times daily.

Pituitary (Whole) (National Drug)
Tablets gr ½......................... Bottles of 100, 500, 1,000
each grain representing gr 5 fresh gland.

Dosage: 1–4 tablets three times daily.

Pituitary (Whole) (Parke, Davis)
Emplets, Enteric coated, gr 1.......... Bottles of 100, 500.
Powder............................. Bottles of 1 oz., ¼ lb.
Tablets gr 1......................... Bottles of 100, 300
representing gr 5 fresh gland.

Dosage: 1–4 gr three times daily.

Pituitary (Whole) (Reed and Carnrick)
Powder............................. Bottles of 1 oz., ¼ lb., 1 lb.
Tablets, Plain, Enteric coated, gr 1...... Bottles of 100, 500, 1,000

Dosage: 1–2 gr three times daily.

Pituitary Substance (Whole) (Rorer)
Capsules gr 1........................ Bottles of 100
Powder............................. Bottles of 1 oz.

Dosage: Gr 1 three times daily.

Glytuitary (Schieffelin)
Pills................................ Bottles of 50
each 5 m of glycerine extract equivalent to gr 1 fresh gland.

Dosage: 1 pill three to four times daily.

Pituitary Nucleoprotein (Schieffelin)
Tablets gr 1......................... Bottles of 100
containing 10% dry nucleoprotein.

Dosage: 1–2 tablets every 3 hr.

Pituitary Substance (Whole) (Searle)
Capsules, desiccated, gr ½............. Bottles of 100, 500
each grain representing about 5 gr fresh gland.

Dosage: 1–2 capsules three times daily.

Pituitary Body, Whole Gland (Sharp and Dohme)
Powder............................. Bottles of 1 oz., ¼ lb.
each grain desiccated substance representing gr 5 fresh gland.

Dosage: Gr 1⁄10–½ three times daily.

Pituitary Extract (Whole) **(United Laboratories)**
Solution.............................. Bottles of 15 cc, 50 cc
each cc representing gr 5 whole gland.

Dosage: 1 cc *intramuscularly*, three to four times weekly.

Pituitary (Whole) **(Wyeth)**
Powder.............................. Bottles of 1, 4 oz.
each grain desiccated substance representing gr 5 fresh gland.

Dosage: Gr ½–1 three times daily.

Pituitary Substance **(Zemmer)**
Tablets, Plain, Keratin coated, gr 1/10.... Bottles of 100, 1,000
each grain desiccated substance representing gr 5 fresh gland.

Dosage: 1 tablet three times daily.

PLACENTAL PRODUCTS

Description: Are available as powdered extracts only; the placenta is thought to contain 3 hormones: Emmenin, with estrogenic qualities; Estrin, and an antero-pituitary-like principle effective in menorrhagia and metrorrhagia.

Action: Is believed to exercise a restraining effect on ovulation and post-pituitary activity; is related to mammary gland hyperplasia during gestation, and to affect the quality and quantity of milk secreted.

Uses: Mainly as galactogogue; in hyperemesis gravidarum to catabolize placental protein waste products; in nursing mothers—to increase growth of their infants; in dysmenorrhea, menorrhagia and metrorrhagia; to regulate flow during nursing period.

Dosage: In accordance with preparation.

Preparations

Placental Substance **(Armour)**
Powder.............................. Bottles of 1, 4, 8, 16 oz.
Tablets gr 5.............................. Bottles of 50, 100

Dosage: 5 gr three times daily at meal time.

Placenta **(Boericke and Tafel)**
Capsules gr 5.............................. Bottles of 60

Dosage: 2 capsules three times daily.

Placenta Substance **(Carnrick, G. W.)**
Capsules gr 5.............................. Bottles of 50, 100
Powder.............................. Bottles of 1 oz.
Tablets gr 3.............................. Bottles of 100, 500, 1,000

Dosage: Gr 3–5 three times daily.

Placenta **(Colwell)**
Crinogen.............................. Bottles of 1 oz.
5 m representing gr 1 desiccated gland.

Dosage: 2–3 gr three times daily.

Placenta Substance **(Colwell)**
Powder.............................. Bottles of 1, 4, 8, 16 oz.
Tablets gr 5.............................. Bottles of 50, 500
1 part desiccated substance representing 5 parts fresh gland.

Dosage: Gr 5 three times daily.

Plestrin Solution **(Harrower)**

Ampules 1 cc representing 50 units..... Boxes of 5
Capsules gr 5 representing 5 units...... Boxes of 40

Dosage: 1 ampule daily ***intramuscularly*** and 1–3 capsules three times daily as supplement.

Placental **(Lafayette Pharmacal)**

Enterocaps, gr 2, gr 5.................. Bottles of 100
each grain desiccated substance representing gr 8 fresh gland.

Dosage: Gr 2–5 three times daily.

Placenta Extract **(Lang)**

Glycerol extract...................... Bottles of ½, 1, 2 oz.
each cc representing 1 Gm fresh gland.

Dosage: 10–60 drops three to four times daily.

Placenta **(Lilly)**

Powder............................. Bottles of 1, 4 oz.
Pulvules gr 5......................... Bottles of 100, 500
Tablets, Enteric coated, gr 5............ Bottles of 100, 500
each grain desiccated substance representing gr 6 fresh gland.

Dosage: Gr 5 three times daily.

Placenta **(Marvell)**

Powdered extract...................... Bottles of 1 oz., ¼ lb., 1 lb.

Dosage: Gr 2–5 three times daily.

Placenta **(Miller)**

Capsules gr 5......................... Bottles of 100, 1,000
Powder............................. Bottles of 1 oz., ¼, 1 lb.
Tablets, Chocolate coated, Enteric coated,
gr 5................................ Bottles of 100, 1,000
1 part desiccated substance representing 7 parts fresh gland.

Dosage: 5 gr three to four times daily.

Placenta Extract **(Miller)**

Ampules 1 cc, 2 cc.................... Boxes of 12, 100
Ampules 5 cc......................... Boxes of 6, 50
each cc containing 25 rat units (Allen-Doisy).

Dosage: 1–5 cc two to three times weekly *intramuscularly.*

Placenta **(Parke, Davis)**

Capsules gr 5......................... Bottles of 100, 500
Emplets, Enteric coated, gr 5.......... Bottles of 100, 500
Powder............................. Bottles of 1 oz., ¼ lb.
each grain representing gr 6 fresh substance.

Dosage: 5 gr three times daily.

Placenta Substance **(Zemmer)**

Tablets, Plain, Keratin coated, gr 5...... Bottles of 100, 1,000

Dosage: 1 tablet three times daily after meals.

PROSTATE PREPARATIONS

Description: Are used as homostimulant to prostate and sex glands; as sedative in prostatic irritability; in testicular atrophy after prostatectomy; in prostatic hypertrophy with pollakiuria and impotence.

Dosage: In accordance with preparation.

Prostate Substance (Armour)
Powder.............................. Bottles of 1, 4, 8, 16 oz.
Tablets gr 2.......................... Bottles of 100, 500, 1,000

Dosage: Gr 2 three times daily.

Prostate Gland (Boericke and Tafel)
Capsules gr 5.......................... Bottles of 60

Dosage: 2 capsules three times daily.

Prostate Gland Substance (Burroughs Wellcome)
Tabloid gr 2½.......................... Bottles of 100, 500

Dosage: 1 tablet three to four times daily.

Prostate Substance (Carnrick, G. W.)
Capsules gr 3.......................... Bottles of 100
Powder.............................. Bottles of 1 oz.
Tablets gr 2.......................... Bottles of 100, 500, 1,000

Dosage: Gr 2–5 three times daily.

Prostate (Colwell)
Crinogen.............................. Bottles of 1 oz.
5 m representing gr 1 desiccated gland.

Dosage: 4–5 gr three times daily.

Prostate Substance (Glandular Laboratories)
Capsules gr 1.......................... Bottles of 25
in physiological salt.

Dosage: 1 capsule three times daily.

Prostate (Lafayette Pharmacal)
Enterocaps, gr 2, gr 5....................Bottles of 100
each grain desiccated substance representing gr 8 fresh gland.

Dosage: Gr 2–5 three times daily.

Prostate Extract (Lang)
Glycerol extract of fresh gland............ Bottles of 2, 8, 16 oz.
each cc representing 1 Gm fresh gland.

Dosage: 15–60 drops three or four times daily after meals.

Prostate Substance (Marvell)
Powdered extract....................... Bottles of 1 oz., ¼, ½, 1 lb.
Tablets gr 2.......................... Bottles of 100

Dosage: Gr 2 three times daily.

Prostate (Miller)
Capsules gr 5.......................... Bottles of 100, 1,000
Powder.............................. Bottles of 1 oz., ¼, 1 lb.
Tablets, Chocolate coated, Enteric coated,
gr 5.................................. Bottles of 100, 1,000
1 part desiccated substance representing 6 parts fresh gland.

Dosage: 5 gr three to four times daily.

Prostate Extract (Miller)
Ampules 1 cc, 2 cc...................... Boxes of 12, 100
Ampules 5 cc.......................... Boxes of 6, 50
Ampule-vials 30 cc...................... Packages of 1

Dosage: 1–5 cc *intramuscularly* two to three times weekly.

Prostate (National Drug)
Tablets gr 2.......................... Bottles of 100, 500, 1,000
each grain representing gr 7 fresh gland.

Dosage: 1–3 tablets three to four times daily.

Prostate (Reed and Carnrick)

Ampacoids 1 cc........................ Boxes of 6
representing sterile aqueous solution of prostatic hormone equivalent to gr 10.

Dosage: 1 cc *subcutaneously* or *intramuscularly*, three to six times weekly, or more as required.

Prostate Substance (Rorer)

Capsules gr 2........................ Bottles of 100
Powder........................ Bottles of 1 oz.
Tablets gr 2........................ Bottles of 100

Dosage: Gr 2 three times daily.

Prostate Substance (Zemmer)

Tablets gr 5........................ Bottles of 100, 1,000
each grain representing gr 6 fresh gland.

Dosage: 1 tablet three times daily after meals.

SPLEEN PREPARATIONS

Description: Are available as dried extracts from fresh animal spleens.

Action: Are stated to stimulate leucocytogenesis, to influence metabolism of calcium and other minerals and to favorably affect skin nutrition.

Uses: In splenomegalia, malaria and trypanosomiasis; in disturbances accompanied by eosinophilia; eczema, urticaria, asthma and other allergic states.

Dosage: As per preparation required.

Spleen Liquid (40%, 150%) (Armour)

Ampules 2 cc, 5 cc........................ Boxes of 12, 50

Dosage: 2 cc *intramuscularly*, three to four times weekly.

Spleen Substance (Armour)

Capsules gr 5........................ Bottles of 50, 500
Powder........................ Bottles of 1, 4, 8, 16 oz.
Tablets gr 1........................ Bottles of 100, 500, 1,000

Dosage: 2–4 gr every 3–4 hr.

Spleen (Boericke and Tafel)

Capsules gr 5........................ Bottles of 60

Dosage: 1 capsule three times daily.

Spleen Substance (Burroughs Wellcome)

Tabloid gr 5........................ Bottles of 100, 500

Dosage: 1–4 tabloids three to four times daily after meals.

Spleen Substance (Carnrick, G. W.)

Capsules gr 5........................ Bottles of 100
Powder........................ Bottles of 1 oz.
Tablets gr 3........................ Bottles of 100, 500, 1,000

Dosage: Gr 3–5 three times daily.

Splenocrin Solution (Harrower)

Ampules 1 cc........................ Boxes of 5
Vials 20 cc........................ Cartons of 1
containing the active fraction from the spleen.

Dosage: 2–20 cc *intramuscularly*, three to five times weekly.

Spleen **(Lafayette Pharmacal)**
Enterocaps, gr 2, gr 5.................. Bottles of 100
each grain desiccated substance representing gr 5½ fresh gland.

Dosage: Gr 2–5 three times daily.

Spleen Extract **(Lang)**
Glycerol extract of fresh gland.......... Bottles of 2, 8 oz., 1 pt.
each cc representing 1 Gm fresh gland.

Dosage: 10–60 drops three to four times daily.

Spleen Substance **(Miller)**
Capsules gr 5......................... Bottles of 100, 1,000
Powder.............................. Bottles of 1 oz., ¼, 1 lb.
Tablets, Compressed, Chocolate coated or
Enteric coated, gr 5.................... Bottles of 100, 1,000
1 part desiccated substance representing 5 parts fresh gland.

Dosage: 15–25 gr before meals.

Spleen Extract **(Miller)**
Ampules 1 cc, 2 cc.................... Boxes of 12, 100
Ampule-vials 30 cc.................. Packages of 1

Dosage: 1–2 cc two to three times weekly, *intramuscularly*.

Spleen Substance **(Rorer)**
Capsules gr 5......................... Bottles of 100
Powder.............................. Bottles of 1 oz.
Tablets, Chocolate coated, Enteric coated,
gr 5................................ Bottles of 100, 1,000
1 part desiccated substance representing 5 parts fresh gland.

Dosage: 15–25 gr after meals.

Spleen Extract **(United Laboratories)**
Ampules 2 cc......................... Boxes of 6, 12, 24, 100

Dosage: 2 cc *intramuscularly*, three to four times weekly.

Spleen Substance **(Zemmer)**
Tablets gr 5......................... Bottles of 100, 1,000
each grain representing gr 8 fresh gland.

Dosage: 1–3 tablets four times daily.

TESTICULAR PRODUCTS

Description: Orchic products are usually prepared from the whole testicle, the spermatogenic and interstitial portions, and are concentrated, 1 part of extract representing 10 parts of fresh glandular substance; some preparations contain Leydig tissue only.

Action and Uses: Contains apparently several hormones which have not been isolated, with the exception of perhaps one. Is known to control development of the male sexual characteristics at maturity; of pelvis, hair, genitals and libido; to determine the mental and physical status of the male; promote sexual desire and activity; influence metabolic exchange. *Used* in hypogonadism, impotence, avirilism, asexualism; in premature senility, chronic prostatitis and dementia praecox.

Dosage: 2–5 gr.

Preparations

Orchic Substance **(Abbott)**
Ampules 1 cc........................ Boxes of 6, 100
containing gr ⅓ soluble fresh testis solids; chlorbutanol 0.5 %.
Dosage: 1 cc daily for several days, *intramuscularly.*

Orchic Substance **(Armour)**
Powder............................. Bottles of 1, 4, 8, 16 oz.
Tablets gr 2......................... Bottles of 100, 500, 1,000
Dosage: Gr 2 three times daily.

Testicles **(Boericke and Tafel)**
Capsules gr 5........................ Bottles of 60
Dosage: 1 capsule four times daily.

Orchic Extract Solution **(Breon)**
Ampules 1 cc........................ Boxes of 12, 100
containing gr 55 fresh gland substance, chlorbutanol gr 1/12.
Dosage: 1 ampule *intramuscularly,* on alternate days.

Didymin **(Burroughs Wellcome)**
Tabloids gr 5........................ Bottles of 100, 500
representing gr 5 orchitic substance.
Dosage: 1–4 tabloids three to four times daily, after meals.

Testogan **(Cavendish)**
Ampules 1 cc........................ Boxes of 12
representing 4 Gm fresh testicle, and containing 1 mg Yohimbin, 2.1 cc.
Tablets............................. Boxes of 40, 100
representing 4 Gm fresh testicle; Yohimbin 6 mg.
Dosage: 3–4 tablets orally, or 1 cc *intramuscularly,* daily.

Orchic Substance **(Carnrick, G. W.)**
Capsules gr 5........................ Bottles of 100
Powder............................. Bottles of 1 oz.
Tablets gr 2......................... Bottles of 100, 500
Dosage: Gr 2–5 three times daily.

Orchic (Testicular) **(Colwell)**
Ampules 1 cc........................ Boxes of 12
representing gr 27½ fresh substance.
Crinogen............................ Bottles of 1 oz.
5 m representing gr 1 desiccated gland.
Dosage: 1–3 gr (Crinogen) or 1 ampule *intramuscularly,* daily.

Orchic (Special Concentration) **(Colwell)**
Ampules 1 cc........................ Boxes of 12
representing water soluble active hormone from gr 60 fresh testicular substance.
Solution............................ Bottles of 1 oz.
1 m representing 1 gr desiccated gland, 1 cc representing gr 60 fresh testicular substance.
Dosage: 5–10 gr (solution) or 1 ampule *intramuscularly,* daily.

Orchic Solution **(Drug Products)**
Ampules (Hyposols) 1 cc.............. Boxes of 12, 100
containing gr 0.33 soluble orchic solids of fresh testicular substance.
Dosage: 1 ampule *intramuscularly,* three to five times weekly.

Orchic Substance (Glandular)

Capsules gr 2........................ Bottles of 25
in physiological salt.

Dosage: 1 capsule three times daily.

Lydin (Harrower)

Capsules............................ Boxes of 40
5 gr representing active principle from gr 108 fresh Leydig cells.
Solution—Ampules 1 cc................ Boxes of 5
representing 100 Gm fresh interstitial cells of Leydig of bovine testes.

Dosage: 1–2 capsules at meals and at bedtime; or 1 ampule *intramuscularly,* every 1–2 days.

Orchic Substance (Harvey-Pittenger)

Capsules gr 2........................ Bottles of 100, 500, 1,000
Powder............................... Bottles of 1, 4, 8 oz., 1 lb.
1 part desiccated substance representing 10 parts fresh gland.

Dosage: 2–4 gr three times daily.

Endo-Orchic Liquid (Intravenous Products)

Ampules 1 cc......................... Boxes of 12, 100
representing gr 2⅓ fresh orchic substance.

Dosage: 1 ampule twice weekly, *intramuscularly.*

Orchic (Lafayette Pharmacal)

Enterocaps, gr 2, gr 5................ Bottles of 100
each grain desiccated substance representing 8 gr fresh gland.

Dosage: Gr 2–5 three times daily.

Orchic Extract (Lang)

Glycerol extract of fresh gland.......... Bottles of 1, 4, 8 oz., 1 pt.

Dosage: 25–60 drops three to four times daily after meals.

Orchic Substance (Lilly)

Powder............................... Bottles of 1, 4 oz.
Tablets, Plain and Enteric coated, gr 5.. Bottles of 100, 500
each grain representing gr 7 fresh gland.

Dosage: 2–10 gr three times daily.

Orchic Substance (Marvell)

Powdered extract...................... Bottles of 1 oz., ¼, ½, 1 lb.
Tablets gr 2.......................... Bottles of 100

Dosage: Gr 2 three times daily.

Orchiben Concentrate (Standardized) (Marvell)

Ampules 1 cc.......................... Boxes of 6

Dosage: 1 cc *intramuscularly,* three to five times weekly.

Orchiben Solution (Marvell)

Ampules 1 cc, representing gr 55 fresh substance........................... Boxes of 12

Dosage: 1 cc *intramuscularly,* three to five times weekly

Testempco (Marvell)

Tablets 0.01.......................... Boxes of 100

Dosage: 1 tablet three times daily.

Testempco Solution (Marvell)

Ampules 1 cc.......................... Boxes of 12
representing gr 27½ fresh testicle.

Dosage: 1 cc *intramuscularly* every 2 days.

Orchic Substance (McNeil)

Capsules, Enteric coated, gr 5........... Bottles of 100, 500
Tablets, Enteric coated, gr 5............ Bottles of 100, 500
Solution—Ampules 1 cc................ Boxes of 6, 100
each cc representing gr 27½ fresh substance.

Dosage: 1 cc *intramuscularly*, every 2–3 days; *orally*—1 capsule or tablet three times daily.

Orcon (Concentrated Solution) (McNeil)

Ampule-vials 5 cc..................... Cartons of 1
each cc representing 227 Gm fresh tissue.
Capsules (pink)...................... Bottles of 100, 500
representing gr 70 fresh tissue.

Dosage: 1–2 capsules; or 1 cc *intramuscularly* every 2 days.

Orchic (Testicular) (Miller)

Capsules gr 2, gr 5..................... Bottles of 100, 500, 1,000
Powder.............................. Bottles of 1 oz., ¼, 1 lb.
Tablets, Compressed, gr 5.............. Bottles of 100, 500, 1,000
Tablets, Enteric coated, gr 5............ Bottles of 100, 500, 1,000
1 part desiccated substance representing 7 parts fresh interstitial testis.

Dosage: 1 capsule or tablet three times daily.

Orchic Extract (Testicular) (Miller)

Ampules 1 cc, 2 cc.................... Boxes of 12, 100
Ampules 5 cc......................... Boxes of 6, 50
Ampule-vials 30 cc................... Packages of 1
each cc representing 55 gr fresh gland.

Dosage: 1–5 cc *intramuscularly*, two to three times weekly.

Orchic Extract (Testicular) (Special Strength) (Miller)

Ampules 1 cc, 2 cc.................... Boxes of 12, 100
Ampules 5 cc......................... Boxes of 6, 50
Ampule-vials 30 cc................... Packages of 1
each cc representing 75 gr fresh interstitial cells of Leydig.

Dosage: 1–5 cc two to three times weekly.

Orchic Substance (National Drug)

Tablets gr 2......................... Bottles of 100, 500, 1,000
each grain representing gr 10 fresh testes.

Dosage: 1–2 tablets three times daily.

Orchic Extract (National Drug)

Ampules 1 cc.
Ampule-vials 25 cc.
each cc representing gr 15 fresh substance.

Dosage: 1 cc, three to five times weekly.

Orchic Substance (Parke, Davis)

Emplets, Enteric coated, gr 5.......... Bottles of 100, 500
Powder.............................. Bottles of 1 oz, ¼ lb.
Tablets, Compressed, gr 5.............. Bottles of 100, 500
each grain representing gr 7 fresh substance.

Dosage: 5–10 gr three times daily.

Ampacoids Testicle (Reed and Carnrick)

Ampacoids 1 cc....................... Boxes of 6
representing gr 30 fresh gland.

Dosage: 1 cc *subcutaneously* or *intramuscularly*, three times daily.

Orchic Substance **(Rorer)**
Capsules gr 2........................ Bottles of 100
Powder.............................. Bottles of 1 oz.
Tablets gr 2......................... Bottles of 100

Dosage: Gr 2 three times daily.

Gleydig **(Schieffelin)**
Pills............................... Bottles of 36
each representing gr 2 fresh glycerine extract of interstitial cells substance.

Dosage: 1 pill two to three times daily.

Orchic Substance Soluble Extract **(Sherman)**
Ampules 1 cc........................ Boxes of 6, 100
containing gr 1/3.

Dosage: 1 cc *intramuscularly*, three to four times weekly.

Orchic Substance **(Searle)**
Tablets, Enteric coated, gr 5............ Bottles of 100, 500
each grain representing gr 9 fresh gland.

Dosage: 1–2 tablets three times daily.

Orchic Solution **(Stoddard)**
Ampules 1 cc........................ Boxes of 6, 100
representing water soluble ingredients of gr 27½ fresh substance; chlorbutanol 0.5%.

Dosage: 1 cc two to three times weekly, *subcutaneously* or *intramuscularly*.

Liporcin **(Stoddard)**
Tablets gr 5......................... Bottles of 100, 500, 1,000
lipoidal extract of testicular substance.

Dosage: 1–2 tablets three times daily.

Orchitic Extract (Heavy Concentrated) **(United Laboratories)**
Ampules 2 cc........................ Boxes of 6, 12, 24, 100
Ampules 5 cc........................ Boxes of 6, 12, 24

Dosage: 2 cc intramuscularly, three times weekly.

Orchic Substance **(Zemmer)**
Tablets, plain and keratin coated........ Bottles of 100, 1,000

Dosage: 1 tablet three to four times daily.

THYMUS PREPARATIONS

Description: Are desiccated products of thymus gland of young animals; concentrated, each grain to represent about 6–8 gr of fresh thymus substance.

Action: Is believed to aid physical and mental development during childhood; to prevent precocious sex development; to influence mineral metabolism (calcium and phosphorus).

Uses: In combination with other endocrines in menorrhagia and metrorrhagia; in calcium demineralization; in osteoarthritis and especially fragilitas ossium; in rickets, chorea, laryngismus stridulus and hemophilia; lately has been advocated in uterine inertia in combination with pituitary substances.

Dosage: 2–5 gr.

Preparations

Thymus Substance (Armour)

Capsules gr 5........................ Bottles of 50, 500
Powder.............................. Bottles of 1, 4, 8, 16 oz.

Dosage: Rickets—2 gr morning and evening. Arthritis deformans—5 gr three times daily, increased by 5 gr every week; used cautiously in uric acid diathesis.

Thymus (Boericke and Tafel)

Capsules gr 5........................ Bottles of 60

Dosage: 1 capsule three times daily.

Thymus (Burroughs Wellcome)

Tabloids gr 5........................ Bottles of 100, 500

Dosage: 1–5 tabloids three times daily after meals.

Thymus Substance (Carnrick, G. W.)

Capsules gr 5........................ Bottles of 100
Powder.............................. Bottles of 1 oz.
Tablets gr 3......................... Bottles of 100, 500, 1,000

Dosage: Gr 3–5 three times daily.

Thymus (Colwell)

Crinogen............................ Bottles of 1 oz.
5 m representing gr 1 desiccated gland.

Dosage: 1–2 gr daily.

Thymus (Drug Products)

Capsules gr 1........................ Bottles of 100
representing gr 6 fresh substance.

Dosage: 1 capsule after meals, increased.

Thymocrin Solution (Harrower)

Ampules 1 cc........................ Boxes of 5
prepared from thymus nucleoprotein.

Dosage: 1 cc *intramuscularly*, daily or every other day.

Thymus Extract (Lang)

Glycerol extract of fresh gland.......... Bottles of ½, 1, 2 oz.
each cc representing 1 Gm fresh gland.

Dosage: 15–30 drops three to four times daily.

Thymus (Lafayette Pharmacal)

Enterocaps, gr 1, gr 2.................. Bottles of 100
each grain desiccated substance representing gr 6 fresh gland.

Dosage: Gr 1–2 three times daily.

Thymus (Lilly)

Powder.............................. Bottles of 1, 4 oz.
Tablets, Chocolate coated, Enteric coated,
gr 2................................ Bottles of 100, 500
each grain desiccated substance representing gr 6 fresh gland.

Dosage: Gr 2 three times daily.

Thymus Extract (Miller)

Ampules 1 cc, 2 cc.................... Boxes of 12, 100
Ampule-vials 30 cc.................... Packages of 1

Dosage: 1–2 cc two to three times weekly, *intramuscularly.*

Thymus Substance (Miller)

Capsules gr 2, gr 5.................... Boxes of 100, 1,000
Powder.................................. Bottles of 1 oz., ¼ lb., 1 lb.
Tablets, Enteric coated, gr 5........... Bottles of 100, 1,000
1 part desiccated substance representing 6 parts fresh gland.

Dosage: 2–5 gr three times daily.

Thymus (National Drug)

Tablets gr 1........................ Bottles of 100, 500, 1,000
representing gr 7 fresh gland.

Dosage: 4–8 tablets three to four times daily, 1 hr. after meals.

Thymus Gland (Parke, Davis)

Emplets, Enteric coated, gr 2........... Bottles of 100, 500
Powder.................................. Bottles of 1 oz., ¼ lb.
Tablets, Chocolate coated, gr 2......... Bottles of 100, 500, 1,000

Dosage: Gr 2 three times daily.

Thymus (Reed and Carnrick)

Powder.................................. Bottles of 1 oz., ¼, 1 lb.
Tablets, plain, Enteric coated, gr 2..... Bottles of 100, 500, 1,000

Dosage: Rickets—2 gr one to three times daily. Arthritis deformans—5–15 gr three times daily.

Thymus Gland (Wyeth)

Powder.................................. Bottles of 1, 4 oz.
each grain representing gr 6 fresh gland.

Dosage: Gr 2–5 three times daily.

Thymus (Zemmer)

Tablets gr 2........................ Bottles of 100, 1,000

Dosage: 1 tablet three to four times daily.

THYROID PRODUCTS

Description: Thyroid preparations are most frequently utilized because of the ramified function of the gland; they are available as powders, liquid extracts and hormones: Thyroxin, Thyractin (Thyroglobulin, Diiodothyrin).

Action: Controls metabolic rate and cell permeability; favors detoxication through its effect on general metabolism and stimulation of immunity factors; influences sex development; speeds up physical and mental growth; is related to puberty, the menstrual process and pregnancy.

Uses: In delayed puberty, amenorrhea, sterility; in hypothyroidism, thyrogenous obesity, non-toxic goitre, cretinism, myxedema; in eczema, ichthyosis and other skin affections; in backward children, delayed dental eruption and certain types of epilepsy and dementia; in enuresis, nephrosis, chronic arthritis.

Dosage: In accordance with preparation.

Preparations

Thyroid Gland "Lowenthal" (American Organotherapy)
Capsules gr 5........................ Boxes of 50
containing gr 1 thyroid gland desiccated U.S.P.

Dosage: 1 capsule before meals.

Thyroid (U.S.P.) (Armour)
Powder............................ Bottles of 1, 4, 8, 16 oz.
Tablets gr 1/10, gr 1/4, gr 1/2, gr 1, gr 2... Bottles of 100, 500, 1,000

Dosage: Gr 1/10–1 three times daily.

Thyroid (Boericke and Tafel)
Capsules gr 5........................ Bottles of 60
containing gr 1 thyroid.

Dosage: 1 capsule three times daily.

Thyroid (Burroughs Wellcome)
Tabloids gr 1/100, gr 1/10, gr 1/4, gr 1/2, gr 1,
gr 1½, gr 2, gr 2½, gr 5............... Bottles of 100, 500
standardized to contain 0.4% iodine; 5 gr representing gr 1 desiccated thyroid substance.

Dosage: Gr 1/100–1/10 three times daily.

Thyroid (U.S.P.) (Carnrick, G. W.)
Capsules gr 1, gr 2, gr 3, gr 5........... Bottles of 100
Powder............................ Bottles of 1 oz.
Tablets gr 1/100, gr 1/10, gr 1/4, gr 1/2, gr 1,
gr 2............................ Bottles of 100, 500, 1,000

Dosage: Gr 1/100–5 one to four times daily.

Thyroid (Colwell)
Crinogen........................... Bottles of 1 oz.
5 m representing gr 1/3 desiccated gland.

Dosage: M 5 three times daily.

Thyroid Solution (Colwell)
Ampules 1 cc........................ Boxes of 12
representing gr 1 desiccated gland.

Dosage: *Use intramusularly*, 1 cc two to three times weekly.

Thyroid (Drug Products)
Capsules gr 1/10, gr 1/5, gr 1............ Bottles of 100
each grain desiccated substance representing gr 5 fresh gland.

Dosage: 1/10 gr three times daily. In eclampsia, rapid thyroidization.

Thyroid Substance (Glandular Laboratories)
Capsules gr 1/4, gr 1/2, gr 1............. Bottles of 25
in physiological salt.

Dosage: 1 capsule three times daily.

Endothyrin (Harrower)
Tablets gr 1........................ Bottles of 50
containing thyroid U.S.P. triple strength gr 1/2.

Dosage: 1/2 tablet three times daily, increased as necessary.

Endothyrin Solution (Harrower)
Ampules 1 cc........................ Boxes of 5
representing the active soluble constituents of gr 20 fresh gland.

Dosage: 1 cc three to four times weekly, *intramuscularly*.

Thyroid (U.S.P.) **(Harvey-Pittenger)**

Capsules gr ¼, gr 1, gr 2.............. Bottles of 100, 500, 1,000
Powder.............................. Bottles of 1, 4, 8 oz., 1 lb.

1 part desiccated substance representing 5 parts fresh gland and containing 0.17–0.23 % iodine in combination.

Dosage: 1–5 gr three times daily.

Thyroid **(Hynson, Westcott and Dunning)**

Powder.............................. Bottles of 1 oz
Tablets gr 1/100, gr 1/50, gr 1/10, gr ¼, gr ½, gr 1, gr 2.......................... Tubes of 100

Dosage: Adults—½–5 gr three times daily. Infants—1/100–1 gr three times daily

Thyroid Extract **(Lang)**

Glycerol extract........................ Bottles of ½, 1, 2 oz.

each cc representing 1 Gm fresh gland.

Dosage: 8–20 drops three to four times daily.

Thyroid **(Lederle)**

Tablets gr 1/10, gr ½, gr 1, gr 2......... Bottles of 100

assayed to contain 0.23 % iodine in organic combination.

Dosage: Adults—beginning with 3–6 gr daily, 1–2 gr daily for maintenance.

Thyroid **(Lafayette Pharmacal)**

Enterocaps, gr 1/10, gr ¼, gr ½, gr 1, gr 2, gr 5........................ Bottles of 100

each grain desiccated substance representing gr 5 fresh gland.

Dosage: Gr 1/10–1 three times daily.

Thyroid **(Lilly)**

Powder.............................. Bottles of 1, 4 oz.
Pulvules gr 1, gr 2.................... Bottles of 100, 500, 1,000
Tablets gr 1/10........................ Bottles of 100, 500, 1,000
Tablets, chocolate coated, gr 1/5......... Bottles of 100, 500, 1,000
Tablets, gr ¼......................... Bottles of 100, 1,000
Tablets, enteric coated, gr ¼............ Bottles of 100, 500, 1,000
Tablets gr ½.......................... Bottles of 100, 500, 1,000
Tablets, enteric coated, gr ½............ Bottles of 100, 500, 1,000
Tablets gr 3/5.......................... Bottles of 100, 1,000
Tablets gr 1........................... Bottles of 100, 500, 1,000
Tablets, chocolate coated, gr 1.......... Bottles of 100, 500, 1,000
Tablets, enteric coated, gr 1............ Bottles of 100, 1,000
Tablets gr 2........................... Bottles of 100, 500, 1,000
Tablets, chocolate coated, gr 2.......... Bottles of 100, 500, 1,000
Tablets, enteric coated, gr 3............ Bottles of 100, 1,000
Tablets, enteric coated, gr 5............ Bottles of 100, 1,000

each grain representing gr 5 fresh gland; containing 0.17 % to 0.23 % iodine.

Dosage: Gr 1/5–1 three times daily.

Thyroid Gland **(Maltbie)**

Tablets gr 1........................... Bottles of 100, 1,000

representing gr 5 fresh gland.

Dosage: 1 tablet three times daily.

Thyroid Substance **(Marvell)**

Tablets gr 1/10, gr ¼, gr ½, gr 1, gr 2.... Bottles of 100

Dosage: Gr 1/10–½ three times daily.

Thyroid Gland (McNeil)

Capsules gr 1, gr 2 .... Bottles of 100, 500, 1,000
Tablets gr 1/4, gr 1/2, gr 1, gr 2 .... Bottles of 100, 500, 1,000

Dosage: 1/4–4 gr one to four times daily.

Thyroid Extract (Miller)

Ampules 1 cc, 2 cc .... Boxes of 12, 100
Ampule-vials 30 cc .... Packages of 1

Dosage: 1–2 cc daily, *intramuscularly.*

Thyroid Substance (Miller)

Tablets gr 1/16, gr 1/12, gr 1/10, gr 1/8, gr 1/6, gr 1/4, gr 1/3, gr 1/2, gr 2/3, gr 3/4, gr 1, gr 2. Bottles of 100, 1,000
Tablets, Chocolate coated, gr 1/4, gr 1, gr 2 Bottles of 100, 1,000
1 part desiccated substance representing 5 parts fresh gland.

Dosage: Gr 1/16–1 three times daily.

Thyroid (National Drug)

Capsules gr 1 .... Bottles of 100, 500, 1,000
Tablets gr 1/10, gr 1/4, gr 1/2, gr 1, gr 2 .... Bottles of 100, 500, 1,000
each grain representing gr 5 fresh gland.

Dosage: 1 capsule or tablet four to five times daily.

Thyroid (Parke, Davis)

Powder .... Vials 1 oz., Bottles 1/4 lb.
Capsules gr 2 .... Bottles of 100, 500
Emplets, Enteric coated, gr 1/4, gr 1/2, gr 1, gr 2, gr 3, gr 5 .... Bottles of 100, 500
Tablets, Compressed, gr 1/10, gr 1/4, gr 1/2, gr 1, gr 2 .... Bottles of 100, 500
Tablets, Chocolate coated, gr 1/5, gr 1/2, gr 1, gr 2 .... Bottles of 100, 500
each grain desiccated substance representing gr 5 fresh gland; assayed to contain 0.3% iodine or 50% above U.S.P.

Dosage: 1/10–5 gr three times daily.

Thyroprotein (Parke, Davis)

Ampules 1 cc .... Boxes of 12, 100
representing gr 1/50 thyroprotein; chloretone 0.5%.
Tablets, Compressed, 1% .... Bottles of 50
representing gr 1/60 thyroprotein.
Tablets, Compressed, 2% .... Bottles of 50
representing gr 1/25 thyroprotein.
Tablets, Compressed, 5% .... Bottles of 50
representing gr 1/10 thyroprotein.

Dosage: 1–5 cc *hypodermatically* two to four times weekly. Oral: Gr 1/50–1/10 two to three times daily.

Thyroid (Reed and Carnrick)

Powder .... Bottles of 1 oz., 1/4, 1 lb.

Thyracoids (Reed and Carnrick)

Tablets gr 1/10, gr 1/4, gr 1, gr 2 .... Bottles of 100
Tablets, Enteric coated, gr 1/10, gr 1/4, gr 1, gr 2 .... Bottles of 100
standardized to represent entire potency desiccated thyroid.

Dosage: Gr 1/10–1 three times daily. *See Chap. I.*

Thyroxine Synthetic (Roche)

Ampules 1.1 cc (1:1,000 solution)....... Boxes of 6 and 12
Crystals.............................. Vials of 100 mg
Liquid................................ Vials of 15 cc
representing 2 mg per cc.
Tablets 1 mg......................... Boxes of 30

Dosage: 2–4 tablets or 1–2 ampules daily. *See Chap. I.*

Thyroid Substance (Rorer)

Capsules gr ¼, gr ½, gr 1, gr 2......... Bottles of 100.
Powder................................ Bottles of 1, 4 oz., 1 lb.
Tablets gr ¼, gr ½, gr 1, gr 2.......... Bottles of 100

Dosage: Gr ¼–½ three times daily.

Thyroid Nucleoprotein (Schieffelin)

Powder 10%........................... Bottles of ½ oz.
Tablets 1%, 2%, 5%................... Bottles of 100

Thyroid Residue (Schieffelin)

Ampules 30 m......................... Boxes of 6
Solution............................. Bottles of ½ oz.
representing 0.05 mg per cc.

Dosage: Hypothyroidism—5–20 m *orally* or *subcutaneously* every 2–3 hr. In postoperative toxemia—20–30 m *subcutaneously* or *intramuscularly* every 2–3 hr.

Glythoid (Schieffelin)

Pills 5 m, 10 m...................... Bottles of 50
each 5 m representing gr 1 fresh gland.

Dosage: M 5 three times daily.

Thyroid Substance (Searle)

Tablets gr 1, gr 2................... Bottles of 100, 500

Dosage: Gr 1–2 three times daily.

Thyroid Substance (U.S.P.) (Searle)

Tablets, enteric coated, gr 1............ Bottles of 100, 500
representing 5 gr fresh gland; contains not less than 0.2% iodine.

Dosage: Gr 1 three times daily.

Thyroid Gland (U.S.P.) (Sharp and Dohme)

Capsules gr 2........................ Bottles of 100
Powder............................... Bottles of 1 oz.
Tablets gr 1/10, gr ⅕, gr 1, gr 2......... Bottles of 100
each gr desiccated substance representing gr 5 fresh gland.

Dosage: Gr 1/10–1 three times daily.

Thyroid Substance (Smith-Dorsey)

Capsules gr 1, gr 2.................. Boxes of 500, 1,000
Tablets gr 1, gr 2................... Bottles of 1,000

Dosage: Gr 1–2 three times daily.

Thyroxin (Squibb)

Crystals............................. Tubes of 10 mg
Tablets gr 1/320, 1/160, 1/80, 1/32......... Bottles of 100

Dosage: 0.4–1 mg daily. *See Chap. I.*

Thyroid (Stoddard)

Tablets gr ½......................... Bottles of 100, 500, 1,000

Dosage: ½–2 tablets daily.

Thyroid Gland (U.S.P.) **(Upjohn)**
Tablets gr ⅛, gr 1, gr 2 .... Bottles of 100, 1,000
each gr representing gr 5 fresh substance, containing 0.17% to 0.25% iodine.

Dosage: 2–5 gr daily.

Thyroid **(Westerfield)**
Tablets, Enteric coated, gr 1/10, gr ¼, gr ½, gr 1 .... Bottles of 100, 500, 1,000

Dosage: ¼–4 gr daily or 1 gr three times daily, increased to 3–4 gr.

Thyroid Gland (U.S.P.) **(Wyeth)**
Powder .... Bottles of 1, 4 oz.
Tablets gr 1, gr 2 .... Bottles of 100, 1,000
each gr desiccated substance representing gr 5 fresh gland.

Dosage: Gr 1–2 three times daily.

Thyroid **(Zemmer)**
Tablets gr 1/10, gr ¼, gr ½, gr 1, gr 2 .... Bottles of 100, 1,000
each gr representing gr 5 fresh gland.

Dosage: 1/10–2 gr three times daily.

Miscellaneous Endocrine Preparations

Products from various organs, the use of which is still in the experimental stage; arrangement is by organs.

Bone Marrow Substance **(Armour)**
Powder .... Bottles of 1, 4, 8, 16 oz.

Dosage: Gr 2–5 three times daily.

Red Bone Marrow (Medullary Glyceride) **(Armour)**
Extract .... Bottles of 16 oz.

Dosage: Adults—1–2 teaspoonfuls three times daily in water or milk;—Infants—in rickets, 4–5 dr. daily.

Brain Substance **(Armour)**
Powder .... Bottles of 4, 8, 16 oz.
Tablets gr 2 .... Bottles of 100, 500, 1,000

Dosage: Gr 2 three times daily.

Cerebrin **(Burroughs Wellcome)**
Tabloids gr 5 .... Bottles of 100, 500

Dosage: 1 tablet three to four times daily, after meals.

Brain Substance **(Carnrick, G. W.)**
Powder .... Bottles of 1 oz.

Dosage: Gr 2 three times daily.

Brain Substance **(Drug Products)**
Capsules gr 1 .... Bottles of 100
representing gr 6 fresh tissue.

Dosage: 1 capsule after meals, increased as indicated.

Brain **(Lafayette Pharmacal)**
Enterocaps, gr 5 .... Bottles of 100
each grain desiccated substance representing gr 10 fresh gland.

Dosage: Gr 5 three times daily.

Brain Substance Extract (Lang)
Glycerol extract.................... Bottles of 4, 16 oz.
each cc representing 1 Gm fresh gland.

Corpus Striatum Extract (Lang)
Glycerol extract.................... Bottles of 4, 16 oz.
each cc representing 1 Gm fresh gland.
Dosage: 1 cc *intramuscularly*, three to five times weekly.

Cardiac Substance (Marvell)
Powdered extract.................... Bottles of 1 oz., ¼, ½, 1 lb.
Dosage: Gr 2 three times daily.

Heart Muscle (Lafayette Pharmacal)
Enterocaps, gr 2.................... Bottles of 100
each grain desiccated substance representing gr 6 fresh gland.
Dosage: 1 capsule three times daily.

Duodenin (Armour)
Tablets gr 1.................... Bottles of 100
Dosage: Gr 1 three times daily.

Duodenal Substance (Carnrick, G. W.)
Powder.................... Bottles of 1 oz.
Dosage: Gr 1 three times daily.

Duodenal Substance (Glandular Laboratories)
Capsules gr 2.................... Bottles of 25
in physiological salt.
Dosage: 1 capsule three times daily.

Duodenal (Lafayette Pharmacal)
Enterocaps, gr 2, gr 5.................... Bottles of 100
each grain desiccated substance representing gr 6 fresh gland.
Dosage: Gr 2–5 three times daily.

Duodenal Substance (Lang)
Glycerol extract.................... Bottles of 4, 16 oz.
each cc representing 1 Gm fresh gland.
Dosage: 1 cc *intramuscularly*, three to five times weekly.

Duodenal Substance (Marvell)
Powdered extract.................... Bottles of 1 oz., ¼, ½, 1 lb.
Dosage: Gr 2 three times daily.

Duodenal Substance (Miller)
Powder.................... Bottles of 1 oz., ¼, 1 lb.
1 part desiccated substance representing 6 parts fresh gland.
Dosage: Gr 2 three times daily.

Kidney Substance (Armour)
Powder.................... Bottles of 4, 8, 16 oz.
Tablets gr 2.................... Bottles of 100, 500, 1,000
Dosage: Gr 2 three times daily.

Kidney Substance (Burroughs Wellcome)
Tabloids gr 5.................... Bottles of 100, 500
Dosage: 1 tablet three times daily.

Kidney Substance (Carnrick, G. W.)
Capsules gr 5........................ Bottles of 100
Powder........................ Bottles of 1 oz.
Tablets gr 2........................ Bottles of 100, 500, 1,000

Dosage: Gr 2–5 three times daily.

Kidney Substance (Drug Products)
Capsules gr 1........................ Bottles of 100
representing gr 6 fresh gland.

Dosage: 1 capsule four times daily, before meals.

Kidney (Lafayette Pharmacal)
Enterocaps, gr 5........................ Bottles of 100
each grain desiccated substance representing gr 6 fresh gland.

Dosage: Gr 5 three times daily.

Kidney Extract (Lang)
Glycerol extract........................ Bottles of 4 oz., 1 pt.
each cc representing 1 Gm fresh gland.

Dosage: 1 Gm fresh gland daily.

Kidney Extract (Renal) (Miller)
Ampules 2 cc........................ Boxes of 12, 100
Ampule-vials 30 cc........................ Packages of 1
each cc representing soluble extractives of gr 55 fresh substance.

Dosage: 2 cc *intramuscularly* every 6 hr.

Kidney Substance (Miller)
Capsules gr 5........................ Bottles of 100, 500, 1,000
Powder........................ Bottles of 1 oz., ¼ lb, 1 lb
Tablets, Compressed, Enteric coated, gr 5. Bottles of 100, 500, 1,000
1 part desiccated substance representing 6 parts fresh gland.

Dosage: 1–3 capsules or tablets every 4 hr.

Nephritin (Reed and Carnrick)
Tablets........................ Bottles of 80, 500, 1,000
contains an extract of normal kidney substance.

Dosage: 2–4 tablets three to four times daily. *See Chap. I.*

Lymphatic Gland (Burroughs Wellcome)
Tabloids gr 5........................ Bottles of 100

Dosage: 1 tabloid three times daily.

Lymphatic Substance (Carnrick, G. W.)
Powder........................ Bottles of 1 oz.
Tablets gr 3........................ Bottles of 100, 500, 1,000

Dosage: Gr 3 three times daily.

Lymphatic (Drug Products)
Capsules gr 1........................ Bottles of 100
representing gr 5 fresh gland.

Dosage: 1–3 capsules three times daily.

Lymphatic (Lafayette Pharmacal)
Enterocaps, gr 2........................ Bottles of 100
each grain desiccated substance representing gr 7 fresh gland.

Dosage: Gr 2 three times daily.

Parotid Substance (Armour)
Powder........................ Bottles of 1, 4, 8, 16 oz.
Tablets gr 2........................ Bottles of 100, 500, 1,000

Dosage: Gr 2 three times daily.

Parotid Gland (Boericke and Tafel)
Capsules gr 5........................ Bottles of 60
Dosage: 1 capsule three times daily.

Parotid (National Drug)
Tablets gr 1........................ Bottles of 100, 500, 1,000
representing gr 7½ fresh gland.
Dosage: 1 tablet three times daily.

Seminal Vesicles (Marvell)
Powdered extract.................... Bottles of 1 oz., ¼, ½, 1 lb.

Spinal Cord Substance (Armour)
Powder.............................. Bottles of 1, 4, 8, 16 oz.
Tablets gr 2........................ Bottles of 100, 500, 1,000
Dosage: Gr 2 three times daily.

Spinal Cord Substance (Carnrick, G. W.)
Powder.............................. Bottles of 1 oz., ¼ lb.
Dosage: Gr 2 three times daily.

Part II

Pluriglandular Products

Some physicians are still of the opinion, that uniglandular therapy is the only rational method of utilizing endocrine preparations; most, however, consider this view erroneous and make extensive use of pluriglandular therapy; they contend, that in the exercise of every function several glands are intimately associated; that affections of one gland must necessarily reflect unfavorably on the others of such functional group. For the latter group of practitioners the following products are presented.

Classification

For the convenience of the clinician and to facilitate his selection of a preparation for a particular purpose, the 246 pluriglandular preparations presented here for treatment of various endocrine syndromes are classified into 30 groups. As the composition of each product differs considerably from the others, in glandular components and dosage, the grouping is necessarily on a broad basis.

Group 1: Pluriglandular preparations in the treatment of hypoadrenia, nerve exhaustion, convalescence, malnutrition and anemia.

7 Splenoid Compound "Lowenthal"
12 Lymphoid Compound 1 "Lowenthal"
13 Lymphoid Compound 2 "Lowenthal"
21 Glandular Compound Male
22 Glandular Compound Female
34 Spleen-Red Bone Marrow Compound
38 Hemoglobin Compound-End. Comp. 1
66 Hemoglobin Co. 1
83 Adreno-Spermin
84 Solution Adreno-Spermin Comp. 1A
94 Adreno-Hypophysis Compound
107 Spermin Hemoglobin Compound
155 Suprarenal Mixture
163 Adrempco Capsules
164 Adrempco 100
165 Atoco Capsules
181 Glandular Compound 5
225 Adrenal Prostate Compound
226 Adrenal Spermin Compound

Group 2: Pluriglandular preparations influencing attacks of bronchial asthma, bronchial spasm and dyspnea.

35 Suprarenal-Pituitary Compound
53 Pituitary-Phosphate Comp. End. Comp. 16
73 Pit-Ren
121 Ephedan
215 Asthmaglands
246 Thyroid Pituitary Compound

Group 3: Corpus luteum combinations influential in the treatment of vomiting of pregnancy, nervous disorders after oophorectomy, female sexual debility, menopausal disturbances.

8 Corpus Luteum Compound "Lowenthal"
20 Corpus Luteum Compound
132 Corluroid
203 Corpus Luteum Compound

Group 4: Preparations of male gonadal organs indicated in the treatment of asexualism, impotence, sexual debility, sex neuroses and premature senility.

1 Orchic Pituitary Compound
5 Yohimbin and Orchic Compound
17 "Tabloid" Glandular Mixture 1
37 Viriligen
52 Gonad-Prostate Compound
108 Gonad Compound
109 Sol. Gonad Compound
123 Glandular Compound 1
126 Orchan
129 Thyorchan
131 Asexualism
135 Gonadrenal
139 Malex
146 Orchiroid 1
147 Orchiroid 2
148 Orchiroid 3
156 Thyorchic
158 Yohimbine and Ovarian Mixture
159 Yohimbine and Orchic Mixture
162 Glandular Compound Male
168 Orchiben Compound
169 Orchic Epinephrine Compound
177 Vesix
186 Orcon Compound 1
187 Orcon Compound 2
190 Orchic Compound 1
191 Orchic Compound 2
192 Orchic Compound 3
201 Pluriglandular Compound 2
204 Orchic Compound
205 Orchic Compound Special
210 Testacoids
212 Forto-Testin
213 Remogland
218 Cerebro-Orchic Compound
222 Homoglands
224 Vitaglands
228 Intesti-Sols Orchic Compound
232 Yohimbine Endocrine Compound
234 Orchi-Himbine Compound
240 Orchic Compound

Group 5: Preparations influencing arterial hypertension in female, menopausal and essential hypertension.

48 Hepatic-Ovary Pancreas Compound
97 Thyro Pancreas Compound with Ovary
171 Pan-Orch-Oid

Group 6: Pluriglandular combinations for use in male hypertension.

57 Spermin-Pancreas Compound-End. Comp. 21

Group 7: Pluriglandular products for use in hepatic and biliary disturbances, as hepatic cirrhosis and insufficiency, toxic hypertension, malarial cachexia and anemia.

89 Hepato Splenic Compound
113 Heparnucleate Liver Extract
114 Solution Heparnucleate Liver Extract
115 Anabolin
116 Anabolin Solution
117 Anabolin Solution Fortior

Group 8: Mammary-placental combinations effective in breast dysfunction; in agalactia, also uterine subinvolution, pelvic congestion and its symptoms.

26 Mammagen
27 Mammary Compound
44 Mammary-Placenta Compound
50 Ovary-Mammary Compound
51 Mammary-Ergotin Compound
69 Mammary Compound
86 Placento-Mammary Compound
98 Mamma-Ovary Compound

99 Chalomen (Mamma-Pituitary Comp.)
122 Galacan
125 Mameran
140 Mammary Mixture
154 Placental Mixture
167 Mammary Compound
182 Glandular Compound 7
183 Glandular Compound 8
188a Mammary Compound 1
189 Mammary Compound 2
230 Mammary Placenta Compound with Pituitary

Group 9: Preparations for use in ovarian dysfunction with sexual apathy and sterility, menstrual disorders, menopausal depressive states, neuroses, melancholia, psychoses.

3 Ovarian Thyroid Compound
4 Ovarian Pituitary Compound
10 Ova Mammoid Compound
29 Ovarian Compound
23 Hormotone
41 Ovarian Compound
61 Endocrine Compound
63 Thy-Ovar Compound
80 Thyovaroids
110 Gonad-Ovarian Compound
123a Glandular Comp. 2
130 Thyovaran
134 Femex
149 Ovaroid 1
150 Ovaroid 2
151 Ovaroid 3
157 Thyovary
173 Polempco 96-Polyglandular Sol.
175 Polempco 102-Polyglandular "T"
178 Glandular Compound 2
194 Ovarian Compound 2
196 Ovarian Residue Compound
207 Ovacoids
229 Intesti-Sols Ovarian Compound
243 Pituitary Ovarian Compound

Group 10: Combinations for ovarian deficiency with thyroidal hypertrophy, nervousness, sympathetic instability, headaches.

73a Pitovaco

Group 11: Ovarian combinations to overcome ovarian insufficiency in sex imbalance, menstrual disorders and climacteric disturbances, hypochondriasis, neurasthenia, melancholia.

2 Ovarian Compound
11 Placentoid Compound
18 "Tabloid" Glandular Mixture 2
65 Corpus-Ovar-1
71 Ovarian Compound 1
77 Thyovaco
87 Menocrin
88 Menocrin Solution
111 Adreno-Ovarian Compound
123a Glandular Compound 2
127 Ovaran
161 Glandular Compound—Female
174 Polempco 101—Polyglandular "O"
180 Glandular Compound 4
193 Ovarian Compound 1
195 Ovarian Compound 3
206 Ovarian Compound
220 Glanditone
223 Ovara-Dysfunction
235 Ovarian-Suprarenal Compound
242 Menovarian
245 Thyroid Ovarian Compound

Group 12: Pancreas-liver combinations for stimulation of enzymatic and motor functions of the respective organs, for use in cholecystitis, jaundice and in intestinal disturbances.

58 Glycocholate-Pancreas Compound
244 Secretin Compound

Group 13: Homostimulating pancreas combinations effecting carbohydrate tolerance for use in diabetes mellitus.

15 Pancrepatine
54 Secretin-Pancreas-Myrtillin Comp.
100 Pan-Secretin
120a Diabetan
144 Oralsulin Mixture
145 Oralsulin with Duodenal Substance
221 Glycosuretics

Group 14: Pituitary-Thymus preparations for stimulating uterine function during pregnancy and labor.

81 Pituthymin Solution
188 Pituitary Thymus
233 Thymo-Pitsin
236 Thymus Pituitary Solution

Group 15: Parathyroid combinations for use in tetany, paralysis agitans, nervous tremors, epileptic and uremic convulsive tendencies.

30 Parathyroid Compound
56 Parathyroid-Spermin Compound
95 Para Spleen Compound
96 Para Spleen Compound Solution
118 Para Calcium Tablets
119 Para Calcium Solution
128 Paracal
197 Parathyroid Compound
216 Calcium Lactate with Parathyroid
231 Parathyroid and Spermin Compound

Group 16: Prostate products for use in prostatic disturbances with hypertrophy, vesical irritation, senility and decreased sex function.

6 Prostoid Compound
28 Orchic-Prostate Compound
47 Prostate-Spermin Compound
103 Prostate Compound
184 Glandular Compound 9
199 Prostatic Compound
239 Prostate Compound

Group 17: Pituitary-Anterior combinations recommended for use in hyperpituitary manifestations with mental disturbances, loss of memory, mental and physical retardation in children, dwarfism, mongolism.

85 Antero-Pituitary Compound
101 Pituitary Compound
227 Anter-Pituitary Compound

Group 18: Pituitary-Posterior combinations for use in posterior pituitary disturbances.

101 Pituitary Compound
102 Solution Pituitary Compound

Group 19: Pineal compounds applicable in the treatment of retarded mental and physical backwardness and mongolism.

31 Pineal Compound Male
32 Pineal Compound Female

Group 20: Pluriglandular remedies stated to be effective in renal disturbances, acute and chronic nephritis, defective renal permeability and function, in the prevention of uremia.

46 Renal-Pancreas Compound
33 Renal-Pancreas Compound
112 Renal Compound

Group 21: Placental compounds are used in placental toxemia, hyperemesis gravidarum.

45 Placenta-Thyroid Compound
104 Placenta-Compound
105 Placenta Luteum Compound

Group 22: Splenic compounds for use in anemias.

34 Spleen Red Bone Marrow Compound
136 Hemo-splenic

Group 23: Thymus combinations employed in the treatment of psoriasis, severe dermatitis.

202 Thymus and Suprarenal Extracts

Group 24: Endocrine combinations stated to be effective in arthritis, rheumatism, rheumatoid arthritis.

36 Thymus Compound
79 Adrosil
106 Thymus-Spermin Compound

Group 25: Pituitary whole gland combinations recommended in delayed bodily and sexual development, hypophyseal obesity, sexual infantilism.

9 Pituitoid Compound
40 Pituitary Thymus Compound
64 Hormones Solutions
74 Pituitary Compound 1
82 Accretin Capsules
198 Pituitary Compound

Group 26: Endocrine compounds employed in pathological thyroids with resulting cretinism, non-toxic goitre, hypothyroidal states, general backwardness.

19 "Tabloid" Thyrovarium
43 Nucleinized Thyro-Iodid Comp.
55 Thyro-Pituitary Compound
76 Thyroid-Ioform Compound
91 Thyroid Compound
92 Iodized Thyroid Compound
219 Cretinglands

Group 27: Combinations for use in thyroidal dysfunction with irritability, tachycardia, cardiac neuroses and moderate thyroidal hypertrophy.

42 Pancreas-Adrenal Compound
90 Pancreas Compound
172 Polempco Capsules

Group 28: Endocrine combinations for homo-stimulating purposes, influencing general metabolism and indicated in asthenia, hypertension, debility, convalescence and other manifestations of hypo adrenia.

16 Iodobesin (Obesity)
24 Incretone
59 Pulmo-Hemoglobin Compound
62 Multicrinogen
67 Lecithin Compound 1
72 Ovarian Comp. 2
124 Hemovarian
138 Leci-Nuclein
141 Morrol with Suprarenal
142 Normalizer 1
143 Normalizer 2
176 Semvesco
178 Glandular Compound 2
200 Pluriglandular Comp. 1
209 Protonuclein
214 Remolysin
217 Cerebro-Lecithin with Nuclein
238 Ovarian Compound

Group 29: Combinations intended for stimulation of digestive organs, in deficient secretory and motor functions of gastro-intestinal tract.

75 Secretin Compound
133 Duobilad
211 Panacoids

Group 30: Lymphoid tissue products for tonic and hematinic effect in lymphadenia, disordered metabolism and neurasthenia.

12 Lymphoid Compound 1
13 Lymphoid Compound 2
14 Lymph Compounds
68 Lymphatic Compound

Pluriglandular Endocrine Preparations

1. Orchic Pituitary Compound—Capsules (Kerakote)—Bottles of 100 and 500 **(Abbott)**

Contains

	Gr	Gm
Suprarenal (entire)	1/4	0.016
Thyroid	1/12	0.005
Anterior pituitary	1	0.064
Orchic substance	1 1/2	0.097
Prostate	1 1/2	0.097
Calcium glycerol comp	2/3	0.042

For use in male hypogonadism, impotence, sexual neurasthenia.

Dosage: 1 capsule three times daily.

2. Ovarian Compound—Capsules (Kerakote)—Bottles of 100 and 500 **(Abbott)**

Contains

	Gr	Gm
Ovarian substance (entire)	4	0.259
Thyroid	1/8	0.008

For use in ovarian insufficiency, infantilism.

Dosage: 1–3 capsules daily after meals.

3. Ovarian Thyroid Compound—Capsules (Kerakote)—Bottles of 100 and 500 **(Abbott)**

Contains	Gr	Gm
Ovarian substance (entire)	2	0.130
Thyroid	1/12	0.005
Pituitary (entire)	1/8	0.008
Calcium glycerol compound	1½	0.055

For use in sexual apathy, sterility, menstrual disorders.

Dosage: 1 capsule four times daily.

4. Ovarian Pituitary Compound—Capsules (Kerakote)—Bottles of 100 and 500 **(Abbott)**

Contains	Gr	Gm
Ovarian substance (entire)	1½	0.097
Thyroid	1/20	0.003
Pituitary anterior	1½	0.097
Pituitary (entire)	3/40	0.004
Calcium glycerol compound	1⅜	0.088

For use in menstrual disorders, functional sterility, neuroses.

Dosage: 1 capsule three times daily after meals.

5. Yohimbin and Orchic Compound—Capsules (Kerakote)—Bottles of 50 and 100 **(Abbott)**

Contains	Gr	Gm
Yohimbin hydrochloride	1/12	0.005
Orchic substance	1½	0.097
Anterior pituitary	1½	0.097
Suprarenal	1½	0.097
Thyroid	1/10	0.006

For use in anaphrodisia, impotency, hypogonadal states.

Dosage: 1–2 capsules three times daily after meals.

6. Prostoid Compound "Lowenthal"—Capsules—Boxes of 50 **(American Organotherapy)**

Contains	Gr	Gm
Prostate gland and Testicular extract	2	0.130
Lactose	3	0.194

For use in hypertrophy of prostate, senility, chronic prostatitis, prostatorrhea, impotence.

Dosage: 1 capsule three times daily.

7. Splenoid Compound "Lowenthal"—Capsules—Boxes of 50 **(American Organotherapy)**

Contains	Gr	Gm
Spleen substance	2	0.130
Suprarenal gland	1/4	0.016
Thyroid gland (U.S.P.)	1/8	0.008
Iron glycerophosphate	1/2	0.032
Sodium and calcium glycerophosphate	2	0.130
Pancreas	1	0.064

For use as adjuvant and supportive in tuberculosis, pernicious anemia, chronic malnutrition, post-influenza, diabetes.

Dosage: 1 capsule before meals.

8. Corpus Luteum Compound "Lowenthal"—Capsules—Boxes of 50 **(American Organotherapy)**

Contains	Gr	Gm
Corpus luteum } Ovarian substance }	3	0.194
Excipient	2	0.130

For use in nervous disorders following oophorectomy, in menopause, hysteria, neurasthenia and as aphrodisiac.

Dosage: 1 capsule three times daily.

9. Pituitoid Compound "Lowenthal"—Capsules—Boxes of 50 **(American Organotherapy)**

Contains

	Gr	Gm
Whole pituitary body	½	0.032
Thymus gland	1	0.064
Thyroid gland (U.S.P.)	⅙	0.012
Sodium and calcium glycerophosphate	2	0.130

For use in mental disturbances, loss of memory, dementia praecox, idiocy and imbecility of children.

Dosage: 1, three times daily before meals.

10. Ova Mammoid Compound "Lowenthal"—Capsules—Boxes of 50 **(American Organotherapy)**

Contains

	Gr	Gm
Ovarian extract	1	0.064
Mammary gland extract	1	0.064
Lactose	3	0.194

For use in menopausal disturbances, neuroses, melancholia, hysteria, functional sterility, sexual apathy in women, amenorrhea, metrorrhagia.

Dosage: 1 capsule before meals.

11. Placentoid Compound "Lowenthal"—Capsules—Boxes of 50 **(American Organotherapy)**

Contains

	Gr	Gm
Desiccated placenta	2	0.130
Mammary gland substance	1	0.064
Sodium and calcium glycerophosphate	2	0.130

For use in nervous disorders following oophorectomy, as aphrodisiac, in menopause, hysteria, neurasthenia.

Dosage: 1 capsule three times daily.

12. Lymphoid Compound 1 "Lowenthal"—Capsules (Soluble elastic)—Boxes of 100 **(American Organotherapy)**

Contains

	Gr	Gm
Lymphatic glands, testes, brain and spinal cord	2	0.130
Iron glycerophosphate	¼	0.016
Sodium and calcium glycerophosphate	2	0.130
Strychnine nitrate	1/60	0.001
Aloin	1/20	0.003

For use as hematinic, tonic and stimulant of nervous and muscular tissues; in neurasthenia, debility, impotency, paralysis, brain disorders.

Dosage: 1, three times daily before meals.

13. Lymphoid Compound 2 "Lowenthal"—Capsules (Soluble elastic)—Boxes of 100 **(American Organotherapy)**

Contains

	Gr	Gm
Lymphatic gland, testes, brain and spinal cord	2	0.130
Iron glycerophosphate	¼	0.016
Sodium and calcium glycerophosphate	2	0.130

For use as hematinic, tonic and stimulant of nervous and muscular tissues; in neurasthenia, debility, impotence, paralysis, brain disorders.

Dosage: 1, three times daily before meals.

14. Lymph Compounds "Lowenthal"—Ampules—8 m (**American Organotherapy**)
Boxes of 12—Bottles of 1 oz.

Contains

Orchitic fluids, lymph gland extracts,
Spinal cord and brain substance
Bichloride of gold and sodium............ gr 1/50 (0.001 Gm) to 10 m
Alcohol less than 1 %

For use in degenerative diseases, neurasthenia, nervous collapse, brain disorders, disordered metabolism.

Dosage: 8–10 drops three times weekly or 1 ampule *intramuscularly*.

15. Pancrepatine Globules (Gluten coated)—Boxes of 100 (**Anglo-French**)
Prepared from pancreas and hepatic hormones, each globule containing 0.25 Gm of active substance.

For use as substitutional therapy in reducing glycosuria and hyperglycemia and relief of symptoms in diabetes mellitus, especially in those averse to insulin hypodermics.

Dosage: Adults—2–4 globules three times daily after meals, increased by 2 globules daily till 12 are taken; dosage maintained till urine is sugar-free.

16. Iodobesin—Dragees—Bottles of 60 (**Anglo-French**)

Each dragee represents

	Gm
Liver extract	0.050
Pituitary extract	0.004
Testicular extract	0.040
Ovarian extract	0.050
Thyroid (deprived of lipoids)	0.005
Suprarenal extract	0.001
Iodalbumin (colloidal)	0.050

For use in controlling metabolism; in obesity of endocrine origin, with headache, faintness, amenorrhea, edematous lower extremities.

Dosage: 2 dragees daily for 10 days, then 3–4 daily for 10 days and rest period of 10 days.

17. 'Tabloid' Glandular Mixture 1 (Male) (**Burroughs Wellcome**)
Bottles of 100 and 500

Contains

	Gr	Gm
Glandula thymicae	2	0.13
Glandula thyroideae	1/5	0.013
Glandula anterior pituitary	1/2	0.032
Glandula suprarenalis	1/4	0.016
Didymini	1/2	0.032
Cerebrini	1/2	0.032

For use in hypotonic and neurasthenic conditions, premature senile changes and hypochondriasis.

Dosage: 1 'Tabloid' three to four times daily after meals, increased if necessary.

18. 'Tabloid' Glandular Mixture 2 (Female)—Bottles of 100 and 500 (**Burroughs Wellcome**)

Contains

	Gr	Gm
Glandula thymicae	2	0.13
Glandula thyroideae	1/5	0.013
Glandula anterior pituitary	1/2	0.032
Glandula suprarenalis	1/4	0.016
Varium	1/2	0.032
Mamos	1/2	0.032
Cerebrini	1/2	0.032

Dosage: 1, three to four times daily after meals, increased if necessary.

For use in hypotonic and neurasthenic conditions, premature senile changes and hypochondriasis; in amenorrhea and menopause.

19. 'Tabloid' Thyrovarium—Bottles of 100 and 500 **(Burroughs Wellcome)**

Contains

	Gr	Gm
Thyroid gland	1/4	0.016
Varium	5	0.324

For use in cretinism, backwardness in children and other hypothyroidism cases.

Dosage: 1, three times daily after meals, gradually increased.

20. Corpus Luteum Compound—Capsules and Tablets—Bottles of 40 and 100 each **(G. W. Carnrick)**

Contains

	Gr	Gm
Corpus luteum	1	0.064
Thyroid	1/10	0.006
Physiological salts	1/4	0.016

For use in vomiting of pregnancy, (hyperemesis gravidarum) menstruation psychosis, mild manic depressive insanity (females).

Dosage: 1–3 every 3 or 4 hr.

21. Glandular Compound Male—Capsules and Tablets—Bottles of 40 and 100 each **(G. W. Carnrick)**

Contains

	Gr	Gm
Thyroid	1/10	0.006
Pituitary	1/40	0.001
Suprarenal	1/4	0.016
Orchic	1/4	0.016
Physiological salts	1/4	0.016

For use in hypoadrenia, asthenia, low blood pressure, fatigue syndrome.

Dosage: 1 or 2, three times daily.

22. Glandular Compound Female—Capsules and Tablets—Bottles of 40 and 100 each **(G. W. Carnrick)**

Contains

	Gr	Gm
Thyroid	1/10	0.006
Pituitary	1/40	0.001
Suprarenal	1/4	0.016
Ovarian	1/4	0.016
Physiological Salts	1/4	0.016

For use in hypoadrenia, asthenia, low blood pressure, fatigue syndrome.

Dosage: 1 or 2, three times daily.

23. Hormotone—Tablets—Bottles of 50 and 100 **(G. W. Carnrick)**

Contains extracts from the anterior and posterior pituitary, follicular and luteal parts of ovary, adrenal gland, and thyroid 1/10 gr per tablet.

For use as uterine tonic in lowered metabolism and suboxidation, in debility and for correcting amenorrhea, dysmenorrhea and menopausal symptoms.

Dosage: 1–3 tablets three times daily.

24. Incretone—Bottles of 6 oz. **(G. W. Carnrick)**

Contains extracts from thyroid, pituitary, ovary and testis, in a bitter tonic vehicle.

For use to stimulate appetite and general metabolism, in asthenia, general debility and convalescence.

Dosage: 1–2 teaspoonfuls three times daily before meals.

25. Kinazyme—Capsules and Tablets—Bottles of 100, 500, 1,000 **(G. W. Carnrick)**

Contains extracts of pancreas, liver, spleen, whole pituitary gr 1/60, with calcium phosphate and parathyroid gr 1/40—per capsule or tablet.

For use as reconstructive tonic in tuberculosis and general malnutrition of children and adults.

Dosage: 2–4 capsules or tablets after meals.

26. Mammagen—Capsules and Tablets—Bottles of 100, 500, 1,000 (G. W. Carnrick)
Contains corpus luteum, placenta, mammary gland, whole pituitary gr ⅛ (0.008 Gm) per tablet or capsule.

For use as galactogogue in agalactia and deficient lactation.

Dosage: 1–2 capsules or tablets after meals, beginning several days before delivery.

27. Mammary Compound—Capsules and Tablets—Bottles of 40 and 100 each (G. W. Carnrick)

Contains	Gr	Gm
Mammary	2	0.130
Post. pituitary	1/10	0.006
Thymus	½	0.032
Placenta	½	0.032
Calcium lactate	1	0.064

For use in menorrhagia, metrorrhagia, sub-involution.

Dosage: 1 or 2, three times daily.

28. Orchic-Prostate Compound—Capsules and Tablets—Bottles of 40 and 100 each (G. W. Carnrick)

Contains	Gr	Gm
Orchic	1	0.064
Prostate	2	0.130
Calcium glycerophosphate	2	0.130

For use in enlarged prostate, sexual neurasthenia, vesical irritation.

Dosage: 2 or 3, three times daily.

29. Ovarian Compound—Capsules and Tablets—Bottles of 40 and 100 each (G. W. Carnrick)

Contains	Gr	Gm
Ovarian	3	0.194
Thyroid	1/10	0.006
Physiological salts	¼	0.016

For use in amenorrhea, ovarian hypofunction, menopause.

Dosage: 1 or 2, three times daily; may be increased to 3 or 4, week before menstrual period.

30. Parathyroid Compound—Capsules and Tablets—Bottles of 40 and 100 each (G. W. Carnrick)

Contains	Gr	Gm
Parathyroid	1/20	0.003
Orchic	1	0.064
Calcium lactate	2	0.130

For use in tetany, uremia, epilepsy, paralysis agitans, nervous tremor of children.

Dosage: 2 or 3, three times daily.

31. Pineal Compound Male—Capsules and Tablets—Bottles of 40 and 100 each (G. W. Carnrick)

Contains	Gr	Gm
Anterior pituitary	⅕	0.013
Thyroid	⅛	0.008
Suprarenal	1	0.064
Orchic	1½	0.097
Pineal	1/30	0.002
Physiological salts	¼	0.016

For use in backward children, mongolism, retarded mental or physical development.

Dosage: 1 or 2, three times daily.

32. Pineal Compound Female—Capsules and Tablets—Bottles of 40 and 100 each (G. W. Carnrick)

Contains

	Gr	Gm
Anterior pituitary	1/5	0.013
Thyroid	1/8	0.008
Suprarenal	1	0.064
Ovarian	1½	0.097
Pineal	1/30	0.002
Physiological salts	¼	0.016

For use in backward children, mongolism, retarded mental or physical development.

Dosage: 1 or 2, three times daily.

33. Renal-Pancreas Compound—Capsules and Tablets—Bottles of 40 and 100 each (G. W. Carnrick)

Contains

	Gr	Gm
Kidney	2	0.130
Pancreas	2	0.130

For use in nephritis and prevention of uremia.

Dosage: 1 or 2, three times daily.

34. Spleen-Red Bone Marrow Compound—Tablets—Bottles of 100 (G. W. Carnrick)

Contains

	Gr	Gm
Spleen	1	0.064
Red bone marrow	1	0.064

For use in secondary anemias.

Dosage: 1–3 tablets three times daily.

35. Suprarenal-Pituitary Compound—Capsules and Tablets—Bottles of 40 and 100 (G. W. Carnrick)

Contains

	Gr	Gm
Suprarenal	2	0.130
Pituitary (whole)	½	0.032
Thyroid	1/10	0.006
Ant. pituitary	1½	0.097
Physiological Salts	¼	0.016

For use in bronchial asthma.

Dosage: 1 or 2, three times daily.

36. Thymus Compound—Capsules and Tablets—Bottles of 40 and 100 (G. W. Carnrick)

Contains

	Gr	Gm
Thymus	3	0.194
Thyroid	1/10	0.006
Pituitary	1/20	0.003

For use in chronic arthritis, rheumatoid arthritis, arthritis deformans.

Dosage: 1 or 2, three times daily.

37. Viriligen—Ampules 1 cc—Boxes of 6—Capsules and Tablets—Bottles of 100 (G. W. Carnrick)

Contains extracts of anterior pituitary, suprarenal cortex, testis, lymph gland, brain and spinal cord tissue, with thyroid 1/10 gr per capsule or tablet.

For use as aphrodisiac in lowered sexual virility and neurasthenia.

Dosage: 1–2 capsules or tablets before meals; 1 ampule every 3 days, *intramuscularly.*

38. Hemoglobin Compound—Capsules—Bottles of 100 (Cole)

Contains

	Gr	Gm
Hemoglobin	5	0.324
Ox gall, desiccated	½	0.032

	Gr	Gm
Spleen substance, desiccated	1½	0.097
Calcium glycerophosphate	q.s.	

For use in anemia, chlorosis, malnutrition.

Dosage: 1–2, three times daily after meals.

39. Suprarenal-Spermin Compound—Capsules—Bottles of 100 (Cole)

Contains

	Gr	Gm
Suprarenal substance	¼	0.016
Thyroid substance	⅛	0.008
Testicular substance (spermin extract)	2	0.130
Calcium phosphate	q.s.	

For use in asthenia, hypotension, neurasthenia, hypoadrenia, nervous debility.

Dosage: 1–2 capsules three times daily before meals.

40. Pituitary-Thymus Compound—Capsules—Bottles of 100 (Cole)

Contains

	Gr	Gm
Pituitary (anterior lobe)	2	0.130
Thymus substance	1½	0.097
Thyroid substance	1/10	0.006
Calcium glycerophosphate	q.s.	

For use in retarded development, (physical or mental) in children, endocrine deficiency (thyroid-pituitary, etc.), rickets and chronic rheumatic conditions.

Dosage: Children under 5 yr., 1, twice daily after meals, older children, 1, three or four times daily.

41. Ovarian Compound 24—Capsules—Bottles of 100 (Cole)

Contains

	Gr	Gm
Whole ovarian substance	⅛	0.008
Pituitary substance	⅛	0.008
Thyroid substance	1/10	0.006
Remineralizing compound 12	q.s.	

For use in amenorrhea, dysmenorrhea, sexual apathy, sterility, irregularities at puberty and menopause.

Dosage: 1, four times daily, after meals and at bedtime.

42. Pancreas-Adrenal Compound—Capsules—Bottles of 100 (Cole)

Contains

	Gr	Gm
Pancreas	3	0.194
Ovarian substance	1½	0.097
Adrenal substance	¼	0.016
Pituitary (total)	½	0.032

For use in sympathetic nerve irritability, hyperthyroidism, toxemia.

Dosage: 1, four times daily after meals; in extreme cases 2 capsules.

43. Nucleinized Thyro-Iodide Compound—Capsules—Bottles of 100 (Cole)

Contains

	Gr	Gm
Thyroid	½	0.032
Ferrous iodide	½	0.032
Nuclein	¼	0.016
Calcium glycerophosphate	1	0.064
Remineralizing comp. 12		

For use in non-toxic goiter, hyperthyroidism in young girls.

Dosage: 1, three times daily between meals, with water.

44. Mammary-Placenta Compound—Capsules—Bottles of 100 (Cole)

Contains

	Gr	Gm
Mammary substance	2	0.130
Placenta substance	2	0.130

	Gr	Gm
Pituitary (total)	1/3	0.024
Calcium glycerophosphate	q.s.	

For use in deficient breast secretion, agalactia, uterine subinvolution.

Dosage: 2, three times daily before meals for first ten days, after delivery then 1 capsule 3 times daily where required.

45. Placenta-Thyroid Compound—Capsules—Bottles of 100 (Cole)

Contains

	Gr	Gm
Placenta substance	5	0.324
Thyroid extract	1/12	0.005
Benzocaine	1/6	0.012
Calcined magnesium	q.s.	

For use in vomiting and nausea of pregnancy.

Dosage: 2, three times daily.

46. Renal-Pancreas Compound—Capsules—Bottles of 100 (Cole)

Contains

	Gr	Gm
Renal substance	4	0.259
Pancreas substance	4	0.259
Gold and sodium chloride	1/12	0.005

For use in acute and chronic nephritis, in impaired renal function.

Dosage: 1, three times daily.

47. Prostate-Spermin Compound—Capsules—Bottles of 100 (Cole)

Contains

	Gr	Gm
Prostate substance	2	0.130
Spermin extract (Leydig cells)	2	0.130
Lymphatic glands	2	0.130
Nucleinic acid	1/4	0.016
Calcium glycerophosphate	q.s.	

For use in prostatorrhea, impotence, senility, post-operative prostatectomy.

Dosage: 1, three times daily—continued as long as required.

48. Hepatic-Ovary-Pancreas Compound—Capsules—Bottles of 100 (Cole)

Contains

	Gr	Gm
Hepatic substance	2	0.130
Pancreas (total)	2	0.130
Ovarian substance	2	0.130
Bile salts	1	0.064
Thyroid	1/10	0.006

For use in arterial hypertension in women.

Dosage: 1, four times daily.

50. Ovary-Mammary Compound—Capsules—Bottles of 100 (Cole)

Contains

	Gr	Gm
Anterior pituitary	1/3	0.024
Mammary substance	3	0.194
Ovarian substance	1	0.064
Thyroid substance	1/10	0.006
Calcium phosphate	q.s.	

For use in menorrhagia.

Dosage: 1, three times daily.

51. Mammary-Ergotin Compound—Capsules—Bottles of 100 (Cole)

Contains

	Gr	Gm
Mammary substance	3	0.194
Ergotin	1/2	0.032
Pituitary (total)	1/4	0.016
Calcium phosphate	q.s.	

For use in menorrhagia, metrorrhagia, uterine fibroids.

Dosage: 1 capsule three times daily; double dosage 3 days before and during flow.

52. Gonad-Prostate Compound—Capsules—Bottles of 100 (Cole)

Contains

	Gr	Gm
Spermin extract (Leydig cells)	3	0.194
Prostate	1	0.064
Adrenal (total)	1	0.064
Pituitary (anterior lobe)	¼	0.016
Yohimbine hydrochloride	⅒	0.006
Extract damiana	¼	0.016

For use in impotence, sexual neurasthenia, hypogonadism, senilty.

Dosage: 1–2 capsules three times daily.

53. Pituitary-Phosphate Compound—Capsules—Bottles of 100 (Cole)

Contains

	Gr	Gm
Pituitary (anterior lobe)	2	0.130
Adrenal substance	1	0.064
Calcium lactate, Calcium phosphate	q.s.	

For use in bronchial asthma.

Dosage: 1 capsule four times daily.

54. Secretin-Pancreas-Myrtillin Compound—Capsules—Bottles of 100 (Cole)

Contains

Pancreas, secretin and vaccinium Myrtillus with remineralization compound 12.

For use as homostimulant to pancreas, to incite secretion of bile and reduce blood sugar; for mild diabetes.

Dosage: 1–2, ½–1 hr. before meals and at bedtime.

55. Thyro-Pituitary Compound—Capsules—Bottles of 100 (Cole)

Contains

	Gr	Gm
Thyroid substance	½	0.130
Pituitary (whole)	⅛	0.008
Phytolacca decandra, apocynum cannabinum and remineralizing compound 12	q.s.	

For use in obesity.

Dosage: 1–2, three or four times daily.

56. Parathyroid-Spermin Compound—Capsules—Bottles of 100 (Cole)

Contains

	Gr	Gm
Parathyroid substance	1/15	0.0042
Spermin extract (Leydig cells)	2	0.130
Ox gall	2	0.130
Spleen substance	1	0.064
Remineralizing comp. 12	q.s.	

For use where calcium therapy is indicated.

Dosage: 1, four times daily between meals.

57. Spermin-Pancreas Compound—Capsules—Bottles of 100 (Cole).

Contains

	Gr	Gm
Hepatic substance	2	0.130
Bile salts	1	0.064
Pancreas (total)	2	0.130
Thyroid	⅒	0.006
Orchic substance	2	0.130
Calcium phosphate	1	0.064

For use in arterial hypertension in men.

Dosage: 1, three or four times daily.

58. Glycocholate-Pancreas Compound—Capsules—Bottles of 100 **(Cole)**

Contains

	Gr	Gm
Purified bile salts, sodium glycotaurocholate	2	0.130
Hepatic substance	1	0.064
Secretin (duodenal substance)	1	0.064
Pancreas	q.s.	

For use in cholecystitis, functional liver deficiency, gall-stones, intestinal indigestion.

Dosage: 1–3, three or four times daily, increased or decreased as required.

59. Pulmo-Hemoglobin Compound—Capsules—Bottles of 100 **(Cole)**

Contains

	Gr	Gm
Pulmonary substance (purified)	5	0.324
Ox gall	1/8	0.008
Hemobin (predigested hemoglobin)	2	0.130
Calcium glycerophosphate	1	0.064

For use in phthisis, anemia, etc.

Dosage: 1, three or four times daily after meals.

60. Ovarian Compound 4—Capsules—Bottles of 100 **(Cole)**

Contains

	Gr	Gm
Orchic concentrate	20	1.296 fresh
Placenta substance	30	1.944 fresh
Suprarenal substance	1/4	0.016
Thyroid substance	1/20	0.003
Nucleinic acid and calcium glycerophosphate.		

For use in impotence, sexual neurasthenia.

Dosage: 1 or 2, three or four times daily.

61. Endocrine Compound 26—Capsules—Bottles of 100 **(Cole)**

Contains

	Gr	Gm
Ovarian substance	2	0.130
Adrenal substance	1	0.064
Pituitary (total)	1/4	0.016
Yohimbine	1/2	0.032
Extract damiana	1/10	0.006
Capsicum and calcium glycerophosphate	q.s.	

For use in frigidity, sexual neurasthenia, hypo-ovarianism.

Dosage: 1, three or four times daily.

62. Multicrinogen (Colwell's Hormone Solution)—Ampules 1 cc—Boxes of 12 **(Colwell)**

Contains

	Gr	Gm
Pituitary (entire body)	1/12	0.005
Thyroid	1/6	0.012
Suprarenal	1/5	0.013
Ovarian substance	1/3	0.024
Testicular substance	1/2	0.032

For use as general metabolic stimulant.

Dosage: 1 ampule *intramuscularly* two to three times weekly.

63. Thy-Ovar Compound—Bottles of 1 oz. **(Colwell)**

5 m equal to gr 1 thyroid and ovarian extracts as follows:

	Gr	Gm
Thyroid	1/6	0.012
Ovarian	5/6	0.060

For use in ovarian dysfunction.

Dosage: 5–15 m two to three times daily.

64. Hormones Solution—Bottles of 4, 8, 16 and 32 oz. **(Colwell)**
Contains entire pituitary, thyroid, suprarenal, gonads, in 90 % water and 10 % glycerine; free from proteins, fats; *For use* in menopausal and menstrual irregularities; in hyperemesis gravidarum, asthenia and hypotension; for backward children and mongolism.

Dosage: 1 teaspoonful three times daily before meals; children in accordance.

65. Corpus-Ova 1—Capsules—Packages of 100 **(Drug Products)**

Contains desiccated	Gr	Gm
Corpus luteum	½	0.032
Ovarian extract (from sow)	½	0.032
Thyroid	1/10	0.006
Pituitary whole gland	⅛	0.008

For use in amenorrhea, dysmenorrhea, menorrhagia, climacteric disorders.

Dosage: 1 capsule three times daily at meals, for 10 days, then 2 capsules three times daily for 10 days before menses, at onset of menses omitted for 10 days, then repeated for several months.

66. Hemoglobin Compound 1—Capsules—Packages of 100 **(Drug Products)**

Contains desiccated	Gr	Gm
Hemoglobin	1	0.064
Spleen substance	¼	0.016
Hepatic substance	1	0.064
Suprarenal whole gland	½	0.032

For use in hemoglobin insufficiency, acute and chronic anemia and chlorosis.

Dosage: 1 capsule after meals, gradually increased as indicated.

67. Lecithin Compound 1—Capsules—Packages of 100 **(Drug Products)**

Contains desiccated	Gr	Gm
Suprarenal whole gland	¼	0.016
Thyroid gland	1/10	0.006
Orchic substance	1	0.064
Lecithin	1	0.064

For use in premature senility, convalescence after infective diseases, asthenia and neurasthenia.

Dosage: 1 capsule before meals and upon retiring, or as indicated.

68. Lymphatic Compound 1—Capsules—Packages of 100 **(Drug Products)**

Contains desiccated	Gr	Gm
Lymphatic gland	1	0.064
Pituitary whole gland	¼	0.016
Thymus gland	¼	0.016
Thyroid gland	1/10	0.006

For use in infantilism, endocrine disorders in the adult, in lymphadenia.

Dosage: 1 capsule after meals, gradually increased as needed.

69. Mammary Compound 1—Capsules—Packages of 100 **(Drug Products)**

Contains desiccated	Gr	Gm
Mammary gland	1	0.064
Ovarian extract (from sow)	1	0.064
Thyroid gland	1/10	0.006

For use in functional menorrhagia and metrorrhagia, ovarian irritability, pelvic congestion; to induce uterine contraction; in deficient lactation, atrophy of breasts.

Dosage: 1 capsule three times daily; double dose 3 days before and during menses; omitted for 1 week, then repeated.

70. Orchic Compound—Capsules—Packages of 100 **(Drug Products)**

Contains desiccated

	Gr	Gm
Orchic substance	1	0.064
Thyroid gland	1/10	0.006
Suprarenal whole gland	1/4	0.016
Pituitary whole gland	1/4	0.016
Acid nucleinic	1/4	0.016

For use in premature senility, sexual asthenia and neurasthenia in men, neuroses due to sexual impotence.

Dosage: 1 capsule three times daily or as indicated.

71. Ovarian Compound 1—Capsules—Packages of 100 **(Drug Products)**

Contains desiccated

	Gr	Gm
Ovarian extract (from sow)	1	0.064
Mammary gland	1/2	0.032
Thyroid gland	1/10	0.006
Pituitary whole gland	1/8	0.008
Suprarenal whole gland	1/2	0.032
Acid nucleinic	1/4	0.016

For use in sexual imbalance, neurasthenia in women, menstrual disturbances, hypochondriasis and melancholia due to ovarian dysfunction, natural or artificial menopause.

Dosage: 1 capsule three times daily or as indicated.

72. Ovarian Compound 2—Capsules—Packages of 100 **(Drug Products)**

Contains desiccated

	Gr	Gm
Ovarian extract (from sow)	1/2	0.032
Pituitary whole gland	1/8	0.008
Suprarenal whole gland	1	0.064
Calcium glycerophosphate	1	0.064
Lecithin	1/4	0.016

For use in asthenia of general nervous system, with anemia.

Dosage: 1 capsule three times daily or as indicated.

73. Pit-Ren—Capsules—Packages of 100; Hyposols—1 cc Packages 12, 25 and 100 **(Drug Products)**

A combination of desiccated hypophysis cerebri and epinephrine hydrochloride.

For use in suitable cases of true allergic asthma, rhinorrhea, hay fever and pneumonia.

Dosage: 1 or 2 capsules every 2–4 hr. or as required, followed with a glass of hot water; in pneumonia or other acute cases hyposols *subcutaneously* or *intramuscularly* are used, *never* intravenously, and followed by capsules.

73a. Pitovaco—Pulvoids—Bottles 100, 1,000 **(Drug Products)**

Each represents

Ovarian fresh gland	gr 1	(0.064 Gm)
Pituitary whole gland	gr 1	(0.064 Gm)
Calcium glycerophosphate	gr 1	(0.064 Gm)
Nucleinic acid solution	m 10	(0.6 cc)
Ferronas	gr 1	(0.064 Gm)
Arsenic trioxide	gr 1/100	(0.65 mg)

For use in ovarian disorders accompanied by headache, constipation, thyroid hypertrophy, nervousness; hot flushes.

Dosage: 1–2 pulvoids three times daily.

74. Pituitary Compound 1—Capsules—Packages of 100 **(Drug Products)**

Contains desiccated

	Gr	Gm
Pituitary whole gland	1/4	0.016
Thymus gland	1/4	0.016
Thyroid gland	1/10	0.006

For use in maldevelopment, cretinism, chorea, epilepsy and retarded mentality in children.

Dosage: 1 capsule at meals for 4 out of every 5 weeks, for 4–6 mo.

75. Secretin Compound—Capsules—Packages of 100 **(Drug Products)**
A combination of the active principles of the stomach, pancreas and duodenum.

For use as gastric and intestinal homostimulant in indigestion, as general alimentary secretory stimulant.

Dosage: 1 capsule with meals three times daily or as indicated; in hypothyroidism with the additional use of ¼ gr fresh thyroid substance.

76. Thyroid-Ioform Compound—Capsules—Packages of 100 **(Drug Products)**
Contains

Thyroid gland desiccated	gr ⅕	(0.013 Gm)
Ioform (organic iodine)	gr ¼	(0.016 Gm)
Nuclein solution	m 5	(0.308 cc)
Ferronas	gr 2½	(0.162 Gm)

For use in goiter, simple thyroid enlargement, hyperthyrosis.

Dosage: 1 capsule with water three times daily between meals, or as indicated.

77. Thyovaco—Pulvoids—Bottles 100, 1,000 **(Drug Products)**

Represents	Gr	Gm
Ovarian fresh gland	1	0.064
Thyroid fresh gland	¼	0.016
Calcium glycerophosphate	1	0.064
Ferronas	1	0.064
Strychnine sulphate	1/120	0.0005
Arsenic trioxide	1/80	0.0008

For use in amenorrhea, dysmenorrhea, menorrhagia, metrorrhagia.

Dosage: 1–2 pulvoids three times daily.

79. Adrosil—Tablets—Bottles of 25 **(Glandular Laboratory)**
Contains extracts of thyroid, thymus, testes, suprarenal with sodium salicylate.

For use in rheumatism.

Dosage: 1–3 tablets after meals.

80. Thyovaroids—Tablets—Bottles of 100 and 1,000 **(Hance)**

Contains	Gr	Gm	
Ovarian substance	1	0.064	equivalent to gr 7½ (fresh gland)
Thyroid substance	⅛	0.008	
Calcium glycerophosphate	1	0.064	
Blaud's mass	1	0.064	
Strychnine sulphate	1/200	0.0003	
Arsenous acid	1/80	0.0008	

For use in amenorrhea, dysmenorrhea, menopause.

Dosage: 1 tablet three times daily.

81. Pituthymin Solution—Ampules—1 cc Boxes of 5 **(Harrower)**
Contains post-pituitary and thymus, 10 International units.

For use similarly to liquor pituitarii.

Dosage: ½–1 cc *intramuscularly*, daily or every other day; later once weekly.

82. Accretin—Capsules—Boxes of 40 **(Harrower)**
Contains active concentrates from anterior lobe of the pituitary and thymus; contains growth stimulating principle with vitamin B.

For use in infantilism, growth dystrophies, shortness of stature.

Dosage: 1–3 capsules three times daily at meals.

83. Adreno-Spermin—Sanitablets and Capsules—Packages of 100 **(Harrower)**

Contains	Gr	Gm
Total adrenal	¼	0.016
Thyroid	1/12	0.005
Spermin extract	2	0.130
Calcium glycerophosphate q.s.		

For use to support depleted adrenal function, stimulate oxidation, raise sympathetic tone; as endocrine tonic in asthenia, hypoadrenia, circulatory insufficiency with hypotension, neurasthenia and convalescence.

Dosage: 1, four times daily, after meals and in the evening.

84. Solution Adreno-Spermin Compound 1A—Ampules 1 cc—Boxes of 5 **(Harrower)**
Contains soluble active constituents of gr 20 (1.296 Gm) fresh gland in proportions—spermin 24, total adrenal 3, thyroid 1; standardized to 0.6 % N content.

For use—as above.

Dosage: Administered every second day, 1 ampule.

85. Antero-Pituitary Compound—Sanitablets 5 gr—Bottles of 100 **(Harrower)**

Contains	Gr	Gm
Anterior pituitary	2	0.130
Thymus	1	0.064
Thyroid	1/12	0.005
Calcium phosphorus compound	5	0.324

For use to stimulate growth in defective development of children of endocrine origin; in retarded mentality, mongolism, dwarfism; also in petit mal, chorea.

Dosage: 1 tablet twice daily, at meals for 4–5 weeks.

86. Placento-Mammary Compound—Sanitablets gr 5—Packages of 100 **(Harrower)**

Contains	Gr	Gm
Desiccated placenta	2	0.130
Mammary substance	1½	0.097
Pituitary	⅓	0.021
Calcium-phosphorus compound q.s.	5	0.324

For use to stimulate function of breasts, encourage uterine involution; is galactogogue in agalactia, hypogalactia, and prophylactic for milk-poor nursing mothers; in uterine subinvolution, infantile malnutrition.

Dosage: 2 tablets, twice daily and at bedtime for 2 weeks, then twice daily.

87. Menocrin—Sanitablets gr 5—Packages of 100 **(Harrower)**

Contains	Gr	Gm
Ovarian concentrate	3	0.194
Thyroid	1/12	0.005
Pituitary (anterior)	¼	0.016
Calcium-phosphorus compound q.s.	5½	0.356

For use to regulate menstrual endocrine control in amenorrhea, dysmenorrhea, sexual neuroses, menopausal disorders, dysovarism.

Dosage: 2 tablets three times daily before meals, 10 days before period, omitted 10 days at onset of menses; 1 tablet three times daily until 10 days before menses; repeated again.

88. Menocrin Solution—Ampules 1 cc—Boxes of 5 **(Harrower)**
Contains above constituents in ampule form of standardized 0.6 % N content; each cc is equal to 20 gr fresh gland in proportions; ovary 36, pituitary 3, thyroid 1.

Dosage: 1 cc intramuscularly every other day.

89. Hepatic Splenic Compound—Sanitablets gr 5—Packages of 100 **(Harrower)**

Contains	Gr	Gm
Liver parenchyma	2½	0.162
Spleen parenchyma	2	0.130

	Gr	Gm
Anabolin	1/4	0.016
Boldine hydrochloride	1/60	0.0010
Calcium phosphorus comp. q.s.	5	0.324

For use in hepatic cirrhosis and insufficiency; in toxicosis of tuberculosis, cachexia, malaria and malnutrition.

Dosage: 1 tablet three times daily and at bedtime; occasionally dosage is doubled.

90. Pancreas Compound—Sanitablets—Packages of 100 **(Harrower)**

Contains	Gr	Gm
Adrenal	1/2	0.032
Pituitary (total)	1/2	0.032
Ovary	1	0.064
Pancreas (total)	3	0.194

For use as a functional antagonist of sympathetic; in thyroidal, irritable, weak and rapid cardiac action; in post-influenzal and toxic asthenia with susceptible thyroid; in moderate hyperthyroidism.

Dosage: 1 tablet after each meal and at bedtime; occasionally the dose is doubled.

91. Thyroid Compound—Sanitablets—Packages of 100 **(Harrower)**

Contains	Gr	Gm
Thyroid	1/4 or 1/2	0.016 or 0.032
Calcium phosphorus comp.	5	0.324

For use in thyroid conditions.

Dosage: 1 tablet three times daily.

92. Iodized Thyroid Compound—Sanitablets—Packages of 100 **(Harrower)**

Contains	Gr	Gm
Thyroid	1/4	0.016
Ferrous iodide	1/4	0.016
Nucleic acid	1/4	0.016
Calcium phosphorus comp. q.s.		

For use the same as thyroid augmented by leucocytogenesis.

Dosage: 1 tablet in water before meals and at bedtime.

93. Bile Salts—Sanitablets gr 5—Packages of 100 **(Harrower)**

Contains	Gr	Gm
Repurified bile salts	3½	0.227
Liver substance q.s.	5	0.324

For use in liver insufficiency, intestinal stasis, gall bladder and duodenal dysfunction, mucous colitis, hepatic cirrhosis.

Dosage: 1 tablet twice daily before meals for 3 days, then 6 tablets for 3 days; with 9 tablets for 3 days, continued until free bile appears in stools; then reduced to 3 a day for several weeks.

94. Adreno-Hypophysis Compound—Sanitablets—Boxes of 100 **(Harrower)**

Contains	Gr	Gm
Adrenal (total)	1/2	0.032
Pituitary (anterior)	2	0.130
Calcium lactate / Calcium phosphate q.s.		

For use in asthenia and hypoadrenalism; also in bronchial asthma and anaphylactic conditions with endocrine basis.

Dosage: 1 tablet four times daily at meals and at bedtime.

95. Para-Spleen Compound—Sanitablets—Packages of 100 **(Harrower)**

Contains	Gr	Gm
Desiccated parathyroid	1/20	0.003
Spermin extract	1	0.064
Spleen substance	2	0.130

Bile salts	½	0.032
Calcium phosphorus comp	q.s.	

For use in parathyroid insufficiency, tetany, chorea, paralysis agitans; in varicose ulcers, gastric and duodenal ulcers, suppurative otitis, ulcerative colitis.

Dosage: 1 tablet at meals and at bedtime.

96. Para Spleen Compound Solution 24A—Ampules—Boxes of 5 **(Harrower)**
Contains standardized solution of 1 cc equals 20 gr fresh glands in proportion of spleen 10, parathyroid 1.

Dosage: 1 cc every other day for 2 months, intramuscularly.

97. Thyro-Pancreas Compound with Spermin / **Thyro-Pancreas Compound with Ovary** } Sanitablets—Boxes of 100 **(Harrower)**

Contains	Gr	Gm
Pancreas (total)	2	0.130
Thyroid	1/12	0.005
or { Spermin extract	2	0.130
or { Ovary	2	0.130
Calcium phosphorus compound	q.s.	

For use to antagonize adrenal irritability and functional hypertension; in menopausal high blood pressure.

Dosage: 1 tablet four times daily.

98. Mamma-Ovary Compound—Sanitablets—Boxes of 100 **(Harrower)**

Contains	Gr	Gm
Mammary substance	2½	0.162
Ovary	1	0.064
Thyroid	⅛	0.008
Calcium phosphorus compound ... q.s. ad	5	0.324

For use as ovarian regulator, to decrease ovarian hyperfunction, in moderate menorrhagia, difficult menstrual onset, dysovarism with irritability and abnormal pelvic congestion (usually in young girls).

Dosage: 1 tablet three times daily before meals; double dose 3 days before and during menses; omitted 1 week and repeated for at least 3 months.

99. Chalomen (Mamma-Pituitary Compound)—Sanitablets and Capsules—Boxes of 100 **(Harrower)**

Contains	Gr	Gm
Mammary substance	3	0.194
Corpus luteum	1	0.064
Luteinizing hormone (antepituitary)	1/40	0.001
Ergotin (Bonjean)	½	0.032
Calcium phosphorus compound	5	0.324

For use as uterine decongestant, muscle tonic and ovarian antagonist; in menorrhagia, metrorrhagia, excessive menstrual or climacteric hemorrhages.

Dosage: 1 capsule three times daily before meals; double dose for 2 weeks beginning at onset of menses; omitted for 1 week and repeated.

100. Pan-Secretin—Sanitablets—Boxes of 100 **(Harrower)**

Contains	Gr	Gm
Pancreas islets (tail)	3½	0.227
Secretin extract (duodenal)	1½	0.097

For use to stimulate pancreas (Langerhansian) function, ferment formation, increase carbohydrate tolerance and reduce blood sugar; does not replace insulin; Used as supplementary treatment in diabetes mellitus.

Dosage: 1-4, three to four times daily.

101. Pituitary Compound—Sanitablets—Boxes of 100 (Harrower)

Contains

	Gr	Gm
Anterior pituitary	2¾	0.178
Posterior pituitary	¼	0.016
Calcium phosphorus compound	q.s.	

For use to stimulate metabolism and gonadal function in essential dyspituitarism; in adiposogenital dystrophy, hypopituitarism, gonadal maldevelopment, pituitary developmental dystrophies.

Dosage: 1 or more tablets four times a day before meals.

102. Solution Pituitary Compound—Ampules—1 cc Boxes of 5 (Harrower)
Standardized to contain 0.5% N; each cubic centimeter equals 18½ gr of fresh anterior lobe and 1 gr of posterior lobe of pituitary gland.

Dosage: 1 cc daily or every other day.

103. Prostate Compound—Sanitablets—Packages of 100 (Harrower)

Contains

	Gr	Gm
Prostate extract	2	0.130
Spermin extract	2	0.130
Nucleic acid	¼	0.016
Calcium phosphorus compound	q.s. ad	

For use as hemostimulant to prostate and sex glands and as prostatic sedative; *For use* in enlarged prostate, prostatism and after prostatic operations.

Dosage: 1 tablet four times daily.

104. Placenta-Compound—Sanitablets—Packages of 100 (Harrower)

Contains

	Gr	Gm
Placental parenchyma	5	0.324
Thyroid	1/24	0.002
Calcium phosphorus compound	q.s.	

For use to relieve placental toxemia and hyperemesis gravidarum.

Dosage: 2 tablets with charged ice water, four times daily, with sedatives to aid retention.

105. Placenta Luteum Compound—Ampules 1 cc—Boxes of 5 (Harrower)
Contents standardized to contain 0.65% N, representing soluble active constituents of fresh glands, in proportions of: placenta 3, corpora lutea 1, for supplementary therapy.

Dosage: 1 cc every 24 hr.

106. Thymus Spermin Compound—Sanitablets—Packages of 100 (Harrower)

Contains

	Gr	Gm
Adreno-Spermin	3	0.194
Thymus	3	0.194

For use to stimulate metabolism in arthritis deformans, chronic forms of arthritis with deficient cell regeneration.

Dosage: 1 tablet four times daily; after each meal and at bedtime; dosage may be increased for few weeks, then reduced.

107. Spermin Hemoglobin Compound—Sanitablets—Packages of 100 (Harrower)

Contains

	Gr	Gm
Adreno-Spermin	3	0.194
Hemoglobin	3	0.194

For use to support depleted adrenal function; to increase sympathetic tone and oxidation; *For use* in hypoadrenalism with anemia, convalescence; chronic invalids.

Dosage: 1 tablet four times daily after meals.

108. Gonad Compound—Sanitablets—Packages of 100 **(Harrower)**

Contains

	Gr	Gm
Adrenal (total)	½	0.032
Thyroid	1/24	0.002
Anterior pituitary	½	0.032
Extract prostate	1½	0.097
Lydin	1½	0.097

For use as general endocrine stimulant, especially of gonads; in functional hypogonadism, aspermia, sterility, asexualism, presenility, sexual neurasthenia.

Dosage: 2 tablets twice daily before meals.

109. Solution of Gonad Compound—Ampules 1 cc—Boxes of 5 **(Harrower)**
Contains a solution of above endocrines; 1 cc = 0.6% N; each cubic centimeter represents 20 Gm fresh gland in proportions of prostate 18, lydin 12, anterior pituitary 12, adrenal 6, thyroid 1.

For use—as above.

Dosage: 1 cc every 24–48 hr., in intramuscular injection.

110. Gonad-Ovarian Compound—Sanitablets—Packages of 100 **(Harrower)**

Contains

	Gr	Gm
Menocrin (thyro-ovarian compound)	3	0.194
Spermin extract	1½	0.097
Anterior pituitary	1½	0.097

For use as ovarian and general cell stimulant; in dysovarism, ovarian insufficiency, asexualism, infantilism.

Dosage: 1, three times daily before meals; 2 tablets, three times daily before meals for 10 days before menses; omitted 10 days; 1 tablet three times daily until 10 days before menses; repeated.

111. Adreno-Ovarian Compound—Sanitablets—Packages of 100 **(Harrower)**

Contains

	Gr	Gm
Menocrin	4	0.259
Adrenal gland	1	0.064

For use as utero-ovarian regulator in ovarian dysfunction, menstrual disorders with hypoadrenalism.

Dosage: 1 tablet three times daily for 10 days; double dosage from 7–10 days before menstruation; omitted for 10 days at onset of menses; repeated.

112. Renal Compound—Sanitablets—Packages of 100 **(Harrower)**

Contains

	Gr	Gm
Desiccated renal glomerular tissue	2½	0.162
Pancreas	2½	0.162

To affect renal permeability, lessen albumin leakage and stimulate renal efficacy;

For use in acute and chronic Bright's disease and essential albuminuria.

Dosage: 1 or more tablets four times daily before meals.

113. Heparnucleate Liver Extract—Tubes of 4½ Gm—Box of 12 **(Harrower)**

Contains

	Gm
Heparhemin	4
Sodium nucleates	0.25
Iron nucleates	0.25

Each dose contains 30 mg of organic iron and 20 mg of organic phosphorus with hemopoietin from 125 Gm of fresh liver.

For use in severe anemias to increase the red blood corpuscles.

Dosage: 1 tube daily with milk, soup (not hot) or orange juice.

114. Solution Heparhemin-Liver Extract—Ampules 5 cc—Boxes of 3 **(Harrower)**
Contains a stable solution of hemopoietic liver principle for *intramuscular* injection,

each 5 cc is equivalent to 100 Gm fresh liver.

For use—in pernicious and secondary anemias where oral liver administration is not tolerated.

Dosage: 5 cc daily.

115. Anabolin Tablets—Vials of 15—Bottles 50 **(Harrower)**

Contains hepatic extract gr 1 (0.064 Gm) equal to 1 cc hepatic solution of defined hypotensive potency; with traces of histamine.

For use to reduce functional hypertension through influence on liver and endocrine catalysis; in toxic and menopausal hypertension.

Dosage: 1 tablet three times daily.

116. Anabolin Solution—Ampules 1 cc—Boxes of 5 **(Harrower)**

Prepared from hepatic parenchyma; contains fractions of proteins and less than 0.01 % histamine.

For use—as above.

Dosage: 1 cc for injection mornings, daily or every second day, *intramuscularly.*

117. Anabolin Solution Fortior—Ampules 1 cc—Boxes of 5 **(Harrower)**

Contains above double strength, for *hypodermic* use in above cases.

118. Paracalcin—Tablets—Vials of 15—Bottles of 50 **(Harrower)**

Contains	Gr	Gm
Parathyroid	1/10	0.006
Calcium lactate	3	0.194
Starch	1	0.064

Standardized each tablet to equal one unit is; not affected by stomach secretions.

For use in decreased calcium metabolism and parathyroid detoxication; in paralysis agitans, chronic septic ulceration and tetany.

Dosage: 1 tablet three times daily.

119. Paracalcin Solution—Ampules 1 cc—Boxes of 5 **(Harrower)**

1 cc equals 10 units; injected *intramuscularly* every other day.

For use to supplement oral tablet medication, in above conditions.

120. Liquor Pituitarii (U.S.P.)—Ampules 1 cc—Boxes of 5 **(Harrower)**

Standardized by oxytocic and pressor methods; 1 cc equals 10 international units.

For use in diabetes insipidus, intestinal paresis, following labor and post-partum hemorrhage; contraindicated in first stage of labor.

Dosage: ½–1 cc *intramuscularly.*

120a. Diabetan—Capsules 5 gr—Boxes of 100, 500 and 1,000 **(Harvey-Pittenger)**

Contains per capsule 2½ gr Islands of Langerhans, desiccated, with alkaline salts;

For use in diabetes mellitus of pancreatic origin; *also used* for control of adrenal excess in hypertension of alimentary origin.

Dosage: 1 or 2 before meals.

121. Ephedan—Capsules 5 gr—Boxes of 100, 500 and 1,000 **(Harvey-Pittenger)**

Presents the antispasmodic and antiasthmatic principles of Ephedra (Ma-Huang), anterior pituitary desiccated and suprarenal desiccated, with alkaline salts.

For use in bronchial asthma, bronchitis, dyspnea.

Dosage: 1 every 3 hr.

122. Galacan—Capsules 5 gr—Boxes of 100, 500 and 1,000 **(Harvey-Pittenger)**

Contains a mixture of endocrine galactagogues represented by mammary substance, desiccated placenta and whole pituitary, with alkaline salts.

For use as a galactagogue in deficient milk secretion and in infantile malnutrition.

Dosage: 2 before meals.

123. Glandular Compound 1 (Male)—Capsules 5 gr—Boxes of 100, 500 and 1,000 **(Harvey-Pittenger)**

Contains

	Gr	Gm
Thyroid desiccated	¼	0.016
Suprarenal desiccated	2	0.130
Orchic substance desiccated	2	0.130
Phosphate compound q.s.	5	0.324

For use as alterative and tonic in sexual and general debility, due to lessened adrenal and genital function; in some forms of borderline neuroses and psychoses resulting from dysfunction of these glands.

Dosage: 1–2 capsules three times daily.

123a. Glandular Compound 2 (Female)—Capsules 5 gr—Boxes of 100, 500 and 1,000 **(Harvey-Pittenger)**

Contains desiccated

	Gr	Gm
Thyroid	¼	0.016
Suprarenal	1	0.064
Corpus luteum	½	0.032
Ovarian substance	1½	0.097
Phosphate compound q.s.	5	0.324

For use as alterative and tonic; in disorders following menopause and in general debility, myxedema, obesity, etc.

Dosage: 1–2 three times daily.

124. Hemovaran—Capsules 5 gr—Boxes of 100, 500 and 1,000 **(Harvey-Pittenger)**
Contains ovarian whole substance desiccated, with lecithin, nucleinic acid and hemoglobin.

For use in anemia, malnutrition, menstrual neuroses and psychoses; in vasomotor disturbances of natural or artificial (surgical) menopause.

Dosage: 1 or 2 before meals.

125. Mameran—Capsules 5 gr—Boxes of 100, 500 and 1,000 **(Harvey-Pittenger)**
Contains a combination of mammary substance desiccated and pituitary whole desiccated, with ergotin (Bonjean) ½ gr and calcium phosphate comp. q.s. 5 gr.

For use in menorrhagia, metrorrhagia and climacteric hemorrhages.

Dosage: 1 three times daily after meals; 2, every 3 hr. in hemorrhage.

126. Orchan—Capsules 5 gr—Boxes of 100, 500 and 1,000 **(Harvey-Pittenger)**
Contains a well balanced combination of desiccated thyroid, suprarenal and orchic substances with alkaline salts q.s. gr 5.

For use in sexual neurasthenia; premature senility, adynamia and systemic nerve depletion.

Dosage: 1, before each meal and on retiring.

127. Ovaran—Capsules gr 5—Boxes of 100, 500 and 1,000 **(Harvey-Pittenger)**
Contains a well balanced combination of desiccated thyroid, suprarenal, corpus luteum and whole ovarian substances with alkaline salts q.s. gr 5.

For use in menopause either natural or surgical; in amenorrhea, dysmenorrhea, etc.

Dosage: 1, or 2 three times daily.

128. Paracal—Capsules gr 4—Boxes of 100, 500 and 1,000 **(Harvey-Pittenger)**

Contains

	Gr	Gm
Parathyroid substance desiccated	1/10	0.006
Calcium lactate	3	0.194
Alkaline salts q.s.	4	0.259

For use in deficient calcium metabolism, rickets, scrofula, locomotor ataxia and in treatment of gastric and duodenal ulcers.

Dosage: 1, four times daily.

129. Thyorchan—Capsules gr 5—Boxes of 100, 500 and 1,000 **(Harvey-Pittenger)**
Contains thyroid desiccated, orchic substance desiccated, suprarenal desiccated with strychnine sulphate gr 1/80, yohimbine hydrochloride gr 1/12 and alkaline salts q.s. 5 gr.

For use in impotence, asexualism, hypogonadism; as active reconstructive and dynamic aphrodisiac.

Dosage: 1, every three hours.

130. Thyovaran—Capsules gr 5—Boxes of 100, 500 and 1,000 **(Harvey-Pittenger)**
Contains thyroid desiccated, ovarian whole desiccated and pituitary whole desiccated with alkaline salts q.s. 5 gr.

For use in amenorrhea, dysmenorrhea, sexual apathy and neuroses connected with the menstrual function.

Dosage: 1, three times daily, double dose 5 days before menses and omitted at onset for 10 days.

131. Asexualism, Male—Enterocaps—Bottles of 100 **(Lafayette Pharmacal)**
Contains extracts:

	Gr	Gm
Orchic	½	0.032
Brain	½	0.032
Pituitary	½	0.032
Suprarenal	¼	0.016
Thyroid	1/10	0.006
Thymus	1	0.064

For use in male asexualism, (for female see 160).

Dosage: 1 capsule before meals and at bedtime.

132. Corluroid—Enterocaps—Bottles of 100 **(Lafayette Pharmacal)**
Contains

	Gr	Gm
Corpus luteum	4	0.259
Thyroid	1/8	0.008

For use as indicated.

Dosage: 1 capsule three times daily.

133. Duobilad—Enterocaps—Bottles of 100 **(Lafayette Pharmacal)**
Contains

	Gr	Gm
Duodenal	3	0.194
Bile	1½	0.097
Suprarenal	¼	0.016
Mineral salts comp.	¾	0.048

For use where indicated.

Dosage: 1 capsule two to three times daily.

134. Femex—Enterocaps—Bottles of 100 **(Lafayette Pharmacal)**
Contains

	Gr	Gm
Ovarian extract	1¾	0.112
Pituitary anterior	½	0.032
Suprarenal	¼	0.016
Thyroid	1/16	0.004
Yohimbine	1/12	0.005
Nux vomica	¼	0.016

For use in frigidity, impotence, moroseness.

Dosage: 1 capsule before meals and at bedtime.

135. Gonadrenal—Enterocaps—Bottles of 100 **(Lafayette Pharmacal)**
Contains

	Gr	Gm
Gonads	1	0.064
Suprarenal	1/3	0.021

	Gr	Gm
Thyroid	1/12	0.005
Lecithin	1	0.064
Calcium glycerophosphate	1	0.064

For use as indicated.

Dosage: 1 capsule three to four times daily.

136. Hemo-Splenic—Enterocaps—Bottles of 100 **(Lafayette Pharmacal)**

Contains

	Gr	Gm
Hemoglobin	4	0.259
Spleen	1	0.064
Nucleinic Acid	½	0.032
Mineral salts compound	q.s.	

For use in conditions indicated.

Dosage: 1 capsule four times daily.

137. Hepato-Bilad—Enterocaps—Bottles of 100 **(Lafayette Pharmacal)**

Contains

	Gr	Gm
Hepatic parenchyma	2	0.130
Spleen substance	2	0.130
Bile salts	½	0.032
Gonadrenal	1	0.064

For use in conditions indicated.

Dosage: 1 capsule, two to three times daily.

138. Leci-Nuclein—Enterocaps—Bottles of 100 **(Lafayette Pharmacal)**

Contains

	Gr	Gm
Lecithin	1½	0.097
Nuclein	1	0.064
Calcium glycerophosphate	2	0.130
Calcium phosphate	2	0.130

For use as indicated.

Dosage: 1 capsule three times daily.

139. Malex—Enterocaps—Bottles of 100 **(Lafayette Pharmacal)**

Contains

	Gr	Gm
Orchic extract	3	0.194
Pituitary anterior	½	0.032
Suprarenal	¼	0.016
Thyroid	1/16	0.004
Yohimbine hydrochloride	1/12	0.005
Nux vomica	¼	0.016

For use in frigidity, impotence, moroseness.

Dosage: 1 capsule before meals and at bedtime.

140. Mammary Mixture—Enterocaps—Bottles of 100 **(Lafayette Pharmacal)**

Contains extracts

	Gr	Gm
Mammary	1½	0.097
Placenta	2	0.130
Pituitary	⅓	0.021

For use in hyperovarism, uterine subinvolution, deficient lactation, uterine hemorrhage of functional origin.

Dosage: 1 or 2 capsules before meals and at bedtime.

141. Morrol with Suprarenal—Enterocaps—Bottles of 100 (Lafayette Pharmacal)

Contains

	Gr	Gm
Morrhugan (concentrate from 50 m cod liver oil)		
Suprarenal	1/4	0.016
Calcium guaiacol sulphonate	1	0.064
Berberine sulphate	1/16	0.004
Nux vomica	1/10	0.006
Ginger	1	0.064

For use as indicated.

Dosage: 1 capsule before meals and at bedtime.

142. Normalizer 1—Enterocaps—Bottles of 100 (Lafayette Pharmacal)

Contains

	Gr	Gm
Pituitary extract	1	0.064
Suprarenal extract	1	0.064
Hemoglobin	1	0.064
Nux vomica	1/10	0.006

For use in malnutrition, low blood pressure, anemia.

Dosage: 1 capsule before meals and at bedtime.

143. Normalizer 2—Enterocaps—Bottles of 100 (Lafayette Pharmacal)

Contains

	Gr	Gm
Pituitary extract	2	0.130
Suprarenal extract	2	0.130
Hemoglobin	1 1/3	0.085
Strychnine sulphate	1/100	0.0006

For use in conditions indicated.

Dosage: 1 capsule three times daily.

144. Oralsulin Mixture—Enterocaps—Bottles of 100 (Lafayette Pharmacal)

Contains

	Gr	Gm
Oralsulin	A	
Thyroid	1/16	0.004
Pituitary	1/8	0.008
Duodenal	1	0.064

For use: See Chap. III.

145. Oralsulin with Duodenal—Enterocaps—Bottles of 100 (Lafayette Pharmacal)

Contains

	Gr	Gm
Oralsulin	A	
Duodenal extract	2	0.130

For use: See Chap. III.

146. Orchiroid 1—Enterocaps—Bottles of 100 (Lafayette Pharmacal)

Contains extracts

	Gr	Gm
Orchic	1/2	0.032
Thyroid	1/32	0.002

For use as cell stimulant, in deficient oxidation, toxemia.

Dosage: 1 capsule with meals and on retiring.

147. Orchiroid 2—Enterocaps—Bottles of 100 (Lafayette Pharmacal)

Contains extracts

	Gr	Gm
Orchic	1	0.064
Thyroid	1/16	0.004

For use as Orchiroid 1.

Dosage: 1 capsule with meals and on retiring.

148. Orchiroid 3—Enterocaps —Bottles of 100 (Lafayette Pharmacal)

Contains extracts

	Gr	Gm
Orchic	2	0.130
Thyroid	⅛	0.008

For use as Orchiroid 1.

Dosage: 1 capsule with meals and on retiring.

149. Ovaroid 1—Enterocaps—Bottles of 100 (LafayettePharmacal)

Contains extracts

	Gr	Gm
Ovarian	½	0.032
Thyroid	1/32	0.002

For use as cell stimulant, in deficient oxidation, toxemia.

Dosage: 1 capsule with meals and on retiring.

150. Ovaroid 2—Enterocaps—Bottles of 100 (Lafayette Pharmacal)

Contains extracts

	Gr	Gm
Ovarian	1	0.064
Thyroid	1/16	0.004

For use as Ovaroid 1.

Dosage: 1 capsule with meals and on retiring.

151. Ovaroid 3—Enterocaps—Bottles of 100 (Lafayette Pharmacal)

Contains extracts

	Gr	Gm
Ovarian	2	0.130
Thyroid	⅛	0.008

For use as Ovaroid 1.

Dosage: 1 capsule with meals and on retiring.

154. Placental Mixture—Enterocaps—Bottles of 100 (Lafayette Pharmacal)

Contains extracts

	Gr	Gm
Placenta	5	0.324
Thyroid	1/24	0.002

For use to promote uterine involution and lactation; in agalactia and nausea of pregnancy.

Dosage: 1 or 2 capsules before meals and at bedtime.

155. Suprarenal Mixture—Enterocaps—Bottles of 100 (Lafayette Pharmacal

Contains extracts

	Gr	Gm
Suprarenal	¼	0.016
Thyroid	1/12	0.005
Gonadal	2	0.130

For use in muscular atony, asthenia, cardiac insufficiency.

Dosage: 1 capsule before meals and at bedtime.

156. Thyorchic—Enterocaps—Bottles of 100 (Lafayette Pharmacal)

Contains extracts

	Gr	Gm
Orchic	2½	0.162
Thyroid	1/16	0.004
Pituitary	1/16	0.004
Calcium glycerophosphate	⅜	0.024

For use in conditions indicated.

Dosage: 1 capsule three times daily.

157. Thyovary—Enterocaps—Bottles of 100 **(Lafayette Pharmacal)**

Contains extracts

	Gr	Gm
Ovarian	2½	0.162
Thyroid	1/12	0.005
Pituitary	⅛	0.008

For use in scanty or irregular menstruation, sterility, sexual apathy.

Dosage: 1 capsule before meals and at bedtime; discontinued during menstrual function.

158. Yohimbine and Ovarian Mixture—Enterocaps—Bottles of 100 **(Lafayette Pharmacal)**

Contains

	Gr	Gm
Yohimbine hydrochloride	1/12	0.005
Ovarian extract	1½	0.097
Corpus luteum	1½	0.097
Pituitary anterior	1½	0.097
Suprarenal	1½	0.097
Thyroid	1/10	0.006

For use in senility, sexual indifference, atrophy.

Dosage: 1 capsule 1, 2 or 3 hr. after meals and on retiring.

159. Yohimbine and Orchic Mixture—Enterocaps—Bottles of 100 **(Lafayette Pharmacal)**

Contains

	Gr	Gm
Yohimbine hydrochloride	1/12	0.005
Orchic extract	1½	0.097
Pituitary anterior	1½	0.097
Suprarenal	1½	0.097
Thyroid	1/10	0.006

For use in senility, sexual indifference, atrophy.

Dosage: 1 capsule 1, 2 or 3 hr. after meals and on retiring.

160. Asexualism Female—Enterocaps—Bottles of 100 **(Lafayette Pharmacal)**

Contains extracts

	Gr	Gm
Ovarian	½	0.032
Mammary	½	0.032
Brain	½	0.032
Thymus	1	0.064
Thyroid	1/10	0.006
Suprarenal	¼	0.016
Pituitary	½	0.032

For use as indicated.

Dosage: 1 capsule before meals and at bedtime.

161. Glandular Compound (Female)—Capsules and Tablets—Bottles of 100 and 1,000 **(Maltbie)**

Contains desiccated—

	Gr	Gm
Thyroid	⅛	0.008
Thymus	½	0.032
Suprarenal	¼	0.016
Ovarian, (whole)	½	0.032

Dosage: 1–2 three times daily after meals.

162. Glandular Compound (Male)—Capsules and Tablets—Bottles of 100 and 1,000 **(Maltbie)**

Contains desiccated—

	Gr	Gm
Thyroid	⅛	0.008
Thymus	½	0.032

Suprarenal	¼	0.016
Orchic	½	0.032

Dosage: 1–2, three times daily after meals.

163. Adrempco—Capsules—Bottles of 50 **(Marvell)**
Contains thyroid gr ⅛ (0.008 Gm), pituitary, ovarian, testicular and adrenal substance.

For use in hypoadrenia, hypotension.

Dosage: 1 capsule three times daily.

164. Adrempco 100—Ampules 1 cc—Boxes of 12 **(Marvell)**
Each cubic centimeter representing Desiccated—

	Gr	Gm
Pituitary (entire)	1/12	0.006
Thyroid	⅙	0.012
Adrenals	⅕	0.014
Ovarian	⅓	0.024
Testicle	½	0.032

For use in asthenia, neurasthenia, premature senility, retarded development, hypotonia.

Dosage: 1 ampule injected *intramusculary* every other day.

165. Atoco—Capsules—Bottles of 50 **(Marvell)**
Contains thyroid gr 1/10 (0.006 Gm), adrenal substance, testicular extract and calcium glycerphosphate.

For use in asthenia, exhaustion, deficient nerve nutrition.

Dosage: 1 capsule three or four times daily.

166. Bilempco—Capsules—Bottles of 50 **(Marvell)**
Contains adrenal gr ¼ (0.016 Gm) bile salts compound gr 2 (0.13 Gm) with duodenal substance and calcium glycerophosphate.

For use in intestinal stasis and as biliary stimulant.

Dosage: 1–2 capsules four times daily between meals.

167. Mammary Compound—Capsules—Bottles of 50 **(Marvell)**
Contains mammary substance, placenta, entire pituitary.

For use as galactogogue.

Dosage: 1–2 capsules three times daily.

168. Orchiben Compound—Capsules—Bottles of 50 **(Marvell)**

	Gr	Gm
Contains testicular extract (concentrated)	3	0.193
Thyroid	1/10	0.006

with anterior pituitary, suprarenal and vitamin E.

For use in asthenia, hypogonadism.

Dosage: 1–2 capsules three times daily after meals.

169. Orchic-Epinephrine Compound—Ampules 1 cc—Boxes of 12 **(Marvell)**
Contains extracts of anterior pituitary, prostate, orchic glands, with 2 m of epinephrine chloride (1:1,000) per ampule.

For use in hypogonadism, hypotonia and sexual neurasthenia.

Dosage: 1 ampule two to three times weekly, *intramusculary*.

170. Ovempco—Capsules—Bottles of 50 **(Marvell)**
Contains thyroid gr 1/12 (0.005 Gm), pituitary, ovarian extract and calcium glycerophosphate.

For use in toxemia of pregnancy, vicarious menstruation, menopause.

Dosage: 1 capsule three times daily.

171. Pan-Orch-Oid—Capsules—Bottles of 50 (Marvell)
Contains thyroid gr 1/15 (0.004 Gm), orchic and pancreas substance.

For use in essential hypertension.

Dosage: 1 capsule three times daily.

172. Polempco—Capsules—Bottles of 50 (Marvell)
Contains thyroid gr 1/8 (0.008 Gm), pituitary, ovarian and testicular extracts.

For use in hysteria, vasomotor atony.

Dosage: 1 capsule three times daily before meals.

173. Polempco 96—Polyglandular Solution—Ampules 1 cc—Boxes of 12 (Marvell)

Represents per cc desiccated	Gr	Gm
Pituitary entire	1/12	0.005
Thyroid	1/6	0.012
Ovary	1/3	0.024
Testicle	1/12	0.005

For use in presenility, neurasthenia, genitourinary disturbances, hyperemesis gravidarum.

Dosage: 1 ampule daily, severe cases twice daily; *intramuscularly.*

174. Polempco 101—Polyglandular "O"—Ampules 1 cc—Boxes of 12 (Marvell)

Represents per cc desiccated	Gr	Gm
Pituitary entire	1/12	0.005
Thyroid	1/6	0.012
Ovarian	1	0.06

For use in presenility, neurasthenia, hyperemesis gravidarum.

Dosage: 1 ampule daily, *intramuscularly.*

175. Polempco 102—Polyglandular "T"—Ampules 1 cc—Boxes of 12 (Marvell)

Represents per cc desiccated	Gr	Gm
Pituitary entire	1/12	0.005
Thyroid	1/6	0.012
Testicle	1	0.06

For use in presenility, neurasthenia, genitourinary disturbances, hyperemesis gravidarum.

Dosage: 1 ampule daily, *intramuscularly.*

176. Semvesco—Capsules—Bottles of 50 (Marvell)
Contains thyroid gr 1/60 (0.001 Gm), suprarenal, anterior pituitary, testicular, prostatic, seminal vesicle extracts.

For use as restorative tonic, in nervous impotency.

Dosage: 1 capsule three times daily.

177. Vesix—Capsules—Bottles of 50 (Marvell)
Contains seminal vesicles substance, prostate, testicle.

For use in sexual impotence, neuroses, prostatic hypertrophy.

Dosage: 1 capsule three times daily.

178. Glandular Compound 2 Female—Capsules and Tablets—Bottles of 100 and 500 (McNeil)

Contains desiccated	Gr	Gm
Thyroid gland	1/2	0.032
Suprarenal gland	1	0.064
Corpus luteum	1/2	0.032
Ovarian substance	1	0.064

For use as alterative in disorders following menopause and in general debility, myxedema, obesity, etc.

Dosage: 1 or 2 capsules or tablets.

179. Glandular Compound 3, Male—Capsules and Tablets—Bottles of 100 and 500 **(McNeil)**

Contains dessicated

	Gr	Gm
Thyroid	½	0.032
Suprarenal	1	0.064
Testicular substance	3	0.194
Calcium glycerophosphate	1	0.064

For use as alterative in general debility of men.

Dosage: 1 or 2 capsules or tablets, three times daily.

180. Glandular Compound 4—Capsules and Tablets—Bottles of 100 and 500 **(McNeil)**

Contains

	Gr	Gm
Thyroid, desiccated	1/12	0.005
Ovarian residue, desiccated	2½	0.162
Pituitary, desiccated	⅛	0.008
Strychnine glycerophosphate	1/200	0.00032
Manganese glycerophosphate	1/14	0.004
Iron glycerophosphate	1/7	0.009
Calcium glycerophosphate	2 1/7	0.139

For use in amenorrhea, dysmenorrhea, neurasthenia, and the disorders following menopause.

Dosage: 1 or 2 capsules or tablets, three times daily.

181. Glandular Compound 5—Capsules—Bottles of 100 and 500 **(McNeil)**

Contains

	Gr	Gm
Suprarenal, desiccated	1	0.064
Thyroid, desiccated	1/12	0.005
Spermin extract	1	0.064
Brain substance, desiccated	1	0.064
Calcium glycerophosphate	2⅔	0.172

For use in asthenia, hypotension and neurasthenia.

Dosage: 1 capsule, three times daily.

182. Glandular Compound 7—Capsules and Tablets—Bottles of 100 and 500 **(McNeil)**

Contains desiccated

	Gr	Gm
Placenta	2	0.130
Mammary substance	1½	0.097
Pituitary	⅓	0.021
Calcium glycerophosphate	1⅔	0.111

For use in deficient milk secretion and malnutrition of nursing infants.

Dosage: 2 capsules or tablets with meals, for 10 days; then 1, three times daily.

183. Glandular Compound 8—Capsules—Bottles of 100 and 500 **(McNeil)**

Contains

	Gr	Gm
Mammary substance, desiccated	2½	0.162
Ergotin	½	0.032
Pituitary, desiccated	¼	0.016
Calcium glycerophosphate	1	0.064

For use in menorrhagia, metrorrhagia, and uterine fibroids.

Dosage: 1 or 2 capsules every 3 hr.

184. Glandular Compound 9—Capsules and Tablets—Bottles of 100 and 500 **(McNeil)**

Contains

	Gr	Gm
Prostate gland, desiccated	1½	0.097
Spermin extract	3	0.194
Lymphatic gland, desiccated	1½	0.097

	Gr	Gm
Sodium nucleinate	1/8	0.008
Calcium glycerophosphate	1 3/8	0.088

For use in prostatic irritability and insufficiency, in senility and following prostatectomy.

Dosage: 1 capsule or tablet three times daily.

185. Glandular Compound 10—Capsules and Tablets—Bottles of 100 and 500 (McNeil)

Contains	Gr	Gm
Prostate gland, desiccated	3	0.194
Thyroid, desiccated	1/4	0.013
Extract cascara sagrada	1	0.064
Papain	1	0.064

For use as alterative and gentle laxative in senility and general debility in men.

Dosage: 1 capsule or tablet three times daily.

186. Orcon Compound 1—Capsules—Bottles of 100 and 500 (McNeil)

Contains Orchic concentrate (equivalent to 70 gr fresh substance)	Gr	Gm
Thyroid gland, desiccated	1/2	0.032
Suprarenal gland, desiccated	1	0.064
Calcium glycerophosphate	1/2	0.032
Sodium glycerophosphate	1/2	0.032

Dosage: 1 or 2 capsules three times daily.

187. Orcon Compound 2—Capsules—Bottles of 100 and 500 (McNeil)

Contains Orchic concentrate (equivalent to gr 28 fresh substance)	Gr	Gm
Pituitary anterior, desiccated	1	0.064
Strychnine glycerophosphate	1/60	0.001
Calcium glycerophosphate	1 1/2	0.097
Sodium glycerophosphate	1 1/2	0.097

Dosage: 1 or 2 capsules three times daily.

188. Pituitary-Thymus—Ampules 1 cc—Vials 10 cc (McNeil)

1/2–1 cc *intramuscularly* according to the occasion.

188a. Mammary Compound 1—Capsules—Bottles of 100, 1,000 (Miller)

Contains	Gr	Gm
Mammary	5	0.324
Whole pituitary	1	0.064
Ergotin (Bonjean)	1/2	0.032

For use in uterine congestion associated with menopause; contraindicated in hypo-ovarianism, amenorrhea, infantilism.

Dosage: 1, before each meal; doubled several days before and during menstruation, discontinued for several days after.

189. Mammary Compound 2—Capsules—Bottles of 100, 1,000 (Miller)

Contains	Gr	Gm
Mammary	2 1/2	0.162
Placenta	2 1/2	0.162
Whole pituitary	1	0.064

For use in agalactia and uterine subinvolution.

Dosage: 1, before each meal, after delivery.

190. Orchic Compound 1—Capsules—Bottles of 100, 1,000 (Miller)

Contains	Gr	Gm
Orchic substance	5	0.324
Suprarenal	1	0.064
Thyroid	1/12	0.005

For use in functional impotence, hypogonadism, sexual neurasthenia, obesity of endocrine origin.

Dosage: 1, before each meal and at bedtime.

191. Orchic Compound 2—Capsules—Bottles of 100, 1,000 **(Miller)**

Contains

	Gr	Gm
Orchic substance	5	0.324
Anterior pituitary	1	0.064

For use in delayed sexual and general development, obesities of sexual infantilism.

Dosage: 1 before each meal and at bedtime.

192. Orchic Compound 3—Capsules—Bottles of 100, 1,000 **(Miller)**

Contains

	Gr	Gm
Orchic substance	5	0.324
Whole pituitary	1	0.064
Thyroid	1/12	0.005

For use in delayed sexual and general development, obesities of sexual infantilism.

Dosage: 1 before each meal and at bedtime.

193. Ovarian Compound 1—Capsules—Bottles of 100, 1,000 **(Miller)**

Contains

	Gr	Gm
Whole ovarian substance	5	0.324
Whole pituitary substance	1	0.064
Thyroid	1/12	0.005

For use in amenorrhea, dysmenorrhea, menopausal disturbances, conditions resulting from hypo-ovarianism.

Dosage: 1 or 2, before each meal and at bedtime.

194. Ovarian Compound 2—Capsules—Bottles of 100, 1,000 **(Miller)**

Contains

	Gr	Gm
Whole ovarian substance	5	0.324
Whole suprarenal substance	1	0.064
Thyroid	1/12	0.005

For use in conditions resulting from hypo-ovarianism and in hypotension.

Dosage: 1 or 2, before each meal.

195. Ovarian Compound 3—Capsules—Bottles of 100 and 1,000 **(Miller)**

Contains

	Gr	Gm
Ovarian substance (whole)	5	0.324
Pituitary substance (whole)	1	0.064
Suprarenal substance (whole)	1	0.064
Thyroid	1/12	0.005

For use in amenorrhea, dysmenorrhea, menopausal disturbances, conditions resulting from hypo-ovarianism and hypotension.

Dosage: 1 capsule before meals.

196. Ovarian Residue Compound—Capsules—Bottles of 100 and 1,000 **(Miller)**

Contains

	Gr	Gm
Ovarian residue substance	5	0.324
Whole pituitary substance	1	0.064
Thyroid	1/12	0.005

For use in amenorrhea, dysmenorrhea, menopausal disturbances, psychoses and neuroses of hypo-ovarianism; in sexual neurasthenia, vasomotor disturbances of decreased ovarian function.

Dosage: 1 or 2, once or twice daily.

197. Parathyroid Compound—Capsules—Bottles of 100, 1,000 (Miller)

Contains	Gr	Gm
Parathyroid	1/20	0.003
Calcium lactate	2	0.130

For use in paralysis agitans, eclampsia, tetany, chronic ulceration, chorea, toxemia, hemophilia.

Dosage: 1, three times daily.

198. Pituitary Compound—Capsules—Bottles of 100, 1,000 (Miller)

Contains	Gr	Gm
Whole pituitary substance	2½	0.162
Whole ovarian substance	2½	0.162
Thyroid	1/12	0.005

For use in delayed sexual and general development, hypopituitary obesity of sexual infantilism.

Dosage: 1 or 2 daily or twice daily.

199. Prostatic Compound—Capsules—Bottles of 100, 1,000 (Miller)

Contains	Gr	Gm
Prostatic substance	2½	0.162
Orchic substance	2½	0.162
Thyroid	1/12	0.005

For use in compensatory prostatic hypertrophy, sexual neurasthenia of decreased prostatic and testicular function.

Dosage: 1, 2 or 3 capsules three or four times daily.

200. Pluriglandular Compound 1—Ampules 1 cc—Boxes of 12, 100 (Miller)
Contains soluble, active principles representing fresh glands:

	Gr	Gm
Ovarian residue	55	3.564
Suprarenal (whole)	6	0.384
Thyroid	1	0.064

Dosage: 1 cc two or three times weekly, *intramuscularly.*

201. Pluriglandular Compound 2—Ampules 1 cc—Boxes of 12, 100 (Miller)

Contains	Gr	Gm
Orchic principle (active)	55	3.564
Suprarenal (whole)	6	0.384
Thyroid	1	0.064

Dosage: 1 cc two or three times weekly, *intramuscularly.*

202. Thymus and Suprarenal Extracts—Ampules 2 cc—Boxes of 12, 100 (Miller)
Contains fractions derived from 50 gr each (3.240 Gm) fresh thymus and suprarenal glands; *used* in psoriasis, other severe types of dermatitis.

Dosage: 2 or 3 weekly, *intramuscularly.*

203. Corpus Luteum Compound—Capsules—Bottles of 100, 500 and 1,000 (National Drug)

Contains	Gr	Gm
Corpus luteum	½	0.032
Thyroid	¼	0.016
Ovarian substance	½	0.032
Suprarenal	1	0.064
Calcium phosphate	q.s.	

For use in menopause, obesity, myxedema, general debility, sterility in women, sexual debility.

Dosage: 1–3 capsules three times daily.

204. Orchic Compound—Capsules and Tablets—Bottles of 100, 500 and 1,000 each **(National Drug)**

Contains

	Gr	Gm
Orchic substance	1	0.064
Thyroid U.S.P.	1/5	0.013
Calcium phosphate compound	5	0.324

For use in sexual and general debility in men, neuroses.

Dosage: 1–2, three times daily.

205. Orchic Compound Special—Tablets—Bottles of 100, 500 and 1,000 **(National Drug)**

Contains

	Gr	Gm
Cannabin concentrated	1/20	0.003
Orchic substance	1	0.064
Yohimbin	1	0.064
Avenin concentrated	1	0.064
Strychnine sulphate	1/50	0.001
Zinc phosphide	1/10	0.006

For use in sexual and general debility of men, in neuroses.

Dosage: 1–2, three times daily.

206. Ovarian Compound—Capsules—Tablets—Bottles of 100, 500 and 1,000 each **(National Drug)**

Contains

	Gr	Gm
Ovarian substance	1	0.064
Thyroid (U.S.P.)	1/4	0.013
Pituitary entire	1/8	0.008
Calcium phosphate compound	q.s.	

For use in menstrual disturbances.

Dosage: 1–2, three times daily, 7–10 days before period.

207. Ovacoids—Tablets—Bottles of 100, 500 and 1,000 **(Reed and Carnrick)**
Contains hormones of fresh ovary and anterior pituitary.

For use in menopause with hot flashes, nervous attacks; in artificial frigidity, arterial hypertension after menopause; in chlorosis, vomiting of pregnancy, psychoses of pregnancy and puerperium.

Dosage: 2–6 tablets three times daily.

208. Pancrobilin—Pills—Bottles of 100, 500 and 1,000 **(Reed and Carnrick)**
Contains pancreatic enzymes and 0.7 gr (0.11 Gm) of pure bile salts representing gr 4 (0.26 Gm) of dehydrated bile.

For use as intestinal secretory and peristaltic stimulant; in chronic indigestion, jaundice and post-operatively.

Dosage: 1–3 pills three times daily.

209. Protonuclein—Tablets—Bottles of 100, 500 and 1,000 **(Reed and Carnrick)**
Contains thyroid, suprarenal, lymphatic, brain, spleen, pancreas, thymus, salivary substances, pepsin and excipients.

For use in malnutrition, debility, neurasthenia and convalescence.

Dosage: 2–4 tablets four times daily.

210. Testacoids—Tablets—Bottles of 100, 500 and 1,000 **(Reed and Carnrick)**

Contains per tablet hormones representing:	Gr	Gm
Testicle (fresh)	25	1.600
Prostate (fresh)	5	0.324

For use in hypo-gonadism.

Dosage: 2–6 tablets three times daily; increased if necessary.

211. Panacoids—Tablets—Bottles of 100, 500 and 1,000 **(Reed and Carnrick)**

Contains per tablet:

	Gr	Gm
Pancreas desiccated	2	0.13
Duodenal substance desiccated	1	0.06

For use in intestinal indigestion and functional disorders of the pancreas.

Dosage: 1–4 tablets.

212. Forto-Testin—Tablets—Bottles of 100 **(Remogland)**

Contains orchic, suprarenal anterior pituitary with nux vomica and dicalcium phosphate.

For use in sex gland insufficiency, disturbed metabolism, asthenia.

Dosage: 1 tablet three times daily after meals.

213. Remogland—Tablets—Boxes of 40 and 100; Ampules—Boxes of 12 **(Remogland)**

Contains extracts of gonads, adrenals, anterior pituitary, thyroid with calcium glycerophosphate and nux vomica.

For use in treatment of sexual impotence, defective testicular secretion.

Dosage: Orally 1–2 tablets three times daily before meals; *intramuscularly* 1 ampule every 2 days.

214. Remolysin—Tablets—Vials of 50 and 100 **(Remogland)**

Contains extracts thyroid, pituitary, pancreas, female generative glands.

For use in stimulating metabolism, tissue oxidation; to decrease weight without systemic disturbances.

Dosage: Orally 1–3 tablets after meals.

215. Asthmaglands—Capsules—Bottles of 100, 500 and 1,000 **(Rorer)**

Contains

	Gr	Gm
Extract Ephedra vulgaris	3	0.194
Anterior pituitary substance	½	0.032
Adrenal substance	1½	0.097

For use as antispasmodic in asthma.

Dosage: 1 capsule every 3 hr.

216. Calcium Lactate with Parathyroid—Capsules—Bottles of 100, 500 and 1,000 **(Rorer)**

Contains

	Gr	Gm
Calcium lactate	3	0.194
Parathyroid	1/20	0.003

For use in calcium deficiency, gastric ulcer, rickets, tuberculosis.

Dosage: 1 capsule two or three times daily.

217. Cerebro-Lecithin with Nuclein—Capsules 7 gr—Bottles of 100 **(Rorer)**

Contains

	Parts
Nuclein	20
Calcium glycerophosphate	20
Extract nux vomica	1¼
Lecithin	5
Brain substance	25

Uses: Aphrodisiac, stimulant, reconstructive.

Dosage: 1 or 2 capsules three times daily.

218. Cerebro-Orchic Compound—Capsules 5 gr—Bottles of 100 **(Rorer)**

Contains

	Parts
Adrenal substance	25
Thyroid	8.33
Testicular substance	100

Brain substance	100
Calcium glycerophosphate	266.67

Uses: Aphrodisiac, reconstructive.

Dosage: 1 capsule before each meal and upon retiring.

219. Cretinglands—Capsules—Bottles of 100 **(Rorer)**
Contains

	Gr	Gm
Anterior pituitary substance	1/4	0.016
Suprarenal (entire)	1	0.064
Pineal (whole gland)	1/40	0.001
Phospho-Calcium Compound with ether	q.s.	
Thyro-Spermin Compound, for male treatment, or	1 3/8	0.088
Thyro-Ovarian Compound, for female treatment	1 3/8	0.088

Uses: Cretinism, maldevelopment.

Dosage: 1 or 2 capsules two or three times daily.

220. Glanditone—Tablets—Bottles of 100 **(Rorer)**
Contains

	Gr	Gm
Anterior pituitary, fresh gland	1/4	0.016
Ovarian substance, fresh gland	1	0.064
Thyroid fresh gland	1/4	0.016
Extract nux vomica	1/20	0.003
Calferrose	2	0.130

Uses: Reconstructive tonic in menstrual disorders.

Dosage: 1 tablet three or four times daily.

221. Glycosuretics—Capsules—Bottles of 100 **(Rorer)**
Contains concentrated extract of splenic part of pancreas.

For use in early cases of glycosuria and diabetes.

Dosage: 2 capsules after meals and at bedtime.

222. Homoglands—Capsules—Bottles of 100 **(Rorer)**
Contains

	Parts
Orchic substance (desiccated)	50
Prostatic substance (desiccated)	25
Calco-lecithin glycerophosphate	56 1/4

Uses: Aphrodisiac, general stimulant.

Dosage: 2 capsules after meals and at bedtime.

223. Ovara-Dysfunction—Capsules—Bottles of 100 **(Rorer)**
Contains

	Gr	Gm
Ovarian substance	2	0.130
Lecithin	1/2	0.032
Hemoglobin	5	0.324
Alkaline salts	q.s.	

For use in ovarian dyshormonism, menstrual neuroses and psychoses, menopausal disturbances.

Dosage: 1 or 2 capsules three times daily.

224. Vitaglands—Capsules—Bottles of 100 **(Rorer)**
Contains

	Gr	Gm
Yohimbin hydrochloride	1/24	0.0026
Phosphorus compound, nuxated	5/24	0.013
Thyroid, desiccated	1/20	0.003
Pituitary anterior	1/4	0.016
Suprarenal substance	1/8	0.008
Orchic substance	1	0.064
Calco-lecithin comp	q.s.	

Uses: Aphrodisiac.

Dosage: 1 or 2 capsules two or three times daily.

225. Adrenal-Prostate Compound—Capsules—Bottles of 100 and 500 (Searle)

Contains

	Gr	Gm
Adrenal substance desiccated	1/4	0.016
Thyroid gland desiccated	1/12	0.005
Pituitary substance-anterior	1	0.064
Prostate gland	1½	0.097
Spermin extract	1½	0.097
Calcium compound base	q.s.	

For use in hypofunction of genital system, asthenia, body depletion following protracted illness; in hypotension.

Dosage: 1 capsule after meals and at bedtime.

226. Adrenal-Spermin Compound—Capsules and Tablets—Bottles of 100 and 500 (Searle)

Contains

	Gr	Gm
Adrenal substance desiccated	1/4	0.016
Thyroid gland desiccated	1/12	0.005
Spermin extract	1	0.064
Lecithin	1	0.064
Calcium compound base	q.s.	

For use as a metabolic stimulant in asthenic states.

Dosage: 1 capsule before meals and at bedtime.

227. Anter-Pituitary Compound—Capsules—Bottles of 100 and 500 (Searle)

Contains

	Gr	Gm
Pituitary anterior desiccated	2	0.130
Thymus substance desiccated	1	0.064
Thyroid gland desiccated	1/12	0.005
Calcium compound base	q.s.	

For use during developmental period for disorders of the osseous, mental, genital and physical systems.

Dosage: 1 capsule three times daily.

228. Intesti-Sols Orchic Compound—Pills (Enteric-coated)—Bottles of 100 and 500 (Searle)

Contains

	Gr	Gm
Orchic substance	1½	0.097
Prostate substance	½	0.032
Thymus substance	1	0.064
Suprarenal substance	1/4	0.016
Thyroid substance	1/6	0.012
Zinc phosphide	1/8	0.008
Strychnine nitrate	1/100	0.0006
Yohimbine HCl	1/12	0.005

For use in deficiencies of male gonads.

Dosage: 1 pill three times daily, varied according to conditions.

229. Intesti-Sols Ovarian Compound—Pills (Enteric-coated)—Bottles of 100 and 500 (Searle)

Contains

	Gr	Gm
Ovarian substance	1½	0.097
Pituitary substance (whole)	1/12	0.005
Thyroid substance	1/6	0.012
Hemoglobin	1	0.064
Zinc phosphide	1/8	0.008
Strychnine nitrate	1/100	0.0006

For use in hypofunction of ovaries, pituitary, thyroid.

Dosage: 1 or 2, three times daily ½ hr. before meals.

230. Mammary-Placenta Compound with Pituitary—Capsules—Bottles of 100 and 500 (Searle)

Contains

	Gr	Gm
Mammary substance	1½	0.097
Placenta substance	2	0.130
Pituitary substance (entire)	⅓	0.021
Calcium compound base	q.s.	

For use as galactogogue to encourage uterine involution.

Dosage: 2 capsules at meals three times daily for 10 days; then 1 capsule three times daily for several weeks.

231. Parathyroid and Spermin Compound—Capsules—Bottles of 100 and 500 (Searle)

Contains

	Gr	Gm
Parathyroid substance desiccated	1/10	0.006
Spermin extract	1	0.064
Bile salts compound	2	0.130
Calcium compound base	q.s.	

For use as tonic, cholagogue.

Dosage: 1 capsule ½ hr. before meals, three times daily, decreasing when possible.

232. Yohimbine-Endocrine Compound—Capsules and Tablets—Bottles of 100 and 500 (Searle)

Contains

	Gr	Gm
Yohimbine HCl	1/12	0.005
Orchic substance	1½	0.097
Suprarenal substance	1/12	0.005
Thyroid substance	1/12	0.005
Extract damiana	½	0.032
Lecithin	⅛	0.008

For use as tonic, aphrodisiac.

Dosage: 1, three times daily for several weeks, then decreasing; rest 2–3 weeks and repeat.

233. Thymo-Pitsin—Ampules ½ cc—Boxes of 10, 25 and 100 (Searle)

Contains oxytocic principle of posterior pituitary with the hormone of the thymus gland.

For use in first stage of labor; *intramuscularly,* ¼–½ cc.

234. Orchi-Himbine Compound—Capsules—Bottles of 100 (Smith-Dorsey)

Contains

	Gr	Gm
Yohimbine hydrochloride	1/16	0.004
Orchic substance	2½	0.16
Ovarian substance	⅓	0.02
Prostate	⅙	0.01
Pituitary entire	1/12	0.005
Suprarenal	⅓	0.02
Thyroid U.S.P.	1/10	0.006
Pituitary anterior	⅓	0.02

For use in senility, asthenia, impotence.

Dosage: 1 capsule three to four times daily.

235. Ovarian-Suprarenal Compound—Capsules—Bottles of 100 (Carroll Dunham Smith)

Contains desiccated	Gr	Gm
Ovarian substance whole	1½	0.097
Corpus luteum substance	½	0.032
Suprarenal	1	0.064
Thyroid	⅛	0.008
Calcium glycerophosphate	1	0.064
Saw palmetto powdered extract	¼	0.016
Nucleinic acid	1/32	0.002

For use in dysmenorrhea, amenorrhea and menorrhagia, when a stimulant action is desired.

Dosage: 1 capsule three times daily for 10 days, double the dose for 7–10 days before menses; omitted at onset for 10 days and repeated.

236. Thymus Pituitary Solution—Ampules ½ cc—Boxes of 6 and 100 **(Stoddard)**
Contains water soluble constituents of gr 10½ fresh thymus gland and equal parts of post-pituitary solution (U.S.P.) with chlorbutanol 5% preservative.

For use where pituitary is indicated.

Dosage: 1 ampule *intramuscularly* or *subcutaneously*, according to the occasion.

237. Epinephrine Compound—Bottles of 1 oz. **(Stoddard)**

Contains	Gr	Gm
Epinephrine chloride	⅖	0.025
Chloretone	2¼	0.144
Normal saline	q.s.	

For use—as for epinephrine.

238. Ovarian Compound—Tablets—Bottles 100, 500 and 1,000 **(Stoddard)**

Contains desiccated	Gr	Gm
Thyroid	1/12	0.005
Ovarian	1	0.064
Suprarenal	¼	0.016
Anterior pituitary	⅛	0.008
Alkaline base, aromatics	q.s.	

For use as tonic in convalescence, asthenia, hypoadrenia, hypotension in female.

Dosage: 1–3 tablets daily; omitted during menses.

239. Prostate Compound—Tablets—Bottles of 100, 500 and 1,000 **(Stoddard)**

Contains desiccated	Gr	Gm
Prostate	2	0.130
Orchic	1	0.064
Alkaline base, aromatics	q.s.	

For use in prostatic hypertrophy, prostatitis (non-gonorrheal), senility.

Dosage: 1–2 tablets three times daily.

240. Orchic Compound—Tablets—Bottles of 100, 500 and 1,000 **(Stoddard)**

Contains desiccated	Gr	Gm
Thyroid	1/12	0.005
Orchic	1	0.064
Suprarenal	¼	0.016
Anterior pituitary	⅛	0.008
Alkaline base, aromatics	q.s.	

For use as tonic in convalescence, asthenia, neurasthenia, hypoadrenia, hypotension in male.

Dosage: 1–3 tablets three times daily.

241. Low-Tone—Tablets (Enteric coated)—Bottles of 100, 500, 1,000 **(Westerfield)**

Contains	Gr	Gm
Adrenal substance	¼	0.016
Thyroid	unstated	
Spermin	"	
Lecithin	"	

For use in hypotension, lethargy, depressed states, neurasthenia.

Dosage: 1–2 tablets three or four times daily.

242. Menovarian—Tablets (Enteric coated)—Bottles of 100, 500, 1,000 **(Westerfield)**

Contains	Gr	Gm
Ovarian substance (whole)	3/4	0.048
Lecithin	1/8	0.008
Ext. cannabis indica	1/8	0.008
Blaud's mass	2 1/2	0.162
Cascarin	1/8	0.008

For use in menstrual disorders with nervous manifestations, functional amenorrhea, dysmenorrhea, menopause.

Dosage: 1–2 tablets two to three times daily.

243. Pituitary Ovarian Compound—Tablets—Bottles 100 and 1,000 **(Zemmer)**

Contains	Gr	Gm
Ovarian substance	1	0.064
Corpus luteum	1	0.064
Thyroid	1/12	0.005
Pituitary	1/8	0.008
Calcium glycerophosphate compound	1 1/12	0.055

For use in menstrual disorders, premature senility, neurasthenia.

Dosage: 1 four times daily.

244. Secretin Compound Tablets—Bottles 100 and 1,000 **(Zemmer)**

Contains	Gr	Gm
Duodenal substance	1/8	0.008
Bile	1/8	0.008
Pancreatin	1/2	0.032
Caro-peptin	1 1/2	0.097
Ext. cascara	1/4	0.016
Hydrastin	1/20	0.003
Ext. taraxacum	1	0.064

For use in constipation, intestinal stasis, gall bladder disorders.

Dosage: 1–3, 1 hr. after meals.

245. Thyroid Ovarian Compound Tablets—Bottles 100 and 1,000 **(Zemmer)**

Contains	Gr	Gm
Thyroid	1/4	0.016
Ovarian substance	2	0.130
Anterior pituitary	1/12	0.005

For use in menstrual disorders, neurasthenia.

Dosage: 1, three times daily.

246. Thyroid Pituitary Compound Tablets—Bottles 100 and 1,000 **(Zemmer)**

Contains	Gr	Gm
Thyroid	1/4	0.016
Anterior pituitary	1/4	0.016
Suprarenal	1/4	0.016
Cerebral substance	1/8	0.008

For use in asthma.

Dosage: 1–3, every 3 hr.

CHAPTER V

HYPODERMIC MEDICAMENTS

This chapter presents 1,563 Ampule medicaments, 630 Intravenous and 933 Subcutaneous and Intramuscular; the arrangement is alphabetical (1) by manufacturer or distributor and (2) by drug.

Parenteral administration of drugs is now quite popular; the introduction of vaccines, sera and allergens, of insulin, dextrose and other products used exclusively by injection has given great impetus to hypodermic therapy. Besides, many drugs formerly prepared for oral use only have now been purified and made available and even preferable for hypodermic administration.

PART I

INTRAVENOUS THERAPY

Advantages—(1) Complete absorption and full dosage of a drug is thus assured; (2) the injected medication is not subjected to changes through gastro-intestinal chemical action as in oral therapy; (3) being introduced directly into circulation, the drug is carried rapidly to every part of the organism, becomes quickly effective at the desired place and exerts there its full therapeutic action.

Disadvantages—Are few where correct medication and technic are employed; intravenous therapy is best avoided in kidney affections with function below 50%, in those with advanced cardiac disease or an idiosyncrasy for the particular drug to be administered.

Dosage—Adults, in accordance with drug injected; children, in proportion to weight, or at age of 10 yr.—½ dosage, 5 yr.—¼, 2½ yr.—⅛, and 1 yr.—1/12 dosage.

Reactions—To overcome "needle shock," usually a psychic reaction, the lowering of the head will usually suffice; in severer reactions with flushing of face, burning sensation, dizziness, nausea or vomiting, urticarial rash, cyanosis, dyspnea—injections of epinephrin 1:1,000, 7-10 m., repeated in 20 min. if necessary, will afford relief.

Technic—Needle and syringe are best sterilized by boiling, surface of ampule by alcohol immersion; the tourniquet is applied about 2 in. above site of injection, which is sterilized with tincture of iodine, alcohol 70%; the vein, usually the median cephalic or basilic, is distended by pressure of forearm or flexing of elbow, or in poorly filling veins by application of heat to forearm. Patient is to be assured of the harmlessness and painlessness of the procedure; the needle is thrust into vein quickly, tourniquet removed, and medication injected slowly, usually 1 min. per cubic centimeter; needle is quickly removed, puncture compressed, bleeding stopped, drop of antiseptic and collodion, if desired, applied. Frequency of injection depends upon the drug used and its period of elimination.

For the convenience of the clinician and to facilitate the ready choice of a hypodermic drug for a particular purpose, the 630 Intravenous Ampules in 1,096 forms are presented here in groups, classified in accordance with their therapeutic functon.

Group 1. Alkalizers—Ampules 24, 94, 193, 223, 286, 361, 420, 431.

Group 2. Amebacides—Ampules 1, 172, 278, 612

Group 3. Analgesics—Ampules 32, 33, 34, 35, 36, 61, 62, 63, 73, 92, 93, 99, 100, 114, 115, 125, 136, 137, 155, 158, 159, 160, 161, 171, 198, 199, 200, 201, 208, 229, 230, 231, 250, 251, 284, 285, 293, 295, 323, 324, 325, 334, 360, 367, 380, 381, 425, 426, 427, 428, 451, 452, 466, 467, 468, 506, 507, 508, 509, 510, 527, 528, 545, 546, 547, 548, 564, 565, 566, 567, 600, 604, 606, 616, 617, 618.

Group. 4. Antiluetics—Ampules 1, 4, 16, 20, 29, 70, 88, 89, 139, 140, 141, 152, 187, 188, 189, 221, 248, 249, 266, 330, 353, 373, 376, 378, 383, 384, 385, 387, 388, 395, 396, 416, 417, 443, 460, 491, 492, 495, 541, 550, 551, 570, 576, 577, 578, 579, 580, 581, 584, 585, 610.

Group 5. Antiseptics—Ampules 3, 15, 17, 51, 78, 87, 122, 126, 186, 265, 340, 352, 404, 415, 442, 494, 609.

Group 6. Arterial Dilators—Ampules 2, 473, 481.

Group 7. Bromine Preparations—Ampules 65, 95, 202, 211, 252, 297, 298, 362, 370.

Group 8. Calcium Therapy Agents—Ampules 5, 6, 7, 42a, 43, 44, 67, 71, 72, 120, 143, 166, 167, 169, 215, 253, 254, 255, 302, 306, 308, 331, 332, 398, 400, 432, 433, 457, 478, 483, 484, 485, 515, 532, 552, 591, 599.

Group 9. Cancer Palliatives—Ampules 41, 123, 124, 128, 274, 349.

Group 10. Chaulmoogra Derivatives—Ampule 571.

Group 11. Cholagogues—Ampule 473.

Group 12. Creosote Products—Ampules 30, 31, 81, 82, 103, 104, 144, 147, 168, 175, 256, 257, 270, 272, 273, 280, 310, 333, 342, 343, 399, 407, 450, 503, 504, 601, 605.

Group 13. Detoxicants—Ampules 37, 38, 64, 101, 162, 209, 232, 296, 326, 368, 390, 429, 453, 469, 511, 529, 549, 568, 587, 588.

Group 14. Dextrose Preparations—Ampules 8, 9, 10, 45, 79, 80, 106, 107, 130, 145, 146, 173, 174, 260, 275, 276, 277, 283, 289, 303, 309, 313, 327, 338a, 338b, 341, 371, 402, 405, 433, 434, 435, 458, 475, 485, 517, 533, 535, 553, 554, 555, 592, 602,

Group 15. Diagnostic Agents—Ampules 178, 237, 243, 244, 246, 247, 259, 268, 345. 374, 375, 480, 582, 595.

Group 16. Digitalis Preparations—Ampules 119, 212, 213, 233, 245, 317, 386, 516.

Group 17. Distilled Waters—Ampules 40, 102, 116, 138, 142, 210, 234, 300, 369, 430, 454, 472, 477, 512, 530, 531, 534, 569, 573, 596, 597, 619.

Group 18. Diuretics—Ampules 238, 239, 240, 389, 479, 481, 572, 583, 586.

Group 19. Ephedrine Preparations—Ampule 377.

Group 20. Gold Preparations—Ampules 11, 301, 335, 393, 401, 488.

Group 21. Gonocidal Preparations—Ampule 574.

Group 22. Hematinics—Ampules 12, 13, 25, 26, 48, 49, 57, 74, 75, 84, 85, 96, 190, 110, 111, 129, 131, 132, 133, 134, 149, 150, 151, 154, 156, 165, 176, 179, 180, 181, 182, 183, 184, 203, 206, 216, 220, 224, 225, 227, 261, 262, 263, 271, 279, 287, 291, 304, 314, 320, 336, 337, 346, 347, 348, 351, 363, 365, 406, 409, 410, 411, 412, 413, 421, 423, 437, 438, 439, 440, 447, 463, 489, 490, 501, 519, 520, 523, 539, 540, 542, 556, 559, 562, 598, 607, 613, 614.

Group 23. Hemostatics—Ampules 117, 305.

Group 24. Iodine Preparations—Ampules 60, 98, 112, 113, 135, 157, 169, 207, 214, 228, 292, 322, 343, 366, 424, 449, 465, 476, 502, 525, 543, 544, 563, 615.

Group 25. Narcotics—Ampule 474.

Group 26. Nucleotides—Ampule 163.

Group 27. Non-Specific Agents—Ampules 83, 235, 382, 392, 498, 589, 590.

Group 28. Parasiticides—Ampules 21, 39, 53, 66, 69, 90, 91, 152, 164, 196, 222, 241, 242, 269, 299, 318, 328, 329, 339, 358, 394, 403, 419, 445, 460, 470, 500, 513, 521, 560.

Group 29. **Pituitary Products**—Ampule 611.

Group 30. **Saline Injections**—Ampules 27, 28, 52, 55, 58, 194, 197, 204, 267, 288, 356, 357, 359, 418, 522.

Group 31. **Sclerosing Agents**—Ampules 22, 54, 127, 195, 294, 319, 372, 379, 446, 462, 499, 505, 561, 593.

Group 32. **Silver Preparations**—Ampule 121.

Group 33. **Stimulating Agents**—Ampules 68, 105, 118, 397, 444, 455, 456, 482, 575.

Group 34. **Suprarenal Products**—Ampules 391, 455, 514.

Group 35. **Synergists**—Ampules 14, 50, 86, 185, 264, 316, 350, 414, 441, 459, 493, 608.

Group 36. **Tin Preparations**—Ampules 59, 290.

Group 37. **Transfusion, Citrates**—Ampules 97, 205, 226, 321, 364, 422, 448, 464, 524, 594.

Group 38. **Urinary Antiseptics**—Ampules 18, 19, 23, 46, 47, 76, 77, 108, 148, 153, 170, 190, 191, 192, 217, 218, 219, 258, 281, 282, 311, 312, 344, 354, 355, 408, 436, 471, 496, 497, 518, 536, 537, 538, 557, 558, 603, 604.

AMPULES

Intravenous

1. **Acetarsone**—Ampules, containing 0.5 and 0.1 Gm acetarsone; Boxes of 25 and 100, with ampules of sodium hydroxide for alkalization; Amoebacide and spirocheticide; *Dosage:* 1 ampule diluted to 20 cc, three times weekly for 7–8 weeks. *See Chap. I.* **(Abbott)**

2. **Acetylcholine Bromide**—Ampules containing 100 and 200 mg; Boxes of 6; Vasodilator; *Dosage:* 0.1–0.3 Gm daily or as required. *See Chap. I.* **(Abbott)**

3. **Acriflavine Powder (Neutral)**—Ampules containing 0.5 and 0.1 Gm; Boxes of 6; Bactericide; *Dosage:* 0.5% solution, 10–50 cc. *See Chap. I.* **(Abbott)**

4. **Arsphenamine**—Ampules of 0.1, 0.2, 0.3, 0.4, 0.5, 0.6, 1.0, 2.0, 3.0 Gm; containing 30% arsenic; Boxes of 1 ampule with "Alkpules" vials of sodium hydroxide for neutralization; Antiluetic; *Dosage:* 0.3–0.4 Gm, one to two times weekly for 8–10 doses. *See Chap. I.* **(Abbott)**

5. **Calcicol**—Ampules 10 cc; Boxes of 6, 25 and 100; containing calcium guaiacol sulphonate gr 10 (0.66 Gm); *For use* in respiratory affections; *Dosage:* 10–20 cc daily, or two to three times weekly. **(Abbott)**

6. **Calcium Chloride**—Ampules 5 and 10 cc; Boxes of 6, 25 and 100; 10% solution; *For use* in calcium deficiencies, hemorrhage; *Dosage:* 1–10 cc, two to three times weekly. **(Abbott)**

7. **Calcium Gluconate**—Ampules 10 cc; Boxes 6, 25 and 100; 10% solution; *For use* in calcium deficiency; *Dosage:* 1 ampule daily, or every 2–3 days. *See Chap. I.* **(Abbott)**

8. **D-Dextrose**—Ampules 10, 20, 50 and 100 cc; Boxes of 6, 25 and 100; 50% solution; *For use* as nutrient, stimulant in shock, hyperinsulinism; *Dosage:* as required. *See Chap. I.* **(Abbott)**

9. **Dextrose-Ringer's Concentrate**—Ampules 100 cc; Boxes of 6, 25 and 100; 5% dextrose; Nutritive; *Dosage:* 500 cc per hour slowly, then 100 cc per hour for several days. *See Chap. I.* **(Abbott)**

10. **Dextrose and Sodium Chloride**—Ampules 5 and 20 cc; Boxes of 6, 25 and 100; For varicose vein obliteration; dextrose 50%, sodium chloride 30%; *Dosage:* 2–10 cc, two to three times weekly. **(Abbott)**

11. **Gold Sodium Thiosulphate**—Ampules 0.01, 0.025, 0.05, 0.1, 0.25 Gm; Boxes of 6; Lupus therapy; *Dosage:* 0.01 Gm increased by 0.01 Gm weekly. *See Chap. I.* **(Abbott)**

12. Iron Cacodylate—Ampules 5 cc; Boxes 6, 25 and 100; containing iron cacodylate gr 1 (0.065 Gm); *For use* in anemia, leukemia, lymphadenitis; *Dosage:* 2–5 cc. **(Abbott)**

13. Iron Arsenic and Phosphorus—Ampules 5 cc; Boxes of 6, 25, and 100; containing iron cacodylate gr 1 (0.065 Gm) and sodium glycerophosphate gr 1½ (0.097 Gm); *For use* as tonic, hematinic; *Dosage:* 2–5 cc, one to two times weekly. **(Abbott)**

14. Magnesium Sulphate 10%—Ampules 20 cc; Boxes of 6, 25 and 100; *For use* in eclampsia; *Dosage:* 5–20 cc every hour or as required. **(Abbott)**

15. Mercuric Oxycyanide—Ampules 5 cc, gr ⅛ (0.008 Gm), gr ¼ (0.016 Gm), gr ⅙ (0.01 Gm); Boxes of 6, 25 and 100; Antiseptic and germicide; *Dosage:* as required. *See Chap. I.* **(Abbott)**

16. Mercury Cyanide—Ampules 1 cc; Boxes 12 and 100; Containing mercury cyanide gr ⅙ (0.01 Gm); *For use* as Antiluetic; *Dosage:* ¼–1 cc daily or every 2–5 days. **(Abbott)**

17. Metaphen—Ampules 10 cc; Boxes of 6, 25 and 100; Antiseptic and germicide; 1:1,000 solution: *Dosage:* as required. *See Chap. I.* **(Abbott)**

18. Methenamine—Ampules 5 cc; Boxes 6, 25 and 100; Containing methenamine U.S.P. gr 15½ (1 Gm), and gr 31 (2 Gm) with C.P. water q.s. 5 cc; *For use* as Urinary Antiseptic; *Dosage:* 2–5 cc, every 2–3 days. **(Abbott)**

19. Methenamine and Sodium Iodide—Ampules 20 cc; Boxes of 6, 25 and 100; Containing methenamine U.S.P. gr 23 (1.5 Gm) and sodium iodide gr 15½ (1.0 Gm); *For use* in gonorrheal epididymitis, orchitis; *Dosage:* 10–20 cc every 2–3 days. **(Abbott)**

20. Neoarsphenamine—Ampules 0.15, 0.3, 0.5, 0.6, 0.75, 0.9, 1.5, 3.0, 4.5 Gm; Boxes of 1 ampule; Antiluetic; *Dosage:* 0.45–0.6 Gm twice weekly for 10–12 doses; *See Chap. I.* **(Abbott)**

21. Quinine Dihydrochloride—Ampules 10 cc; Boxes of 6, 25 and 100; Containing quinine dihydrochloride gr 7½ (0.5 Gm) and C.P. water q.s. 10 cc; *For use* in malaria; *Dosage:* 1 ampule twice daily. **(Abbott)**

22. Quinine and Urethane—Ampules 2 cc; Boxes of 12 and 100; Containing quinine hydrochloride gr 4.1 (0.26 Gm) and urethane gr 2.05 (0.13 Gm); C.P. water q.s. 2 cc; *For use* in varicose vein obliteration; *Dosage:* 1–2 cc at 1 sitting. **(Abbott)**

23. Salihexin—Ampules 10 cc; Boxes of 6, 25 and 100; Urinary antiseptic; *Dosage:* 1 ampule daily or every 2 days, for 15 doses. *See Chap. I.* **(Abbott)**

24. Sodium Bicarbonate—Ampules 20 cc; Boxes 6, 25 and 100; Containing sodium bicarbonate gr 23 (1.5 Gm), C.P. water q.s. 20 cc; *For use* in acidosis, vomiting; *Dosage:* 10–20 cc daily. *See Chap. I.* **(Abbott)**

25. Sodium Cacodylate—Ampules 5 cc; Boxes 6, 25 and 100; Containing sodium cacodylate gr 5 (0.324 Gm) or gr 7½ (0.5 Gm), C.P. water q.s. 5 cc; *For use* in anemia, leukopenia, neurasthenia; *Dosage:* 2–5 cc, two to three times weekly. **(Abbott)**

26. Sodium Cacodylate—Ampules 10 cc; Boxes of 6, 25 and 100; Containing sodium cacodylate gr 15½(1 Gm); *Use* and *dosage* same as above. **(Abbott)**

27. Sodium Chloride—Ampules 20 cc; Boxes of 6, 25 and 100; Containing sodium chloride 4.25 Gm, C.P. water q.s. 20 cc; For preparing physiological salt solution to make 500 cc. **(Abbott)**

28. Sodium Chloride—Ampules 5 cc; Boxes 6, 25 and 100; *For use* in varicose vein obliteration. **(Abbott)**

29. Sodium Iodide—Ampules 10 cc; Boxes of 6, 25 and 100; Containing sodium iodide gr 31 (2 Gm) or 15½ gr (1 Gm), C.P. water q.s. 10 cc; *For use* in asthma, goitre, syphilis; *Dosage:* 5–10 cc every 2–6 days. **(Abbott)**

30. Sodium Iodide and Guaiacol—Ampules 20 cc; Boxes of 6, 25 and 100; Containing sodium iodide gr 31 (2 Gm) and guaiacol gr ¾ (0.049 Gm), C.P. water q.s. 20 cc; *For use* in respiratory affections; *Dosage:* 10–20 cc every 2–4 days. **(Abbott)**

31. Sodium Iodide, Guaiacol and Creosote—Ampules 20 cc; Boxes 6, 25 and 100; Containing sodium iodide gr 31 (2 Gm), guaiacol gr ¾ (0.05 Gm), creosote gr ⅔ (0.043 Gm), C.P. water q.s. 20 cc; *Dosage:* 10–20 cc every 2–4 days. **(Abbott)**

32. Sodium Salicylate—Ampules 5, 10 and 20 cc: Boxes of 6, 25 and 100; Containing respectively, sodium salicylate gr 15½ (1 Gm), gr 31 (2 Gm), gr 31 (2 Gm), C.P. water q.s. to each; *For use* in rheumatism, myalgia, neuralgia; *Dosage:* 2–5 cc every 3–4 hr. **(Abbott)**

33. Sodium Salicylate—Ampule 5 cc; Boxes of 6, 25 and 100; 40 % solution; *For use* in varicose vein obliteration; *Dosage:* 3–5 cc, two to three times weekly. **(Abbott)**

34. Sodium Salicylate and Iodide—Ampules 20 cc; Boxes of 6, 25 and 100; Containing sodium salicylate gr 15½ (1 Gm), sodium iodide gr 15½ (1 Gm), C.P. water q.s. 20 cc; *For use* in rheumatism; *Dosage:* 10–20 cc every 2–4 days. **(Abbott)**

35. Sodium Salicylate and Iodide with Colchicine—Ampules 20 cc; Boxes 6, 25 and 100; Containing sodium salicylate gr 15½ (1 Gm), sodium iodide gr 15½ (1 Gm), colchicine gr 1/100 (0.65 mg), C.P. water q.s. 20 cc; *For use* in arthritis, gout; *Dosage:* 10–20 cc daily. **(Abbott)**

36. Sodium Salicylate and Iodide with Colchicine—Ampules 20 cc; Boxes 6, 25 and 100: Containing sodium salicylate gr 31 (2 Gm), sodium iodide gr 31 (2 Gm), colchicine gr 1/100 (0.65 mg). *Use* and *dosage* as above. **(Abbott)**

37. Sodium Thiosulphate—Ampules 10 cc; Boxes 6, 25 and 100; Containing sodium thiosulphate gr 15½ (1 Gm), C.P. water q.s. 10 cc; *For use* in metallic poisoning; *Dosage:* 0.5–1.0 Gm daily. *See Chap. I.* **(Abbott)**

38. Sodium Thiosulphate—Ampules 5 cc; Boxes of 6, 25 and 100; Containing sodium thiosulphate gr 7½ (0.5 Gm), C.P. water q.s. 5 cc; *Use* and *dosage* as above. **(Abbott)**

39. Tartar Emetic—Ampules 10 cc; Boxes 6, 25 and 100; Containing antimony potassium tartrate gr 1⅗ (0.1 Gm), C.P. water q.s. 10 cc; *For use* in granuloma inguinale, Vincent's angina, kala-azar, bilharziasis, trypanosomiasis; *Dosage:* 5–12 cc every 2 days. **(Abbott)**

40. C.P. Water—Ampules 5, 10, 20, 50 and 100 cc; Boxes of 6, 25 and 100. **(Abbott)**

---

41. Lead Selenide—Ampules 5, 10 and 15 cc; Cancer therapy; *Dosage:* 5–15 cc with glucose weekly, for 8–12 doses. *See Chap. I.* **(Anglo-French)**

42. Orargol—Ampules 5 and 10 cc; Boxes of 2 and 6. Alterative; *Dosage:* 5–20 cc daily or every 2 days. **(Anglo-French)**

42a. Calcium Chloride—Ampules 5 cc; Boxes of 6, 25 and 100; Either 5 % solution gr 3¾, or 10 % solution, gr 7½; Calcium therapy; *For use* in paralysis agitans, tetany, epilepsy, chorea; with oral administration of parathyroid extracts. **(Berwyn)**

43. Calcium Chloride—Ampules 10 cc; Boxes of 6, 25 and 100; 10 % solution gr 15½; *For use* as above; *Usual dosage:* 1 ampule every 2–3 days. **(Berwyn)**

44. Calcium Lactate—Ampules 5 cc; Boxes of 6, 25 and 100; Calcium therapy; *For use* in intestinal and pulmonary tuberculosis; *Dosage:* 2–10 cc, two to three times weekly. **(Berwyn)**

45. Glucose Solution—Ampules 5, 10, 20, 50 and 100 cc; Boxes of 6, 25 and 100; 50 and 100 cc also in boxes of 1; *For use* in carbohydrate metabolic disturbances, post-operative shock and acidosis, severe toxemias, acidosis, hypoglycemia from excessive insulin intake. *See Chap. I.* **(Berwyn)**

46. Hexamethylenamine—Ampules 5 cc; Boxes of 6, 25 and 100; gr 15½ or gr 31; *For use* in cystitis, pyelitis, urethritis, acute nephritis, bronchitis, pneumonia and certain septicemias, also dysuria and anuria; *Dosage:* usually from 15½–31 gr; Urine must be kept acid in reaction. **(Berwyn)**

47. **Hexamethylenamine and Sodium Iodide**—Ampules 20 cc; Boxes of 6, 25 and 100; *For use* in infections of G.U. tract as gonorrhea and preventative against renal infections; Urine must be kept acid in reaction. (Berwyn)

48. **Iron Cacodylate**—Ampules 5 cc; Boxes of 6, 25 and 100; *For use* in anemia, chlorosis, malnutrition; *Dosage:* ½–2½ gr as indicated. (Berwyn)

49. **Iron Cacodylate and Glycerophosphate**—Ampules 5 cc; Boxes of 6, 25 and 100; Containing iron cacodylate gr 1, sodium glycerophosphate gr 2; *For use* in anemia. (Berwyn)

50. **Magnesium Sulphate**—Ampules 10 and 20 cc; Boxes of 6, 25 and 100; 10 cc ampules of 25% solution, 20 cc of 10% solution; May be used with morphine, producing prolonged analgesic action, and to relieve spasmodic symptoms in tetany and eclampsia; *Usual dosage:* 1 ampule as required. (Berwyn)

51. **Mercurochrome**—Ampules of 5, 10 and 20 cc; Boxes of 6, 25 and 100; 1% solution: *For use* in septicemia, bacteremia, gonorrheal arthritis and epididymitis, chronic specific infections; *Usual dosage:* 0.5 cc per kilo body weight, twice weekly. *See Chap. I.* (Berwyn)

52. **Physiological Salt Solution**—Ampules 20, 50 and 100 cc: Boxes of 1, 25, 6 and 100; *For use* as diluent for intravenous solutions. (Berwyn)

53. **Quinine Dihydrochloride**—Ampules 20 cc; Boxes of 6, 25 and 100; Containing gr 10; *For use* in malarial fever, lobar pneumonia and as tonic; *Usual dosage:* 1 ampule, two or three times weekly. (Berwyn)

54. **Quinine Hydrochloride and Urethane**—Ampules 2 cc; Boxes of 12 and 100; Containing quinine hydrochloride 0.266 Gm, urethane 0.133 Gm; For the treatment of varicose veins. *See Chap. II.* (Berwyn)

55. **Ringer's Physiological Saline Solution**—Ampules 50 and 100 cc; Boxes of 1, 6, 25 and 100; Where indicated. (Berwyn)

56. **Sodium Bromide**—Ampules 10 cc; Boxes of 6, 25 and 100; Boxes of 6, 25 and 100; Containing gr 15½; Sedative. (Berwyn)

57. **Sodium Cacodylate**—Ampules 5 cc (gr 3), 5 cc (gr 7½), 10 cc (15½ gr); Boxes of 6, 25 and 100; *For use* in malarial cachexia, neurasthenia, psoriasis, anemia, leukemia and pellagra; *Usual dosage:* ¾–15½ gr. (Berwyn)

58. **Sodium Chloride**—Ampules 5 cc; Boxes of 6, 25 and 100: Either 20 or 30% Solutions; *For use* as indicated. (Berwyn)

59. **Sodium Citrate**—Ampules 50 cc; Boxes 1, 6, 25 and 100; 2½% Solution; *For use* in blood transfusions. (Berwyn)

60. **Sodium Iodide**—Ampules 10 cc (15½ gr) and 20 cc (31 gr); Boxes of 6, 25 and 100; *For use* in asthma, arteriosclerosis, simple goiter, systemic conditions of gonorrheal origin; *Usual dosage:* 7¾–31 gr, two or three times weekly. (Berwyn)

61. **Sodium Salicylate**—Ampules 5 cc (15½ gr), 20 cc (20 gr); Boxes of 6, 25 and 100; *For use* in arthritis of pyogenic origin, streptococcic tonsillitis, neuralgia, myalgia; *Dosage:* 1 ampule daily as indicated. (Berwyn)

62. **Sodium Salicylate Compound**—Ampules 20 cc; Boxes of 6, 25 and 100; Containing sodium salicylate gr 15½, sodium iodide gr 15½, colchicine gr 1/100; *For use* in acute and chronic arthritis, sciatica, lumbago, other rheumatic conditions; *Dosage:* 10–20 cc every 2–4 days. (Berwyn)

63. **Sodium Salicylate and Iodide**—Ampules 20 cc; Boxes of 6, 25 and 100; Containing sodium salicylate gr 15½ and sodium iodide gr 15½; *For use* in acute and chronic arthritis, sciatica, bronchial asthma; also where complicated by lues. *Dosage:* 1 ampule, two to three times weekly. (Berwyn)

64. **Sodium Thiosulphate**—Ampule 10 cc; Boxes of 6, 25 and 100; *For use* in overcoming toxic reactions of arsenic, bismuth, mercury; Containing gr 7½; *Dosage:* gr 3¾ daily increasing to 15½ gr as indicated. *See Chap. I.* (Berwyn)

65. **Strontium Bromide**—Ampule 10 cc; Boxes of 6, 25 and 100; Containing gr 15½; *For use* as sedative. (Berwyn)

66. Tartar Emetic—Ampules 5 cc; Boxes of 6, 25 and 100; 1 % Solution; *For use* in granuloma inguinale (tropical ulcer); *Dosage:* 5 cc at 3 or 4 day intervals. (Berwyn)

---

67. Afenil—Ampules 10 cc; Boxes of 1; 10 % aqueous solution of calcium chloride-urea; *Dosage:* 1 ampule once or twice daily. *See Chap. I.* (Bilhuber-Knoll)

---

68. Alpha Lobelin—Ampules 1 cc (infant); Boxes of 6, 12 and 100; crystalline alkaloid isolated from Lobelia inflata, gr 3/20 (0.01 Gm); Respiratory stimulant; *Dosage:* ½–1 ampule as required. *See Chap. I.* (Bischoff)

---

69. Antimony and Potassium Tartrate—Ampules 5 cc; Boxes of 6 and 25; Containing gr ¾ (0.05 Gm) antimony and potassium tartrate per 5 cc; *For use* in bilharziasis, granuloma inguinale and Vincent's infections; *Dosage:* tolerance tested by first dose of 1 cc, then increased daily by 1 cc until 7–15 cc are given; 12–15 injections constitute a course. (Breon)

70. Arseno-Mer-Sodide—Ampules 20 cc; Boxes of 6 and 25; Containing sodium dimethylarsenate gr 22½ (1.46 Gm), mercury oxycyanide gr ⅛ (0.008 Gm), sodium iodide gr 15 (0.97 Gm).
Ampules 10 cc; Boxes of 6 and 25; Containing half above strength; *For use* as antiluetic with tonic effect; *Dosage:* initial injection 10 cc, then 20 cc at 2–4 day intervals, 12–24 injections constituting a course. (Breon)

71. Calcium Chloride—Ampules 5 cc; Boxes of 6 and 25; Containing gr 4 (0.26 Gm), 5 % solution;
Ampules 10 cc; Boxes of 6 and 25; Containing gr 15½ (1 Gm), 10 % solution; *For use* in calcium therapy of asthma, anaphylactic reactions, hemoptysis, magnesium and oxalic acid poisoning, tetany, tuberculosis; *Dosage:* 5 cc of 5 % solution, occasionally 10 cc of 10 % solution, daily or alternate days for 3 weeks; course repeated after 1–2 weeks. (Breon)

72. Calcium-Glucosan—Ampules 30 cc; rubber-stoppered vials; Containing anhydrous dextrose in combination with calcium hydroxide gr 15½ (1 Gm) or calcium chloride gr 31 (2 Gm); *For use* in calcium therapy of asthma, tuberculosis; *Dosage:* initial 10 cc, if tolerated 20 cc following day, subsequently 30 cc every 2–3 days. (Breon)

73. Cincosal Compound—Ampules 20 cc; Boxes of 6 and 25; Containing sodium cinchophen gr 15½ (Gm 1), sodium salicylate gr 15½ (1 Gm), sodium iodide gr 7¾ (0.5 Gm).
Ampules 10 cc; Boxes of 6 and 25; Containing half above strength; *For use* in uric acid excretion, as antipyretic and analgesic; *Dosage:* 10 cc daily for several injections, then on alternate days; course of 10 or more doses. (Breon)

74. Ferro-Arsen—Ampules 10 cc; Boxes of 6 and 25; Containing sodium dimethylarsenate gr 5 (0.32 Gm), ferric chloride gr 2¼ (0.15 Gm), calcium chloride, potassium chloride, sodium chloride aa q.s. to adjust solution; triple distilled water q.s. 10 cc.
Ampules 5 cc; Same strength solution; *For use* in anemia, chlorosis, convalescence, chorea and other conditions where tonic alterative is indicated; *Dosage:* initial dose 5 cc, increased after first few weeks to 10 cc, at 2–3 day intervals, as indicated. (Breon)

75. Ferro-Guai-Arsen—Ampules 10 cc; Boxes of 6 and 25; Containing sodium dimethylarsenate gr 4 (0.26 Gm), ferric chloride gr 1⅛ (0.07 Gm), guaiacol gr ⅝ (0.04 Gm), Creosote gr ⅝ (0.04 Gm), calcium chloride, sodium chloride, potassium chloride, triple distilled water q.s. 10 cc; *For use* in anemias incident to tuberculosis and bronchitis, *Dosage:* 1 ampule every 3–4 days. (Breon)

76. Formodide—Ampules "A" 20 cc; Boxes of 6 and 25; Containing methenamine gr 7 (0.45 Gm); sodium iodide gr 15½ (1 Gm).
Ampules "B" 20 cc; Boxes of 6 and 25; Containing methenamine gr 15½ (1 Gm), sodium iodide gr 31 (2 Gm); *For use* in cystitis, epididymitis, orchitis, pyelitis and

toxemias; *Dosage:* "A" for 2–3 injections, at 24 hr. intervals as indicated; after desired effect "B" at 3 day intervals. **(Breon)**

77. **Formotone**—Ampules 5 cc; Boxes of 6 and 25; Containing methenamine U.S.P., gr 7 (0.45 Gm), gr 15 (0.97 Gm), gr 31 (2 Gm); *For use* as urinary antiseptic; Contraindicated in acute and chronic nephritis; *Dosage:* initial, gr 7 (0.45 Gm), repeated in 12–24 hr.; then gr 15 (0.97 Gm) to gr 31 (2 Gm) as indicated. **(Breon)**

78. **Gentian Violet**—Ampules 10 cc; Boxes of 6 and 25; Containing 1% solution; *For use* in general septicemia and inaccessible local infections of gram-positive organisms; *Dosage:* 5 mg per kilogram (2.2 lb.) of body weight. *See Chap. I.* **(Breon)**

79. **Glucose**—Ampules 20, 50 and 100 cc; Boxes of 6 and 25; Containing 50% solution; *For use* in acidosis of starvation, anuria, resistant eczema, as glucose tolerance test; *Dosage:* initial dose 75 Gm, 50 Gm subsequently, warmed to 100 or 110°F; 3 of the 50 cc ampules diluted in equal quantity of pure distilled water makes 75 Gm of 25% solution.
Ampules 5 and 10 cc; Boxes of 6 and 25; Containing 50% (by weight) solutions; *For use* in varicose veins (small or thin walled veins). *See Chap. I.* **(Breon)**

80. **Glucose-Chloride**—Ampules 10 cc; Boxes of 6 and 25; Containing glucose 50%, sodium chloride 30%; *For use* in varicose veins; *Dosage:* 2–10 cc, not more than 20 cc at 1 sitting. **(Breon)**

81. **Guaisodide**—Ampules 20 cc; Boxes of 6 and 25; Containing guaiacol gr ⅝ (0.04 Gm), creosote gr ⅝ (0.04 Gm), sodium iodide gr 32 (2.07 Gm), glucose gr 37⅗ (2.4 Gm).
Ampules 10 cc; Boxes of 6 and 25; Containing same strength; *For use* in bronchial affections, bronchial pneumonia and certain asthma cases; Contraindicated in tuberculosis, and hypersensitiveness to iodides; *Dosage:* initial dose 10 cc; in 12–24 hr. give 20 cc and same, daily, as indicated. (Breon)

82. **Gui-Calcium**—Ampules 20 cc; Boxes of 6 and 25; Containing gr 10 (0.65 Gm); *For use* in tuberculosis and other pulmonary diseases; Contraindicated in heart inflammation, blood pressure dysfunction and nephritis; *Dosage:* 10 cc first 1 or 2 injections, subsequently 20 cc daily for 30 injections, course may be repeated. **(Breon)**

83. **Hydrochloric Acid**—Ampules 10 cc; Boxes of 6 and 25; Containing 1:1,500 solution; *For use* in stimulating production of antibodies and phagocytes; *Dosage:* 1 injection every 2–3 days, in severe cases daily for several days; then intervals extended. **(Breon)**

84. **Iron and Arsenic (Iron Cacodylate)**—Ampules 5 cc; Boxes of 6 and 25; Containing gr 1 (0.065 Gm); *For use* as hematinic; *Dosage:* 1 ampule every second day. **(Breon)**

85. **Iron, Arsenic and Phosphorus**—Ampules 5 cc; Boxes of 6 and 25; Containing iron cacodylate gr 1 (0.065 Gm), sodium glycerophosphate gr 1½ (0.097 Gm); *For use* in anemia, neurasthenia, osteomalacia, rickets and certain skin conditions; *Dosage:* 1 ampule every 2–3 days for 12–24 ampules. (Breon)

86. **Magnesium Sulphate**—Ampules 20 cc; Boxes of 6 and 25; Containing 10% solution; *For use* as anticonvulsive, anesthetic, tissue dehydrant, sedative in eclampsia, pulmonary edema, hydrophobia, intracranial tension, etc.; *Dosage:* 1 ampule in mild cases, severe 8 injections within 24 hr. may be given as indicated. **(Breon)**

87. **Mercurochrome**—Ampules 10 and 20 cc; Boxes of 6 and 25; Containing 1% solution; *For use* in general, local and urinary infections; *Dosage:* 10 cc of 1% solution per 100 lb. body weight, in desperate cases 6 mg per kilo of body weight or 23 cc per 100 lb. *See Chap. I.* **(Breon)**

88. **Mercury Oxycyanide**—Ampules 5 cc; Boxes of 6 and 25; Containing gr ⅛ (0.008 Gm), gr ⅙ (0.01 Gm), or gr ¼ (0.16 Gm) of mercury oxycyanide of reagent quality in triple distilled water; *For use* as antiluetic; *Dosage:* gr ¼ (0.16 Gm) daily for 3–4 weeks, or every 2–3 days as indicated, or as alterative. *See Chap. I.* **(Breon)**

89. Mer-Sodide—Ampules 20 cc; Boxes of 6 and 25; Containing mercury oxycyanide gr 1/6 (0.01 Gm), sodium iodide gr 31 (2 Gm).
Ampules 10 cc; Boxes of 6 and 25; Containing half strength; *For use* as antiluetic; *Dosage:* 20 cc daily for 10 days after initial dose of 10 cc, then 10 cc every 2–3 days, and 20 cc at 3–4 day intervals for 10–24 doses. **(Breon)**

90. Quinarsen—Ampules 20 cc; Boxes of 6 and 25; Containing quinine dihydrochloride gr 10 (0.65 Gm), sodium dimethylarsenate gr 7¾ (0.5 Gm), urethane gr 3 (0.19 Gm); *For use* in malarial infections; *Dosage:* initial dose 10 cc, then 20 cc every 2–3 hr. preceding expected paroxysm. *See Chap. II.* **(Breon)**

91. Quinine Dihydrochloride—Ampules 5 cc; Boxes of 6 and 25; Containing gr 7½ (0.49 Gm);
Ampules 20 cc; Boxes of 6 and 25; Containing gr 10 (0.65 Gm); *For use* in malaria, influenza; *Dosage:* 1 ampule daily, in extreme cases twice daily. **(Breon)**

92. Salsocol—Ampules 20 cc; Boxes of 6 and 25; Containing sodium salicylate and sodium iodide gr 32 (2.07 Gm) each, sodium dimethylarsenate gr 5 (0.32 Gm), colchicine gr 1/100 (0.0006 Gm);
Ampules 10 cc; Boxes of 6 and 25; *For use* in rheumatism and gout; *Dosage:* initial dose 5 cc; then 20 cc at 1–4 day intervals as indicated. **(Breon)**

93. Salsodide—Ampules 20 cc; Boxes of 6 and 25; Containing sodium salicylate gr 25 (1.62 Gm), sodium dimethylarsenate gr 3 (0.19 Gm), sodium iodide gr 15 (0.97 Gm);
Ampules 10 cc; Boxes of 6 and 25; Same strength; *For use* in rheumatism and other streptococcic infections; *Dosage:* initial dose 10 cc followed by 20 cc daily or every 2–3 days as indicated. **(Breon)**

94. Sodium Bicarbonate—Ampules 20 cc; Boxes of 6 and 25; Containing gr 23 (1.5 Gm); *For use* in acidosis; *Dosage:* diabetes 100–200 cc of 7.5%, in postoperative acidosis about 300 cc of 7.5%. *See Chap. I.* **(Breon)**

95. Strontium Bromide—Ampules 10 cc; Boxes of 6 and 25; Containing gr 15½ (1 Gm); *For use* in eczema, pemphigus pruriginosus, herpes zoster; *Dosage:* initially, 3–5 cc, then 10 cc every second day, up to 15 injections as indicated. **(Breon)**

96. Sodium Cacodylate—Ampules 5 cc; Boxes of 6 and 25; Containing gr 3 (0.19 Gm), gr 5 (0.32 Gm), gr 7 (0.45 Gm) or gr 15 (0.97 Gm); *For use* as hematinic. **(Breon)**

97. Sodium Citrate—Ampules 50 cc; Boxes of 6 and 25; Containing 2.5% solution or gr 19.4 (1.25 Gm); *For use* in blood transfusion; *Dosage:* 1 ampule for 500 cc of blood. **(Breon)**

98. Sodium Iodide—Ampules 10 and 20 cc; Boxes of 6 and 25; Containing gr 31 (2 Gm);
Ampules 10 cc; Boxes of 6 and 25; Containing gr 15½ (1 Gm); *For use* in iodine therapy; *Dosage:* 1 ampule as indicated. **(Breon)**

99. Sodium Salicylate—Ampules 10 cc; Boxes of 6 and 25; Containing gr 15½ (1 Gm);
Ampules 20 cc; Boxes of 6 and 25; Containing gr 31 (2 Gm); *For use* as antirheumatic; *Dosage:* 20 cc every 12–24 hr. then every 2–3 days for a month or 6 weeks as indicated.
Ampules 5 cc; Boxes of 6 and 25; Containing 20% (white label), 30% (buff label), 40% solution (pink label); Each box containing 3 concentrations; *For use* in varicose veins, especially large varices of the long saphenous system. **(Breon)**

100. Sodium Salicylate with Sodium Iodide—Ampules 20 cc; Boxes of 6 and 25; Containing gr 15½ (1 Gm) each; *For use* in rheumatism and other bacterial infections; *Dosage:* severe cases, 20 cc every 24 hr. until symptoms are under control, then 20 cc every 2–4 days as indicated. **(Breon)**

101. Sodium Thiosulphate—Ampules 10 cc; Boxes of 6 and 25; Containing gr 15½ (1 Gm);
Ampules 20 cc; Boxes of 6 and 25; Containing gr 64 (4.15 Gm); *For use* in metallic poisoning and accumulation; *Dosage:* 10 cc daily for 3 days, fourth day and

sixth 1.3 Gm, eighth day 2 Gm; severe cases, 4 Gm daily for 3–4 days, then at 2–4 day intervals. *See Chap. I.* **(Breon)**

102. Triple Distilled Water—Ampules of 5, 10, 20, 50 and 100 cc; Boxes of 6 and 25; *For use* in preparing solutions for injection. **(Breon)**

---

103. Anastil—Ampules 1 cc; Boxes of 6 and 10; Plain; Containing gr 0.05 guaiacol; with novocain; *Dosage:* 1 ampule every 2–3 days. *See Chap. I.* **(Cavendish)**

104. Anastil—Ampules 1 cc; Boxes of 3 and 6; Reinforced; Containing gr 0.075 guaiacol; with novocain; Expectorant; *Dosage:* 1 ampule every 2–3 days. *See Chap. I.* **(Cavendish)**

---

105. Caffeine Sodio-Benzoate—Ampules 2 cc; Boxes of 12, 25 and 100; Containing gr 7½ (0.5 Gm); *For use* as cardiac stimulant; or gr 3¾ (0.25 Gm); *For use* as cerebral, respiratory and circulatory stimulant. **(Cheplin)**

106. Glucose (Dextrose U.S.P.)—Ampules 50 cc + 2 cc Buffer solution; Boxes of 1; Containing 25 Gm dextrose. *See Chap. I.* **(Cheplin)**

107. Glucose (Dextrose U.S.P.)—Ampules 20 cc; Boxes of 6; Containing 10 Gm. *See Chap. I.* **(Cheplin)**

108. Hexamethylenamine—Ampules 5 cc; Boxes of 6; Containing gr 31 (2.0 Gm); Urinary antiseptic. **(Cheplin)**

109. Iron Cacodylate—Ampules 5 cc; Boxes of 6; Containing gr 1 (0.065 Gm); Tonic and alterative. **(Cheplin)**

110. Sodium Cacodylate—Ampules 5 cc; Boxes of 6; Containing 7½ (0.5 Gm). **(Cheplin)**

111. Sodium Cacodylate—Ampules 10 cc; Boxes of 6; Containing 15½ gr (1.0 Gm); *For use* in syphilis, dermatologic conditions, anemia. **(Cheplin)**

112. Sodium Iodide—Ampules 10 cc; Boxes of 6; Containing 15½ gr (1.0 Gm); Antisyphilitic. **(Cheplin)**

113. Sodium Iodide—Ampules 20 cc; Boxes of 6; Containing gr 31 (2.0 Gm); *For use* in chronic rheumatism, syphilis, asthma, chronic bronchitis. **(Cheplin)**

114. Sodium Iodide and Sodium Salicylate—Ampules 20 cc; Boxes of 6; Containing sodium iodide gr 15½ (1.0 Gm), sodium salicylate gr 15½ (1.0 Gm); *For use* in chronic and acute rheumatism. **(Cheplin)**

115. Sodium Salicylate—Ampules 5 cc; Boxes of 6; Containing gr 15½ (1.0 Gm); Antirheumatic. **(Cheplin)**

116. Triple Distilled Water (Sterilized)—Ampules 5 cc; Boxes of 6. **(Cheplin)**

---

117. Coagulen—Ampules 1.5 and 5 cc; Cartons of 5; 3% sterile solution;
Ampules 20 cc; Cartons of 1; 3% sterile solution; Physiological hemostat; *Dosage:* 2–3 cc several times daily. *See Chap. I.* **(Ciba)**

118. Coramine—Ampules 1.1 cc; Cartons of 5, 20, 100 and 500;
Ampules 5.5 cc; Cartons of 3 and 13; Circulatory and respiratory stimulant; *Dosage:* 1–2 ampules as required. *See Chap. I.* **(Ciba)**

119. Digifoline—Ampules 1.1 cc; Cartons of 5, 20, 100 and 500;
Ampules 5.0 cc; Cartons of 1; Digitalis therapy; *Dosage:* 0.03 cc per pound of body weight, then every 2 hr. ⅛ m per pound of body weight. *See Chap. I.* **(Ciba)**

---

120. Calcium Levulinate—Ampules 10 cc; Boxes of 6; Containing 1.31% calcium, equivalent to 1.82% calcium oxide; 10% aqueous solution; Calcium therapy; *Dosage:* 10–20 cc as required. *See Chap. I.* **(Crookes)**

121. Collosol Argentum—Ampules 2, 5, 10 and 20 cc; Boxes of 6; Containing metallic silver 1:2,000, or 0.05%; colloidal silver; *For use* as systemic germicide in sepsis and septicemia; *Dosage:* 1 ampule two to three times weekly. *See Chap. I.* **(Crookes)**

122. Collosol Chrysarobin—Ampules 2 cc; Boxes of 6; Containing colloidal chrysarobin 1:500 solution; *Dosage:* as required. *See Chap. I.* (Crookes)

123. Collosol Lead M.A.—Ampules 5, 10 and 20 cc; Boxes of 3; Cancer therapy; Containing suspension of lead, mercury; *Dosage:* as required. *See Chap. XII.* (Crookes)

124. Collosol Selenium—Ampules 1 and 5 cc; Boxes of 6; 0.05% solution; Palliative in malignant diseases, especially inoperable; *Dosage:* 5–10 cc two to three times weekly. *See Chap. I.* (Crookes)

125. Lithium Salicylate—Ampules 2 and 5 cc; Boxes of 6; Containing lithium salicylate 30% with tutocaine 1%; Sclerosing solution; *Dosage:* 1–4 cc per injection. *See Chap. II.* (Crookes)

126. Mercurochrome (Collosol Brand)—Ampule 25 cc; Box of 1 with isotonic glucose solution 25 cc; Containing scales 0.1 Gm: Antiseptic; Non-colloidal. (Crookes)

127. Sodium Morrhuate—Collosol Brand—Ampules 2 and 15 cc; Boxes of 6; Containing sodium salts of fatty acids of cod liver oil with high iodine content; 5% solution; Sclerosing agent; *Dosage:* 0.5–1 cc per injection, up to a total of 10 cc at 1 sitting. *See Chap. I.* (Crookes)

128. Tetanol—Collosol—Ampules 5, 10 and 20 cc; Containing 13% calcium; *For use* in tetany; *Dosage:* 1 ampule as necessary. *See Chap. I.* (Crookes)

---

129. Coliron—Ampules 1 cc; Boxes of 12 and 100; Containing gr ½ (0.03 Gm) colloidal iron cacodylate;
Ampules 2 cc; Boxes of 12 and 100; Containing gr 1 (0.065 Gm);
Ampules 5 cc; Boxes of 12 and 100; Containing gr 2½ (0.16 Gm); Iron and arsenic therapy; *For use* in secondary anemias, tuberculosis, syphilis, convalescence; *Dosage:* 12 injections, ½–2½ gr at 1–4 day intervals; Injected very slowly. (Cutter)

130. Glucose Solution—Ampules 20 cc; Boxes of 6, 25 and 100; Containing 50% solution; gr 154;
Ampules 50 cc; Boxes of 1, 6, 25 and 100; Containing 50% solution; gr 385;
Ampules 100 cc; Boxes of 1, 6, 25 and 100; Containing 50% solution; gr 770; *For use* in shock, severe acute infections, diabetic coma, pernicious vomiting; *Dosage:* 50–75 Gm (1 cc—½ Gm). *See Chap. I.* (Cutter)

131. Glycero-Coliron—Ampules 1 cc; Boxes of 12 and 100; Containing colloidal iron cacodylate gr ⅓ (0.02 Gm), sodium glycerophosphate gr 1½ (0.1 Gm) strychnine sulphate gr 1/128 (0.0005 Gm);
Ampules 2 cc; Boxes of 12 and 100; Containing colloidal iron cacodylate gr ⅔ (0.04 Gm), sodium glycerophosphate gr 3 (0.2 Gm), strychnine sulphate gr 1/64 (0.001 Gm); *For use* as hematinic and tonic; *Dosage:* 1–2 cc at 2–7 day intervals; Injected very slowly. (Cutter)

132. Glycerophosphate Compound—Ampules 1 cc; Boxes of 12 and 100; Containing sodium glycerophosphate gr 1½ (0.1 Gm), sodium cacodylate gr 1 (0.065 Gm), iron cacodylate gr ⅙ (0.011 Gm), strychnine sulphate gr 1/128 (0.0005 Gm); *For use* as hematinic and tonic; *Dosage:* 1–2 cc at 2–7 day intervals; Injected very slowly. (Cutter)

133. Iron Cacodylate—Ampules 1 cc; Boxes of 12 and 100; Containing gr ½ (0.032 Gm);
Ampules 2 cc; Boxes of 12 and 100; Containing gr 1 (0.065 Gm);
Ampules 5 cc; Boxes of 12 and 100; Containing gr 2½ (0.16 Gm); *For use* in secondary anemias, tuberculosis, syphilis and convalescence; *Dosage:* 12 injections, 1½ gr, at 2–3 day intervals; Injected slowly. (Cutter)

134. Sodium Cacodylate—Ampules 1 cc; Boxes of 12 and 100; Containing gr 3 (0.194 Gm), or gr 5 (0.32 Gm); *For use* in syphilis, anemia, tuberculosis, neuralgia, dry scaly skin conditions; *Dosage:* gr ¾ initially, gradually increased; Injected slowly, diluted with 2 parts salt solution. (Cutter)

135. Sodium Iodide—Ampules 10 cc; Boxes of 6 and 100; Containing gr 15½ (1 Gm), or gr 31 (2 Gm); *For use* in syphilis, goiter, gonorrhea, arthritis and arteriosclerosis; *Dosage:* initially ⅓–½ of 1 Gm ampule, injected very slowly, with gradually increased dosage. **(Cutter)**

136. Sodium Salicylate—Ampules 5 cc; Boxes of 12 and 100; Containing gr 15½ (1 Gm); *For use* as antirheumatic; *Dosage:* 15 gr every 8–12 hr., injected slowly. **(Cutter)**

137. Saliciodide—Ampules 5 cc; Boxes of 6 and 100; Containing sodium salicylate and sodium iodide gr 15½ (1 Gm) each; *For use* as antirheumatic and in streptococcic infections; Contraindicated in tuberculosis and nephritis; *Dosage:* 10 cc twice daily to 10 cc twice weekly as indicated. **(Cutter)**

138. Triple Distilled Water—Ampules 5, 10, 20 cc; Boxes of 6 and 100; Ampules 50 cc; Boxes of 1, 6 and 50; *For use* in preparing solutions for injection. **(Cutter)**

---

139. Diarsenol—Ampules of 0.1, 0.2, 0.3, 0.4, 0.5, 0.6, 1.0, 2, 3 Gm. A brand of arsphenamine U.S.P.; *For use* in syphilis. *See Chap. I.* **(Diarsenol)**

140. Neodiarsenol—Ampules of 0.15, 0.3, 0.45, 0.6, 0.75, 0.9 Gm; A brand of neoarsphenamine U.S.P.; *For use* in syphilis. *See Chap. I.* **(Diarsenol)**

141. Sodium Diarsenol—Ampules of 0.15, 0.3, 0.45, 0.6, 0.75, 0.9 Gm; A brand of arsphenamine N.N.R.; *For use* in syphilis. *See Chap. I.* **(Diarsenol)**

---

142. Aqua Double Distilled De-aerated—Ampules 5, 10 and 20 cc; Boxes of 12 and 100; *For use* in preparing solutions for injection. **(Drug Products)**

143. Calcium Gluconate—Ampules 10 cc; Boxes of 12, 25 and 100; Containing 10% solution; *For use* in calcium therapy; may be used intramuscularly, deep. *See Chap. I.* **(Drug Products)**

144. Calcium Guaiacol Sulphonate—Ampules 20 cc; Boxes of 12, 25 and 100; Containing gr 5 (0.0324 Gm), or gr 10 (0.643 Gm). **(Drug Products)**

145. Dextrose Anhydrous Pure (d-Glucose)—20 and 50 cc; Boxes of 12, 25 and 100; Containing 50% solution. *See Chap. I.* **(Drug Products)**

146. Dextrose-Sodium—Ampules 10 cc; Boxes of 12, 25 and 100; Containing dextrose anhydrous C.P. (D-Glucose) 25%, sodium chloride C.P. 15%, aqua double distilled de-aerated q.s.; *For use* in varicose veins. **(Drug Products)**

147. Guaiacol and Iodide—Ampules 20 cc; Boxes of 12, 25 and 100; Containing guaiacol calcium sulphonate gr 5 (0.324 Gm), sodium iodide gr 15½ (1 Gm), aqua double distilled de-aerated q.s.; *For use* in bronchial asthma, bronchitis and bronchial pneumonia. **(Drug Products)**

148. Hexaphan—Ampules 10 cc; Boxes of 12, 25 and 100; Containing methenamine gr 35 (2.268 Gm), cinchophen gr 5 (0.324 Gm), aqua double distilled de-aerated q.s.; *For use* in pyelitis, rheumatic arthritis, gonorrheal rheumatism. **(Drug Products)**

149. Iron Colloidal—Ampules 5 cc; Boxes of 12, 25 and 100; Containing colloidal iron gr ⅛ (0.008 Gm) in isotonic solution. **(Drug Products)**

150. Iron Cacodylate (Colloidal)—Ampules 5 cc; Boxes of 12, 25 and 100; Containing gr 1 (0.065 Gm) in isotonic solution. **(Drug Products)**

151. Iron Cacodylate Compound (Colloidal)—Ampules 5 cc; Boxes of 12, 25 and 100; Containing iron cacodylate colloidal gr 1 (0.065 Gm), sodium glycerophosphate gr 2 (0.13 Gm), aqua double distilled de-aerated q.s. **(Drug Products)**

152. Mercury Oxycyanide—Ampules 5 cc; Boxes of 12, 25 and 100; Containing gr ⅙ (.01 Gm); *For use* in lues and yaws; *Dosage:* 5 cc every 3–4 days or as indicated; preferable to mix 5 cc of solution with 15 cc of patient's blood in 20 cc syringe, injecting slowly. **(Drug Products)**

153. Methenamine—Ampules 5 cc; Boxes of 12, 25 and 100; Containing gr 31 (2 Gm). **(Drug Products)**

154. **Sodium Cacodylate**—Ampules 5 cc; Boxes of 12, 25 and 100; Containing gr 7½ (0.5 Gm). (Drug Products)

155. **Sodium-Cinchophen Compound**—Ampules 20 cc; Boxes of 12, 25 and 100; Containing cinchophen gr 7½ (0.5 Gm), sodium iodide and sodium salicylate gr 15½ (1 Gm) each, colchicine gr 1/100 (0.00065 Gm), aqua double distilled de-aerated q.s. (Drug Products)

156. **Sodium-Ferro Cacodylate (Colloidal)**—Ampules 5 cc; Boxes of 12, 25 and 100; Containing sodium cacodylate gr 3 (0.194 Gm), iron cacodylate colloidal gr 1 (0.065 Gm), aqua double distilled de-aerated q.s. isotonic. (Drug Products)

157. **Sodium Iodide**—Ampules 10 cc; Boxes of 12, 25 and 100; Containing gr 15½ (1 Gm);
Ampules 20 cc; Boxes of 12, 25 and 100; Containing gr 31 (2 Gm). (Drug Products)

158. **Sodium Iodide Compound**—Ampules 20 cc; Boxes of 12, 25 and 100; Containing sodium iodide and sodium salicylate gr 15½ (1 Gm) each, colchicine gr 1/100 (0.00065 Gm), aqua double distilled de-aerated q.s. (Drug Products)

159. **Sodium Iodide-Salicylate**—Ampules 20 cc; Boxes of 12, 25 and 100; Containing sodium iodide gr 22½ (1.458 Gm), sodium salicylate gr 15½ (1 Gm), aqua double distilled de-aerated q.s. (Drug Products)

160. **Sodium Salicylate**—Ampules 5 cc; Boxes of 12, 25 and 100; Containing gr 15½ (1 Gm). (Drug Products)

161. **Sodium Salicylate Compound**—Ampules 10 cc; Boxes of 12, 25 and 100; Containing sodium salicylate and methenamine each gr 15½ (1 Gm), aqua double distilled de-aerated q.s. (Drug Products)

162. **Sodium Thiosulphate, C.P.**—Ampules 10 cc; Boxes of 12, 25 and 100; Containing 10% solution; *For use* in metallic poisoning and arsphenamine dermatitis. *See Chap. I.* (Drug Products)

---

163. **Adenine Sulphate**—Ampules 20 cc, 0.5 Gm in 20 cc saline; *For use* in increasing polymorphonuclear cells; *Dosage:* injected twice daily. *See Chap. I.* (Eastman)

---

164. **Antimony and Potassium Tartrate**—Ampules 10 cc; Boxes of 12; Containing (0.10 Gm); *For use* in granuloma inguinale; *Dosage:* 1 ampule every 4–5 days as indicated. (Fitch)

165. **Arsenic and Phosphorus**—Ampules 5 cc; Boxes of 12; Containing sodium dimethylarsenate and sodium glycerophosphate gr 1 (0.065 Gm) each; *For use* as hematinic and tonic; *Dosage:* 1 ampule every 2–3 days. (Fitch)

166. **Calcium Chloride**—Ampules 10 cc; Boxes of 12; Containing 5% solution; *For use* as calcium therapy; *Dosage:* 10 cc every 2–3 days as indicated, observing tolerance. (Fitch)

167. **Calcium Gluconate**—Ampules 5 cc; Boxes of 12; Containing 0.50 Gm;
Ampules 10 cc; Boxes of 12; Containing gr 15½ (1 Gm); *For use* in calcium therapy; *Dosage:* 5–10 cc as indicated every 3–4 days. *See Chap. I.* (Fitch)

168. **Calcium Guaiacol Sulphonate**—Ampules 20 cc; Boxes of 12; Containing 2% solution; *For use* in phthisis and night sweats; *Dosage:* 20 cc every 2–3 days. 10 cc as initial dose. (Fitch)

169. **Calcium Iodide**—Ampules 10 cc; Boxes of 12; Containing gr 10 (0.65 Gm); *For use* as calcium therapy with the benefit of iodine; *Dosage:* 10 cc injected slowly every 2–3 days as indicated, testing tolerance with 5 cc as initial dose. (Fitch)

170. **Cinchomethenamine**—Ampules 10 cc; Boxes of 12; Containing cinchophen gr 7 (0.5 Gm) and methenamine gr 31 (2 Gm) per 10 cc; *For use* as antirheumatic; *Dosage:* 10 cc slowly injected every 2 or 3 days as indicated. (Fitch)

171. **Cinchophenate and Salicylate**—Ampules 10 cc; Boxes of 12; Containing sodium phenylcinchoninate 0.50 Gm and sodium salicylate Gm 0.65; *For use* in arthritis,

gout, lumbago and sciatica; *Dosage:* 10 cc injected slowly every 2 or 3 days as indicated. **(Fitch)**

172. **Emethalogan**—Ampules 6 cc; Boxes of 12; Containing 1 or 2% solutions; *For use* in gastrointestinal ulcerations, amebic dysentery and hepatic abscess; *Dosage:* 1 ampule every 2 or 3 days for 4–6 injections preceded by bicarbonate of soda orally. **(Fitch)**

173. **Glucose**—Ampules 5, 10, 20, 50 and 100 cc; Boxes of 12; *For use* in acidosis, coma, convulsions, in hypoglycemia of insulin overdosage; in diabetes mellitus during strict diet;
Ampules 500 cc; Boxes of 10 and 12; 1% solution. Injected slowly, as indicated.
Ampules 5 and 10 cc; *For use* in varicose veins; 50% solution. *See Chap. I.* **(Fitch)**

174. **Glucose and Sodium Chloride**—Ampules 10 cc; Boxes of 12; Containing glucose 5 cc (50%) and sodium chloride 5 cc (30%); *For use* in varicose veins. **(Fitch)**

175. **Guaiacol and Iodide**—Ampules 20 cc; Boxes of 12; Containing sodium iodide gr 7½ (0.5 Gm) potassium guaiacol sulphonate gr 5 (0.30 Gm); *For use* in pneumonia, bronchitis, etc.; *Dosage:* 20 cc every 2 or 3 days as indicated. **(Fitch)**

176. **Hemoglobin**—Ampules 5 cc; Boxes of 12; Containing gr 1 (0.065 Gm); *For use* as hematinic; *Dosage:* 5 cc every 2–3 days. **(Fitch)**

177. **Indigo Carmine Solution**—Ampules 10 cc; Boxes of 12; Containing gr 6 (0.389 Gm); *For use* as kidney function test. **(Fitch)**

178. **Invert Sugar**—Ampules 10 cc; Boxes of 12; Containing 60% solution; *For use* in varicose veins. **(Fitch)**

179. **Iron Arsenic and Glycerophosphate**—Ampules 5 cc; Boxes of 12; Containing iron dimethylarsenate gr 1 (0.065 Gm), sodium glycerophosphate gr 2 (0.13 Gm); *For use* as hematinic and tonic; *Dosage:* 5 cc injected slowly every 2–3 days as indicated. **(Fitch)**

180. **Iron Arsenic and Glycerophosphate Special**—Ampules 10 cc; Boxes of 12; Contents as above. **(Fitch)**

181. **Iron Arsenic and Glycerophosphate (Large)**—Ampules 10 cc; Boxes of 12; Double strength, as above; *Dosage:* 10 cc every 2–3 days as indicated, testing tolerance at initial dose with 2–3 cc only. **(Fitch)**

182. **Iron Cacodylate**—Ampules 5 cc; Boxes of 12; Containing gr 1 (0.065 Gm); *For use* as hematinic; *Dosage:* 5 cc injected slowly every 2–3 days. **(Fitch)**

183. **Iron Colloidal (Plain)**—Ampules 5 cc; Boxes of 12; Containing gr ⅛ (8 mg), or gr ¼ (16 mg); *For use* as hematinic where arsenic is poorly tolerated; *Dosage:* 5–10 cc as indicated. **(Fitch)**

184. **Iron Colloidal with Arsenic**—Ampules 5 cc; Boxes of 12; Containing iron in colloidal form 8 mg, arsenic 10 mg; *For use* as hematinic; *Dosage:* 5 cc every 2–3 days as indicated;
Ampules 10 cc; Boxes of 12; Double dosage. **(Fitch)**

185. **Magnesium Sulphate**—Ampules 20 cc; Boxes of 12; Containing Gm 2 in distilled water q.s.; *For use* in eclampsia, toxemia of pregnancy and puerperal infection; *Dosage:* 20 cc, injected slowly, as indicated. **(Fitch)**

186. **Mercurochrome**—Ampules 20 cc; Boxes of 12; Containing 1% solution; *For use* in septicemia; *Dosage:* 10–20 cc as indicated. *See Chap. I.* **(Fitch)**

187. **Mercury and Arsenic**—Ampules 5 cc; Boxes of 12; Containing mercury biniodide gr 1/12 (5 mg), sodium dimethylarsenate gr 15½ (1 Gm); *For use* as antiluetic; *Dosage:* 5 cc every 4–6 days, alternating with sodium iodide. **(Fitch)**

188. **Mercury and Arsenic with Phosphorus**—Ampules 5 cc; Boxes of 12; Containing mercury biniodide gr 1/12 (5 mg), sodium dimethylarsenate gr 15½ (1 Gm), phosphorus gr 1/100 (0.6 mg); *For use* as antiluetic; *Dosage:* 5 cc every 3–4 days alternating with sodium iodide. **(Fitch)**

189. Mercury Oxycyanide—Ampules 5 cc; Boxes of 12; Containing gr 1/8 (8 mg); Ampules 20 cc; Boxes of 12; Containing gr 1/6 (12 mg); *For use* as antiluetic; *Dosage:* 20 cc every 3–4 days. *See Chap. I.* (Fitch)

190. Methenamine—Ampules 5 cc; Boxes of 12; Containing gr 15½ (1 Gm); Ampules 10 cc; Boxes of 12; Containing gr 31 (2 Gm); *For use* as urinary tract antiseptic; *Dosage:* 5 cc every 2–3 days as indicated. (Fitch)

191. Methenamine and Iodide—Ampules 20 cc; Boxes of 12; Containing methenamine gr 23 (1.5 Gm) and sodium iodide gr 15½ (1 Gm); *For use* in toxemia of pneumonia, in cystitis, orchitis and pyelitis; *Dosage:* 20 cc every 2–3 days as indicated. (Fitch)

192. Methenamine and Salicylate—Ampules 20 cc; Boxes of 12; Containing methenamine and sodium salicylate gr 15½ (1 Gm) each; *For use* in pyelitis, otitis media, pneumonia and pleurisy with effusion; *Dosage:* 20 cc every 2–3 days as indicated. (Fitch)

193. Natrium Bicarbonate—Ampules 20 cc; Boxes of 12; Containing gr 23 (1.5 Gm); *For use* in acidosis; *Dosage:* 20 cc as indicated. (Fitch)

194. Physiological Salt Solution—Ampules 20, 50 and 100 cc; Boxes of 12; Ampules 500 cc; Boxes of 1. (Fitch)

195. Quinine and Urethane—Ampules 2 cc; Boxes of 12; *For use* in varicose veins. *See Chap. II.* (Fitch)

196. Quinine Dihydrochloride—Ampules 5 cc; Boxes of 12; Containing gr 4½ (0.3 Gm);
Ampules 10 cc; Boxes of 12; Containing gr 10 (0.65 Gm); *For use* as antimalarial; *Dosage:* initial tolerance dose 2–3 cc, then 5 cc, as indicated. (Fitch)

197. Ringer's Solution—Ampules 100 cc; Boxes of 12; Ampules 500 cc; Boxes of 1. (Fitch)

198. ℞ 272—Ampules 20 cc; Boxes of 12; Containing sodium salicylate gr 17 (1.10 Gm), sodium iodide gr 15 (1 Gm), guaiacol glyceryl ester gr 1½ (0.097 Gm), lithium benzoate gr 1 (0.065 Gm), colchicine gr 1/100 (0.00065 Gm), sodium citrate gr 2 (0.13 Gm); *For use* in muscular or articular streptococcic infections; *Dosage:* 20 cc every 2–3 days. (Fitch)

199. Salicylate and Iodide—Ampules 20 cc; Boxes of 12; Containing gr 15½ (1 Gm) each; *For use* in streptococcic infections, pneumonia, pleurisy; *Dosage:* 20 cc every 2–3 days. (Fitch)

200. Salicylate and Iodide with Colchicine—Ampules 20 cc; Boxes of 12; Containing gr 15½ (1 Gm) each of salicylate and iodide, colchicine gr 1/10 % (0.00065 Gm); *For use* as antirheumatic and in gout; *Dosage:* 20 cc; every 2–3 days, then every second day.
Ampules 20 cc; Boxes of 12; Containing sodium salicylate gr 31 (2 Gm), sodium iodide gr 15½ (1 Gm), colchicine gr 1/100 (0.6 mg);
Ampules 20 cc; Boxes of 12; Double first strength. (Fitch)

201. Salicylate Combination—Ampules (4) containing 20 % solution; 30 % solution, 40 % solution; *For use* in varicose veins. (Fitch)

202. Sodium Bromide—Ampules 10 cc; Boxes of 12; Containing gr 15½ (1 Gm); *For use* in eczemas; *Dosage:* 10 cc twice weekly as indicated. (Fitch)

203. Sodium Cacodylate—Ampules 5 cc; Boxes of 12; Containing 0.20 or 0.50 Gm; Ampules 10 cc; Boxes of 12; Containing 1.0 or 1.5 Gm; *For use* in anemia, syphilis; *Dosage:* 5–10 cc every 2–3 days as indicated. (Fitch)

204. Sodium Chloride—Ampules 5 cc; Boxes of 12; Containing 20 or 30 % solutions. (Fitch)

205. Sodium Citrate—Ampules 20 cc; Boxes of 12; Containing gr 31 (2 Gm); Ampules 20 cc; Boxes of 12; Containing 2½ % solution; *For use* in blood transfusions. (Fitch)

206. Sodium Glycerophosphate—Ampules 5 cc; Boxes of 12; Containing 0.20 Gm; Ampules 10 cc; Boxes of 12; Containing 0.80; *For use* as hematinic and tonic; *Dosage:* 5 cc every 2 or 3 days as indicated. **(Fitch)**

207. Sodium Iodide—Ampules 10 cc; Boxes of 12; Containing gr 15½ (1 Gm);
Ampules 20 cc; Boxes of 12; Containing gr 31 (2 Gm);
Ampules 30 cc; Boxes of 12; Containing gr 46.3 (3 Gm); *For use* in arthritis, asthma, arteriosclerosis, bronchitis, goitre, and syphilis; *Dosage:* 10, 20 or 30 cc every 2–3 days as indicated. **(Fitch)**

208. Sodium Salicylate—Ampules 5 cc; Boxes of 12; Containing gr 15½ (1 Gm);
Ampules 10 cc; Boxes of 12; Containing gr 31 (2 Gm); *For use* as analgesic in streptococcic infections; *Dosage:* 5 cc daily or as indicated;
Ampules 2 cc; Boxes of 12; 25% solution; *For use* in varicose veins;
Ampules 5 cc; Boxes of 12; 20, 30 or 40% solutions; Varicose veins. **(Fitch)**

209. Sodium Thiosulphate—Ampules 10 cc; Boxes of 12; Containing gr 15½ (1 Gm); *For use* in arsenical, bismuth, lead and mercury poisoning; *Dosage:* 10 cc as indicated. *See Chap. I.* **(Fitch)**

210. Sterile Triple Distilled Water—Ampules of 5, 10, 20, 30, 50 and 100 cc; Boxes of 12;
Ampules of 500 cc; Boxes of 1. **(Fitch)**

211. Strontium Bromide—Ampules 10 cc; Boxes of 12; Containing 10% solution; *For use* in various forms of dermatitis; *Dosage:* 10 cc twice weekly or as indicated. **(Fitch)**

---

212. Digitaline "Nativelle"—Ampules 1 cc; Containing 0.2 mg (gr 1/300); Digitalis therapy; *Dosage:* 1 ampule daily for 3–4 days. *See Chap. I.* **(Fougera)**

213. Ouabaine "Arnaud"—Ampules 1 cc; Boxes of 6; Containing gr 1/240 (0.25 mg); Cardiac stimulant; *For use* in acute heart failure, arrhythmia, nephritic heart; *Dosage:* 1–2 ampules daily for 3–5 days. *See Chap. I.* **(Fougera)**

---

214. Neo Riodine "Astier"—Ampules 5 cc; Boxes of 10 and 50; Containing 44% iodine; *For use* in cardiovascular lesions with fibrous changes, aortitis, angina pectoris, coronary sclerosis, arterial hypertension, lues; *Dosage:* 1–5 cc three to four times weekly for 6–10 doses. *See Chap. I.* **(Gallia)**

---

215. Calcium Chloride—Swab-Seal 30 cc; Containing gr 3⅞ (0.251 Gm) per 5 cc; *For use* in tuberculosis and in calcium deficiency; *Dosage:* 5 cc, as indicated. **(Harvey-Pittenger)**

216. Glycerophosphate Compound 1—Swab-Seal 30 cc; Containing sodium glycerophosphate gr 2 (0.130 Gm), iron cacodylate gr 1 (0.065 Gm) per 5 cc; *For use* as hematinic and tonic; *Dosage:* 5 cc. **(Harvey-Pittenger)**

217. Hexamethylenamine—Swab-Seals 30 cc; Containing gr 23 (1.49 Gm) per 5 cc; *For use* as urinary tract antiseptic; in tuberculosis, meningitis, influenza, and puerperal septicemia; *Dosage:* 5 cc as indicated. **(Harvey-Pittenger)**

218. Hexamethylenamine and Sodium Iodide—Swab-Seals 120 cc; Containing hexamethylenamine gr 23 (1.49 Gm), sodium iodide gr 15½ (1 Gm) per 20 cc; *For use* in colon infections, persistent type; pyelitis, acute infections of biliary system, cystitis, toxemia of pneumonia; *Dosage:* 20 cc. **(Harvey-Pittenger)**

219. Hexamethylenamine and Sodium Salicylate—Swab-Seals 60 cc; Containing hexamethylenamine gr 15½ (1 Gm) and sodium salicylate gr 15½ (1 Gm); *For use* in otitis media, pyelitis, mastoid involvement, pneumonia and pleurisy with effusion; *Dosage:* 10 cc as indicated. **(Harvey-Pittenger)**

220. Iron Cacodylate—Swab-Seals 30 cc; Containing gr 1 (0.065 Gm) per 5 cc; *For use* as tonic and hematinic; *Dosage:* 5 cc as indicated. **(Harvey-Pittenger)**

221. Mercury Oxycyanide—Swab-Seals 30 cc; Containing gr ⅙ (0.01 Gm) per 5 cc; *For use* in syphilis and yaws; *Dosage:* 5 cc as indicated. **(Harvey-Pittenger)**

222. Quinine Dihydrochloride—Swab-Seals 60 cc; Containing gr 7¾ (0.502 Gm) per 10 cc; *For use* as antimalarial; *Dosage:* maximum gr 7½ (0.502 Gm) per 100 lb. of body weight; susceptibility tested by small doses at onset. **(Harvey-Pittenger)**

223. Sodium Bicarbonate—Swab-Seals 120 cc; Containing gr 15½ (1 Gm) per cubic centimeter; *For use* in acidosis; *Dosage:* 20 cc. *See Chap. I.* **(Harvey-Pittenger)**

224. Sodium Cacodylate—Swab-Seals 60 cc; Containing gr 15½ (1 Gm) per 10 cc; *For use* in chronic infectious endocarditis, postencephalitic Parkinsonian syndromes; *Dosage:* 10 cc. **(Harvey-Pittenger)**

225. Sodium Cacodylate and Mercuric Iodide—Swab-Seals 30 cc; Containing sodium cacodylate gr 31 (2 Gm) mercuric iodide gr 1/12 (0.005 Gm); *For use* in psoriasis, yaws, late syphilis; *Dosage:* 5 cc as indicated. **(Harvey-Pittenger)**

226. Sodium Citrate—Swab-Seals 120 cc; Containing gr 75 (4.86 Gm) per 20 cc; *For use* in hemorrhage, by increasing prothrombin factors of blood; *Dosage:* 20 cc. **(Harvey-Pittenger)**

227. Sodium Glycerophosphate—Swab-Seals 30 cc; Containing gr 5 (0.324 Gm) per 5 cc; *For use* as hematinic and tonic; *Dosage:* 5 cc as indicated. **(Harvey-Pittenger)**

228. Sodium Iodide—Swab-Seals 60 cc; Containing gr 31 (2 Gm) per 20 cc; *For use* in stimulating respiratory mucosa, liquefying mucous secretions, favoring elimination of toxins in bronchial asthma, aortitis, chronic bronchitis, arthritis, arteriosclerosis, tertiary syphilis; *Dosage:* 20 cc. **(Harvey-Pittenger)**

229. Sodium Salicylate—Swab-Seals 30 cc; Containing gr 15½ (1 Gm) per 5 cc; *For use* in streptococcal infection, including tonsillitis, arthritis; is analgesic and antipyretic; *Dosage:* 5 cc as indicated. **(Harvey-Pittenger)**

230. Sodium Salicylate and Sodium Iodide—Swab-Seals 120 cc; Containing gr 15½ (2 Gm) each per 20 cc; *For use* in bronchial or lobar pneumonia, influenza, as antirheumatic, in septicemia; *Dosage:* 20 cc as indicated. **(Harvey-Pittenger)**

231. Sodium Salicylate and Sodium Iodide with Colchicine—Swab Seals 120 cc; Containing sodium salicylate and sodium iodide gr 15½ (1 Gm) each, colchicine gr 1/100 (0.00065 Gm) per 20 cc; *For use* as antirheumatic; *Dosage:* 20 cc as indicated. **(Harvey-Pittenger)**

232. Sodium Thiosulphate—Swab-Seals 60 cc; Containing gr 15½ (1 Gm) per 10 cc; *For use* in arsenical, lead, bismuth and other metallic poisoning, in checking salvarsan dermatitis; *Dosage:* 10 cc as indicated. *See Chap. I.* **(Harvey-Pittenger)**

233. Strophanthin—Swab-Seals 30 cc; Containing gr 1/65 (0.0011 Gm) per 5 cc; *For use* in cases requiring immediate digitalis therapy; *Dosage:* 1 cc as indicated. **(Harvey-Pittenger)**

234. Distilled Water—Swab-Seals 60 cc; *For use* in preparing solutions for injection. **(Harvey-Pittenger)**

---

235. Caseosan—Ampules 1 cc; Boxes of 10; Ampules 5cc, Boxes of 6;
Ampules 10 cc; Boxes of 5; Containing 5% casein solution; Non-specific protein therapy; *Dosage:* 0.25–2.0 cc at 1–3 day intervals. *See Chap. I.* **(Heyden)**

237. Thorotrast—Ampules 25 cc; Boxes of 3;
Ampules 12 cc; Boxes of 2, 10; *For use* in splenohepatography and arteriography, and cystography; *Dosage:* 8–75 cc, depending on the part radiographed. *See Chap. I.* **(Heyden)**

---

238. Metaphyllin (Aminophyllin)—Ampules 10 cc; Boxes of 5; Containing 0.24 Gm; Cardiotonic and diuretic; *Dosage:* 1 ampule one to three times daily. *See Chap. I.* **(Hurst)**

239. Metaphyllin with Calcium—Ampules 10 cc; Boxes of 5; *For use* in cardiorenal edema, insufficiency, arterial diseases, hypertension; *Dosage:* 1 ampule one to three times daily. *See Chap. I.* **(Hurst)**

240. Metaphyllin with Calcium and Iodine—Ampules 10 cc; Cartons of 5; *For use* in angina pectoris, cardiac and bronchial asthma, arteriosclerosis, hypertension, cardiac insufficiency; *Dosage:* 2–3 injections daily. *See Chap. I.* **(Hurst)**

---

241. Antimony Sodium Thioglycollate (C.A.)—Ampules 10 and 20 cc; Boxes of 12; Containing not less than 37% antimony; 0.5% solution; Trypanosomicide; *For use* in trypanosomiasis, kala-azar, filiariasis; *Dosage:* intramuscularly or intravenously, 1–2 ampules in 10–20 cc sterile water, twice weekly for 15–25 injections. *See Chap. I.* **(Hynson, Westcott and Dunning)**

242. Antimony Thioglycollamide—Ampules 10 and 20 cc; Boxes of 12; Containing not less than 30% antimony; 0.4% solution; Trypanosomicide; *For use* as above; *Dosage:* 1–2 gr in 10–20 cc sterile water, twice weekly for 15–25 injections; intramuscularly or intravenously. *See Chap. I.* **(Hynson, Westcott and Dunning)**

243. Bromsulphalein—Ampules 3 cc; Boxes of 6; Containing 37% of bromine; 5% solution; *For use* in liver function diagnosis. *For dosage: see Chap. I.* **(Hynson, Westcott and Dunning)**

244. Flumerin-H—Ampules 5 cc; Boxes of 12; Antisyphilitic; *Dosage:* 2–5 mg per kilogram of body weight, in 2% solution, every 3–4 days. *See Chap. I.* **(Hynson, Westcott and Dunning)**

245. Ouabain—Ampules of 0.5 mg; Boxes of 4; Cardiac stimulant; *Dosage:* intravenously or intramuscularly, 1 ampule in 4,000–8,000 cc of saline every 24 hr. *See Chap. I.* **(Hynson, Westcott and Dunning)**

246. Phenolsulphonphthalein—Ampules 1 cc; Boxes of 10; Renal function test; *For uses, dosage, interpretation, see Chap. I.* **(Hynson, Westcott and Dunning)**

247. Phenoltetrachlorphthalein—Ampules 2 cc; Boxes of 8; Containing 50 mg of phenoltetrachlorphthalein; Liver function test; *For use, dosage, interpretation, see Chap. I.* **(Hynson, Westcott and Dunning)**

---

248. Endoarsan—Ampules 5 cc; Boxes of 6, 25 and 100; Containing sodium dimethyl-arsenate gr 15½ (1.0 Gm), mercury gr 1/12 (0.005 Gm), phosphorus gr 1/100 (0.0006 Gm);
Ampules 5 cc; Boxes of 6, 25 and 100; Containing sodium dimethyl-arsenate gr 31 (2.0 Gm), mercury gr 1/12 (0.005 Gm), phosphorus gr 1/100 (0.0006 Gm);
Ampules 10 cc; Boxes of 6, 25 and 100; Containing sodium dimethyl-arsenate gr 15½ (1.0 Gm), mercury gr 1/12 (0.005 Gm), phosphorus gr 1/100 (0.0006 Gm);
Ampules 20 cc; Boxes of 6, 25 and 100; Containing sodium dimethyl-arsenate gr 15½ (1.0 Gm); mercury gr 1/12 (0.005 Gm), phosphorus gr 1/100 (0.0006 Gm);
For use in luetic, paretic and tabetic cases; also shingles (herpes zoster). **(Intravenous Products)**

249. Endoarsenide—Ampules 10 cc; Boxes of 6, 25 and 100; Containing sodium dimethyl-arsenate gr 15½ (1.0 Gm), mercury gr 1/16 (0.00405 Gm), iodide gr 11¼ (0.75 Gm);
Ampules 20 cc; Boxes of 6, 25 and 100; Containing sodium dimethyl-arsenate gr 31 (2.0 Gm), mercury gr ⅛ (0.008 Gm), iodide gr 22½ (1.5 Gm); *For use* in syphilis. **(Intravenous Products)**

250. Endo-Atosal—Ampules 10 cc; Boxes of 6, 25 and 100; Containing solution cinchophen and sodium salicylate gr 7½ (0.5 Gm) each; *For use* in rheumatism, sciatica, neuritis and neuralgia. **(Intravenous Products)**

251. Endo-Atosal and Iodide—Ampules 20 cc; Boxes of 6, 25 and 100; Containing cinchophen gr 7½ (0.5 Gm), salicylate gr 15½ (1.0 Gm), iodide gr 7½ (0.5 Gm); *For use* in severe neuritis, rheumatism and gout. **(Intravenous Products)**

252. Endo-Bromide Compound—Ampules 20 cc; Boxes of 6, 25 and 100; *For use* in epilepsy, nervous disorders and alcoholism. **(Intravenous Products)**

253. Endo-Calcium Chloride—Ampules 10 cc; Boxes of 6, 25 and 100; Containing gr 10 (0.643 Gm); *For use* in calcium deficiency and diarrhea. **(Intravenous Products)**

254. Endo-Calcium Gluconate—Ampules 10 cc; Boxes of 6, 25 and 100; Containing calcium chloride gr 10 (0.643 Gm), glucose 20%; *For use* in calcium therapy. **(Intravenous Products)**

255. Endo-Calcium Gluconate—Ampules 10 cc; Boxes of 6, 25 and 100; Containing 10% solution; *For use* in asthma, hay fever, urticaria and dermatoses. **(Intravenous Products)**

256. Endo-Calcium Guaiacol Sulphonate—Ampules 20 cc; Boxes of 6, 25 and 100; Containing calcium gr 1 (0.065 Gm), guaiacol gr 6 (0.384 Gm); *For use* in pulmonary tuberculosis, bronchitis. **(Intravenous Products)**

257. Endocaodin Special—Ampules 20 cc; Boxes of 6, 25 and 100; Containing calcium iodide gr 10 (0.643), guaiacol sulphonate gr 5 (0.324 Gm); *For use* in pulmonary conditions. **(Intravenous Products)**

258. Endo-Hexamethylenamine and Sodium Iodide—Ampules 20 cc; Boxes of 6, 25 and 100; Containing gr 15½ (1.0 Gm) each; *For use* in pleurisy and pyelitis. **(Intravenous Products)**

259. Endo-Indigo Carmine—Ampules 5 cc; Boxes of 6, 25 and 100; Containing 0.4 Gm; *For use* in kidney function test. **(Intravenous Products)**

260. Endo-Invert Sugar—Ampules 10 cc; Boxes of 6, 25 and 100; 50%, 60%, 75% Solutions; *For use* in varicose veins. **(Intravenous Products)**

261. Iron and Arsenic (Endoferarsan)—Ampules 5 cc; Boxes of 6, 25 and 100; Containing colloidal iron cacodylate gr 1 (0.065 Gm), sodium dimethylarsenate gr 3 (0.2 Gm); *For use* as hematinic and tonic. Ampules 10 cc; double strength. **(Intravenous Products)**

262. Iron, Arsenic and Glycerophosphate (Endoferarsan and Glycerophosphate)—Ampules 5 cc; Boxes of 6, 25 and 100; Containing double strength. **(Intravenous Products)**

263. Endo-Iron Cacodylate—Ampules 5 cc; Boxes of 6, 25 and 100; Containing gr 1 (0.065 Gm); *For use* in anemic conditions and as tonic. **(Intravenous Products)**

264. Endo-Magnesium Sulphate—Ampules 5 cc; Boxes of 6, 25 and 100; Containing gr 7½ (0.5 Gm);
Ampules 10 cc; Boxes of 6, 25 and 100; Containing gr 15½ (1.0 Gm);
Ampules 20 cc; Boxes of 6, 25 and 100; Containing gr 31 (2.0 Gm). **(Intravenous Products)**

265. Endo-Mercurochrome—(H.,W. and D.)—Ampules 5 cc; Boxes of 6, 25 and 100; Gr ¾ (0.04860 Gm);
Ampules 10 cc; Boxes of 6, 25 and 100; Gr 1½ (0.097 Gm);
Ampules 20 cc; Boxes of 6, 25 and 100; Gr 3 (0.194 Gm); 1% solution. **(Intravenous Products)**

266. Endo-Mercury Oxycyanide—Ampules 5 cc; Boxes of 6, 25 and 100; Containing gr ⅛ (8 mg), or gr ⅙ (12 mg). *See Chap. I.* **(Intravenous Products)**

267. Endo-Physiological Saline—Ampules 10, 20 and 50 cc; *For use* in preparing solutions for injection. **(Intravenous Products)**

268. Endo-Pyelographic Solution—Ampules 20 cc; Boxes of 6, 25 and 100; Containing sodium iodide gr 37 (2.392 Gm), indigo carmine gr 5 (0.324 Gm); Special shaped ampule for pyelography. **(Intravenous Products)**

269. Endoquin—Ampules 5 cc; Boxes of 6, 25 and 100; Containing gr 7½ (0.5 Gm); *For use* in acute and chronic malaria. **(Intravenous Products)**

270. Endocaodin—Ampules 20 cc; Boxes of 6, 25 and 100; Containing calcium iodide gr 10 (0.643 Gm), Guaiacol gr ¾ (0.04860 Gm); *For use* in pulmonary conditions. **(Intravenous Products)**

271. Endo-Ciagen—Ampules 5 cc; Boxes of 6, 25 and 100; Containing copper colloidal 0.1 mg, iron cacodylate 0.065 Gm, sodium cacodylate 0.2 Gm; *For use* in anemias, leukemias. **(Intravenous Products)**

272. Endocreocol—Ampules 20 cc; Boxes of 6, 25 and 100; Containing sodium iodide gr 15½ (1.0 Gm), guaiacol and creosote gr ⅝ each; *For use* in bronchial affections. **(Intravenous Products)**

273. Endocreodin—Ampules 20 cc; Boxes of 6, 25 and 100; Containing sodium iodide gr 22½ (1.5 Gm), guaiacol gr ¾ (0.04860 Gm); *For use* in bronchitis, pneumonia, asthma. **(Intravenous Products)**

274. Endo-Dermol—Ampules 10 cc; Boxes of 6, 25 and 100; Containing calcium-strontiobromide 10%; *For use* in dermatitis of various forms, eczemas, itching. **(Intravenous Products)**

275. Endo-Dextrose (Glucose, C.P.)—Ampules 20 cc; Boxes of 6, 25 and 100; Containing gr 154 (10 Gm), 50% solution; *For use* in acidosis, toxemias of pregnancy, eclampsia, edema, surgical shock. *See Chap. I.* **(Intravenous Products)**

276. Endo-Dextrose (Glucose, C.P.)—Ampules 50 cc; Boxes of 6, 25 and 100; Containing gr 385 (25 Gm), 50% solution; *For use* as above. *See Chap. I.* **(Intravenous Products)**

277. Endo-Dextrose (Glucose, C.P.)—Ampules 100 cc; Boxes of 6, 25 and 100; Containing gr 770 (50 Gm), 50% solution; *For use* as above. *See Chap. I.* **(Intravenous Products)**

278. Endo-Emetine Hydrochloride—Ampules 5 cc; Boxes of 6, 25 and 100; Containing gr ½ (0.032 Gm); *For use* in amebic infections. **(Intravenous Products)**

279. Endoglobin—Ampules 5 and 10 cc; Boxes of 6, 25 and 100; A colloidal solution of hemoglobin; *For use* in anemia, chlorosis. **(Intravenous Products)**

280. Endo-Guaiacol—Ampules 20 cc; Boxes of 6, 25 and 100; Containing guaiacol gr 3 (0.194 Gm), iodine gr ⅔ (0.045 Gm); *For use* in incipient phthisis, bronchitis. **(Intravenous Products)**

281. Endo-Hexamethylenamine—Ampules 10 cc; Boxes of 6, 25 and 100; Containing gr 31 (2.0 Gm); *For use* as urinary tract antiseptic. **(Intravenous Products)**

282. Endo-Hexamethylenamine and Sodium Iodide—Ampules 10 cc; Boxes of 6, 25 and 100; Containing hexamethylenamine gr 22 (1.4 Gm), sodium iodide gr 15½ (1.0 Gm); *For use* in pleurisy, pyelitis, otitis media and gonorrheal rheumatism. **(Intravenous Products)**

283. Endo-Quinine Dihydrochloride—Ampules 10 cc; Boxes of 6, 25 and 100; Containing gr 15½ (1.0 Gm); *For use* in malaria. **(Intravenous Products)**

284. Endosal—Ampules 20 cc; Boxes of 6, 25 and 100; Containing sodium iodide and sodium salicylate gr 15½ (1.0 Gm) each, colchicine gr 1/100 (0.00065 Gm);
Ampules 10 cc; Boxes of 6, 25 and 100; Containing sodium iodide gr 15½ (1.0 Gm), sodium salicylate gr 7½ (0.5 Gm), colchicine gr 1/100 (0.00065 Gm);
Ampules 20 cc; Boxes of 6, 25 and 100; Containing sodium iodide gr 15½ (1.0 Gm), sodium salicylate gr 31 (2.0 Gm), colchicine gr 1/100 (0.00065 Gm); *For use* in severe rheumatic conditions. **(Intravenous Products)**

285. Endosal with Iron—Ampules 20 cc; Boxes of 6, 25 and 100; Containing sodium iodide and salicylate gr 15½ (1.0 Gm) each, colchicine gr 1/100 (0.00065 Gm), ferric salicylate;
Ampules 20 cc; Double strength; *For use* in rheumatism, arthritis complicated with anemia. **(Intravenous Products)**

286. Endo-Sodium Bicarbonate—Ampules 20 cc; Boxes of 6, 25 and 100; Containing gr 15½ (1.0 Gm); *For use* in acidosis. **(Intravenous Products)**

287. Endo-Sodium Cacodylate—Ampules 5 cc; Boxes of 6, 25 and 100; Containing gr 7½ (0.5 Gm), gr 15½ (1.0 Gm) or gr 31 (2.0 Gm). **(Intravenous Products)**

288. Endo-Sodium Chloride—Ampules 5 and 10 cc; Boxes of 6, 25 and 100; 20% solutions; *For use* in varicose veins. **(Intravenous Products)**

289. Endo-Sodium Chloride and Dextrose—Ampules 10 cc; Boxes of 6, 25 and 100; Containing dextrose 50%, sodium chloride 30%, equal parts;
Ampules 20 cc; Rubber stoppered vials; *For use* in varicose veins. **(Intravenous Products)**

290. **Endo-Sodium Citrate**—Ampules 20 cc; Boxes of 6, 25 and 100; Containing gr 77½ (5.0 Gm);
Ampules 50 cc; Boxes of 6, 25 and 100; Containing 2½ %; *For use* in hemorrhage, hemoptysis and blood transfusion. **(Intravenous Products)**

291. **Endo-Sodium Glycerophosphate**—Ampules 5 cc; Boxes of 6, 25 and 100; Containing gr 12 (0.8 Gm); *For use* in neurasthenia, osteomalacia and rickets. **(Intravenous Products)**

292. **Endo-Sodium Iodide**—Ampules 10 and 20 cc; Boxes of 6, 25 and 100; Containing gr 31 (2.0 Gm);
Ampules 10 cc; Boxes of 6, 25 and 100; Containing gr 15½ (1.0 Gm). **(Intravenous Products)**

293. **Endo-Sodium Iodide and Salicylate**—Ampules 20 cc; Boxes of 6, 25 and 100; Containing sodium iodide gr 22 (1.426 Gm), salicylate gr 15½ (1.0 Gm); *For use* in streptococcic infections, pneumonia and pleurisy. **(Intravenous Products)**

294. **Endo-Sodium Morrhuate**—Ampules 2 and 5 cc; Boxes of 6, 25 and 100; 5% solution; *For use* in varicose veins. **(Intravenous Products)**

295. **Endo-Sodium Salicylate**—Ampules 5 cc; Boxes of 6, 25 and 100; Containing gr 15½ (1.0 Gm), gr 22 (1.5 Gm), gr 31 (2.0 Gm), gr 37½ (2.5 Gm);
Ampules 10 cc; Boxes of 6, 25 and 100; Containing gr 22 (1.5 Gm); *For use* as analgesic or antipyretic. **(Intravenous Products)**

296. **Endo-Sodium Thiosulphate**—Ampules 5 cc; Boxes of 6, 25 and 100; Containing gr 7½ (0.5 Gm);
Ampules 10 cc; Boxes of 6, 25 and 100; Containing gr 15½ (1.0 Gm); *For use* in varied metallic toxicoses, checking salvarsan dermatitis. **(Intravenous Products)**

297. **Endo-Strontium Bromide**—Ampules 10 cc; Boxes of 6, 25 and 100; Containing gr 15½ (1.0 Gm); *For use* in eczema, psoriasis, urticaria, acne and pruritus. **(Intravenous Products)**

298. Endo-Strontium Bromide—Ampules 10 cc; Boxes of 6, 25 and 100; Containing gr. 15½ and gr 31 (2.0 Gm) glucose; *For use* in hay fever, neuritis and skin conditions. **(Intravenous Products)**

299. **Endo-Tartar Emetic**—Ampules 10 cc; Boxes of 6, 25 and 100; Containing antimony potassium tartrate gr 1½ (0.1 Gm); *For use* in trench mouth, granuloma inguinale, tropical diseases, chancroid, chronic eye inflammation. **(Intravenous Products)**

300. **Triple Distilled Water**—Ampules 5, 10, 20, 30, 50, 100 cc; Boxes of 6, 25 and 100; *For use* in preparing solutions for injection. **(Intravenous Products)**

---

301. **Collodaurum**—Ampules 2 and 5 cc; Boxes of 12; Colloidal gold; *For use* as hematinic, in anemia, malnutrition; as analgesic, as prophylactic in cancer surgery; *Dosage:* 2–5 cc two to three times weekly. *See Chap. III.* **(Kahlenberg)**

---

302. **Calcium Chloride**—Ampules 10%; Boxes of 6 and 25. **(Lakeside)**

303. **Dextrose (d-Glucose)**—Ampules 10 Gm, 20 cc, 25 Gm, 50 cc; Boxes 6 and 25. *See Chap. I.* **(Lakeside)**

304. **Sodium Cacodylate**—Ampules 0.243 Gm (3¾ gr), 5 cc; Boxes 6 and 25. **(Lakeside)**

---

305. **Acacia**—Ampules 100 cc; Boxes of 1, 6 and 25; Containing acacia 30 Gm and sodium chloride 4.5 Gm; *For use* as hemostatic. **(Lilly)**

306. **Calcium Chloride, U.S.P.**—Ampules 10 cc; Boxes of 6 and 25; Containing 7½ gr (0.5 Gm), or 15½ gr (1.0 Gm); Calcium therapy; *For use* in tuberculosis, epididymitis, asthma, hay fever. **(Lilly)**

308. Gluco-Calcium—Ampule (vial) 30 cc; Package of 1; Calcium therapy, as above. (Lilly)

309. Glucose—Ampules 20 cc; Boxes of 6, 25 and 100; Buffered; 1/10 % cresol; 10 Gm Glucose;
Ampules 50 cc; Boxes of 1, 6, 25 and 100; Buffer separate; No preservative; 25 Gm glucose;
Ampules 50 cc; Boxes of 1, 6, 25 and 100; Unbuffered; No preservative; 25 Gm glucose;
Ampules 50 cc; Boxes of 1, 6, 25 and 100; Buffered; No preservative; 25 Gm glucose;
Ampules 100 cc; Boxes of 1, 6, 25 and 100; Buffer separate; no preservative; 50 Gm glucose; *For use* in metabolic carbohydrate deficiency, post-operative shock and acidosis, severe toxemias, hypoglycemia from insulin overdosage. *See Chap. I.* (Lilly)

310. Guaiacol and Sodium Iodide—Ampules 20 cc; Boxes of 6 and 25; Containing sodium iodide gr 22 (1.5 Gm), potassium guaiacol sulphonate representing guaiacol gr 3/4 (0.05 Gm); *For use* in pulmonary tuberculosis. (Lilly)

311. Hexamethylenamine (Methenamine)—Ampules 5 cc; Boxes of 6 and 25; Containing gr 31 (2.0 Gm) Urinary antiseptic. (Lilly)

312. Hexamethylenamine (Methenamine) and Sodium Iodide—Ampules 20 cc; Boxes of 6 and 25; Containing methenamine gr 23 (1.5 Gm), sodium iodide gr 15½ (1.0 Gm). (Lilly)

313. Invert Sugar—Ampules of 10 cc; Boxes of 6 and 25; Containing 5, 6 or 7½ Gm; *For use* in treatment of varicose veins. (Lilly)

314. Iron Cacodylate—Ampules 5 cc; Boxes of 6 and 25; Containing gr 1 (0.065 Gm); *For use* in anemia and dry skin affections. (Lilly)

316. Magnesium Sulphate—Ampules 20 cc; Boxes of 6 and 25; 10% Solution; Ampules 10 cc; Boxes of 6 and 25; 25% Solution; Antispasmodic. (Lilly)

317. Ouabain—Ampules 2 cc; Boxes of 12; Containing gr 1/128 (0.0005 Gm) in buffered sterile normal saline solution; Cardiac stimulant for emergencies only. *See Chap. I.* (Lilly)

318. Quinine Dihydrochloride—Ampules 5 cc; Boxes of 6 and 25; Containing gr 7½ (0.5 Gm);
Ampules 20 cc; Boxes of 6 and 25; Containing gr 10 (0.65 Gm); *For use* as antimalarial, antipyretic and tonic. (Lilly)

319. Quinine Hydrochloride and Urethane—Ampules 2 cc; Boxes of 12; Containing quinine hydrochloride 0.266 Gm, urethane 0.133 Gm; *For use* in treatment of varicose veins. *See Chap. II.* (Lilly)

320. Sodium Cacodylate—Ampules 5 cc; Boxes of 6 and 25; Containing gr 3 (0.2 Gm);
Ampules 5 cc; Boxes of 6 and 25; Containing gr 5 (0.325 Gm)
Ampules 5 cc; Boxes of 6 and 25; Containing gr 7½ (0.5 Gm);
Ampules 10 cc; Boxes of 6 and 25; Containing gr 15½ (1 Gm);
Ampules 5 cc; Boxes of 6 and 25; Containing gr 15½ (1 Gm); An organic arsenical. (Lilly)

321. Sodium Citrate—Ampules 5 cc; Boxes of 6 and 25; Containing gr 18 (1.17 Gm);
Ampules 50 cc; Boxes of 6 and 25; Containing 2½% Solution; *For use* in blood transfusions. (Lilly)

322. Sodium Iodide—Ampules 10 cc; Boxes of 6 and 25; Containing 15½ gr (1 Gm);
Ampules 10 cc; Boxes of 6 and 25; Containing gr 31 (2 Gm);
Ampules 20 cc; Boxes of 6 and 25; Containing gr 31 (2 Gm); *For use* in asthma, simple goiter, scrofula, syphilitic gummata and arteriosclerosis. (Lilly)

323. Sodium Iodide and Sodium Salicylate—Ampules 20 cc; Boxes of 6 and 25; Containing sodium iodide gr 15½ (1 Gm), sodium salicylate 15½ (1 Gm); Antirheumatic, especially in luetic cases. (Lilly)

324. Sodium Salicylate—Ampules 5 cc; Boxes of 6 and 25; Containing gr 15½ (1 Gm);
Ampules 10 cc; Boxes of 6 and 25; Containing gr 31 (2 Gm); Antirheumatic, antiseptic. (Lilly)

325. Sodium Salicylate and Iodide with Colchicine 1—Ampules 20 cc; Boxes of 6 and 25; Containing sodium salicylate gr 15½ (1 Gm), sodium iodide gr 15½ (1 Gm), colchicine gr 1/100 (0.00065 Gm); Antirheumatic and in uric acid diathesis. (Lilly)

326. Sodium Thiosulphate—Ampules 10 cc; Boxes of 6 and 25; Containing gr 7½ (0.5 Gm); *For use* in metallic poisoning. (Lilly)

327. Solutions of Invert Sugar—Ampules 10 cc; Containing Gm 5, 6 or 7.5; *For use* as sclerosing agent. (Lilly)

328. Tartar Emetic—Ampules 5 cc; Boxes of 6 and 25; 1% Solution; *For use* in Vincent's angina, chancroidal infections and its complications. (Lilly)

---

329. Antimony Potassium Tartrate—Ampules 10 cc; Boxes of 6, 25 and 50; Containing gr 1½ (100 mg); *For use* in granuloma inguinale, tropical diseases and chancroids. (Loeser)

330. Bismuth—Ampules 5 cc; Boxes of 6, 25, 50 and 100; Containing 15 mg; *For use* in syphilis, yaws, as spirillicide. (Loeser)

331. Calcium Chloride—Ampules 5 cc; Boxes of 6, 50 and 100; Containing 250 mg; *For use* in intestinal tuberculosis, tetany, asthma, hay fever and hemorrhage. (Loeser)

332. Calcium Gluconate—Ampules 10 cc, 10% solution. Packages 6, 25, 50 and 100. *See Chap. I.* (Loeser)

333. Calcium Guaiacol Sulphonate—Ampules 20 cc; Boxes of 6, 25 and 50; Containing calcium 60 mg, guaiacol approximately 360 mg; *For use* in pulmonary affections, tuberculous and non-tuberculous. (Loeser)

334. Colchicine, Salicylate and Iodide—Ampules 20 cc; Boxes of 6, 25 and 50; Containing colchicine gr 1/120 (0.0005 Gm), sodium salicylate and sodium iodide gr 15½ (1 Gm) each; *For use* in rheumatism and arthritis. (Loeser)

335. Colloidal Gold—Ampules 10 cc; Boxes of 6, 25 and 50; Containing 1 mg; *For use* in tuberculosis and cancer. (Loeser)

336. Colloidal Iron—Ampules 5 cc; Boxes of 6, 25 and 50; Containing metallic iron 8 mg; *For use* as hematinic and in low blood pressure. (Loeser)

337. Cupiron-Ampules—5 cc; Containing copper and colloidal iron cacodylate. Packages 6, 25, 50 and 100; *For use*—as hematinic. (Loeser)

338. Dextrose (d-Glucose)—Ampules 20, 50 and 100 cc; Boxes of 6, 25, 50 and 100; Containing 50% solution by volume; *For use* in eclampsia, vomiting of pregnancy, infections. *See Chap. I.* (Loeser)

338a. Dextrose—Ampules, 50%, 5 and 10 cc. Packages of 12, for varicose vein injection. *See Chap. I.* (Loeser)

338b. Dextrose—Ampules, 10 cc 50%; sodium chloride 30%. Packages of 12, for varicose vein injections. *See Chap. I.* (Loeser)

339. Emetine Hydrochloride—Ampule 5 cc 32 mg. Packages of 6, 25, 50 and 100. (Loeser)

340. Gentian Violet—Ampules 20 cc; Boxes of 6; Containing gr 1½ (100 mg); 5% solution; *For use* in septicemias. *See Chap. I.* (Loeser)

341. Glucose—See Dextrose. (Loeser)

342. Guaiacalx—Ampule 20 cc; Contains guaiacol 0.4 Gm, calcium 90 mg. Packages 6, 25 and 50. (Loeser)

343. Guaiacol and Iodine—Ampules 20 cc; Boxes of 6, 25 and 50; Containing gr 3 (0.2 Gm) guaiacol, gr ⅔ (45 mg) iodine; *For use* in pulmonary tuberculosis, bronchitis, influenza, pneumonia. **(Loeser)**

344. Hexamethylenamine—See Methenamine. **(Loeser)**

344a. Hydrochloric Acid—Ampules 10 cc; Boxes of 6, 25 and 100; Containing HCl C.P. 1:1,500 or 1:1,000; *For use* as non-specific therapy agent and for correction of acid base balance in allergic states—asthma, hay fever, epilepsy, sinusitis and others; *Dosage:* initial 3–5 cc, increased to 10 cc, slowly and cautiously, every 3–5 days. **(Loeser)**

345. Indigo Carmine—Ampules 10 cc; Boxes of 6, 25 and 100; Containing 0.04 Gm, 4% solution; *For use* as renal function test. **(Loeser)**

346. Iron and Arsenic—Ampules 5 cc; Boxes of 6, 25, 50 and 100; Containing gr 1 (0.065 Gm) colloidal iron cacodylate; *For use* as hematinic. **(Loeser)**

347. Iron, Arsenic and Phosphorus—Ampules 5 cc; Boxes of 6, 25, 50 and 100; Containing colloidal iron cacodylate 3 mg, sodium glycerophosphate gr 3 (0.2 Gm); *For use* as hematinic. **(Loeser)**

348. Iron Glycerophosphate—Colloidal—Ampules 5 cc. Packages 6, 50, 100. **(Loeser)**

349. Lead—Ampules 10 cc, 50 mg. Packages of 6. **(Loeser)**

350. Magnesium Sulphate—Ampules 20 cc; Boxes of 6, 25 and 50; Containing 10% solution; *For use* in eclampsia, tetany, puerperal infection, as anesthesia. **(Loeser)**

351. Manganese Chloride—Ampules 10 cc; Boxes of 6, 25 and 50; Containing 25 mg; *For use* as hematinic, in schizophrenia and other psychoses. **(Loeser)**

352. Mercurochrome—Ampules 5, 10 and 20 cc; Boxes of 6, 25 and 50; Containing 1% solutions; *For use* in septicemias and infections. *See Chap. I.* **(Loeser)**

353. Mercury Oxycyanide—Ampules 5 cc; Boxes of 6, 25 and 50; Containing gr ⅛ (8 mg), or gr ⅙ (12 mg); *For use* as antisyphilitic. **(Loeser)**

354. Methenamine—Ampules 5 cc; Boxes of 6, 25 and 50; Containing 1.5 Gm; *For use* in toxemias, cystitis, pyelitis, bronchitis, pneumonia. **(Loeser)**

354a. Methylene Blue—Ampules 50 cc; Packages of 1, 6, 25 and 100. *For use* in Carbon monoxide and cyanide poisoning. **(Loeser)**

355. Methenamine and Sodium Iodide—Ampules 20 cc; Boxes of 6, 25 and 50; Containing methenamine gr 15½ (1 Gm), sodium iodide gr 15½ (1 Gm); *For use* in toxemia, pneumonia, bronchitis and other infections. **(Loeser)**

356. Physiological Salt Solution—Ampules of 50, 100 and 250 cc; Boxes of 6, 25 and 50; Containing 0.85% solution; *For use* in preparing solutions for injection. **(Loeser)**

357. Physiological Salt Solution—Concentrated—Ampules 20 cc; Boxes of 6, 25 and 50; 20 cc added to 480 cc distilled water making 500 cc of 0.85% physiological salt solution; *For use* as above. **(Loeser)**

358. Quinine Dihydrobromide—Ampules 10 cc; Boxes of 6, 25 and 50; Containing gr 10 (0.65 Gm) or gr 7½ (0.5 Gm); *For use* as antimalarial. **(Loeser)**

359. Ringer's Physiological Saline Solution—Ampules 50, 100 and 250 cc; Boxes of 6, 25 and 50; Containing 0.7% sodium chloride, 0.03% potassium chloride, 0.025% calcium chloride. **(Loeser)**

360. Salicylate and Iodide—Ampules 20 cc; Boxes of 6, 25 and 50; Containing gr 15 (1 Gm) each of the sodium salts; *For use* in chronic and subacute arthritis, all streptococcus infections. **(Loeser)**

361. Sodium Bicarbonate—Ampules 20 cc; Boxes of 6, 25 and 50; Containing 1.5 Gm; *For use* in acidosis. **(Loeser)**

362. Sodium Bromide—Ampules 10 cc; Boxes of 6, 25 and 50; Containing gr 15 (1 Gm); *For use* in eczemas and various skin affections. **(Loeser)**

363. Sodium Cacodylate—Ampules 5 cc; Boxes of 6, 25 and 50; Containing gr 24 (1.5 Gm), or gr 15 (1 Gm), or gr 7½ (0.5 Gm) sodium dimethylarsenate (cacodylate). (Loeser)

364. Sodium Citrate—Ampules 20 cc; Boxes of 6, 25 and 50; Containing gr 31 (2 Gm); *For use* in blood transfusions, hemorrhage, endarteritis obliterans. (Loeser)

365. Sodium Glycerophosphate—Ampules 5 cc; Boxes of 6, 25 and 50; Containing gr 12 (0.8 Gm), or gr 3 (0.2 Gm); *For use* in neurasthenia and anemia. (Loeser)

366. Sodium Iodide—Ampules 10 cc; Boxes of 6, 25 and 50; Containing gr 15 (1 Gm); Ampules 20 cc; Boxes of 6, 25 and 50; Containing gr 31 (2 Gm); *For use* in asthma, bronchitis, pneumonia, syphilis, goitre, arthritis. (Loeser)

366a. Sodium Morrhuate—Ampules 2 cc; Packages of 12, 25 and 100; Containing sodium morrhuate 5% and 10%; *For use* as sclerosing agent in varicose veins; *Dosage:* 0.5 cc of 5% solution, increased to 1.5 cc at 24–48 hr. intervals; 10% solution whenever required. *See Chap. I.* (Loeser)

367. Sodium Salicylate—Ampules 5 cc; Boxes of 6, 25 and 50; Containing gr 15 (1 Gm);
Ampules 10 cc; Boxes of 6, 25 and 50; Containing gr 31 (2 Gm); *For use* as antirheumatic. (Loeser)

368. Sodium Thiosulphate—Ampules 10 cc; Boxes of 6, 25 and 50; Containing gr 15 (1 Gm); *For use* in arsphenamine dermatitis, metallic poisoning and skin conditions. *See Chap. I.* (Loeser)

369. Sterilized Distilled Water—Ampules 5 cc; Boxes of 6, 50 and 100;
Ampules 10, 20, 30, 50 and 100 cc; Boxes of 6, 25 and 50; *For use* in preparing solutions for injection. (Loeser)

370. Strontium Bromide—Ampules 10 cc; Boxes of 6, 25 and 50; Containing gr 15 (1 Gm); *For use* in skin diseases, tabes, nerve disturbances. (Loeser)

371. Invert Sugar—Ampules 5 cc, 60%, Packages of 12, for varicose vein injection. (Loeser)

372. Quinine and Urethane—Ampules 2 cc, Packages of 12, for varicose vein injection. *See Chap. II.* (Loeser)

---

373. Arsphenamine—Ampules 0.1, 0.2, 0.3, 0.4, 0.5, 0.6, 1.0 Gm; Antiluetic; By gravity method; *Dosage:* 0.3–0.4 Gm once or twice weekly. *See Chap. I.* (Mallinckrodt)

374. Iodeikon—Ampules 3.5 mg; Boxes of 5; Radiopaque medium for x-ray study; *Dosage:* 55 mg per kilogram of body weight, total not to exceed 3½ Gm, diluted to 200 cc with Ringer's solution; radiography 10 hr. later. *See Chap. I.* (Mallinckrodt)

375. Iso-Iodeikon—Ampules 2.5 Gm; Boxes of 5; Combined liver function and cholecystography; *Dosage:* 40 mg per kilogram body weight, total not to exceed 2.5 Gm, diluted to 150 cc with Ringer's solution; radiography 10 hr. later. *See Chap. I.* (Mallinckrodt)

376. Neoarsphenamine—Ampules 0.15, 0.3, 0.45, 0.6, 0.75, 0.9, 1.5 Gm; Antiluetic; *Dosage:* 0.45–0.6 Gm, diluted to 10 cc, once or twice weekly. *See Chap. I.* (Mallinckrodt)

---

377. Ephedrine Hydrochloride—Ampules 1 cc and Vials of 10 cc; Cartons of 1; Containing gr ¾ (0.05 Gm); *For use* as circulatory stimulant; *Dosage:* ½–1 cc. *See Chap. I.* (McNeil)

378. Mercury Oxycyanide—Ampules 5 cc; Boxes of 6; Containing gr ⅙ (0.011 Gm); *For use* as antisyphilitic; *Dosage:* 2½–5 cc as indicated. *See Chap. I.* (McNeil)

379. Quinine-Urethane—Ampules 2 cc; Boxes of 6 and 100; Containing quinine hydrochloride gr 2 (0.133 Gm), urethane gr 1 (0.066 Gm); *For use* in varicose veins; *Dosage:* 2 cc. *See Chap. II.* (McNeil)

380. **Sodium Salicylate**—Ampules 5 cc; Boxes of 6; Containing per cubic centimeter, gr 3.1 (0.198 Gm); *For use* as analgesic, antipyretic and antiseptic; *Dosage:* 1¼–5 cc, one to four times daily. **(McNeil)**

381. **Sodium Salicylate Compound**—Ampules 10 cc; Cartons of 1; Containing per cubic centimeter, sodium salicylate, sodium iodide gr 1 (0.065 Gm) each, sodium cacodylate gr ¼ (0.01620 Gm), colchicine gr 1/1000; *For use* as analgesic and alterative in rheumatism and gout; *Dosage:* 10–20 cc daily as indicated. **(McNeil)**

---

382. **Citrosalven**—Ampules 50 and 100 cc; Containing sodium citrate, sodium chloride, and buffer salts; Antacid; *Dosage:* 50–100 cc two to three times weekly. *See Chap. III.* **(Medicinal Products)**

---

383. **Arsphenamine**—Ampules of 0.1, 0.2, 0.3, 0.4, 0.5, 0.6 Gm; Antisyphilitic; By gravity method only; *Dosage:* 0.3–0.4 Gm twice weekly. *See Chap. I.* **(Merck)**

384. **Neoarsphenamine**—Ampules of 0.15, 0.3, 0.45, 0.6, 0.75, 0.9 Gm; Boxes of 1 with a 10 cc ampule distilled water; Boxes of 10 with ten 10 cc ampules distilled water; Syringe method; *Dosage:* 0.45–0.6 Gm weekly. *See Chap. I.* **(Merck)**

385. **Tryparsamide**—Ampules of 1, 2 and 3 Gm.; Antiluetic; Also in trypanosomiasis; *Dosage:* 0.04–0.05 Gm per kilogram of body weight, once weekly for 8–16 doses. *See Chap. I.* **(Merck)**

386. **Digitan**—Ampules 1 cc, 1½ grs; Boxes of 6. **(Merck)**

---

387. **Neosalvarsan**—Ampules of 0.15, 0.3, 0.45, 0.6, 0.75, 0.9 Gm; Single dosage; with or without 10 cc ampule of triple distilled water;
Ampules of 1.5, 1.8, 3.0, 4.5 Gm: Multiple dosage; Antisyphilitic; *Dosage:* 0.45–0.6 Gm twice weekly. *See Chap. I.* **(Metz)**

388. **Salvarsan**—Ampules of 0.1, 0.2, 0.3, 0.4, 0.5, 0.6 Gm; Single dosage;
Ampules of 1, 1.2, 2.0, 3.0 Gm; Antisyphilitic; by gravity method only; *Dosage:* 0.3–0.4 Gm weekly. *See Chap. I.* **(Metz)**

389. **Salyrgan**—Ampules 1 cc; Boxes of 5;
Ampules 2 cc; Boxes of 10; Powerful diuretic; Containing not less than 37.6% of mercury; 10% aqueous solution; *Dosage:* 0.5–1.0 cc daily. *See Chap. I.* **(Metz)**

390. **Sulfactol**—Ampules gr 10 (0.6 Gm); Boxes of 10; Sterile crystals;
Ampules gr 15 (1.0 Gm); Boxes of 10; Sterile crystals;
Ampules gr 15 (1.0 Gm); Boxes of 5 with 5 (10 cc) ampules sterile triple distilled water; *For use* in prevention and treatment of toxic reactions in syphilis from arsenic, bismuth, mercury, and other poisoning; in eczema. *See Chap. I.* **(Metz)**

391. **Suprarenin**—Ampules 1 cc; Boxes of 20; Vasoconstrictor and hemostatic; *Dosage:* 0.5–1.0 cc daily. *See Chap. I.* **(Metz)**

392. **Synodal**—Ampules 6 cc; Boxes of 5; Non-specific therapy; Containing lipoproteins with emetine, gr 1 per cubic centimeter; *Dosage:* 1 ampule twice weekly. *See Chap. I.* **(Metz)**

393. **Triphal**—Ampules of 0.025 and 0.1 Gm; Lupus therapy; Containing 44% gold; *Dosage:* 1 ampule twice weekly. *See Chap. I.* **(Metz)**

---

394. **Antimony Potassium Tartrate**—Ampules 5 cc; Boxes of 6 and 50; Containing gr ¾ (0.05 Gm)
Ampules 10 cc; Boxes of 6 and 50; Containing gr 1½ (0.10 Gm) *For use* in granuloma inguinale (tropical ulcer), chancroid (Ducrey) infections, in Vincent's angina; *Dosage:* 5 cc every 3–4 days, gradually increasing to 10 cc. **(Miller)**

395. **Arsenic and Mercury**—Ampules 5 cc; Boxes of 6 and 50; Containing gr 10.8 (0.7 Gm) of sodium dimethyl-arsenate and gr 1/12 (0.006 Gm) of mercury oxycyanide; Antisyphilitic; *Dosage:* 1 ampule every 3–4 days. **(Miller)**

396. Arsenic, Mercury and Iodine—Ampules 10 cc; Boxes of 6 and 50; Containing sodium dimethylarsenate gr 10.8 (0.7 Gm), mercury oxycyanide gr 1/6 (0.004 Gm), sodium iodide gr 7½ (0.5 Gm); Antisyphilitic; *Dosage:* 1 ampule every 3–4 days. (Miller)

397. Caffeine Sodium Benzoate—Ampules 1 cc; Boxes of 12 and 100; Containing gr 3¾ (0.25 Gm)
Ampules 2 cc; Boxes of 12 and 100; Containing gr 7½ (0.5 Gm); *For use* as cardio-renal stimulant in chronic nephritis, cardiac dropsy, collapse, pneumonia; *Dosage:* as frequently as desired. (Miller)

398. Calcium Chloride—Ampules 5 cc; Boxes of 6 and 50; 5 and 10% solutions;
Ampules 10 cc; Boxes of 6 and 50; 5 and 10% solutions; *For use* as calcium therapy with parathyroid extract in chorea, epilepsy, paralysis agitans, tetany, hemorrhage due to hemophilia, varicose ulcer and in tuberculosis; *Dosage:* 1 ampule every 2–3 days. (Miller)

399. Calcium Guaiacol Sulphonate—Ampules 10 cc; Boxes of 6 and 50; Containing gr 5 (0.32 Gm) *For use* in tuberculosis and certain respiratory diseases; *Dosage:* 1 ampule every 3–4 days. (Miller)

400. Calcium Lactate—Ampules 2 cc; Boxes of 12 and 100; Containing gr 2 (0.13 Gm); *For use* in intestinal and pulmonary tuberculosis, for calcium therapy; *Dosage:* 1 ampule every 3 days. (Miller)

401. Colloidal Gold—Ampules 5 and 10 cc; Boxes of 6 and 50; Glass stoppered bottle 4 oz.; package of 1; *For use* in lupus erythematosus; *Dosage:* 5–10 cc, two to three times weekly; 10 cc may be daily given. (Miller)

402. Dextrose—Ampules 10 cc; Boxes of 6 and 50; Containing gr 77½ (5.0 Gm) dextrose (Glucose)
Ampules 20 cc; Boxes of 6 and 50; Containing gr 155 (10.0 Gm) dextrose (Glucose)
Ampules 50 cc; Boxes of 6 and 50; Containing gr 387 (25.0 Gm) dextrose (Glucose)
Ampules 100 cc; Boxes of 6 and 50; Containing gr 775 (50.0 Gm) dextrose (Glucose)
Ampules, double ended and rubber capped, 50 cc; Boxes of 6 and 50; Containing gr 387 (25.0 Gm) dextrose (Glucose); *For use* in carbohydrate metabolic disturbances, post-operative shock and acidosis, thyrotoxicosis, pyogenic processes, acute chorea or eclampsia etc. *See Chap. I.* (Miller)

403. Emetine Hydrochloride—Ampule 1 cc; Boxes of 12 and 100; Containing gr ½ (0.032 Gm)
Ampules 1 cc; Boxes of 12 and 100; Containing gr 1 (0.065 Gm)
Ampules 5 cc; Boxes of 6 and 50; Containing gr ½ (0.032 Gm)
Ampules 5 cc; Boxes of 6 and 50; Containing gr 1 (0.065 Gm) *For use* in protozoan infections and particularly in amebic dysentery and amebic hepatitis; *Dosage:* ½–1 gr, 1 or 2 daily until 8 gr are given. (Miller)

404. Gentian Violet—Ampules 10 cc; Boxes of 6 and 50; Containing 1.0% solution;
Ampules 20 cc; Boxes of 6 and 50; Containing 1.0% solution;
Ampules 50 cc; Boxes of 6 and 50; Containing 1.0% solution; *For use* in bacteremias and septicemias; as specific for tularemia; *Dosage:* 0.5 cc per kilogram (2.2 lb.) body weight, twice weekly. *See Chap. I.* (Miller)

405. Glucose-Calcium—Ampules 30 cc; Boxes of 6 and 50; Containing calcium equivalent to 1 Gm of calcium hydroxide; *For use* in tuberculosis, asthma, hay fever; *Dosage:* 10–15 cc, three times weekly. (Miller)

406. Glycerophosphate Compound—Ampules 5 cc; Boxes of 6 and 50; Containing sodium glycerophosphate gr 1½ (0.1 Gm), iron cacodylate gr 1/6 (0.012 Gm), strychnine cacodylate gr 1/125 (0.0005 Gm); *For use* as hematinic and tonic; *Dosage:* 1 ampule every 2–3 days. (Miller)

407. Guaiacol and Iodine—Ampules 20 cc; Boxes of 6 and 50; Containing guaiacol gr 3 (0.20 Gm) and sodium iodide gr 23 (1.50 Gm); *For use* in respiratory diseases, asthma, bronchial affections, pneumonia and infections associated with pulmonary tuberculosis; *Dosage:* 1 ampule every 3–5 days. **(Miller)**

408. **Hexamethylenamine (Formin)**—Ampules 5 cc; Boxes of 6 and 50; Containing gr 15½ (1.0 Gm), or gr 31 (2.0 Gm); *See Chap. I.*
Ampules 10 cc; Boxes of 6 and 50; Containing gr 31 (2.0 Gm); *For use* as genitourinary antiseptic, in acute nephritis, bronchitis, pneumonia, spirochetosis, certain septicemias, dysuria and anuria; *Dosage:* 15½–31 gr daily; urine must be kept acid. **(Miller)**

409. **Iron Cacodylate**—Ampules 2 cc; Boxes 12 and 100; Containing gr 1 (0.065 Gm); Ampules 5 cc; Boxes of 6 and 50; Containing gr 1 (0.065 Gm), gr 2 (0.13 Gm) or gr 3 (0.20 Gm); *For use* as hematinic and tonic and in dry scaly skin conditions; *Dosage:* ½–3 gr as indicated. **(Miller)**

410. **Iron Cacodylate Compound**—Ampules 2 cc; Boxes of 12 and 100; Containing iron cacodylate gr ½ (0.032 Gm), sodium cacodylate gr 2 (0.13 Gm), strychnine cacodylate gr 1/37 (0.002 Gm), sodium glycerophosphate gr 2 (0.13 Gm); *For use* as hematinic and tonic; *Dosage:* 1 ampule every 2–3 days. **(Miller)**

411. **Iron Cacodylate and Phosphorus**—Ampules 5 cc; Boxes of 6 and 50; Containing iron cacodylate gr 1 (0.065 Gm), sodium glycerophosphate gr 1 (0.065 Gm); *For use* as hematinic and tonic; *Dosage:* 1 ampule every 3–4 days. **(Miller)**

412. **Iron Cacodylate and Strychnine**—Ampules 5 cc; Boxes of 6 and 50; Containing iron cacodylate gr 1 (0.065 Gm), strychnine sulphate gr 1/128; *For use* as hematinic and tonic; *Dosage:* 1 ampule every 2–3 days. **(Miller)**

413. **Iron Glycerophosphate Compound**—Ampules 1 cc; Boxes of 12 and 100; Containing iron citrate gr ½ (0.032 Gm), sodium glycerophosphate gr 1 (0.065 Gm), sodium cacodylate (dimethylarsenate) gr ½ (0.032 Gm); *For use* as hematinic and tonic; *Dosage:* 1 ampule every 2–3 days. **(Miller)**

414. **Magnesium Sulphate**—Ampules 1 cc; Boxes of 12 and 100; 25 or 50% solution; gr 3¾ (0.25 Gm) or gr 7½ (0.50 Gm);
Ampules 2 cc; Boxes of 12 and 100; 25 or 50% solution; Gr 7½ (0.50 Gm) or 15½ (1.0 Gm);
Ampules 10 cc; Boxes of 6 and 50; 10% solution; gr 15½ (1.0 Gm);
Ampules 20 cc; Boxes of 6 and 50; 10% solution; gr 31 (2.0 Gm); *For use* with morphine for prolonged effect, as antispasmodic in tetany and eclampsia; *Dosage:* 1 ampule as indicated. **(Miller)**

415. **Mercurochrome**—Ampules 5, 10 and 20 cc; Boxes of 6 and 50; 1% Solution; *For use* in septicemia, bacteremia, gonorrheal arthritis, epididymitis; either straight or with equal volume 50% dextrose (glucose); *Dosage:* 0.5 cc per kilogram (2.2 lb.) body weight, twice weekly. *See Chap. I.* **(Miller)**

416. **Mercury Oxycyanide**—Ampules 5 cc; Boxes of 6 and 50; Containing gr ⅛ (0.008 Gm), gr ⅙ (0.012 Gm), or gr ¼ (0.016 Gm); Antisyphilitic; *Dosage:* ⅛–¼ gr three times weekly. *See Chap. I.* **(Miller)**

417. **Mercury and Iodine**—Ampules 5 cc; Boxes of 6 and 50; Containing gr ⅛ (0.008 Gm) of mercury oxycyanide and gr 7½ (0.50 Gm) sodium iodide; Antisyphilitic; *Dosage:* 1 ampule every 3–4 days. **(Miller)**

418. **Physiological Salt Solution**—Ampules 50 and 100 cc; Boxes of 6 and 50; 0.85% of sodium chloride in triple glass distilled water. **(Miller)**

419. **Quinine Dihydrochloride**—Ampules 10 cc; Boxes of 6 and 50; Containing gr 5 (0.325 Gm);
Ampules 20 cc; Boxes of 6 and 50; Containing gr 10 (0.65 Gm); *For use* as antimalarial, antiperiodic, antipyretic and tonic; *Dosage:* 1 ampule two or three times weekly as indicated. **(Miller)**

420. **Sodium Bicarbonate**—Ampules 10 cc; Boxes of 6 and 50; Containing gr 11½ (0.75 Gm);
Ampules 20 cc; Boxes of 6 and 12; Containing gr 23 (1.50 Gm); *For use* in severe acidosis; to prevent alkalosis, repeated CO_2 and pH determinations of blood should be made. *See Chap. I.* **(Miller)**

421. Sodium Cacodylate—Ampules 5 cc; Boxes of 6 and 50; Containing gr 7¾, 15½, 23, or 31; *For use* in anemia, chlorosis, malarial cachexia, leukemia, pellagra and psoriasis; *Dosage:* 1 ampule two to three times weekly as indicated. (Miller)

422. Sodium Citrate—Ampules 20 cc; Boxes of 6 and 50; Containing gr 31 (2.0 Gm); *For use* in blood transfusions; *Dosage:* 1 ampule in about 900 cc of blood. (Miller)

423. Sodium Glycerophosphate—Ampules 5 cc; Boxes of 6 and 50; Containing gr 12 (0.80 Gm); *For use* in rachitis, osteomalacia, general muscular and nervous debility; *Dosage:* 1 ampule every 2 or 3 days. (Miller)

424. Sodium Iodide—Ampules 5 cc; Boxes of 6 and 50; Containing gr 7¾ (0.50 Gm) C.P. sodium iodide; or gr 15½ (1.0 Gm);
Ampules 10 cc; Boxes of 6 and 50; Containing gr 15½ (1.0 Gm) or gr 31 (2.0 Gm);
Ampules 20 cc; Boxes of 6 and 50; Containing gr 31 (2.0 Gm); *For use* in asthma, arteriosclerosis, simple goiter, syphilitic gummata, dermatitis, systemic gonorrheal infections; *Dosage:* gr 7¾–31, two to three times weekly. (Miller)

425. Sodium Salicylate—Ampules 5 cc; Boxes of 6 and 50; Containing gr 5 (0.325 Gm) or gr 15½ (1.0 Gm);
Ampules 10 cc; Boxes of 6 and 50; Containing gr 23 (1.5 Gm) or gr 31 (2.0 Gm); *For use* in arthritis of pyogenic origin, streptococcic tonsillitis, myalgia; *Dosage:* 1 ampule daily as indicated. (Miller)

426. Sodium Salicylate and Sodium Iodide—Ampules 10 cc; Boxes of 6 and 50; Containing gr 7¾ (0.50 Gm) each of sodium salicylate, and sodium iodide.
Ampules 20 cc; Boxes of 6 and 50; Containing gr 15½ each of sodium salicylate and sodium iodide; *For use* in acute and chronic arthritis, sciatica, bronchial asthma; *Dosage:* 1 ampule two to three times weekly. (Miller)

427. Sodium Salicylate, Sodium Iodide and Colchicine—Ampules 20 cc; Boxes of 6 and 50; Containing sodium salicylate and sodium iodide gr 15½ each (1.0 Gm); *For use* in acute and chronic arthritis, sciatica, lumbago and other rheumatic conditions; *Dosage:* 10–20 cc every 2–4 days. (Miller)

428. Sodium Salicylate, Sodium Iodide and Sodium Cacodylate—Ampules 20 cc; Boxes of 6 and 50; Containing sodium salicylate gr 25 (1.65 Gm), sodium iodide; gr 15½ (1.0 Gm), sodium cacodylate gr 3 (0.2 Gm); *For use* in acute and chronic arthritis of pyogenic processes of streptococcic and gonococcic origin; *Dosage:* 10–20 cc every 2–4 days. (Miller)

429. Sodium Thiosulphate—Ampules 5 cc; Boxes of 6 and 50; Containing gr 3¾ (0.25 Gm) or gr 7¾ (0.50 Gm);
Ampules 10 cc; Boxes of 6 and 50; Containing gr 15½ (1.0 Gm); *For use* in arsenic, bismuth, mercury and other metallic poisoning; *Dosage:* gr 3¾ daily increased to gr 15½ as indicated. *See Chap. I.* (Miller)

430. Water (Triple Distilled)—Ampules of 5, 10, 20, 50 and 100 cc; Boxes of 6 and 50; Rubber capped ampule-vial 10 cc; Boxes 6 and 50. (Miller)

---

431. Buffer Solution—Ampules 1 cc; Boxes of 12, 25 and 100; Containing dibasic sodium phosphate, anhydrous gr 3½ (0.225 Gm), potassium biphosphate, anhydrous gr 9⁄16 (0.035 Gm) in triple distilled water; each cubic centimeter contains buffer solution sufficient for 50 cc dextrose 50%;
Ampules 2 cc; Boxes of 12, 25 and 100; Double strength; each 2 cc containing sufficient solution for 100 cc of dextrose 50%. (National Drug)

432. Calcium Chloride—Ampules 10 cc; Boxes of 6, 12, 25 and 100; Containing gr 15½ (1.0 Gm);
Ampules 5 cc; Boxes of 12, 25 and 100; 5% solution; *For use* in calcium therapy, hay fever, asthma, tetany, paralysis agitans, chorea, varicose veins, ulcers. (National Drug)

433. Calcium Gluconate—Ampules 10 cc; Boxes of 6, 12, 25 and 100; 10% solution: Ampule-vials 25 cc; Boxes of 1; 10% solution. *See Chap. I.* (National Drug)

434. Dextrose C.P. (d-Glucose)—Ampules 20 cc; Boxes of 6, 12, 25 and 100; 50% solution.
Ampule-vials 50 cc; With or without Buffer; 50% solution; Boxes of 1, 12, 25 and 100;
Ampule-vials 100 cc; Boxes of 1, 12, 25 and 100; With or without buffer solution; *For use* in shock, post-operative acidosis, eclampsia, toxemias of pregnancy, to overcome hypoglycemia following excessive doses of insulin. *See Chap. I.* **(National Drug)**

435. Dextrose and Sodium Chloride—Ampules 10 cc; Boxes of 6, 12, 25 and 100; Containing dextrose, C.P. (Anhydrous) 2.5 Gm, sodium chloride C.P. 1.5 Gm, in triple distilled water q.s.
Ampule-vials 25 cc; Boxes of 6; Containing per cubic centimeter dextrose C.P. (anhydrous) .25 Gm, sodium chloride C.P. .15 Gm, in triple distilled water q.s. *For use* in varicose veins and ulcers. **(National Drug)**

436. Hexamethylenamine—Ampules 10 cc; Boxes of 12, 25 and 100; Containing gr 31 (2.0 Gm) in triple distilled water q.s. 10 cc; *For use* as urinary tract antiseptic. **(National Drug)**

437. Iron, Arsenic and Phosphorus—Ampules 2 cc; Boxes of 12, 25 and 100; Containing iron cacodylate gr 1 (0.065 Gm), sodium glycerophosphate gr 2 (0.130 Gm), triple distilled water q.s. 2 cc; *For use* as hematinic. **(National Drug)**

438. Iron, Arsenic and Strychnine—Ampules 2 cc; Boxes of 12, 25 and 100; Containing iron cacodylate gr 1 (0.065 Gm), strychnine phosphate gr 1/64 (0.001 Gm), in triple distilled water q.s. *For use* as hematinic and tonic. **(National Drug)**

439. Iron Arsenite—Ampules 1 cc; Boxes of 12, 25 and 100; Containing iron arsenite (soluble) gr 1 (0.065 Gm), procaine 0.2%, in triple distilled water, q.s. 1 cc; *For use* as hematinic, in pseudo-leukemia or Hodgkin's disease. **(National Drug)**

440. Iron Cacodylate—Ampules 5 cc; Boxes of 12, 25 and 100; *For use* as hematinic and tonic. Containing gr 1 (0.065 Gm) in triple distilled water. **(National Drug)**

441. Magnesium Sulphate C.P.—Ampules 20 cc; Boxes of 12, 25 and 100; 10% solution; *For use* in eclampsia, toxemia of pregnancy, as depletant and sedative. **(National Drug)**

442. Mercurochrome—Ampule-vials 30 and 100 cc; Boxes of 12; 1% solution; *For use* in puerperal and general septicemia, streptococcic and staphylococcic infections, erysipelas, post-operative genito-urinary infections, arthritis and rheumatic conditions. *See Chap. I.* **(National Drug)**

443. Mercury Oxycyanide—Ampules 5 cc; Boxes of 12, 50 and 100; Containing gr 1/6 (0.012 Gm) in triple distilled water q.s. 5 cc; *For use* in mercury therapy. *See Chap. I.* **(National Drug)**

444. Pilocarpine and Sparteine Compound—Ampules 2 cc; Boxes of 12, 25 and 100; Containing pilocarpine hydrochloride gr 1/10 (0.006 Gm), sparteine sulphate gr 1/2 (0.032 Gm), caffeine and sodium benzoate gr 1/2 (0.032 Gm); *For use* in acute diabetic and uremic coma, eclampsia. **(National Drug)**

445. Quinine and Urea Hydrochloride—Ampules 2 cc; Boxes of 12, 25 and 100; Containing gr 15 1/2 (1.0 Gm); *For use* in malaria. *See Chap. I.* **(National Drug)**

446. Quinine-Urethane—Ampules 2 cc; Boxes of 12, 25 and 100; Containing quinine hydrochloride gr 4 (0.26 Gm), urethane gr 2 (0.13 Gm), distilled water q.s.; Ampule-vials 25 cc; Boxes of 1; Half strength; *For use* in varicose veins. *See Chap. I.* **(National Drug)**

447. Sodium Cacodylate—Ampules 10 cc; Boxes of 12, 25 and 100; Containing gr 10 (0.65 Gm) in physiologic salt solution q.s. 10 cc; *For use* as antirheumatic. **(National Drug)**

448. Sodium Citrate—Ampule-vials 30 cc; Boxes of 6; Containing 2 1/2% solution; *Dosage:* 1 ampule for each 270 cc of blood, in transfusions. **(National Drug)**

449. Sodium Iodide—Ampules 10 cc; Boxes of 12, 25 and 100; Containing gr 15½ (1.0 Gm);
Ampules 20 cc; Boxes of 12, 25 and 100; Containing gr 31 (2.0 Gm); *For use* as antisyphilitic. **(National Drug)**

450. Sodium Iodide and Guaiacol—Ampules 20 cc; Boxes of 6, 12, 25 and 100; Containing sodium iodide gr 31 (2.0 Gm), guaiacol gr ¾ (0.05 Gm); *For use* as antispasmodic in chronic coughs, bronchitis and asthma; *Dosage:* injected slowly at 1–3 day intervals. **(National Drug)**

451. Sodium Salicylate—Ampules 5 cc; Boxes of 12, 25 and 100; 20 or 30 % solutions; *For use* as antirheumatic, in gout, arthritis, acute articular rheumatism;
Ampules 5 cc; Boxes of 12, assorted solutions of 20, 30 and 40 %;
Ampules 10 cc; Boxes of 12, 25 and 100; Containing gr 31 (2.0 Gm);
Ampule-vials 25 cc; Boxes of 1; 20, 30 or 40 % solutions; *For use* in varicose veins. **(National Drug)**

452. Sodium Salicylate and Iodide with Colchicine 1—Ampules 20 cc; Boxes of 6, 12, 25 and 100; Containing sodium salicylate gr 15½ (1.0 Gm), sodium iodide gr 15½ (1.0 Gm), colchicine gr 1/100 (0.0006 Gm); *For use* in arthritis, gout, sciatica and rheumatism, neuritis. Number 2—Half strength. **(National Drug)**

453. Sodium Thiosulphate—Ampules 10 cc; Boxes of 6, 12, 25 and 100; Containing gr 7½ (0.5 Gm); *For use* in arsenical, bismuth, lead, mercury and other metallic poisoning. *See Chap. I.* **(National Drug)**

454. Water (Triple Distilled)—Ampules 5, 10 and 20 cc; Boxes of 12, 25 and 100;
Ampule-vials 30 cc; Boxes of 6, 12, 25 and 100;
Ampule-vials 100 cc; Boxes of 6, 12 and 25; *For use* in preparing solutions for injection. **(National Drug)**

---

455. Adrenalin Chloride Solution (I.C.C.)—Ampules 1 cc; Boxes of 12; Adrenalin 1–100,000, may be given as saline intravenous infusion, in cases of shock; *Dosage:* 8–15 m as required. *See Chap. I.* **(Parke, Davis)**

456. Caffeine Sodio-Benzoate—Ampules 2 cc; Boxes of 12 and 100; Containing gr 7½ (0.5 Gm) in distilled water; *For use* in heart failure, cardiac dropsy, chronic nephritis, collapse, pneumonia of aged; *Dosage:* 1–2 cc as indicated. **(Parke, Davis)**

457. Calcium Chloride—Ampules 10 cc; Boxes of 6 and 25; Containing gr 15½ (1 Gm) in aqueous solution; *For use* for calcium supply; in paralysis agitans, tetany, epilepsy, chorea, tuberculosis; with parathyroid in varicose ulcer and chronic ulcerative diseases; seepage may cause sloughing; *Dosage:* 10 cc at 1–3 day intervals. **(Parke, Davis)**

458. Glucose (Dextrose U.S.P.)—Ampules 20 cc; Boxes of 6 and 25; Containing 10 Gm;
Ampules 50 cc; Boxes of 1, 6 and 25; Containing 25 Gm;
Ampules 100 cc; Boxes of 1, 6 and 25; Containing 50 Gm; Buffered; *For use* in metabolic carbohydrate deficiency, toxemia of pregnancy, chorea and eclampsia, postoperative shock, acidosis, hyperthyroidism, hypoglycemia from overdose of insulin; *Dosage:* ampule solution is diluted to twice its volume by addition of sterile distilled water. *See Chap. I.* **(Parke, Davis)**

459. Magnesium Sulphate—Ampules 10 cc; Boxes of 6 and 25; Containing 25 % solution; *For use* as antispasmodic in eclampsia and tetanus, as central nervous system depressant; *Dosage:* 5–10 cc, repeated hourly if necessary. **(Parke, Davis)**

460. Mercurosal—Ampules 0.1 Gm, 5 cc; Boxes of 12 and 100; Antiluetic; *Dosage:* 1 ampule twice a week. *See Chap. I.* **(Parke, Davis)**

461. Quinine Dihydrochloride—Ampules 10 cc; Boxes of 6 and 25; Containing gr 5 (0.3 Gm);
Ampules 20 cc; Boxes of 6 and 25; Containing gr 10 (0.65 Gm) in physiologic salt solution; *For use* in malarial fever, lobar pneumonia, as tonic in convalescence. **(Parke, Davis)**

462. Quinine Hydrochloride and Urethane—Ampules 2 cc; Boxes of 12 and 100; Containing quinine hydrochloride Gm 0.266, urethane 0.133 Gm, distilled water q.s.; *For use* in varicose veins; Detail dosage, contraindications, technique of administration supplied with each package. (Parke, Davis)

463. Sodium Cacodylate—Ampules 5 cc; Boxes of 6 and 25; Containing gr 3 (0.2 Gm) or gr 7 (0.45 Gm);
Ampules 10 cc; Boxes of 6 and 25; Containing gr 15½ (1 Gm); *For use* as tonic or alterative; *Dosage:* gr ¾ (0.05 Gm) to gr 15½ (1 Gm) for adults, children relatively smaller doses. (Parke, Davis)

464. Sodium Citrate—Ampules 50 cc; Boxes of 1 and 6; 2.5 % aqueous solution; *For use* in blood transfusions; *Dosage:* 1 ampule for prevention of coagulation of 500 cc of blood. (Parke, Davis)

465. Sodium Iodide—Ampules 10 cc; Boxes of 6 and 25; Containing gr 15½ (1 Gm); Ampules 20 cc; Boxes of 6 and 25; Containing gr 31 (2 Gm) in distilled water q.s.; *For use* in gonorrheal sequelae, asthma, simple goiter, scrofula, syphilitic gummata and arteriosclerosis; *Dosage:* 10–20 cc daily or on alternate days; in syphilitic lesions dose rapidly increased to tolerance. (Parke, Davis)

466. Sodium Iodide and Sodium Salicylate—Ampules 20 cc; Boxes of 6 and 25; Containing gr 15½ (1 Gm) each sodium iodide and sodium salicylate in distilled water q.s.; *For use* in acute and chronic arthritis, especially of luetic origin, bronchial asthma, lumbago, sciatica; *Dosage:* 10–20 cc at 2–4 day intervals as indicated. (Parke, Davis)

467. Sodium Salicylate—Ampules 10 cc; Boxes of 6 and 25; Containing gr 20 (1.3 Gm), distilled water q.s.; *For use* as antipyretic and analgesic in tonsillitis and arthritis of streptococcus origin; *Dosage:* gr 20 daily for 5 days, then alternate days. (Parke, Davis)

468. Sodium Salicylate and Iodide with Colchicine—Ampules 20 cc; Boxes of 6 and 25; Containing gr 15½ (1 Gm) each of sodium salicylate and sodium iodide, colchicine gr 1/100 (0.00065 Gm), distilled water q.s.;
Ampules 20 cc; Boxes of 6 and 25; Containing gr 31 (2 Gm) each of sodium salicylate and sodium iodide, colchicine gr 1/500 (0.00130 Gm), distilled water q.s.; *For use* as antirheumatic, in gout; *Dosage:* 10–20 cc at 2–4 day intervals. (Parke, Davis)

469. Sodium Thiosulphate—Ampules 10 cc; Boxes of 6 and 25; Containing gr 7½ (0.5 Gm), distilled water q.s.; *For use* in arsenical poisoning; in bismuth and mercurial poisoning doubtfully; *Dosage:* 0.3, 0.45, 0.60, 0.75 Gm on successive days, then 0.9, 1.2, 1.8 Gm on alternate days; may be repeated if indicated. *See Chap. I.* (Parke, Davis)

470. Tartar Emetic—Ampules 5 cc; Boxes of 6 and 25; Containing antimony and potassium tartrate gr ¾ (0.05 Gm), distilled water q.s.; *For use* in granuloma inguinale (tropical ulcer), Vincent's angina, chancroidal infections and complications; *Dosage:* 5 cc at 3–4 day intervals, or 2 cc initially and gradually increased to 10 cc. (Parke, Davis)

471. Uritone—Ampules 5 cc; Boxes of 6 and 25; Containing uritone gr 31 (2 Gm); distilled water q.s.; 40 % solution; *For use* in pyelitis, acute nephritis, spirochetosis; in anuria and dysuria; *Dosage:* 5 cc, may be given daily, continued as indicated. (Parke, Davis)

472. Water—Double Distilled—Ampules 5, 10 and 20 cc; Boxes of 6 and 25; *For use* in preparation of solutions for injection. (Parke, Davis)

---

473. Decholin Sodium—Ampules 10 cc; Boxes of 3 and 20; in 5 or 20 % solutions; Choleretic; *For use* and *dosage, see Chap. I.* (Riedel-de Haen)

473a. Aminophyllin—Ampule 10 cc; Boxes of 6; Containing theophyllin 75%, ethylenediamine 25%; each ampule gr 4 (0.24 Gm); Cardiotonic, vasodilator of coronaries. *Dosage:* 1–3 ampules daily. *See Chap. I.* (Pharmedic)

474. Pernoston—Ampules 1.1 cc; 2.2 cc; Boxes of 10;
Ampules 2.2 cc; Boxes of 50; Each cubic centimeter containing 0.1 Gm (1½ gr); Hypnotic; *For use* in psychiatry, surgery and obstetrics; *see Chap. I.* **(Riedel-de Haen)**

---

475. Glucose (Dextrose C.P.)—Ampules 20–50 cc; Boxes of 1, 6, 12, 25 and 100; 50% Solution; *For use* in toxemias of pregnancy, eclampsia, also varicose veins. *See Chap. I.* **(Rorer)**

475a. Methylene Blue—Ampule 50 cc; Packages of 1 and 6; *For use* in carbon monoxide and cyanide poisoning. *See Chap. I.* **(Rorer)**

476. Sodium Iodide—Ampules 10 cc; Boxes of 6 and 12; Containing gr 15 (0.972 Gm); *For use* in bronchial asthma, adenitis, arthritis, orchitis and gonorrheal epididymitis; *Dosage:* 5–10 cc, slowly injected. **(Rorer)**

477. Water—Double Distilled—Ampules 5, 10, 20 and 50 cc; Boxes of 6, 12 and 100; *For use* in preparing solutions for injection. **(Rorer)**

---

478. Calglucon—Ampules 10 cc; Boxes of 5, 20 and 100; Calcium gluconate; 10% solution;
Ampules 5 cc; Boxes of 10 and 150; 10% solution; *Dosage:* 2–10 cc every 1–3 days. *See Chap. I.* **(Sandoz)**

479. Scillaren B—Ampules 1 cc; Boxes of 6, 12 and 50; Containing total glucosidal principles of squills gr 1/130 (0.0005 Gm); Cardiodiuretic; *Dosage:* 1 cc daily. *See Chap. I.* **(Sandoz)**

---

480. Neo-Iopax—Ampules 20 cc; Boxes of 1; Containing Gm 15 of substance dissolved in 20 cc of 10% solution of invert sugar; Radiopaque medium for the G. U. tract; *Dosage:* 1 ampule; radiography in 20–30 min. *See Chap. I.* **(Schering)**

---

481. Aminophyllin—Ampules 10 cc; Boxes of 6, 25 and 100; Containing theophyllin 75%, ethylenediamine 25%; each ampule gr 4 (0.24 Gm); Cardiotonic, vasodilator of coronaries; *Dosage:* 1–3 ampules daily. *See Chap. I.* **(Searle)**

482. Caffeine Sodium Benzoate—Ampules 2 cc; Boxes of 12, 25 and 100; Containing gr 7½ (0.5 Gm); Cerebral, cardiac stimulant and diuretic. **(Searle)**

483. Calcium Chloride—5 cc; Boxes of 6, 25 and 100; Containing 5% Solution; Calcium therapy; *For use* in tetany. **(Searle)**

484. Calcium Chloride—Ampules 10 cc; Boxes of 6, 25 and 100; Containing gr 15½ (1.0 Gm); 10% Solution. *For use* in tetany. **(Searle)**

485. Calcium Gluconate—Ampules 10 cc; Boxes of 6, 25 and 100; 10% Solution; *For use* in calcium therapy; effective in tetany, spasmophilia, dermatologic conditions, eclampsia. *See Chap. I.* **(Searle)**

486. Dextrose—Ampules 20 and 50 cc; Boxes of 6, 25 and 100; Also 50 cc, Box of 1; 20 cc represents 10 Gm d-Glucose U.S.P. buffered with 0.4 Gm sodium lactate; 50 cc represents 25.0 Gm d-Glucose U.S.P. buffered with 1.0 Gm sodium lactate. *See Chap. I.* **(Searle)**

487. Dextrose and Sodium Chloride Stable Solution—Ampules 20 cc; Boxes of 6, 25 and 100; Containing equal parts of 50% solution dextrose, 30% sodium chloride and benzyl alcohol for local anesthetic effect; *For use* in varicose veins. **(Searle)**

488. Gold Sodium Thiosulphate—Ampules 1 cc; Boxes of 12 and 25; Containing 10 mg of the salt;
Ampules 2 cc; Boxes of 6, 25; Containing 25 mg;
Ampules 5 cc; Boxes of 6, 25; Containing 50 mg of the salt; solution contains gold 37%; *For use* in inhibiting growth of tubercle bacillus; *see Chap. I.* **(Searle)**

489. Iron, Arsenic and Phosphorus—Ampules 5 cc; Boxes of 6, 25 and 100; Containing sodium glycerophosphate gr 2 (0.13 Gm), sodium cacodylate gr 1¼ (0.081 Gm), iron cacodylate gr ⅔ (0.043 Gm); *For use* as hematinic. **(Searle)**

490. **Iron Cacodylate**—Ampules 5 cc; Boxes of 6, 25 and 100; Containing gr 1 (0.065 Gm); *For use* as hematinic. (Searle)

491. **Arsphenamine**—Ampules of 0.1, 0.2, 0.3, 0.4 Gm; Arsenical; *For use* as antisyphilitic. *See Chap. I.* (Searle)

492. **Neoarsphenamine**—Ampules of 0.15, 0.3, 0.45, 0.6 Gm; Arsenical; *For use* as antisyphilitic. *See Chap. I.* (Searle)

493. **Magnesium Sulphate**—Ampules 20 cc; Boxes of 6, 25 and 100; 10% solution; *For use* in controlling convulsions of eclampsia. (Searle)

494. **Mercurochrome 220**—Ampules 10 and 20 cc; Boxes of 6, 25 and 100; 1% solution stabilized with 0.18% of ammonium hydroxide; *For use* as systemic antiseptic in sepsis and septicemia; *Dosage:* 0.4% solution, 5 mg per kilogram of body weight. *See Chap. I.* (Searle)

495. **Mercury Oxycyanide**—Ampules 5 cc; Boxes of 6, 25 and 100; Containing gr ⅙ (0.011 Gm); Antiluetic. *See Chap. I.* (Searle)

496. **Methenamine**—Ampules 5 cc; Boxes of 6, 25 and 100; Containing gr 15½ (1.0 Gm) or gr 31 (2.0 Gm); Urinary antiseptic; its use to be proceeded by acidifier, as acid sodium phosphate. (Searle)

497. **Methenamine and Sodium Iodide**—Ampules 20 cc; Boxes of 6, 25 and 100; Containing methenamine gr 23 (1.5 Gm) and sodium iodide gr 15½ (1.0 Gm); *For use* in gonorrheal infections, acute and chronic cystitis, epididymitis, orchitis, pyelitis and toxemias. (Searle)

498. **Proteolac**—Ampules 1 and 2 cc; Boxes of 12, 25 and 100;
Ampules 5 and 10 cc; Boxes of 6, 25 and 100; Non-specific milk protein therapy agent; *Dosage:* 0.5–10 cc every 2–5 days. *See Chap. I.* (Searle)

499. **Quinine and Urethane**—Ampules 2 cc; Boxes of 12, 25 and 100; Containing quinine hydrochloride gr 4 (0.266 Gm) and urethane gr 2 (0.133 Gm); *For use* in varicose veins and hemorrhoids. *See Chap. II.* (Searle)

500. **Quinine Dihydrochloride**—Ampules 5 and 20 cc; Boxes of 6, 25 and 100; *For use* as anti-antimalarial, antipyretic and tonic; Containing either gr 15½ (1.0 Gm) in 5 cc; or gr 10 (0.648 Gm). (Searle)

501. **Sodium Cacodylate**—Ampules 5 cc; Boxes of 6, 25 and 100; Containing gr 7½ (0.50 Gm), or gr 15½ (1.0 Gm); *For use* as hematinic, in pellagra, malarial cachexia, neurasthenia, psoriasis. (Searle)

502. **Sodium Iodide**—Ampules 10 cc; Boxes of 6, 25 and 100; Containing gr 15½ (1.0 Gm);
Ampules 10 cc; Boxes of 6, 25 and 100; Containing gr 31 (2.0 Gm);
Ampules 20 cc; Boxes of 6, 25 and 100; Containing gr 31 (2.0 Gm); *For use* in arteriosclerosis, gonorrheal sequelae, asthma, simple goitre. (Searle)

503. **Sodium Iodide, Creosote and Guaiacol**—Ampules 20 cc; Boxes of 6, 25 and 100; Containing sodium iodide gr 31 (2.0 Gm); creosote gr ⅝ (0.04 Gm), guaiacol gr ⅝ (0.04 Gm); Expectorant, especially bronchial. (Searle)

504. **Sodium Iodide with Guaiacol**—Ampules 20 cc; Boxes of 6, 25 and 100; Containing sodium iodide gr 31, (2.0 Gm), guaiacol gr ¾ (0.048 Gm); *For use* as above. (Searle)

505. **Sodium Morrhuate 5% with Benzyl Alcohol**—Ampules 5 cc; Boxes of 6, 25 and 100; For varicose vein therapy; *Dosage:* 0.5–2 cc per vein, total at 1 sitting not to exceed 5 cc; given at 2–7 day intervals. *See Chap. I.* (Searle)

506. **Sodium Salicylate**—Ampules 5 cc; Boxes of 6, 25 and 100; Containing gr 15½ (1.0 Gm);
Ampules 5 cc; Boxes of 6, 25 and 100; Containing gr 31 (2.0 Gm);
Ampules 10 cc; Boxes of 6, 25 and 100; Containing gr 31 (2.0 Gm); *For use* as antirheumatic; in sepsis and pneumonia; as analgesic. (Searle)

507. **Sodium Salicylate and Iodide**—Ampules 20 cc; Boxes of 6, 25 and 100; Containing gr 15½ (1.0 Gm) each; *For use* in acute and chronic arthritis, especially with luetic history.
Ampules 20 cc; Boxes of 6, 25 and 100; Containing gr 31 (2.0 Gm). (Searle)

508. Sodium Salicylate and Iodide with Colchicine—Ampules 20 cc; Boxes of 6, 25 and 100; Containing gr 15½ (1.0 Gm) or gr 31 (2.0 Gm) each of the sodium salts and colchicine gr 1/100; *For use* in gout, elimination of urates and uric acid. (Searle)

509. Sodium Salicylate, Iodide and Cacodylate—Ampules 20 cc; Boxes of 6, 25 and 100; Containing sodium salicylate gr 25 (1.62 Gm), sodium iodide gr 15 (1.0 Gm), sodium cacodylate gr 3 (0.194 Gm). (Searle)

510. Sodium Salicylate, Iodide and Cacodylate with Colchicine—Ampules 20 cc; Boxes of 6, 25 and 100; Containing sodium salicylate gr 31 (2.0 Gm), sodium iodide gr 31 (2.0 Gm), sodium cacodylate gr 15 (0.324 Gm), Colchicine gr 1/100 (0.00065 Gm). (Searle)

511. Sodium Thiosulphate—Ampules 5 cc; Boxes of 6, 25 and 100; Containing gr 7½ (0.50 Gm);
Ampules 10 cc; Boxes of 6, 25 and 100; Containing gr 15½ (1.0 Gm); *For use* in mercurial, arsenical, bismuth and other metallic poisoning. *See Chap. I.* (Searle)

512. Sterile Double Distilled Water—Ampules 5, 10 and 20 cc; Boxes of 6, 25 and 100; *For use* in preparing arsenicals and other preparations for injection. (Searle)

513. Tartar Emetic—Ampules 10 cc; Boxes of 6, 25 and 100; 1% solution; Containing antimony potassium tartrate U.S.P. gr 1⅗ (0.1 Gm); *For use* in tropical diseases as bilharziasis, trypanosomiasis, kala-azar. (Searle)

---

514. Adrin Solution—Ampules 1 cc; Boxes of 6 and 100; An epinephrine hydrochloride solution 1:1,000; *For use* as vasoconstrictor; *Dosage:* 0.5–1 cc as necessary. *See Chap. I.* (Sharp and Dohme)

515. Calcium Chloride—Ampules 10 cc; Boxes of 6; Containing 1.0 Gm in 10% solution;
Ampule-vials 10 cc; Boxes of 6; Containing 1.0 Gm in 10% solution; *For use* in increasing coagulability of blood, in stabilizing calcium metabolism. (Sharp and Dohme)

516. Digitos—Ampules of 1 and 5 cc; Boxes of 4 and 12 respectively; Digitalis therapy; *Dosage:* 5–60 m every 24–48 hr. *See Chap. I.* (Sharp and Dohme)

517. Glucose (Dextrose U.S.P.)—Ampules 20, 50 and 100 cc; Boxes of 6; Containing 50% solution; the 50 and 100 cc ampules have additional ampules of buffer solution which if added to 100 cc of glucose solution, produces same hydrogen-ion concentration as blood. *See Chap. I.* (Sharp and Dohme)

518. Hexamethylenamine—Ampules 5 cc; Boxes of 6; Containing gr 31 (2 Gm); *For use* as urinary tract antiseptic. (Sharp and Dohme)

519. Iron, Arsenic and Phosphorus—Ampules 5 cc; Boxes of 6; Containing iron cacodylate gr 1 (0.065 Gm), sodium glycerophosphate gr 2 (0.125 Gm), in sterile solution; *For use* as hematinic and tonic. (Sharp and Dohme)

520. Iron Cacodylate—Ampules 2 cc; Boxes of 12; Containing gr ½ (0.032 Gm);
Ampules 5 cc; Boxes of 12; Containing gr 1 (0.065 Gm); *For use* as hematinic, tonic and alterative. (Sharp and Dohme)

521. Quinine Dihydrochloride—Ampules 10 cc; Boxes of 6; Containing gr 5 (0.324 Gm), or gr 10 (0.65 Gm);
Ampules 5 cc; Boxes of 6; Containing gr 7½ (0.5 Gm);
Ampules 20 cc; Boxes of 6; Containing gr 10 (0.65 Gm); *For use* in quinine therapy of malarial toxemia. (Sharp and Dohme)

522. Ringer's Solution, Concentrated—Ampule-vials 25 cc; Boxes of 1; Contents of 1 ampule-vial mixed with distilled water 1 liter will make 1,000 cc Ringer's solution. (Sharp and Dohme)

523. Sodium Cacodylate—Ampules 5 cc; Boxes of 6; Containing gr 3 (0.2 Gm), gr 5 (0.324), gr 7½ (0.5 Gm);
Ampule-vials 5 cc; Boxes of 6; Containing gr 7½ (0.5 Gm);
Ampules 10 cc; Boxes of 6; Containing gr 15½ (1.0 Gm);

Ampule-vials 10 cc; Boxes of 6; Containing gr 15½ (1.0 Gm); *For use* in syphilitic conditions, anemias, psoriasis and pellagra. **(Sharp and Dohme)**

524. Sodium Citrate—Ampules 50 cc; Boxes of 6; Containing 2½% solution; *For use* in blood transfusions. **(Sharp and Dohme)**

525. Sodium Iodide—Ampules 10 cc; Boxes of 6; Containing gr 15½ (1.0 Gm);
Ampule-vials 10 cc; Boxes of 6; Containing gr 15½ (1.0 Gm);
Ampules 20 cc; Boxes of 6; Containing gr 31 (2.0 Gm);
Ampule-vials 20 cc; Boxes of 6; Containing gr 31 (2.0 Gm). **(Sharp and Dohme)**

526. Sodium Iodide and Sodium Salicylate—Ampules and Ampule-vials 20 cc; Boxes of 6; Containing gr 15½ (1.0 Gm) each. **(Sharp and Dohme)**

527. Sodium Salicylate—Ampules 5 cc; Boxes of 6; Containing gr 15½ (1.0 Gm);
Ampules 10 cc; Boxes of 6; Containing gr 20 (1.3 Gm);
Ampule-vials 10 cc; Boxes of 6; Containing gr 20 (1.3 Gm);
Ampules 20 cc; Boxes of 6; Containing gr 30 (1.944 Gm);
Ampule-vials 20 cc; Boxes of 6; Containing gr 30 (1.944 Gm); *For use* as antirheumatic. **(Sharp and Dohme)**

528. Sodium Salicylate and Iodide with Colchicine—Ampules 20 cc; Containing sodium salicylate and sodium iodide gr 15 (1.0 Gm) each, colchicine gr 1/100 (0.0006 Gm);
Ampule-vials 20 cc; Contents as above. **(Sharp and Dohme)**

529. Sodium Thiosulphate—Ampules 10 cc; Boxes of 6; Containing gr 15 (1 Gm);
Ampule-vials 10 cc; Boxes of 6; Containing gr 15 (1 Gm); *For use* in arsenic, mercury and other metallic poisoning. *See Chap. I.* **(Sharp and Dohme)**

530. Water, Double Distilled, Sterilized—Ampules 5, 10, 20 and 50 cc; Boxes of 6; *For use* in preparing solutions for injection. **(Sharp and Dohme)**

531. Water, Triple Distilled, Sterilized—Ampules 5 cc; Boxes of 6; *For use* as above. **(Sharp and Dohme)**

---

532. Calcium Chloride—Ampules 5 and 10 cc; Boxes of 6, 25 and 100; Solutions of 5 or 10%; *For use* in paralysis agitans, tetany, epilepsy, chorea. **(Sherman)**

533. Dextrose and Sodium Chloride—Ampules 5 cc and 10 cc; Boxes of 6 and 25 and 100; Containing equal parts of dextrose C.P. 50% and sodium chloride C.P. 30%; *For use* in treating varicose veins. **(Sherman)**

534. Double Distilled Water—Ampules 5, 10, 20, 50 and 100 cc; Boxes of 6, 25 and 100. **(Sherman)**

535. Glucose—Ampules 20 and 50 cc; Boxes of 6, 25 and 100. *See Chap. I.* **(Sherman)**

536. Hexamethylenamine—Ampules 5 cc; Boxes of 6, 25 and 100; Containing gr 31 (2.0 Gm); *For use* in urinary infections, liver disturbances, acute nephritis, septicemia, anuria, dysuria. **(Sherman)**

537. Hexamethylenamine and Sodium Iodide—Ampules 10 cc; Boxes of 6, 25 and 100; Containing hexamethylenamine gr 12 (0.77 Gm) and sodium iodide gr 7½ (0.49 Gm); *For use* in preventing kidney involvement in general septic conditions. **(Sherman)**

538. Hexamethylenamine and Sodium Iodide—Ampules 20 cc; Boxes of 6, 25 and 100; Containing hexamethylenamine gr 24 (1.54 Gm) and sodium iodide gr 15½ (1.0 Gm); *For use* in preventing kidney involvement in general septic conditions. **(Sherman)**

539. Iron and Arsenic—Ampules 5 cc; Boxes of 6, 25 and 100; Containing iron cacodylate gr 1 (0.06 Gm); *For use* in anemia, lymphadenitis, leukemia, as general tonic. **(Sherman)**

540. Iron Arsenic and Phosphorus—Ampules 5 cc; Boxes of 6, 25 and 100; Containing iron cacodylate gr 1 (0.6 Gm) and sodium glycerophosphate gr 2 (0.13 Gm); *For use* in anemia, neurasthenia, rachitis, osteomalacia, convalescence. **(Sherman)**

541. **Mercury Oxycyanide**—Ampules 5 cc; Boxes of 6, 25 and 100; Containing gr 1/8 (0.008 Gm) or gr 1/6 (0.012 Gm), or gr 1/4 (0.016 Gm); Antisyphilitic. *See Chap. I.* **(Sherman)**

542. **Sodium Cacodylate**—Ampules 5 cc; Boxes of 6, 25 and 100; Containing gr 7, (0.45 Gm) or gr 15½ (1.0 Gm); *For use* in anemia, malaria, non-parasitic chronic skin diseases. **(Sherman)**

543. **Sodium Iodide**—Ampules 10 cc; Boxes of 6, 25 and 100; Containing gr 15½ (1.0 Gm) or gr 31 (2.0 Gm); *For use* in bronchial asthma, simple goitre, glandular hypertrophy, arteriosclerosis. **(Sherman)**

544. **Sodium Iodide**—Ampules 20 cc; Boxes of 6, 25 and 100; Containing gr 31 (2.0 Gm) *For use* as above. **(Sherman)**

545. **Sodium Salicylate**—Ampules 10 cc; Boxes of 6, 25 and 100; Containing gr 20 (1.3 Gm) or gr 31 (2.0 Gm); *For use* in acute rheumatism, gout, sciatica, chronic arthritis, streptococcus infections. **(Sherman)**

546. **Sodium Salicylate**—Ampules 20 cc; Boxes of 6, 25 and 100; Containing gr 31 (2.0 Gm); *For use* as above. **(Sherman)**

547. **Sodium Salicylate and Iodide**—Ampules 20 cc; Boxes of 6, 25 and 100; Containing sodium salicylate gr 15 (0.97 Gm), sodium iodide gr 15 (0.97 Gm); *For use* in chronic rheumatism with thickening of synovial membrane. **(Sherman)**

548. **Sodium Salicylate and Sodium Iodide with Colchicine**—Ampules 20 cc; Boxes of 6, 25 and 100; Containing sodium salicylate gr 15 (0.97 Gm), sodium iodide gr 15 (0.97 Gm), colchicine gr 1/100 (0.00065 Gm); *For use* in painful arthritis and gout. **(Sherman)**

549. **Sodium Thiosulphate**—Ampules 10 cc; Boxes of 6, 25 and 100; Containing gr 15½ (1.0 Gm); *For use* in arsenic, mercury, lead, bismuth, copper poisoning. *See Chap. I.* **(Sherman)**

---

550. **Arsphenamine**—Ampules of 0.1, 0.2, 0.3, 0.4, 0.5, 0.6 Gm; *For use* as antiluetic; *Dosage:* 0.3–0.4 Gm, diluted to 10 cc, every 5 days. *See Chap. I.* **(Squibb)**

551. **Neoarsphenamine**—Ampules of 0.15, 0.30, 0.45, 0.60, 0.75, 0.9, 3.0, 4.5 Gm; with 10 cc ampule of double distilled water; *For use* in primary and secondary syphilis; *Dosage:* 0.45–0.6 Gm diluted to 10 cc every 5 days. *See Chap. I.* **(Squibb)**

---

552. **Calcium Chloride**—Ampules 10 cc; Boxes of 6; Containing gr 15½ (1 Gm); *For use* in tetany, paralysis agitans, epilepsy, chorea, tuberculosis; *Dosage:* 5–10 cc at 2–3 day intervals, injected very slowly; sloughs subcutaneous tissue. **(Upjohn)**

553. **Dextrose**—See Glucose. **(Upjohn)**

554. **Glucose (Dextrose) U.S.P.**—Ampules 20 cc; Boxes of 6; Containing gr 155 (10 Gm); 50% solution.
Ampules 50 cc; Boxes of 6; Containing gr 386 (25 Gm); 50% solution.
Ampules 100 cc; Boxes of 6; Containing gr 772 (50 Gm); 50% solution with a buffer salt to prevent acidity development; *Dosage:* 50–100 cc of 50% solution, repeated one to three times daily as indicated; may be diluted with sterile double distilled water. *See Chap. I.* **(Upjohn)**

555. **Glucose and Sodium Chloride with Benzyl Alcohol**—Vials 30 cc; Rubber-capped; Containing per cc glucose (Dextrose U.S.P.) 0.25 Gm (25%), sodium chloride 0.15 Gm (15%), benzyl alcohol 0.015 Gm (1.5%) to lessen cramping sensation; *For use* in varicose veins. **(Upjohn)**

556. **Glycerophosphate Compound, ℞ A, Double Strength**—Ampules 5 cc; Boxes of 6; Containing sodium glycerophosphate gr 3 (0.194 Gm), strychnine cacodylate gr 1/65 (0.001 Gm), iron cacodylate gr 1/3 (0.02 Gm) with chlorbutanol gr 1/12 (0.005 Gm) per cubic centimeter; *For use* as hematinic and tonic; *Dosage:* 5–10 cc at 1–2 day intervals. **(Upjohn)**

557. Hexamethylenetetramine (Methenamine) and Sodium Iodide—Ampules 20 cc; Boxes of 6; Containing gr 15½ (1 Gm) each drug; *For use* as urinary tract antiseptic; *Dosage:* 20 cc at 1 or 2 day intervals. (Upjohn)

558. Hexamethylenetetramine (Methenamine)—Ampules 10 cc; Boxes of 6; Containing gr 31 (2 Gm) per 10 cc; *For use* as above; *Dosage:* 5–10 cc at 1–2 day intervals. (Upjohn)

559. Iron Cacodylate—Ampules 2 and 5 cc; Boxes of 6 (5 cc) and 12 (2 cc); Containing gr 1 (0.065 Gm) per ampule; *For use* in anemias and dry scaly skin conditions; *Dosage:* small initial doses, repeated and increased as indicated. (Upjohn)

560. Quinine Dihydrochloride—Ampules 10 cc; Boxes of 6; Containing gr 5 (0.32 Gm) per 10 cc;
Ampules 20 cc; Boxes of 6; Containing gr 10 (0.65 Gm) per 20 cc; *For use* as antimalarial, in lobar pneumonia and as tonic in convalescence. (Upjohn)

561. Quinine Hydrochloride and Urethane—Ampules 2 cc; Boxes of 12; Containing quinine hydrochloride gr 4 (0.26 Gm), and urethane (ethyl carbamate) gr 2 (0.13 Gm) in distilled water; *For use* in varicose veins. *See Chap. II.* (Upjohn)

562. Sodium Cacodylate—Ampules 5 cc; Boxes of 6; Containing gr 7 (0.45 Gm);
Ampules 10 cc; Boxes of 6; Containing gr 15½ (1 Gm); *For use* as tonic or alterative action of arsenic; *Dosage:* gr 5 (0.3 Gm) at 3–5 day intervals. (Upjohn)

563. Sodium Iodide—Ampules 10 cc; Boxes of 6; Containing gr 15½ (1 Gm) per ampule;
Ampules 20 cc; Boxes of 6; Containing gr 31 (2 Gm) per ampule; *For use* in syphilitic gummata, arteriosclerosis, asthma and simple goiter; *Dosage:* 10–20 cc at 2–4 day intervals. (Upjohn)

564. Sodium Salicylate—Ampules 10 cc; Boxes of 6; Containing gr 15½ (1 Gm) per ampule;
Ampules 20 cc; Boxes of 6; Containing gr 31 (2 Gm) per ampule; *For use* as antirheumatic; *Dosage:* 10–20 cc daily for 3 or 4 days. (Upjohn)

565. Sodium Salicylate and Iodide—Ampules 20 cc; Boxes of 6; Containing gr 15½ (1 Gm) each; *For use* in arthritis, acute and chronic, particularly with luetic history *Dosage:* 10–20 cc daily for 3–4 days. (Upjohn)

566. Sodium Salicylate and Iodide with Colchicine 1—Ampules 20 cc; Boxes of 6; Containing sodium salicylate and sodium iodide gr 15½ (1 Gm) each, colchicine gr 1/100 (0.00065 Gm); *For use* as antirheumatic and in gout. (Upjohn)

567. Sodium Salicylate and Iodide with Colchicine 2—Ampules 20 cc; Boxes of 6; Containing sodium salicylate and sodium iodide gr 31 (2 Gm) each, colchicine gr 1/100 (0.00065 Gm); *For use* as above; *Dosage:* 10–20 cc at 1–3 day intervals. (Upjohn)

568. Sodium Thiosulphate—Ampules of 1 Gm; Boxes of 10; *For use* in arsenical, mercury and other metallic poisoning; *Dosage:* gr 7½–15½ (0.5–1 Gm) at intervals of 4 hr. to 1–2 days, as indicated; supplemented by oral administration of gr 15½ (1 Gm) in solution three times daily. *See Chap. I.* (Upjohn)

569. Water, Sterile Double Distilled—Ampules 5, 10 and 20 cc; Boxes of 6; *For use* in preparing solutions for injection. (Upjohn)

---

570. Arsphenamine-Hoechst—Ampules of 0.1, 0.2, 0.3, 0.4, 0.5, 0.6 Gm. (Winthrop)

571. Chaulmestrol—Ampules 1 and 3 cc; Boxes of 10; Leprosy remedy; *Dosage:* 0.5–6 cc weekly. *See Chap. I.* (Winthrop)

572. Cymarin—Ampules of gr 1/60 (0.001 Gm) solution; Boxes of 10; *For use* as cardiotonic and diuretic; *Dosage:* gr 1/120–1/60 daily. *See Chap. I.* (Winthrop)

573. Distilled Water—Ampules of 10 and 20 cc; Boxes of 5; *For use* in preparing solutions for injection. (Winthrop)

574. Gono-Yatren—Ampules 2.5 cc; Boxes of 6; Containing 50, 100, 150, 200, 300, 400 million gonococci; *For use* in gonorrheal therapy; *Dosage:* 0.1–1 cc every 2–4 days. *See Chap. VI.* (Winthrop)

575. **Homocamfin**—Ampules 1 cc; Boxes of 5; 1 % solution; Cardio-respiratory stimulant; *Dosage:* 0.3–1 cc, as necessary. *See Chap. I.* (Winthrop)

576. **Isopule**—See Neosalvarsan. (Winthrop)

577. **Neoarsphenamine-Hoechst**—Ampules of 0.15, 0.3, 0.45, 0.6, 0.75, 0.9 Gm; *See Chap. I.* (Winthrop)

578. **Neoarsphenamine-Hoechst in Iso-Double Ampule**—Ampule (half containing) 0.15, 0.3, 0.45, or 0.6 Gm of neoarsphenamine; (other half respectively) 3.5, 5, 7.5, 10 cc distilled water; *See Chap. I.* (Winthrop)

579. **Neosalvarsan**—Ampules of 0.15, 0.3, 0.45, 0.6, 0.75, 0.9, 1.5, 1.8, 3.0, 4.5 Gm; Brand of neoarsphenamine. *See Chap. I.* (Winthrop)

580. **Neosalvarsan with Distilled Water**—Ampules of 0.15, 0.3, 0.45, 0.6, 0.75, 0.9 Gm each with 10 cc ampule of sterile distilled water;
Ampules 0.15, 0.3, 0.45, 0.6, 0.75, 0.9 Gm; Boxes of 5 with 5 (10 cc) ampules sterile distilled water. *See Chap. I.* (Winthrop)

581. **Neosalvarsan in Isopule (Double Ampule)**—Ampule of 0.45 Gm neosalvarsan with 7.5 cc water;
Ampule of 0.6 Gm neosalvarsan with 10 cc water. *See Chap. I.* (Winthrop)

582. **Neoskiodan**—Ampules of 20 cc; Containing gr 7; *For use* in urography; *Dosage:* 1 ampule; radiography in 30 min.; *See Chap. I.* (Winthrop)

583. **Novasurol**—Ampules 1.2 cc; Boxes of 5; Containing 10 % neutral sterile solution; *For use* as powerful diuretic; *Dosage:* 1–2 cc once or twice weekly. *See Chap. I.* (Winthrop)

584. **Salvarsan**—Ampules of 0.1, 0.2, 0.3, 0.4, 0.5, 0.6, 1.0, 1.2, 3.0, 4.0 Gm; Brand of arsphenamine. *See Chap. I.* (Winthrop)

585. **Salvarsan Glucose Solution**—Ampules 3 cc; Boxes of 10; Containing 5 % salvarsan base. *See Chap. I.* (Winthrop)

586. **Salyrgan**—Ampules of 1 cc; Boxes of 5;
Ampules of 2 cc; Boxes of 10; *For use* as diuretic; *Dosage:* 1 ampule twice weekly. *See Chap. I.* (Winthrop)

587. **Sodium Thiosulphate**—See Sulfactol. (Winthrop)

588. **Sulfactol**—Ampules of 0.6 and 1.0 Gm; Boxes of 10; Containing sterile crystals; Ampules of 1.0 Gm; Boxes of 5 with 5 ampules (10 cc) of distilled water. *See Chap. I.* (Winthrop)

589. **Yatren-Casein (Strong)**—Ampules 1 cc; Boxes in 6; *For use* in foreign protein therapy. *See Chap. I.* (Winthrop)

590. **Yatren-Casein (Weak)**—Ampules 1 cc; Boxes of 6; *For use* in foreign protein therapy; *Dosage:* 1 cc every 3 days. *See Chap. I.* (Winthrop)

---

591. **Calcium Chloride**—Ampules 10 cc; Boxes of 6 and 25; Containing calcium chloride, anhydrous, gr 15½ (1 Gm) in distilled water; is equivalent to calcium chloride crystals 2 Gm; *For use* in calcium deficiency, anaphylaxis, asthma, hay fever, tetany, tuberculosis, hemoptysis, epididymitis, paralysis agitans. (Wyeth)

592. **Glucose (Dextrose U.S.P.)**—Ampules 50 cc; Boxes of 1, 6 and 25; Containing 50 % solution; *For use* in metabolic disturbances, in toxemias of pregnancy, chorea, eclampsia, acidosis of starvation, post operative shock, insulin overdosage, diluted with equal amount distilled sterile water;
Ampule undiluted—for varicose vein injection. *See Chap. I.* (Wyeth)

593. **Quinine Hydrochloride and Urethane**—Ampules 2 cc; Boxes of 12; Containing quinine hydrochloride gr 4 (0.266 Gm), urethane gr 2 (0.133 Gm), distilled water q.s.; *For use* in varicose veins and ulcers; *Dosage:* 1 cc in 1 varix or pocket; not more than 6 or 7 injections at a time. *See Chap. II.* (Wyeth)

594. **Sodium Citrate**—Ampules 50 cc; Boxes of 1 and 6; Containing 2½ % solution; *For use* in blood transfusions to prevent coagulation—1 ampule prevents coagulation of 500 cc blood. (Wyeth)

595. Phenolsulphonphthalein—Ampules 1 cc; Boxes of 12; Containing monosodium salt gr 1/10 (0.006 Gm) in distilled water; *For use* in testing renal function. *See Chap. I.* (Wyeth)

596. Sterile Water, Double Distilled—Ampules 10 and 20 cc; Boxes of 6 and 25. (Wyeth)

597. Sterile Water, Triple Distilled—Ampules 5 cc; Boxes of 6 and 25. (Wyeth)

---

598. Cacodylates Glycerophosphate Compound—Ampules 5 cc; Boxes of 6, 25 and 100; Containing iron cacodylate gr ½ (0.032 Gm), sodium cacodylate gr 5 (0.324 Gm), sodium glycerophosphate gr 1½ (0.097 Gm) in distilled water; *For use* as hematinic and tonic; *Dosage:* 2–5 cc, injected slowly, every 3 days. (Zemmer)

599. Calcium Chloride—Ampules 5 cc; Boxes of 6, 25 and 100; 5% solution in distilled water;
Ampules 10 cc; Boxes of 6, 25 and 100; 10% solution in distilled water; *For use* in calcium therapy; *Dosage:* 2–10 cc, two to three times weekly. (Zemmer)

600. Colchicine Sal-Iodide Compound—Ampules 20 cc; Boxes of 6, 25 and 100; Containing gr 15½ each sodium salicylate and sodium iodide, gr 1/100 (0.0006 Gm) colchicine, in distilled water; *For use* as antirheumatic; *Dosage:* ½–1 ampule daily until relieved, then 1 ampule two to three times weekly. (Zemmer)

601. Creohex—Ampules 5 cc; Boxes of 3, 6 and 12 complete treatments; Containing creosote solution gr 1.60, sodium salicylate gr 1.28, iron phosphate gr 1.28, hexamine gr 1/28 in normal saline solution; *For use* in pulmonary infections; *Dosage:* 3–5 cc as indicated—Solution A is drawn into syringe then injected into Solution B and desired amount withdrawn for use. (Zemmer)

602. Dextrose (Glucose)—Ampules 10 and 50 cc; Boxes of 6, 25 and 100; 50% solution; *For use* in toxemias of pregnancy, acidosis and shock. *See Chap. I.* (Zemmer)

603. Hexamethylenamine—Ampules 5 cc; Boxes of 6, 25 and 100; Containing gr 15½ (1 Gm) or gr 21 (1.4 Gm) or gr 31 (2.0 Gm) in normal saline solution; *For use* as genitourinary antiseptic; urine to be kept acid; *Dosage:* 1 ampule every 2–3 days. (Zemmer)

604. Hexa-Sal—Ampules 10 cc; Boxes of 6, 25 and 100; Containing hexamethylenamine gr 15½ (1.0 Gm), sodium salicylate gr 15½ (1.0 Gm), in distilled water; *For use* as urinary antiseptic; *Dosage:* 5–10 cc every 2 or 3 days. (Zemmer)

605. Intravenous Cresote Compound—See Creohex. (Zemmer)

606. Iodo-Salicylate Compound—Ampules 10 and 20 cc; Boxes of 6, 25 and 100; Containing sodium salicylate and sodium iodide gr 15½ (1.0 Gm) each in normal saline solution; *For use* in glandular disturbances, rheumatism, as analgesic and antipyretic; *Dosage:* ½–1 ampule every 2–4 days. (Zemmer)

607. Iron Cacodylate—Ampules 5 cc; Boxes of 6, 25 and 100; Containing gr 1 (0.065 Gm) in normal saline; *For use* as hematinic; *Dosage:* ½–1 ampule every 2–3 days. (Zemmer)

608. Magnesium Sulphate—Ampules 20 cc; Boxes of 6, 25 and 100; Containing 10% solution; *For use* in controlling convulsions of eclampsia. (Zemmer)

609. Mercurochrome—Ampules 10 and 20 cc; Boxes of 6, 25 and 100; Containing 1% solution; *For use* in septicemia, pyemia, puerperal infection, furunculosis, carbuncle and inaccessible abscesses. *See Chap. I.* (Zemmer)

610. Mercury Oxycyanide—Ampules 5 cc; Boxes of 6, 25 and 100; Containing gr ⅛ (0.00810 Gm) in distilled water; *For use* in syphilitic conditions and glandular enlargement. *See Chap. I.* (Zemmer)

611. Pituitary Extract—Ampules ½ and 1 cc; Boxes of 6, 25 and 100; *Dosage:* ½ or 1 cc intramuscularly, in severe instances—intravenously; another injection may follow after 30 min. *See Chap. I.* (Zemmer)

612. Quinine Dihydrochloride—Ampules 10 cc; Boxes of 6, 25 and 100; Containing gr 7½ (0.05 Gm); *For use* in malaria and as antiperiodic, antipyretic and tonic. (Zemmer)

613. Sodium Cacodylate—Ampules 5 cc; Boxes of 6, 25 and 100; Containing gr 7 (0.452 Gm), or gr 15 (1.0 Gm);
Ampules 10 cc; Boxes of 6, 25 and 100; Containing gr 31 (2.0 Gm); Arsenic therapy. (Zemmer)

614. Sodium Cacodylate Compound—Ampules 5 cc; Boxes of 6, 25 and 100; Containing sodium cacodylate gr 10 (0.65 Gm), red mercury iodide gr 1/10 (0.0065 Gm), sodium iodide gr ½ (0.032 Gm) in normal saline solution; *For use* as antisyphilitic. (Zemmer)

615. Sodium Iodide—Ampules 10 cc; Boxes of 6, 25 and 100; Containing gr 15½ (1.0 Gm), or gr 31 (2.0 Gm);
Ampules 20 cc; Boxes of 6, 25 and 100; Containing gr 31 (2.0 Gm); *For use* in asthma, bronchitis, pneumonia, acute and chronic nephritis, syphilis, goiter, arthritis; *Dosage:* ½–1 ampule every 2–6 days, as indicated. (Zemmer)

616. Sodium Salicylate—Ampules 5 cc; Boxes of 6, 25 and 100; Containing gr 15½ (1.0 Gm);
Ampules 10 cc; Boxes of 6, 25 and 100; Containing gr 31 (2.0 Gm); in distilled water; *For use* as antirheumatic; *Dosage:* ½–1 ampule repeated in 3–4 hr. as indicated. (Zemmer)

617. Sodium Salicylate and Iodide—See iodo-salicylate compound. (Zemmer)

618. Sodium Salicylate and Iodide Compound with Colchicine—See colchicine saliodide compound. (Zemmer)

619. Sterile Double Distilled Water—Ampules 5, 10 and 20 cc; Boxes of 6, 25 and 100; *For use* in making solutions for injections. (Zemmer)

Part II

Intramuscular and Subcutaneous Therapy

Advantages: *Intramuscular* injections are used particularly in introducing metallic and oily solutions; they are more rapidly absorbed than subcutaneous, though less readily than intravenous. Site of injection: for heavy and oily solutions the buttocks, alternated at each injection, are used; for light aqueous liquids—the deltoid region may be employed.

Drugs *subcutaneously* introduced are less rapidly absorbed than intramuscular or intravenous; otherwise the advantages are the same. Only watery solutions are here to be used; any site where skin may be lifted from underlying tissue may be utilized for the injection; sterilization and technic—as for intramuscular method.

Technic: Needles—non-breakable, stainless, 1½–1¾ gauge, 1½–2 in. long. Medication is warmed previous to filling syringe, needle is quickly introduced with a thrust, medicament injected, site lightly massaged, antiseptic applied with collodion dressing where necessary. Heavy oily medication is best drawn up from ampule with one needle and the injection made with another; pain caused by the hypodermic procedure may be relieved by hot applications.

For the convenience of the clinician and to facilitate the ready choice of a hypodermic drug for a particular purpose, the 933 Intramuscular and Subcutaneous Ampules in 1,478 forms here to be described are presented in groups, classified in accordance with their therapeutic function:

Group 1. Amebacides—Ampules 57, 107, 138, 414, 449, 563, 779, 915.

Group 2. Analgesics—Ampules 128, 200, 203, 276, 278, 455, 457, 540, 931, 932, 933.

Group 3. Antiluetics—Ampules 1, 2, 3, 16, 17, 18, 19, 20, 21, 27, 28, 29, 33, 39, 51, 52, 73, 74, 75, 76, 77, 78, 79, 118, 119, 120, 121, 127, 131, 134, 146, 171, 184, 185, 225, 255, 277, 283, 288, 322, 323, 324, 325, 342, 347, 352, 353, 354, 355, 356, 402, 403, 435, 436, 437, 438, 458, 459, 469, 474, 476, 480, 486, 487, 488, 523, 535, 536, 537, 538, 542, 546, 546a, 547, 550, 557, 580, 581, 582, 583, 595, 610, 629, 630, 631, 649, 679, 681, 682, 683, 684, 701, 709, 738, 752, 766, 770, 792, 793, 794, 795, 806, 823, 826, 827, 829, 837, 838, 851, 852, 853, 854, 876, 878, 888, 902, 911, 924, 945, 947, 948, 949.

Group 4. Antiseptics—Ampules 227, 392, 422, 452, 729, 791, 907, 953.

Group 5. Antispasmodics—Ampules 36, 48, 49, 128, 143, 152, 210, 228, 311, 345, 609, 713, 732.

Group 6. Aphrodisiacs—Ampules 169, 391, 506, 507, 508, 509, 510, 705.

Group 7. Arterial Dilators—Ampules 34, 275, 398, 706, 885.

Group 8. Bromine Preparations—Ampule 642.

Group 9. Calcium Therapy Agents—Ampules 54, 232, 233, 238, 239, 246, 257a, 313, 405, 559, 560, 733, 740, 772, 773, 774.

Group 10. Cancer Palliatives—Ampule 229.

Group 11. Chaulmoogra Derivatives—Ampules 409, 864.

Group 12. Creosote Products—Ampules 163, 164.

Group 13. Dextrose Preparations—Ampule 158.

Group 14. Diagnostic Agents—Ampules 124, 187, 284, 351, 380, 470, 502, 671, 708, 726, 798, 867, 918, 926.

Group 15. Detoxicants—Ampules 129, 196.

Group 16. Digitalis Preparations—Ampules 137, 204, 213, 280, 412, 655, 707, 777, 778.

Group 17. Distilled Waters—Ampules 97, 197, 198, 413, 765.

Group 18. Diuretics—Ampules 341, 548, 576, 737, 865, 880, 887.

Group 19. Endocrine Homostimulants—Ampules 477, 505.

Group 20. Ephedrine Preparations—Ampules 58, 59, 108, 139, 176, 361, 415, 416, 417, 513, 564, 615, 652, 667, 780, 842, 916, 937.

Group 21. Ergot Preparations—Ampules 142, 316, 362, 565, 566, 616, 668, 734, 781.

Group 22. General Anesthetics—Ampule 410.

Group 23. Gold Preparations—Ampules 35, 744, 906.

Group 24. Gonocidal Preparations—Ampules 31, 227, 228, 243, 254, 263, 363 "G," 396, 531, 641, 695, 761, 804, 866.

Group 25. Hematinics—Ampules 8, 10, 11, 12, 61, 62, 63, 64, 65, 66, 67, 68, 69, 70, 71, 93, 94, 95, 96, 103, 110, 111, 112, 113, 130, 145, 153, 173, 179, 180, 181, 182, 191, 192, 193, 215, 223, 224, 236, 240, 241, 242, 247, 248, 249, 250, 251, 252, 253, 259, 260, 261, 262, 269, 270, 271, 272, 281, 286, 317, 318, 319, 320, 321, 334, 335, 359, 364, 365, 366, 367, 368, 369, 387, 393, 418, 419, 420, 423, 424, 425, 426, 427, 428, 429, 430, 453, 462, 464, 465, 466, 467, 473, 485, 489, 514, 516, 517, 518, 519, 520, 532, 567, 570, 571, 572, 573, 574, 575, 601, 602, 617, 618, 619, 620, 621, 622, 623, 624, 625, 643, 653, 670, 672, 673, 674, 675, 676, 677, 696, 697, 718, 719, 720, 721, 722, 730, 745, 746, 747, 748, 749, 762, 763, 764, 782, 783, 784, 785, 786, 787, 788, 789, 805, 811, 812, 813, 814, 815, 821, 843, 844, 845, 846, 847, 848, 849, 862, 884, 889, 917, 919, 920, 921, 922, 929, 939, 940, 941, 942, 943, 952.

Group 26. Hemostatics—Ampules 201, 539, 905.

Group 27. Hypotensors—Ampules 9, 282, 292, 521, 577, 648, 769, 944.

Group 28. Intestinal Peristaltics—Ampules 206, 712.

Group 29. **Iodine Preparations**—Ampules 226, 285, 289, 290, 422, 533, 645, 930, 953.

Group 30. **Liver Products**—Ampules 42, 159, 170, 209, 296, 372, 373, 432, 680.

Group 31. **Local Anesthetics**—Ampules 30, 88, 89, 128B, 188, 189, 205, 221, 222, 268, 331, 384, 446, 447, 448, 451, 471, 472, 479, 490, 491, 528, 529, 543, 544, 585, 599, 637, 638, 639, 728, 754, 755, 756, 758, 801, 835, 858, 860, 868, 881, 882, 908, 951.

Group 32. **Magnesium Synergists**—Ampules 15, 72, 116, 183, 374, 433, 434, 468, 522, 579, 628, 678, 723, 750, 790, 817, 874, 875, 923, 946.

Group 33. **Narcotics**—Ampules 80, 81, 98, 147, 212, 218, 219, 326, 327, 439, 632, 633, 685, 710, 711, 877.

Group 34. **Non-specific Agents**—Ampules 13, 14, 44, 50, 100, 114, 115, 117, 231, 244, 245, 272A, 273, 274, 337, 338, 340, 363 "A" and "U", 371, 373, 375, 388, 397, 492, 524, 545, 722A, 751, 757, 824, 825, 883, 904, 909, 910.

Group 35. **Nucleotides**—Ampules 148, 686, 822.

Group 36. **Oral Amebacides**—Ampule 779.

Group 37. **Orchic Preparations**—Ampules 22, 122, 162, 165, 167, 298, 304, 376, 390, 494, 495, 496, 497, 525, 586, 704, 818, 831.

Group 38. **Ovarian Products**—Ampules 6, 23, 41, 43, 56, 82, 83, 106, 123, 156, 161, 168, 186, 194, 199, 207, 258, 264, 265, 295, 300, 305, 308, 314, 328, 329, 346, 348, 349, 360, 377, 378, 411, 441, 442, 483, 498, 499, 500, 515, 526, 562, 587, 588, 613, 634, 654, 669, 687, 688, 700, 702, 717, 735, 742, 776, 796, 797, 809, 830, 832, 850, 855, 914, 925, 936.

Group 39. **Pancreas Products**—Ampule 589.

Group 40. **Parasiticides**—Ampules 90, 91, 92, 129, 190, 315, 332, 343, 344, 385, 530, 597, 598, 608, 666, 693, 694, 759, 760, 802, 803, 841, 859, 869.

Group 41. **Parathyroid Products**—Ampules 24, 299, 306, 379, 443, 450, 501, 590, 635.

Group 42. **Pituitary Products**—Ampules 25, 26, 45, 85, 86, 87, 125, 126, 144, 149, 150, 160, 208, 267, 293, 297, 301, 307, 330, 381, 382, 383, 395, 444, 445, 503, 504, 527, 556, 591, 592, 593, 626, 627, 636, 689, 690, 691, 692, 724, 727, 753, 767, 799, 800, 819, 820, 828, 833, 834, 856, 857, 863, 872, 927, 950.

Group 43. **Placental Products**—Ampules 308, 594.

Group 44. **Phosphorus Products**—Ampule 879.

Group 45. **Prostate Products**—Ampules 596, 703.

Group 46. **Saline Injections**—Ampules 421, 454, 600, 644.

Group 47. **Sclerosing Agents**—Ampules 128A, 151, 216, 217, 333, 386, 599, 640, 861.

Group 48. **Silver Preparations**—Ampules 31, 235, 254, 396, 452, 531, 641, 695, 729, 761, 804.

Group 49. **Soporifics**—Ampules 725, 873.

Group 50. **Spinal Anesthetics**—Ampules 541, 549, 584, 870, 886, 900, 901.

Group 51. **Spleen Products**—Ampules 46, 302, 306.

Group 52. **Stimulating Agents**—Ampules 4, 5, 55, 96, 99, 101, 102, 132, 136, 154, 155, 166, 172, 174, 175, 202, 211, 256, 257, 287, 312, 336, 350, 357, 358, 399, 400, 404, 407, 408, 431, 440, 456, 460, 461, 463, 481, 482, 511, 512, 558, 561, 578, 603, 611, 612, 646, 650, 651, 698, 715, 716, 739, 741, 771, 775, 807, 808, 839, 840, 871, 912, 913, 934, 935.

Group 53. **Suprarenal Products**—Ampules 47, 60, 109, 133, 141, 157, 177, 214, 266, 291, 303, 310, 381, 389, 394, 478, 484, 551, 552, 553, 554, 555, 604, 614, 627, 647, 652, 731, 743, 768, 810, 903, 938.

Group 54. **Thymus Products**—Ampules 309, 605.

Group 55. **Thyroid Products**—Ampules 294, 606, 699, 714, 736.

Group 56. Tin Preparations—Ampules 38, 230.
Group 57. Urinary Antiseptics—Ampules 568, 569.

AMPULES

Subcutaneous and Intramuscular

1. **Bismarsen**—Ampules 0.1, 0.2 Gm; Boxes of 10 and 100; Antisyphilitic; *Intramuscular use*; *Dosage:* 0.1–0.2 Gm weekly. *See Chap. I.* **(Abbott)**
2. **Bismo-Cymol**—Ampules 1 and 2 cc; Boxes of 12 and 100; Each ampule containing 100 mg bismuth; *Intramuscular use;* Antisyphilitic; *Dosage:* 2 cc twice weekly for 6–8 weeks. *See Chap. I.* **(Abbott)**
3. **Bismuth Subsalicylate**—Ampules 1 cc; Boxes of 12 and 100; Containing bismuth subsalicylate gr 2 (0.13 Gm), camphor 10%, eugenol 1%, neutral vegetable oil q.s. 1 cc; *For use* in neurosyphilis, arsenic-fast syphilis; *Dosage:* 1 cc every 3–7 days. **(Abbott)**
4. **Caffeine Sodio-Benzoate**—Ampules 2 cc; Boxes of 12 and 100; Containing caffeine sodio-benzoate gr 7½ (0.5 Gm); *For use* as cardiac stimulant, and diuretic; *Dosage:* 1–2 cc, twice daily, if necessary. **(Abbott)**
5. **Camphor in Oil**—Ampules 1 cc; Boxes of 12 and 100; Containing camphor gr 3 (0.2 Gm), neutral vegetable oil q.s. 1 cc; *For use* as stimulant; *Dosage:* 1–2 cc every 3–4 hr. **(Abbott)**
6. **Corpora Lutea**—Ampules 1 cc; Boxes of 6 and 100; Containing soluble corpora lutea in saline gr ⅓, chlorbutanol gr 1/12; *For use* in sterility, menstrual disorders; *Dosage:* 1 cc daily, or two to three times weekly. *See Chap. IV.* **(Abbott)**
7. **Epinephrine Hydrochloride**—Ampules 1 cc; Boxes of 12 and 100; Containing epinephrine hydrochloride 1:1,000—1 cc, chlorbutanol 0.5%; *For use* in asthma; *Dosage:* ⅓–1 cc, when necessary. **(Abbott)**
8. **Glycerophosphate Compound**—Ampules 1 cc; Boxes of 12 and 100; Containing sodium glycerophosphate gr 1½ (0.097 Gm), iron and ammonium citrate gr 3/10 (19.4 mg), strychnine citrate gr 1/80 (0.81 mg), sodium cacodylate gr ½ (32.4 mg); *For use* in anemia, neurasthenia; *Dosage:* 1 cc daily. **(Abbott)**
9. **Hepasol**—Ampules 1 cc; Boxes of 12 and 100; 1 cc representing gr 25 fresh liver tissue; *For use* in hypertension; *Dosage:* 1 cc daily. **(Abbott)**
10. **Iron Arsenite**—Ampules 1 cc; Boxes of 12 and 100; Containing iron arsenite and ammonium citrate gr 1 (0.065 Gm), quinine and urea hydrochloride 0.5%; *For use* in anemia, chlorosis; *Dosage:* ¼–1 cc daily. **(Abbott)**
11. **Iron Arsenite and Strychnine**—Ampules 1 cc; Boxes of 12 and 100: Containing iron arsenite and ammonium citrate gr 1 (0.065 Gm), strychnine nitrate gr 1/65 (0.001 Gm) quinine and urea hydrochloride 0.5%; *For use* in anemia, chlorosis; *Dosage:* ¼–1 cc daily. **(Abbott)**
12. **Iron Cacodylate**—Ampules 1 cc; Boxes of 12 and 100; Containing iron cacodylate gr ½ (0.032 Gm); *For use* in anemia, lymphadenitis, leukemia; *Dosage:* ¼–1 cc daily. **(Abbott)**
13. **Lactigen**—Ampules 5 and 10 cc; Boxes of 6, 25 and 100; *Intramuscular;* Protein therapy; *Dosage:* 1–10 cc every 3–5 days. *See Chap. I.* **(Abbott)**
14. **Mangatrate**—Ampules 1.5 cc; Boxes of 12 and 100; Containing manganese butyrate 1%, chlorbutanol 0.5%; *For use* in furunculosis, acute gonorrhea; *Dosage:* 1 cc followed by 1.5 cc in 4–5 days. **(Abbott)**
15. **Magnesium Sulphate 50%**—Ampules 2 cc; Boxes of 12 and 100; *For use* in obstetric anesthesia, as synergist; *Dosage:* 2 cc with or without morphine. **(Abbott)**
16. **Mercury Biniodide**—Ampules 1 cc; Boxes of 12 and 100; Containing 0.01 Gm (gr ⅙). *See Chap. I.* **(Abbott)**

17. **Mercuric Potassium Iodide**; Containing potassium iodide 0.01 Gm, red mercuric iodide, 0.01 Gm; Boxes of 12 and 100. *See Chap. I.* (Abbott)

18. **Mercuric Salicylate**—Ampules 1 cc; Boxes of 12 and 100; Containing mercury salicylate gr 1 (0.065 Gm), eugenol 1%, camphor 10%, vegetable oil q.s. 1 cc; *For use* as antiluetic; *Dosage:* 1 cc every 7–10 days; *Intramuscular.* (Abbott)

19. **Mercuric Salicylate**—Ampules 1 cc; Boxes of 12 and 100; mercury salicylate gr 1½ (0.097 Gm), eugenol 1%, camphor 10%, vegetable oil q.s. 1 cc; *For use* and *dosage* as above; *intramuscular.* (Abbott)

20. **Mercury Succinimide**—Ampules 1 cc; Boxes of 12 and 100; Containing mercury succinimide gr ⅙ (0.01 Gm); *For use* as antiluetic; *Dosage:* 0.25–1 cc daily or every 2–5 days; *Intramuscular* injections. *See Chap. I.* (Abbott)

21. **Mercury Benzoate**—Ampules 1 cc; Boxes of 12 and 100; 2% solution; gr ⅓ of mercury benzoate in 2½% sodium chloride solution per ampule; Antisyphilitic, gonocide; *Dosage:* 1 ampule every 2 days, *Intramuscularly. See Chap. I.* (Abbott)

22. **Orchic Substance**—Ampules 1 cc; Boxes of 6 and 100; Containing soluble fresh testes solids gr ⅓, chlorbutanol 0.5%; *For use* as substitution therapy; *Dosage:* 1 cc daily for several days. *See Chap. IV.* (Abbott)

23. **Ovarian Substance**—Ampules 1 cc; Boxes of 12 and 100; Containing soluble fresh ovaries (entire) gr 22½; *For use* in menopausal disorders; *Dosage:* 1 cc every 2–3 days. *See Chap. IV.* (Abbott)

24. **Parathyrin**—Ampules 1 cc; Boxes of 6 and 100; Representing gr 1/10 fresh gland, chlorbutanol 0.5%; *For use* in calcium deficiency, tetany, chorea. *Dosage:* 1 ampule, twice daily. *See Chap. IV.* (Abbott)

25. **Pituitary Extract Obstetrical**—Ampules ½ and 1 cc; Boxes of 6 and 100; *For use* in labor for control of hemorrhage, intestinal and vesical atony; *Dosage:* ⅕–2 cc as required. *See Chap. I.* (Abbott)

26. **Pituitary Extract Surgical**—Ampules 1 cc; Boxes of 6 and 100; *For use* in surgical shock, intestinal paresis, flatulence; *Dosage:* ½–1 cc immediately after operation; repeated as required. *See Chap. I.* (Abbott)

27. **Potassium Bismuth Tartrate**—Ampules 2 cc; Boxes of 10 and 100; Containing potassium bismuth tartrate, 0.1 Gm. *See Chap. I.* (Abbott)

28. **Potassium Bismuth Tartrate with Butyn**—Ampules 2 cc; Boxes of 10 and 100; Containing potassium bismuth tartrate 0.1 Gm, butyn 0.012 Gm, suspended in almond oil;—or containing potassium bismuth tartrate 0.2 Gm, butyn 0.012 Gm;—or potassium bismuth tartrate 0.1 Gm, butyn 0.6%, metaphen 0.01%; Antisyphilitic; *Dosage:* 0.1–0.2 Gm every 4–7 days till 3 Gm have been given; *Intramuscular* injections only; *see Chap. I.* (Abbott)

29. **Potassium Mercuric Iodide**—Ampules 1 cc; Boxes of 12 and 100; Containing gr ¼ (0.016 Gm) of potassium mercuric iodide; Antisyphilitic; *Dosage:* 1 ampule every 3 days, *Intramuscularly. See Chap. I.* (Abbott)

30. **Procaine-Epinephrin**—Ampules 1 cc; Boxes of 10; Containing procaine 0.02 Gm (gr ⅓) Epinephrin gr 1/1,600. *See Chap. I.* (Abbott)

31. **Solution Silver Nitrate 1%**—Wax ampules; Boxes of 12 and 100; *For use* in prophylaxis of ophthalmia neonatorum. (Abbott)

32. **Sodium Cacodylate**—Ampules 1 cc; Boxes of 12 and 100; Containing sodium cacodylate gr ¾ (0.05 Gm), gr 3 (0.2 Gm), gr 5 (0.324 Gm) or gr 7 (0.454 Gm). (Abbott)

33. **Sulpharsphenamine**—Ampules 0.2, 0.3, 0.4, 0.6 Gm; Antisyphilitic; *Dosage:* 0.1–0.6 Gm twice weekly. *See Chap. I.* (Abbott)

33a. **Homiodin**—Ampules 1 cc; Boxes of 10, 50, 100; *For use* in vasomotor rhinitis, and protracted rhino-pharyngitis. *See Chap. II.* (American Bio-Chemical)

34. **Acecoline**—Ampules 0.1, 0.2, 0.5 Gm; Crystalline powder—with a 5 cc ampule of distilled water; Cartons of 6; Vasodilator; *Dosage:* 0.05–0.2 Gm as required, subcutaneously or intramuscularly, *Not* intravenously. *See Chap. I.* (Anglo-French)

35. **Allochrysine**—Ampules of 2 cc; Boxes of 2 ampules for a single injection; Containing 0.05, 0.1 and 0.2 Gm of Allochrysine—with 8 cc ampule artificial serum; *For use* to relieve fever, cough, expectoration, improve general condition in tuberculosis; *Dosage:* 2 cc once or twice weekly for 10–15 weeks, *intramuscularly. See Chap. I.* (Anglo-French)

36. **Anti-Asthmatic "Heckel"**—Ampules 5 cc; Boxes of 12; Antispasmodic; *Dosage:* ½ ampule subcutaneously two or three times daily. *See Chap. II.* (Anglo-French)

37. **Bacte-Dysenteri-Phage**—Ampules 2 cc; Boxes of 10 and 50.
Bacte-Intesti-Phage—Ampules 2 cc; Boxes of 10 and 50.
Bacte-Coli-Phage—Ampules 1 and 10 cc; Boxes of 50 and 5 respectively.
Bacte-Pyo-Phage—Ampules 2 and 50 cc; Boxes of 1 and 10.
Bacte-Staphy-Phage—Ampules 2 and 50 cc; Boxes of 10, 1 and 10 respectively.
Bacte-Rhino-Phage—Ampules 2 cc; Boxes of 10 and 50. *For use, dosage and administration, see Chap. VI.* (Anglo-French)

38. **Stannoxyl**—Ampules 1 cc; Boxes of 8; Anti-infective; *Dosage:* 1–2 cc daily, *intramuscularly. See Chap. I.* (Anglo-French)

39. **Sulfarsenol**—Ampules—0.06, 0.12, 0.18, 0.03, 0.42, 0.60, Gm. *See Chap. I.* (Anglo-French)

---

40. **Anterior Pituitary Liquid**—Ampules 1 cc; Boxes of 6; *For use* in hypopituitarism, in stimulating skeletal growth in pituitary dwarfs, restoring menstrual function in amenorrhea of pituitary origin, preventing delayed puberty. *See Chap. IV.* (Armour)

41. **Corpus Luteum**—Ampules 1 cc; Boxes of 6; *For use* in relief of symptoms of artificial and natural menopause. *See Chap. IV.* (Armour)

42. **Liver Liquid**—Ampules 1 cc; Boxes of 6; *For use* in pernicious anemia. *See Chap. IV.* (Armour)

43. **Ovarian Substance**—Ampules 1 cc; Boxes of 6; *For use* in treating dysmenorrhea; *Dosage:* 2–5 gr, three times daily for a few days prior to period. *See Chap. IV.* (Armour)

44. **Peptone Solution**—Ampules 1 and 2 cc; Boxes of 12, 50 and 100; Foreign protein therapy; 5% sterile, isotonic solution; *Intramuscular* injection; *For use and dosage, see Chap. I.* (Armour)

45. **Pituitary Liquid**—Obstetrical; Ampules 0.5 and 1 cc; Boxes of 6, 50 and 100; Surgical; Ampules 1 cc; Boxes of 6, 50 and 100; Double strength; Obstetrical or Surgical; Ampules 1 cc; Boxes of 6, 50 and 100; *For use* and *dosage, see Chap. I.* (Armour)

46. **Spleen Liquid**—Ampules 2 cc; Boxes of 12 and 50; Ampules 5 cc; Boxes of 12; Astringent in eczema, urticaria, angioneurotic edema. *See Chap. IV.* (Armour)

47. **Suprarenalin**—Ampules 1 cc; Boxes of 6, 50 and 100; Solutions of 1:1,000 and 1:10,000; Vasoconstrictor. *See Chap. I.* (Armour)

---

48. **Asthmolysin**—Ampules 1 cc; Boxes of 10; Antispasmodic; *Dosage:* 1–3 ampules as necessary. *See Chap. III.* (Beisner)

49. **Spasmolysin**—Ampules 1 cc; Boxes of 10; Antispasmodic; *Dosage:* 1–2 ampules as necessary. *See Chap. III.* (Beisner)

50. **Terpichin**—Ampules 1 cc; Boxes of 10; Non-specific therapy; 15% purified turpentine oil with quinine ½%, anesthesin ½% in olive oil 84%; *Dosage:* 1–2 cc every 2 days, *intragluteally See Chap. II.* (Beisner)

51. **Bismuth Salicylate**—Ampule 1 cc; Boxes of 12, 100 and 500; Containing gr 2; Antisyphilitic; *Intramuscular; For use* in intolerance or resistance to arsenicals and mercurials; *Dosage:* 1–2 gr weekly for about 14 injections. (Berwyn)

52. **Bismuth Sodium Tartrate**—Ampules 2 cc; Boxes of 12, 100 and 500; Containing 1½ % bismuth sodium tartrate. (Berwyn)

53. **Caffeine Sodio-Benzoate**—Ampules 2 cc (gr 3¾), or 2 cc (gr 7½); Boxes of 12, 100, 500; Cardiac, respiratory and cerebral stimulant, diuretic in cardiac failure, collapse, neuralgia and pneumonia. (Berwyn)

54. **Calcium Cacodylate**—Ampules 2 cc; Boxes of 12, 100 and 500; *For use* in tuberculosis. (Berwyn)

55. **Camphor in Oil**—Ampules 1 cc; Containing gr 3; Boxes of 12, 100 and 500; Ampules 5 cc; Containing gr 10; Boxes of 6, 25, and 100; Ampules 10 cc; Containing gr 36; Boxes of 6, 100 and 500; *For use* as heart stimulant in nervous depression, hysteria, convalescence, adynamic fevers. (Berwyn)

56. **Corpus Luteum Extract**—Ampules 1 cc; Boxes of 6, 100 and 500; Containing 3 gr per cubic centimeter; *For use* in nervous disturbances of menopause, nausea during pregnancy. *See Chap. IV.* (Berwyn)

57. **Emetine Hydrochloride**—Ampules ½ cc (gr ⅓); Boxes of 6, 100, 500; Ampules 1 cc (gr ½); Boxes of 6, 100, 500; Ampules 1 cc (gr 1); Boxes of 6, 100, 500; *For use* in amebic dysentery, hepatitis and other Endameba manifestations. (Berwyn)

58. **Ephedrine Sulphate**—Ampules 1 cc; Boxes of 12, 100 and 500; *For use* in asthma and hay fever. (Berwyn)

59. **Epinephrine-Ephedrine Compound**—Ampules 1 cc; Boxes of 12, 100 and 500; Containing epinephrine hydrochloride 1:2,500, ephedrine hydrochloride 3 %, chlorbutanol 0.5 %; Antispasmodic; *For use* in asthma. (Berwyn)

60. **Epinephrine Hydrochloride**—Ampules 1 cc; Boxes of 12, 100 and 500; Solutions of 1:1,000 or 1:10,000; Antispasmodic; *For use* in asthma. (Berwyn)

61. **Glycerophosphates Compound**—Ampules 1 cc; Boxes of 12, 100 and 500; Containing sodium glycerophosphate gr 1½, strychnine cacodylate gr 1/125, iron cacodylate gr ½, chlorbutanol 0.5 %; *For use* in chlorosis, anemia, neurasthenia and convalescence. (Berwyn)

62. **Glycerophosphates Compound (Double Strength)**—Ampules 1 cc; Boxes of 12, 100 and 500; Containing sodium glycerophosphate gr 3, strychnine cacodylate gr 1/65, iron cacodylate gr ⅛, chlorbutanol 0.5 %; *For use* as above. (Berwyn)

63. **Iron Arsenite**—Ampules 1 cc; Boxes 12, 100 and 500; Containing gr ⅙ or gr 1; with quinine and urea hydrochloride 0.5 %; *For use* in cutaneous diseases, pernicious anemia, chlorosis. (Berwyn)

64. **Iron Arsenite and Manganese**—Ampules 1 cc; Boxes of 12, 100 and 500; Containing iron arsenite gr ¾, manganese citrate gr 1/100, quinine and urea hydrochloride 0.5 %; *For use* in chlorosis and anemia. (Berwyn)

65. **Iron Arsenite and Strychnine 1**—Ampules 1 cc; Boxes of 12, 100 and 500; Containing iron arsenite gr 1, strychnine nitrate gr 1/65, quinine and urea hydrochloride 0.5 %. (Berwyn)

66. **Iron Arsenite and Strychnine 2**—Ampules 1 cc; Boxes of 12, 100 and 500; Containing iron arsenite gr ⅜, strychnine nitrate gr 1/65, quinine and urea hydrochloride 0.5 %. (Berwyn)

67. **Iron Arsenite and Strychnine 3**—Ampules 1 cc; Boxes of 12, 100 and 500; Containing iron arsenite gr ¼, strychnine nitrate gr 1/100, quinine and urea hydrochloride 0.5 %. (Berwyn)

68. **Iron Arsenite and Strychnine 4**—Ampules 1 cc; Boxes of 12, 100 and 500; Containing iron arsenite gr ¾, strychnine nitrate 1/65, quinine and urea hydrochloride 0.5 %; *For use* in the treatment of atonic dyspepsia with anemia, chlorosis, malnutrition, in convalescence. (Berwyn)

69. Iron Cacodylate—Ampules 1 cc; Boxes of 12, 100 and 500; *For use* in anemias and leukemia. (Berwyn)

70. Iron Citrate (Green)—Ampules 1 cc; Boxes of 12, 100 and 500; Containing iron and ammonium citrate gr 1/4, gr 3/4 or gr 1 1/2 with quinine and urea hydrochloride 0.5%; *For use* in anemia. (Berwyn)

71. Iron Citrate and Manganese—Ampules 1 cc; Boxes of 12, 100 and 500; Containing iron citrate gr 3/4, manganese citrate gr 1/100, quinine and urea hydrochloride 0.5%. (Berwyn)

72. Magnesium Sulphate—Ampules 2 cc; Boxes of 12, 100 and 500; 50% Solution; *For use* with morphine for prolonged effect. (Berwyn)

73. Mercury Cyanide—Ampule 1 cc; Boxes of 12, 100; Containing gr 1/6; *For use* in syphilis. *See Chap. I.* (Berwyn)

74. Mercury Iodide (Red)—Ampules 1 cc; Boxes of 12, 100 and 500; Containing mercuric iodide (red) gr 1/6, potassium iodide solution q.s., chlorbutanol 2%, oil q.s. 1% in oil. *See Chap. I.* (Berwyn)

75. Mercury Iodide (Red)—Ampules 1 cc; Boxes of 12, 100 and 500; Containing mercuric iodide (red) gr 1/6, sodium iodide gr 1/6, physiological salt solution q.s. 1% in water. *See Chap. I.* (Berwyn)

76. Mercury Iodide (Red)—Ampules 1 cc; Boxes of 12, 100 and 500; Containing mercuric iodide (red) gr 1/3, sodium iodide gr 1/3; 2% in water; *For use* in syphilitic conditions. *See Chap. I.* (Berwyn)

77. Mercury Salicylate—Ampules 1 cc; Boxes of 12, 100 and 500; Containing mercury salicylate, gr 1 and quinine and urea hydrochloride 0.5%; in oil. (Berwyn)

78. Mercury Salicylate—Ampules 1 cc; Boxes of 12, 100 and 500; Containing mercury salicylate gr 2, quinine and urea hydrochloride 0.5%; in oil. *For use* in syphilis. (Berwyn)

79. Mercury Succinimide—Ampules 1 cc; Boxes of 12, 100 and 500; Containing gr 1/6; *For use* in syphilitic conditions. *See Chap. I.* (Berwyn)

80. Morphine Sulphate—Ampules 2 cc; Boxes of 12; Containing morphine sulphate gr 1/8 or gr 1/4 with magnesium sulphate 25%; *For use* to prolong action and lessen dosage of morphine. (Berwyn)

81. Morphine and Atropine—Ampules 1 cc; Boxes of 12; Containing morphine sulphate gr 1/4, atropine sulphate gr 1/100, physiological salt solution q.s. *For use* to increase analgesia, lessen depression. (Berwyn)

82. Ovarian Extract (Entire)—Ampules 1 cc; Boxes of 12, 100 and 500; equivalent of gr 10 fresh ovarian substance;
Ampules 1 cc; Boxes of 12, 100 and 500; equivalent of gr 31; *For use* in disorders of menopause and deficient ovarian secretion. *See Chap. IV.* (Berwyn)

83. Ovarian Residue Extract—Ampules 1 cc; Boxes of 12, 100 and 500; Each cubic centimeter containing substance equal to gr 31 of fresh ovarian without corpus luteum; *For use* in menstrual irregularities and dysmenorrhea. *See Chap. IV.* (Berwyn)

84. Physiological Salt Solution—Ampules 1 cc; Boxes of 12, 100 and 500; *For use* as indicated. (Berwyn)

85. Pituitary Anterior Lobe—Ampules 1 cc; Boxes of 6, 100 and 500; *For use* in promoting growth. *See Chap. IV.* (Berwyn)

86. Pituitary Extract U.S.P. Obstetrical—Ampules 1/2 and 1 cc; Boxes of 6, 100 and 500; *For use* in stimulating muscular contractions of uterus, intestines, bladder, raising and maintaining blood pressure in shock, pneumonia, diphtheria. *See Chap. I.* (Berwyn)

87. Pituitary Extract Surgical (Double Strength)—Ampules 1 cc; Boxes of 6, 100 and 500; *For use* in obviating surgical shock and as above; not in obstetrical cases. *See Chap. I.* (Berwyn)

88. **Procaine Solution**—Ampules 2 cc; Boxes of 12, 100 and 500; ½% solution; Ampules 1 cc; Boxes of 12, 100 and 500; 1 or 2% solutions; Ampules 5 cc; Boxes of 6, 25 and 100; 2% solution; Ampules 10 cc; Boxes of 6, 25 and 100; 2% solution; *For use* as local anesthetic. *See Chap. I.* **(Berwyn)**

89. **Procaine 2% with Epinephrine**—Ampules 1 cc; Boxes of 12, 100 and 500; Containing procaine gr ⅓, epinephrine hydrochloride gr 1/3,200; *For use* as local anesthetic. **(Berwyn)**

90. **Quinine Dihydrochloride**—Ampules 1 cc; Boxes of 12, 100 and 500; Containing either gr 3¾ or gr 7½. **(Berwyn)**

91. **Quinine Dihydrochloride**—Ampules 2 cc; Boxes of 12, 100 and 500; Containing gr 15½. *For use* in malarial fevers, lobar pneumonia, as tonic during convalescence. **(Berwyn)**

92. **Quinine and Urea Hydrochloride**—Ampules 2 cc; Boxes of 12, 100 and 500; 1 or 5% Solutions; Ampules 1 cc; Boxes of 12, 100 and 500; gr 7½; Ampules 2 cc; Boxes of 12, 100 and 500; gr 15½; *For use* in the treatment of malaria. *See Chap. II.* **(Berwyn)**

93. **Sodium Cacodylate**—Ampules 1 cc; Boxes of 12, 100 and 500; Containing gr ¾, 1½, 2, 3, 5 or 7. **(Berwyn)**

94. **Sodium Cacodylate**—Ampules 2 cc; Boxes of 12, 100 and 500; Containing gr 15½; *For use* in treatment of cachexia of malaria, anemia, leukemia, neurasthenia, non-parasitic chronic skin diseases. **(Berwyn)**

95. **Sodium Glycerophosphate**—Ampules 1 cc; Boxes of 12, 100 and 500; *For use* in muscular and nervous debility, rachitis, osteomalacia. **(Berwyn)**

96. **Strychnine Sulphate**—Ampules 1 cc; Boxes of 12, 100 and 500; *For use* in acute collapse and shock, faintness, as antidote in chloroform or chloral hydrate poisoning. **(Berwyn)**

97. **Water, Double Distilled**—Ampules 5, 10 and 20 cc; Boxes of 6, 25, 100 and 500. **(Berwyn)**

---

98. **Dilaudid**—Ampules 1 cc; gr 1/32 (0.0025 Gm); Boxes of 6; Crystalline morphine derivative; *Dosage:* gr 1/32 as required. *See Chap. I.* **(Bilhuber-Knoll)**

99. **Metrazol**—Ampules 1 cc; Boxes of 6 and 20; Cardiotonic; *Dosage:* 1–2 ampules *subcutaneously*, two to three times daily. *See Chap. I.* **(Bilhuber-Knoll)**

---

100. **Activin**—Ampules 1 cc; Boxes of 6 and 12; Non-specific protein therapy, an organic iodine; *Dosage:* 0.5–1 cc twice weekly, *intramuscularly*. *See Chap. I.* **(Bischoff)**

101. **Alpha Lobelin**—Ampules 1 cc; Boxes of 6, 12 and 100; Respiratory stimulant, crystalline alkaloid, gr 3/20 (0.01 Gm); *Dosage:* ½–1 ampule as required. *See Chap. I.* **(Bischoff)**

102. **Camphogen**—Ampules 1 or 2 cc; Boxes of 6; Containing water soluble camphor 2%, acetdiethylamid 25%, sodium salicylate 15%, water 58%; *Dosage:* 0.5–1 cc as required. *See Chap. II.* **(Bischoff)**

---

103. **Cacodylates-Strychnine Compound Solution**—Ampules 1 cc; Boxes of 12 and 100; Containing iron cacodylate gr ¼ (0.016 Gm), sodium cacodylate gr ¾ (0.049 Gm), strychnine nitrate gr 1/100 (0.006 Gm), sodium glycerophosphate gr 2 (0.13 Gm); *For use* as hematinic and tonic; *Dosage:* 1 ampule at 2–4 day intervals. **(Breon)**

104. **Caffeine and Sodium Benzoate**—Ampules 2 cc; Boxes of 12 and 100; Containing gr 7½ (0.49 Gm); *For use* as cardiac, cerebral and respiratory stimulant; *Dosage:* ½–1 ampule as indicated. **(Breon)**

105. **Camphor in Olive Oil**—Ampules 1 cc; Boxes of 12 and 100; Containing gr 3 (0.19 Gm);
Ampules 10 cc; Boxes of 12 and 100; Containing gr 36¼ (2.35 Gm); *For use* as cardiac stimulant in pneumonia, typhoid fever and in acute septic affections; *Dosage:* 1–2 cc every 2–4 hr.; in severe cases, 10 cc may be given and repeated at 12 hr. intervals. (Breon)

106. **Corpus Luteum Solution**—Ampules 1 cc; Boxes of 12 and 100; Containing gr ⅓ (0.022 Gm) soluble extractives with chlorbutanol gr 1/12; *For use* in menstrual dysfunction, nausea of pregnancy, abortion without demonstrable cause, sterility; *Dosage:* 1–2 ampules daily as indicated for 12 injections. *See Chap. IV.* (Breon)

107. **Emetine Hydrochloride**—Ampules 1 cc; Boxes of 6 and 100; Containing gr 1 (0.065 Gm); *For use* in amebic dysentery, hemorrhages; *Dosage:* 1 ampule daily, *intramuscularly* injected. (Breon)

108. **Ephedrine Hydrochloride**—Ampules 1 cc; Boxes of 6 and 100; Containing gr ¾ (50 mg); *For use* in asthma, hay fever and nasal congestions. *See Chap. I.* (Breon)

109. **Epinephrin Solution**—Ampules 1 cc; Boxes of 12 and 100; Containing 1:1,000 solution; *For use* in asthma, hemorrhage, cardiovascular collapse; *Dosage:* For relief of asthmatic attacks 5–10 m, for hemorrhage control in lungs 7–10 m every 20–30 min. *See Chap. I.* (Breon)

110. **Iron and Arsenic**—Ampules 2 cc; Boxes of 12 and 100; Containing gr 1 (0.065 Gm) of iron cacodylate; *For use* as hematinic and tonic. (Breon)

111. **Iron Arsenite**—Ampules 1 cc; Boxes of 12 and 100; Containing gr 1 (0.065 Gm) iron arsenite; *For use* as hematinic; *Dosage:* 1 ampule on alternate days. (Breon)

112. **Iron Citrate Compound with Nuclein**—Ampules 1 cc; Boxes of 12 and 100; Containing iron citrate gr ¾ (0.049 Gm), potassium arsenite gr 1/64 (0.001 Gm), strychnine sulphate gr 1/64 (0.001 Gm), sodium nucleinate gr ⅛ (0.008 Gm); *For use* as tonic; *Dosage:* 1 ampule on alternate days, *intramuscularly* injected. (Breon)

113. **Iron Citrate, Green**—Ampules 1 cc; Boxes of 12 and 100; Containing gr 1 (0.065 Gm); *For use* as tonic; *Dosage:* 1 ampule every 2 days. (Breon)

114. **Lacmanese**—Ampules 10 cc; Boxes of 6 and 25; Containing Lactpro 8.5 cc and manganese butyrate solution 1% 1.5 cc, benzyl alcohol 0.3%;
Ampules 5 cc; Boxes of 6 and 25; Same strength as above; *For use* as foreign protein therapy, in gonorrhea and sequelae, acne, eye infections, inflammatory rheumatism, arthritis, puerperal fever; Contraindications—heart dysfunction, diabetes, alcoholism, asthmatic individuals; *Dosage:* 5 cc initially, 10 cc at 3–5 day intervals, *intragluteally* injected. (Breon)

115. **Lactpro**—Ampules 2, 5, 10 cc; Boxes of 6 and 100; *For use* in foreign protein therapy; *Dosage:* initial adult 5 cc then 10 cc *intramuscularly* into upper buttocks, children 2–5 cc, slightly older and frail adults 5–8 cc, every 3–5 days. (Breon)

116. **Magnesul**—Ampules 2 cc; Boxes of 12 and 50; Containing 50% solution of magnesium sulphate with procain 2½%; Intramuscular injection; *For use* in muscular relaxation and with morphine sulphate for prolonged effect. (Breon)

117. **Manganese Butyrate**—Ampules 1 and 1.5 cc; Boxes of 12 and 100, half of 1 cc (white label), and half of 1.5 cc (green label);
Ampules 2 cc; Boxes of 12 and 100; Containing manganese butyrate 1.0%, benzyl alcohol 2.0%; *For use* in infections as gonorrhea, acne, boils, carbuncles; *Dosage:* Initially 1 cc, 4 days later 1½–2 cc. (Breon)

118. **Mercuric Iodide, Red, in Almond Oil**—Ampules 1 cc; Boxes of 12 and 100; Containing gr ⅙ (0.01 Gm) or 44% metallic mercury; *For use* as antiluetic with involvement of bones and joints; *Intramuscularly* injected; *Dosage:* 1 ampule at 3–5 day intervals. *See Chap. I.* (Breon)

119. Mercury Bichloride in Oil—Ampules 1 cc; Boxes of 12 and 100; Containing gr 1/6 (0.01 Gm); *For use* as antiluetic; *Dosage:* 1 ampule at 6–7 day intervals. **(Breon)**

120. Mercury Salicylate with Quinine and Urea—Ampules 1 cc; Boxes of 12 and 100; Containing 60% metallic mercury and 1% quinine and urea; *Dosage:* 1 ampule at 5–7 day intervals, *intramuscularly* injected. **(Breon)**

121. Mercury Succinimide—Ampules 1 cc; Boxes of 12 and 100; Containing gr 1/6 (0.01 Gm); 50%; *For use* as antiluetic; *Dosage:* 1 cc every 1–2 days, may be increased to 1½ cc (¼ gr). *See Chap. I.* **(Breon)**

122. Orchic Extract Solution—Ampules 1 cc; Boxes of 12 and 100; Containing gr 55 (3.6 Gm) fresh gland substance with chlorbutanol gr 1/12; *For use* in impotence, asthenia, neurasthenia and melancholia; *Dosage:* 1 ampule on alternate days, *intramuscularly. See Chap. IV.* **(Breon)**

123. Ovarian Extract Solution—Ampules 1 cc; Boxes of 12 and 100; Containing gr 40 (2.6 Gm), fresh whole gland substance, with chlorbutanol gr 1/12; *For use* in menopausal disorders, retarded or imperfect female development, nausea and vomiting of pregnancy; *Dosage:* 1 ampule, *intramuscularly,* every 2–3 days. *See Chap. IV.* **(Breon)**

124. Phenolsulphonephthalein—Ampules 1 cc; Boxes of 12 and 100; Containing gr 1/100 (0.006 Gm); *For use* as renal function test. *See Chap. I.* **(Breon)**

125. Pituitary Solution, Anterior—Ampules 1 cc; Boxes of 6 and 100; Containing gr 18.5 with chlorbutanol gr 1/12; *For use* in promoting skeletal growth; *Dosage:* 1 cc every 1–2 days, *intramuscularly* and *intravenously.* **(Breon)**

126. Pituitary Extract—Ampules ½ and 1 cc; Boxes of 6 and 100; Obstetrical; Containing posterior lobe with chlorbutanol gr 1/12 per cubic centimeter; *Dosage:* 1/5–2 cc; *For use* in hastening second stage of labor in normal pelvis, increasing intestinal peristalsis, in surgical shock and circulatory failure;
Ampules 1 cc; Boxes of 6 and 100; Surgical, Double strength; *Dosage:* ½–1 cc immediately after or 4 hr. after operation, as indicated. *See Chap. I.* **(Breon)**

127. Potassium-Sodium Bismuth Tartrate—Ampules 2 cc; Boxes of 12 and 100; Containing potassium sodium bismuth tartrate gr 3.1 (0.2 Gm), benzyl alcohol 2%, in vegetable oil emulsion q.s.; *For use* as antiluetic; Contraindicated in nephritis; *Dosage:* 1–2 cc every 5–7 days as tolerated; course not to exceed 3 Gm of drug, with 4–6 weeks rest. *See Chap. I.* **(Breon)**

128. Quinine and Urea Hydrochloride—Ampules 2 cc; Boxes of 12 and 100; 5% solution; *For use* in treatment of hemorrhoids; *Dosage:* 1–4 cc at a time, at 5–7 day intervals;
Ampules 1 cc; Boxes of 12 and 100; 1% solution; *For use* as local anesthetic, *subcutaneously* injected;
Ampules 2 cc; Boxes of 12 and 100; Containing gr 7½ (0.49 Gm); *For use* in malarial infection, pneumonia, sciatica and whooping cough; *Dosage:* 1 ampule as indicated. *See Chap. I.* **(Breon)**

129. Quinine Dihydrochloride—Ampules 1 cc; Boxes of 12 and 100; Containing gr 7½ (0.49 Gm); *For use* in malaria, influenza; *Dosage:* 1 ampule every 4 hr. as indicated. **(Breon)**

130. Sodium Cacodylate—Ampules 1 cc; Boxes of 12 and 100; Containing gr 1 (0.065 Gm); gr 2 (0.13 Gm), gr 3 (0.19 Gm), gr 5 (0.32 Gm), gr 7 (0.45 Gm), Ampules 2 cc; gr 15 (0.98 Gm); *For use* as tonic; warmed slightly before injecting. **(Breon)**

131. Solu-Bismuth—Ampules 2 cc; Boxes of 12 and 100; Containing potassium sodium bismuth tartrate gr 3/5 (0.04 Gm), 64% of the salt or 25 mg in each 2 cc; *For use* as antiluetic; *Dosage:* 1 cc, *intragluteally,* to test tolerance, then 2 cc at 2–3 day intervals, course is 30 injections; 4–6 weeks rest, then course repeated. **(Breon)**

132. Strychnophos—Ampules 1 cc; Boxes of 12 and 100; Containing sodium glycerophosphate gr 1½ (0.1 Gm), strychnine cacodylate gr 1/130 (0.0005 Gm); *For use* in neurasthenia; *Dosage:* 1 ampule *intramuscularly* every 1–2 days. **(Breon)**

133. Suprarenal Chloride Solution (Epinephrin)—Ampules 1 cc; Boxes of 12 and 100; Containing 1:1,000 solution; *For use* in asthma, hemorrhage, cardiovascular collapse; *Dosage:* for asthmatic attacks 5–10 m at onset if possible; for hemorrhage control (pulmonary) 7–10 m at 20–30 min. intervals. *See Chap. I.* **(Breon)**

---

134. Bismuth Metal—Hypoloids 5, 10 and 25 cc; Boxes of 10; Rubber-capped; Containing gr 3 (0.194 Gm) in sterile isotonic glucose solution. **(Burroughs Wellcome)**

135. Caffeine Sodio-Benzoate—Hypoloids 1 cc; Boxes of 10 and 100; Containing gr 3¾ (0.25 Gm) or gr 7½ (0.5 Gm). **(Burroughs Wellcome)**

136. Camphor in Olive Oil—Hypoloids 1 cc; Boxes of 10 and 100; Containing gr 1½ (0.1 Gm) or gr 3 (0.2 Gm). **(Burroughs Wellcome)**

137. Digitalin—Hypoloids 1 cc; Boxes of 10; Containing gr 1/140 (0.001 Gm); Digitalis therapy; *Dosage:* gr 1/100 to gr 1/30 as required. *See Chap. I.* **(Burroughs Wellcome)**

138. Emetine Hydrochloride—Hypoloids 1 cc; Boxes of 6 and 10; Containing gr ⅓ (0.02 Gm), gr ½ (0.03 Gm), gr 1 (0.065 Gm). **(Burroughs Wellcome)**

139. Ephedrine—Hypoloids 1 cc; Boxes of 10; Containing ephedrine hydrochloride gr ½ (0.03 Gm); Vasoconstrictor; *Dosage:* 1–4 ampules *subcutaneously,* as required. *See Chap. I.* **(Burroughs Wellcome)**

140. Epinephrine—Hypoloids 1 cc; Boxes of 10 and 100; *Dosage:* hypodermic injection 5–15 m; *intravenous* injection 1–500 cc normal saline. *See Chap. I.* **(Burroughs Wellcome)**

141. Epinine—Hypoloid Epinine Hydrochloride 1 cc; Boxes of 10; Vasoconstrictor; *Dosage:* 0.5–1 cc as required. *See Chap. I.* **(Burroughs Wellcome)**

142. Ernutin—Hypoloids 1 cc; Boxes of 6 and 100; Containing 0.1% stable salt of ergotoxine; Uterine stimulant; *Dosage:* 0.3–0.6 cc as required. *See Chap. III.* **(Burroughs Wellcome)**

143. Hyoscine Hydrobromide—Hypoloids 1 cc; Boxes of 10 and 100; Containing gr 1/130 (0.0005 Gm). **(Burroughs Wellcome)**

144. Infundin—Hypoloids 0.5 cc; Boxes of 6 and 100; Original strength; 10 international units;
Hypoloids 1 cc; Boxes of 6 and 100; Original strength; 10 international units;
Hypoloids 0.5 cc; Boxes of 6; 5 international units;
Hypoloids 1 cc; Boxes of 6; 5 international units; Pituitary extract, posterior lobe; *Dosage:* 0.5–1 cc as required. *See Chap. I.* **(Burroughs Wellcome)**

145. Iron and Arsenic—Hypoloids 1 cc; Boxes of 10 and 100; Containing iron and ammonium citrate gr ¾ (0.05 Gm), sodium arsenate exsiccated gr 1/32 (0.002 Gm), water q.s. 1 cc. **(Burroughs Wellcome)**

146. Mercury Salicylate without Creosote—Hypoloids 1 cc; Boxes of 10 and 100; Containing gr 1½ (0.1 Gm). **(Burroughs Wellcome)**

147. Morphine Hydrochloride—Hypoloids 1 cc; Boxes of 10; Containing gr ⅙ (0.01 Gm) or gr ⅓ (0.02 Gm). **(Burroughs Wellcome)**

148. Nuclein—Hypoloids 1 cc; Boxes of 10; Containing gr ½ (0.032 Gm); Leucocyte stimulant; *Dosage:* 1 ampule daily, *subcutaneously; See Chap. II.* **(Burroughs Wellcome)**

149. Pituitary Extract, Posterior Lobe—See Infundin. **(Burroughs Wellcome)**

150. Pituitary Extract, Whole Gland—Hypoloids 1 cc; Boxes of 10; Containing gr ⅙ (0.01 Gm) and gr ⅓ (0.02 Gm). *See Chap. I.* **(Burroughs Wellcome)**

151. Quinine and Urethane—Hypoloid 2 cc; Boxes of 5; Sclerosing agent; *Dosage:* 0.5–1 cc per vein. *See Chap. II.* **(Burroughs Wellcome)**

152. Scopolamine Hydrobromide—Hypoloids 0.5 cc; Boxes of 10; Containing gr 1/450 (0.00014 Gm) or gr 1/150 (0.00043 Gm). *See Chap. I.* **(Burroughs Wellcome)**

153. Sodium Cacodylate—Hypoloids 1 cc; Boxes of 10 and 100; Containing gr ¾ (0.05 Gm), gr 1½ (0.1 Gm), gr 3 (0.2 Gm), gr 5 (0.324 Gm), gr 7 (0.454 Gm). **(Burroughs Wellcome)**

154. Strophanthin—Hypoloids 1 cc; Boxes of 10; Containing gr 1/100 (0.00065 Gm). **(Burroughs Wellcome)**

155. Strychnine Sulphate—Hypoloids 1 cc; Boxes of 10; Containing gr 1/32 (0.002 Gm). **(Burroughs Wellcome)**

---

156. Corpus Luteum—Ampules 1 cc; Boxes of 6; Containing 20% solution. *See Chap. IV.* **(G. W. Carnrick)**

157. Epinephrine—Ampules 1 cc; Boxes of 6; Containing 1:10,000 solution. *See Chap. I.* **(G. W. Carnrick)**

158. Glycogen—Ampules 2 cc; Boxes of 6. **(G. W. Carnrick)**

159. Liver Extract (Erythgen Brand)—Ampules 2.5 cc; Boxes of 6; Representing Gm 50 fresh liver, per ampule; *Dosage:* 2 ampules daily for 3–4 days, then 2 ampules weekly. *See Chap. I.* **(G. W. Carnrick)**

160. Posterior Pituitary—Ampules ½ and 1 cc; Boxes of 6; Obstetrical; Ampules 1 cc; Boxes of 6; Surgical. *See Chap. IV.* **(G. W. Carnrick)**

161. Thelestrin—Standardized Ovarian Hormone—Ampules 1 cc; Boxes of 6; Representing 25 rat units per cubic centimeter; *For action* and *uses see Chap. I.* **(G. W. Carnrick)**

162. Viriligen—Ampules 1 cc; Boxes of 6; Containing extracts of anterior pituitary, suprarenal cortex, testes, lymph glands, brain and spinal cord tissue, with thyroid 1/10 gr per ampule; *For use* as aphrodisiac in lowered sexual virility and neurasthenia; *Dosage:* 1 ampule every 3 days. *See Chap. IV.* **(G. W. Carnrick)**

---

163. Anastil—Ampules 1 cc; Boxes of 6 and 10; Plain; Containing gr 0.05 guaiacol; Intramuscular; with novocain; Expectorant; *Dosage:* 1 cc every 2–3 days. *See Chap. I.* **(Cavendish)**

164. Anastil—Ampules 1 cc; Boxes of 3 and 6; Reinforced; Containing gr 0.075 guaiacol; Intramuscular; with novocain; Expectorant; *Dosage:* 1 cc every 2 or 3 days. *See Chap. I.* **(Cavendish)**

165. Lipolysin—Ampules 1 cc; Packages of 12 and 100; Containing:
Masculine—testicular extract, pancreatic hormone, ferments, enzymes and pituitary gland;
Feminine—Extracts of ovaries with pancreatic hormones, ferments, enzymes and pituitary gland; *For use* in obesity, to regulate sugar metabolism; *Dosage:* 1 ampule two to three times weekly, *intramuscularly.* *See Chap. III.* **(Cavendish)**

166. Myoston—Ampules 1 cc; Boxes of 12; Cardiac stimulant; *Dosage:* 1 ampule *subcutaneously,* as required. *See Chap. III.* **(Cavendish)**

167. Testogan—Ampules 1.1 cc; Boxes of 12; Containing mg 1 yohimbin; Male aphrodisiac; *Dosage:* 1 ampule every 2 days. *See Chap. IV.* **(Cavendish)**

168. Thelygan—Ampules 1.1 cc; Boxes of 12; Containing mg 1 yohimbin; Female aphrodisiac; *Dosage:* 1 ampule every 2 days. *See Chap. IV.* **(Cavendish)**

169. Yohimbin—Ampules 1 cc; Boxes of 12; Containing m 15 of 1% solution; Aphrodisiac; *Dosage:* 1 ampule as required. *See Chap. III.* **(Cavendish)**

---

170. Liver Extract—Ampules 2.5 cc; Boxes of 12; Containing condensed principle from 25 Gm liver; *For use* in pernicious anemia; *Dosage:* 2.5 cc daily during remission; for maintenance 2.5 cc weekly. *See Chap. I.* **(Chappel)**

---

171. Bismuth Subsalicylate—Ampules 1 cc; Boxes of 12; Containing bismuth subsalicylate 0.13 Gm, camphor 0.1 Gm, creosote 0.1 Gm, in olive oil; Antisyphilitic; *Intramuscular.* **(Cheplin)**

172. **Caffeine Sodio-Benzoate**—Ampules 2 cc; Boxes of 12, Containing gr 3¾ (0.25 Gm), or gr 7½ (0.5 Gm); *used* as Cardiac cerebral, respiratory and circulatory stimulant; *Intramuscular.* **(Cheplin)**

173. **Calcium Cacodylate**—Ampules 2 cc; Boxes of 12; Containing gr 1½ (0.1 Gm) of 5% solution; *Intramuscular; For use* in anemia, pellagra, cachexia. **(Cheplin)**

174. **Camphor in Oil**—Ampules 1 cc; Boxes of 12; Containing gr 1½ (0.1 Gm) or gr 3 (0.2 Gm); Circulatory stimulant; *Intramuscular.* **(Cheplin)**

175. **Camphor in Oil**—Ampules 10 cc; Boxes of 6; Containing gr 36 (2.33 Gm); Circulatory stimulant; *For use* in typhoid fever, pneumonia, quick heart stimulant in shock and collapse; *Intramuscular.* **(Cheplin)**

176. **Ephedrine Sulphate**—Ampules 1 cc; Boxes of 12; Containing gr ¾ (0.05 Gm); *For use* in relief of arterial hypotension. *See Chap. I.* **(Cheplin)**

177. **Epinephrine Hydrochloride**—Ampules 1 cc; Boxes of 12; 1:1,000 Solution; *For use* in shock, surgical heart failure, collapse following hemorrhage. *See Chap. I.* **(Cheplin)**

178. **Glycerophosphate Compound**—Ampules 1 cc; Boxes of 12; Containing sodium glycerophosphate gr 1½ (0.1 Gm), strychnine cocodylate gr 1/125 (0.0005 Gm), iron cacodylate gr ⅙ (0.01 Gm); *For use* in neurasthenia, anemia, functional nervous disorders; *Intramuscular.* **(Cheplin)**

179. **Iron Arsenite**—Ampules 1 cc; Boxes of 12; Containing 0.5% quinine and urea hydrochloride; *For use* in anemia, chlorosis, leucocythemia, malarial anemia, pellagra, dry scaly cutaneous diseases; *Intramuscular.* **(Cheplin)**

180. **Iron Arsenite with Strychnine**—Ampules 1 cc; Boxes of 12; Containing soluble iron arsenite gr 1 (0.065 Gm) strychnine nitrate gr 1 (0.001 Gm), quinine and urea hydrochloride 0.5%; *Intramuscular; For use* in neurasthenia, anemia, malnutrition. **(Cheplin)**

181. **Iron Cacodylate**—Ampules 1 and 2 cc; Boxes of 12; Containing gr ½ (0.032 Gm); *Intramuscular; For use* in anemia, malnutrition, pellagra. **(Cheplin)**

182. **Iron Citrate (Green)**—Ampules 1 cc; Boxes of 12; Containing iron and ammonium citrate green gr ¾ (0.05 Gm), 0.5% quinine and urea hydrochloride; *Intramuscular; For use* in anemia, chlorosis. **(Cheplin)**

183. **Magnesium Sulphate**—Ampules 2 cc; Boxes of 12; Containing magnesium sulphate 1.0 Gm in 50% aqueous solution, sterilized; *Intramuscular; For use* in obstetrics with morphine and ether anesthesia, in tetanus, chorea minor, eclampsia, puerperal sepsis. **(Cheplin)**

184. **Mercury Salicylate**—Ampules 1 cc; Boxes of 12; Containing gr 1 (0.065 Gm); Antisyphilitic; *Intramuscular.* **(Cheplin)**

185. **Mercury Succinimide**—Ampules 1 cc; Boxes of 12; Containing gr ⅙ (0.01 Gm) Antisyphilitic; *Intramuscular. See Chap. I.* **(Cheplin)**

186. **Ovarian Substance**—Ampules 1 cc; Boxes of 12; Containing soluble substances derived from 40 gr fresh ovarian substance; *For use* in disorders of menopause, or female reproductive development. *See Chap. IV.* **(Cheplin)**

187. **Phenolsulphonphthalein**—Ampules 1 cc; Boxes of 12; Containing gr 6 mg monosodium salt, *For use* in renal function tests; *Intramuscular. See Chap. I.* **(Cheplin)**

188. **Procaine Hydrochloride**—Ampules 1 cc; Boxes of 12; Containing gr 3/10 (0.02 Gm); aqueous 2% solution; Local anesthetic in minor surgery and dentistry. *See Chap. I.* **(Cheplin)**

189. **Procaine and Adrenalin**—Ampules 1 cc; Boxes of 12; Containing procaine hydrochloride gr ⅓ (0.02 Gm), adrenalin 1/1600 gr (0.00004 Gm), 0.5% chlorbutanol, in sterile solution; *For use* as local anesthetic, the adrenalin prolonging anesthetic effect of procaine. *See Chap. I.* **(Cheplin)**

190. **Quinine and Urea Hydrochloride**—Ampules 2 cc; Boxes of 12; Containing gr 15½ (1.0 Gm), Antimalarial. *See Chap. II.* **(Cheplin)**

191. Sodium Cacodylate—Ampules 1 cc; Boxes of 12; Containing gr ¾ (0.05 Gm) or gr 1½ (0.1 Gm); *Intramuscular.* (Cheplin)

192. Sodium Cacodylate—Ampules 2 cc; Boxes of 12; Containing gr 15½ (1.0 Gm); *Intramuscular.* (Cheplin)

193. Sodium Citrate—Ampules 50 cc; Boxes of 1; 2½% Solution; *For use* in blood transfusions to prevent coagulation. (Cheplin)

194. Solution Corpus Luteum—Ampules 1 cc; Boxes of 6; Containing soluble solids gr ⅓ of fresh corpus luteum; *For use* in general disorders of menopause. *See Chap. IV.* (Cheplin)

195. Solution Pituitary, Obstetrical U.S.P.X.—Ampules 1 cc; Boxes of 6; *For use* in post-partum hemorrhage, subinvolution, uterine inertia. *See Chap. I.* (Cheplin)

196. Sodium Thiosulphate—Ampules 10 cc; Boxes of 6; Containing gr 15½ (1.0 Gm); *For use* in overcoming toxic reactions of arsenic, bismuth, mercury. *See Chap. I.* (Cheplin)

197. Double Distilled Water (Sterilized)—Ampules 5, 10 and 20 cc; Boxes of 6; Ampules 50 cc; Boxes of 1. (Cheplin)

198. Triple Distilled Water (Sterilized)—Ampules 5 cc; Boxes of 6; *For Intravenous Use.* (Cheplin)

---

199. Agomensin—Ampules 1.1 cc; Cartons of 5 and 20; Containing gr ¾ (0.04 Gm); Hydrosoluble ovarian substance; *For use* in ovarian hypofunction; *Dosage:* 1–4 ampules every 2–3 days. *See Chap. I.* (Ciba)

200. Cibalgine—Ampules 2.3 cc; Boxes of 5; Containing gr 3½ (0.23 Gm) amidopyrin, gr ½ (0.03 Gm) dial; Analgesic, antipyretic, sedative; *Dosage:* 1–2 cc, repeated in 4–6 hr. *See Chap. II.* (Ciba)

201. Coagulen—Ampules 1.5 and 5 cc; Cartons of 5; 3% sterile solution;
Ampules 20 cc; Cartons of 1; 3% sterile solution; Physiological hemostatic; *Dosage:* 1.5–5 cc as preoperative prophylactic; postoperatively up to 20 cc. *See Chap. I.* (Ciba)

202. Coramine—Ampules 1.1 cc; Cartons of 5, 20, 100 and 500;
Ampules 5.5 cc; Cartons of 3 and 12; Circulatory and respiratory stimulant; *Dosage:* 1–2 ampules as necessary. *See Chap. I.* (Ciba)

203. Dial (C.A.)—Ampules 1 cc; Cartons of 5; Containing gr 1½ (0.09 Gm), urethane gr 6 (0.35 Gm);
Ampules 2.3 cc; Cartons of 5, 20 and 100; *For use* as hypnotic, sedative; *Dosage:* 2–4 cc as required. *See Chap. I.* (Ciba)

204. Digifoline (C.A.)—Ampules 1.1 cc; Cartons of 5, 20, 100 and 500;
Ampules 5.0 cc; Cartons of 1; Digitalis therapy; *Dosage:* 1 cc one to four times daily. *See Chap. I.* (Ciba)

205. Nupercaine (C.A.)—Ampules 2 cc; Cartons of 10; Containing 1:200 solution in buffered salt; *For use* in spinal anesthesia;
Ampules 5 cc; Cartons of 10; Containing 1:1,000 in physiological salt solution; *For injection* anesthesia (not spinal);
Ampules 25 cc; Cartons of 1; Containing 1:1,000, in physiological salt solution; *For injection* anesthesia (not spinal);
Ampules 2 or 5 cc; Cartons of 10; Containing Nupercaine 1:1,000 with epinephrine 1:100,000; *For use* in injection anesthesia (not spinal); *Dosage:* 7.5–10 mg dissolved in 2–5 cc solution. *See Chap. I.* (Ciba)

206. Peristaltine—Ampules 1.5 cc; Cartons of 5 and 20; Containing gr 2½; Standardized cascara preparation; *Dosage:* 1 ampule as required. *See Chap. I.* (Ciba)

207. Sistomensin—Ampules 1.1 cc; Cartons of 5 and 20; Containing 0.05 Gm Sistomensin in sterile oily solution; Ovarian hormone; *Dosage:* 1–2 ampules three times weekly. *See Chap. I.* (Ciba)

---

208. Anteri-Cole—Ampules 5 and 15 cc; Boxes of 6; Anterior pituitary; *For use* in secondary amenorrhea, ovarian hypofunction, climacterium; *Dosage:* 1 cc once or twice daily for 8–10 days after menses. *See Chap. I.* (Cole)

209. Hepati-Cole—Ampules 5 cc; Boxes of 6; Hematopoietic; Containing substance equivalent to Gm 20 fresh liver tissue; *Dosage:* 1–2 cc daily, *intramuscularly. See Chap. I.* **(Cole)**

---

210. Atropine Sulphate—Cartridges 1 cc; Boxes of 10; Containing gr 1/50 (0.0013 Gm), or gr 1/100 (0.00065 Gm). **(Cook)**

211. Caffeine Sodium Benzoate—Cartridges 1 cc; Boxes of 10; Containing gr 3¾ (0.25 Gm) or gr 7½ (0.50 Gm). **(Cook)**

212. Codein Sulphate—Cartridges 1 cc; Boxes of ten; Containing gr ½ (0.032 Gm); *For use* as narcotic. **(Cook)**

213. Digitalin (German)—Cartridges 1 cc; Boxes of 10; Containing gr 1/60 (0.001 Gm). *See Chap. I.* **(Cook)**

214. Epinephrin—Cartridges 1 cc; Boxes of 10; Containing 1:1,000 solution. **(Cook)**

215. Glycerophosphate Compound 1—Cartridges 1 cc; Boxes of 10; Containing sodium glycerophosphate gr 1½ (0.1 Gm), strychnine cacodylate gr 1/25 (0.0005 Gm), iron cacodylate gr ⅙ (0.01 Gm). **(Cook)**

216. Montague 1—Cartridges 1 and 5 cc; Boxes of (1 cc) 10, (5 cc) 10 and 100; Containing quinine and urea hydrochloride 5%, epinephrin gr 1/3,000; *For use* in hemorrhoids. **(Cook)**

217. Montague 2—Cartridges 1 and 5 cc; Boxes of (1 cc) 10, (5 cc) 10 and 100; Containing cresylic acid 10% in glycerin base; *For use* in hemorrhoids. **(Cook)**

218. Morphin Sulphate—Cartridges 1 cc; Boxes of 10; Containing gr ½ (0.032 Gm), gr ¼ (0.016 Gm), gr ⅛ (0.008 Gm). **(Cook)**

219. Morphin and Atropin—Cartridges 1 cc; Boxes of 10; Containing morphin gr ½ (0.032 Gm) and atropin gr 1/75 (0.0008 Gm), or morphin gr ½ (0.032 Gm) and atropin gr 1/150 (0.0004 Gm), or morphin gr ¼ (0.016 Gm) and atropin gr 1/150 (0.0004 Gm). **(Cook)**

220. Morphin and Hyoscin—Cartridges 1 cc; Boxes of 10; Containing morphine gr ⅙ (0.011 Gm), hyoscine hydrobromide gr 1/150 (0.0004 Gm). **(Cook)**

221. Procain and Epinephrin—Cartridges 5 cc; Boxes of 10 and 100; Containing procain gr ⅓ (0.02 Gm) and epinephrin gr 1/1,200 (0.00005 Gm), or procain gr ⅙ (0.01 Gm) and epinephrin gr 1/1,200 (0.00005 Gm), or procain gr ⅓ (0.02 Gm) and epinephrin gr 1/3,000 (0.00002 Gm), or procain gr ⅙ (0.01 Gm) and epinephrin gr 1/3,000 (0.00002 Gm); *For use* as local anesthetic. **(Cook)**

222. Procain—Cartridges 5 cc; Boxes of 10 and 100; Containing gr ⅓ (0.02 Gm), 2% solution;
Cartridges 5 cc; Boxes of 10 and 100; Containing gr ⅙ (0.01 Gm), 1% solution; *For use* as local anesthetic. *See Chap. I.* **(Cook)**

---

223. Collosol Ferro-Manganese—Arsenic—Ampules 0.5, 1 and 2 cc; Boxes of 6; Containing iron as hydroxide and arsenite 1:4,000; manganese arsenite 1:1,000, arsenic 1:2,000; *For use* in anemias, chronic skin diseases; *Dosage:* 1–2 cc twice weekly. *See Chap. I.* **(Crookes)**

224. Collosol Ferro-Manganese—Ampules 1 and 5 cc; Boxes of 6; Containing colloidal iron 1:1,200, colloidal manganese 1:1,000; *For use* as hematinic, in menstrual disorders, some skin disorders; *Dosage:* 1–2 cc, *intramuscularly,* every 4 days. *See Chap. I.* **(Crookes)**

225. Collosol Hydrargyrum—Ampules 3 cc; Boxes of 6; Containing colloidal mercury 1%; Antisyphilitic; *Dosage:* 1 ampule three times weekly. *See Chap. I.* **(Crookes)**

226. Collosol Iodine—Ampules 1 cc; Boxes of 6; Containing 1%; Iodine therapy; *Intramuscular;*
Ampules 5, 10, 20, 25 cc; Boxes of 6; Containing 0.2% iodine;
Ampules 10 cc; Boxes of 6; Containing 0.4% iodine;

Ampules 1 cc; Boxes of 6; Containing 0.8% iodine; *Dosage:* 1 cc every 4 days. *See Chap. I.* (Crookes)

227. Collosol Manganese—Ampules 0.5, 1 and 2 cc; Boxes of 6; Containing manganese 0.25% in emulsoid; *For use* as general antiseptic; *Dosage:* 0.5–1 cc *intramuscularly* every 2–3 days. *See Chap. I.* (Crookes)

228. Collosol Palladium—Ampules 0.5 and 1 cc; Boxes of 6; Containing colloidal metallic palladium 1:2,000; *For use* in gonorrheal and coccogenic infections, epilepsy; *Dosage:* 0.5–1 cc *intramuscularly*, as required. *See Chap. I.* (Crookes)

229. Collosol Selenium—Ampules 1, 5 and 10 cc; Boxes of 6; Containing 0.05% solution, colloidal form; Palliative in malignant, inoperable cases; *Dosage:* 5 cc twice weekly, intramuscularly. *See Chap. I.* (Crookes)

230. Collosol Stannum—Ampules 1 and 2 cc; Boxes of 6; Containing stannum oleate 1:2,000; *For use* in furunculosis; *Dosage:* 1 cc *intramuscularly* every 2–3 days. *See Chap. I.* (Crookes)

231. Collosol Sulphur—Ampules 1, 2, 5 and 10 cc; Boxes of 6; Colloidal sulphur; Containing 0.1% sulphur solution; *Dosage:* 1–2 cc *intramuscularly* twice weekly. *See Chap. I.* (Crookes)

232. Calcium Levulinate—Ampules 2 and 10 cc; Boxes of 6; Containing 1.31% calcium, equivalent to 1.82% calcium oxide; 10% aqueous solution; Calcium therapy; *Dosage:* 2 cc *intramuscularly*, as necessary. *See Chap. I.* (Crookes)

234. Collosol Antimony—Ampules 0.5, 1, 2, 5, 10 cc; Boxes of 6; Containing antimony sulphide 0.04%; Colloidal antimony; *Dosage:* 2–10 cc one or two times weekly, *intramuscularly*, *See Chap. I.* (Crookes)

235. Collosol Argentum—Ampules 2, 5 and 10 cc; Boxes of 6; Colloidal silver 1:2,000 or 0.05%; *Dosage:* 1 ampule two to three times weekly, *intramuscularly. See Chap. I.* (Crookes)

236. Collosol Arsenic—Ampules 1 and 2 cc; Boxes of 6; Colloidal arsenic; Containing 0.0013 Gm arsenic acid (1/15 gr); *Dosage:* 1 cc twice weekly, *intramuscularly. See Chap. I.* (Crookes)

237. Collosol Aurum—Ampules 1 and 2 cc; Boxes of 6; Metallic gold 0.05% aqueous colloidal suspension 1:8,000; *Dosage:* 1 ampule every 2–4 days, *intramuscularly. See Chap. I.* (Crookes)

238. Collosol Calcium—Ampules 0.5, 1 and 2 cc; Boxes of 6; Colloidal calcium; Containing calcium 0.05%, aqueous solution 0.85%; *Dosage:* 1 cc two to three times weekly. *See Chap. I.* (Crookes)

239. Collosol Calcium with Lecithin—Ampules 0.5, 1 and 2 cc; Boxes of 6; Containing collosol calcium with lecithin 1%; *For use* in nervous debility, emotional disturbances; *Dosage:* 0.5–2 cc daily. *See Chap. I.* (Crookes)

240. Collosol Ferro-Arsenicum—Ampules 1 and 2 cc; Boxes of 6; Containing colloidal iron hydroxide 0.05%, colloidal arsenic sulphide 0.033%; *For use* in anemias, as hematinic; *Dosage:* 2 cc once or twice weekly. *See Chap. II.* (Crookes)

241. Collosol Ferro-Arsenicum and Strychnine 0.1%—Ampules 1 and 2 cc; Boxes of 6; *Use, dosage* and *content* as above. *See Chap. II.* (Crookes)

242. Collosol Ferrum—Ampules 1 and 2 cc; Boxes of 6; Containing ferric hydroxide; 1:2,000 solution; Colloidal iron; *Dosage:* 2 cc once or twice weekly. *See Chap. I.* (Crookes)

243. Collosol Trimine—Ampules 1 cc; Boxes of 6; Containing colloidal iron, manganese hydroxide, zinc hydroxide; *For use* in subacute recurrent urethritis, gonorrheal ophthalmia; *Dosage:* 0.5–1.5 cc *intramuscularly* every 3 days till 6 cc are injected. *See Chap. I.* (Crookes)

244. Colsul—Ampules 1, 2, 5, 10 cc; Boxes of 6; Containing 1% solution of elementary sulphur in water *or* olive oil; Pyrexia therapy; *Dosage:* 0.5–5 cc as required. *See Chap. I.* (Crookes)

245. Manganese Butyrate—Ampules 1 cc; Boxes of 6; *For use* in acute streptococcal infections; *Dosage:* 1 ampule as required. *See Chap. I.* **(Crookes)**

246. Tetanol-Collosol—Ampules 2 cc; Boxes of 6; Containing 13% calcium; *Dosage:* 1 ampule *intramuscularly* as required. *See Chap. I.* **(Crookes)**

247. Collosol Cuprum—Ampules 1, 2, 3 and 5 cc; Boxes of 6; Colloidal copper; Containing 0.05% colloidal suspension of copper; *Dosage:* 3 cc intramuscularly every 3 days. *Combinations*—Collosol Cuprum et Ferrum; Containing cuprum 1:20,000;
Ampules 1 and 2 cc; Boxes of 6—Collosol Cuprum et Ferro-Arsenicum; Containing cuprum 1:20,000;
Ampules 1 and 2 cc; Boxes of 6—Collosol Cuprum et Ferro-Manganese; Containing cuprum 1:20,000;
Ampules 1 and 2 cc; Boxes of 6. *See Chap. I.* **(Crookes)**

---

248. Coliron—Ampules 1 cc; Boxes of 12 and 100; Containing gr ½ (0.03 Gm); Colloidal iron cacodylate;
Ampules 2 cc; Boxes of 12 and 100; Containing gr 1 (0.065 Gm);
Ampules 5 cc; Boxes of 12 and 100; Containing gr 2½ (0.16 Gm); Iron and arsenic therapy, *for use* in secondary anemias, tuberculosis, syphilis, convalescence; *Dosage:* 12 injections, ½–2½ gr at 1–4 day intervals; *intramuscularly.* **(Cutter)**

249. Glycero-Coliron—Ampules 1 cc; Boxes of 12 and 100; Containing colloidal iron cacodylate gr ⅓ (0.02 Gm), sodium glycerophosphate gr 1½ (1 Gm), strychnine sulphate gr 1/128 (0.0005 Gm);
Ampules 2 cc; Boxes of 12 and 100; Containing colloidal iron cacodylate gr ⅔ (0.04 Gm), sodium glycerophosphate gr 3 (0.2 Gm), strychnine sulphate gr 1/64 (0.001 Gm); *For use* as hematinic and tonic; *Dosage:* 1–2 cc at 2–7 day intervals; *Intramuscularly.* **(Cutter)**

250. Glycerophosphate Compound—Ampules 1 cc; Boxes of 12 and 100; Containing sodium glycerophosphate gr 1½ (1 Gm), sodium cacodylate gr 1 (0.065 Gm), iron cacodylate gr ⅙ (0.011 Gm), strychnine sulphate gr 1/128 (0.0005 Gm); *For use* as hematinic and tonic; *Dosage:* 1–2 cc at 2–7 day intervals; *Intramuscularly.* **(Cutter)**

251. Iron Arsenite and Strychnine Sulphate—Ampules 1 cc; Boxes of 12 and 100; Containing iron arsenite gr 1 (0.065 Gm) and strychnine sulphate gr 1/64 (0.001 Gm); *For use* as cardiac stimulant and hematinic. **(Cutter)**

252. Iron Cacodylate—Ampules 1 cc; Boxes of 12 and 100; Containing gr ½ (0.032 Gm);
Ampules 2 cc; Boxes of 12 and 100; Containing gr 1 (0.065 Gm);
Ampules 5 cc; Boxes of 12 and 100; Containing gr 2½ (0.16 Gm); *For use* in secondary anemias, tuberculosis, syphilis and convalescence; *Dosage:* 12 injections, 1½ gr, at 2–3 day intervals; *intramuscularly.* **(Cutter)**

253. Sodium Cacodylate—Ampules 1 cc; Boxes of 12 and 100; Containing gr 3 (0.194 Gm), or gr 5 (0.32 Gm); *For use* in syphilis, anemia, tuberculosis, neuralgia, dry scaly skin conditions; *Dosage:* gr ¾ initially, gradually increase. **(Cutter)**

254. Silver Nitrate Solution—Beeswax ampules—1% (0.02 cc) for ophthalmia prevention. *Dosage:* 2 drops in each eye. Boxes of 12 and 100. **(Cutter)**

---

255. Bi-Na-Gluconate—Ampules 2 cc; Boxes of 12, 25 and 100; Containing metallic bismuth gr ¼ (0.016 Gm) with 2% benzylic alcohol as local anesthetic; *For use* in tertiary and congenital syphilis, interstitial keratitis; *Intragluteally* injected. **(Drug Products)**

256. Caffeine and Sodium Benzoate—Ampules 2 cc; Boxes of 12 and 100; Containing gr 7½ (0.5 Gm). **(Drug Products)**

257. Camphor—Ampules 1 cc; Boxes of 12 and 100. **(Drug Products)**

257a. Colloidal Calcium Malate—Hyposols 5 cc; Boxes of 12, 25 and 100; Containing elemental calcium 0.05 Gm in double distilled deaerated water; *For use* in calcium therapy; *Dosage:* intragluteally or intramuscularly 2 to 3 times weekly. (Drug Products)

258. Corpteum—Ampules 1 cc; Boxes of 12 and 100; Representing gr 3 (0.194 Gm) dessicated corpus luteum substance. (Drug Products)

259. Iron and Ammonium Citrate—Ampules 1 cc; Boxes of 12 and 100; Containing gr 1½ (0.097 Gm). (Drug Products)

260. Iron Arsenite and Strychnine—Ampules 1 cc; Boxes of 12 and 100; Containing metallic iron gr ⅙ (0.01 Gm), arsenic trioxide gr 1/10 (0.008 Gm), strychnine nitrate gr 1/65 (0.001 Gm). (Drug Products)

261. Iron Cacodylate—Ampules 1 cc; Boxes of 12 and 100; Containing colloidal iron cacodylate gr ½ (0.032 Gm). (Drug Products)

262. Iron and Nuclein Compound—Ampules 1 cc; Boxes of 12 and 100; Containing iron and ammonium citrate gr ¾ (0.05 Gm), sodium arsenate gr 1/65 (0.001 Gm), strychnine sulphate gr 1/65 (0.001 Gm), nuclein solution m 10 (0.61 cc). (Drug Products)

263. Man-Glu-Col—Ampules 1 cc; Boxes of 12, 25 and 100; Containing metallic manganese 0.003 Gm, benzylic alcohol 2% as local anesthetic, distilled (double) water q.s.; *For use* in staphylococcus and gonococcus infections; *Dosage:* in staphylococcus infections, acne, boils—0.5 cc on first day, gradually increased every fourth day until 2 cc are given; in gonococcus infections—first, third and fifth day 0.5 cc, seventh day 1.0 cc; *Intramuscularly* only. (Drug Products)

264. Orchic Solution—Ampules 1 cc; Boxes of 12 and 100; Containing gr ⅓ soluble solids from fresh testicular substance. *See Chap. IV.* (Drug Products)

265. Ovarian Solution—Ampules 1 cc; Boxes of 12 and 100; Representing gr 40 (2.59 Gm) fresh whole ovary substance. *See Chap. IV.* (Drug Products)

266. Pit-Ren—Double ampule—Amber portion containing ½ cc epinephrin hydrochloride 1:1,000, chlorbutanol, with sterile normal saline; Flint glass portion contains ½ cc pituitary solution; each portion may be used independently or combined, as indicated. (Drug Products)

267. Pituitary Solution—Ampules ½ cc; Boxes of 12 and 100; Containing 5 units;
Ampules 1 cc; Boxes of 12 and 100; Containing 10 units; *For surgical or obstetrical use;*
Ampules 1 cc; Boxes of 12 and 100; Containing 20 units; *For surgical use* only. *See Chap. I.* (Drug Products)

268. Procaine Solution—Ampules 2 cc; Boxes of 12 and 100; Containing 2% procaine. *See Chap. I.* (Drug Products)

269. Sodium Cacodylate—Ampules 1 cc; Boxes of 12 and 100; Containing gr ¾ (0.048 Gm), gr 1½ (0.097 Gm), gr 3 (0.197 Gm), gr 5 (0.324 Gm). (Drug Products)

270. Sodium Glycerophosphate Compound 1—Ampules 1 cc; Boxes of 12 and 100; Containing iron cacodylate colloidal gr ⅙ (0.01 Gm), strychnine cacodylate gr 1/125 (0.0005 Gm), sodium glycerophosphate gr 1½ (0.097 Gm); *For use* in chlorosis, neurasthenia and anemia. (Drug Products)

271. Sodium Glycerophosphate Compound 2—Ampules 1 cc; Boxes of 12 and 100; Containing iron cacodylate colloidal gr ⅓ (0.02 Gm), strychnine cacodylate gr 1/65 (0.001 Gm), sodium glycerophosphate gr 3 (0.194 Gm); *For use* as above. (Drug Products)

272. Sodium Glycerophosphate Compound 3—Ampules 1 cc; Boxes of 12 and 100; Containing sodium glycerophosphate gr 1½ (0.097 Gm), strychnine cacodylate gr 1/125 (0.0005 Gm); *For use* as above. (Drug Products)

272a. Sulphur Colloidal Isotonic—Hyposols 1 cc; Boxes of 10, 25 and 100; Containing colloidal sulphur 10 mg., isotonic solution q.s. 1 cc; *For use* in arthritis, rheumatism, neuritis, and dermatologic affections; *Dosage:* 1 hyposol twice weekly for 25 to 30 injections, intramuscularly, also intravenously. **(Drug Products)**

---

273. Aolan—Ampules 5 and 10 cc; Boxes of 5 and 100; Containing lactalbumin in colloidal form; Protein therapy; *Intramuscular; Dosage:* 5–10 cc every 2–5 days; Children, 1–3 cc. *See Chap. I.* **(Duke)**

274. Aolan—Ampules 1 cc; Boxes of 5 and 100; Contents as above; *Intradermal; Dosage:* 0.2–0.3 cc daily. *See Chap. I.* **(Duke)**

---

275. Acetyl Choline Bromide—Ampules of 0.1 Gm; Bottles of 1, 3, 5 and 01 Gm; Vasodilator; *Dosage:* 0.05–0.1 Gm daily. *See Chap. I.* **(Eastman)**

---

276. Ampoules "Reipar"—Ampules 1 cc; Boxes of 10; Salicylic acid injection therapy; *For use* as analgesic; *Dosage:* 1–10 cc as required, injected over most painful points. *See Chap. II.* **(Fougera)**

277. Bismuthoidol (Robin)—Ampules 2 cc; Boxes of 10 and 50; Containing gr ⅛ metallic bismuth; Colloidal metallic bismuth; *For use* in syphilis; *Dosage:* 1 ampule *intramuscularly* every 2–3 days. *See Chap. I.* **(Fougera)**

278. Camphro-Salyl Ampules "Fraisse"—Ampules 5 cc; Boxes of 6; Containing benzyl salicylate gr 0.50, camphor gr 0.10, pure olive oil 5 cc; Analgesic; *Dosage:* 1 ampule every 2–3 days injected over most painful areas. *See Chap. II.* **(Fougera)**

279. Delbiase (Gelodelbiase)—Ampules 5 cc; Boxes of 6; Biological stimulant; *Intramuscular; Dosage:* 1 ampule every other day. *See Chap. III.* **(Fougera)**

280. Digitaline "Nativelle"—Ampules 1 cc; Containing 0.25 Gm in oil; Digitalis therapy; *Dosage:* 1 ampule daily, *intramuscularly,* for 3–4 days. *See Chap. I.* **(Fougera)**

281. Ferruginous Compound "Fraisse"—Ampules 1 cc; Boxes of 12 and 50; Containing iron cacodylate gr ⅙ (0.011 Gm), sodium glycerophosphate gr 1½ (0.10 Gm), strychnine cacodylate gr 1/120 (0.0005 Gm); Hematinic; *Dosage:* 1 ampule daily for 12 days. *See Chap. II.* **(Fougera)**

282. Hypotens "Fraisse"—Ampules 2 cc; Boxes of 12; *For use* in arterial hypertension, arteriosclerosis, angina pectoris, Bright's disease; *Dosage:* 1 ampule daily for 12 days. *See Chap. III.* **(Fougera)**

283. Iodo-Bismuthate of Quinine "Fraisse"—Ampules 4 cc; Boxes of 6 and 25; Containing 0.2 Gm in olive oil;
Ampules 3 cc; Boxes of 6 and 25; Containing 0.3 Gm in olive oil; Antiluetic; *Dosage:* 0.2–0.3 Gm, *intramuscularly,* every 3–5 days for 20 injections. *See Chap. I.* **(Fougera)**

284. Lipiodol "Lafay"—Ampules 1 cc; Boxes of 12.
Ampules 2 cc; Boxes of 8.
Ampules 3 cc; Boxes of 6.
Ampules 5 cc; Boxes of 4; *For use* as X-Ray contrast medium; *Dosage:* intratracheal injections, 1–5 cc as required. *See Chap. I.* **(Fougera)**

285. Naiodine "Logeais"—Ampules 5, 10 and 20 cc; Boxes of 6; Containing sodium iodide gr ⅙; *For use* as an antispasmodic and general sedative; *Dosage: intramuscularly,* 20–40 cc two to three times daily. *See Chap. I.* **(Fougera)**

286. Neusthenic—Ampules 1 cc; Boxes of 12 and 50; Containing sodium glycerophosphate gr 1½ (0.09 Gm), strychnine cacodylate gr 1/120 (0.0005 Gm); *For use* as dynamic stimulant; *Dosage:* 1 ampule daily for 12 days. *See Chap. II.* **(Fougera)**

287. Ouabaine "Arnaud"—Ampules 2 cc; Boxes of 6; *For use* in acute heart failure, arrhythmia, nephritic heart; Containing gr 1/120 (0.50 mg); *Dosage:* 1–2 ampules daily for 3–5 days; *intramuscularly. See Chap. I.* **(Fougera)**

288. Sol-Bi "Fraisse"—Ampules 2 cc; Packages of 6 and 25; Containing 0.08 Gm; *For use* as Spirocheticide and antiluetic; (4% metallic bismuth) *Dosage: intramuscularly*, 1 ampule every 3 days. *See Chap. I.* (Fougera)

289. Tiodine "Cognet"—Ampules 1 cc; Boxes of 12; Containing gr 0.20; *For use* as iodine-sulphur therapy; *Dosage: intramuscularly*, 1 ampule every 2 days. *See Chap. I.* (Fougera)

---

290. Neo Riodine "Astier"—Ampules 5 cc; Boxes of 10 and 50; Containing 44% iodine; *For use* in cardiovascular lesions with fibrous changes, aortitis, angina pectoris, coronary sclerosis, arterial hypertension, lues; *Dosage: intramuscularly*, 2–5 cc two to three times weekly. *See Chap. I.* (Gallia)

---

291. Adreno-Cortin—Ampules 1 cc; Boxes of 5; Representing 5 Gm adrenal cortex; *For use* in hypoadrenia, Addison's disease, cachexia and fatigue syndrome; *Dosage:* 1 ampule daily. *See Chap. IV.* (Harrower)

292. Anabolin and Anabolin Fortior—Ampules 1 cc; Boxes of 5; Representing 1 gr (0.064 Gm) hepatic extract; *For use* in hypertension, menopause; *Dosage:* 1 ampule daily. Anabolin Fortior—double strength. *See Chap. I.* (Harrower)

293. Apestrin—Ampules 1 cc; Boxes of 5; Representing the anterior pituitary estrin; *For use* where estrin is indicated; *Dosage:* 1 ampule daily or every other day. *See Chap. IV.* (Harrower)

294. Endothyrin—Ampules 1 cc; Boxes of 5; Representing 20 gr (1.296 Gm) fresh thyroid gland and 0.05% of titratable iodine; *For use* in hypothyroidism, suboxidation, obesity; *Dosage:* 1 ampule daily or every other day. *See Chap. IV.* (Harrower)

295. Endovarin—Ampules 1 cc; Boxes of 5; Representing 23 gr (1.490 Gm) ovarian substance; *For use* in hypo-ovarism, menopause, scanty menstruation, asexualism; *Dosage:* 1 ampule every other day for 3 days, beginning 10 days before period, then 3–5 days prior to menstruation; injected daily *intramuscularly. See Chap. II.* (Harrower)

296. Heparhemin—Ampules 5 cc; Boxes of 5; Representing 100 Gm fresh liver; *For use* in pernicious anemia and severe secondary anemias; *Dosage:* 1 ampule *intramuscularly*, daily, then 1–2 injections weekly. (Harrower)

297. Liq. Pituitarii—Ampules 1 cc; Boxes of 5; Representing 10 I.U.; *For use* where Pituitrin is indicated; *Dosage:* ½–1 ampule *intramuscularly* as required. *See Chap. I.* (Harrower)

298. Lydin Solution—Ampules 1 cc; Boxes of 5; Representing 100 Gm male interstitial tissue; *For use* in hypogonadism, impotence, asexualism, presenility; *Dosage:* 1 ampule intramuscularly, daily. (Harrower)

299. Paracalcin—Ampules 1 cc; Boxes of 5; Representing 10 units, standardized; *For use* in parathyroid insufficiency and calcium metabolism disorders; *Dosage:* 1 ampule every 1–2 days. *See Chap. IV.* (Harrower)

300. Plestrin—Ampules 1 cc; Boxes of 5; Representing 50 rat units placental estrin; *For use* in ovarian insufficiency, infantilism, primary amenorrhea, sterility; *Dosage:* 1 ampule intramuscularly, daily. *See Chap. I.* (Harrower)

301. Pituthymin—Ampules 1 cc; Boxes of 5; Representing 10 I.U. of posterior pituitary and thymus; *For use* where Liq. Pituitarii is indicated; *Dosage:* ½–1 ampule intramuscularly every 1–2 days. *See Chap. IV.* (Harrower)

302. Splenocrin—Ampule-vials 20 cc; Representing the active fraction of the spleen, influencing mineral balance and skin nutrition; *For use* in splenomegaly, eosinophilia, eczema, urticaria; *Dosage:* 2–20 cc *intramuscularly*, repeated as necessary. *See Chap. IV.* (Harrower)

303. Solution Adreno-Spermin—Ampules 1 cc; Boxes of 5; Representing 20 gr (1.296 Gm) fresh glands in proportions of: spermin 24, total adrenal 3, thyroid 1; *For use* in deficient oxidation, fatigue syndrome, hypotension, neurosis; *Dosage:* 1 ampule every second day. (Harrower)

304. **Solution Gonad Compound**—Ampules 1 cc; Boxes of 5; Representing 20 gr (1.296 Gm) in proportions: prostate 18, lydin 12, anterior pituitary 12, adrenal 6, thyroid 1; *For use* in functional impotence, aspermia, sexual neurasthenia; *Dosage:* 1 ampule daily or every other day. **(Harrower)**

305. **Solution Menocrin**—Ampules 1 cc; Boxes of 5; Representing 20 gr (1.296 Gm) glandular substance in proportions: ovary 36, pituitary 3, thyroid 1; *For use* in amenorrhea, dysmenorrhea, sexual apathy, neuroses and psychoses; *Dosage:* 1 ampule every second day. **(Harrower)**

306. **Solution Para-Spleen Compound**—Ampules 1 cc; Boxes of 5, Representing 20 gr (1.296 Gm) fresh glands in proportions: spleen 10, parathyroid 1; *For use* in parathyroid insufficiency and where calcium is indicated; *Dosage:* 1 ampule every other day for 2 mo. **(Harrower)**

307. **Solution Pituitary Compound**—Ampules 1 cc; Boxes of 5; Representing 18½ gr (1.199 Gm) anterior lobe and 1 gr (0.064 Gm) posterior lobe; *For use* in adiposogenital dystrophy, infantilism, gonadal maldevelopment; *Dosage:* 1 ampule every 1–2 days. **(Harrower)**

308. **Solution Placento-Luteum Compound**—Ampules 1 cc; Boxes of 5; Representing 20 gr (1.296 Gm) fresh glands in proportions: placenta 3, corpora lutea 1; *For use* in vomiting and nausea of pregnancy; *Dosage:* 1 ampule every 12–24 hr. **(Harrower)**

309. **Thymocrin**—Ampules 1 cc; Boxes of 5; Representing thymus nucleoprotein; *For use* in certain dermatoses, psoriasis and arthritis; *Dosage:* 1 cc *intramuscularly* every 1–2 days. **(Harrower)**

---

310. **Adrenapit**—Swab-Seals 15 cc; Containing epinephrin chloride 1:1,000 solution; *For use* in raising blood pressure in shock and in anesthetic accidents; *Dosage:* small initial dose, increased as necessary. **(Harvey Pittinger)**

311. **Atropine Sulphate**—Swab-Seals 15 cc; Containing gr 1/100 per cubic centimeter; *For use* in checking secretions, to relieve spasm, stimulate circulation and respiration; *Dosage:* 1 cc, as indicated. **(Harvey Pittinger)**

312. **Caffeine and Sodium Benzoate**—Swab-Seals 15 cc; Containing gr 3⅞ per cubic centimeter; *For use* as diuretic, cerebral stimulant, cardiac stimulant in cardiac dropsy, senile pneumonia; *Dosage:* 2 cc, as indicated. **(Harvey Pittinger)**

313. **Calcium Cacodylate**—Swab-Seals 15 cc; Containing gr ¾ (0.04860 Gm) per cubic centimeter; *For use* as hematinic and tonic. **(Harvey Pittinger)**

314. **Corpus Luteum Extract**—Swab-Seals 6 and 15 cc; Containing gr 3 (0.194 Gm) per cubic centimeter; *For use* in functional and surgical menopause, functional disorders of generative female organs, habitual abortion; *Dosage:* 1 cc when indicated. *See Chap. IV.* **(Harvey Pittinger)**

315. **Emetine Hydrochloride**—Swab-Seals 15 cc; Containing gr 1/12 (0.005 Gm); *For* dental *use* in pyorrhea alveolaris.
Swab-Seals 15 cc; Containing gr ½ (0.032 Gm); *For use* in amaebic dysentery, hepatitis; *Dosage:* 1 cc. **(Harvey Pittinger)**

316. **Ergopit**—Swab-Seals 6 cc; Containing gr 38 (2.5 Gm) Concentrated ergot; *For use* in uterine inertia and hemorrhage; in pneumonia, peritonitis, meningitis, uterine fibroids; *Dosage:* 15–30 m as indicated. **(Harvey Pittinger)**

317. **Glycerophosphate Compound 2**—Swab-Seals 15 cc; Containing sodium glycerophosphate gr 1½ (0.097 Gm), strychnine cacodylate gr 1/125, iron cacodylate gr ⅙ (0.1 Gm) per cubic centimeter; *For use* as hematinic and tonic; *Dosage:* 1 cc as indicated. **(Harvey Pittinger)**

318. **Iron Arsenite**—Swab-Seals 15 cc; Containing gr 1 (0.065 Gm) per cubic centimeter; *For use* in anemia, chlorosis, dry scaly cutaneous diseases, malarial intoxication, leucocythemia and pseudoleukemia, pellagra and chorea; *Dosage:* 1 cc as indicated. **(Harvey Pittinger)**

319. Iron Arsenite and Strychnine—Swab-Seals 15 cc; Containing iron arsenite gr ¾ (0.04860 Gm) and strychnine nitrate gr 1/64 (0.001 Gm); *For use* as hematinic and tonic; *Dosage:* 1 cc as indicated. **(Harvey Pittinger)**

320. Iron Cacodylate—Swab-Seals 15 cc; Containing gr ½ (0.032 Gm) per cubic centimeter; *For use* as tonic, hematinic and alterative; *Dosage:* 1 cc as indicated. **(Harvey Pittinger)**

321. Iron Citrate—Swab-Seals 15 cc; Containing gr 1 (0.065 Gm) per cubic centimeter; *For use* as tonic and hematinic; *Dosage:* 1 cc as indicated. **(Harvey Pittenger)**

322. Mercury Cacodylate—Swab-Seals 15 cc; Containing gr 1 (0.065 Gm) per cubic centimeter; *For use* as antisyphilitic; *Intragluteally.* **(Harvey Pittenger)**

323. Mercuric Chloride—Swab-Seals 15 cc; Containing gr 1/20 (0.0032 Gm); *For use* as antisyphilitic, in chronic skin affections; chronic rheumatism, as alterative; *Dosage:* 1 cc as indicated. **(Harvey Pittenger)**

324. Mercuric Iodide (Red)—Swab-Seals 15 cc; Containing gr ⅙ (0.01 Gm) per cubic centimeter; *For use* in scrofula and syphilis; *Dosage:* 1 cc as indicated. *See Chap. I.* **(Harvey Pittenger)**

325. Mercury Succinimide—Swab-Seals 15 cc; Containing gr 1/12 (0.005 Gm) per cubic centimeter; *For use* in syphilis, pyorrhea alveolaris; *Dosage:* 1 cc as indicated. *See Chap. I.* **(Harvey Pittenger)**

326. Morphine Sulphate—Swab-Seals 15 cc; Containing gr ¼ (.016 Gm); *For use* in lessening pain, inducing sleep, to check peristalsis and for suppressing cough; *Dosage:* 1 cc as indicated. **(Harvey Pittenger)**

327. Morphine and Atropine 2—Swab-Seals 15 cc; Containing morphine sulphate gr ¼ (0.016 Gm) and atropine sulphate gr 1/150 per cubic centimeter; *For use* as above; *Dosage:* 1 cc as indicated. **(Harvey Pittenger)**

328. Ovarian Extract (Whole)—Swab-Seals 6 cc; Containing gr 3 (0.194 Gm) per cubic centimeter; *For use* in diminished ovarian function; *Dosage:* 1 cc as indicated. *See Chap. IV.* **(Harvey Pittenger)**

329. Ovarian Residue Extract—Swab-Seals 6 and 15 cc; Containing gr 3 (0.194 Gm) per cubic centimeter; *For use* in nausea of pregnancy, types of habitual abortion, diminished ovarian function, natural and surgical. *Chap. IV.* **(Harvey Pittenger)**

330. Pituitary Extract—Swab-Seals 6 and 15 cc; Obstetrical; *For use* in uterine inertia, surgical shock, intestinal and bladder paralysis post-operatively, enuresis; *Dosage:* 1 cc as indicated. *See Chap. I.* **(Harvey Pittenger)**

331. Procaine—Swab-Seals 15 and 60 cc; Containing gr ⅓ (0.0215 Gm) per cubic centimeter; 2% solution; *For use* as local anesthetic. *See Chap. I.* **(Harvey Pittenger)**

332. Quinine Dihydrochloride—Swab-Seals 15 cc; Containing gr 3⅞ (0.251 Gm) per cubic centimeter; *For use* as antimalarial; *Deep intramuscular* injection; *Dosage:* 1 cc as indicated. **(Harvey Pittenger)**

333. Quinine and Urea Hydrochloride—Swab-Seals 30 cc; Containing gr ⅙ (0.01 Gm) per cubic centimeter; *For use* as local anesthetic, 1%, in injection treatment of internal hemorrhoids and as antimalarial in chronic malaria. *See Chap. II.* **(Harvey Pittenger)**

334. Sodium Cacodylate—Swab-Seals 15 cc; Containing gr 1 (0.065 Gm) per cubic centimeter.
Swab-Seals 15 cc; Containing gr 5 (0.324 Gm) per cubic centimeter; *For use* in anemia, chlorosis, chorea, syphilis, malarial cachexia, neurasthenia; *Dosage:* 1 cc as indicated. **(Harvey Pittenger)**

335. Strophanthin—Swab-Seals 30 cc; Containing gr 1/65 (0.001 Gm) per cubic centimeter; *For use* as cardiac stimulant; *Dosage:* 1 cc as indicated. **(Harvey Pittenger)**

336. Strychnine Sulphate—Swab-Seals 15 cc; Containing gr 1/65 (0.001 Gm) per cubic centimeter; *For use* as tonic stimulant to central nervous system, as respiratory stimulant in shock, respiratory depression, narcotic poisoning, alcoholism; *Dosage:* 1 cc as indicated. **(Harvey Pittenger)**

---

337. Siliform—Ampules 1 cc; Boxes of 5 and 100; *For use* as non-specific protein therapy; *Dosage: intragluteally,* 3 ampules every 4–5 days, over painful areas. *See Chap. III.* **(Heilkraft)**

---

338. Caseosan—Ampules 1 cc; Boxes of 10.
Ampules 10 cc; Boxes of 5. Containing 5 % casein solution; *For use* as non-specific protein therapy; *Dosage:* 0.5–2 cc *intramuscularly; intracutaneously*—0.3–1 cc every 1–3 days. *See Chap. I.* **(Heyden)**

340. Sufrogel—Ampules 1 cc; Boxes of 3; Containing finely divided sulphur 0.3 % in gelatin; *For use* in intramuscular sulphur therapy; *Dosage:* 0.2–0.4 cc, *intragluteally,* every 8 days. *See Chap. I.* **(Heyden)**

---

341. Metaphyllin (Aminophyllin)—Ampules 2 cc; Boxes of 6; Containing 0.48 Gm; *For use* as cardiotonic and diuretic; *Dosage: intramuscularly,* 1 ampule as required. *See Chap. I.* **(Hurst)**

---

342. Iodo-Bismuth of Quinine—Ampules 2 cc; Boxes of 10 and 100; Containing 0.04 cgm metalloid bismuth per cubic centimeter; *For use* as antiluetic; *Dosage: intramuscularly,* 1 ampule every 5 days. *See Chap. I.* **(Huxley)**

---

343. Antimony Sodium Thioglycollate (C.A.)—Ampules 10 and 20 cc; Boxes of 12; Containing not less than 37 % antimony; 0.5 % solution; *For use* as trypanosomicide; *Dosage: Intramuscularly,* 1–2 Gm in 10–20 cc sterile water twice weekly for 15–25 injections. *See Chap. I.* **(Hynson, Westcott and Dunning)**

344. Antimony Thioglycollamide—Ampules 10 and 20 cc; Boxes of 12; Containing not less than 30 % antimony; 0.4 % solution; *For use* as trypanosomicide; *Dosage: intramuscularly,* 1–2 gr in 10–20 cc sterile water, twice weekly for 15–25 injections. *See Chap. I.* **(Hynson, Westcott and Dunning)**

345. Benzyl Benzoate—Ampules 1 cc; Boxes of 10; Containing benzyl benzoate 0.5 cc in olive oil; *For use* as antispasmodic; *Dosage: intramuscularly,* 1 ampule as required. *See Chap. I.* **(Hynson, Westcott and Dunning)**

346. Lutein Solution (Corpus Luteum)—Ampules 1 cc; Boxes of 6; Containing water soluble extract 0.2 Gm per cubic centimeter; *For use* in functional ovarian disorders, not anatomical, in retarded ovarian function and development, in sterility; *Dosage:* deep intramuscular injection; in nausea of pregnancy 1 cc daily; in pernicious vomiting 1 cc twice daily. *See Chap. IV.*
(Hynson, Westcott and Dunning)

347. Mercury Salicylate (C.A.)—Ampules gr 1, 1½ and 2; Boxes of 12; *For use* as antiluetic; *Intramuscular*—20 gauge needle; *Dosage:* 1 ampule twice weekly. *See Chap. I.* **(Hynson, Westcott and Dunning)**

348. Ovarian Residue Solution—Ampules 1 cc; Boxes of 6; *For use* in functional ovarian disorders; in retarded ovarian function and development, sterility; Deep *intramuscular* injection; *Dosage:* average case of nausea or vomiting of pregnancy, 1 cc daily for 5 days; severe—1 cc daily for 15 days; pernicious 1 cc twice daily. *See Chap. IV.* **(Hynson, Westcott and Dunning)**

349. Ovarian (Whole) Solution—Ampules 1 cc; Boxes of 6; Containing water soluble extractives of 0.2 Gm; *For use* in delayed menstruation and mal-developement of sexual organs, in influencing general metabolism and fatty tissues; *Intramuscular;* 1 ampule—every 1–2 days. *See Chap. IV.* **(Hynson, Westcott and Dunning)**

350. Ouabain—Ampules of 0.5 mg; Boxes of 4; *For use* as cardiac stimulant; *Dosage: intramuscularly,* 1 ampule in 4,000–8,000 cc saline daily. *See Chap. I.*
(Hynson, Westcott and Dunning)

351. **Phenolsulphonphthalein**—Ampules 1 cc; Boxes of 10; *For use* as renal function test; *Dosage:* with bladder empty, 1 cc is injected, preceded ½ hr. by the drinking of ½–1 glass of water; urine collected in 70 min. and again after 2 hr.; excretion determined colorimetrically. Normal: 1 hr.—50%, 2 hr.—85%. *See Chap. I.* **(Hynson, Westcott and Dunning)**

352. **Red Mercuric Iodide**—Ampules 1 cc; Boxes of 10; Containing gr ⅙ (0.001 Gm) in neutral fatty oil; *For use* as antiseptic and antisyphilitic; *Dosage: intramuscularly,* 1 ampule twice weekly. *See Chap. I.* **(Hynson, Westcott and Dunning)**

---

353. **Endo-Bisarphen**—Ampules 2 cc; Boxes of 12, 25 and 100; Containing bismuth 44 mg, arsenic 16 mg; *For use* in Wassermann-fast syphilis. **(Intravenous Products)**

354. **Endo-Bismulate**—Ampules 2 cc; Boxes of 12, 25 and 100; Containing bismuth salicylate in oil. **(Intravenous Products)**

355. **Endo-Bismuth Soluble**—Ampules 2 cc; Boxes of 12, 25 and 100; Containing neutral water soluble bismuth in 1.5% solution. **(Intravenous Products)**

356. **Endo-Bismuth Suspension**—Ampules 4 cc; also concentrated in 2 cc. Boxes of 12, 25 and 100; Containing quinine-iodo-bismuthate gr 3 (0.194 Gm). **(Intravenous Products)**

357. **Endo-Caffeine Sodium Benzoate**—Ampules 2 cc; Boxes of 12 and 100; Containing gr 7½ (0.5 Gm). **(Intravenous Products)**

358. **Endo-Camphor in Oil**—Ampules 1 and 2 cc; Boxes of 12 and 100; Containing 0.2 Gm.
Ampules 10 cc; Boxes of 12 and 100; Containing 2.35 Gm. **(Intravenous Products)**

359. **Copfersan**—Ampules 2 cc; Boxes of 12 and 100; Containing colloidal copper 0.04 mg, iron cacodylate 0.026 Gm, sodium cacodylate 0.08 Gm.
Ampules 1 cc; Boxes of 12 and 100; Half strength. **(Intravenous Products)**

360. **Endo-Corpus Luteum**—Ampules 1 cc; Boxes of 12 and 100; Containing gr 3 (0.194 Gm). **(Intravenous Products)**

361. **Endo-Ephedrine Sulphate**—Ampules 1 cc; Boxes of 12 and 100; Containing gr ¾ (0.04860 Gm). **(Intravenous Products)**

362. **Endo-Ergot**—Ampules 1 cc; Boxes of 12 and 100. **(Intravenous Products)**

363. **Endogen**—Ampules "A" 2 cc; Boxes of 12, 25 and 100; *For use* in arthritis.
Ampules "G" 2 cc; Boxes of 12, 25 and 100; *For use* in gonorrhea.
Ampules "U" 2 cc; Boxes of 12, 25 and 100; *For use* in ulcer. **(Intravenous Products)**

364. **Endo-Glycerophosphate Compound**—Ampules 1 cc; Boxes of 12 and 100. **(Intravenous Products)**

365. **Endo-Iron Arsenite**—Ampules 1 cc; Boxes of 12 and 100; Containing iron arsenite gr 1 (0.065 Gm), ammonium citrate 0.1. **(Intravenous Products)**

366. **Endo-Iron Arsenite and Strychnine**—Ampules 1 cc; Boxes of 12 and 100. **(Intravenous Products)**

367. **Endo-Iron Cacodylate**—Ampules 1 cc; Boxes of 12 and 100; Containing gr ½ (0.03 Gm), or gr 1 (0.065 Gm). **(Intravenous Products)**

368. **Endo-Iron Citrate**—Ampules 1 cc; Boxes of 12 and 100; Containing gr 1 (0.065 Gm). **(Intravenous Products)**

369. **Endo-Iron Citrate Compound with Nuclein**—Ampules 1 cc; Boxes of 12 and 100. **(Intravenous Products)**

370. **Endolac**—Ampules 5 and 10 cc; Boxes of 6, 25 and 100; Contains sterile milk. **(Intravenous Products)**

371. **Endolac Soluble**—Ampules 5 and 10 cc; Boxes of 5, 25 and 100; Contains fat-free milk. **(Intravenous Products)**

372. **Endo-Liver Extract**—Ampules 1 cc; Boxes of 12, 25 and 100; Containing 50 Gm fresh, refined and concentrated liver; *For use* in pernicious anemia. (Intravenous Products)

373. **Endo-Livolipins**—Ampules 1 cc; Boxes of 12, 25 and 100; Containing liver lipins. Ampules 2 cc; Boxes of 12, 25 and 100; Triple strength. (Intravenous Products)

374. **Endo-Magnesium Sulphate**—Ampules 2 cc; Boxes of 12 and 100; Containing gr 15½ (1.0 Gm). (Intravenous Products)

375. **Manganese Butyrate**—Ampules 1 and 1½ cc; Boxes of 12 and 100; 1 % Solutions. (Intravenous Products)

376. **Endo-Orchic Liquid**—Ampules 1 cc; Boxes of 12 and 100; Contains orchic substance. (Intravenous Products)

377. **Endo-Ovalipins**—Ampules 1 cc; Boxes of 6, 12 and 25; Contains ovarian lipins. (Intravenous Products)

378. **Endo-Ovarian Liquid**—Ampules 1 cc; Boxes of 12 and 100; Contains ovarian substance. (Intravenous Products)

379. **Endo-Paradin**—Ampules 1 cc; Boxes of 12 and 100; Contains parathyroid substance. (Intravenous Products)

380. **Endo-Phenolsulphonphthalein**—Ampules 1 cc; Boxes of 12 and 100; Containing 6 mg. (Intravenous Products)

381. **Endo-Pitrenalin**—Ampules 1 cc; Boxes of 12 and 100; Contains epinephrin-pituitary extracts. (Intravenous Products)

382. **Endo-Pituitary Liquid**—Ampules ½ and 1 cc; Boxes of 12 and 100; *For use* in obstetrics.
Ampules 1 cc; Boxes of 12 and 100; *For surgical use.* (Intravenous Products)

383. **Endo-Pituitary Liquid (Anterior)**—Ampules 1 cc; Boxes of 12 and 100. (Intravenous Products)

384. **Endo-Procaine**—Ampules 2 cc; Boxes of 12 and 100; Containing gr ⅔ (0.04 Gm). (Intravenous Products)

385. **Endo-Quinine Dihydrochloride**—Ampules 1 cc; Boxes of 12 and 100; Containing gr 3¾ (0.243 Gm), or gr 7½ (0.05 Gm).
Ampules 2 cc; Boxes of 12 and 100; Containing gr 15½ (1.0 Gm). (Intravenous Products)

386. **Endo-Quinothane**—Ampules 2 cc; Boxes of 12, 25 and 100; Containing quinine and urethane. (Intravenous Products)

387. **Endo-Sodium Cacodylate**—Ampules 1 cc; Boxes of 12 and 100; Containing gr 1 (0.065 Gm), gr 2 (0.13 Gm), gr 3 (0.2 Gm), gr 5 (0.3 Gm) or gr 7½ (0.5 Gm).
Ampules 2 cc; Boxes of 12 and 100; Containing gr 7½ (0.5 Gm), or gr 15½ (1.0 Gm). (Intravenous Products)

388. **Endo-Solulac Compound**—Ampules 5 and 10 cc; Boxes of 6, 25 and 100; Containing solution endolac 0.75 cc, manganese butyrate 1 %. (Intravenous Products)

389. **Endo-Suprarenalin**—Ampules 1 cc; Boxes of 12 and 100; 1:1,000 Solution. (Intravenous Products)

390. **Endo-Testolipins**—Ampules 1 cc; Boxes of 6, 12 and 25; Contains orchic lipins, gonadal male hormone. (Intravenous Products)

391. **Endo-Yohimbine and Spermin Compound**—Ampules 1 cc; Boxes of 12 and 100; *For use* in neurasthenia and as an aphrodisiac. (Intravenous Products)

---

392. **Chlorine Gas "Roehling"**—Ampules 10 cc; Containing 0.85 Gm chlorine; *For use* as inhalant antiseptic; *Dosage:* by inhalation, 1 ampule opened in 700 cu. ft. room space, room sealed; given once daily. *See Chap. I.* (Lakeside)

393. **Sodium Cacodylate**—Ampules 5 cc, 3¾ gr (0.243 Gm) Boxes 6, 25, 50 and 100. (Lakeside)

394. Epinephrin Hydrochloride—Ampules 1 cc; Boxes of 12; Containing active principle of suprarenal medulla 1:1,000, physiologically standardized; *Dosage:* 0.5–1 cc *intramuscularly*, as required. *See Chap. I.* **(Lederle)**

395. Pituitary Extract (Posterior)—Ampules 1 cc (White); Boxes of 6 and 100; 5 international units.
Ampules 1 cc (Yellow); Boxes of 6 and 100; 10 international units.
Ampules 1 cc (Red); Boxes of 6 and 100; 20 international units. *Dosage:* 0.5–1 cc as required. *See Chap. I.* **(Lederle)**

396. Solution Silver Nitrate 1%—Beeswax Ampules 0.2 cc. Boxes of 12 and 100. *For use* in ophthalmia neonatorum. *Dosage:* 2 drops in each eye. **(Lederle)**

---

397. Amfetin—Ampules 50 cc; Packages of 1, 6 and 25; *For use* in stimulating normal tissue repair in abdominal operations; *Dosage:* Injection by syringe through catheter, of 50–200 cc at body temperature, into peritoneal cavity before closing last suture. *See Chap. I.* **(Lilly)**

398. Amyl Nitrite (Aspirols)—Ampules 3 and 5 m; Boxes of 12; *For use* as vasodilator in angina pectoris, asthma, some forms of migraine; as *inhalant only.* **(Lilly)**

399. Ammonia, Aromatic (Aspirols)—Boxes of 12; *For use* as cardiac stimulant in acute cardiac failure, in syncope; for *inhalation only.* **(Lilly)**

400. Aromatic Spirits of Ammonia—Ampules 2 cc; Boxes of 12; *For use* as respiratory and cardiac stimulant; For *oral* administration only. **(Lilly)**

401. Antimeningococcic Serum—*See Chap. VI.* **(Lilly)**

402. Bismoid—Ampules 1 cc; Boxes of 6; Containing bismuth gr ⅜ (0.25 Gm); *For use* as antiluetic; *Dosage: intramuscularly*, 1 ampule twice weekly. *See Chap. I.* **(Lilly)**

403. Bismuth Salicylate—Ampules of 1 cc; Boxes of 12; Containing gr 2 (0.13 Gm), camphor oil 10%, creosote 10% in vegetable oil; *Intramuscular; For use* as antisyphilitic. **(Lilly)**

404. Caffeine Sodio-Benzoate—Ampules of 2 cc; Boxes of 12; Containing gr 3¾ (0.25 Gm), or gr 7½ (0.5 Gm); *For use* as respiratory stimulant. **(Lilly)**

405. Calcium Cacodylate—Ampules 1 cc; Boxes of 12; Containing gr ¾ (0.05 Gm); *For use* in calcium therapy. **(Lilly)**

407. Camphor in Oil—Ampules 1 cc; Boxes of 12; Containing either gr 1½ (0.1 Gm) or gr 3 (0.2 Gm). *For use* as cardiac stimulant. **(Lilly)**

408. Camphor in Oil—Ampules 5 cc; Boxes of 6; Containing gr 10 (0.65 Gm). *For use* as cardiac stimulant. **(Lilly)**

409. Chaulmoogra Oil Ethylated—Ampules of 1, 3 and 5 cc; Boxes (1 cc) of 12; Boxes of (3, 5 cc) of 6 and 25; *For use* in leprosy. **(Lilly)**

410. Chloroform—Ampules of 30 Gm; Boxes of 6; Convenient dropper container for inhalation. *For use* as anesthetic. **(Lilly)**

411. Corpus Luteum Extract—Ampules 1 cc; Boxes of 6; Representing gr 3 (0.2 Gm) desiccated corpus luteum; *For use* in ovarian dysfunction. *See Chap. IV.* **(Lilly)**

412. Digiglusin—Ampules 1 cc; Boxes of 6; Each cubic centimeter representing 15 m of potent tincture; *For use* and *dosage see Chap. I.* **(Lilly)**

413. Distilled Water—Ampules 5, 10, 20, 50 and 100 cc; Boxes of 6 and 25; Especially processed *for use* in preparing solutions for injection. **(Lilly)**

414. Emetine Hydrochloride—Ampules 1 cc; Boxes of 6 and 12; Containing either gr ⅓ (0.02 Gm), gr ½ (0.032 Gm), gr 1 (0.065 Gm); *For use* in amebic dysentery. **(Lilly)**

415. Ephedrine Sulphate—Ampules 1 cc; Boxes of 6; Containing gr ¾ (0.05 Gm); *For use* as vasconstrictor; *Dosage:* 1 ampule as required. *See Chap. I.* **(Lilly)**

416. **Ephedrine and Caffeine**—Ampules 2 cc; Boxes of 12; Formula A—containing ephedrine sulphate gr ⅜ (0.025 Gm), caffeine sodio-benzoate gr 7½ (0.5 Gm). **(Lilly)**

417. **Ephedrine and Caffeine**—Ampules 4 cc; Boxes of 6; Formula B—containing ephedrine sulphate gr ¾ (0.05 Gm), caffeine sodio-benzoate gr 15½ (1.0 Gm). **(Lilly)**

418. **Glycerophosphate Compound**—Ampules 1 cc; Boxes of 12; Formula A— Containing sodium glycerophosphate gr 1½ (0.1 Gm), strychnine cacodylate gr 1/128 (0.0005 Gm), iron cacodylate gr ⅙ (0.01 Gm); *For use* as hematinic and tonic. **(Lilly)**

419. **Glycerophosphate Compound**—Ampules 1 cc; Boxes of 12; Formula B—containing sodium glycerophosphate gr 1½ (0.1 Gm), strychnine cacodylate gr 1/128 (0.0005 Gm), sodium cacodylate gr ¾ (0.05 Gm). *For use* as tonic. **(Lilly)**

420. **Glycerophosphate Compound**—Ampules 1 cc; Boxes of 12; Formula C—containing sodium glycerophosphate gr 1 (0.065 Gm), iron cacodylate gr ¼ (0.016 Gm), strychnine sulphate gr 1/120 (0.00055 Gm). *For use* as tonic. **(Lilly)**

421. **Hartmann's Solution (Physiological Buffer Solution)**—Ampules 10 and 20 cc; Boxes of 6 and 25. **(Lilly)**

422. **Iodine Tincture, U.S.P.**—Ampules 1 cc; Boxes of 6; With brush for *topical use.* **(Lilly)**

423. **Iron Arsenite, Soluble**—Ampules 1 cc; Boxes of 12; Containing gr ¾ (0.05 Gm), Equivalent to arsenic trioxide gr 1/90 (0.0007 Gm) and iron gr ⅛ (0.008 Gm); *For use* in anemia, and dry scaly skin conditions. **(Lilly)**

424. **Iron Arsenite and Strychnine, 1**—Ampules 1 cc; Boxes of 12; Containing iron arsenite gr ⅜ (0.025 Gm), equivalent to arsenic trioxide gr 1/180 (0.00035 Gm), iron gr 1/16 (0.004 Gm), strychnine nitrate gr 1/64 (0.001 Gm). *For use* as tonic. **(Lilly)**

425. **Iron Arsenite and Strychnine, 2**—Ampules 1 cc; Boxes of 12; Containing iron arsenite gr ¾ (0.05 Gm) equivalent to arsenic trioxide gr 1/90 (0.0007 Gm), iron gr ⅛ (0.008 Gm), strychnine nitrate gr 1/64 (0.001 Gm). *For use* as tonic. **(Lilly)**

426. **Iron Arsenite and Strychnine, 3**—Ampules 1 cc; Boxes of 12; Containing iron arsenite gr 1 (0.065 Gm); equivalent to arsenic trioxide gr 1/70 (0.009 Gm), iron gr ⅙ (0.01 Gm), strychnine nitrate gr 1/64 (0.001 Gm). *For use* as tonic. **(Lilly)**

427. **Iron Cacodylate**—Ampules 1 cc; Boxes of 12; Containing gr ½ (0.032 Gm).
Ampules 1 cc; Boxes of 12; Containing gr ¾ (0.05 Gm).
Ampules 2 cc; Boxes of 12; Containing gr 1 (0.065 Gm) *For use* as hematinic. **(Lilly)**

428. **Iron Citrate (Green) (Iron and Ammonium Citrate, Green)**—Ampules 1 cc; Boxes of 12; Containing gr ¾ (0.05 Gm).
Ampules 1 cc; Boxes of 12; Containing gr 1 (0.065 Gm).
Ampules 1 cc; Boxes of 12; Containing gr 1½ (0.1 Gm); *For use* in anemias and chlorosis. **(Lilly)**

429. **Iron Citrate and Manganese**—Ampules 1 cc; Boxes of 12; Containing iron citrate gr ¾ (0.05 Gm), manganese citrate gr 1/100 (0.00065 Gm) with ½% quinine and urea hydrochloride; *For use* as hematinic. **(Lilly)**

430. **Iron and Arsenic.**—Ampules 1 cc; Boxes of 12; Containing iron and ammonium citrate, green gr ¾ (0.05 Gm); *For use* as hematinic. **(Lilly)**

431. **Lobeline Sulphate**—Ampules 1 cc; Boxes of 12; Containing gr 1/20 (0.003 Gm); *For use* as dental local anesthetic. **(Lilly)**

432. **Liver Extract**—Ampules 10 cc; Rubber-capped; Boxes of 1 ampule; Containing mammalian liver; standardization—3 or 4 Gm representing 100 Gm fresh liver. *For use* as hematinic; *Dosage:* 2 cc daily. *See Chap. I.* **(Lilly)**

433. Magnesium Sulphate—Ampules 2 cc; Boxes of 12; 25% Solution; *For use* in prolonging effect of morphine sulphate. **(Lilly)**

434. Magnesium Sulphate—Ampules 2 cc; Boxes of 12; 50% Solution; *For use* as antispasmodic in tetany, eclampsia. **(Lilly)**

435. Mercuric Iodide (Red)—Ampules 1 cc; Boxes of 12; 1% aqueous solution; *For use* as antisyphilitic. *See Chap. I.* **(Lilly)**

436. Mercury Cyanide—Ampules 1 cc; Boxes of 12; Containing gr 1/6 (0.01 Gm) with procaine 1/2%; *For use* as antisyphilitic. *See Chap. I.* **(Lilly)**

437. Mercuric Salicylate—Ampules 1 cc; Boxes of 12; Containing gr 1 (0.065 Gm) with quinine and urea hydrochloride 1/2%.
Ampules 1 cc; Boxes of 12; Containing gr 1 1/2 (0.1 Gm) with quinine and urea hydrochloride 1/2%.
Ampules 1 cc; Boxes of 12; Containing gr 2 (0.13 Gm) with quinine and urea hydrochloride 1/2%; *For use* as antisyphilitic. *See Chap. I.* **(Lilly)**

438. Mercury Succinimide—Ampules 1 cc; Boxes of 12; Containing gr 1/6 (0.01 Gm); *For use* as antisyphilitic. *See Chap. I.* **(Lilly)**

439. Morphine Sulphate with Magnesium Sulphate—Ampules 2 cc; Boxes of 12; Containing morphine sulphate gr 1/8 with magnesium sulphate 25%.
Ampules 2 cc; Boxes of 12; Containing morphine sulphate gr 1/4 with magnesium sulphate 25%. *For use* in prolonging effect of morphine. **(Lilly)**

440. Ouabain—Ampules 2 cc; Boxes of 12; Containing gr 1/128 (0.0005 Gm); Buffered sterile solution; *For use* as cardiac stimulant of strophanthin type. *Dosage:* 1 ampule diluted, daily. *See Chap. I.* **(Lilly)**

441. Ovarian Extract (Whole)—Ampules 1 cc; Boxes of 6 and 12; Representing gr 10 (0.65 Gm) or gr 31 (2 Gm) fresh ovarian substance including corpus luteum, *For use* in ovarian dysfunction. *See Chap. IV.* **(Lilly)**

442. Ovarian Residue Extract—Ampules 1 cc; Boxes of 12; Representing gr 31 (2 Gm) fresh ovarian substance without corpus luteum; *For use* in ovarian dysfunction. *See Chap. IV.* **(Lilly)**

443. Para-Thor-Mone—Ampules 1 cc; Boxes of 6; Containing 20 units; *For use* as parathyroid therapy; *Dosage:* 20–60 units daily, as required. *See Chap. I.* **(Lilly)**

444. Pituitary Extract, Obstetrical U.S.P.—Ampules 1/2 and 1 cc; Boxes of 6; *For use* in uterine inertia, prevention of post-partum hemorrhage. *See Chap. I.* **(Lilly)**

445. Pituitary Extract, Surgical U.S.P.—Ampules 1/2 and 1 cc; Boxes of 12; *For use* in post-operative intestinal stasis, hemorrhage, shock, enuresis. *See Chap. I.* **(Lilly)**

446. Procaine—Ampules of 1 cc; Boxes of 12; Containing gr 1/6 (0.01 Gm); 1% solution; or gr 1/3 (0.02 Gm) 2% solution; *For use* as local anesthetic. *See Chap. I.* **(Lilly)**

447. Procaine—Ampules of 5 cc; Boxes of 6 and 25; Containing gr 1.3 (0.02 Gm); 2% solution; *For use* as local anesthetic. *See Chap. I.* **(Lilly)**

448. Procaine and Adrenalin—Ampules 1 cc; Boxes of 12; Containing procaine gr 1/3 (0.02 Gm), adrenalin gr 1/1,600 (0.00004 Gm) in Ringer's solution. *For use* as anesthetic. *See Chap. I.* **(Lilly)**

449. Propyl-Cephaeline—Ampules 1 cc; Boxes of 12; Containing gr 1/2 (0.032 Gm); A synthetic ipecac alkaloid; *For use* as amebacide. **(Lilly)**

450. Quinine Dihydrochloride—Ampules 1 cc; Boxes of 12; Containing gr 3 3/4 (0.25 Gm) or gr 7 1/2 (0.5 Gm); *For use* as antimalarial, antipyretic.
Ampules 2 cc; Boxes of 12; Containing gr 15 1/2 (1.0 Gm); For similar purposes. **(Lilly)**

451. Quinine and Urea Hydrochloride—Ampules 1 and 2 cc; Boxes of 12; 5% Solution; *For use* as local anesthetic; Ampules 1 and 2 cc; Boxes of 12; Containing gr 7 1/2 (0.5 Gm), or gr 15 1/2 (1 Gm); *For same use.* **(Lilly)**

452. **Silver Nitrate Solution**—1 and 2% solutions in wax ampules; *For use* in prevention and treatment of ophthalmia neonatorum; expel 2 drops in outer canthus of each eye, lids kept apart; Packages of 24 (in 12 enameled tin boxes). **(Lilly)**

453. **Sodium Cacodylate**—Ampules 1 cc; Boxes of 12; Containing gr ¾ (0.05 Gm); or gr 1½ (0.1 Gm); or gr 2 (0.13 Gm); or gr 3 (0.2 Gm); or gr 7 (0.45 Gm); or gr 5 (0.325 Gm);
Ampules 2 cc; Boxes of 12; Containing gr 15½ (1 Gm); *For use* in anemia, leukemia, pellagra, malarial cachexia. **(Lilly)**

454. **Sodium Chloride**—Ampules 10 cc; Boxes of 6 and 25; Containing gr 31 (2 Gm). **(Lilly)**

455. **Sodium Salicylate**—Ampules 5 cc; Boxes of 6 and 25; Containing gr 31 (2 Gm). *For use* as antirheumatic. **(Lilly)**

456. **Strychnine Sulphate**—Ampules 1 cc; Boxes of 12; Containing gr 1/64 (0.001 Gm); *For use as* respiratory stimulant. **(Lilly)**

457. **Sodium Amytal** —Ampules 0.25 Gm (3¾ gr) 0.5 Gm (7½ gr) 1.0 Gm (15½ gr) with ampule distilled water. Boxes of 1. *For use* as sedative. *See Chap. I.* **(Lilly)**

---

458. **Bismuth in Oil**—Ampules 1 cc; Packages of 12 and 100; Bottles of 30 and 100 cc; Containing 0.1 Gm in 1 cc. **(Loeser)**

459. **Bismuth Tartrate Soluble "Cowleys"**—Ampules 1 cc; Boxes of 12 and 100; Vials 15 cc; Containing 25 mg per cubic centimeter. **(Loeser)**

460. **Caffeine Sodium Benzoate**—Ampules 2 cc; Boxes of 12 and 100; Containing gr 7½ (0.5 Gm). **(Loeser)**

461. **Camphor in Oil**—Ampules 1 cc; Boxes of 12 and 100; Containing 0.2 Gm per cubic centimeter. **(Loeser)**

462. **Copper, Iron and Manganese**—Ampules 1 cc; Boxes of 12 and 100. **(Loeser)**

463. **Ether in Oil**—Ampules 2 cc; Boxes of 12 and 100; Containing 50% each. **(Loeser)**

464. **Iron Arsenite**—Ampules 1 cc; Boxes of 12 and 100; Containing 30 mg. **(Loeser)**

465. **Iron Arsenite and Strychnine**—Ampules 1 cc; Boxes of 12 and 100; Containing iron arsenite 30 mg, strychnine 0.5 mg. **(Loeser)**

466. **Iron Cacodylate**—Ampules 1 cc; Boxes of 12 and 100; Containing 60 mg. **(Loeser)**

467. **Iron Citrate**—Ampules 1 cc; Boxes of 12 and 100; Containing 60 mg. **(Loeser)**

468. **Magnesium Sulphate**—Ampules 2 cc; Boxes of 12 and 100; Containing 50% solution. **(Loeser)**

469. **Mercury Cyanide**—Ampules 1 cc; Boxes of 12 and 100; Containing 30 mg. **(Loeser)**

470. **Phenolsulphonphthalein**—Ampules 1 cc; Boxes of 12 and 100; Containing 6 mg. **(Loeser)**

471. **Procaine Hydrochloride with Suprarenin**—Ampules 1 cc; Boxes of 12 and 100; Containing 2% solution. **(Loeser)**

472. **Quinine and Urea Hydrochloride**—Ampules 1 cc; Boxes of 12 and 100; Containing 0.25 Gm. **(Loeser)**

473. **Sodium Cacodylate**—Ampules 1 cc; Boxes of 12 and 100; Containing 0.1 or 0.3 Gm, or 0.5 Gm. **(Loeser)**

---

474. **Arsphenamine**—Ampules 0.1, 0.2, 0.3, 0.4, 0.5, 0.6, 1.0 Gm; *For use* as antiluetic; *Dosage:* 0.3–0.45 Gm twice weekly, *intramuscularly. See Chap. I.* **(Mallinckrodt)**

475. **Calcium Gluconate**—Bottle of 4 oz.; Containing normal calcium salt of gluconic acid 10% solution; *Dosage:* 1–2 ampules daily. *See Chap. I.* **(Mallinckrodt)**

476. Sulpharsphenamine—Ampules 0.15, 0.3, 0.45, 0.75, 0.9, 1.5 Gm; *For use* as antiluetic; *Dosage:* intragluteally, 0.45–0.6 Gm twice weekly. *See Chap. I.* **(Mallinckrodt)**

---

477. Adrempco—Ampules 1 cc; Boxes of 12; Containing pituitary (entire) gr 1/12 (0.005 Gm), thyroid gr 1/6 (0.012 Gm), adrenals gr 1/5 (0.014 Gm), ovarian gr 1/3 (0.02 Gm), testicular gr 1/2 (0.032 Gm); *For use* in underdevelopment, asthenia, neurasthenia and premature senility. **(Marvell)**

478. Adrenal Cortex Solution—See Interrenin. **(Marvell)**

479. Benacol Solution—Ampules 3 cc; Boxes of 6 and 25; Containing 5 parts each ethacaine and phenmethylol in 90 parts pure sweet almond oil. *For use* as analgesic. *Dosage:* 1 ampule *subcutaneously* in fan-shaped manner, around painful area. *See Chap. II.* **(Marvell)**

480. Bisempco Cream—Ampules 1 cc; Boxes of 12; 10 % solution bismuth subsalicylate in hydrogenated oil; *For use* in syphilis, and as topical application in Vincent's angina; *Dosage:* *intramuscularly,* 1 ampule twice weekly. *See Chap. I.* **(Marvell)**

481. Caffein Sodium Benzoate—Ampules 2 cc; Boxes of 12; Containing 0.50 Gm; *For use* in cardiac dropsy, renal insufficiency, narcotic intoxication, neuralgias. **(Marvell)**

482. Camphor—Ampules 1 cc; Boxes of 12; Containing gr 3 (0.2 Gm); *For use* as rapid circulatory stimulant in adynamic fevers as typhoid and pneumonia. **(Marvell)**

483. Corpus Luteum Solution—Ampules 1 cc; Boxes of 12; Containing gr 3 of desiccated corpora lutea, 1/2 % chlorbutanol; *For use* in vomiting of pregnancy, aberrations of menstruation, natural or artificial. *See Chap. IV.* **(Marvell)**

484. Interrenin—Ampules 1 cc; Boxes of 6 and 12; Each cubic centimeter representing 5 Gm fresh adrenal gland; *For use* in hyperthyroidism preparatory for surgical intervention, in Addison's disease, hypoadrenia and loss of weight; *Dosage:* 1–3 cc, *intramuscularly,* daily. *See Chap. IV.* **(Marvell)**

485. Iron Arsenite—Ampules 1 cc; Boxes of 12; Containing gr 1 (0.06 Gm) iron arsenite and 0.06 ammonium citrate, equivalent to gr 1/6 metallic iron and gr 1/10 arsenic trioxide with strychnine nitrate 0.001 Gm; *For use* as hematinic with nerve and cardiac stimulation. **(Marvell)**

486. Mercury Bichloride—Ampules 1 cc; Boxes of 12; Containing gr 1/6 (0.01 Gm); *For use* as antisyphilitic and alterative. **(Marvell)**

487. Mercury Cacodylate—Ampules 1 cc; Boxes of 12; Containing gr 1/2 (0.03 Gm); *For use* as antisyphilitic and alterative. **(Marvell)**

488. Mercury Salicylate (Salempco)—Ampules 1 cc; Boxes of 12; Containing benzocain 2 %, mercury salicylate gr 1 (0.065 Gm), gr 1 1/2 (0.10 Gm), or gr 2 (0.13 Gm) in hydrogenated oil; *For use* as antisyphilitic; *Intramuscularly.* **(Marvell)**

489. Neurempco—Ampules 1 cc; Boxes of 12; 3, containing iron citrate 0.03 Gm, sodium glycerophosphate 0.10 Gm, sodium cacodylate 0.06 Gm, strychnine sulphate 0.001 Gm.

Ampules 1 cc; Boxes of 12; "4," containing iron cacodylate 0.02 Gm, strychnine cacodylate 0.0005 Gm, sodium arsenate 0.001 Gm, sodium glycerophosphate 0.03 Gm.

Ampules 1 cc; Boxes of 12; "8," containing iron cacodylate 0.01 Gm, sodium glycerophosphate 0.065 Gm, strychnine cacodylate 0.0005 Gm, chlorbutanol 1/2 %. *For use* as hematinic and tonic; *Dosage:* *intramuscularly,* 1 ampule two or three times weekly. *See Chap. II.* **(Marvell)**

490. Novocain—Ampules 1 cc; Boxes of 12; Containing 1 or 2 % solution; *For use* as local anesthetic. *See Chap. I.* **(Marvell)**

491. Novocain in Solution Epinephrin—Ampules 1 cc; Boxes of 12; Containing novocain 1 or 2 % solution in epinephrin 1:20,000; *For use* as local anesthetic. *See Chap. I.* **(Marvell)**

492. Oil of Turpentine—Ampules 1 cc; Boxes of 12; Containing 0.20 cc in olive oil; *For use* in epidydimitis; *Dosage:* 1 ampule, *intramuscularly*, alternate days. **(Marvell)**

493. Olive Oil—Ampules 10 cc; Boxes of 6; *For use* in lubrication of ureters. **(Marvell)**

494. Orchiben Concentrate—Ampules 1 cc; Boxes of 6; *For use* in premature senility, in neurasthenia, poor development, sterility, mild mental affections, hypochondria. *See Chap. IV.* **(Marvell)**

495. Orchiben Solution—Ampules 1 cc; Boxes of 12; Containing gr 55 (3.5636 Gm) fresh orchic gland; *For use* as above described. *See Chap. IV.* **(Marvell)**

496. Orchic-Epinephrine Compound—Ampules 1 cc; Boxes of 12; Containing pituitary (anterior lobe), prostate, orchic and 2 m of solution epinephrine chloride 1:1,000. *See Chap. IV.* **(Marvell)**

497. Orchic Solution—See Testempco. **(Marvell)**

498. Ovamone (Ovarialhormone Solution)—Ampules 1 cc; Boxes of 6; Standardized to 25 rat units; *For use* in hypofunctioning of ovaries, artificial and natural; *Intramuscular. See Chap. IV.* **(Marvell)**

499. Ovarialhormon Folliculin Menformon Solution—Ampules 1 cc; Boxes of 3; Standardized to 40 mouse units; Containing 0.1 mg dry substance, sodium chloride; *Dosage:* 1 injection daily increased to twice daily as indicated; may be administered *intravenously. See Chap. IV.* **(Marvell)**

500. Ovarian Solution—Ampules 1 cc; Boxes of 12; *For use* in infantilism, ovarian dysfunction, artificial and natural. *See Chap. IV.* **(Marvell)**

501. Parathyroid Solution—Ampules 1 cc; Boxes of 12; Representing gr 2 fresh parathyroid gland; *For use* in epilepsy, eclampsia, psoriasis, eczema, in conditions due to calcium deficiency, tetany, uremia, varicose ulcer. *See Chap. IV.* **(Marvell)**

502. Phenolsulphonphthalein Solution—Ampules 1 cc; Boxes of 10; Containing gr 1/10 (0.006 Gm); *For use* as kidney function test; *intramuscularly* or *intravenously. See Chap. I.* **(Marvell)**

503. Pituitary (Anterior Lobe) Solution—Ampules 1 cc; Boxes of 12; Representing gr 18½ fresh anterior pituitary; *For use* in obesity, enuresis, retarded development, mental deficiency, sexual non-development. *See Chap. IV.* **(Marvell)**

504. Pituitary (Entire) Solution—Ampules 1 cc; Boxes of 12; Representing gr 15.43 whole pituitary gland; *For use* in asthma, exophthalmic goitre, uterine fibroids, obesity of pituitary origin. *See Chap. IV.* **(Marvell)**

505. Polempco (Polyglandular Solution)—Ampules 1 cc; Boxes of 12; Containing pituitary (entire) gr 1/12 (0.005 Gm), thyroid gr ⅙ (0.012 Gm), ovarian gr ⅓ (0.02 Gm), testicular gr 1/12 (0.005 Gm); *For use* in physical and sexual retarded development, pre-senility, neurasthenia. *See Chap. IV.* **(Marvell)**

506. Polyglandular "O"—Ampules 1 cc; Boxes of 12; Containing pituitary (entire) gr 1/12 (0.005 Gm), thyroid gr ⅙ (0.012 Gm), ovarian gr 1 (0.065 Gm). *See Chap. IV.* **(Marvell)**

507. Polyglandular "T"—Ampules 1 cc; Boxes of 12; Containing pituitary (entire) gr 1/12 (0.005 Gm), thyroid gr ⅙ (0.012 Gm), testicular gr 1 (0.065 Gm). *See Chap. IV.* **(Marvell)**

508. Semvesco Solution—Ampules 1 cc; Boxes of 12; Containing seminal vesicle gr ⅙ (0.012 Gm), pituitary (anterior) gr 1/12 (0.005 Gm), thyroid gr ⅙ (0.012 Gm), adrenal gr 1/12 (0.005 Gm), orchic gr ⅓ (0.02 Gm), prostate gr ⅙ (0.012 Gm); *For use* in sexual impotence, as tonic in neuroses and in hypertrophy of prostate. *See Chap. IV.* **(Marvell)**

509. Testempco Solution—Ampules 1 cc; Boxes of 12; Representing gr 27½ fresh testicular substance; *For use* in premature senility, sterility, arrested growth. *See Chap. IV.* **(Marvell)**

510. Yohimbin Hydrochloride—Ampules 1 cc; Boxes of 12; Containing gr 1/12 (0.005 Gm). *For use* as aphrodisiac. (Marvell)

---

511. Caffeine Sodio-Benzoate—Ampules 2 cc; Boxes of 6 and 100; Containing gr 7½ (0.5 Gm); *For use* as cardiac and respiratory stimulant and diuretic; *Dosage:* 1–2 cc as indicated. (McNeil)

512. Camphor in Oil—Ampules 1 cc; Boxes of 6 and 100; Containing gr 1½ (0.1 Gm) or gr 3 (0.2 Gm); *For use* as circulatory stimulant; *Dosage:* 1 cc, repeated, *intramuscularly*, as indicated. (McNeil)

513. Ephedrine Hydrochloride—Ampules 1 cc and Vials 10 cc; Cartons of 1 each; Containing gr ¾ (0.05 Gm); *For use* as circulatory stimulant; *Dosage:* ½ cc as indicated. *See Chap. I.* (McNeil)

514. Glycerophosphate Compound—Ampules 1 cc and Vials 10 cc; Cartons of 1; Containing sodium glycerophosphate gr 1½ (0.1 Gm), iron cacodylate gr ⅙ (0.12 Gm), strychnine sulphate gr 1/125; *For use* as tonic in neurasthenia and anemia; *Dosage:* 1 cc as indicated. (McNeil)

515. Corpus Luteum—Ampules 1 cc; Boxes of 6 and 100; Containing gr 3 (0.2 Gm) desiccated substance with gr 1/12 (0.006 Gm) chlorbutanol; *Dosage:* 1 cc every 2 days. *See Chap. IV.* (McNeil)

516. Iron Arsenite—Ampules 1 cc and Vials 10 cc; Cartons of 1; Containing gr 1 (0.065 Gm); *For use* as alterative, hematinic and general tonic; *Dosage:* ¼–1 cc as indicated. (McNeil)

517. Iron Arsenite Compound—Ampules 1 cc and Vials 10 cc; Cartons of 1; Containing per cubic centimeter, iron arsenite gr 1 (0.065 Gm), strychnine nitrate gr 1/64 (0.00101 Gm); *For use* as alterative, hematinic and general tonic; *Dosage:* 1 cc as indicated. (McNeil)

518. Iron Cacodylate—Vials 1 cc and Vials 10 cc; Cartons of 1; Containing gr ½ (0.03 Gm); *For use* as alterative and hematinic; *Dosage:* 1 cc as indicated. (McNeil)

519. Iron Citrate—Ampules 1 cc and Vials 10 cc; Cartons of 1; Containing gr 1 (0.065 Gm); *For use* as hematinic; *Dosage:* 1–2 cc as indicated. (McNeil)

520. Iron Citrate-Nuclein Compound—Ampules 1 cc and Vials 10 cc; Cartons of 1; Containing per cubic centimeter, iron citrate soluble gr ¾ (0.04860 Gm), sodium arsenate gr 1/64 (0.00101 Gm), strychnine sulphate gr 1/64 (0.00101 Gm), sodium nucleinate gr ⅛ (0.00810 Gm); *For use* as hematinic and reconstructive tonic; *Dosage:* 1 cc as indicated. (McNeil)

521. Liver Solution (Concentrated)—Ampules 1 cc; Boxes of 6 and 100; *For use* in hepatic insufficiency and high blood pressure; *Dosage:* ½–1 cc, *intramuscularly*, once to twice daily. *See Chap. I.* (McNeil)

522. Magnesium Sulphate—Ampules 2 cc; Boxes of 6 and 100; 50% solution; *For use* as sedative and analgesic, to prolong effect of morphine; *Dosage:* 2 cc as indicated. (McNeil)

523. Mercury Succinimide—Ampules 5 cc; Boxes of 6 and 100; Containing gr ⅙ (0.012 Gm); *For use* as antisyphilitic; *Dosage:* ¼–1 cc, *intramuscularly*, at 1–5 day intervals. (McNeil)

524. Nuclein Solution—Ampules 1 cc; Boxes of 6 and 100; 5% solution; Containing sodium salt of nucleinic acid; *For use* in leucopenia; *Dosage:* 1 cc one to four times daily as indicated. (McNeil)

525. Orchic Solution—Ampules 1 cc; Boxes of 6 and 100; Representing gr 27½ fresh orchic substance; *Dosage:* 1 cc every 2–3 days as indicated, *intramuscularly*. *See Chap. IV.* (McNeil)

526. Ovarian Substance—Ampules 1 cc; Boxes of 6 and 100; Representing gr 23 (1.490 Gm) fresh whole ovarian substance; *Dosage:* 1 cc every 2–3 days, *intramuscularly*. *See Chap. IV.* (McNeil)

527. Pituitary Solution, U.S.P.X.—Ampules ½ and 1 cc; Boxes of 6; Vials 10 cc; Containing active principle of posterior lobe of pituitary gland; *For use* in uterine inertia, pulmonary hemorrhage, cerebral anemia, shock, and as diuretic; *Dosage:* ½–1 cc as indicated. *See Chap. I.* **(McNeil)**

528. Procaine with Epinephrine—Ampules 1 cc; Vials of 10 cc; Containing per cubic centimeter, procaine gr ⅓ (0.02 Gm), epinephrine hydrochloride gr 1/1,620 (0.00004 Gm); *For use* as local anesthetic; *Dosage:* 1 cc as indicated. *See Chap. I.* **(McNeil)**

529. Quinine and Urea Hydrochloride—Ampules 5 cc; Boxes of 6; 1% solution; *For use* as local anesthetic; *Dosage:* 5 cc *subcutaneously*, as indicated. *See Chap. II.* **(McNeil)**

530. Quinine Dihydrochloride—Ampules 1 cc and Vials of 10 cc; Cartons of 1; Containing gr 7½ (0.5 Gm); *For use* as tonic, antipyretic and antimalarial; *Dosage:* ½–1 cc *intramuscularly*, once or twice daily. **(McNeil)**

531. Silver Nitrate—Ampules of wax; 1% solution; *For use* in new born to prevent ophthalmia neonatorum; 2 drops into each eye; in cold weather ampule to be slightly warmed. **(McNeil)**

532. Sodium Cacodylate—Ampules 1 cc and Vials of 10 cc; Containing gr 1½ (0.1 Gm), gr 3 (0.2 Gm), gr 5 (0.33 Gm), gr 7½ (0.5 Gm); *For use* as alterative; *Dosage:* 1 cc every other day. **(McNeil)**

533. Sodium Iodide—Ampules 10 cc; Cartons of 1; Containing gr 15½ (1 Gm). Ampules 20 cc; Cartons of 1; Containing gr 31 (2 Gm); *For use* as alterative. **(McNeil)**

---

535. Bismosol—Ampules 1 cc; Boxes of 10; Containing potassium sodium bismuthotartrate Gm 10, piperazine Gm 0.3, aqueous solution of glucose q.s. 100 cc; *For use* as antisyphilitic; *Dosage: intramuscularly*, 1 ampule twice weekly. *See Chap. II.* **(Merck)**

536. Neoarsphenamine—Ampules of 0.15, 0.3, 0.45, 0.6, 0.75, 0.9 Gm; Box of 1 with a 10 cc ampule distilled water; Boxes of 10 with ten 10 cc ampules distilled water; *For use* as antisyphilitic; *Dosage:* 0.45–0.6 Gm twice weekly, by syringe method; occasionally intramuscularly. *See Chap. I.* **(Merck)**

537. Sulpharsphenamine—Ampules of 0.1, 0.2, 0.3, 0.4, 0.5, 0.6 Gm; Single doses; antisyphilitic; *Dosage:* 0.45–0.6 Gm twice weekly, *intramuscularly. See Chap. I.* **(Merck)**

538. Tryparsamide—Ampules of 1, 2 and 3 Gm; *For use* as antiluetic, also in trypanosomiasis (African sleeping sickness); *Dosage:* 0.04–0.05 Gm per kilogram of body weight, for 8–16 doses. *See Chap. I.* **(Merck)**

---

539. Fibrogen Subcutaneous—Ampules 2 cc; Packages of 4; ampules 1 cc, packages of 6; *For use* as hemostatic; *Dosage:* 2–4 cc as required. *See Chap. I.* **(Merrell)**

540. Natural Salicylates—Ampules of 20% sodium salicylate.
Ampules of sodium salicylate (natural) 15½ gr, sodium iodide 15½ gr; *For use* as antirheumatic. *See Chap. I.* **(Merrell)**

---

541. Gravocain—Ampules 0.75 cc; Packages of 5; Containing 40% solution of novocain and small amount of strychnin; *For use* in obstetric spinal anesthesia; *Dosage:* ½–1 ampule *intraspinally*, on full cervial dilatation. *See Chap. I.* **(Metz)**

542. Neosalvarsan—Ampules of 0.15, 0.3, 0.45, 0.6, 0.75, 0.9 Gm; Single dosage; with or without 10 cc ampule triple distilled water;
Ampules of 1.5, 1.8, 3.0, 4.5 Gm; Multiple dosage; *For use* as antisyphilitic; *Dosage:* 0.45 to 0.6 Gm twice weekly. *See Chap. I.* **(Metz)**

543. Novocain—Ampules of 50, 100, 120, 150, 200, 300, 500 mg; Boxes of 10; Vials of 5 Gm and 1 oz; Boxes of 10.
Ampules of 2 and 5 cc each; Solutions 1% without Suprarenin.

Ampules of 1½ and 5 cc each; Solutions 20% without Suprarenin; *For use* as local anesthetic. *See Chap. I.* (Metz)

544. Novocain-Suprarenin Solutions (N.S.)—Ampules 1 cc; Boxes of 20.
Ampules 3 cc; Boxes of 10 and 100.
Ampules 6 cc; Boxes of 10; Solution (isotonic) "E" Containing Novocain 2%, Suprarenin 1:20,000.
Ampules 2 and 6 cc; Boxes of 10; Solution (isotonic) "T," Novocain 2%, Suprarenin 1:50,000.
Ampules 1 cc; Boxes of 20.
Ampules 3 cc; Boxes of 10 and 100; Solution (isotonic) "T," Novocain 2%, Suprarenin 1:50,000.
Ampules 1.5 and 5 cc; Boxes of 10; Concentrated; Novocain 20%, Suprarenin 1:9,009.
For use as anesthetic; *Dosage:* 0.5–5 cc as required. *See Chap. I.* (Metz)

545. Omnadin—Ampules 2 cc; Boxes of 5; *For use* as lipo-protein therapy; *Dosage:* intramuscularly, 1 ampule daily. *See Chap. I.* (Metz)

546. Salvarsan—Ampules 0.1, 0.2, 0.3, 0.4, 0.5, 0.6 Gm; Single dosage;
Ampules 1, 1.2, 2.0, 3.0 Gm, Multiple dosage; *For use* as antisyphilitic; *Dosage:* 0.3–0.45 Gm twice weekly. *See Chap. I.* (Metz)

546a. Salvarsan Glucose Solution—Ampules 3 cc; Boxes of 10; A preparation of 5% aqueous glucose in salvarsan base; *For use* as antisyphilitic; *Dosage:* 0.3–0.45 Gm twice weekly. *See Chap. I.* (Metz)

547. Silver-Salvarsan—Ampules 0.1, 0.15, 0.2, 0.25, 0.3 Gm; Single dosage;
Ampules 0.6 Gm; Multiple dosage; *For use* as antisyphilitic; *Dosage:* 0.1–0.3 Gm every 4 days. *See Chap. I.* (Metz)

548. Salyrgan—Ampules 1 cc; Boxes of 5;
Ampules 2 cc; Boxes of 10; *For use* as powerful diuretic; Containing not less than 37.6% of mercury; Used only in 10% solution; *Dosage: intramuscularly,* 1 ampule daily. *See Chap. I.* (Metz)

549. Spinocain—Ampules 2 cc; Boxes of 10; Containing novocain 10%, strychnine sulphate 1.1 mg to 1 cc; *For use* as spinal anesthetic; also
Ampules 1 cc; Boxes of 10; Ephedrine Novocaine Solution; Containing ephedrine hydrochloride 5% and Novocaine 1%; *Dosage:* as per special pamphlet supplied. *See Chap. II.* (Metz).

550. Sulpharsphenamine—Ampules 0.1, 0.15, 0.3, 0.45, 0.6, 0.75, 0.9 Gm; Single doses; with or without 10 cc ampule triple distilled water;
Ampules 3.0 Gm; Multiple doses; *For use* as antisyphilitic; *Dosage:* 0.45–0.6 Gm daily. *See Chap. I.* (Metz)

551. Suprarenin—Ampules 1 cc; Boxes of 20; *For use* as vasoconstrictor and hemostatic; *Dosage: intramuscularly,* 0.5–1 cc daily. *See Chap. I.* (Metz)

---

552. Adrenalin (Epinephrin)—Ampules 1 cc; Boxes of 12 and 100; Containing suprarenal medulla, 1:1,000 solution; *For use* as vasoconstrictor. *See Chap. I.* (Miller)

553. Adrenalin Cortex—Ampules 1 cc; Boxes of 12 and 100; Concentrated extract of fresh suprarenal cortex; *For use* in hypoadremia. (Miller)

554. Adrenal (Whole)—Ampules 1 cc; Boxes of 12 and 100; *Intramuscular; Dosage:* 1 or 2 cc, two or three times weekly, as indicated. (Miller)

555. Adrenal Medulla—Ampules 1 cc; Boxes of 12 and 100; 1:1,000 Solution of fresh suprarenal medulla. *For use* as vasoconstrictor. (Miller)

556. Anterior Pituitary—Ampules 1 cc; Boxes of 12 and 100; each cubic centimeter represents 45 gr fresh gland substance; 0.5% chlorbutanol; *For use* in delayed development, sexual and general, also in hypopituitary obesities; *Dosage:* 1 cc *intramuscular,* two to three times weekly. *See Chap. IV.* (Miller)

557. Bismuth Salicylate—Ampules 1 cc; Boxes of 12 and 100; Containing gr 2 (0.13 Gm).

Ampules 2 cc; Boxes of 12 and 100; Containing gr 4 (0.26 Gm). Bottle 30 cc; Boxes of 12. The suspension in oil also contains novocain, anesthesin and camphor; Intramuscular; *For use* in neurosyphilis in the intolerant to arsenicals and mercurials; 1 ampule, once or twice weekly for 15 injections. *See Chap. I.* **(Miller)**

558. **Caffeine Sodium Benzoate**—Ampules 1 cc; Boxes of 12 and 100; Containing gr 3¾ (0.25 Gm).
Ampules 2 cc; Boxes of 12 and 100; Containing gr 7½ (0.5 Gm). *For use* as cardiorenal stimulant in chronic nephritis, cardiac dropsy, pneumonia; *Intramuscular.* **(Miller)**

559. **Calcium Cacodylate**—Ampules 2 cc; Boxes of 12 and 100; 5% Solution; *For use* in tuberculosis; *Dosage:* 1 ampule every 3–4 days. **(Miller)**

560. **Calcium Iodide**—Ampules 2 cc; Boxes of 12 and 100; Containing gr 3 (0.2 Gm); *For use* in calcium deficiency; *Dosage:* 1 ampule every 3–4 days. **(Miller)**

561. **Camphor in Oil**—Ampules 1 cc; Boxes of 12 and 100; Containing gr 3 (0.2 Gm).
Ampules 5 cc; Boxes of 6 and 50; Containing gr 15½ (1.0 Gm).
Ampules 10 cc; Boxes of 6 and 50; Containing gr 31 (2.0 Gm); *For use* as cardiac and general stimulant; *Dosage:* 3–10 gr; pneumonia crisis gr 31 every 10 hr. *Intramuscular.* **(Miller)**

562. **Corpus Luteum Extract**—Ampules 1 cc; Boxes of 12 and 100; Representing gr 25 fresh gland substance.
Ampule-vial 30 cc; Boxes of 1; Representing gr 25 fresh gland substance per cubic centimeter; Containing 0.5% chlorbutanol. *See Chap. IV.* **(Miller)**

563. **Emetine Hydrochloride**—Ampules 1 cc; Boxes of 12 and 100; Containing gr ½ (0.032 Gm).
Ampules 5 cc; Boxes of 6 and 50; Containing gr ½ (0.032 Gm).
Ampules 1 cc; Boxes of 12 and 100; Containing gr 1 (0.065 Gm).
Ampules 5 cc; Boxes of 6 and 50; Containing gr 1 (0.065 Gm); *For use* in amebic dysentery and amebic hepatitis; *Dosage:* ½–1 gr, once or twice daily—until 8 gr are given; *Intramuscular.* **(Miller)**

564. **Ephedrine**—Ampules 1 cc; Boxes of 12 and 100; Containing gr ¾ (0.05 Gm); *For use* in bronchial asthma and hay fever; *Dosage:* 1 ampule every 4 hr., as indicated. *See Chap. I.* **(Miller)**

565. **Ergamine**—Ampules 1 cc; Boxes of 12 and 100; Containing ergamine 1:10,000 in normal saline with 0.5% chlorbutanol. *See Chap. I.* **(Miller)**

566. **Ergot**—Ampules 1 cc; Boxes of 12 and 100; *For use* in post-partum hemorrhage, uterine inertia; *Dosage:* 1 cc, as indicated. **(Miller)**

567. **Glycerophosphate Compound**—Ampules 1 cc; Boxes of 12 and 100; Containing sodium glycerophosphate gr 1½ (0.1 Gm), iron cacodylate gr ⅙ (0.012 Gm), strychnine cacodylate gr 1/125 (0.0005 Gm); *For use* as hematinic and tonic. **(Miller)**

568. **Hexamethylenamine and Sodium Iodide**—Ampules 10 cc; Boxes of 6 and 50; Containing hexamethylentetramine gr 15½ (1.0 Gm) and sodium iodide gr 7¾ (0.5 Gm). **(Miller)**

569. **Hexamethylenamine and Sodium Iodide**—Ampules 20 cc; Boxes of 6 and 50; Containing hexamethylentetramine gr 31 (2.0 Gm) and sodium iodide gr 15½ (0.1 Gm); *For use* in genitourinary infections and as prophylactic; urine must be kept acid. **(Miller)**

570. **Iron Arsenite**—Ampules 1 cc; Boxes of 12 and 100; Containing gr ½ (0.032 Gm).
Ampules 1 cc; Boxes of 12 and 100; Containing gr 1 (0.065 Gm); *For use* in dry scaly cutaneous diseases, anemias; *Dosage:* ½–1 gr, *intramuscular.* **(Miller)**

571. **Iron Cacodylate**—Ampules 1 cc; Boxes of 12 and 100; Containing gr ½ (0.032 Gm) or gr ¾ (0.05 Gm); combined with a suitable local anesthetic; also Ampules 1 cc; Boxes of 12 and 100; Containing gr 1 (0.065 Gm); *For use* as hematinic and tonic; *Dosage:* ½–3 gr as indicated; Intramuscular. **(Miller)**

572. **Iron Cacodylate Compound**—Ampules 2 cc; Boxes of 12 and 100; Containing iron cacodylate gr ½ (0.032 Gm), sodium cacodylate gr 2 (0.13 Gm), strychnine cacodylate gr 1/37 (0.002 Gm), sodium glycerophosphate gr 2 (0.13 Gm); *For use* in atonic conditions, malnutrition; *Dosage:* 1 ampules every 2 or 3 days; *Intramuscularly.* (Miller)

573. **Iron Cacodylate and Strychnine**—Ampules 1 cc; Boxes of 12 and 100; Containing iron cacodylate gr 1 (0.065 Gm) and strychnine sulphate gr 1/128; *For use* as general tonic; *Intramuscularly.* (Miller)

574. **Iron Citrate** (Green)—Ampules 1 cc; Boxes of 12 and 100; Containing gr ½ (0.032 Gm).
Ampules 1 cc; Boxes of 12 and 100; Containing gr 1 (0.065 Gm).
Ampules 1 cc; Boxes of 12 and 100; Containing gr 1½ (0.10 Gm). *For use* in anemias and as tonic; *Dosage:* 1 ampule *intramuscularly,* every other day. (Miller)

575. **Iron Glycerophosphate Compound**—Ampules 1 cc; Boxes of 12 and 100; Containing iron citrate gr ½ (0.032 Gm), sodium glycerophosphate gr 1 (0.065 Gm), sodium cacodylate (dimethylarsenate) gr ½ (0.032 Gm); *For use* as hematinic and tonic; *Dosage:* 1 ampule every 2–3 days. (Miller)

576. **Kidney (Renal) Extract**—Ampules 2 cc; Boxes of 12 and 100; Each cubic centimeter representing gr 55 fresh interstitial kidney substance; *For use* in kidney insufficiency; *Dosage:* 1 ampule *intramuscularly,* not less than every 6 hr. *See Chap. IV.* (Miller)

577. **Liver Extract (Hypotensive)**—Ampules 1 and 5 cc; Boxes of 1 cc—12 and 100; 2 cc—6 and 50.
Ampule-vial 30 cc; Boxes of 1; *For use* in pernicious anemia; *Intramuscular; Dosage:* 1 cc daily or bi-daily until blood pressure is reduced, in severe cases to 5 cc daily. (Miller)

578. **Lobeline Sulphate**—Ampules 1 cc—Boxes of 12 and 100; Containing gr 1/20 (0.003 Gm) or gr 1/6 (0.01 Gm); *For use* as respiratory stimulant; *Dosage:* gr 1/20 at short intervals, children gr 1/6; *Intramuscular.* (Miller)

579. **Magnesium Sulphate**—Ampules 1 cc; Boxes of 12 and 100; 50% Solution; gr 7½ (0.50 Gm).
Ampules 1 cc; Boxes of 12 and 100; 25% Solution; gr 3¾ (0.25 Gm).
Ampules 2 cc; Boxes of 12 and 100; 50% Solution; gr 15½ (1.0 Gm).
Ampules 2 cc; Boxes of 12 and 100; 25% Solution; gr 7½ (0.50 Gm).
Ampules 10 cc; Boxes of 6 and 50; 10% Solution; gr 15½ (1.0 Gm).
Ampules 20 cc; Boxes of 6 and 50; 10% Solution; gr 31 (2.0 Gm). *For use* with morphine for prolonged effect; *Dosage:* 1 ampule as necessary. (Miller)

580. **Mercury Iodide (Red)**—Ampules 1 cc; Boxes of 12 and 100; Containing gr 1/6 (0.012 Gm) or gr 1/3 (0.02 Gm); *For use* as antisyphilitic; *Dosage:* 1/6–1/3 gr, three times weekly, *intramuscularly. See Chap. I.* (Miller)

581. **Mercury Iodide (Red) in Oil**—Ampules 1 cc; Boxes of 12 and 100; Containing gr 1/3 (0.02 Gm) in neutral vegetable oil; *For use* as antisyphilitic where slow absorption is indicated; *Dosage:* 1 cc, three times weekly, *intramuscularly. See Chap. I.* (Miller)

582. **Mercury Salicylate**—Ampules 1 cc; Boxes of 12 and 100; Containing gr 1½ (0.1 Gm), in neutral vegetable oil with local anesthetic; *Dosage:* 1 cc three times weekly, *intramuscularly; For use* as antisyphilitic. *See Chap. I.* (Miller)

583. **Mercury Succinimide**—Ampules 1 cc; Boxes of 12 and 100; Containing gr 1/6 (0.01 Gm); *For use* as antisyphilitic; *Dosage:* ½–1 cc daily as indicated, *intramuscularly. See Chap. I.* (Miller)

584. **Novocain (Intraspinal) Crystals**—Ampules of 50 mg; Boxes of 6 and 50;
Ampules of 100 mg; Boxes of 6 and 50
Ampules of 125 mg; Boxes of 6 and 50
Ampules of 150 mg; Boxes of 6 and 50
Ampules of 200 mg; Boxes of 6 and 50

Ampules of 250 mg; Boxes of 6 and 50
Ampules of 300 mg; Boxes of 6 and 50. Prepared for solution with cerebrospinal fluid, injected according to accepted technic for spinal anesthesia. *See Chap. I.* **(Miller)**

585. Novocain—Ampules 2 cc; Boxes of 12 and 100; 1 or 2% Solutions
Ampules 5 cc; Boxes of 6 and 50; ½, 1 or 2% Solutions
Ampules 10 cc; Boxes of 6 and 50; ½, 1 or 2% Solutions
Ampule-vial 10 cc Rubber-capped; Boxes of 6 and 50; 1 or 2% Solutions;
Ampules 15 cc; Boxes of 6 and 50; 1 or 2% Solutions
Ampules 20 cc; Boxes of 6 and 50; 1 or 2% Solutions
Ampules 30 cc; Boxes of 6 and 50; 1 or 2% Solutions
Ampules 50 cc; Boxes of 6 and 50; 1 or 2% Solutions
Ampule-vial 50 cc Rubber-capped; Boxes of 6 and 50; 1 or 2% Solutions; *For use* in nerve block or local anesthesia. *See Chap. I.* **(Miller)**

586. Orchic (Testicular) Extract—Ampules 1 cc; Boxes of 12 and 100;
Ampules 2 cc; Boxes of 12 and 100;
Ampules 5 cc; Boxes of 12 and 100;
Ampule-vial 30 cc; Box of 1. **Each cubic centimeter represents gr 55 of fresh interstitial substance;** *For use* **in stimulating other glands of internal secretion,** in functional impotence, obesity and hypogonadism. *Dosage:* 1–5 cc, two to three times weekly, *intramuscularly. See Chap. IV.* **(Miller)**

587. Ovarian Extract (Whole)—Ampules 1–2 and 5 cc; Boxes of 12 and 100;
Ampule-vial 30 cc; Boxes of 1; Each cubic centimeter represents 25 rat (Allen Doisy) units; *For use* in hypo-ovarism; *Dosage:* 1–5 cc *intramuscularly*, two to three times weekly, as indicated. *See Chap. IV.* **(Miller)**

588. Ovarian Residue Extract—Ampules 1, 2 cc; Boxes of 12 and 100;
Ampules 5 cc; Boxes of 6 and 50;
Ampule-vial 30 cc; Boxes of 1; Each cubic centimeter represents 25 rat (Allen and Doisy) units; *Dosage:* 1–5 cc, *intramuscularly*, two to three times weekly. *See Chap. IV.* **(Miller)**

589. Pancreatic Extract—Ampules 1 cc; Boxes of 12 and 100; Each cubic centimeter represents gr 30 of fresh pancreatic tissue; *For control* of carbohydrate metabolism, and as possible antagonistic agent toward function of suprarenals and thyroid through sympathetic; *Dosage:* 1 cc *Intramuscularly*, two to three times weekly. *See Chap. IV.* **(Miller)**

590. Parathyroid Extract—Ampules 1 cc; Boxes of 12 and 100;
Ampule-vial 30 cc; Boxes of 1. *For use* with calcium in certain cases of arthritis, paralysis agitans, eclampsia, tetany; *Dosage:* Adults from 0.2–0.4 cc, *intramuscularly* every 12 hr., for not more than 10 days. *See Chap. IV.* **(Miller)**

591. Pituitary Extract—Ampules 1 cc; Boxes of 12 and 100;
Ampule-vial 30 cc; Boxes of 1; Each cubic centimeter represents 10 International units; *For obstetrical use* in uterine inertia, post-partum hemorrhage and shock; *Dosage:* 0.5–1.0 cc *Intramuscularly*, as indicated. *See Chap. I.* **(Miller)**

592. Pituitary Extract (Double Strength)—Ampules 1 cc; Boxes of 12 and 100;
Ampule-vial 30 cc; Rubber-capped; Boxes of 1; Each cubic centimeter represents 20 international units; *For surgical use* in shock and post-operative treatment; *Dosage:* 0.5–1.0 cc *Intramuscularly. See Chap. I.* **(Miller)**

593. Pituitary (Whole Gland) Extract—Ampules 1 cc; Boxes of 12 and 100;
Ampule-vial 30 cc; Rubber-capped; Boxes of 1; *For use* in obesities; *Dosage:* 1 cc, two to three times weekly. *See Chap. IV.* **(Miller)**

594. Placenta Extract—Ampules 1 and 2 cc; Boxes of 12 and 100;
Ampules 5 cc; Boxes of 6 and 50;
Ampule-vial 30 cc; Rubber stoppered; Boxes of 1; *For use* as galactagogue, especially with mammary substance, in nausea of pregnancy, in functional hypo-ovarianism; *Dosage:* 1–5 cc, two to three times weekly. **(Miller)**

595. **Potassium Bismuth Tartrate**—Ampules 2 cc; Boxes of 12 and 100; Containing gr 3 (0.2 Gm) in neutral vegetable oil with suitable local anesthetic; *For use* as antisyphilitic; *Dosage:* 1 ampule two to three times weekly, *intramuscularly*. *See Chap. I.* (Miller)

596. **Prostatic Extract**—Ampules 1 and 2 cc; Boxes of 12 and 100;
Ampules 5 cc; Boxes of 6 and 50;
Ampule-vial 30 cc; rubber-stoppered; Boxes of 1; *For use* in types of prostatic hypertrophy of compensatory nature; *Dosage:* 1–5 cc *intramuscularly*, two to three times weekly. *See Chap. IV.* (Miller)

597. **Quinine Dihydrochloride**—Ampules 1 cc; Boxes of 12 and 100; Containing gr 7½ (0.50 Gm), or gr 3¾ (0.25 Gm);
Ampules 2 cc; Boxes of 12 and 100; Containing gr 15½ (1.0 Gm). *For use* as antimalarial, antipyretic and tonic. *Dosage:* 1 ampule two to three times weekly, *intramuscularly*. (Miller)

598. **Quinine and Urea Hydrochloride**—Ampules 1 cc; Boxes of 12 and 100; Containing gr 7¾ (0.5 Gm).
Ampules 2 cc; Boxes of 12 and 100; Containing gr 15½ (1 Gm). *For use* as antimalarial; *Dosage:* 1 ampule *intramuscularly*, three times weekly. *See Chap. II.* (Miller)

599. **Quinine and Urea**—Ampules 2 cc; Boxes of 12 and 100; 1 and 5% Solutions;
Ampules 5 cc; Boxes of 6 and 50; 1% Solution;
Ampules 30 cc; Boxes of 6 and 50; 5% Solution; Rubber-capped ampule-vial. *For use* as local anesthetic in submucous surgery, injection obliteration of internal hemorrhoids. *See Chap. II.* (Miller)

600. **Ringer's Solution**—Ampules 10 cc; Boxes of 6 and 50; An isotonic Ringer's Solution. (Miller)

601. **Sodium Cacodylate**—Ampules 1 cc; Boxes of 12 and 100; Following strengths—gr ¾, 1½, 2, 3, 5 or 7¾; *For use intramuscularly* in anemia, chlorosis, malarial cachexia, leukemia, pellagra, psoriasis; *Dosage:* 1 ampule two to three times weekly as indicated; children according to weight and age. (Miller)

602. **Sodium Glycerophosphate**—Ampules 1 cc; Boxes of 12 and 100; Containing gr 1½ (0.01 Gm)
Ampules 2 cc; Boxes of 12 and 100; Containing gr 3 (0.20 Gm); *For use* in osteomalacia, rachitis, general muscular and nervous debility and neurasthenia; *Dosage:* 1 ampule every 2–3 days, *intramuscularly*. (Miller)

603. **Strychnine Sulphate**—Ampules 1 cc; Boxes of 12 and 100; Containing gr 1/64 (0.001 Gm) or gr 1/32 (0.002 Gm); *For use* in collapse and shock, general debility, as antidote in chloral hydrate and chloroform poisoning; *intramuscularly; Dosage:* 1 ampule as indicated. (Miller)

604. **Suprarenal Extract (Whole Gland)**—Ampules 1 and 2 cc; Boxes of 12 and 100; *For use* in chronic toxemias, defective oxidation, fatigue and diminished sympathetic tone; *Dosage:* 1 or 2 cc, two to three times weekly, *intramuscularly*. (Miller)

605. **Thymus Extract**—Ampules 1 and 2 cc; Boxes of 12 and 100; *For use* in sexual hyperactivity or precocity, arthritis, and as leucocytic stimulant; Also Ampule-vial 30 cc; Boxes of 1; *Dosage:* 1 or 2 cc two or three times weekly. *See Chap. IV.* (Miller)

606. **Thyroid Extract**—Ampules 1 and 2 cc; Boxes of 12 and 100;
Ampule-vial 30 cc; Boxes of 1; Containing not less than 0.30% of iodine; Each cubic centimeter contains active extractives of gr 5 of fresh gland substance; *For use* in myxedema, cretinism, obesity of hypothyroid origin, dry scaly skin diseases, simple goitre, enuresis; *Dosage:* 1 ampule daily as indicated, *intramuscularly*. *See Chap. IV.* (Miller)

---

608. **Antimony and Potassium Tartrate**—Ampules 5 cc; Boxes of 1, 25 and 100; 1% solution. (National Drug)

609. Atropine Sulphate—Ampule-vial 25 cc; Boxes of 1; contains gr 1/100 per cubic centimeter. (National Drug)

610. Bismol—Ampules 1 cc; Boxes of 1, 25 and 100; Containing bismuth subsalicylate gr 2 (0.13 Gm) in colloidal suspension with sodium ricinoleate, oil base q.s., with benzocaine 1% and guaiacol ½% for local anesthetic effect; *Intramuscular;* Ampules 2 cc; Boxes of 1, 25 and 100; Containing bismuth subsalicylate gr 4 (0.26 Gm) in colloidal suspension with sodium ricinoleate, oil base, and above local anesthetic;
Ampule-vials 25 cc; Boxes of 1; Containing bismuth subsalicylate gr 2 (0.13 Gm), benzocaine 1%, guaiacol ½%, sodium ricinoleate ¼%, oil sesame q.s. 1 cc; *See Chap. II.* (National Drug)

611. Caffeine and Sodium Benzoate—Ampules 2 cc; Boxes of 1, 25 and 100; Containing gr 7¾ (0.50 Gm) in triple distilled water;
Ampule-vials 25 cc; Boxes of 1; Containing gr 3⅞ (0.250 Gm), with procaine 0.2% in triple distilled water per cubic centimeter; *For use* as powerful respiratory, cardiac and renal stimulant. (National Drug)

612. Camphor in Oil—Ampules 1 cc; Boxes of 1, 25 and 100; Containing gr 3 (0.2 Gm) in purified olive oil q.s. per cubic centimeter; *Intramuscular.*
Ampule-vials 25 cc; Boxes of 1; Containing gr 3 (0.2 Gm) in olive oil q.s. per cubic centimeter; *For use* as powerful respiratory and cardiac stimulant. (National Drug)

613. Corpus Luteum—Ampules 1 cc; Boxes of 6, 12, 25 and 100; Representing gr 18 (1.166 Gm) fresh gland, or gr 3 (0.194 Gm) of dessicated substance.
Ampule-vials 15 and 25 cc; Boxes of 1; Representing gr 3 (0.194 Gm) dessicated substance; *For use* in menstrual dysfunction, vomiting of pregnancy (4–8 m *intramuscularly*, every 2–3 hr) and as symptomatic remedy in hyperthyroidism and functional high blood pressure. *See Chap. IV.* (National Drug)

614. Epinephrine U.S.P.—Ampules 1 cc; Boxes of 12, 25 and 100; Containing 1:1,000 solution;
Ampule-vials 25 cc; Boxes of 1; Containing 1:1,000 Solution. *See Chap. I.* (National Drug)

615. Ephedrine—Ampule-vials 25 cc; Boxes of 1; Containing gr ¾ (0.04860 Gm). *See Chap. I.* (National Drug)

616. Ergosol—Ampules 1 cc; Boxes of 12, 25 and 100; Containing gr 2½ (0.1524 Gm) per minim of active extract of ergot.
Ampule-vials 25 cc; Boxes of 1; Representing gr 2.5 per cubic centimeter. (National Drug)

617. Glycerophosphate Compound—Ampules 1 cc; Boxes of 12, 25 and 100; Containing sodium glycerophosphate gr 1 1/12 (0.1 Gm), strychnine cacodylate gr 1/125 (0.0005 Gm), iron cacodylate gr ⅙ (0.01 Gm), triple distilled water q.s.
Ampule-vials 25 cc; Boxes of 1; Contains the above with procaine 0.2%; *For use* in neurasthenia, chronic malaria, and as hematinic and sustaining tonic. (National Drug)

618. Glycerophosphate Compound 2—Ampules 5 cc; Boxes of 12, 25 and 100; Containing sodium glycerophosphate gr 1½ (0.1 Gm), strychnine cacodylate gr 1/125 (0.0005 Gm), iron cacodylate gr ⅙ (0.01 Gm), triple distilled water q.s. 5 cc; *For use* as above. (National Drug)

619. Iron Arsenite—Ampules 1 cc; Boxes of 12, 25 and 100; Containing gr 1 (0.065 Gm), procaine 0.2% in triple distilled water q.s. 1 cc;
Ampule-vials 25 cc; Boxes of 1: same strength; *Intramuscular.* (National Drug)

620. Iron Arsenite and Strychnine—Ampules 1 cc; Boxes of 12, 25 and 100; Containing per cubic centimeter iron arsenite gr ¾ (0.05 Gm), strychnine nitrate gr 1/64 (0.001 Gm), procaine 0.2%, distilled water q.s.
Ampule-vials 25 cc; Boxes of 1; Same strength; *For use* as hematinic, tonic and for dry scaly forms of eczema; *Intramuscular.* (National Drug)

621. Iron Cacodylate—Ampules 1 cc; Boxes of 12, 25 and 100; Containing gr ½ (0.032 Gm) in triple distilled water; *Intramuscular.*
Ampule-vials 25 cc; Boxes of 1; Same strength; *For use* as hematinic, and tonic in chronic malaria, and in scaly cutaneous affections. **(National Drug)**

622. Iron Cacodylate Compound, 2—Ampules 5 cc; Boxes of 12, 25 and 100; Containing iron cacodylate gr 1 (0.065 Gm), sodium glycerophosphate gr 2 (0.130 Gm), in triple distilled water.
Ampule-vials 25 cc; Boxes of 1; Half strength; *Intramuscular.* **(National Drug)**

623. Iron Citrate—Ampules 1 cc; Boxes of 12, 25 and 100; Containing per cubic centimeter gr 1 (0.065 Gm) with Procaine 0.2% in triple distilled water q.s.
Ampule-vials 25 cc; Boxes of 1; Same strength. **(National Drug)**

624. Iron Cacodylate and Strychnine—Ampule-vials 25 cc; Boxes of 1; Containing per cubic centimeter iron cacodylate gr ½ (0.325 Gm), strychnine phosphate gr 1/129 (0.0005 Gm), in triple distilled water q.s. **(National Drug)**

625. Iron Citrate Compound—Ampules 1 cc; Boxes of 12, 25 and 100; Containing per cubic centimeter iron citrate gr ¾ (0.05 Gm), sodium arsenate gr 1/64 (0.001 Gm), strychnine sulphate gr 1/64 (0.001 Gm), procaine 0.2%, triple distilled water q.s.
Ampule-vials 25 cc; Boxes of 1; Same strength; *For use* as hematinic and tonic. **(National Drug)**

626. Liquor Pituitary, U.S.P.X. Obstetrical—Ampules ½ and 1 cc; Boxes of 6, 12, 25 and 100;
Ampule-vials 25 cc; Boxes of 1; Standardized, 10 units;
Ampule-vials 15 cc; Boxes of 1; Standardized, 10 units; *For use* in uterine inertia, in third stage of labor, in menorrhagia, shock, pneumonia, asthma; *Intramuscular. See Chap. I.* **(National Drug)**

627. Liquor Pituitary and Epinephrine—Ampules 1 cc; Boxes of 6, 12, 25 and 100; Containing liquor pituitary ½ cc, epinephrine U.S.P. 1:1,000 solution ½ cc;
Ampule-vials 25 cc; Boxes of 1; Same strength; Intramuscular. *For use* as vaso-constrictor in asthma, pneumonia, hay fever; *Dosage:* 1–2 cc at 12–48 hr. intervals. *See Chap. I.* **(National Drug)**

628. Magnesium Sulphate C.P.—Ampules 2 cc; Boxes of 12, 25 and 100; 50% solution procaine 0.2%;
Ampule-vials 25 cc; Boxes of 1; Same strength; Procaine 0.2%; *For use* as analgesic, or with morphine for prolonged effect. **(National Drug)**

629. Mercuric Iodide (Red)—Ampules 1 cc; Boxes of 12, 25 and 100; Containing gr 1/6 (0.01 Gm), sodium iodide gr 1/6 (0.01 Gm); *For use* in scrofula and syphilis; *Intramuscular. See Chap. I.* **(National Drug)**

630. Mercury Cacodylate—Ampules 1 cc; Boxes of 12, 25 and 100; Containing gr ½ (0.032 Gm);
Ampule-vials 25 cc; Boxes of 1; Same strength; In triple-distilled water.
Ampules 1 cc; Boxes of 12, 25 and 100; Containing gr 1 (0.065 Gm), or gr 1½ (0.1 Gm); *Intragluteally; For use* in syphilis. **(National Drug)**

631. Mercury Salicylate—Ampules 1 cc; Boxes of 12, 25 and 100; Containing gr 1 (0.065 Gm), or gr 2 (0.13 Gm) in special oil base; Deep *intramuscular* injection. *See Chap. I.* **(National Drug)**

632. Morphine Sulphate—Ampules 1 cc; Boxes of 12, 25 and 100; Containing gr ¼ (0.016 Gm) in triple-distilled water.
Ampule-vials 25 cc; Boxes of 1; Same strength. **(National Drug)**

633. Morphine and Atropine ℞ B—Ampules 1 cc; Boxes of 12, 25 and 100; Containing per cubic centimeter morphine sulphate gr ¼ (0.016 Gm), atropine sulphate gr 1/150 (0.0004 Gm), triple-distilled water q.s.
Ampule-vials 25 cc; Boxes of 1; Same strength. **(National Drug)**

634. Ovarian Extract—Ampules 1 cc; Boxes of 12, 25 and 100; Representing gr 31 (2.0 Gm) fresh ovarian (entire) substance.

Ampule-vials 15 and 25 cc; Boxes of 1; Same strength; *For use* in controlling nervous manifestations of menopause, supplying deficient ovarian secretion; *Dosage:* 1 cc, intramuscularly daily for 1 week, then on alternate days as indicated. *See Chap. IV.* (National Drug)

635. **Parathyroidin Solution**—Ampules 1 cc; Boxes of 6, 12, 25 and 100; Representing gr 3⅓ (0.215 Gm) per 16 minims; *For use* with intravenous injections of calcium chloride in chronic gastritis, gastric ulcer, asthma, hay fever, varicose veins and chronic indolent ulcers; in diabetes with symptoms of acetonuria and convulsions, in adiposis dolorosa; *Intramuscular.* (National Drug)

636. **Pituitary Extract (Anterior)**—Ampules 1 cc; Boxes of 6, 12, 25 and 100; Representing gr 7½ (0.05 Gm) to 16 minims; *For use* in exophthalmic goitre, fibroid growths and benign tumors. (National Drug)

637. **Procaine Solution**—Ampules 2 cc; Boxes of 12, 25 and 100; ½ % solution; Ampules 1, 5 and 10 cc; Boxes of 12, 25 and 100; 2 % solutions; Ampule-vials 25 cc; Boxes of 1; ½ and 2 % Solutions; Ampule-vials 100 cc; Boxes of 1; 2 % solution; *For use* as local anesthetic. *See Chap. I.* (National Drug)

638. **Procaine and Epinephrine** (Strong)—Ampules 1 cc; Boxes of 12, 25 and 100; Containing epinephrine gr 1/250 (0.000052 Gm), procaine gr ⅓ (0.02 Gm) in triple distilled water.
Ampule-vials 25 cc; Boxes of 1; Containing procaine 2 %, epinephrine chloride 1:20,000; *For use* as local anesthetic; *Dosage:* 25–50 cc of 2 % solution usually sufficient for extensive operation. *See Chap. I.* (National Drug)

639. **Procaine and Epinephrine** (Mild)—Ampules 1 cc; Boxes of 12, 25 and 100; Containing procaine gr ⅓ (0.02 Gm), epinephrine hydrochloride gr 1/6250 (0.00001 Gm), in triple-distilled water.
Ampule-vials 25 cc; Boxes of 1; Same strength; *For use* as local anesthetic. *See Chap. I.* (National Drug)

640. **Quinine and Urea Hydrochloride**—Ampules 5 cc; Boxes of 12, 25 and 100; Containing gr ¾ (0.05 Gm); gr 3⅞ (0.251 Gm); gr 7¾ (0.496 Gm).
Ampule-vials 25 cc; Boxes of 1; Containing gr 3⅞ (0.251 Gm) in triple-distilled water. *For use* as local anesthetic, 1 % solution; for treating chronic internal hemorrhoids. *See Chap. I.* (National Drug)

641. **Silver Nitrate**—Wax ampules of 6 drops; Boxes of 6, 12, 25 and 100; *For use* in treatment of eyes of new born; ampule pricked with needle, expressing 2 drops into each eye, after washing with sterile warm water. *See Chap. I.* (National Drug)

642. **Sodium Bromide**—Ampules 10 cc; Boxes of 12, 25 and 100; Containing gr 15⅖ (1 Gm). *For use* as for all bromides. (National Drug)

643. **Sodium Cacodylate**—Ampules 1 cc; Boxes of 12, 25 and 100; Containing gr ¾ (0.05 Gm), gr 3 (0.2 Gm), gr 5 (0.33 Gm), gr 7 (0.45 Gm);
Ampules 5 cc; Boxes of 12, 25 and 100; Containing gr 10 (0.65 Gm), gr 5 (0.33 Gm);
Ampules 10 cc; Boxes of 12, 25 and 100; Containing gr 7¾ (0.5 Gm), gr 15½ (1.0 Gm);
Ampules 20 cc; Boxes of 12, 25 and 100; Containing sodium cacodylate gr 5 (0.33 Gm), sodium iodide gr 32 (2.0 Gm), sodium salicylate gr 32 (2.0 Gm), colchicine salicylate gr 1/100 (0.00065 Gm);
Ampule-vials 25 cc; Boxes of 1; Containing gr 3 (0.2 Gm), or gr 7 (0.45 Gm) with procaine 0.2 %, in triple-distilled water; Hematinic; *For use* in chronic malaria, neurasthenia, neuralgia, and anemias. (National Drug)

644. **Sodium Chloride**—Ampule-vials 25 cc; Boxes of 1; 20 or 30 % solutions. (National Drug)

645. **Sodium Iodide**—Ampules 10 cc; Boxes of 12, 25 and 100; Containing gr 31 (2.0 Gm). (National Drug)

646. **Strychnine Sulphate**—Ampules 1 cc; Boxes of 12, 25 and 100; Containing gr 7½ (0.5 Gm). (National Drug)

647. Adrenalin Chloride Solution—Ampules 1 cc; Boxes of 12 and 100; 1:1,000 solution;
Ampules 1 cc; Boxes of 12 and 100; 1:10,000 solution;
Ampules 1 cc; Boxes of 12 and 100; 1:2,600 solution; *For use* as vasoconstrictor and stimulant; *Dosage:* 0.5–1 cc as required. *See Chap. I.* (Parke, Davis)

648. Amyl Nitrite—Ampules 5 m; Tin boxes of 12 and 100; For inhalation only. (Parke, Davis)

649. Bismuth Salicylate—Ampules 1 cc; Boxes of 12 and 100; Containing bismuth salicylate gr 2 (0.13 Gm), chloretone (chlorbutanol) 3 %, oil base q.s.; *For use* as antisyphilitic; *Dosage: intramuscularly* only, 1 Ampule twice weekly. *See Chap. I.* (Parke, Davis)

650. Caffeine Sodio-Benzoate—Ampules 2 cc; Boxes of 12 and 100; Containing caffeine sodio-benzoate gr 7½ (0.5 Gm), distilled water q.s.; *For use* as cardiac stimulant in cardiac dropsy, chronic nephritis, collapse and pneumonia in the aged; *Dosage:* 1–2 cc, repeated as indicated. (Parke, Davis)

651. Camphor in Oil—Ampules 1 cc; Boxes of 12 and 100; Containing pure camphor gr 3 (0.2 Gm), vegetable oil q.s.;
Ampules 5 cc; Containing gr 10 (0.65 Gm) vegetable oil q.s.;
Ampules 10 cc; Containing camphor gr 36 (2.35 Gm), vegetable oil q.s.; Boxes of 6 each; *Intramuscular; For use* as cardiac stimulant in nervous depression, hysteria, convalescence from acute or chronic disease and in crisis of lobar pneumonia; *Dosage:* gr 3–10; repeated as indicated; in pneumonia gr 36 every 12 hr. if required. (Parke, Davis)

652. Adrephine—Ampules 1 cc; Boxes of 12 and 100; Containing adrenalin 1:2,500, ephedrine hydrochloride 3 %, chloretone 0.5 %, distilled water q.s. *See Chap. I.* (Parke, Davis)

653. Calcium Cacodylate—Ampules 2 cc; Boxes of 12; Containing calcium cacodylate 5%; *For use* as general tonic in tuberculosis, and to prevent hemorrhage. (Parke, Davis)

654. Corpora Lutea—Ampules 1 cc; Boxes of 6 and 100; Containing soluble extract gr 3⁄10 (0.02 Gm), chloretone 0.5 %; *For use* in nausea of pregnancy; *Dosage:* 1 ampule two to three times weekly. *See Chap. IV.* (Parke, Davis)

655. Digitalone—Ampules 1 cc; Boxes of 12 and 100; Containing equivalent of same amount of tincture of digitalis U.S.P. per cubic centimeter, chloretone 0.5 %; *For use* as Digitalis Therapy; *Dosage:* ½–1 cc as indicated. (Parke, Davis)

666. Emetine Hydrochloride—Ampules ½ cc; Boxes of 6; Containing gr ⅓ emetine hydrochloride, physiological salt solution q.s.
Ampules 1 cc; Containing gr ½ or gr 1; *For use* in amebic dysentery, amebic hepatitis and for other tissues similarly invaded; *Dosage:* gr ⅓–1, two to three times daily for not more than gr 8. *See Chap. I.* (Parke, Davis)

667. Ephedrine Sulphate—Ampules 1 cc; Boxes of 12 and 100; Containing gr ¾ (0.048 Gm) in distilled water q.s.; *For use* as decongestive; *Dosage:* ½–1 ampule as required. *See Chap. I.* (Parke, Davis)

668. Ergot Aseptic—Ampules 1 cc; Boxes of 3, 6 and 100; Each cubic centimeter equivalent to Gm 1 of prime ergot; Containing chloretone 0.5 %, but no alcohol, *For use* in preventing post-partum hemorrhage, in the non-pregnant uterus to check bleeding in menorrhagia and metrorrhagia; *Dosage:* 1–2 cc, *intramuscularly* as indicated. *See Chap. I.* (Parke, Davis)

669. Estrogen—Ampules 1 cc; Boxes of 6; Ovarian follicular hormone standardized, Doisy and Allen 25 rat units per cubic centimeter; *For use* in functional amenorrhea, surgical menopause, sexual frigidity, delayed puberty; *Dosage:* 1–2 cc, *intramuscularly;* daily for 6–8 days; may be repeated each month. *See Chap. IV.* (Parke, Davis)

670. Glycerophosphate Compound—Ampules 1 cc; Boxes of 12; Containing sodium glycerophosphate gr 1½ (0.1 Gm), strychnine cacodylate gr 1⁄125 (0.0005 Gm), iron cacodylate gr 1/6 (0.01 Gm), chloretone (chlorbutanol) 0.5%, distilled water q.s.; *For use* as hematinic and tonic; *Dosage:* 1 ampule at 1–3 day intervals. **(Parke, Davis)**

671. Histamine Phosphate—Ampules 1 cc; Boxes of 12; Containing histamine phosphate 1:1,000 solution; *For use* in diagnosis of pernicious anemia; Directions accompany package. *See Chap. I.* **(Parke, Davis)**

672. Iron Arsenite—Ampules 1 cc; Boxes of 12 and 100; Containing iron arsenite gr 1/6 (0.01 Gm), quinine and urea hydrochloride 0.5%, distilled water, q.s.; or iron arsenite gr 1 (0.065 Gm), quinine and urea hydrochloride 0.5%, distilled water q.s.; *For use* in anemia, malarial intoxication, pellagra and chorea; *Dosage:* initial dose small and gradually increased; *Intramuscularly.* **(Parke, Davis)**

673. Iron Arsenite and Manganese—Ampules 1 cc; Boxes of 12 and 100; Containing iron arsenite gr 3/4 (0.05 Gm), manganese citrate gr 1/100 (0.00065 Gm), quinine and urea hydrochloride 0.5%, distilled water q.s. *For use* as hematinic and tonic, particularly when accompanied by skin lesions; *Dosage:* initial dose small, gradually increased; *Intramuscularly.* **(Parke, Davis)**

674. Iron Arsenite and Strychnine—Ampules 1 cc; Boxes of 12 and 100; Containing iron arsenite gr 1 (0.065 Gm), strychnine nitrate gr 1/65 (0.001 Gm), quinine and urea hydrochloride 0.5%, distilled water q.s.; or iron arsenite gr 3/4 (0.05 Gm), strychnine nitrate gr 1/65 (0.001 Gm), quinine and urea hydrochloride (0.5%, distilled water, q.s.; or iron arsenite gr 1/4 (0.015 Gm), strychnine nitrate gr 1/100 (0.00065 Gm), quinine and urea hydrochloride 0.5%, distilled water q.s. *For use* as hematinic and tonic; *Dosage:* initial dose small, gradually increased, *Intramuscularly.* **(Parke, Davis)**

675. Iron Cacodylate—Ampules 1 cc; Boxes of 12 and 100; Containing iron cacodylate gr 1/2 (0.03 Gm), distilled water q.s.; *For use* as hematinic; *Dosage:* gr 1/2 *intramuscularly,* gradually increased to limit of tolerance. **(Parke, Davis)**

676. Iron Citrate (Green)—Ampules 1 cc; Boxes of 12 and 100; Containing quinine and urea hydrochloride 0.5%, distilled water q.s., and iron and ammonium citrate either gr 1/4 (0.015 Gm), gr 3/4 (0.05 Gm), or gr 1 1/2 (0.1 Gm); *For use* as hematinic; *Dosage:* 1/4–1 1/2 gr daily or on alternate days, *intramuscularly* preferred, according to tolerance of patient. **(Parke, Davis)**

677. Iron Citrate and Manganese—Ampules 1 cc; Boxes of 12 and 100; Containing iron citrate gr 3/4 (0.05 Gm), manganese citrate gr 1/100 (0.00065 Gm), quinine and urea hydrochloride 0.5%, distilled water, q.s.; *For use* as hematinic; *Dosage:* 1 cc *Intramuscularly* preferred. **(Parke, Davis)**

678. Magnesium Sulphate—Ampules 2 cc; Boxes of 12 and 100; Containing 50% Solution; gr 15 1/2 (1 Gm), distilled water q.s.; *For use* with morphine for prolonged effect, requiring half amount of morphine; combined morphine and magnesium sulphate injection reduces risk in inhalation anesthesia. **(Parke, Davis)**

679. Mercuric Iodide (Red)—Ampules 1 cc; Boxes of 12 and 100; Containing mercuric iodide, red gr 1/6 (0.01 Gm), sodium iodide gr 1/6 (0.01 Gm), physiologic salt solution q.s.; 1% aqueous solution; or
Ampules 1 cc; Boxes of 12 and 100; Containing mercuric iodide, red, gr 1/3 (0.02 Gm), sodium iodide gr 1/3 (0.02 Gm), distilled water q.s.; 2% aqueous solution; or
Ampules 1 cc; Boxes of 12 and 100; Containing mercuric iodide, red, gr 1/6 (0.01 Gm), potassium iodide q.s., chloretone 2%, pure vegetable oil q.s.; *For use* as Antisyphilitic; *Dosage:* 1 cc at 2 day intervals, *Intragluteally. See Chap. I.* **(Parke, Davis)**

680. Liver Extract—Ampules 2 cc; Packages of 6; *For use* as hematopoietic; *For use* and *dosage, see Chap. I; Intramuscularly. See Chap. I.* **(Parke, Davis)**

681. Mercury Cyanide—Ampules 1 cc; Boxes of 12 and 100; Containing gr 1/6 (0.01 Gm) of mercury cyanide, 0.5% apothesine, physiologic salt solution q.s.; *For use* as antisyphilitic. *See Chap. I.* **(Parke, Davis)**

682. **Mercury Salicylate**—Ampules 1 cc; Boxes of 12 and 100; Containing basic apothesine 1 %, oil base q.s., mercury salicylate either gr 2 (0.13 Gm), or gr 1 (0.065 Gm); *For use* as antisyphilitic; *Dosage:* 1–2 gr, *intramuscularly*, at weekly intervals. *See Chap. I.* **(Parke, Davis)**

683. **Mercurosal**—Ampules 0.5 Gm; Boxes of 12 and 100. *See Chap. I.* **(Parke, Davis)**

684. **Mercury Succinimide**—Ampules 1 cc; Boxes of 12 and 100; Containing mercury succinimide gr 1/6, apothesine 0.5 %, distilled water q.s., *For use* in mercury therapy; *Intramuscular* injection preferable; *Dosage:* 1/2–1 cc every 3 days, or as indicated. *See Chap. I.* **(Parke, Davis)**

685. **Morphine and Atropine ℞ "A"**—Ampules 1 cc; Boxes of 12 and 100; Containing morphine sulphate gr 1/4 (0.015 Gm), atropine sulphate gr 1/100 (0.00065 Gm), physiologic salt solution q.s.; *For use* in morphine therapy; *Dosage:* as indicated. **(Parke, Davis)**

686. **Nuclein Solution, 1**—Ampules 1 cc; Boxes of 12 and 100; 5 % solution of nucleinic acid with 0.5 % chloretone; *For use* in septic and anemic conditions, suppurative tonsillitis, chronic bronchial catarrh, neurasthenia; *Dosage:* 1 cc daily, or on alternate days. **(Parke, Davis)**

687. **Ovarian Residue**—Ampules 1 cc; Boxes of 12 and 100; Containing soluble extract gr 3/5 (0.04 Gm), chloretone 0.5 %; *For use* in menstrual irregularities, nervous disturbances of menopause; *Intramuscularly. See Chap. IV.* **(Parke, Davis)**

688. **Ovarian Substance (Whole)**—Ampules 1 cc; Boxes of 12 and 100; Containing gr 3/5 (0.04 Gm), with corpus luteum, chloretone 0.5 %; *For use* in hyposecretion of ovaries; *Intramuscularly. See Chap. IV.* **(Parke, Davis)**

689. **Pitocin**—Ampules 0.5 and 1 cc; Boxes of 6 and 100; *For use* in obstetrics for uterine inertia, increase of blood pressure not being desirable; *Dosage:* 1/2–1 ampule on full cervical dilatation, *intramuscularly. See Chap. I.* **(Parke, Davis)**

690. **Pitressin**—Ampules 1 cc; Boxes of 6 and 100; Containing the pressor and anti-diuretic principles of the pituitary gland, 20 units per cubic centimeter; *Dosage: intramuscularly*, 1/2–1 ampule as required. *See Chap. I.* **(Parke, Davis)**

691. **Pituitrin (Posterior Lobe)**—Ampules 0.5 and 1 cc; Boxes of 6 and 100; with chloretone (chlorbutanol) 0.5 %; *Dosage:* 1/2–1 ampule as required. *See Chap. I.* **(Parke, Davis)**

692. **Pituitary Body (Anterior Lobe)—Antuitrin**—Ampules 1 cc; Boxes of 6 and 100; Containing chloretone (chlorbutanol), 0.5 %; *For use* in stimulating skeletal development, at time of puberty, to activate reproductive system; *Dosage:* 1 cc daily. *See Chap. IV.* **(Parke, Davis)**

693. **Quinine Dihydrochloride**—Ampules 1 cc; Boxes of 12 and 100; Containing gr 3 3/4 (0.25 Gm)
Ampules 1 1/2 cc; Boxes of 12 and 100; Containing gr 7 1/2 (0.5 Gm) with distilled water, q.s.; *For use* as tonic in malarial fever, lobar pneumonia; *Intramuscular.*
Ampules 2 cc; Boxes of 12 and 100; Containing gr 15 1/2 (0.1 Gm). *See Chap. I.* **(Parke, Davis)**

694. **Quinine and Urea Hydrochloride**—Ampules 5 cc; Boxes of 6; 1 % aqueous solution; *Local* use;
Ampules 2 cc; Boxes of 12 and 100; 1 % aqueous solution; Local use;
Ampules 1 1/2 cc; Boxes of 12 and 100; Gr 7 1/2 (0.5 Gm); *Intramuscular* use;
Ampules 2 cc; Boxes of 12 and 100; Gr 15 1/2 (1 Gm); *Intramuscular* use; *For use* as local anesthetic particularly for submucous tissues; and as *intramuscular* injections for treatment of malaria. *See Chap. I.* **(Parke, Davis)**

695. **Silver Nitrate Solution**—Capsules of wax; Boxes of 2; 1 % solution; *For use* as local application by instillation into newborn infants' eyes as preventive for gonorrheal ophthalmia; Needle prick 1 end, compress between fingers, expressing 2 drops into each eye. *See Chap. I.* **(Parke, Davis)**

696. Sodium Cacodylate—Ampules 1 cc; Boxes of 12 and 100; Containing either gr ¾ (0.05 Gm), gr 1½ (0.1 Gm), gr 2 (0.13 Gm), gr 3 (0.2 Gm), gr 5 (0.3 Gm), or gr 7 (0.45 Gm); also
Ampules 2 cc; Boxes of 12 and 100; Containing gr 15½ (1 Gm); *For use* in malarial cachexia, neurasthenia, psoriasis, anemia, leukemia and pellagra; *Dosage:* Gr ¾ (0.05 Gm) to gr 15½ (1 Gm) for adults; children relatively smaller doses. **(Parke, Davis)**

697. Sodium Glycerophosphate—Ampules 1 cc; Boxes of 12 and 100; Containing gr 1½ (0.1 Gm); *For use* in muscular and nervous debility, rachitis, osteomalacia; to accelerate metabolism, while retarding elimination of organic phosphorus; *Dosage:* 1 cc daily or on alternate days, as indicated. **(Parke, Davis)**

698. Strychnine Sulphate—Ampules 1 cc; Boxes of 12 and 100; Containing either gr 1/64 (0.001 Gm), or gr 1/32 (0.002 Gm) in physiologic salt solution; *For use* in acute collapse and shock, faintness, weakened circulation and as antidote for chloroform or chloral hydrate poisoning. **(Parke, Davis)**

699. Thyroprotein—Ampules 1 cc; Boxes of 12 and 100; Containing thyroprotein gr 1/50 (0.00125 Gm) in physiologic salt solution with 0.5% chloretone (chlorbutanol); Adjusted to contain organic iodine 0.33%; *For use* in thyroid therapy; *Dosage:* gr 1/50 at intervals indicated by patient's response. **(Parke, Davis)**

700. Theelin—Ampules 1 cc; Boxes of 6 and 100; Representing 50 rat units. *For use* in crystalline ovarian follicular hormone therapy; *Dosage:* 1–2 ampules daily. *See Chap. I.* **(Parke, Davis)**

701. Thio-Bismol—Ampules 2 cc; Boxes of 12 and 100; Containing gr 3 (0.194 Gm) in aqueous solution; *For use* as Antisyphilitic; *Dosage:* 0.5–2 cc twice weekly. *See Chap. I.* **(Parke, Davis)**

---

702. Ampacoids Ovary—Ampules 1 cc; Boxes of 6; Representing gr 31 (2.0 Gm) fresh ovary, equivalent in oestrus producing potency to 10 rat units; *For use* in amenorrhea, dysmenorrhea, sexual neurasthenia, all forms of hypo-ovarism; *Dosage:* 1 ampule three to six times weekly. *See Chap. I.* **(Reed and Carnrick)**

703. Ampacoids Prostate—Ampules 1 cc; Boxes of 6; Representing gr 10 (0.65 Gm) fresh gland substance; *For use* in prostatic hypertrophy, impotence, neurasthenia; *Dosage:* 1 ampule three to six times weekly. *See Chap. I.* **(Reed and Carnrick)**

704. Ampacoids Testicle—Ampules 1 cc; Boxes of 6; Representing gr 30 (2.0 Gm) fresh testicular substance; *For use* in impotence, sexual neurasthenia, all forms of hypogonadism; *Dosage:* 1 ampule three to six times weekly. *See Chap. I.* **(Reed and Carnrick)**

---

705. Remogland—Ampules 1 cc; Boxes of 12; Containing extracts of gonads, adrenals, anterior pituitary and thyroid gland gr 1/10 (0.006 Gm), with calcium glycerophosphate gr ⅛ (0.008 Gm) and nux vomica; *For use* in impotence and defective testicular hormone secretion; *Dosage:* *Intramuscularly,* 1 ampule every 2 days. *See Chap. III.* **(Remogland)**

---

706. Acetylcholine—Ampules of 0.1 Gm acetylcholine chloride crystals; Packages of 6 with 2 cc ampule sterile, double distilled water; *For use* as vasodilator; *Dosage:* 0.05–0.2 Gm daily, as 5% solution. *See Chap. I.* **(Roche)**

707. Digalen "Cloetta"—Ampules 2.1 cc; Boxes of 6 and 12; 2 cc equal 1 cat unit; Contains the glucosidal complex of digitalis; *Dosage:* 1 ampule every 6–8 hr. *See Chap. I.* **(Roche)**

708. Histamine—Ampules 1.1 cc; Boxes of 6; Containing 1:1,000 solution; *For use* as vagotropic; *Dosage:* 1 ampule for diagnosis. *See Chap. I.* **(Roche)**

709. Oleo-Bi—Ampules 2 cc; Boxes of 12; Containing equivalent to 0.1 Gm Bi; *For use* as bismuth antisyphilitic; *Dosage:* 1 ampule two to three times weekly; deep *intragluteal* injections. *See Chap. I.* **(Roche)**

710. Pantopon—Ampules 1.1 cc; Cartons of 6 and 12; Containing gr 1/3 (0.02 Gm); *For use* as injectable opium; *Dosage:* 1 ampule as required. *See Chap. I.* (Roche)

711. Papaverine Sulphate—Ampules 1.1 cc; Cartons of 6; Containing gr 2/3 (0.043 Gm); *For use* as Antispasmodic; *Dosage:* 1/2–1 1/3 gr several times daily. *See Chap. I.* (Roche)

712. Prostigmin—Ampules 1 1 cc; Boxes of 6; Containing 0.05% solution; *For use* as injectable Peristaltic; *Dosage:* 1 ampule, repeated in 4–5 hr. *See Chap. I.* (Roche)

713. Scopolamine—Ampules 1.2 cc; Boxes of 12 and 100; Containing scopolamine hydrobromide—gr 1/100 or gr 1/200 (obstetrical); *For use* as cerebral sedative; *Dosage:* 1 ampule as required. *See Chap. I.* (Roche)

714. Thyroxine Synthetic—Ampules 1.1 cc; Boxes of 6 and 12; Containing 1:1,000 solution; *For use* as thyroid therapy; *Dosage:* 1–2 ampules daily. *See Chap. I.* (Roche)

---

715. Caffeine Sodio-Benzoate—Ampules 2 cc; Boxes of 6, 25 and 100; Containing gr 7 1/2 (0.05 Gm); *For use* as cardiac, respiratory and cerebral stimulant and diuretic; *Dosage:* 1/2–1 ampule. (Rorer)

716. Camphor in Olive Oil—Ampules 1 cc; Boxes of 6, 12 and 100; Containing either gr 1 (0.065 Gm), gr 2 (0.13 Gm) or gr 3 (0.194 Gm); *For use* as powerful cardiac stimulant, in surgical shock, depressed circulation, sunstroke, toxemia; *Dosage:* gr 3, *intramuscularly.* (Rorer)

717. Corpora Lutea—Ampules 1 cc; Boxes of 6, 12 and 100; Containing gr 3 (0.194 Gm); *For use* in menstrual disorders, sterility, nervous and mental states associated with pelvic congestion; *Dosage:* 1 ampule twice weekly. *See Chap. IV.* (Rorer)

718. Glycerophosphate Compound—Ampules 1 cc; Boxes of 6, 12 and 100; Containing iron cacodylate gr 1/6 (0.012 Gm), sodium glycerophosphate gr 1 1/2 (0.09 Gm), strychnine cacodylate gr 1/120; *For use* as tonic in anemia, neurasthenia; *Dosage:* 1 ampule daily or as indicated. (Rorer)

719. Iron Arsenite—Ampules 1 cc; Boxes of 6, 12 and 100; Containing gr 1 with quinine and urea hydrochloride; *For use* as hematinic and tonic; *Dosage:* 1/4–1 ampule, daily or as indicated. (Rorer)

720. Iron Arsenite and Strychnine—Ampules 1 cc; Boxes of 6, 25 and 100; Containing gr 1 iron arsenite and gr 1/65 strychnine nitrate; *For use* as hematinic and tonic; *Dosage:* 1/4–1 ampule daily or as indicated. (Rorer)

721. Iron Citrate (Green)—Ampules 1 cc; Boxes of 6, 12 and 100; Containing gr 1 with quinine and urea hydrochloride; *For use* as Hematinic; *Dosage:* 1/4–1 ampule daily, or as indicated. (Rorer)

722. Iron Citrate and Strychnine—Ampules 1 cc; Boxes of 6, 12 and 100; Containing iron citrate gr 1 and strychnine nitrate gr 1/60; *For use* as Hematinic; *Dosage:* 1/4–1 ampule daily or as indicated. (Rorer)

722a. Lacto-Protein—Ampules 1, 5, 10 cc; Packages of 6, 12 and 100; Containing sterile milk proteins with fat content largely removed; *For use* as non-specific therapy agent; *Dosage:* initial 1–1.5 cc intramuscularly every 3–4 days, cautiously increased to 5–10 cc for 10–20 injections. (Rorer)

723. Magnesium Sulphate—Ampules 2 cc; Boxes of 6, 12 and 100; 50% solution by weight; *For use* as sedative, analgesic, and for prolonging action of morphine; *Dosage:* 2 cc. (Rorer)

724. Neonataline—Ampules 1/2 and 1 cc; Boxes of 6 and 12; Containing thymus and pituitary extract; by combining, the pituitary action is made smoother, more rhythmical, and more prolonged; Contraindications similar to pituitary. (Rorer)

725. Paraldehyde—Ampules 2 cc; Boxes of 6, 12 and 100; *For use* as soporific where pain is not present. (Rorer)

726. Phenolsulphonphthalein—Ampules 1 cc; Boxes of 6, 12 and 100; Containing gr 1/10 (0.006 Gm); *For use* as kidney function test; *Intramuscular.* *See Chap. I.* (Rorer)

727. Pituitary Extract (Obstetrical)—Ampules ½ and 1 cc; Boxes of 6, 12 and 100; assayed physiologically and standardized; *For use* as Oxytocic; Contraindicated in nephritis, myocarditis, arteriosclerosis or where anatomical impediment to normal delivery exists; *Dosage:* 1/5–2 cc as indicated. *See Chap. I.* (Rorer)

728. Procaine—Ampules 1 cc; Boxes of 6, 12 and 100; Containing gr ¾ (0.04860 Gm); *For use* as local anesthetic. *See Chap. I.* (Rorer)

729. Silver Nitrate—Ampules of wax; 1% solution; *For use* as prophylactic in gonorrheal ophthalmia in new born; express 2 drops into each eye. *See Chap. I.* (Rorer)

730. Sodium Cacodylate—Ampules 1 cc; Boxes of 6, 12 and 100; Containing gr 1 (0.065 Gm), gr 2 (0.130 Gm), gr 3 (0.194 Gm), gr 5 (0.324 Gm); *For use* in anemia, skin conditions, neurasthenia, and as general alterative; *Dosage:* to be gradually increased; cumulative action to be watched for. (Rorer)

731. Supranephrin—Ampules 1 cc; Boxes of 6, 12 and 100; 1:1,000 solution; *For use* as powerful astringent and hemostatic, raises blood pressure in collapse, shock, internally for pernicious vomiting of pregnancy; *Dosage:* 5–15 m. (Rorer)

---

732. Bellafoline—Ampules 1 cc; Boxes of 6 and 20; Containing gr 1/125 (0.0005 Gm); *For use* as vagus depressor; *Dosage:* 0.5–2 cc daily. *See Chap. I.* (Sandoz)

733. Calcium Gluconate (Calglucon)—Ampules 10 cc, 10% and 20% solution; Boxes of 5, 20 and 100; Calcium gluconate. (Rorer)
Ampules 5 cc, 10% and 20% solution; Boxes of 10, 50 and 150; Ampules 2 cc, 10% sol, Boxes 3, 10, 50. *Dosage:* *Intramuscularly,* 10 cc every 1–3 days. *See Chap. I.* (Sandoz)

734. Gynergen—Ampules 1 cc; Boxes of 6, 12, 50 and 100; Containing 0.0005 Gm; Ampules 0.5 cc; Boxes of 6 and 50; Containing 0.00025 Gm specific alkaloid of ergot; *Dosage:* 0.5–1 cc as required. *See Chap.* I. (Sandoz)

---

735. Progynon—Ampules 1 cc; Boxes of 12; Containing 25 Allen-Doisy units of female sex hormone; *Dosage:* 1 ampule once or twice daily. *See Chap. I.* (Schering)

---

736. Thyroid Residue—Ampules 30 m; Boxes of 6; Containing 0.05 mg iodine per cubic centimeter; *For use* as thyroid therapy in hypertension, in acute toxemic post-operative cases of hyperthyroidism; *Dosage:* 20–30 m every 2 hr. (Schieffelin)

---

737. Aminophyllin—Ampules 2 cc; Boxes of 6, 25 and 100; Gr 7½ (0.48 Gm); *For use* as cardiotonic; Containing theophyllin content 75%, ethylenediamine content 25%; *Dosage:* 1–3 ampules daily, *intramuscularly. See Chap. I.* (Searle)

738. Bismuth Sodium Tartrate—Ampules 2 cc; Boxes of 12, 25 and 100; 1.5% solution; Containing 74% metallic bismuth; *For use* as Antiluetic; *Dosage:* 1 ampule twice weekly, *intramuscularly. See Chap. I.* (Searle)

739. Caffeine Sodium Benzoate—Ampules 2 cc; Boxes of 12, 25 and 100; Gr 7½ (0.5 Gm); *For use* as cerebral stimulant and diuretic. (Searle)

740. Calcium Gluconate—Ampules 10 cc; Boxes of 6, 25 and 100; 10% Solution; *For use* as calcium therapy in tetany, spasmophilia, dermatologic conditions, eclampsia; *Dosage:* 10 cc *intravenously* in A.M., 10 cc *intramuscularly* in P.M. *See Chap. I.* (Searle)

741. Camphor in Oil—Ampules 1 cc; Boxes of 12, 25 and 100; Containing gr 3 (0.20 Gm); *For use* as quick cardiac stimulant; *Intramuscular.* (Searle)

742. Corpus Luteum—Ampules 1 cc; Boxes of 12, 25 and 100; Containing gr 3 (0.2 Gm); *For use* in "morning sickness," hyperemesis gravidarum, menstrual and menopausal dysfunction; *Intramuscular. See Chap. IV.* (Searle)

743. Epinephrin—Ampules 1 cc; Boxes of 12, 25 and 100; 1:1,000 Solution; Active principle of suprarenal gland in normal saline; *For use* as powerful vasoconstrictor in dyspnea of asthma, in urticaria and to prolong anesthesia. *See Chap. I.* (Searle)

744. Gold Sodium Thiosulphate—Ampules 1 cc; Boxes of 12 and 25; 10 mg of salt;
Ampules 2 cc; Boxes of 6 and 25; 25 mg of salt;
Ampules 5 cc; Boxes of 6 and 25; 50 mg of salt; Solution containing 37 % of gold; *For use* in inhibiting growth of tubercle bacillus and in lupus erythematosus. *See Chap. I.* (Searle)

745. Iron and Ammonium Citrate—Ampules 1 cc; Boxes of 12, 25 and 100; 1½ gr (0.10 Gm); *For use* as Hematinic; *Intramuscular.* (Searle)

746. Iron, Arsenic and Phosphorus, 1—Ampules 1 cc; Boxes of 12, 25 and 100; Containing sodium glycerophosphate 1½ gr (0.10 Gm), strychnine cacodylate gr 1/125 (0.0005 Gm), iron cacodylate gr 1/6 (0.011 Gm); *Intramuscular; For use* as hematinic, and for chronic malaria, neurasthenia. (Searle)

747. Iron, Arsenic and Phosphorus, 2—Ampules 2 cc; Boxes of 12, 25 and 100; Containing sodium glycerophosphate gr 3 (0.2 Gm), sodium cacodylate gr 2 (0.13 Gm), iron cacodylate gr 2/3 (0.043 Gm), strychnine nitrate gr 1/33 (0.002 Gm) *Intramuscular; For use* as Hematinic. (Searle)

748. Iron Arsenite—Ampules 1 cc; Boxes of 12, 25 and 100; Containing gr 1 (0.065 Gm); *Intramuscular; For use* as Hematinic. (Searle)

749. Iron Cacodylate—Ampules 1 cc; Boxes of 12, 25 and 100; Containing gr 1 (0.065 Gm); *Intramuscular; For use* in anemia and dry skin affections. (Searle)

750. Magnesium Sulphate—Ampules 2 cc; Boxes of 12, 25 and 100; 50 % Solution; *For use* in prolonging effects of morphine, as analgesic, sedative and hypnotic. (Searle)

751. Manganese Butyrate—Ampules 1 and 1½ cc; Boxes of 12, 25 and 100; Containing manganese butyrate gr 1/6 (0.01 Gm), benzyl alcohol gr 1/3 (0.02 Gm); *Intramuscular; For use* in furunculosis, staphylococcus infections; acute gonorrhea; *Dosage:* 1 cc, 4 or 5 days later 1½ cc. *See Chap. I.* (Searle)

752. Mercury Succinimide—Ampules 1 cc; Boxes of 12, 25 and 100; Containing gr 1/6 (0.011 Gm); *For use* as Antiluetic; *Intramuscular. See Chap. I.* (Searle)

753. Pituitary Solution—Ampules ½ and 1 cc; Boxes of 12, 25 and 100; Posterior lobe; *For use* in obstetrics for uterine inertia. *See Chap. I.* (Searle)

755. Procaine and Epinephrin—Ampules 5 cc; Boxes of 6, 25 and 100; Containing procaine gr 1⅔ (0.108 Gm), epinephrin 1:6,000; *For use* as local anesthetic. (Searle)

757. Proteolac—Ampules 1 cc; Boxes of 12, 25 and 100; *Intramuscular* or *intradermal;*
Ampules 2 cc; Boxes of 12, 25 and 100;
Ampules 5 cc; Boxes of 6, 25 and 100; *Intragluteal;*
Ampules 10 cc; Boxes of 6, 25 and 100; *Intragluteal;* Composed of defatted milk specially processed for use as non-specific protein therapy agent; stimulates leucocytosis and antibody formation to build body resistance, in arthritis, gonorrheal complications, pelvic inflammations, skin affections; also for testing tolerance. *See Chap. I.* (Searle)

758. Quinine and Urea Hydrochloride—Ampules 2 cc; Boxes of 12, 25 and 100; 1 % Solution; *For use* as local anesthetic. *See Chap. I.* (Searle)

759. Quinine and Urea Hydrochloride—Ampules 2 cc; Boxes of 12 and 25; Intramuscular; Containing gr 15½ (1.0 Gm): *For use* as antipyretic and antimalarial. *See Chap. I.* (Searle)

760. **Quinine Dihydrochloride**—Ampules 2 cc; Boxes of 12, 25 and 100; Containing gr 15½ (1.0 Gm); *For use* as tonic, antimalarial, antipyretic. *See Chap. I.* (Searle)

761. **Silver Nitrate**—Ampules 0.70 cc (10 m); Boxes of 12; 1% Solution; Special eye dropper; *For use* as prophylactic against ophthalmia neonatorum, in ophthalmic surgery and therapy, and as caustic and astringent antiseptic. *See Chap. I.* (Searle)

762. **Sodium Cacodylate**—Ampules 1 cc; Boxes of 12, 25 and 100; Containing gr ¾ (0.048 Gm); *Intramuscular; For use* as Hematinic, in the cachexia of malaria and syphilis. (Searle)

763. **Sodium Cacodylate**—Ampules 1 cc; Boxes of 12, 25 and 100; Containing gr 1½ (0.10 Gm) *Intramuscular; For use* as Hematinic. (Searle)

764. **Sodium Cacodylate**—Ampules 1 cc; Boxes of 12, 25 and 100; Containing gr ¾ (0.048 Gm);
Ampules 1 cc; Boxes of 12, 25 and 100; Containing gr 3 (0.20 Gm);
Ampules 1 cc; Boxes of 12, 25 and 100; Containing gr 5 (0.324 Gm);
Ampules 1 cc; Boxes of 12, 25 and 100; Containing gr 7½ (0.50 Gm);
Ampules 2 cc; Boxes of 12, 25 and 100; Containing gr 15½ (1.0 Gm); *For use* as above stated. (Searle)

765. **Sterile Double Distilled Water**—Ampules of 5, 10 and 20 cc; Boxes of 6, 25 and 100; *For use* in preparing solutions of arsenicals and other preparations for injection. (Searle)

766. **Sulpharsphenamine**—Ampules of 0.1, 0.2, 0.3, 0.4, 0.5, 0.6 Gm; *for use* as Antisyphilitic; *Intramuscular. See Chap. I.* (Searle)

767. **Thymo-Pitsin**—Ampules 0.5 cc; Boxes of 10, 25 and 100; contains the oxytoccic principle of post-pituitary with thymus gland hormone; *For use* in obstetrics. *See Chap. III.* (Searle)

---

768. **Adrin Solution**—Ampules 1 cc; Boxes of 6 and 100; Contains epinephrine hydrochloride solution 1:1,000; *For use* as Vasoconstrictor; *Dosage:* 0.5–1 cc as required. *See Chap. I.* (Sharp and Dohme)

769. **Amyl Nitrate**—Ampules of 5 m; Boxes of 12; Hermetically sealed and enclosed in absorbent and protective fabric. (Sharp and Dohme)

770. **Bismuth Salicylate**—Ampules 1 cc; Boxes of 12; Containing bismuth salicylate gr 1½ (0.1 Gm), camphor gr 1½ (0.1 Gm), creosote, suspended in oil; Intramuscular. *See Chap. I.* (Sharp and Dohme)

771. **Caffeine Sodio-Benzoate**—Ampules 2 cc; Boxes of 12; Containing gr 3¾ (0.25 Gm), or gr 7½ (0.5 Gm); *For use* in cardiac failure, collapse, neuralgia, dropsy of cardiac origin, chronic nephritis and pneumonia of the aged. (Sharp and Dohme)

772. **Calcium Cacodylate**—Ampules 2 cc; Boxes of 12; Containing 5% solution. (Sharp and Dohme)

773. **Calcium Lactate**—Ampules 5 cc; Boxes of 6; Containing 5% sterile solution; *For use* in calcium therapy; also Ampule-vials of 5 cc. (Sharp and Dohme)

774. **Calcium Chloride**—Ampule-vials 10 cc; Boxes of 6. (Sharp and Dohme)

775. **Camphor in Oil**—Ampules of 1 cc; Boxes of 12; Containing gr 1½ (0.1 Gm) or gr 3 (0.2 Gm);
Ampules of 10 cc; Boxes of 6; Containing gr 36 (2.33 Gm); *For use* in typhoid fever, pneumonia, as a quick heart stimulant in shock and collapse. (Sharp and Dohme)

776. **Corpus Luteum Extract**—Ampules 1 cc; Boxes of 6; Representing gr 3 (0.2 Gm) desiccated corpus luteum per cubic centimeter; *For use* in various general disorders of menopause. *See Chap. IV.* (Sharp and Dohme)

777. **Digitalis, Tincture Purified**—Ampules 1 cc; Boxes of 12; *For use* in digitalis therapy. *See Chap. I.* (Sharp and Dohme)

778. Digitos—Ampules 1 cc; Boxes of 12;
Ampules 5 cc; Boxes of 4; *For use* in digitalis therapy; *Dosage: intramuscularly,* 1 cc every 6–8 hr. *See Chap. I.* (Sharp and Dohme)

779. Emetine Hydrochloride—Ampules 1 cc; Boxes of 6; Containing gr ⅓ (0.02 Gm), gr ½ (0.03 Gm), or gr 1 (0.065 Gm); *For use* in the local injection of pyorrheal pockets; *Dosage:* once daily, or on alternate days. *See Chap. I.* (Sharp and Dohme)

780. Ephedrine Sulphate—Ampules of 1 cc; Boxes of 6; Containing gr ¾ (0.05 Gm); Pink colored capsules only. *See Chap. I.* (Sharp and Dohme)

781. Ergotole—Ampules 1 cc; Boxes of 6; Contains liquid extract of ergot of rye; *For use* in ergot therapy. (Sharp and Dohme)

782. Ferrous Iodide Concentrated—Ampules ½ fl. oz.; Boxes of 2; 1 ampule added to 7½ fl. oz. of syrup, makes 8 fl. oz. syrup ferrous iodide U.S.P. (Sharp and Dohme)

783. Glycerophosphate Compound ℞ A—Ampules 1 cc; Boxes of 12; Containing sodium glycerophosphate gr 1½ (0.1 Gm), strychnine cacodylate gr 1/125 (0.0005 Gm), iron cacodylate gr ⅙ (0.01 Gm) in sterile solution. (Sharp and Dohme)

784. Glycerophosphate Compound ℞ B—Ampules 1 cc; Boxes of 12; Containing sodium glycerophosphate gr 1½ (0.1 Gm), sodium cacodylate gr ¾ (0.05 Gm), strychnine cacodylate gr 1/128 (0.0005 Gm), in sterile solution; *For use* as tonic. (Sharp and Dohme)

785. Iron Arsenite—Ampules 1 cc; Boxes of 12; Containing gr ¾ (0.05 Gm) soluble iron arsenite with 0.5% quinine and urea hydrochloride; or gr 1 (0.065 Gm) soluble iron arsenite with 0.5% quinine and urea hydrochloride; *For use* in anemias. (Sharp and Dohme)

786. Iron Arsenite with Strychnine 1—Ampules 1 cc; Boxes of 12; Containing iron arsenite gr 1 (0.065 Gm), strychnine nitrate gr 1/65 (0.001 Gm), quinine and urea hydrochloride 0.5%. (Sharp and Dohme)

787. Iron Arsenite with Strychnine 2—Ampules 1 cc; Boxes of 12; Containing iron arsenite gr ⅜ (0.025 Gm), strychnine nitrate gr 1/65 (0.001 Gm), quinine and urea hydrochloride 0.5%; *For use* in chlorosis and other types of anemia. (Sharp and Dohme)

788. Iron Cacodylate—Ampules 1 cc; Boxes of 12; Containing gr ½ (0.03 Gm), or gr ¾ (0.05 Gm); *For use* as tonic, alterative and hematinic (Sharp and Dohme)

789. Iron Citrate (Green)—Ampules 1 cc; Boxes of 12; Containing iron and ammonium citrate green gr ¾ (0.05 Gm), gr 1 (0.065 Gm), or gr 1½ (0.1 Gm) with quinine and urea hydrochloride 0.5%; *For use* in secondary anemias of the adult and child. (Sharp and Dohme)

790. Magnesium Sulphate Solution—Ampules 2 cc; Boxes of 12; Containing 25 or 50% solutions. (Sharp and Dohme)

791. Mercuric Chloride Corrosive—Ampules 1 cc; Boxes of 12; Containing gr ⅙ (0.01 Gm). (Sharp and Dohme)

792. Mercury Cyanide—Ampules 1 cc; Boxes of 12; Containing gr ⅙ (0.01 Gm). *See Chap. I.* (Sharp and Dohme)

793. Mercuric Iodide Red—Ampules 1 cc; Boxes of 12; Containing mercury iodide red and sodium iodide gr ⅙ (0.01 Gm) each; *For use* as Antisyphilitic. *See Chap. I.* (Sharp and Dohme)

794. Mercury Salicylate—Ampules 1 cc; Boxes of 12; Containing gr 1 (0.065 Gm), or gr 2 (0.13 Gm) with quinine and urea hydrochloride 0.5% in a neutral base; *For use* in secondary syphilis. *See Chap. I.* (Sharp and Dohme)

795. Mercury Succinimide—Ampules 1 cc; Boxes of 12; Containing gr ⅙ (0.01 Gm) in sterile solution. *See Chap. I.* (Sharp and Dohme)

796. Ovarian Extract (Whole Ovary)—Ampules 1 cc; Boxes of 12; Containing gr 10 (0.65 Gm), or gr 31 (2 Gm) fresh ovarian substance including corpus luteum;

For use in disorders of menopause, and in mal-development of female reproductive system. *See Chap. IV.* (Sharp and Dohme)

797. **Ovarian Residue Extract**—Ampules 1 cc; Boxes of 12; Containing gr 31 (2 Gm) fresh ovarian extract, minus corpus luteum; *For use* in menstrual irregularities and dysmenorrhea. *See Chap. IV.* (Sharp and Dohme)

798. **Phenolsulphonphthalein**—Ampules 1 cc; Boxes of 12; Containing gr 1/10 (0.006 Gm) monosodium salt.
Ampule-vial 1 cc; Boxes of 12; *For use* in renal function test. *See Chap. I.* (Sharp and Dohme)

799. **Pituitary Extract**—Ampules ½ and 1 cc; Boxes of 6; Biologically standardized fresh posterior lobe of pituitary gland; *For use* in post-partum hemorrhage, subinvolution of uterus, uterine inertia; Obstetrical strength.
Ampules 1 cc; Boxes of 6; Double strength; *For use* post-operatively.
See Chap. I. (Sharp and Dohme)

800. **Pituitary Extract**—Ampules 1 cc; Boxes of 6; anterior lobe of pituitary gland. *See Chap. I.* (Sharp and Dohme)

801. **Procaine Hydrochloride Solution**—Ampules 1 cc; Boxes of 12; Containing 1 or 2% solutions; *For use* as local anesthetic. *See Chap. I.* (Sharp and Dohme)

802. **Quinine Dihydrochloride**—Ampules 1 cc; Boxes of 12; Containing gr 7½ (0.5 Gm).
Ampules 2 cc; Boxes of 12; Containing gr 15½ (1 Gm); *For use* in quinine therapy of malaria. *See Chap. I.* (Sharp and Dohme)

803. **Quinine and Urea Hydrochloride**—Ampules 5 cc; Boxes of 6; Containing gr ¾ (0.05 Gm); *For use* as local anesthetic.
Ampules 1 cc; Boxes of 12; Containing gr 7½ (0.5 Gm).
Ampules 2 cc; Boxes of 12; Containing gr 15½ (1 Gm). *For use* in malarial and other toxic conditions. *See Chap. I.* (Sharp and Dohme)

804. **Silver Nitrate**—Ampules of wax; Boxes of 2; Containing 1% solution. *See Chap. I.* (Sharp and Dohme)

805. **Sodium Cacodylate**—Ampules 1 cc; Boxes of 12; Containing gr ¾ (0.05 Gm), gr 1½ (0.1 Gm), gr 2 (0.13 Gm), gr 3 (0.2 Gm), gr 5 (0.324 Gm), gr 7 (0.45 Gm).
Ampule-vial 5 cc; Boxes of 6; Containing gr 7½ (0.5 Gm).
Ampules 2 cc; Boxes of 12; Containing gr 15½ (1 Gm).
Ampule-vials 10 cc; Boxes of 6; Containing gr 15½ (1 Gm); *For use* in syphilitic conditions; marked anemia, psoriasis, pellagra. (Sharp and Dohme)

---

806. **Bismuth Salicylate**—Ampules 1 cc; Boxes of 12 and 100; Containing bismuth subsalicylate gr 2 (0.13 Gm), camphor 10%, creosote 10%, in neutral vegetable oil; *For use* as Antisyphilitic. *See Chap. I.* (Sherman)

807. **Caffeine Sodio-Benzoate**—Ampules 2 cc; Boxes of 12 and 100; Containing gr 7½ (0.48 Gm); *For use* in neuralgia, heart failure, chronic nephritis, collapse, pneumonia in the aged. (Sherman)

808. **Camphor in Oil**—Ampules 1 cc; Boxes 12 and 100; Containing gr 3 (0.19 Gm); *For use* in heart failure, hysteria, nervous depression. (Sherman)

809. **Corpus Luteum**—Ampules 1 cc; Boxes 6 and 100; Containing soluble extract from gr 3 (0.19 Gm) desiccated gland; *For use* in hyperemesis gravidarum, menopausal disorders; contraindicated in pregnancy complicated by goitre. *See Chap. IV.* (Sherman)

810. **Epinephrin Chloride**—Ampules 1 cc; Boxes of 12 and 100; Vials of 1 oz; 1:1,000 solution; *For use* as Vasoconstrictor. *See Chap. I.* (Sherman)

811. **Glycerophosphate Compound**—Ampules 1 cc; Boxes of 12 and 100; Containing sodium glycerophosphate gr 1½ (0.09 Gm), iron citrate gr 1 (0.06 Gm), sodium cacodylate gr ½ (0.03 Gm), strychnine sulphate gr 1/128; *For use* in anemia, torpid liver, convalescence, chlorosis. (Sherman)

812. **Glycerophosphate Compound**—Ampules 1 cc; Boxes of 12 and 100; Formula "B," sodium glycerophosphate gr 1½ (0.09 Gm), strychnine cacodylate gr 1/25, iron cacodylate gr 1/6 (0.012 Gm) chlorbutanol 0.5%; *For use* as above. (Sherman)

813. **Iron, Arsenic and Strychnine**—Ampules 1 cc; Boxes of 12 and 100; Containing iron citrate gr 1 (0.06 Gm), sodium arsenate gr 1/64 (0.001 Gm), strychnine sulphate gr 1/128; *For use* in atonic dyspepsia with anemia, chlorosis, malnutrition, convalescence. (Sherman)

814. **Iron Arsenite**—Ampules 1 cc; Boxes of 12 and 100; Containing gr 1 (0.06 Gm); Ampules 1 cc; Boxes of 12 and 100; Containing gr ½ (0.03 Gm). *For use* in pellagra, anemia, dry and scaly cutaneous diseases. (Sherman)

815. **Iron Citrate (Green)**—Ampules 1 cc; Boxes of 12 and 100; Containing gr 1 (0.06 Gm); *For use* as Tonic. (Sherman)

816. **Mercury Iodide (Red) Aqueous**—Ampules 1 cc; Boxes of 12 and 100; Containing gr 1/6 (0.012 Gm); *For use* as Antisyphilitic. *See Chap. I.* (Sherman)

817. **Magnesium Sulphate**—Ampules 2 cc; Boxes of 12 and 100; 50% Solution; *For use* to prolong effects of morphine. (Sherman)

818. **Orchic Substance Soluble Extract**—Ampules 1 cc; Boxes of 6 and 100; Containing gr 1/3 (0.02 Gm); *For use* in neurasthenia and asthenia from approaching sexual exhaustion. (Sherman)

819. **Pituitary Extract (Obstetrical)**—Ampules ½ and 1 cc; Boxes of 6 and 100; Post pituitary. *See Chap. I.* (Sherman)

820. **Pituitary Extract (Surgical)**—Ampules 1 cc; Boxes of 6 and 100; *For use* in prevention of post-operative shock, intestinal and vesical paresis, hemorrhage. *See Chap. I.* (Sherman)

821. **Sodium Cacodylate**—Ampules 1 cc; Boxes of 12 and 100; Containing gr 1 (0.06 Gm).
Ampules 1 cc; Boxes of 12 and 100; Containing gr 3 (0.19 Gm).
Ampules 1 cc; Boxes of 12 and 100; Containing gr 5 (0.32 Gm).
Ampules 1 cc; Boxes of 12 and 100; Containing gr 7 (0.045 Gm).
Ampules 2 cc; Boxes of 12 and 100; Containing gr 15½ (1.0 Gm). *For use* in anemia, malaria, non-parasitic chronic skin diseases. (Sherman)

---

822. **Pentnucleotide**—Ampules 10 cc; Boxes of 12; Contains mixture of sodium salts of pentose nucleotides; *Dosage: intragluteally,* 10 cc twice daily. *See Chap. I.* (Smith, Kline and French)

---

823. **Quicamphol**—Ampules 1.2 cc; Boxes of 6; Containing anhydrous basic quinine 0.03 Gm, camphor 0.025 Gm, eucalyptol 0.18 Gm, menthol 0.08 Gm; *For use* in parenteral quinine therapy; *Dosage:* 1–2 cc daily for 1–2 weeks, *intramuscularly. See Chap. II.* (Spicer)

824. **Quiniobine**—Ampules 2 cc; Boxes of 6; Containing bismuth 0.030 Gm, iodine 0.075 Gm, quinine 0.03 Gm, lecithin 0.22 Gm per cubic centimeter; *For use* as Antiluetic; *Dosage: intragluteally,* 1–2 cc two to three times weekly. *See Chap. I.* (Spicer)

825. **Solvochin**—Ampules 2.2 cc; Boxes of 3 and 12; Containing 25% quinine solution; *Dosage:* 0.5–2 cc once or twice daily, *intramuscularly. See Chap. I.* (Spicer)

826. **Tartro-Quiniobine**—Ampules 2 cc; Boxes of 6; Containing metallic bismuth 0.030 Gm, iodine 0.037 Gm, quinine 0.022 Gm; *For use* as Antiluetic; *Dosage: intragluteally,* 1–2 cc two to three times weekly. *See Chap. II.* (Spicer)

---

827. **Iodobismitol**—Ampules 2 cc; Boxes of 10 and 100.
Vials of 50 cc; Boxes of 1; Containing sodium iodobismuthite gr 2 (0.13 Gm), sodium iodide gr 4 (0.259 Gm), ethylene glycol (containing 0.1% acetic acid) 2 cc; *For use* as Antiluetic; *Dosage: intramuscularly,* 1 ampule two to three times weekly. *See Chap. II.* (Squibb)

828. **Pituitary Solution**—Ampules 1 cc; Boxes of 6 and 100; Containing 5 or 10 units; Obstetrical.
Ampules 1 cc; Boxes of 6 and 100; Containing 10 units; Surgical; *Dosage:* 0.5–1 cc as required. *See Chap. I.* **(Squibb)**

829. **Sulpharsphenamine**—Ampules of 0.1 Gm dissolved in 0.3 cc water.
Ampules of 0.2 Gm dissolved in 0.6 cc water.
Ampules of 0.3 Gm dissolved in 0.9 cc water.
Ampules of 0.4 Gm dissolved in 1.2 cc water.
Ampules of 0.5 Gm dissolved in 1.5 cc water.
Ampules of 0.6 Gm dissolved in 1.8 cc water. *For use* as Antiluetic, especially in neurosyphilis; *Dosage:* 0.45–0.6 Gm once or twice weekly. *See Chap. I.* **(Squibb)**

---

830. **Corpus Luteum Solution**—Ampules 1 cc; Boxes of 6 and 100; Representing gr 3 (0.194 Gm) desiccated corpus luteum in physiologic salt solution with ½% of chlorbutanol; *For use* in relief of nervous symptoms of natural or artificial menopause, nausea of early pregnancy, sterility; *Dosage:* 1 cc two to three times weekly. *See Chap. IV.* **(Stoddard)**

831. **Orchic Solution**—Ampules 1 cc; Boxes of 6 and 100; Representing gr 27½ (1.76 Gm) fresh orchic substance in physiologic salt solution and ½% chlorbutanol; *For use* in premature senility, hypogonadism and as reconstructive tonic during convalescence; *Dosage:* 1 cc two to three times weekly. **(Stoddard)**

832. **Ovarian Solution**—Ampules 1 cc; Boxes of 6 and 100; Representing gr 23 (1.490 Gm) fresh ovarian (whole) substance; in physiologic salt solution. with ½% chlorbutanol; *Dosage:* 1 cc two or three times weekly. *See Chap. IV.* **(Stoddard)**

833. **Pituitary Solution (Posterior Lobe)**—Ampules ½ and 1 cc; Boxes of 6 and 100; Containing water soluble ingredients in physiological solution with ½% chlorbutanol; *For use* in uterine inertia, post-partum hemorrhage; Contraindicated where anatomical impediment to normal delivery exists, nephritis, myocarditis, arteriosclerosis; *Dosage:* 1 cc as indicated. *See Chap. I.* **(Stoddard)**

834. **Thymus Pituitary Solution**—Ampules ½ cc; Boxes of 6 and 100; Representing watery extract of gr 10½ (0.675 Gm) of fresh thymus gland, with equal parts pituitary solution U.S.P.X. and ½% chlorbutanol; *Dosage:* ½ cc as indicated; *For use* in labor at end of first stage or beginning of second, where pituitary solution is contraindicated. **(Stoddard)**

---

835. **A.L.A.**—Ampules 2 cc; Packages of 6; Containing per fluid ounce para-aminobenzoic acid ethylester 3.0%, phenmethylol 5.0%, ether 10%, olive oil 82%; *For use* as local anesthetic; *Dosage:* 0.1–0.5 cc injected over painful area, in fan-shaped manner. *See Chap. II.* **(Sutliff and Case)**

---

837. **Biliposol Solution**—Ampules 2 cc. Packages 12; containing Biliposol in olive oil, with 2% benzyl alcohol, 1.5% ethyl aminobenzoate and 1.5% butyl aminobenzate per cubic centimeter. *See Chap. I.* **(Ulmer)**

---

838. **Bismuth Salicylate**—Ampules 1 cc; Boxes of 12; Containing bismuth salicylate (subsalicylate) gr 2 (0.13 Gm) with camphor and creosote 10% each; *Dosage:* 1–2 cc, *intramuscularly*, at 5–7 day intervals. *See Chap. I.* **(Upjohn)**

839. **Caffeine and Sodium Benzoate**—Ampules 2 cc; Boxes of 12; Containing caffeine and sodium benzoate gr 7½ (0.5 Gm), equivalent to caffeine gr 3¾ (0.25 Gm); *Dosage:* 1–2 cc, one or two times daily, as indicated. **(Upjohn)**

840. **Camphor in Oil**—Ampules 1 cc; Boxes of 12; Containing gr 3 (0.2 Gm) in neutral sweet almond oil; *Dosage:* 1–2 cc, *intramuscularly*, as indicated. **(Upjohn)**

841. **Emetine Hydrochloride**—Ampules 1 cc; Boxes of 6; Containing gr ½ (0.032 Gm) in physiological salt solution; *Dosage:* 1 cc twice daily, as indicated. *See Chap. I.* **(Upjohn)**

842. Ephedrine Sulphate—Ampules 1 cc; Boxes of 12; Containing gr ¾ (0.05 Gm); *Dosage:* ½–1 cc as indicated; generally at 4–24 hr. intervals. *See Chap. I.* (Upjohn)

843. Glycerophosphate Compound ℞ A—Ampules 1 cc; Boxes of 12; Containing sodium glycerophosphate gr 1½ (0.1 Gm), strychnine cacodylate gr 1/125 (0.0005 Gm), iron cacodylate gr ⅙ (0.01 Gm) with chlorbutanol gr 1/12 (0.005 Gm); *Dosage:* 1 cc at 24 hr. intervals as indicated. (Upjohn)

844. Glycerophosphate Compound, ℞ A (Double Strength) the above. (Upjohn)

845. Iron Arsenite, Soluble—Ampules 1 cc; Boxes of 12; Containing iron arsenite, soluble gr 1 (0.065 Gm), approximating metallic iron gr ⅙ (0.01 Gm), arsenic trioxide gr 1/65 (0.001 Gm); *Dosage:* ¼–1 cc as indicated; *Intramuscular.* (Upjohn)

846. Iron Arsenite, Soluble, and Manganese—Ampules 1 cc; Boxes of 12; Containing iron arsenite (soluble) gr ¾ (0.05 Gm), manganese citrate gr 1/100 (0.0006 Gm), quinine and urea hydrochloride 0.5%; *Dosage:* 1 cc, *intramuscularly,* at 1 or 2 day intervals. (Upjohn)

847. Iron Arsenite, Soluble, and Strychnine Nitrate—Ampules 1 cc; Boxes of 12; Containing iron arsenite gr ¾ (0.05 Gm), and strychnine nitrate gr 1/65 (0.001 Gm); also Ampules with iron arsenite gr 1 (0.065); *Dosage:* 1 cc, *intramuscularly,* at 1–2 day intervals. (Upjohn)

848. Iron Cacodylate—Ampules 1 cc; Boxes of 12; Containing gr ½ (0.032 Gm); *Dosage:* gauged by tolerance of patient, initial dose small, gradually increased, *intramuscularly.* (Upjohn)

849. Iron Citrate (Green)—Ampules 1 cc; Boxes of 12; Containing gr ¾ (0.05 Gm), or gr 1½ (0.1 Gm) iron and ammonium citrate; *Dosage:* ¼–1 cc, intramuscularly, either strength, at 2–3 day intervals. (Upjohn)

850. Luthorm—Ampules 1 cc; Boxes of 12; Each cubic centimeter representing 0.02 Gm extractive of corpora lutea of pregnant hogs, equivalent to gr 5–7 of fresh gland substance; *Dosage:* 1 cc, *intramuscularly,* daily or on alternate days for 5–10 doses. (Upjohn)

851. Mercuric Iodide (Red)—Ampules 1 cc; Boxes of 12; Containing gr ⅙ (0.01 Gm) in potassium iodide solution; *Dosage:* 1 cc daily, *intramuscularly. See Chap. I.* (Upjohn)

852. Mercury Salicylate—Ampules 1 cc; Boxes of 12; Containing gr 1 (0.065 Gm) in neutral sweet almond oil base with quinine and urea hydrochloride as local anesthetic; *Intramuscular. See Chap. I.* (Upjohn)

854. Mercury Succinimide—Ampules 1 cc; Boxes of 12; Containing gr ⅓ (0.02 Gm) in distilled water; *Dosage:* 1 cc, *intramuscularly,* at 2 or more days interval. *See Chap. I.* (Upjohn)

855. Ovarian Extract (Whole Ovary)—Ampules 1 cc; Boxes of 12; Containing extractives from gr 31 (2 Gm) fresh pork ovaries, including corpora lutea; *Dosage:* 1 cc intramuscularly, at 2 or more day intervals. *See Chap. IV.* (Upjohn)

856. Pitamin, Obstetrical—Ampules ½ and 1 cc; Boxes of 6; Contains the water soluble principles of posterior pituitary lobe; *For use* in uterine inertia; *Dosage:* 0.5–1.0 cc as indicated. (Upjohn)

857. Pitamin, Surgical—Ampules 1 cc; Boxes of 6; Double strength; *For use* in postoperative shock, hemorrhage, temporary bladder and intestinal paralysis. (Upjohn)

858. Procaine—Ampules 5 cc; Boxes of 6; Containing gr ⅖ (0.025 Gm), with adrenalin hydrochloride solution 1:1,000, ½ m in physiological salt solution.
Ampules 3 cc; Boxes of 12; Containing gr 0.9 (0.06 Gm), with adrenalin hydrochloride solution 1:20,000 in physiological salt solution.
Ampules 1 cc; Boxes of 12; Containing gr ⅓ (0.02 Gm), with adrenalin hydrochloride solution 1:20,000 in physiological salt solution.

Vials 30 cc; Rubber-capped; Containing gr 1/3 (0.02 Gm) in physiological salt solution.

Vials 30 cc; Rubber-capped; Containing gr 1/3 (0.02 Gm) with adrenalin, in physiological salt solution; *For use* as local anesthetic. *See Chap. I.* (Upjohn)

859. Quinine Dihydrochloride—Ampules 1½ cc; Boxes of 12; Containing gr 7½ (0.5 Gm); *For use* in lobar pneumonia, malarial fever, as tonic during convalescence; Intramuscular. *See Chap. I.* (Upjohn)

860. Quinine and Urea Hydrochloride—Ampules 1½ cc; Boxes of 12; Containing gr 7½ (0.5 Gm); *For use* as local anesthetic. *See Chap. I.* (Upjohn)

861. Quinine and Urea Hydrochloride with Procaine—Vials 30 cc; Containing quinine and urea hydrochloride 5% and procaine 2%; Vials, rubber-capped; *For use* in injection treatment of internal hemorrhoids. *See Chap. II.* (Upjohn)

862. Sodium Cacodylate—Ampules 1 cc; Boxes of 12; Containing gr ¾ (0.05 Gm), gr 1½ (0.1 Gm), gr 3 (0.194 Gm), gr 5 (0.324 Gm), gr 7 (0.45 Gm).

Ampules 2 cc; Boxes of 12; Containing gr 15 (0.97 Gm); *For use* in malarial cachexia, neurasthenia, psoriasis, anemia, leukemia and pellagra; *Dosage:* gr 5 (0.3 Gm) at 3–5 day intervals. (Upjohn)

---

863. Antophysin—Ampules 100 rat units; Boxes of 5 with 5 ampules distilled water; Contains anterior pituitary hormone; *For use* in ovarian hypofunction, infantilism, functional amenorrhea and dysmenorrhea; in deficient lutein stimulation, sterility, menopausal disorders; *Administered: intramuscularly. See Chap. I.* (Winthrop)

864. Chaulmestrol—Ampules 1 and 3 cc; Boxes of 10; *For use* as leprosy remedy; *For use* and *dosage, see Chap. I.* (Winthrop)

865. Cymarin—Ampules in Boxes of 10; Containing gr 1/60 (0.001 Gm); *For use* as cardiotonic and diuretic; *For use* and *dosage, see Chap. I.* (Winthrop)

866. Gono-Yatren—Ampules 2.5 cc; Boxes of 6; Containing 50, 100, 150, 200, 300 or 400 million gonococci; 3% yatren added to solutions; *For use* as gonococcus vaccine; *Dosage:* 0.5–4 cc every 2–4 days, *intramuscularly. See Chap. I.* (Winthrop)

867. Entodon—Ampules 2 cc; Boxes of 10; Brand of Propiodal. (Winthrop)

868. Ephedrin-Novocain Solution—Ampules 1 and 2 cc; Boxes of 10 and 100; *For use* as local anesthetic. *See Chap. II.* (Winthrop)

869. Germanin—Ampules of 1.0 Gm; Boxes of 5; (Bayer 205). (Winthrop)

870. Gravocain with Ephedrin-Novocain Solution—Ampules 1 cc; Boxes of 5. Ephedrin-Novocain solution with 5 ampules (0.75 cc) Gravocain. *See Chap. II.* (Winthrop)

871. Homocamfin—Ampules 2 cc; Boxes of 5; Containing 10% solution; *For use* as cardiorespiratory stimulant; *Dosage: intramuscularly,* 1.5–2 cc as required. *See Chap. I.* (Winthrop)

872. Hypophysin—Ampules 0.5 and 1 cc; Boxes of 10; Contains pituitary extract, Posterior Lobe. (Winthrop)

873. Luminal-Sodium—Ampules of 2 and 5 gr; Boxes of 5 and 100 (Hospital use); Brand of Phenobarbital-Sodium. *See Chap. I.* (Winthrop)

874. Magnesium Sulphate—Ampules 2 and 6 cc; Boxes of 10; 25 or 50% Solutions. Ampules 2 and 6 cc; Boxes of 50; 25 or 50% Solutions. (Winthrop)

875. Magnesium Sulphate with Novocain—Ampules 2 and 6 cc; Boxes of 10 and 50; Containing magnesium sulphate 50%, novocain 2½%. (Winthrop)

876. Neosilverarsphenamine—Ampules of 0.1, 0.2, 0.3, 0.4, 0.45 Gm. *See Chap. I.* (Winthrop)

877. **Magnesium Sulphate with Novocain and Morphine**—Ampules 2 and 6 cc; Boxes of 10; Containing magnesium sulphate 50 %, Novocain 2½ %, morphine gr ⅛ per ampule. **(Winthrop)**

878. **Mesurol**—Ampules 1 cc; Boxes of 10; Containing 54–57 % bismuth; *For use* as Antisyphilitic; *Dosage:* deep *intramuscular* injection of 0.5–1 cc once or twice weekly. *See Chap. I.* **(Winthrop)**

879. **Neofosfan**—Ampules 1 cc; Boxes of 10; Containing 11 % phosphorus; *For use* in neurasthenia, psychoneuroses, convalescence from acute infections, early pulmonary tuberculosis; *Dosage:* 1 ampule daily for 30–40 doses. *See Chap. I.* **(Winthrop)**

880. **Novasurol**—Ampules 1 cc; Boxes of 5; Containing 10 % neutral sterile solution of Novasurol; *For use* as powerful diuretic; *Dosage:* 0.5–2 cc; once or twice weekly. *See Chap. I.* **(Winthrop)**

881. **Novocain**—Ampules of crystals of 50, 100, 120, 150, 200, 300, 500 mg: Boxes of 10.
Ampules 2 and 6 cc; Boxes of 10; 1 % solution (without suprarenin).
Ampules 1.5 and 5 cc; Boxes of 10; 20 % (concentrated) without suprarenin. *See Chap. I.* **(Winthrop)**

882. **Novocain-Suprarenin Solution**—Ampules 1 cc; Boxes of 20.
Ampules 3 cc; Boxes of 10 and 100.
Ampules 6 cc; Boxes of 10; Containing novocain 2 %, suprarenin 1:20,000.
Ampules 2 and 6 cc; Boxes of 10; Containing novocain 1 %, suprarenin 1:50,000.
Ampules 1 cc; Boxes of 20.
Ampules 3 cc; Boxes of 10 and 100; Containing novocain 2 %, suprarenin 1:50,000.
Ampules 1.5 and 5 cc; Boxes of 10; Containing novocain 20 %, suprarenin 1:9,000 (approximately). *See Chap. II.* **(Winthrop)**

883. **Omnadin**—Ampules 2 cc; Boxes 5 and 100; Brand of Prolipin. **(Winthrop)**

884. **Optarson**—Ampules 1.2 cc; Boxes of 12; Containing ammonium heptenchlorarsonate gr ⅙ (0.01 Gm) with strychnine nitrate gr 1/64 (0.001 Gm); *For use* as tonic and reconstructive; *Dosage:* 1 ampule every 2 days. *See Chap. II.* **(Winthrop)**

885. **Padutin**—Ampules 1 cc; Boxes of 5; Containing 2 biologic units of pancreas derivative; *For use* as hormonal vasodilator; *Dosage:* *intramuscularly,* 0.5–1 cc twice daily for 10–14 doses. *See Chap. III.* **(Winthrop)**

886. **Pantocain**—Ampules 2 cc; Boxes of 10; Containing 1 % solution; *For use* as spinal anesthetic; *Dosage:* 1–2 cc, 1 % solution, *intraspinally; For use* in surface anesthesia—¼–2 % solution. *See Chap. I.* **(Winthrop)**

887. **Salyrgan**—Ampules 1 cc; Boxes of 5;
Ampules 2 cc; Boxes of 10; *Intramuscular. For use* as Diuretic. *See Chap. I.* **(Winthrop)**

888. **Silver-Salvarsan**—Ampules of 0.1, 0.15, 0.2, 0.25, 0.3, 0.6 Gm; Brand of Silver-Arsphenamine; Intramuscular; *For use* as Antisyphilitic. *See Chap. I.* **(Winthrop)**

889. **Solarson**—Ampules 1 cc; Boxes of 10; Containing chlorarsenol 0.01 Gm corresponding to gr 1/16 (0.004 Gm) of arsenous acid per cubic centimeter; *For use* as tonic and alterative; *Dosage:* 1 ampule every 1–3 days. *See Chap. I.* **(Winthrop)**

900. **Spinocain**—Ampules 2 and 3 cc; Boxes of 10 and 100; *For use* as Spinal Anesthetic—*See Chap. II.* **(Winthrop)**

901. **Spinocain with Ephedrine-Novocain Solution**—Ampules 2 cc; Boxes of 5; Containing spinocain 1 cc, ephedrin hydrochoride 5 %, novocain 1 % solution.
Ampules 3 cc; Boxes of 5; Containing spinocain 2 cc in ephedrin novocain solution. *See Chap. II.* **(Winthrop)**

902. **Sulpharsphenamine**—Ampules of 0.1, 0.15, 0.3, 0.45, 0.6, 0.75, 0.9, 3.0 Gm; Pure Form.

Ampules 10 cc; Containing 0.15, 0.3, 0.45, 0.6 Gm; in distilled water. *See Chap. I.* (Winthrop)

903. Suprarenin—Ampules 1 cc; Boxes of 20; Containing 1:1,000 solution. Ampules of 0.091 Gm of Suprarenin Bitartrate; Boxes of 1. *See Chap. I.* (Winthrop)

904. Synodal—Ampules 6 cc; Boxes of 5; Brand of Emetabol. *See Chap. I.* (Winthrop)

905. Tenamin—Ampules 1.2 cc; Boxes of 10; *For use* as uterine hemostatic. *See Chap. II.* (Winthrop)

906. Triphal—Ampules of 0.025 and 0.1 Gm; Boxes of 1; Brand of Aurothiol. *For use* in lupus erythematosus. *See Chap. I.* (Winthrop)

907. Trypaflavin—Ampules of 10 cc; Boxes of 5; Containing 2% solution; Brand of Acriflavine. *See Chap. I.* (Winthrop)

908. Tutocain—Ampules 3 cc; Boxes of 10; Brand of Butamin; Solution of 1% with suprarenin 1:20,000. *See Chap. I.* (Winthrop)

909. Yatren-Casein (Strong)—Ampules 1 cc; Boxes of 6; *For use* as foreign protein therapy. *See Chap. I.* (Winthrop)

910. Yatren-Casein (Weak)—Ampules 1 cc; Boxes of 6; *For use* as foreign protein therapy; *Dosage:* 1–3 cc every 2–5 days. *See Chap. I.* (Winthrop)

---

911. Bismuth Salicylate—Ampules 1 cc; Boxes of 12; Containing bismuth salicylate gr 2 (0.13 Gm), camphor gr 1½ (0.1 Gm), creosote gr 1½ (0.1 Gm), oil base q.s.; *For use* as Antisyphilitic; *Dosage:* 1 ampule every 3–4 days, *intramuscularly, See Chap. I.* (Wyeth)

912. Caffeine Sodio-Benzoate—Ampules 2 cc; Boxes of 12; Containing gr 3¾ (0.25 Gm) in distilled water, q.s.; *For use* as cardiac and cerbral stimulant and diuretic; or gr 7½ (0.5 Gm). (Wyeth)

913. Camphor in Oil—Ampules 1 cc; Boxes of 12; Containing gr 3 (0.2 Gm) in bland vegetable oil; *For use* as diffusible heart stimulant in nervous depression, hysteria, convalescence, persistent hiccough, crisis of lobar pneumonia with weak heart; Intramuscular. (Wyeth)

914. Corpus Luteum Extract (Soluble)—Ampules 1 cc; Boxes of 6; Containing corpora lutea powder gr 3 (0.2 Gm) in physiologic salt solution; *For use* in functional ovarian disorders, incidental disturbances of menopause natural or surgical, nausea of pregnancy. (Wyeth)

915. Emetine Hydrochloride—Ampules 1 cc; Boxes of 6; Containing gr ⅓ (0.02 Gm), or gr ½ (0.03 Gm); in distilled water; *For use* in amebic dysentery and amebic hepatitis; *Dosage:* ½–1 gr daily. (Wyeth)

916. Ephedrine Sulphate—Ampules 1 cc; Boxes of 12 and 100; Containing gr ¾ (0.04860 Gm) in distilled water q.s.; *For use* in asthma and hay fever. (Wyeth)

917. Glycerophosphate Compound—Ampules 1 cc; Boxes of 12; Containing sodium glycerophosphate gr 1½ (0.1 Gm), strychnine cacodylate gr 1/125 (0.0005 Gm), iron cacodylate gr ⅙ (0.01 Gm); *For use* in chlorosis, anemia, neurasthenia, rachitis, torpid liver, convalescence. (Wyeth)

918. Histamine Phosphate—Ampules 1 cc; Boxes of 12; Containing gr 1/65 (0.001 Gm) in distilled water; *For use* as diagnostic test for presence of hydrochloric acid in stomach during digestive cycle. (Wyeth)

919. Iron Arsenite—Ampules 1 cc; Boxes of 12; Containing gr 1 (0.065 Gm) in distilled water q.s.; *For use* in dry scaly cutaneous diseases, anemia, malarial intoxication, pellagra and chorea. (Wyeth)

920. Iron Arsenite and Strychnine—Ampules 1 cc; Boxes of 12; Containing gr 1 (0.065 Gm) iron arsenite with ammonium citrate, gr 1/65 (0.001 Gm) strychnine nitrate; *For use* in atonic dyspepsia with anemia, malnutrition. (Wyeth)

921. Iron Cacodylate—Ampules 1 cc; Boxes of 12; Containing gr ½ (0.03 Gm). Ampules 5 cc; Boxes of 6 and 25; Containing gr 1 (0.065 Gm) in distilled water q.s.; *For use* as tonic and alterative in anemia, dry skin affections. **(Wyeth)**

922. Iron Citrate (Green)—Ampules 1 cc; Boxes of 12; Containing gr 1 (0.065 Gm); in distilled water, q.s.; *For use* as Hematinic. **(Wyeth)**

923. Magnesium Sulphate—Ampules 2 cc; Boxes of 12; Containing gr 7½ (0.5 Gm) in distilled water q.s.; *For use* as synergist to morphine sulphate; *Intramuscular.* **(Wyeth)**

924. Mercury Salicylate—Ampules 1 cc; Boxes of 12; Containing mercury salicylate gr 1 (0.065 Gm), quinine and urea hydrochloride ½ % in neutral oil base; Intramuscular. *For use* as Antisyphilitic. *See Chap. I.* **(Wyeth)**

925. Ovarian Substance—Ampules 1 cc; Boxes of 12; Containing whole ovary gr 3 (0.2 Gm) representing gr 15 fresh substance; *For use* in generative organ dysfunction, compensatory goiter of young women, disturbances of menopause. *See Chap. IV.* **(Wyeth)**

926. Phenolsulphonphthalein—Ampules 1 cc; Boxes of 12; Containing monosodium salt gr 1/10 (0.006 Gm) in distilled water q.s.; *For use* as renal function test; Intragluteally. *See Chap. I.* **(Wyeth)**

927. Pituitary Extract (Obstetrical)—Ampules ½ and 1 cc; Boxes of 6; Posterior lobe of pituitary body; *For use* in uterine inertia, low blood pressure, shock, intestinal and bladder paralysis following operation; *Dosage:* ¼–1 cc, repeated as indicated. *See Chap. I.* **(Wyeth)**

929. Sodium Cacodylate—Ampules 1 cc; Boxes of 12; Containing gr ¾ (0.05 Gm), gr 1½ (0.1 Gm), gr 3 (0.2 Gm), gr 5 (0.32 Gm), gr 7½ (0.5 Gm) in distilled water q.s.; *For use* in psoriasis, malarial cachexia, anemias, leukemia, pellagra, secondary syphilitic lesions of skin. **(Wyeth)**

930. Sodium Iodide—Ampules 10 cc; Boxes of 6 and 25; Containing gr 15½ (1 Gm). Ampules 20 cc; Boxes of 6 and 25; Containing gr 31 (2 Gm) in distilled water q.s.; *For use* in adenitis, simple goiter, secondary and tertiary syphilis, bronchial asthma, arteriosclerosis, hepatic cirrhosis. **(Wyeth)**

931. Sodium Salicylate—Ampules 10 cc; Boxes of 6; Containing gr 15½ (1 Gm). Ampules 10 cc; Boxes of 6 and 25; Containing gr 31 (2 Gm); *For use* as Antirheumatic. **(Wyeth)**

932. Sodium Salicylate and Sodium Iodide—Ampules 20 cc; Boxes of 6 and 25; Containing gr 15½ (1 Gm) each, in distilled water q.s.; *For use* as Antirheumatic, in bacterial infections, bronchial asthma, lumbago, sciatica. **(Wyeth)**

933. Sodium Salicylate and Sodium Iodide with Colchicine—Ampules 20 cc; Boxes of 6 and 25; Containing sodium salicylate and sodium iodide gr 15½ (1 Gm) each, colchicine gr 1/100 (0.00065 Gm) in distilled water, q.s.; *For use* in gout. **(Wyeth)**

---

934. Caffeine Sodio-Benzoate—Ampules 2 cc; Boxes of 12 and 100; Containing caffeine sodio benzoate gr 7½ (0.5 Gm), distilled water q.s.; *For use* as cardiac and cerebral stimulant; *Dosage:* 1–2 cc; *Intramuscularly,* twice daily. **(Zemmer)**

935. Camphor in Oil—Ampules 1 cc; Boxes of 12 and 100; Containing gr 3 (0.194 Gm); *For use* as cardiac stimulant; *Dosage:* 1–2 cc, *intramuscularly,* as indicated. **(Zemmer)**

936. Corpus Luteum—Ampules 1 cc; Boxes of 6, 25 and 100; Containing gr 3 (0.194 Gm); *For use* in nausea and vomiting of pregnancy, menopausal disorders; *Dosage: Intramuscularly,* as indicated. *See Chap. IV.* **(Zemmer)**

937. Ephedrine Hydrochloride—Ampules 1 cc; Boxes of 6, 25 and 100; Containing gr ¾ (0.04860 Gm); *For use* in asthma, hay fever; *Dosage:* ½–1 cc in evening. **(Zemmer)**

938. Epinephrine Chloride—Ampules 1cc ; Boxes of 12 and 100; 1:1,000 Solution; *For use* in allergic reactions and shock; *Dosage:* 1 cc, intramuscularly, as indicated. **(Zemmer)**

939. Glycerophosphate Compound—Ampules 1 cc; Boxes of 12 and 100; Containing sodium glycerophosphate gr 1½ (0.1 Gm), strychnine cacodylate gr 1/25 (0.0005 Gm), iron cacodylate gr 1/6 (0.01 Gm), procaine 1%, distilled water q.s.; *For use* in anemia, neurasthenia; *Dosage:* 1 cc as indicated. **(Zemmer)**

940. Iron Arsenite and Ammonium Citrate—Ampules 1 cc; Boxes of 12 and 100; Containing iron arsenite and ammonium citrate gr 1 (0.065 Gm), soluble quinine and urea hydrochloride, 5%, q.s.; *For use* in anemia and chlorosis; *Dosage:* ¼–1 cc, as indicated. **(Zemmer)**

941. Iron Arsenite and Strychnine—Ampules 1 cc; Boxes of 12 and 100; Containing iron arsenite and ammonium citrate gr 1 (0.065 Gm), strychnine nitrate gr 1/65 (0.001 Gm), soluble quinine and urea hydrochloride, 5%, q.s.; *For use* in anemias; *Dosage:* ¼–1 cc, *intramuscularly* as indicated. **(Zemmer)**

942. Iron Cacodylate—Ampules 1 cc; Boxes of 12 and 100; Containing gr ½ (0.03 Gm), soluble quinine and urea hydrochloride, 5%, q.s.; *For use* as Hematinic and tonic; *Dosage:* 1 cc, *intramuscularly*, as indicated. **(Zemmer)**

943. Iron and Ammonium Citrate—Ampules 1 cc; Boxes of 12 and 100; Containing gr 1 (0.065 Gm) iron and ammonium citrate gr 1 (0.065 Gm) soluble quinine and urea hydrochloride, 5%, q.s.
Ampules 1 cc; Boxes of 12 and 100; Containing gr 2 (0.13 Gm), soluble quinine and urea hydrochloride 1%, q.s. *Dosage:* single strength—1–2 cc, *Intramuscularly*, as indicated; double strength ½–1 cc. *For use* in anemias; **(Zemmer)**

944. Liver Substance Solution—Ampules 1 cc; Boxes of 12 and 100; Representing gr 25 fresh liver substance; *For use* in hypertension; *Dosage:* 1 cc daily. *See Chap. I.* **(Zemmer)**

945. Mercury Cyanide—Ampules 1 cc; Boxes of 12 and 100; Containing gr 1/6 (0.012 Gm) in normal saline; *For use* in secondary syphilis and some skin conditions; *Dosage:* ¼–1 ampule, *intramuscularly* daily or at 2–5 day intervals. *See Chap. I.* **(Zemmer)**

946. Magnesium Sulphate Solution—Ampules 2 cc; Boxes of 12 and 100; 50% solution; *For use* with morphine for prolonged effect; as analgesic, sedative and hypnotic, in controlling convulsions in eclampsia. **(Zemmer)**

947. Mercury Cyanide—Ampules 1 cc; Boxes of 12 and 100; Containing gr 1/6 (0.01 Gm) in normal saline; *For use* in secondary syphilis and certain skin conditions; *Dosage:* ¼–1 ampule daily or 2–5 day intervals. *See Chap. I.* **(Zemmer)**

948. Mercury Iodide—Ampules 1 cc; Boxes of 12 and 100; Containing mercuric iodide, red gr 1/6 (0.01 Gm), potassium iodide gr 1/6 (0.01 Gm) in distilled water; *For use* as Antisyphilitic; *Dosage:* ½–1 cc, *intramuscularly*, increased as indicated. *See Chap. I.* **(Zemmer)**

949. Mercuric Iodide 1% in Oil—Ampules 1 cc; Boxes of 12 and 100; Containing mercuric iodide, red gr 1/6 (0.01 Gm), potassium iodide gr 1/6 (0.01 Gm), anesthesin gr 1/6 (0.01 Gm), pure olive oil q.s.; *For use* as Antisyphilitic; *Dosage:* ½–1 cc, increased as indicated. **(Zemmer)**

950. Pituitary Extract (Infundibular)—Ampules ½ and 1 cc; Boxes of 6, 25 and 100; *Dosage:* 1 cc, *intramuscularly;* in severe shock, *intravenously. See Chap. I.* **(Zemmer)**

951. Quinine and Urea Hydrochloride—Ampules 2 cc; Boxes of 12 and 100; Containing gr 1/3 (0.02 Gm), in distilled water; *For use* as local anesthetic in rectal, anorectal, urethral and other minor operations. *See Chap. I.* **(Zemmer)**

952. Sodium Cacodylate—Ampules 1 cc; Boxes of 12 and 100; Containing gr ¾ (0.05 Gm), gr 2 (0.13 Gm), gr 3 (0.20 Gm), gr 5 (0.324 Gm) or gr 7 (0.452 Gm); *For use* as Antisyphilitic, and as Hematinic in anemia, skin conditions; *Dosage:* gr ¼ to gr 15 as indicated. **(Zemmer)**

953. Tincture Iodine U.S.P.—Ampules 2 cc; Boxes of 12 and 100: For local application. **(Zemmer)**

CHAPTER VI

BIOLOGICALS

This chapter makes available 535 biologic products in 985 forms, for use in the diagnosis, immunization and treatment of infectious diseases. Each group of preparations is preceded by a brief general description including methods of application. The arrangement in each group is alphabetical by manufacturer of products.

Description: Biological therapy is but an imitation of nature's method of fighting infection; it is based upon the phenomena of natural immunity, the resistance of body cells against bacterial invasion; this includes—first, phagocytosis, the ability of the wandering leukocytes and fixed cells to surround and digest bacteria; and second, the antibody defense, comprising agglutinins, precipitins, alexins, antitoxins, bacteriotropins and others, each with a definite function.

The substantial advances made during the past several decades in bacteriology, serology and immunology have stimulated the production of helpful biologic preparations; it is now possible through the medium of animals to produce immune bodies and by their introduction into the organism substitute nature's method of preventing and curing infectious diseases, formerly beyond the scope of the practitioner.

Sera, Antitoxins: Curative sera are obtained from blood serum of immunized animals, and after treatment in a special manner, are purified, concentrated and carefully tested. Some sera, as those for tetanus and diphtheria, contain only antitoxins which neutralize toxins; others, like the meningococcic or pneumococcic sera, contain specific bactericidal antibodies destructive to the organisms and endotoxins liberated upon their annihilation. Sera are most commonly used for passive immunization and in acute infections.

Vaccines: Vaccines are suspensions of killed bacteria in suitable media, and are prepared and tested in a special manner; their introduction into the body results in the production of specific antibodies not only sufficient to overcome local effects at the site of injection, but also to permeate the rest of the organism, influence the living specific bacteria elsewhere if present, and protect the individual against future infection. Vaccines are used mostly for active immunization and in the treatment of chronic diseases: they offer immunity of considerably longer duration than sera and are prepared as *monovalent* vaccines—from a single strain of bacteria, as *polyvalent*—from a number of different strains of one type of organism, or as *mixed* vaccines—from several different types of bacteria.

Administration: In the administration of biologicals it is essential that an accurate bacteriologic diagnosis be established before any vaccine or serum is administered. It is also best, where obtainable, to use only highly refined and concentrated products, with the least amount of preservative, to avoid anaphylaxis. Undesirable reactions are also avoided by careful dosage, proper intervals between injections and correct technic.

Anaphylaxis: In some individuals, despite the application of the above mentioned precautions, the injection of horse serum may be followed by serum sickness. This occurs from a few hours to 8–10 days after injection, and consists of redness, itching, swelling and pain at site of injection, or of systemic reactions consisting of fever, urticaria, adenitis, hoarseness and cough, nausea and vomiting, vertigo and other symptoms lasting for a considerable period. At times, acute shock and collapse with severe dyspnea, marked drop in blood pressure and other alarming symptoms may occur soon after injection.

Desensitization: In those sensitive to biologic products, desensitization may be accomplished by several injections of diluted (10%) serum, beginning with 1 cc and followed after several minutes by another 3 cc; after 10 min. intervals 10 cc and 25 cc are administered; the undiluted serum in full dosage may then be injected subcutaneously, several hours thereafter. In urgent cases, both desensitization and the therapeutic dose may be given intravenously.

In vaccine therapy, if properly administered, local and general reactions are not common or less pronounced, seldom demanding special treatment; a local or focal manifestation, especially where accompanied by general clinical improvement, is indeed desirable.

Dosage: Dosage and frequency of administration are dependent upon the individual product and its concentration; directions will be found accompanying each preparation hereafter described.

ACNE VACCINOTHERAPY

Description: Acne vaccines are suspensions of killed Bacillus Acne in physiologic salt solution. *Simple acne vaccines* are prepared from several strains of acne bacillus only, obtained from typical acne cases and preserved by the addition of a mild antiseptic, as tricresol; they are available in several strengths and are indicated in cases of simple, non-suppurating comedones. *Mixed acne vaccines* contain, in addition to the bacillus acne also staphylococcus albus and aureus, ordinarily associated with superficial skin infections; the mixed vaccines are mostly employed in the pustular types of acne.

Administration: Before beginning vaccine therapy it is advisable to express existing comedones and open all pustules, after alcohol and antiseptic cleansing. Initial dosage—five to twenty million acne bacilli; dose is then gradually increased; is administered *subcutaneously* or *intramuscularly*, every 3–5–7 days, guarding against undue reaction. Treatment is continued for several months. Three days after each injection the lesions are treated by hot toweling, comedones are extracted and pustules evacuated. Attention to the gastrointestinal tract, constitutional therapy, ultraviolet and Roentgen ray, and acidophilus preparations may be used in conjunction with acne vaccinotherapy.

PREPARATIONS

Acne Bacterin **(Abbott)**
Contains per cc
Acne bacillus.......... 500 million
Staph. epidermidis albus.......... 5000 million

Supply: Packages of 6, 20 cc.

Dosage: 3–5 m increased to 1 cc every 3–5 days.

Acne Bacillus Vaccine (C.A.) **(Cutter)**
Contains per cc
Bac. acne.......... 50 million

Supply: Bottles of 5 cc

Dosage: 0.1 cc, cautiously increased.

Staph-Acne Vaccine (Acne Combined Bacterin) **(Cutter)**
Contains per cc
Bac. acne.......... 50 million
Staphylococcus.......... 500 million

Supply: Bottles of 5 cc

Dosage: 0.05 cc as initial dose, increased.

Staph-Acne Vaccine (Acne Combined Bacterin No. 4) **(Cutter)**
Contains per cc 2750 million bacteria.

Supply: Bottles of 5 cc.

Dosage: 0.05 cc as initial dose, increased.

Acne Bacillus Vaccine (C.A.) (Hollister-Stier)
Contains per cc
Bac. acne.................................... 200 million

Supply: Bottles of 5 cc, 20 cc.

Dosage: 0.1 cc cautiously increased.

Staphylococcus Acne Vaccine (Hollister-Stier)
Contains per cc
Bac. acne.................................... 200 million
Staph. aureus.................................... 500 million
Staph. albus.................................... 500 million

Supply: Bottles of 5 cc, 20 cc.

Dosage: 0.1 cc increased.

Acne Vaccine (Polyvalent) (C.A.) (Lederle)
Contains per cc
Bac. acne (Dilution 4).................................... 40 million

Supply: Vials 5 cc, 10 cc, 20 cc—Packages of 4 vials or syringes containing respectively 5, 10, 20, 40 million per cc.

Dosage: 0.12 cc increased.

Acne Combined Vaccine (Polyvalent) (Lederle)
Contains per cc
Bac. acne.................................... 40 million
Staph. aureus.................................... 200 million
Staph. albus.................................... 200 million

Supply: Vials 5 cc, 20 cc.

Dosage: 0.12 cc increased.

Acne Mixed Vaccine (Lilly)
Contains per cc
Bac. acne.................................... 250 million
Staph. aureus.................................... 1,250 million
Staph. albus.................................... 1,250 million

Supply: Vials 5 cc, 20 cc.

Dosage: 2–4 m.

Acne Bacterin (Acne Vaccine Polyvalent) (C.A.) (Mulford)
Contains
Dosage A—Acne bacillus.................................... 25 million
Dosage B—Acne bacillus.................................... 50 million
Dosage C—Acne bacillus.................................... 100 million
Dosage D—Acne bacillus.................................... 200 million

Supply: Packages of 4 syringes—Dosages A, B, C, D; Vials 5 cc D strength per cc.

Dosage: Initial, 5–25 million bacteria.

Acne Serobacterin (Sensitized, Polyvalent) (Mulford)
Contains
Dosage A—Killed sensitized bacteria.................................... 100 million
Dosage B—Killed sensitized bacteria.................................... 200 million
Dosage C—Killed sensitized bacteria.................................... 400 million
Dosage D—Killed sensitized bacteria.................................... 800 million

Supply: Packages of 4 syringes—Dosages A, B, C, D; Vials 5 cc D strength per cc.

Dosage: Initial 100 million bacteria.

Acne Bacterin Mixed (Mulford)

Contains per cc	A	B	C	D
Acne bacillus	25	50	100	200 million
Staph. aureus	125	250	500	1,000 million
Staph. albus	125	250	500	1,000 million

Supply: Packages of 4 syringes—Dosages A, B, C, D.

Dosage: 50–275 million bacteria, initial dose.

Acne Serobacterin Mixed (C.A.) **(Mulford)**

Contains per cc

	A	B	C	D
Staph. aureus	250	500	1,000	2,000 million
Staph. albus	250	500	1,000	2,000 million
Acne bacillus	100	200	400	800 million

Supply: Packages of 4 syringes—Dosages A, B, C, D.

Dosage: 600 million bacteria, initial dose.

Acne Combined Vaccine (Acne Bacterin) **(National Drug)**

Contains per cc

Bac. acne	250 million
Bac. coli	250 million
Staph. albus	500 million
Staph. aureus	500 million

Supply: Ampule-vials 5 cc, 15 cc, 30 cc.

Dosage: Initial ⅛ cc (2 m) increased by ⅛ cc at 2–5 day intervals.

Acne Vaccine (Combined) **(Parke, Davis)**

Contains per cc

Bac. acne	100 million
Acne diplococcus	100 million
Staph. albus	1,200 million
Staph. aureus	600 million

Supply: Bulbs 1 cc—Packages of 4; Vials 5 cc, 20 cc.

Dosage: 0.1 cc increased by 0.1 cc at intervals of 5–7 days; maximum dose 1 cc.

Acne Vaccine **(Sherman)**

Contains per cc

Bac. acne	40 million
Staph. albus	1,000 million

Supply: Vials 5 cc, 12½ cc.

Dosage: 0.3 cc increased by 0.1 cc at 2–3 day intervals until 1 cc is reached, for 20–25 injections.

Acne Vaccine **(Sherman)**

Contains per cc

Bac. acne	40 million
Bac. coli	300 million
Staph. albus	1,000 million

Supply: Vials 5 cc, 12½ cc.

Dosage: 0.2 cc increased.

Furunculosis Vaccine **(Sherman)**

Contains per cc

Staph. aureus	1,000 million
Staph. albus	1,000 million

Supply: Vials of 5 cc, 12½ cc.

Dosage: Initial 0.3 cc, gradually increased.

Staphylo-Acne Vaccine **(Squibb)**

Contains per cc

	First	Second	Third	Fourth	concentrations.
Staph. albus	125	250	375	500	million
Staph. aureus	125	250	375	500	million
Bac. acne	125	250	375	500	million

Supply: Packages of 4 ampules in above concentrations; Vials 5 cc, 20 cc—highest strength per cc.

Acne Vaccine (C.A.) **(Squibb)**
Contains per cc.
Bac. acne.. 1,000 million

Supply: Vials 5 cc, 20 cc; Packages of 4 ampules containing respectively 250, 500, 750, 1,000 million bacilli.

Dosage: Initial 250–1,000 million.

Acne Vaccine **(U. S. Standard Products)**
Contains per cc.
Bac. acne.. 40 million

Supply: Vials 5 cc, 20 cc.

Dosage: Initial 0.3 cc, gradually increased.

ANTHRAX SEROTHERAPY

Description: Antianthrax Sera are prepared by the immunization of healthy horses against the Bacillus Anthracis; are used effectively in the treatment of anthrax, malignant pustule or woolsorters' disease.

Administration: Should be administered as early as possible, from 50–200 cc, *intravenously;* repeated in 8–10 hr. in severe cases, or where results obtained are not satisfactory.

PREPARATIONS

Antianthrax Serum (C.A.) **(Lederle)**

Supply: 50 cc intravenous outfit.

Dosage: 100–200 cc *intravenously*, repeated in 8 hr. if necessary.

Antianthrax Serum (C.A.) **(Mulford)**

Supply: Packages of one 20 cc syringe or two 10 cc syringes; Packages of one 50 cc double ended vial with outfit for intravenous use.

Dosage: Initial—80–100 cc *intravenously.*

Antianthrax Serum (C.A.) **(Parke, Davis)**

Supply: 50 cc syringe container with needle and gravity tube.

Dosage: 50–100 cc *intravenously*, repeated in 6 hr. or more.

ARTHRITIS VACCINOTHERAPY

Description: The *Simple Vaccines* for use in arthritis are broth cultures, prepared from pure strains of the Cecil type Streptococcus Hemolyticus, isolated from typical cases of rheumatoid arthritis. The *Mixed Vaccines* are combinations of the streptococcus with other bacteria commonly associated in infectious arthritis and rheumatoid disease.

Administration: Administration and dosage in accordance with each preparation; generally, is injected at 3–4 day intervals, *intramuscularly* or *intravenously*, guarding against undue reaction. In addition to vaccine therapy, all foci of infection must be disclosed and eliminated, wherever possible.

Bibliography: *See Chap. XII.*

PREPARATIONS

Rheumatic Bacterin **(Abbott)**
Contains per cc
Pneumococcus.. 25 million
Bac. Friedlander.. 25 million
Streptococcus (polyvalent).. 450 million

Supply: Bulk packages 6 cc, 20 cc.

Dosage: 3–15 m two to three times weekly.

Rheumatoid Arthritis Vaccine (Intramuscular) **(Lederle)**
Prepared from typical strains of hemolytic streptococcus.

Supply: Vials 5 cc—1 (100 million per cc); Vials 5 cc—2 (1,000 million per cc).

Dosage: *Intramuscularly*, first dose 50 million; second 100 million, increased by 100 million twice weekly till a maximum dosage of 1,000 million is reached; repeated as long as necessary.

Rheumatoid Arthritis Vaccine (Intravenous) **(Lederle)**
Prepared from typical strains of hemolytic streptococcus.

Supply: Vials 5 cc—1 (1 million per cc), 2 (10 million per cc), 3 (100 million per cc), 4 (1,000 million per cc).

Dosage: *Intravenously*, beginning with 100 thousand, increasing at weekly intervals till 1 billion is reached in about 14 injections; continued at 1 billion or increased to 3 billion.

Pneumococcus Mixed Vaccine (Rheumatic) **(Lilly)**
Contains per cc

Pneumococcus	400 million
Streptococcus	200 million
Staph. aureus	200 million
Staph. albus	200 million

Supply: Vials 5 cc, 20 cc.

Dosage: Initial 2–4 m.

Streptococcus Vaccine (Intravenous) **(Lilly)**
Contains per cc

	1	2
Streptococcus viridans (Rheumatic)	100	400 million

Supply: Each—vials 20 cc.

Dosage: Initial 100 million, increased every 3–4 days.

S-C-A Soluble Antigen **(Mulford)**
Prepared from streptococcus cardioarthritidis (small).

Supply: Ampule-vials 5 cc—dilutions 1 containing 1 billion, 2–100 million, 3–10 million, 4–1 million bacteria.

Dosage: Beginning with low count, gradually and cautiously increased.

Staphylo-Bacterin Mixed (Staphylococcic Vaccine Mixed) **(Mulford)**
Contains per cc

	A	B	C	D
Staph. aureus	50	100	200	400 million
Staph. albus	50	100	200	400 million
Strept. hemolyticus, non-hemolyticus, viridans	12.5	25	50	100 million
Bac. coli	25	50	100	200 million
Pneumococcus I, II, III	25	50	100	200 million

Supply: Packages of 4 syringes—strengths A, B, C, D; Vials 5 cc, 20 cc—strength D.

Dosage: Initial—10–50 million bacteria.

Staphylo-Serobacterin Mixed **(Mulford)**
Contains per cc

	A	B	C	D
Staph. aureus	250	500	1,000	2,000 million
Staph. albus	250	500	1,000	2,000 million
Strept. hemolyticus, non-hemolyticus, viridans	250	500	1,000	2,000 million
Bac. coli	250	500	1,000	2,000 million
Pneumococcus I, II, III	250	500	1,000	2,000 million

Supply: Packages of 4 syringes—strengths A, B, C, D; Vials 5 cc—strength D.

Dosage: Initial—contents of syringe A.

Pneumo-Strep-Serobacterin (Pneumococcic-Streptococcic Vaccine, Sensitized) (Mulford)

Contains per cc	A	B	C	D
Pneumococcus I, II, III	250	500	1,000	2,000 million
Strep. hemolyticus, non-hemolyticus, viridans	250	500	1,000	2,000 million

Supply: Packages of 4 syringes—strengths A, B, C, D; Vials 5 cc of strength D.

Dosage: Initial—contents of syringe A.

Rheumatism Phylacogen (Parke, Davis)

Culture filtrate of streptococci from rheumatic infection (75%), with staph. aureus and albus.

Supply: Vials 10 cc, rubber-diaphragm-capped.

Dosage: *Subcutaneously*—1 cc, increased gradually to 10 cc; daily injections.
Intravenously—initial 2–4 m, increased gradually to 5 cc; daily injections.

BACILLUS ACIDOPHILUS THERAPY

Description: Acidophilus Cultures are broth or whey products of viable Bacillus Acidophilus or Lactobacillus Acidophilus, containing at the time of manufacture about 200 million living bacteria per cc, and at expiration date at least 50% of viable organisms. Bacillus Bulgaricus Cultures are used mostly for the preparation of fermented milk. Acidophilus preparations are used in putrefactive conditions of the intestinal canal to change offensive intestinal flora into the helpful aciduric types: in mucous colitis, fermentative diarrhea, ulcerative colitis, constipation; in systemic disorders associated with or due to intestinal intoxication.

Administration: Given three to four times daily, in dosages in accordance with strength of culture, in water, milk or fruit juices, with simultaneous administration of lactose or dextrose, 200–300 Gm per day. Preparations should not be used after expiration date.

Bibliography: *See Chap. XII.*

PREPARATIONS

Bacid Culture (Arlington)

An active culture of Bac. acidophilus in liquid form.

Supply: Bottles of 6 oz.

Dosage: ½–1 tablespoonful three times a day before meals, in milk.

Neocultol (Arlington)

Bacillus acidophilus culture incorporated in mineral oil jelly, flavored with chocolate.

Supply: Jars 6 oz.

Dosage: 1–3 teaspoonfuls daily and on retiring.

Bacillus Acidophilus Culture (C.A.) (B. B. Culture)

A pure aqueous suspension of Bac. acidophilus, having an acidity of about 1% lactic acid; contains 100 million viable organisms per cc at time of sale.

Supply: Bottles of 120 cc (4 oz.).

Dosage: 10–15 cc four times daily.

Bac. Bulgaricus Culture (C.A.) (B. B. Culture)

A pure culture of Bac. bulgaricus for the preparation of fermented milk.

Supply: Bottles of 120 cc (4 oz.).

Dosage: Ad libitum.

Culture Lactobacillus **(Bloomfield)**
Contains several strains of Bac. acidophilus, at least 250 million viable bacilli per cc; viability retained for 3 mo.

Supply: Bottles of 16 oz.

Dosage: In accordance with requirements, 1–2 tablespoonfuls after meals.

Bacillus Acidophilus Liquid (C.A.) **(Cheplin)**
Contains 250 million Bac. acidophilus per cc.

Supply: Bottles of 400 cc.

Dosage: 500–1,000 cc daily, given in 3 doses for 6–12 weeks; retention enema—3–4 oz., for colon implantation.

Bacillus Acidophilus **(Cutter)**
Contains fresh high count cultures of pure, viable Bac. acidophilus.

Supply: Bottles of 100 cc—Bottles of 7–10 cc—Packages of 100.

Dosage: 7–10 cc daily.

Bacillus Acidophilus Culture (C.A.) **(Hollister-Stier)**
A pure culture containing 150 million viable organisms per cc at time of issue.

Supply: Bottles of 200 cc.

Dosage: 15–30 cc in milk with lactose, three times daily.

Bacillus Acidophilus and Lactose-Dextrin Mixture **(Hollister-Stier)**
For colon implantation.

Supply: Bottles of 200 cc—Packages of ½ lb.

Dosage: 4–6 oz. as high enema.

Bacillus Bulgaricus Culture **(Lederle)**
Broth culture of Bac. bulgaricus of Metchnikoff.

Supply: Packages of twenty 5 cc vials.

Dosage: As required.

Virilus **(Mt. Vernon Laboratories)**
A culture of living Virilus bacilli, about 550 million per cc; is claimed to remain viable for several years and not affected by gastric juices upon oral administration.

Supply: Ampules—Boxes of 12.

Dosage: 1 ampule three to five times daily, plain or in warm milk.

Acidophilus Blocks (M.A.B.) (C.A.) **(Mulford)**
Blocks each containing 150 billion viable Bac. acidophilus (X-strain) in a 2% agar jelly base, with milk powder, lactose, d-glucose and sucrose and covered with chocolate.

Supply: Boxes of 12 blocks.

Dosage: 3–4 blocks daily, 2 hr. after meals.

Bacillus Acidophilus Liquid (C.A.) **(Mulford)**
Contains a whey culture of pure living Lactobacillus acidophilus, 50 million per cc at time of sale.

Supply: Bottles of 3 oz., 16 oz.

Dosage: 1–2 tablespoonfuls in a glass of milk, with 2 teaspoonfuls of lactose, three times daily, 2–3 hr. after meals.

Acados **(National Drug)**
Standardized, active Bac. acidophilus culture in whey medium, containing maximum of 4,000 million bacilli per cc.

Supply: Bottles of 8 oz.

Dosage: 1–2 tablespoonfuls in milk or water three or four times daily; after active implantation, once or twice daily.

Neo-Acidophilus (Sherman)
A broth culture of Bac. acidophilus.

Supply: Bottles of 3 oz., 1 pt.

Dosage: 1–2 teaspoonfuls three times daily, in fruit juices, milk, grape juice or ginger ale.

Bacillus Bulgaricus (C.A.) (Squibb)
A pure whey culture of Bac. bulgaricus for the preparation of fermented milk.

Supply: Tubes of 12 cc—Packages of 12.

Dosage: Ad libitum.

Condensed Acidophilus (United Laboratories)
Concentrated pure culture of Bac. acidophilus in modified milk medium.

Supply: Bottles of 4 oz.

Dosage: 1 tablespoonful morning and night.

Culture Bacillus Acidophilus (C.A.) (United Laboratories)
A pure culture containing 600 million viable organisms per cc at time of issue.

Supply: Bottles of 120 cc.

Dosage: 15 cc diluted with water, two times daily, followed by lactose.

Culture Bacillus Acidophilus (C.A.) (Vitalait Laboratories)
A pure culture, containing 800 million viable organisms per cc at time of issue.

Supply: Bottles of 120 cc.

Dosage: 15 cc diluted with water, two times daily, followed by lactose.

BUBONIC PLAGUE VACCINOTHERAPY

Description: Bubonic Plague Vaccines are prepared for immunization against bubonic plague from killed Bacillus Pestis, 1,000 million to 5,000 million per cc.

Administration: Where rapid immunity is desired immunization may be accomplished by 1 single injection of comparatively high dosage; in ordinary cases repeated inoculations, two or three, are given in graded dosage; immunity attained is generally highest 14 days after the last injection. Curative therapy is not available.

PREPARATIONS

Plague (Bubonic) Vaccine (C.A.) (Prophylactic, Polyvalent) (Lederle)
Contains per cc
Bac. pestis.. 5,000 million

Supply: Vials 1 cc (1 immunization); Vials 10 cc (10 immunizations).

Dosage: IMMUNIZATION—Single—1 cc, for immediate immunization; multiple—½–⅓ cc at 5–7 day intervals, 2 or 3 injections.

Plague Vaccine Prophylactic (Antipest Vaccine) (C.A.) (Lilly)
Double Vaccination
Contains per cc
Bac. pestis............................ 1,000 million and 2,000 million

Supply: Packages of two 1 cc vials, 1 of each of above strengths (1 double immunization); Vials of 2,000 million per cc in packages of ten; Vials, 1.5 cc for 10 double immunizations.

Dosage: 2 injections—1,000 million and 2,000 million bacteria at 10 days' interval.

Plague Vaccine, Prophylactic (Antipest Vaccine) (C.A.) (Lilly)
Single Vaccination
Contains per cc
Bac. pestis.. 5,000 million

Supply: Packages of three 1 cc vials (3 complete immunizations); Vials 20 cc (20 complete immunizations).

Dosage: 1 injection of 5,000 million bacteria.

Plague Bacterin (Haffkine's Vaccine for Bubonic Plague; Antiplague Vaccine, Antipest Vaccine) (C.A.) **(Mulford)**
Contains per cc
Bac. pestis.. 5,000 million

Supply: Vials 1 cc (1 vaccination); Vials 10 cc (10 vaccinations); Packages of two 1 cc vials (double vaccination); Packages of two 10 cc vials (10 double vaccinations); Packages for 3 dose immunizations containing three 1 cc vials—1,000, 2,000, 5,000 million bacteria.

Dosage: 2 injections—1,000 million and 2,000 million bacteria at 10 days interval.

CATARRHAL-RESPIRATORY VACCINOTHERAPY

Description: Vaccines for the prophylaxis and treatment of catarrhal infections of the upper respiratory tract are prepared from cultures of all the common bacteria associated with respiratory infections: Staphylococcus, Micrococcus catarrhalis, Pneumococcus, Bacillus influenzae, etc. They are used for the production of immunity and in the treatment of those subject to colds, catarrhs, bronchitis, influenza, pharyngitis, laryngitis, coryza and similar conditions. Immunity, where produced, may last from several months to 1 yr.

Administration: For active immunization vaccines are best given during the month of October and repeated in January, February and March; administered subcutaneously, every 2, 3, 5 days, in dosage in accordance with preparation used. For therapeutic purposes is administered in graduated dosage, every 2–3 days, guarding against undue reactions.

Bibliography: *See Chap. XII.*

PREPARATIONS

Respiratory Bacterin (Catarrhal) **(Abbott)**
Contains per cc

Micrococcus catarrhalis	500 million
Bac. Friedlander	500 million
Pneumococcus	80 million
Streptococcus	60 million
Staph. aureus	200 million
Staph. albus	200 million

Supply: Packages 6 cc, 20 cc.

Dosage: Initial 0.25–0.5 cc every 6 days.

Mixed Vaccine—Respiratory Infections—"M.V.R.I." **(Cutter)**
Contains per cc

Staph. aureus	250 million
Staph. albus	250 million
Streptococcus	100 million
Pneumococcus	100 million
Mic. catarrhalis	100 million
Bac. Friedlander	100 million
Bac. influenzae	100 million

Supply: Bottles of 5 cc, 20 cc.

Dosage: Initial 0.5, then 1–2 cc every 5–7 days.

Mixed Vaccine—Respiratory Infections—"M.V.R.I." 4 Count **(Cutter)**
Contains per cc
Double dosage of above,

Supply: Bottles of 5 cc, 20 cc.

Dosage: 0.25–1 cc every 5–7 days.

Respiratory Infections—Prophylactic—"M.V.R.I." (Cutter)

Supply: Syringe containing 1 full immunizing treatment with 3 needles.

Dosage: 3 injections—500, 1,000, 2,000 million bacteria.

Catarrhalis Vaccine, Mixed (Gilliland)

Contains per cc	1	2	3	4
Mic. catarrhalis	25	50	100	200 million
Bac. Friedlander	37	75	150	300 million
Streptococcus	12	25	50	100 million
Pneumococcus	12	25	50	100 million
Staphylococcus	37	75	150	300 million

Supply: Packages of 4 vials 1 cc—strengths 1, 2, 3, 4; Vials 5 cc, 10 cc—strength 4.

Dosage: Initial 0.1 cc of strength 4 every 24–48 hr. in acute cases; in chronic, increased every 3–7 days.

Mixed Vaccine—Respiratory Infections (Low Count) **(Hollister-Stier)**

Contains per cc	
Staph. aureus	400 million
Staph. albus	400 million
Streptococcus	100 million
Pneumococcus	100 million
Mic. catarrhalis	100 million
Bac. Friedlander	100 million
Bac. influenzae	100 million

Supply: Bottles of 5 cc, 20 cc.

Dosage: 0.5, 1, 2 cc every 5–7 days; initial curative 0.1 cc.

Mixed Vaccine—Respiratory Infections (High Count) **(Hollister-Stier)**

Contains per cc	
Staph. aureus	600 million
Staph. albus	600 million
Streptococcus	200 million
Pneumococcus	150 million
Mic. catarrhalis	150 million
Bac. Friedlander	150 million
Bac. influenzae	150 million

Supply: Bottles of 5 cc, 20 cc.

Dosage: Half quantity of above low count.

Catarrhalis Combined Vaccine (Polyvalent) **(Lederle)**

Contains per cc	
Dilution No. 4:	
Mic. catarrhalis	200 million
Bac. Friedlander	200 million
Pneumococcus I, II, III	200 million
Strept. hemolyticus and viridans	200 million
Staph. albus	200 million
Staph. aureus	200 million

Supply: Vials 5 cc, 20 cc Dilution 4; Packages of 4 syringes or 4 vials, graduated dosage.

Dosage: ⅛, ¼, ½, 1 cc of fourth dilution every 3–5 days.

Catarrhal Vaccine Combined (Respiratory Mixed) **(Lilly)**

Contains per cc	1	2	3	4
Mic. catarrhalis	25	50	100	200 million
B. Friedlander	25	50	100	200 million

Pneumococcus	12.5	25	50	100 million
Streptococcus	12.5	25	50	100 million
Staph. aureus	50	100	200	400 million
Staph. albus	25	50	100	200 million

Supply: Vials of 5 cc, 20 cc of 4; Packages of four 1 cc vials of 1, 2, 3, 4.

Dosage: PROPHYLACTIC—Mixtures 1, 2, 3, 4, 4, 4 at intervals of 3–5 days.
THERAPEUTIC—Initial 2–4 m of mixture 4.

Catarrh "Cold" Bacterin Mixed (Mulford)

Contains per cc	A	B	C	D
Mic. catarrhalis	12.5	25	50	100
Pneumococcus I, II, III	12.5	25	50	100
Bac. Friedlander	12.5	25	50	100
Staph. aureus	50	100	200	400
Staph. albus	50	100	200	400
Strept. hemolyticus, non-hemolyticus, viridans	12.5	25	50	100

Supply: Packages of 4 syringes or 4 vials of A, B, C, D strengths; Vials 5 cc, 20 cc—D strength.

Dosage: Initial—contents of syringe A.

Catarrh "Cold" Serobacterin Mixed (Mulford)

Contains per cc	A	B	C	D
Mic. catarrhalis	125	250	500	1000 million
Pneumococcus I, II, III	125	250	500	1000 million
Bac. Friedlander	125	250	500	1000 million
Staph. aureus	125	250	500	1000 million
Staph. albus	125	250	500	1000 million
Strept. hemolyticus, non-hemolyticus, viridans	125	250	500	1000 million

Supply: Packages of 4 syringes of A, B, C, D strengths; Vials 5 cc, 20 cc of D strength; Syringes of D strength.

Dosage: Initial—contents of syringe A.

Catarrhal Vaccine (Cold and Respiratory Bacterin) (National Drug)

Contains per cc

Mic. catarrhalis	200 million
Staph. aureus and albus	200 million
Strept. hemolyticus and viridans	500 million
Bac. Pfeiffer	500 million
Pneumococcus I, II, III, IV	500 million
Bac. Friedlander	100 million

Supply: Ampule-vials 5 cc, 15 cc, 30 cc.

Dosage: Initial 0.25 cc increased every 2–4 days for 4–6 doses.

Catarrhal Vaccine (Respiratory) (Parke, Davis)

Contains per cc

Mic. catarrhalis	50 million
Bac. Friedlander	50 million
Pneumococcus Types I, II, III, IV	100 million
Streptococcus hemolyticus, non-hemolyticus	100 million
Pseudo-diphtheria bacillus	100 million
Bac. influenzae	100 million
Staph. albus	350 million
Staph. aureus	350 million

Supply: Packages of four 1 cc bulbs; Vials 5 cc, 20 cc.

Dosage: PROPHYLACTIC—Beginning with 0.1–0.25 cc gradually increased to 1 cc every 2–5 days, for 4–6 doses.
THERAPEUTIC—As above for 6–10 doses.

Bronchitis Vaccine (Sherman)

Contains per cc

Bac. Friedlander	300 million
Pneumococcus	100 million
Streptococcus	100 million
Mic. catarrhalis	200 million
Staphylococcus	400 million

Supply: Vials 5 cc, 12½ cc.

Dosage: 1 cc every 12 hr. till temperature drops, then every 24 hr. for 2–3 days; in chronic—0.3 cc increased by 0.2 cc every 2–4 days until 1 cc is given, then twice weekly.

Laryngitis Vaccine (Sherman)

Contains per cc

Pneumococcus	100 million
Streptococcus	100 million
Mic. catarrhalis	200 million
Staphylococcus	400 million

Supply: Vials 5 cc, 12½ cc.

Dosage: ACUTE—1–1.5 cc every 6 hr. till temperature drops, continued 1 cc every 12–24 hr.
CHRONIC—0.3 cc increased by 0.2 cc every 48 hr.

Catarrhal Vaccine Combined (Squibb)

Contains per cc

Bac. influenzae	300	million
Streptococcus	300	million
Pneumococcus	300	million
Bac. Friedlander	300	million
Mic. catarrhalis	200	million
Staph. albus	500	million
Staph. aureus	500	million

Supply: Vials 5 cc, 20 cc of fourth strength.

Dosage: PROPHYLACTIC—Initial 0.5 cc increased to 1 cc for 3 injections.
THERAPEUTIC—0.3 cc or more according to reaction.

Catarrhalis Immunogen Combined (Parke, Davis)

An extract of
Micrococcus catarrhalis,
Bac. influenza,
Staph. aureus,
Strept. hemolyticus and non-hemolyticus,
Pneumococci I, II, III.

Supply: Vials 10 cc, rubber-diaphragm capped.

Dosage: Initial 0.5 cc *intramuscularly* or 0.1–0.2 cc *subcutaneously;* gradually increased, avoiding severe reaction; daily or on alternate days; maximum dosage 2 cc or possibly 5 cc.

CHOLERA VACCINES

Description: Cholera Vaccines are prepared from killed organisms of Cholera Vibrio suspended in physiologic saline solution, 500–800 million per cc. *Used* as prophylactic against cholera, stimulating the production of immune bodies; gives mild reaction, offering immunity for 3–6 mo.

Administration: 2 or 3 *subcutaneous* injections of graduated dosage as available, every 5–10 days.

PREPARATIONS

Cholera Vaccine (Polyvalent) (C.A.) (Lederle)
Contains per cc

	1	2
Cholera spirilla	4,000	8,000 million

Supply: Packages of two 1 cc vials for 1 immunization; Packages of two 10 cc vials for 10 immunizations.

Dosage: 1 cc of respective dilutions at 5–7 day intervals.

Cholera Vaccine, Prophylactic (C.A.) (Lilly)
Contains per cc
Cholera vibrios.......................... 500 million, 1,000 million

Supply: 3 Vials 1 cc in single immunization package. 10 complete immunizations in 10 vials, hospital size.

Dosage: Initial 500 million, second and third, 1,000 million of bacteria in 7–10 day intervals, of bulk package 0.5 cc and 1 cc.

Cholera Bacterin (Cholera Vaccine) (C.A.) (Mulford)
Cholera spirilla........................ 500 million and 1,000 million

Supply: Vials 20 cc 1,000 million strength; Package, 3 syringes of 500, 1,000 and 1,000 million bacteria.

Dosage: *Subcutaneously* 3 injections, at 10 day intervals of above strengths.

Cholera Serobacterin (C.A.) (Sensitized Cholera Vaccine) (Mulford)
Contains per cc
500, 1,000 and 2,000 million sensitized bacteria.

Supply: 3 Syringes with 500, 1,000 and 2,000 million bacteria.

Dosage: Injected every 3–5 days.

COLON VACCINOTHERAPY

Description: Bacillus Coli Vaccines are prepared from cultures of various strains of Bacillus Coli Communis only; the *Combined vaccine* (National Drug) contains in addition other toxin-producing microorganisms. Used for the production of immunity and neutralization of toxins in bacillus coli infections: cystitis, fistulae and catarrhal jaundice.

Administration: *Prophylactic—subcutaneously,* at weekly intervals, and small dosage in the beginning, then gradually increased in accordance with resulting reactions, administered every 3–5 days.
Therapeutic—same method; dosage is to be cautiously graded and reactions avoided; course consists of about 10 injections.

PREPARATIONS

Colon Bacillus Vaccine (Coli Bacterin) (Cutter)
Contains per cc
Bac. coli.. 1,000 million

Supply: Bottles of 5 cc;

Dosage: Initial 0.05–0.1 cc, gradually increased every 3–5 days.

Colon Bacilli Vaccine (Hollister-Stier)
Contains per cc
Bac. coli.. 500 million

Supply: Bottles of 5 cc, 20 cc.

Dosage: Initial 25–50 million bacteria, gradually increased.

Coli Bacterin (Bacillus Coli Vaccine) (Mulford)

Contains per cc

	A	B	C	D
Bac coli (Polyvalent)....................	50	100	200	400 million

Supply: Packages of 4 syringes of A, B, C, D strengths; Vials 5 cc, of D strength.

Dosage: Initial 10–50 million bacteria.

Coli Serobacterin (Sensitized B. Coli Vaccine) (Mulford)

Contains per cc

	A	B	C	D
Bac. coli (Polyvalent, sensitized)....	250	500	1,000	2,000 million

Supply: Packages of 4 syringes of A, B, C, D strengths.

Dosage: Initial—contents of syringe A.

Coli Combined Vaccine (B. Coli Mixed Bacterin) (National Drug)

Contains per cc

Bac. coli.. 500 million
Bac. typhosus.................................... 500 million
Bac. paratyphosus A.............................. 250 million
Staph. albus..................................... 250 million
Strept. hemolyticus.............................. 250 million
Strept. viridans................................. 250 million

Supply: Ampule-vials 5 cc, 15 cc, 30 cc.

Dosage: Initial ⅛ cc increased by ⅛ cc every 2–5 days.

Colon Vaccine (Squibb)

Contains per cc

Bac. coli.. 5,000 million

Supply: Vials 5 cc, 20 cc.

Dosage: Initial 250 million, increased to 500 and 100 bacteria every 3–5 days.

Bacillus Coli Communis Vaccine (Squibb)

Contains per cc

Bac. coli communis (polyvalent)......................5,000 million

Supply: Vials 5 cc, 10 cc, 20 cc—Packages of 4 syringes—Packages of 4 syringes with 4 ampules.

Dosage: Prophylactic—0.1 cc subcutaneously, increased every 3 days.
Therapeutic—0.1 cc subcutaneously, increased every 3 days, for 10 injections; repeated in 3–6 mo.

DIPHTHERIA BIOTHERAPY

In diphtheria the biologicals used in diagnosis, immunization and therapy are Antitoxins or Sera, Toxin-Antitoxins and Toxoids.

1. DIAGNOSIS

Schick Test: For the diagnosis of susceptibility to diphtheria, the Schick Test is employed, using diphtheria toxin preparations. After thorough cleansing of the inner arm, 0.1 cc equivalent to 1/50 M.L.D. of toxin properly diluted is injected, *intradermally* only. Observation is made 18–24 hr. later: an area of redness with elevated surface two or more centimeters wide, surrounding the site of injection, persisting for 7–14 days and leaving a scaly, slightly pigmented area—indicates a positive reaction, i.e. absence of free antitoxin in the blood and susceptibility of the individual to diphtheria; the absence of above symptoms means a negative reaction.

Positive reactions must be differentiated from pseudo-reactions; the latter appear earlier, are the size of a dime, more infiltrated, of dusky redness and disappear in 36–48 hr. without scaling; these indicate the presence of abundant antitoxin in the system. Positive Schick tests are obtained most frequently in children up to 3 yr. of age, declining in frequency after that age. Combined reactions where positive and pseudo-reactions are superimposed indicate absence of immunity.

SCHICK TEST PREPARATIONS

Diphtheria Toxin for the Schick Test (C.A.) **(Cutter)**

Supply: Packages of 2 vials—1 of toxin and 1 of salt solution, for 10 or 50 tests.

Dosage: 0.1 cc *intracutaneously.*

Diluted Schick Test **(Cutter)**

Supply: Packages for 10 tests, diluted and ready for use.

Schick Test Control (For detecting pseudo reactions) **(Cutter)**

Supply: Packages for 10 or 50 tests.

Diphtheria Schick Test Toxin (Diluted) (C.A.) **(Gilliland)**

Supply: Packages for 10, 25 or 50 tests.

Dosage: 0.1 cc *intradermally.*

Schick Test (C.A.) **(Gilliland)**

Supply: Packages containing 1 vial of toxin and one 10 cc vial of salt solution—for 50 tests.

Dosage: 0.2 cc *intradermally.*

Schick Test Control (Heated Diphtheria Toxin) (C.A.) **(Gilliland)**

Supply: Packages for 50 tests.

Schick Test (Diluted) **(Hixson)**

Supply: Packages of 1 vial containing diluted toxin without peptones—for 10, 25 or 50 tests.

Diphtheria Toxin for Schick Test (In Peptone Solution) (C.A.) **(Lederle)**

Supply: Packages of 1 syringe for 1 test (diluted); Packages of 1 vial for 10 tests (diluted).

Schick Test Control (Heated Diphtheria Toxin diluted with Peptone Solution) (C.A.) **(Lederle)**

Supply: Packages of 1 syringe for 1 control test; Packages of 1 vial for 10 control tests.

Schick Test (C.A.) **(Lederle)**

Supply: Packages of 1 vial with diluent—for 50 or 100 tests.

Diphtheria Toxin for Schick Test (Diluted) (C.A.) **(Lilly)**

Supply: Packages of 1 vial for 10 or 100 tests.

Dosage: 0.1 cc *intracutaneously.*

Schick Test Control (Toxin heated to destroy specific exotoxins.) **(Lilly)**

Supply: Packages for 10 tests.

Diphtheria Toxin for the Schick Test (C.A.) **(Mulford)**

Supply: Packages containing two 5 cc vials or two 10 cc vials, 1 of toxin and 1 of diluent—for 50 or 100 tests.

Dosage: 0.1 cc.

Diphtheria Toxin for Schick Test Control (C.A.) **(Mulford)**

Supply: Packages of one 5 cc vial or one 10 cc vial for 50 or 100 tests.

Schick Test, Peptone Diluent (C.A.) **(National Drug)**

Supply: Packages of one 1 cc vial, one 5 cc vial or one 10 cc vial, for 10, 50 or 100 tests.

Schick Test Control **(National Drug)**

Supply: Packages for 10 or 50 tests.

Diphtheria Toxin Diluted for Schick Test (C.A.) **(Parke, Davis)**

Supply: Vials of 1 cc or 10 cc for 10 or 100 tests.

Dosage: 0.1 cc.

Diphtheria Toxin Control (Diluted Heated Diphtheria Toxin) (C.A.) **(Parke, Davis)**

Supply: Vials for 50 tests.

Diphtheria Toxin for Schick Test (Diluted with Peptone Solution) (C.A.) **(Squibb)**

Supply: Packages for 10 or 100 tests.

Dosage: 0.1 cc *intracutaneously.*

Schick Test Control **(Squibb)**

Supply: Packages for 100 tests.

Diphtheria Toxin for Schick Test (C.A.) **(U. S. Standard)**

Supply: Packages of undiluted toxin with diluent for 10, 50 or 100 tests.

Diphtheria Toxin for Schick Test Control (C.A.) **(U. S. Standard)**

Supply: Packages for 10, 50 or 100 tests.

---

2. IMMUNIZATION

A. Diphtheria Toxin-Antitoxin

Description: For active immunization Diphtheria Toxoids and Toxin-Antitoxins are employed. The latter are mixtures of concentrated antitoxin and diphtheria toxin, aged and standardized; are stable and potent for 1 yr. and generally cause but slight reaction. *Used* for protection against diphtheria of children from 6 mo. to 5 yr., especially in schools, institutions, asylums, and of adults in contact with children; immunity appears somewhat late but is thought to be permanent.

Administration: Is usually administered *subcutaneously,* 3 injections, at weekly intervals, of same dosage for all ages; infants under 6 mo.—half quantity. Immunity is tested for by the Schick Test 6 mo. after immunization.

Bibliography: *See Chap. XII.*

TOXIN-ANTITOXIN PREPARATIONS

Diphtheria Toxin-Antitoxin Mixture (C.A.) **(Cutter)**

Supply: Packages of three 1 cc ambots for 1 immunization; Bottles of 30 cc for 10 immunizations.

Dosage: 3 *intramuscular* or *subcutaneous* injections of 1 cc each at 7–10 day intervals.

Diphtheria Toxin-Antitoxin Mixture (Goat) (C.A.) **(Cutter)**

Supply: Packages of three 1 cc ambots for 1 immunization; Bottles of 30 cc for 10 immunizations.

Dosage: 3 *intramuscular* or *subcutaneous* injections of 1 cc each at 7–10 day intervals.

Diphtheria Toxin-Antitoxin Mixture (Goat) (C.A.) **(Gilliland)**

Supply: Packages of three 1 cc syringes or vials for 1 immunization; Packages of thirty 1 cc vials for 10 immunizations; Vials 10 cc or 30 cc for 3 or 10 immunizations.

Dosage: 3 *intramuscular* or *subcutaneous* injections of 1 cc each at 7–10 day intervals.

Diphtheria Toxin-Antitoxin (Horse or Sheep) (C.A.) **(Hixson)**

Supply: Packages of three or thirty 1 cc vials for 1 or 10 immunizations; Vials 5 cc—Packages of one or three 10 cc vials for 3 or 10 immunizations—Vials 30 cc for 10 complete immunizations.

Dosage: 3 *intramuscular* or *subcutaneous* injections of 1 cc each at 7–10 day intervals.

Diphtheria Toxin-Antitoxin Mixture (Horse) (C.A.) (1/10th L + Dose) **(Lederle)**

Supply: Packages of 3 vials for 1 immunization—Packages of 30 cc vials for 10 immunizations.

Dosage: 3 *intramuscular* or *subcutaneous* injections of 1 cc each at 7–10 day intervals.

Diphtheria Toxin-Antitoxin Mixture (Goat) (C.A.) **(Lederle)**

Supply: Packages of 3 vials for 1 immunization—Packages of 30 cc vials for 10 immunizations.

Dosage: 3 *intramuscular* or *subcutaneous* injections of 1 cc each at 7–10 day intervals.

Diphtheria Toxin-Antitoxin Mixture (C.A.) (Diphtheria Prophylactic) **(Lilly)** (Sheep)

Contains per cc.

0.1 L + dose of toxin, neutralized with the required amount of antitoxin.

Supply: Packages of three 1 cc vials for 1 complete immunization; Packages of 10 vials for 10 complete immunizations; Vials 30 cc for 10 complete immunizations.

Dosage: 3 *intramuscular* or *subcutaneous* injections of 1 cc each at 7–10 day intervals.

Diphtheria Toxin-Antitoxin Mixture (New Formula (C.A.) **(Mulford)**

Supply: Packages of three or thirty 1 cc ampule-vials for 1 or 10 complete immunizations—Packages of one 10 cc vial or one 30 cc vial for 3 or 10 immunizations.

Dosage: 3 *intramucular* or *subcutaneous* injections of 1 cc each at 7–10 day intervals.

Diphtheria Toxin-Antitoxin Mixture (Goat) **(Mulford)**

Supply: Packages of three or thirty 1 cc ampule-vials for 1 or 10 complete immunizations—Packages of one 10 cc vial or one 30 cc vial for 3 or 10 immunizations.

Dosage: 3 *intramuscular* or *subcutaneous* injections of 1 cc each at 7–10 day intervals.

Toxin-Antitoxin (Diphtheria Toxin-Antitoxin Mixture) (C.A.) **(National Drug)**

Supply: Packages of three or thirty 1 cc ampule-vials for 1 or 10 immunizations. Ampule-vials 15 cc or 30 cc for 5 or 10 immunizations.

Dosage: 3 *intramuscular* or *subcutaneous* injections of 1 cc each at 7 day intervals.

Diphtheria Toxin-Antitoxin Mixture (C.A.) **(Parke, Davis)**

Supply: Packages of three or thirty 1 cc bulbs, 0.1 L + dose of toxin in each cc—for 1 or 10 immunizations; Vials 30 cc, rubber-diaphragm capped, of same strength.

Dosage: 3 *intramuscular* or *subcutaneous* injections of 1 cc each at 7 day intervals.

Diphtheria Toxin-Antitoxin Mixture (New Formula) (C.A.) **(Squibb)**

Supply: Packages of three 1 cc ampules; Vials 10 cc.

Dosage: 3 *intramuscular* or *subcutaneous* injections of 1 cc each at 7–10 day intervals.

Diphtheria Toxin-Antitoxin Mixture (New Formula) (Sheep) (C.A.) **(Squibb)**

Supply: Packages of three 1 cc ampules-vials 10 cc, 30 cc.

Dosage: Three intramuscular, or subcutaneous injections of 1 cc each at 7–10 day intervals.

Diphtheria Toxin-Antitoxin Mixture (C.A.) **(U. S. Standard)**

Supply: Packages of three or thirty 1 cc vials; Vials 30 cc.

Diphtheria Toxin-Antitoxin Mixture (Goat) (C.A.) **(U. S. Standard)**

Supply: Packages of three 1 cc vials; Vials 10 cc, 30 cc.

Diphtheria Toxin-Antitoxin Mixture (Sheep) (C.A.) **(U. S. Standard)**

Supply: Packages of three or thirty 1 cc vials; Vials of 30 cc.

B. Diphtheria Toxoids

Description: Toxoids are prepared from diphtheria toxin treated with formaldehyde by the method of Ramon to reduce or destroy its toxic properties; is stable and non-toxic; develops active immunity promptly and in a shorter period than toxin-antitoxin; is now used more generally in the immunization of children against diphtheria than is toxin-antitoxin mixture; contains no serum and thus produces no serum reactions.

Administration: Is usually administered in two, occasionally three *subcutaneous* injections, at intervals of 3–4 weeks. Sensitivity to toxoids is first determined by the intradermal injection of 0.1 cc of the diluted toxoid; where present sensitivity is shown by a wide area of induration and redness surrounding the site of injection and is accompanied by general malaise, headache and fever. Where such redness more than a half inch in diameter develops within 3 days, it is best to avoid the injection of toxoids, but use instead toxin-antitoxin (goat serum). Sensitiveness is seldom present in children under 6 yr. of age.

Diphtheria Antitoxin in dosage of 1,000 units may also be used in prophylaxis.

Bibliography: *See Chap. XII.*

TOXOID PREPARATIONS

Diphtheria Toxoid (Anatoxine Ramon) (Formalin Treated) (C.A.) **(Cutter)**

Supply: Packages of three or thirty 1 cc ambots for 1 or 10 immunizations; Bottles of 45 cc for 15 immunizations.

Dosage: 2–3 injections of 1 cc each, at 3 week intervals. Infants—0.5 cc.

Toxoid for the Reaction Test **(Cutter)**

Supply: Packages for 1, 10 or 15 tests.

Diphtheria Toxoid (Anatoxine-Ramon) (C.A.) **(Gilliland)**

Supply: Packages of two or twenty 1 cc vials for 1 or 10 immunizations; Vials 30 cc for 15 immunizations.

Dosage: Two *subcutaneous* injections of 1 cc each at monthly intervals; a vial of diluted diphtheria toxoid for skin reaction test where desired.

Diphtheria Toxoid (Anatoxine-Ramon) (C.A.) **(Hixson)**

Supply: Packages of two or twenty 1 cc vials for 1 or 10 complete immunizations; Vials of 10 or 30 cc for 5 or 15 complete immunizations. Obtainable also with potassium alum where specified.

Dosage: Two *subcutaneous* injections of 1 cc each at monthly intervals.

Diphtheria Toxoid (Anatoxine-Ramon) (C.A.) **(Lederle)**

Supply: Packages of two syringes or vials for 1 immunization; Vials 30 cc for 15 immunizations; Syringe of 1:20 diluted Diphtheria Toxoid for 1 sensitivity test—Vials for 5, 10 or 100 sensitivity tests.

Dosage: Two *subcutaneous* injections of 1 cc each at intervals of 3–4 weeks.

Diphtheria Toxoid (C.A.) **(Lilly)**

Supply: Packages of two 1 cc vials for 1 complete immunization; Vials 30 cc for 15 complete immunizations.

Dosage: Two *subcutaneous* injections of 1 cc each at intervals of 3–4 weeks.

Diphtheria Toxoid (Anatoxine-Ramon) (C.A.) **(Mulford)**

Supply: Packages of two or twenty 1 cc ampule-vials for 1 or 10 immunizations; Vials 30 cc for 15 immunizations.

Dosage: Two subcutaneous injections of 1 cc each at intervals of 3 or 4 weeks.

Diphtheria Toxoid (Anatoxine-Ramon) (C.A.) **(National Drug)**

Supply: Packages of two or twenty 1 cc vials for 1 or 10 immunizations; Vials of 10, 20 or 30 cc for 5, 10 or 15 immunizations.

Dosage: Two injections of 1 cc each *subcutaneously* at 2–4 week intervals; small children or infants—0.5 cc followed by 1 cc.

Diphtheria Toxoid (Anatoxine-Ramon) (Formaldehyde Treated) (C.A.) **(Parke, Davis)**

Supply: Packages of 1 bulb of dilute toxoid for sensitivity test, and two 1 cc bulbs of prophylactic toxoid for 1 immunization; Packages of thirty 1 cc bulbs; Vials 30 cc, rubber-diaphragm-capped, containing per cc 0.1 L + dose of toxin; Vials 0.5 cc, 5 cc dilute toxoid for Reaction Test.

Dosage: Two injections of 1 cc each, *subcutaneously*, at 2–4 week intervals; infants under 1 yr.—half dosage.

Diphtheria Toxoid (Anatoxine-Ramon) (Formaldehyde Treated) (C.A.) **(Squibb)**

Supply: Packages of two 1 cc vials for 1 complete immunization.
Packages of twenty 1 cc vials for 10 complete immunizations; Vials 30 cc.

Dosage: Two injections of 1 cc each, *subcutaneously*, at 2–4 week intervals; a third injection is given if Schick test is positive after 8 weeks; infants under 1 yr.—half dosage.

Diphtheria Toxoid **(U. S. Standard)**

Supply: Packages of two and twenty 1 cc vials; Vials of 20 cc.

Dosage: Two injections of 1 cc each, *subcutaneously*, at 2–4 week intervals; a third injection is given if the Schick test is positive after 8 weeks.

---

3. THERAPEUTIC

Diphtheria Antitoxins

Description: For treatment of diphtheria, antitoxins are used; these are highly refined and concentrated products, prepared from serum of healthy horses immunized by repeated and increased injections of diphtheria toxin; they are water-clear fluids, practically free from proteins, serum albumins, euglobins and inert solids producing undesirable reactions; they are concentrated into a relatively small bulk, are quickly absorbed and non-irritating; they neutralize unattached diphtheria toxins and are thus specifics in the treatment of diphtheria.

Administration: Best used *intramuscularly*, also administered *subcutaneously;* in severe, late or laryngeal cases often *intravenously*. Sensitiveness to serum reaction is first determined by intracutaneous injection of 2 or 3 drops of the serum, or of normal horse serum; if found sensitive, desensitization is first accomplished by very small and gradually increased intramuscular doses, at half hour intervals, changing cautiously to the intravenous method if the case be urgent; adrenalin given subcutaneously will assist in overcoming sensitivity. *Dosage*—mild cases 5,000 units, moderate 5,000 to 10,000 units, severe and laryngeal cases 20,000 units and over. Children under 60 lbs.—5,000 to 10,000 units, over 15 yr.—10,000 to 15,000 units; in malignant cases—double dosage. Repeated administrations where indicated; at times combined intramuscular and intravenous injections are necessary.

ANTITOXIN PREPARATIONS

Diphtheria Antitoxin (Concentrated Globulin) (C.A.) **(Cutter)**

Supply: Syringes of 1,000, 5,000, 10,000 or 20,000 units.

Dosage: PROPHYLACTIC—Average dose 1,000 units, at times up to 5,000 units.
THERAPEUTIC—20,000 units or more repeated every 6 hr.; in severe neglected or laryngeal cases 40,000 units *intravenously*, repeated every 6 hr. if necessary.

Diphtheria Antitoxin (Concentrated and Refined) (C.A.) **(Gilliland)**

Supply: Packages of 1 syringe or vial containing 1,000, 5,000, 10,000 or 20,000 units.

Dosage—IMMUNIZING—1,000 units *subcutaneously*.
THERAPEUTIC—Initial 10,000 units, repeated and doubled if necessary in 6 hr.

Diphtheria Antitoxin (C.A.) **(Hixson)**

Supply: Packages of 1 syringe or vial containing 1,000, 3,000, 5,000, 10,000, 20,000 units; Packages of 1 syringe or vial containing 1,000 units sheep antitoxin.

Dosage: IMMUNIZING—1,000 units.
THERAPEUTIC—Initial 10,000 units, repeated in 6–8 hr. if necessary.

Diphtheria Antitoxin (Refined and Concentrated) (C.A.) **(Lederle)**

Supply: Packages of one syringe of 1,000, 5,000, 10,000, 20,000 or 40,000 units.

Dosage: IMMUNIZING—1,000 units *subcutaneously*.
THERAPEUTIC—Total dosage intended, as one injection.

Diphtheria Antitoxin (Purified Concentrated Globulin) (C.A.) **(Lilly)**

Supply: Syringes of 1,000, 5,000, 10,000 or 20,000 units.

Dosage: IMMUNIZING—1,000 units subcutaneously.
THERAPEUTIC—10,000 units subcutaneously or intramuscularly, repeated where necessary.

Diphtheria Antitoxin (Superconcentrated) (C.A.) **(Mulford)**

Supply: Syringes of 1,000 or 5,000 units (prophylactic)—Syringes of 10,000, 20,000 or 40,000 units (therapeutic).

Dosage: IMMUNIZING—1,000 units *subcutaneously*.
THERAPEUTIC—10,000 units *subcutaneously* or *intramuscularly*, repeated where necessary.

Diphtheria Antitoxin (Bovine) **(Mulford)**

Supply: Ampule-vials 30 cc—5,000 units.

For use in those who exhibit hypersensitiveness to horse serum.

Diphtheria Antitoxin (Extra Concentrated and Refined) **(National Drug)**

Supply: Syringes of 1,000, 5,000, 10,000, 20,000 or 40,000 units; Ampules of 1,000, 5,000, 10,000 or 20,000 units.

Dosage: Initial 10,000–20,000 units *intramuscularly* or *intravenously*, repeated every 8–12 hr. as long as necessary; laryngeal and late cases—40,000–50,000 units intravenously, repeated in 6–12 hr.

Diphtheria Antitoxin (Highly Concentrated and Purified) (C.A.) **(Parke, Davis)**

Supply: Syringes of 1,000, 5,000, 10,000 or 20,000 units.

Dosage: PROPHYLACTIC—10,000 units *subcutaneously.*
THERAPEUTIC—10,000–20,000 units *intramuscularly* or *intravenously,* repeated as necessary. Severe cases: 20,000–100,000 units, every 6–12 hr.

Diphtheria Antitoxin (C.A.) **(Squibb)**

Supply: Packages of 1,000, 5,000, 10,000 or 20,000 units.

Dosage: IMMUNIZING—1,000 units.
THERAPEUTIC—5,000–20,000 units, mild; late severe or laryngeal cases—20,000–100,000 units or more, repeated in 6–8 hr. if necessary. Prophylaxis: 1,000–5,000 units *intramuscularly.* Malignant cases: combined *intravenous* and *intramuscular* injections are given.

DYSENTERY SEROTHERAPY

Description: Antidysenteric Sera are polyvalent antitoxins, containing antibacterial substances and antibodies obtained from the blood of horses inoculated with living cultures of Bacillus Dysenteriae of Shiga-Kruse, Flexner and Hiss-Y strains; are *used* in prophylaxis and therapeusis of bacillary dysentery.

Administration: *Prophylactic*—10 cc *subcutaneously.*
Therapeutic—50–100 cc *intravenously,* repeated in 4–8 hr. and guided by the number of diarrheal stools and general symptomatology.

PREPARATIONS

Antidysenteric Serum (Polyvalent) (C.A.) **(Lederle)**

Supply: 50 cc intravenous outfit.

Dosage: PROPHYLACTIC—10 cc *subcutaneously.*
THERAPEUTIC—100 cc *intravenously,* repeated where necessary, in 4 hr.

Antidysenteric Serum (Polyvalent) (C.A.) **(Mulford)**

Supply: Packages containing one 20 cc syringe; Packages containing one double end 50 cc vial with or without intravenous injection outfit.

Dosage: 50–100 cc every 8 hr. until 400 cc are given.

Antidysenteric Serum (C.A.) **(Parke, Davis)**

Supply: Bottles of 20 cc; Syringes of 20 cc.

Dosage: PROPHYLACTIC—Initial 10 cc.
THERAPEUTIC—Initial 60–100 cc *intravenously.*

ERYSIPELAS BIOTHERAPY

Description: Erysipelas Antitoxins are refined and concentrated specific sera, containing antibodies and antibacterial properties of Streptococcus Erysipelatis; are obtained from the blood of horses immunized against toxins and living cultures of streptococcus hemolyticus, isolated from lesions of human virulent erysipelas. *Used* in the treatment of erysipelas and its complications; is most helpful in facial erysipelas.
Erysipelas Vaccines are prepared in the usual manner from the Streptococcus Erysipelatis; they are less popular and used in a manner as described in the individual preparations, mostly in prophylaxis.

Administration: Administered *intramuscularly;* in extreme cases *intravenously;* treatment best instituted immediately upon diagnosis; in doses from 10–20 cc, repeated at intervals of 6–12 hr., as many times as indicated, this depending upon duration of disease, virulence of infection, parts involved and individual's resistance; average number in ordinary cases 2–3 injections, in severe or late cases 5–6; is continued until flush and edema disappear.

Bibliography: *See Chap. XII.*

1. ERYSIPELAS ANTITOXINS

Erysipelas Streptococcus Antitoxin (Refined and Concentrated) (C.A.) **(Lederle)**

Supply: Packages of 1 syringe of therapeutic dose.

Dosage: 1 syringe repeated at intervals of 24 hr. until flush and edema disappear.

Antistreptococcic Serum (Erysipelas Concentrated) (C.A.) **(Lilly)**

Supply: Packages of 1 syringe of therapeutic dose.

Dosage: 1–4 doses, *intramuscularly* or *intravenously.*

Erysipelas Streptococcus Antitoxin (Concentrated) (C.A.) **(Mulford)**

Supply: Packages of one 10 cc syringe (500,000 units).

Dosage: 10–20 cc *intramuscularly* only.

Antistreptococcus Erysipelas Serum (C.A.) **(National Drug)**

Supply: Packages of one 10 cc sterile perfected syringe with chromium steel intravenous needle.

Dosage: Initial 10–20 cc, *intravenously* or *intramuscularly* repeated until disease is under control; severe or late cases—20 cc *intravenously* every 8–10 hr.

Erysipelas Streptococcus Antitoxin (Refined and Concentrated) (C.A.) **(Parke, Davis)**

Supply: Packages of one 10 cc or 20 cc syringe with sterile double-pointed needle.

Dosage: 10–100 cc *intramuscularly,* repeated if necessary, at 6–12 hr. intervals.

Erysipelas Streptococcus Antitoxin (Concentrated) (C.A.) **(Squibb)**

Supply: Packages of 1 syringe of therapeutic dose.

Dosage: 1 dose, repeated every 12–24 hr., *intramuscularly* or *intravenously.*

2. VACCINE PREPARATIONS

Erysipelas Bacterin **(Abbott)**

Contains per cc

Strept. erysipelatis	100 million
Staph. albus	500 million

Supply: Bulk packages 6 cc, 20 cc.

Dosage: 1 cc every 6–12 hr.

Erysipelas Vaccine (Erysipelas Bacterin) **(National Drug)**

Contains per cc

Strept. erysipelatis	200 million

Supply: Ampule-vials 5 cc, 15 cc, 30 cc.

Dosage: Initial 0.25 cc, increased by 0.25 cc every 6–12 hr.; in subacute states—1 cc at 2–4 day intervals.

Erysipelas Streptococcus Immunogen **(Parke, Davis)**

An extract of hemolytic streptococci from erysipelas.

Supply: Vials 10 cc, rubber-diaphragm-capped.

Dosage: Initial 0.5 cc *intramuscularly* or 0.1–0.2 cc *subcutaneously;* gradually increased, avoiding severe reaction; daily or on alternate days; maximum dosage 2 cc or possibly 5 cc.

Erysipelas Phylacogen **(Parke, Davis)**

Culture filtrates of streptococcus hemolyticus and non-hemolyticus, and staphylococcus albus and aureus—from erysipelas cases.

Supply: Vials 10 cc, rubber-diaphragm-capped.

Dosage: *Subcutaneously*—1 cc, increasing gradually to 10 cc; daily injections.
Intravenously—Initial 2–4 m increasing gradually to 5 cc; daily injections.

Erysipelas Vaccine **(Sherman)**
Contains per cc
Strept. erysipelatis.. 100 million
Staph. albus.. 200 million

Supply: Vials 5 cc, 12½ cc.

Dosage: PROPHYLACTIC—Initial 0.5 cc, followed by 1 cc in 24 hr., then 3 injections of 1 cc each at 2–4 day intervals.

FURUNCULOSIS VACCINOTHERAPY

Description: Vaccines for the treatment of furunculosis are prepared from various strains of Staphylococcus Pyogenes Aureus et Albus, the common infective agents; are *used* to raise immunity against these organisms in simple furunculosis and pustular acne; also to prevent their common recurrences and hasten sluggish healing.

Administration: Given *subcutaneously,* beginning with small dose, increased at each injection, every 2–5 days, and guarding against undue reactions.

PREPARATIONS

Furunculosis Bacterin Mixed (C.A.) **(Abbott)**
Contains per cc
Staph. aureus.. 1,000 million
Staph. albus.. 1,000 million

Supply: Bulk packages of 6 cc, 20 cc.

Dosage: 3–5 m at 4 day intervals.

Furunculosis Vaccine (C.A.) **(Parke, Davis)**
Contains per cc.
Staph. aureus.. 2,000 million

Supply: Packages of four 1 cc bulbs—Vials of 5 cc, 20 cc.

Dosage: Initial 0.1 cc, increased to 1 cc at 3–5 day intervals.

GAS-GANGRENE SEROTHERAPY

Description: Antitoxins for the treatment of gas-gangrene are obtained by immunizing horses with toxins of Bac. Perfringens, Vibrion Septique, Bac. Oedematiens, Bac. Sordelli and Bac. Histolyticus; the products are refined, concentrated and potent in the treatment of wounds contaminated with gas forming organisms, by counteracting their toxins. They are *used* principally in inoperable cases of gas-gangrene; also as accessory to surgical treatment in operable cases, as in intestinal obstruction and appendectomy.

Administration: *Prophylactic*—A prophylactic dose is to be given within 12 hr. after injury; where interval is greater or wound is contaminated with dirt and other foreign matter, dosage is repeated in 5–7 days; is also repeated where the possibility of infection is still present after that period.
Therapeutic—Initial injection 1–4 minimum therapeutic doses, *intravenously,* often preceded with a dose of tetanus antitoxin; repeated in 4–6 hr. where necessary or warranted by symptoms; is supplemented during convalescence with 1 therapeutic dose, *subcutaneously,* every 24–48 hr. Intravenous injections are to be given very slowly and precautions taken against possible anaphylaxis.

Bibliography: *See Chap. XII.*

PREPARATIONS

Gas-Gangrene Antitoxin (Polyvalent Anaerobic Antitoxin) (C.A.) **(Lederle)**
Contains per therapeutic dose—refined and concentrated:

Perfringens antitoxin	10,000 units
Vibrion septique antitoxin	10,000 units
Oedematiens antitoxin	200 units
Sordelli antitoxin	200 units
Histolyticus antitoxin	25 units

Supply: Refined and Concentrated—Vials containing 1 therapeutic dose. Unrefined—Vials containing 1 therapeutic dose about 100 cc.

Dosage: Intravenously, 1–4 therapeutic doses, repeated every 4–6 hr. as necessary; preceded with 1,500 units Tetanus Antitoxin.

Gas-Gangrene Antitoxin (Combined) (C.A.) (Lilly)
Concentrated and refined for B. Perfringens (B. Welchii) and Vibrion septique.

Supply: Packages of 1 syringe containing 10,000 units perfringens antitoxin and 10,000 units vibrion septique antitoxin.

Dosage: Intravenously, 1 syringe or more, repeated in 8–24 hr. as required.

Perfringens Antitoxin (Unconcentrated) (C.A.) **(Mulford)**

Supply: Bottles 100 cc containing 100 antitoxic units—Bottles 50 cc containing 100 antitoxic units.

Perfringens Antitoxin (Concentrated) (C.A.) **(Mulford)**

Supply: Syringes 20 cc containing 100 antitoxin units.

Dosage: PROPHYLACTIC—2,500 units.
THERAPEUTIC—4,000–10,000 units *intramuscularly* and 4,000 units *intravenously* followed by 4,000–8,000 units *intramuscularly* daily.

Gas-Gangrene Antitoxin (Combined) (C.A.) **(Parke, Davis)**

Supply: Syringes of 1 therapeutic dose containing 10,000 units perfringens and 10,000 units vibrion septique.

Dosage: Intravenously, 1 syringe, repeated in 8–24 hr.

GONOCOCCUS VACCINOTHERAPY

Description: The *Simple Gonococcus Vaccines* and Bacterins are prepared from pure strains of the Gonococcus obtained from specific sources; the *Mixed Vaccines* contain in addition other bacteria commonly associated with the gonococcus. The Simple vaccines, by raising immunity, are intended to shorten the course of the disease and lessen complications; the Mixed are preferred in the treatment of complications: epididymitis, orchitis, salpingitis, endocervicitis, prostatitis and seminal vesiculitis; in gonorrheal ophthalmia and rheumatism.
Antigonococcus serum is intended for acute systemic infections: gonorrheal arthritis, gonorrheal endocarditis; is administered *intravenously.*

Administration: *Subcutaneously,* in quantities as per concentration of individual preparation, every 5–7 days; treatment continued for several weeks after symptoms have subsided.

Bibliography: *See Chap. XII.*

1. SIMPLE VACCINES

Gonorrhea Bacterin **(Abbott)**

Supply: Bulk packages of 6 cc, 20 cc.

Dosage: 0.5–1 cc every 1–2 days.

Gonococcus Vaccine (Special High Count) **(Abbott)**
Contains per cc
Gonococcus .... 2,000 million

Supply: Bottles of 5 cc.

Dosage: As above.

Gonococcic Vaccine (Neisser Bacterin) **(Cutter)**
Contains per cc
Gonococcus.. 500 million

Supply: Bottles of 5 cc.

Dosage: Acute—0.05–0.2 cc, increased every 2–4 days.

Gonococcic Vaccine **(Gilliland)**

Contains per cc	1	2	3	4
Gonococcus........................	250	500	1,000	2,000 million

Supply: Packages of 4 vials 1 cc each of strengths 1, 2, 3, 4; Vials 5 cc, 10 cc of strength 4.

Dosage: 50–250 million bacteria rapidly increased every 1–3 days; chronic resistant cases—1,000–2,000 million bacteria.

Gonococcic Vaccine **(Hollister-Stier)**
Contains per cc
Gonococcus.. 500 million

Supply: Bottles of 5 cc, 20 cc

Dosage: Acute—0.05–0.25 cc every 3–4 days.

Gonococcus Vaccine (Neisser Vaccine, Polyvalent) **(Lederle)**
Contains per cc
Gonococci.. 1,200 million

Supply: Packages of 4 vials of doses 1–4—Vials 5 cc.

Dosage: ⅛, ¼, ½, 1 cc at 3–5 day intervals.

Gonococcus Glycerol Vaccine (Neisser Glycerol Vaccine, Polyvalent) **(Lederle)**

Supply: Packages of 15 doses, beginning with 100 million gonococci, ending with 1,500 million, each 0.1 cc, serially numbered to represent millions; Packages—Series A (Doses 1–5), Series B (Doses 6–10), Series C (Doses 11–15) with Ampule 4.5 cc diluent, saline solution; Packages—Series D, containing 5 doses—1,600, 1,700 1,800, 1,900, 20,000 million gonococci, for follow-up treatment.

Dosage: 15 graduated doses at intervals of 3–5 days.

Gonococcus Vaccine (Neisser) **(Lilly)**
Contains per cc
Gonococcus.. 1,000 million

Supply: Bottles of 5 cc, 20 cc.

Dosage: Initial 2–4 m.

Neisser Bacterin (Gonococcic Vaccine) **(Mulford)**

Contains per cc	A	B	C	D
Gonococcus...........................	50	100	200	400 million

Supply: Packages of 4 syringes of A, B, C, D strengths; Vials of 5 cc, 20 cc of D strength.

Dosage: Initial 10–50 million bacteria.

Neisser Serobacterin (Gonococcic Vaccine, Sensitized) **(Mulford)**

Contains per cc	A	B	C	D
Gonococcus........................	250	500	1,000	2,000 million

Supply: Packages of 4 syringes of A, B, C, D strengths; Vials of 5 cc of D strength.

Dosage: Initial—contents of syringe A.

Neisser Vaccine (Neisser Bacterin) **(National Drug)**
Contains per cc
Gonococcus.. 2,000 million

Supply: Ampule-vials 5 cc, 15 cc, 30 cc.

Dosage: ACUTE—0.25 cc increased by 0.25 cc at 2–5 day intervals until 1 cc is given.
CHRONIC—0.125–0.25 cc increased by 0.125 cc every 2–5 days, until 2 cc or more are given.

Gonococcus Immunogen **(Parke, Davis)**
An extract of the gonococcus.

Supply: Vials 10 cc, rubber-diaphragm-capped.

Dosage: Initial 0.5 cc *intramuscularly* or 0.1–0.2 cc *subcutaneously*, gradually increased, avoiding severe reaction; daily or on alternate days; maximum dosage 2 cc or possibly 5 cc.

Gonococcus Vaccine (Bacterial Vaccine) (Squibb)

Contains per cc	1	2	3	4
Gonococcus	250	500	750	1,000 million

Supply: Packages of 4 ampules of strengths 1, 2, 3, 4; Vials 5 cc, 20 cc of strength 4.

Dosage: Initial 250 million, increased to 1,000 million every 3–5 days, and continued for several weeks after symptoms have ceased.

Gonococcus Vaccine **(Upjohn)**
Contains per cc
Gonococcus .... 1,000 million

Supply: Ampules 1 cc in packages of 6.

Dosage: Initial 0.25 cc increased to 1 cc every 3–5 days.

2. COMBINED VACCINES

Neisser Bacterin (Gonorrhea Compound) **(Abbott)**
Contains per cc

Gonococcus	3,000 million
Streptococcus	100 million
Pneumococcus	100 million
Bac. coli	200 million
Staph. aureus	1,000 million
Staph. albus	1,000 million

Supply: Bulk packages of 6 cc, 20 cc.

Dosage: 0.25 cc increased to 1 cc every 24 hr.; in arthritis—every 3–6 days.

Urethritis Bacterin **(Abbott)**
Contains per cc

Gonococcus	100 million
Streptococcus	200 million
Pneumococcus	200 million
Staph. aureus	500 million
Staph. albus	500 million
Mic. catarrhalis	100 million
Bac. coli	500 million
Bac. pseudodiphtheriae	300 million

Supply: Bulk packages of 6 cc, 20 cc.

Dosage: Initial 5 m increased to 50 m every 3–5 days.

Mixed Vaccine—Gonorrhea (M.V.G.) (Neisser and Mixed Bacterins) **(Cutter)**
Contains per cc

Gonococcus	50 million
Staph. albus and aureus	250 million
Streptococcus	50 million
Bac. pseudodiphtheriae	50 million
Bac. coli	100 million

Supply: Bottles of 5 cc, 20 cc. Mixed Vaccine (4 Count) 2,500 million per cc—Bottles of 5 cc, 20 cc.

Dosage: Initial 0.1–0.5 cc.

Gonococcic Vaccine Mixed (Gilliland)

Contains per cc	1	2	3	4
Gonococcus	62.5	125	250	500 million
Staph. albus	62.5	125	250	500 million
Bac. pseudo-diphtheriae	62.5	125	250	500 million
Bac. coli	62.5	125	250	500 million

Supply: Packages of four 1 cc vials of strengths 1, 2, 3, 4; Vials 5 cc, 10 cc of strength 4.

Mixed Vaccine—Gonorrhea (Hollister-Stier)

Contains per cc	
Gonococcus	400 million
Staph. albus	400 million
Staph. aureus	400 million
Streptococcus	100 million
Diphtheroids	300 million
Bac. coli	400 million

Supply: Bottles of 5 cc, 20 cc.

Dosage: Initial 0.05–0.25 cc.

Gonococcus Combined Vaccine (Neisser Combined Vaccine, Polyvalent) **Dilution 4** (Lederle)

Contains per cc	
Gonococcus	600 million
Bac. coli	400 million
Strep. hemolyticus, viridans	600 million
Staph. albus, aureus, citreus	2,400 million

Supply: Packages of 4 vials, graduated doses—Vials 5 cc, 20 cc of Dilution 4.

Dosage: 1/8, 1/4, 1/4, 1 cc every 3–5 days.

Urethritis Treatment Vaccine (Polyvalent) **Dilution 4** (Lederle)

Contains per cc	
Gonococcus	400 million
Streptococcus	400 million
Staphylococcus	1,200 million
Bac. coli	400 million
Mic. catarrhalis	400 million
Bac. pseudo-diphtheriae	400 million

Supply: Vials 5 cc, Dilution 4.

Dosage: 1/8, 1/4, 1/2, 1 cc at intervals of 3–5 days.

Gonococcus Mixed Vaccine (Neisser Mixed) (Lilly)

Contains per cc	1	2	3	4	5
Gonococcus	50	100	200	400	1,200 million
Bac. coli	50	100	200	400	600 million
Streptococcus	50	100	200	400	400 million
Staph. aureus	100	200	400	800	1,200 million
Staph. albus	100	200	400	800	1,200 million

Supply: Vials 5 cc, 20 cc of strength 4; Vials 5 cc of strengths 1, 2, 3, 4; Packages of 1 cc vials—1 each of above strengths.

Dosage: Initial—mixture 1; of vials—2–4 m.

Neisser Bacterin Mixed (Gonococcic Vaccine Mixed) **(Mulford)**

Contains per cc	A	B	C	D
Gonococcus	50	100	200	400 million
Staph. aureus	50	100	200	400 million
Staph. albus	50	100	200	400 million
Streptococcus hemolyticus, non-hemolyticus, viridans	50	100	200	400 million
Bac. coli	50	100	200	400 million
Diphtheroids	50	100	200	400 million

Supply: Packages of four 1 cc vials of A, B, C, D strengths; Vials 5 cc, 20 cc of D strength; Single syringes of D strength.

Dosage: Initial content of syringe A.

Neisser Serobacterin Mixed (Gonococcic Vaccine Mixed, Sensitized) **(Mulford)**

Contains per cc	A	B	C	D
Gonococcus	125	250	500	1,000 million
Staph. aureus	125	250	500	1,000 million
Staph. albus	125	250	500	1,000 million
Streptococcus hemolyticus, non-hemolyticus, viridans	125	250	500	1,000 million
Bac. coli	125	250	500	1,000 million
Diphtheroids	125	250	500	1,000 million

Supply: Packages of four 1 cc vials of A, B, C, D strengths; Vials 5 cc, 20 cc of D strength; Single syringes of D strength; Single syringes of E strength and double strength of E.

Dosage: Initial—content of syringe A.

Neisser Combined Vaccine (Neisser Bacterin Combined) **(National Drug)**

Contains per cc	
Gonococcus	1,500 million
Staph. albus and aureus	500 million
Diphtheroids	250 million
Bac. coli	250 million
Strep. hemolyticus and viridans	500 million

Supply: Ampule-vials of 5 cc, 15 cc, 30 cc.

Dosage: Acute—initial 0.25 cc increased by 0.25 cc every 2–5 days till 1 cc is given.
Chronic—until 2 cc are given.

Gonorrheal Vaccine (Combined) (Urethritis Combined). **(Parke, Davis)**

Contains per cc	
Gonococcus	1,000 million
Staph. albus	1,200 million
Staph. aureus	800 million
Mic. catarrhalis	100 million
Bac. coli	500 million
Strept. hemolyticus and non-hemolyticus	200 million
Bac. pseudo-diphtheriae	200 million

Supply: Packages of four 1 cc bulbs; Vials 5 cc, 20 cc.

Dosage: Initial 0.1 cc, increased to 1 cc every 3–5 days.

Gonococcus Immunogen Combined **(Parke, Davis)**

An extract of micrococcus gonorrhoeae, staph. aureus and albus.

Supply: Vials 10 cc, rubber-diaphragm-capped.

Dosage: Initial 0.5 cc *intramuscularly* or 0.1–0.2 cc *subcutaneously*, gradually increased, avoiding severe reaction; daily or on alternate days; maximum dosage 2 cc or possibly 5 cc.

Gonorrhea Phylacogen (Parke, Davis)

Culture filtrates of gonococcus (50%), mixed staphylococcus albus and aureus, streptococcus hemolyticus and non-hemolyticus.

Supply: Vials 10 cc, rubber-diaphragm-capped.

Dosage: *Subcutaneously*—1 cc, increasing gradually to 10 cc; daily injections.
Intravenously—initial 2–4 m, increasing gradually to 5 cc; daily injections.

Gonorrhea Vaccine (Sherman)

Contains per cc

Gonococcus	1,000 million
Streptococcus	100 million
Pneumococcus	100 million
Bac. coli	200 million
Bac. pseudo-diphtheriticus	300 million
Staph. albus	1,000 million

Supply: Vials 5 cc, 12½ cc.

Dosage: ACUTE—0.3 cc increased by 0.2 cc daily until 1 cc is given, then 1 cc every 2–4 days for 20–25 injections.
SUBACUTE AND CHRONIC—At intervals of 2–3 days.

Gonococcus Vaccine Combined (Bacterial Vaccine) (Squibb)

Contains per cc	First	Second	Third	Fourth	
Gonococcus	250	500	750	1000	million
Staph. albus	125	250	375	500	million
Staph. aureus	125	250	375	500	million
Bac. coli	125	250	375	500	million
Diphtheroids	75	150	225	300	million
Streptococcus	25	50	75	100	million
Pneumococcus	25	50	75	100	million

Supply: Packages of 4 ampules of strengths 1, 2, 3, 4; Vials 5 cc, 20 cc of strength 4.

Dosage: Initial 0.3 cc, increased to 1 cc, at 5–7 day intervals.

Gonococcus Mixed Vaccine (Upjohn)

Contains per cc

Gonococcus	1,000 million
Bac. coli	400 million
Diphtheroids	300 million
Streptococcus	200 million
Staph. albus	500 million
Staph. aureus	500 million

Supply: Ampules 1 cc in packages of 6; Vials of 5 cc, 20 cc.

Dosage: 0.2 cc, increased.

Antigonococcic Serum (Mulford)

Supply: Packages of one 50 cc double end vial with intravenous injection outfit.

Dosage: One vial as required.

INFLUENZA VACCINOTHERAPY

Description: Vaccines for use in influenzal infections are prepared from various strains of Pneumococcus, Streptococcus and Staphylococcus in addition to the Bacillus Influenzae, as isolated from cases suffering from this disease; they are used to produce immunity and to increase resistance in those subject to attacks of influenza, grippe, bronchitis or laryngitis.

Administration: *Immunization*—generally 3 injections, administered at 3–5 day intervals, *subcutaneously,* will produce immunity lasting for 1 yr. or over.

Curative—is administered in dosages indicated in each case and individual preparation, until temperature drops to about normal; in threatened pneumonia, influenza-pneumonia prophylactic vaccines are employed.

1. PREPARATIONS

Influenza Bacterin **(Abbott)**

Contains per cc

Bac. influenzae	200 million
Bac. Friedlander	100 million
Bac. pseudo-diphtheriae	100 million
Mic. catarrhalis	100 million
Mic. tetragenus	100 million
Streptococcus	100 million
Pneumococcus	100 million
Staph. aureus	100 million
Staph. albus	100 million

Supply: Bulk packages of 6 cc, 20 cc.

Dosage: PROPHYLACTIC—0.25 cc followed by 0.5 cc at 7–10 day intervals.
THERAPEUTIC—Initial 0.3 cc, cautiously increased.

Mixed Vaccine-Influenza (Rosenow Combination) **(Cutter)**

Contains per cc

Pneumococcus 4 types	3,000 million
Strept. viridans	3,000 million
Strept. hemolyticus	1,000 million
Bac. influenzae	500 million
Staph. aureus	500 million

Supply: Bottles of 5 cc.

Dosage: PROPHYLACTIC—Initial 0.5 cc, followed by 1 cc at 5–7 day intervals for 4 injections.

Influenza Vaccine Mixed **(Gilliland)**

Contains per cc	1	2	3	4
Bac. influenzae	125	250	500	1000
Pneumococcus	125	250	500	1000
Streptococcus	125	250	500	1000

Supply: Packages of four 1 cc vials of strengths 1, 2, 3, 4; Vials 5 cc, 10 cc of strength 4.

Dosage: Initial 50–100 million bacteria, increased.

Mixed Vaccine Influenza (Rosenow Combination) **(Hollister-Stier)**

Contains per cc

Pneumococcus all types and allied streptococci	3,000 million
Strept. hemolyticus	1,000 million
Bac. influenzae	500 million
Staph. albus	250 million
Staph. aureus	250 million

Supply: Bottles of 5 cc, 20 cc.

Dosage: Initial 0.5 cc as prophylaxis; as treatment—0.05–0.1 cc, increased.

Catarrhalis Influenza Vaccine **(Lederle)**

Contains per cc

Mic. catarrhalis	200 million
Bac. influenzae	200 million
Bac. Friedlander	200 million
Strep. hemolyticus	100 million
Strep. viridans	100 million

Staph. albus	200 million
Staph. aureus	200 million
Pneumococcus I, II, III	200 million

Supply: Vials 5 cc, 20 cc.

Dosage: PROPHYLACTIC—0.2 cc increased to 1 cc, at 3–5 day intervals.

Influenza Combined Vaccine (Polyvalent) (Lederle)

Contains per cc

Dilution 4

Bac. influenzae	1,000 million
Pneumococcus I, II, III	1,000 million
Strep. hemolyticus	1,000 million

Supply: Vials 5 cc, Dilution 4.

Dosage: ⅛, ¼, ½, 1 cc at 3–5 day intervals.

Catarrhalis-Influenza Glycerol Vaccine (Lederle)

Contains per cc	1	2	3	4	5
Mic. catarrhalis	50	100	200	400	800 million
Bac. influenzae	50	100	200	400	800 million
Bac. Friedlander	50	100	200	400	800 million
Pneumococcus I, II, III	50	100	200	400	800 million
Strep. hemolyticus and viridans	50	100	200	400	800 million
Staph. albus	50	100	200	400	800 million
Staph. aureus	50	100	200	400	800 million

Supply: Packages of 5 vials for 1 treatment, with vials of sterile diluent.

Dosage: In serial order, first three at 3 day intervals, last two at 5 day intervals.

Influenza Mixed Vaccine (Lilly)

Contains per cc	1	2	3	4
Bac. influenzae	50	125	250	500 million
Mic. catarrhalis	12.5	25	50	100 million
Pneumococcus	150	375	750	1,500 million
Streptococcus	50	125	250	500 million
Staph. aureus	50	125	250	500 million
Staph. albus	50	125	250	500 million

Supply: Packages of four 1 cc vials of strengths 1, 2, 3, 4; Vials 5 cc, 20 cc of strength 4.

Dosage: PROPHYLACTIC—Initial, mixture 1 followed by 2, 3, 4 at 3 day intervals.
THERAPEUTIC—Initial, mixture 1 increased every 1–2 days; or 2–4 m from bulk vials.

Influenza "Cold" Bacterin Mixed (Mulford)

Contains per cc	A	B	C	D
Bac. influenzae	12.5	25	50	100 million
Staph. aureus	50	100	200	400 million
Staph. albus	50	100	200	400 million
Strep. hemolytic, non-hemolytic, viridans	12.5	25	50	100 million
Pneumococcus I, II, III	12.5	25	50	100 million
Mic. catarrhalis	12.5	25	50	100 million
Bac. Friedlander	12.5	25	50	100 million

Supply: Packages of four 1 cc vials of strengths A, B, C, D; Vials 5 cc, 20 cc of strength D—Single syringes of strength D.

Dosage: Initial—contents of syringe A.

Influenza "Cold" Serobacterin Mixed (Mulford)

Contains per cc	A	B	C	D
Bac. influenzae	125	250	500	1,000 million
Bac. Friedlander	125	250	500	1,000 million

Staph. albus	125	250	500	1,000 million
Staph. aureus	125	250	500	1,000 million
Strept. hemolyticus, non-hemolyticus, viridans	125	250	500	1,000 million
Pneumococcus I, II, III	125	250	500	1,000 million
Mic. catarrhalis	125	250	500	1,000 million

Supply: Packages of four 1 cc vials of strengths A, B, C, D; Vials 5 cc, 20 cc of strength D—Single syringes of strength D.

Dosage: Initial—contents of syringe A.

Influenza Combined Vaccine (Influenza Bacterin Mixed) **(National Drug)**

Contains per cc

Bac. influenzae	500 million
Strept. hemolyticus and viridans	500 million
Pneumococcus 4 types	500 million
Mic. catarrhalis	500 million

Supply: Ampule-vials of 5 cc, 15 cc, 30 cc.

Dosage: PROPHYLACTIC—initial $\frac{1}{8}$–$\frac{1}{2}$ cc at 3–5 day intervals, increased to $\frac{1}{2}$ and 1 cc every 1–3 mo. to maintain immunity.
THERAPEUTIC—Initial $\frac{1}{8}$–$\frac{1}{2}$ cc increased to 1 cc at 1–5 day intervals.

Influenza Vaccine Combined **(Parke, Davis)**

Contains per cc

Bac. influenzae	400 million
Strept. non-hemolyticus	300 million
Mic. catarrhalis	100 million
Pneumococcus 4 types	400 million

Supply: Packages of four 1 cc bulbs—Vials 5 cc, 20 cc.

Dosage: Initial 0.1–0.5 cc, rapidly increased to 1 cc or more at 3–5 day intervals.

Influenza Vaccine **(Squibb)**

Contains per cc	1	2	3	4
Bac. influenzae	250	500	750	1,000

Supply: Packages of 4 ampules of strengths 1, 2, 3, 4; Vials 5 cc, 20 cc of strength 4.

Dosage: PROPHYLACTIC—Initial 0.5 cc, second and third doses—1 cc.
THERAPEUTIC—0.3 cc increased.

Influenza Vaccine Combined (Rosenow Combination) **(Squibb)**

Contains per cc	1	2	3	4
Bac. influenzae	125	250	375	500
Pneumococcus	750	1,500	2,250	3,000
Streptococcus	250	500	750	1,000
Staph. aureus	125	250	375	500

Supply: Packages of 4 ampules of strengths 1, 2, 3, 4; Vials 5 cc, 20 cc of strength 4, also Packages of 4 ampules.

Dosage: PROPHYLACTIC—Initial 0.5 cc, followed by 1 cc for 2 doses.
THERAPEUTIC—0.3 cc, increased.

Uses: For prevention of influenza, grippe, pneumonia, colds, bronchitis, laryngitis.

Influenza Mixed Vaccine **(Upjohn)**

Contains per cc

Bac. influenzae	400 million
Pneumococcus 4 types (100 million each)	400 million
Strept. hemolyticus	100 million
Strept. viridans	100 million
Mic. catarrhalis	100 million
Staph. albus	250 million
Staph. aureus	250 million

Supply: Ampules 1 cc in packages of 6—Vials 5 cc, 20 cc.

Dosage: PROPHYLACTIC—Initial 0.3 cc, increased to 1 cc, 3 injections.
THERAPEUTIC—0.3 cc, increased.

2. INFLUENZA-PNEUMONIA PROPHYLAXIS VACCINES

Influenza-Pneumonia Vaccine **(Lilly)**

Contains per cc

Pneumococcus, Types I, II, III	1,500 million
Pneumococcus Type IV and allied diplostreptococcus	1,500 million
Strept. hemolyticus	1,000 million
Staph. aureus	500 million
Bac. influenzae	500 million

Supply: Vials 5 cc.

Dosage: Initial 0.5 cc, increased to 1 and 1.5 cc at 7 day intervals.

Influenza-Pneumonia Vaccine **(Parke, Davis)**

Contains per cc

Pneumococcus 4 types, Type IV predominating	3,000 million
Strept. hemolyticus	1,000 million
Bac. influenzae	500 million
Staph. aureus	500 million

Supply: Packages of 3 bulbs—0.5, 1.0, 1.5 cc—Vials of 20 cc.

Dosage: Contents of 1 bulb every 7 days.

MENINGOCOCCUS BIOTHERAPY

Description: Antimeningococcus Sera are prepared from the serum of horses immunized by repeated injections of Meningococcus cultures, of various strains to assure a well balanced serum. They are refined, concentrated and treated generally by the Banzhaf method. Are used in the specific therapy of meningococcus meningitis and other meningococcus infections, mostly for therapeusis, as immunization is not yet thoroughly established; where used for latter purpose the vaccines are employed.

Administration: Sera should be administered as soon as the diagnosis by lumbar puncture is made; given *intraspinally*, after withdrawal of sufficient spinal fluid to reduce the pressure to about 10 mm Hg.

Dosage: Adults—20–30 cc, infants—15 cc; in epidemics—larger doses, 30–100 cc; repeated every 12–24 hr. for 3–4 days, in accordance with severity of case, and discontinued with disappearance of organisms from spinal fluid; in fulminating cases given *intravenously* and *intraspinally;* in obstruction between ventricular and subarachnoid spaces is administered *intraventricularly* or cisternally. Shock with cessation of breathing during administration, may be overcome by raising of head, abstracting fluid from spinal canal, artificial respiration, epinephrin and stimulants.

Bibliography: *See Chap. XII.*

1. SERUM PREPARATIONS

Antimeningococcic Serum (Combined Types) (C.A.) **(Gilliland)**

Agglutinates meningococci of the regular, irregular and intermediate groups, and Gordon types.

Supply: Packages containing one or two 15 cc vials with gravity injecting outfit.

Dosage: 30 cc or more for adults; 5–15 cc for children, *intraspinally*, daily for 4–6 days or longer. *Intravenously* as supplementary treatment—30–60 cc at 12–24 hr. intervals.

Antimeningococcic Serum (C.A.) **(Lederle)**

Supply: Packages of one or two 15 cc intraspinal cylinders; Packages of one 30 cc intraspinal cylinder.

Dosage: Adults—30 cc or more *intraspinally*. Children—5–15 cc. Severe cases supplemented by 60–90 cc *intravenously*.

Antimeningococcic Serum (Concentrated and Refined) Banzhaf (C.A.) **(Lilly)**
Contains various strains of the meningococcus.

Supply: Ampules 10 cc with intraspinal injection apparatus.

Dosage: 20 cc *intraspinally* every 24 hr. (also cisternal or ventricular methods).

Antimeningococcic Serum (Polyvalent) (C.A.) **(Mulford)**

Supply: Packages of two 15 cc vials with special needle for intraspinal injection; Packages of one 30 cc container with intraspinal and intravenous injection outfits.

Dosage: 1 vial every 12–24 hr. *intraspinally;* supplementary injection 30 cc *intravenously*.

Antimeningococcic Serum (Polyvalent) (C.A.) **(National Drug)**

Supply: Packages of two 15 cc syringes with gravity injection outfit; Ampule-vials 30 cc with special intravenous and intraspinal needles and gravity outfit.

Dosage: Adults 30 cc. Children 10–15 cc *intraspinally* or *intradurally;* supplementary injection 30 cc *intravenously*.

Antimeningococcic Serum (C.A.) **(Parke, Davis)**

Supply: Packages of two 15 cc syringes with flexible gravity tube and special intravenous and intraspinal needles; Packages of one 30 cc syringe with flexible gravity tube and special intravenous and intraspinal needles.

Dosage: 30–150 cc *intravenously; intraspinally*—15–30 cc.

Antimeningococcic Serum (Polyvalent) (C.A.) **(Squibb)**

Supply: Packages of two 15 cc special gravity containers complete with needles, rubber tubing, bulb, etc.

Dosage: SUBDURAL—Adults 15 cc repeated as necessary; children 5–15 cc.
INTRAVENOUS—50–100 cc in earlier stages and severe attacks.—Average case: repeated 8–24 hr. for 3–4 days; severe—every 12 hr. for 3–4 days, then every 24 hr. During epidemics—30–100 cc, *intravenously*.

Antimeningococcus Serum (Polyvalent) (C.A.) **(U. S. Standard)**

Supply: 1 and 2 double-ended 15 cc vials with outfit.

Dosage: 1 vial every 12–24 hr., *intraspinally;* supplemented by 30 cc *intravenously*.

2. VACCINE PREPARATIONS

Meningo-Bacterin (Meningococcic Vaccine) **(Mulford)**

Supply: Packages of 3 syringes containing 500, 1,000, 1,000 million bacteria, for 1 immunization—Packages of 30 vials for 10 immunizations.

Dosage: 500, 1,000, 1,000 million bacteria at 10 day intervals. Children, half dosage.

Meningococcic Vaccine (Polyvalent) **(National Drug)**
Contains per cc

Meningococcus (Gordon Types 1 and 2)	1,500 million
Meningococcus (Gordon Types 3 and 4)	500 million

Supply: Ampule-vials 5 cc, 15 cc, 30 cc.

Dosage: PROPHYLACTIC—4 injections—¼, ½, ¾, 1 cc at 4–5 day intervals.

Epidemic Meningitis Vaccine **(Sherman)**
Contains per cc

Meningococci	1,000 million

Supply: Vials 5 cc, 12½ cc.

Dosage: PROPHYLACTIC—Initial 0.3 cc, in 3–4 days 0.6 cc, in 5 more days 1 cc, with 2 additional injections of 1 cc at 5 day intervals.

PERTUSSIS VACCINOTHERAPY

Description: *Simple Pertussis Vaccines* are prepared in the usual manner from Bacillus Pertussis, in concentrations from 2,000 million to 8,000 million per cc; most available vaccines are of high antigenic power, uniform, stable and used in whooping cough not only as prophylactic, but also to lessen the severity of paroxysms, duration and intensity of the disease and the probability of complications. *Mixed Pertussis vaccines* are of greater benefit in persistent cases of whooping cough, generally due to associated infection; they contain in addition to the Bacillus Pertussis also the common organisms found in infections of the respiratory tract—Bacillus Influenzae, Pneumococcus, Staphylococcus, Micrococcus catarrhalis, etc.
Immunization often establishes a high positive immunity and is useful in checking the spread of the disease during epidemics.

Administration: Pertussis vaccines may be used in children 1 yr. and over, as here they cause but little reaction. *For immunization* generally 3 graduated doses, at 3 day intervals are administered *subcutaneously*, or into the buttocks or anterior abdominal wall; same dosage for all ages except infants under 1 yr., half dosage. *For treatment*—daily administration of gradually increasing doses, in strengths in accordance with individual products.

Bibliography: *See Chap. XII.*

1. VACCINES

Pertussis Bacterin (Prophylactic) **(Abbott)**
Contains per cc
Bac. pertussis (Bordet) .... 5,000 million

Supply: Bulk packages of 6 cc, 20 cc.

Dosage: THERAPEUTIC—Initial 3 m, increased to 1 cc at 3 day intervals; PROPHYLACTIC—3, 6 and 15 m at 3 day intervals.

Pertussis Vaccine (Bordet-Gengou) **(Cutter)**
Contains per cc Bac. pertussis (Bordet-Gengou)
Low Count .... 2,000 million
Special High Count .... 7,500 million
Fresh High Count (Made up fresh on order only.) .... 7,500 million

Supply: Bottles of 5 cc.

Dosage: PROPHYLACTIC—Initial 0.1–0.2 cc *subcutaneously*, rapidly increased at 40 and 72 hr. intervals.
THERAPEUTIC—Daily injections of 0.2, 0.4, 0.8, 0.16, and 2.0 cc.

Pertussis Prophylactic Vaccine **(Cutter)**
Contains Bac. Bordet-Gengou in suspension.

Supply: One syringe and 3 needles for 1 immunizing treatment.

Dosage: 500 million, 1,000 million, 2,000 million bacteria—3 injections at 5–7 day intervals.

Pertussis Vaccine **(Gilliland)**

Contains per cc	1	2	3	4
Bac. pertussis	250	500	1,000	2,000 million

Supply: Packages of four 1 cc vials of strengths 1, 2, 3, 4; Vials 5 cc, 10 cc of strength 4.

Dosage: Initial 250–500 million bacteria, repeated at 1, 2 or 3 day intervals.

Pertussis Vaccine (Hollister-Stier)
Contains per cc
Bac. pertussis (Low Count) .... 2,000 million
Bac. pertussis (High Count) .... 7,500 million

Supply: Bottles of 5 cc, 20 cc (Low Count)—Bottles of 5 cc (High Count).

Dosage: 0.05–0.5 cc every 3–4 days.

Pertussis Glycerol Vaccine (Lederle)

Contains per cc	1	2	3	4	5
Bac. pertussis (Bordet)....	1,000	2,000	4,000	6,000	8,000 million

Supply: Packages of five 1 cc vials of strengths 1, 2, 3, 4, 5; Vial of strength 5 with vial of saline diluent.

Dosage: PROPHYLACTIC—3 *subcutaneous* injections at 3 day intervals.
THERAPEUTIC—Injected daily or every second day; dosage of vial dilution—⅛, ¼, ½, ¾ and 1 cc.

Pertussis Vaccine (Polyvalent) (Lederle)

Contains per cc	1	2	3
Bac. pertussis (Bordet).................	2,000	4,000	4,000 million

Supply: Packages of 3 syringes or 3 vials of strengths 1, 2, 3; Vials 5 cc of strength 2.

Dosage: PROPHYLACTIC—3 consecutive injections at 3 day intervals, or bulk—⅛, ¼, ½ and 1 cc at 1–5 day intervals.

Pertussis Vaccine (Whooping Cough) (Lilly)
Contains Bac. pertussis

Supply: Packages of four 1 cc vials—2,500 million bacteria per cc; Vials 5, 20 cc—2,500 million bacteria per cc; Vials 5 cc—5,000 million bacteria per cc; Packages of four 1 cc vials—250, 500, 1,000, 2,500 million bacteria per cc.

Dosage: PROPHYLACTIC—Initial 2,500 million, second and third injection—5,000 million bacteria at 3 day intervals.
THERAPEUTIC—Initial 2,500 million.

Pertussis Bacterin (Pertussis Vaccine) (Mulford)

Contains per cc	A	B	C	D
Bac. pertussis.....................	250	500	1,000	2,000 million

Supply: Packages of four syringes of strengths A, B, C, D; Vials 5 cc of strength D.

Dosage: One-fifth to entire contents of syringe A, initial dose.

Pertussis Serobacterin (Pertussis Vaccine Sensitized) (Mulford)

Contains per cc	A	B	C	D
Bac. pertussis.....................	250	500	1,000	2,000 million

Supply: Packages of four syringes of strengths A, B, C, D; Vials 5 cc, 20 cc of strength D.

Dosage: Initial one-fifth to entire contents of syringe A.

Pertussis Vaccine (Whooping Cough Bacterin) (National Drug)
Contains per cc
Bac. pertussis.. 4,000 million

Supply: Ampule-vials 5 cc, 15 cc, 30 cc.

Dosage: PROPHYLACTIC—½ cc, ¾ cc, 1 cc, 1½ cc at 2–4 day intervals (3 or 4 doses).
THERAPEUTIC—Same dosage, continued from 1 cc; infants—½ dosage.

Pertussis Vaccine (Parke, Davis)
Contains per cc
Bac. pertussis.. 4,000 million

Supply: Packages of four 1 cc bulbs; Vials 5 cc, 20 cc.

Dosage: PROPHYLACTIC—0.25, 0.5, 0.75, 1 cc at 2 day intervals.

Pertussis Immunogen **(Parke, Davis)**
An extract of Bac. pertussis.

Supply: Vials 10 cc, rubber-diaphragm-capped.

Dosage: Initial 0.5 cc *intramuscularly* or 0.1–0.2 cc *subcutaneously*, gradually increased, avoiding severe reaction; daily or on alternate days; maximum dosage 2 cc or possibly 5 cc.

Whooping Cough Vaccine (Bacterial Vaccine) **(Squibb)**
Contains per cc

Bac. pertussis	4,000 million and 10,000 million

Supply: Vials 5 cc and 20 cc.

Dosage: PROPHYLACTIC—Strengths 1, 2 and 4 at 3–5 day intervals, *subcutaneously*, THERAPEUTIC—Initial 1,000 bacteria, increased every second day.

2. COMBINED VACCINES

Whooping Cough Bacterin **(Abbott)**
Contains per cc

Bac. pertussis	4,000 million
Bac. influenzae	200 million
Mic. catarrhalis	200 million
Pneumococcus	200 million
Streptococcus	200 million
Staph. aureus	100 million

Supply: Bulk packages of 6 cc, 20 cc.

Dosage: 6, 10, 15 and 15 m at 3 day intervals, as treatment.

Pertussis Mixed Vaccine (Pertussis Bacterin Mixed) **(Cutter)**
Contains per cc

Bac. pertussis	1,000 million
Staph. albus	250 million
Staph. aureus	250 million
Streptococcus	100 million
Pneumococcus	100 million
Bac. influenzae	100 million
Mic. catarrhalis	100 million
Bac. Friedlander	100 million

Supply: Bottles of 5 cc—Bottles of 5 cc 4 Count—double strength.

Dosage: Initial 0.1 cc regular count or 0.5 cc 4 count.

Pertussis Vaccine (Mixed) **(Gilliland)**

Contains per cc	1	2	3	4
Bac. pertussis	500	1,000	2,000	4,000 million
Bac. influenzae	50	100	200	400
Pneumococcus	50	100	200	400
Streptococcus	50	100	200	400

Supply: Packages of four 1 cc vials of strengths 1, 2, 3, 4; Vials 5 cc, 10 cc of strength 4.

Dosage: INITIAL PROPHYLACTIC—½–1 cc every 3–5 days.
THERAPEUTIC—Every 24–48 hr.

Pertussis Mixed Vaccine **(Hollister-Stier)**

Bac. pertussis	2,000 million
Staph. albus	200 million
Staph. aureus	200 million
Streptococcus	100 million
Pneumococcus	100 million
Bac. influenzae	100 million
Mic. catarrhalis	100 million

Supply: Bottles of 5 cc, 20 cc.

Dosage: Initial 0.05–0.1 cc.

Pertussis Combined Vaccine (Polyvalent) (Lederle)

Contains per cc

Bac. pertussis	4,000 million
Bac. influenzae	200 million
Pneumococcus I, II, III	200 million
Strept. hemolyticus, viridans	200 million
Staph. albus and aureus	200 million
Mic. catarrhalis	200 million

Supply: Packages of four vials of graduated doses; Vials 5 cc, 20 cc of above strength.

Dosage: 1/8, 1/4, 1/2, 1 cc at intervals of 1–5 days.

Pertussis Mixed Vaccine (Lilly)

Contains per cc	1	2	3	4
Bac. pertussis	500	1,000	2,000	4,000 million
Bac. influenzae	25	50	100	200 million
Streptococcus	12.5	25	50	100 million
Pneumococcus	25	50	100	200 million
Mic. catarrhalis	12.5	25	50	100 million
Staph. aureus	50	100	200	400 million
Staph. albus	12.5	25	50	100 million

Supply: Packages of four 1 cc vials of strengths 1,2, 3, 4—Packages of four 1 cc vials of strength 4; Vials 5 cc, 20 cc of strength 4.

Dosage: PROPHYLACTIC—Initial—strength 4 repeated on alternate days for 3 doses. THERAPEUTIC—Initial, strength 4.

Pertussis Bacterin Mixed (Mulford)

Contains per cc	A	B	C	D
Bac. pertussis	250	500	1,000	2,000 million
Bac. influenzae	25	50	100	200 million
Strept. hemolyticus, non-hemolyticus, viridans	12.5	25	50	100 million
Pneumococcus I, II, III	12.5	25	50	100 million
Mic. catarrhalis	12.5	25	50	100 million
Staph. aureus	12.5	25	50	100 million
Staph. albus	12.5	25	50	100 million

Supply: Packages of four 1 cc vials or four syringes, of strengths A, B, C, D; Vials 5 cc, 20 cc of strength D.

Dosage: Initial—contents of syringe A.

Pertussis Serobacterin Mixed (Pertussis Vaccine Mixed, Sensitized) (Mulford)

Contains per cc	A	B	C	D
Bac. pertussis	500	1,000	2,000	4,000 million
Bac. influenzae	50	100	200	400 million
Strept. hemolyticus, non-hemolyticus, viridans	25	50	100	200 million
Pneumococcus I, II, III	25	50	100	200 million
Mic. catarrhalis	25	50	100	200 million
Staph. aureus	25	50	100	200 million
Staph. albus	25	50	100	200 million

Supply: Packages of 4 syringes of strengths A, B, C, D; Vials 5 cc, 20 cc of strength D.

Dosage: Initial—one-fifth to entire contents of syringe A.

Pertussis Combined Vaccine (Whooping Cough Bacterin Mixed, Polyvalent) **(National Drug)**

Contains per cc

Bac. pertussis	4,000 million
Strep. hemolyticus, viridans	250 million
Pneumococcus I, II, III, IV	500 million
Bac. influenzae	250 million

Supply: Ampule-vials 5 cc, 15 cc, 30 cc.

Dosage: PROPHYLACTIC—¼, ½, 1, 1 cc at 2–4 day intervals—3 or 4 doses. THERAPEUTIC—As above, continued at 1 cc if necessary. Infants—½ dosage.

Pertussis Vaccine Combined **(Parke, Davis)**

Contains per cc

Bac. pertussis	4,000 million
Staph. aureus	500 million
Strept. hemolyticus, non-hemolyticus	100 million
Mic. catarrhalis	40 million
Bac. influenzae	160 million
Pneumococcus I, II, III, IV	200 million

Supply: Packages of four 1 cc bulbs—Vials 5 cc, 20 cc.

Dosage: THERAPEUTIC—0.1–0.2 cc increased at intervals of 3–5 days.

Pertussis Immunogen Combined **(Parke, Davis)**

An extract of Bac. pertussis, Staph. aureus and albus.

Supply: Vials 10 cc, rubber-diaphragm-capped.

Dosage: Initial 0.5 cc *intramuscularly* or 0.1–0.2 cc *subcutaneously*, gradually increased, avoiding severe reaction; daily or on alternate days; maximum dosage 2 cc or possibly 5 cc.

Whooping Cough Vaccine **(Sherman)**

Contains per cc

Bac. pertussis	3,000 million
Pneumococcus	40 million
Streptococcus	30 million
Mic. catarrhalis	100 million

Supply: Vials 5 cc, 12½ cc.

Dosage: PROPHYLACTIC—4 injections—0.25, 0.5, 1, 1 cc at 3 and 5 day intervals.

Whooping Cough Vaccine Combined **(Sherman)**

Contains per cc	1	2	3	4
Bac. pertussis	1,000	2,000	3,000	4,000 million
Staph. albus	50	100	150	200 million
Staph. aureus	50	100	150	200 million
Mic. catarrhalis	50	100	150	200 million
Bac. influenzae	25	50	75	100 million
Streptococcus	25	50	75	100 million
Pneumococcus	50	100	150	200 million

Supply: Packages of 4 ampules of strengths 1, 2, 3, 4; Vials 5 cc, 20 cc of strength 4

Dosage: THERAPEUTIC—Initial 0.3 cc, increased.

Whooping Cough Vaccine Combined **(Squibb)**

Contains per cc

B. pertussis	1,000	2,000	3,000	4,000 million
Staph. albus	50	100	150	200 million
Staph. aureus	50	100	150	200 million
Mic. catarrhalis	50	100	150	200 million
B. influenzae	25	50	75	100 million

Streptococcus....................	25	50	75	100 million
Pneumococcus..................	50	100	150	200 million

Supply: Packages of 4 ampules of strengths 1, 2, 3, 4; Vials 5 cc, 20 cc of strength 4.

Dosage: 4 injections—0.3, 0.5, 1 and 1 cc at 2-3 day intervals; infants—half dosage

---

PLANT POISONING BIOTHERAPY

Description: Preparations for plant poisoning are solutions of specific toxic principles of Rhus Toxicodendron and Rhus Diversiloba, in alcohol, or olive oil or almond oil; stimulate antibody formation and immunity to the specific toxins and are highly potent; *used* for immunization and treatment of plant poison dermatitis, ivy and oak.

Administration: *Prophylactic—intramuscular* injections, 3 to 4 doses at 1 to 3 day intervals, in dosages in accordance with preparation.
Therapeutic—1 to 3 injections at 8–24 hr. intervals, in strengths in accordance with individual preparations. Also administered orally.

Caution: To avoid severe irritation, care must be exercised while injecting a preparation to prevent its dropping on the skin; in accidental contact, the skin must immediately be cleansed with alcohol, petroleum, ether or toluene, using fresh pledgets of cotton for each sponging. The surface of the needle must be wiped free from the extract and site of injection is not to be massaged.

Bibliography: *See Chap. XII.*

IVY POISONING PRODUCTS

Toxivi (Poison Ivy Treatment) 1:10,000 solution (alcohol) (Cutter)

Supply: Packages of 1 syringe with sterile needles, of 3 doses for 1 treatment; Ambots 1 cc.

Dosage: PROPHYLACTIC—1 cc *intramuscularly* every 3–4 days for 3 doses. Therapeutic—1–3 injections every 24 hr.

Poison Ivi (Poison Ivy Prophylactic) 1:2,000 dilution (Cutter)

Supply: Bottles of 100 cc.

Dosage: For internal use only.
PROPHYLACTIC—4–20 drops in water after meals. Therapeutic ½–1 oz. in water on alternate days.

Poison Ivy Extract (In Almond Oil) (C.A.) (Lederle)

Supply: Packages of one or four 1 cc syringes.

Dosage: THERAPEUTIC 1 cc *intramuscularly,* second or third dose at 24 hr. intervals, if necessary;

Ivyol-Poison Ivy Extract (C.A.) (Mulford)
A solution in olive oil of the extracts of rhus toxicodendron.

Supply: Poison Ivy Extract—Packages of 4 hypo-units, each 1 dose.

Dosage: *Intramuscularly,* 1 hypo-unit daily for 4 doses; in susceptible individuals, beginning with ¼–½ unit, for prophylaxis.

Rhus Venenata Antigen (40% Alcoholic Solution with 0.4% Procaine) (National Drug)

Supply: Packages of four 1 cc ampules; Tincture (Oral) in vials of 1 oz.

Dosage: 0.5, 0.75, 1, 1.5 cc *intramuscularly,* every 3–4 days, for immunization; during attack—0.3–0.5 cc on 2 successive days, then 0.3–0.7 cc every 2–3 days, two to three times, then 1 cc daily four times.

Poison Ivy Extract (Rhus Tox) **(Squibb)**

Supply: Preseasonal—Vials 3 cc; Seasonal—Vials 0.3 cc with two 1 cc vials of physiologic saline.

Dosage: Preseasonal—10 subcutaneous injections of gradually increased dosage at weekly intervals for 5 injections, then at 2 or 3 week intervals. Seasonal—2–5 injections daily of 1 cc with 1 cc diluent.

OAK POISONING PRODUCTS

Toxok (Poison Oak Treatment, Intramuscular) 1:10,000 solution (alcohol) **(Cutter)**

Supply: Packages of 1 syringe with sterile needles, of 3 doses for 1 treatment; Packages of two 1 cc ambots.

Dosage: PROPHYLACTIC—1 cc *intramuscularly* three times, every 3–4 days. Therapeutic—1–3 injections every 24 hr.

Poisonok (Poison Oak Prophylactic, Internal) 1:2,000 dilution **(Cutter)**

Supply: Bottles 100 cc, for complete treatment.

Dosage: PROPHYLACTIC—4–20 drops in water after meals, till bottle is finished. THERAPEUTIC—½–1 oz. in water, after breakfast, on alternate days.

Poison Oak-Ivy Treatments **(Hollister-Stier)**

Supply: PROPHYLACTIC—5 graduated doses, 1 treatment. Seasonal—5 equal doses, 1 treatment. Seasonal, Concentrated—5 equal double strength doses.

Poison Oak Extract (In Almond Oil) (C.A.) **(Lederle)**

Supply: Packages of one or four 1 cc syringes.

Dosage: Therapeutic 1 cc *intramuscularly;* second or third dose at 24 hr. intervals if necessary.

Ivyol—Poison Oak Extract (A solution in olive oil) (C.A.) **(Mulford)**

Supply: Packages of 4 hypo-units, each 1 dose.

Dosage: *Intramuscularly,* 1 hypo-unit daily for 4 doses; in susceptible individuals to begin with ¼–½ unit.

Rhus Toxicodendron Antigen (40% Alcoholic Solution with 0.4% Procaine) **(National Drug)**

Supply: Packages of four 1 cc ampules; Ampule-vials 1 cc for 10 diagnostic skin tests; Tincture in vials of 1 oz.

Dosage: As above.

Poison Oak Extract (Rhus Diversiloba) **(Squibb)**

Supply: Preseasonal—Vials 3 cc; Seasonal—Vials 0.3 cc with two 1 cc vials of physiologic saline.

Dosage: Preseasonal—10 subcutaneous injections of gradually increased dosage at weekly intervals for 5 injections, then at 2 or 3 week intervals. Seasonal—2–5 injections.

PNEUMONIA BIOTHERAPY

Description: Most of the Antipneumococcus Sera are highly refined and superconcentrated products, containing all the specific antibacterial and antitoxic substances, bacteriotropins, opsonins, agglutinins and antibodies, effective in the treatment of pneumococcus infections. They are prepared from the serum of horses injected with gradually increasing doses of live Pneumococci, of either type I, or I and II, or all types, resulting in monovalent, bivalent and polyvalent sera. *Used* in specific therapy of lobar pneumonia; cause few complications and but seldom reactions.

Administration: *Antipneumococcic Sera* must be given early, during the first 3 days of the disease, *intravenously,* slowly and at body temperature, 100,000 to 200,000 units in 24 hr.; in intramuscular injections—larger doses are demanded; in early bacteremia—double dosage should be given. Before administering sera, the sensitization test for susceptibility should be made, and if positive the serum should be administered in small doses, every half hour until sensitization is overcome; in severe anaphylactic reactions adrenalin, 1 cc, is given.

Pneumococcus Vaccines are recommended for immunization and for treatment of other pneumococcus infections, as chronic rhinitis, sinusitis and unresolved pneumonia; they are prepared in the usual manner from actively growing cultures of Pneumococci, types I, II, III or all four types and administered in accordance with the individual preparations available.

Bibliography: *See Chap. XII.*

1. ANTIPNEUMOCOCCIC SERA

Antipneumococcic Serum (Types I and II) (C.A.) **(Gilliland)**
Contains high antibody content for both types.

Supply: Packages containing one 50 cc vial with gravity injecting outfit; Vials 50 cc, 100 cc.

Dosage: Initial 50 cc *intravenously,* repeated in accordance with results obtained.

Antipneumococcic Serum (Type I) (Refined and Concentrated) (C.A.) **(Lederle)**
Contains high antibody content for Type I.

Supply: Packages containing syringes of 10,000 or 20,000 units.

Dosage: 40,000–50,000 units in moderate cases, 80,000–100,000 units in severe or toxic cases, *intravenously* within first 24 hr.

Antipneumococcic Serum (Type II) (Refined and Concentrated) (C.A.) **(Lederle)**
Contains high antibody content for Type II.

Supply: Packages containing syringes of 10,000 or 20,000 units.

Dosage: 40,000–50,000 units in moderate cases, 80,000–100,000 units in severe or toxic cases, *intravenously* within first 24 hr.

Antipneumococcic Serum (Type I and II) (C.A.) (Refined and Concentrated) Bivalent. **(Lederle)**
Contains high antibody content for Types I and II.

Supply: Packages containing syringes of 10,000 or 20,000 units.

Dosage: 40,000–50,000 units in moderate cases, 80,000–100,000 units in severe or toxic cases, *intravenously* within first 24 hr.

Antipneumococcic Serum (Type VII) (Refined and Concentrated) **(Lederle)**
Contains high antibody content for Type VII.

Supply: Packages containing syringes of 10,000 or 20,000 units.

Dosage: 40,000–50,000 units in moderate cases, 80,000–100,000 units in severe or toxic cases, *intravenously* within first 24 hr.

Antipneumococcic Serum (Type I) (C.A.) **(Mulford)**

Supply: Packages of one double-end 50 cc vial with intravenous injection outfit.

Dosage: As above.

Antipneumococcic Serum (Types I and II Combined) **(Mulford)**

Supply: Packages of one double-end 50 cc vial with intravenous injection outfit.

Dosage: As above.

Pneumococcus Antibody Globulin (Type I) (C.A.) (Felton, Concentrated) **(Mulford)**

Supply: Syringes of 10 cc containing 10,000 units, or 20 cc containing 20,000 units.

Dosage: Initial—10,000 units; 1 hr. later 20,000 units, repeated every 4–8 hr. until temperature drops.

Pneumococcus Antibody Solution (Types I and II Combined) **(Mulford)**
Contains specific antibodies and free from proteins.

Supply: Packages of one or four 50 cc double end vials with injection outfit.

Antipneumococcic Sera (Refined and Extra Concentrated) **(National Drug)**
Contains per cc 700 Felton antibody units.

Supply: Syringe 10 cc—Type I (monovalent) (C.A.); Syringe 10 cc—Types I and II (bivalent); Syringe 10 cc—Types I, II and III (polyvalent).

Dosage: 10–20 cc repeated every 6–8 hr. as necessary.

Antipneumococcic Serum (Felton, Highly Refined and Concentrated) (C.A.) **(Parke, Davis)**

Supply: Syringes—10,000 units Type I; Syringes—20,000 units Type I; Syringes—10,000 Felton units of each type (I and II); Syringes—20,000 Felton units of each type (I and II).

Dosage: Contents of syringe container repeated in 4 hr. if necessary; in severe cases—adequate dosage, intramuscularly or intravenously.

Antipneumococcic Serum (Types I and II, Concentrated) Felton(C.A.) **(Squibb)**

Supply: Packages of 1 syringe for 1 therapeutic dose, 10,000 units each of Types I, II.

Dosage: 10–20 therapeutic doses repeated in 24 hr. or oftener in severe cases, given *intravenously;* if given intramuscularly, double dosage.

2. PNEUMOCOCCUS VACCINES

Pneumococcic Vaccine **(Gilliland)**

Contains per cc	1	2	3	4	5
Pneumococci I, II, III	250	500	1,000	2,000	5,000

Supply: Packages of four 1 cc vials of strengths 1, 2, 3, 4; Vials 5 cc, 10 cc of strength 5.

Dosage: Immunization—250, 500, 1,000, 2,000 million bacteria at 5–7 day intervals increased if necessary.
Therapeutic—50–250 million *intravenously* every 24–48 hr.

Pneumococcus Vaccine (Polyvalent, Prophylactic) **(Lederle)**

Contains per cc	1	2	3
Pneumococcus Type I	1,500	3,000	3,000 million
Pneumococcus Type II	1,500	3,000	3,000 million
Pneumococcus Type III	1,500	3,000	3,000 million

Supply: Packages of 3 vials for 1 immunization; Vials 5 cc, 20 cc of strength 3, for 2 and 8 immunizations.

Dosage: 3 injections—strengths 1, 2 and 3, at 7 day intervals.

Pneumococcus Antigen **(Lilly)**
Contains per cc
Pneumococcus I, II, III, IV .... 20,000 million

Supply: Vials 5 cc.

Dosage: Therapeutic—1 cc *subcutaneously* at 24 hr. intervals; in severe cases at 4–8 hr. intervals; children—0.25 cc increased with age.

Pneumococcus Vaccine, Prophylactic **(Lilly)**
Contains per cc
Pneumococcus I, II, III, IV .... 5,000 million

Supply: Vials 5 cc.

Dosage: Initial 0.5 cc, second and third—1 cc, at 5–7 day intervals.

Pneumococcus Vaccine (Pneumo-Bacterin) **(National Drug)**
Contains per cc
Pneumococcus I, II, III, IV .... 5,000 million

Supply: Ampule-vials 5 cc, 15 cc, 30 cc.

Dosage: PROPHYLACTIC—½ cc, 1 cc, 1 cc at 5–7 day intervals.
THERAPEUTIC—Initial ¼ cc followed by ½–1 cc at 8–12 hr. intervals as long as temperature is above 101°; subsequent dosage at 24 hr. intervals.

Pneumococcus Immunogen **(Parke, Davis)**
An extract of diplococcus pneumoniae types I, II and III.

Supply: Vials 10 cc, rubber-diaphragm-capped.

Dosage: Initial 0.5 cc *intramuscularly* or 0.1–0.2 cc *subcutaneously*, gradually increased, avoiding severe reaction; daily or on alternate days; maximum dosage 2 cc or possibly 5 cc.

Pneumococcus Vaccine (Bacterial Vaccine) **(Squibb)**

Contains per cc	1	2	3	4
Pneumococcus	750	1,500	2,250	3,000 million

Supply: Packages of 4 ampules and syringes of strengths 1, 2, 3, 4; Vials 5 cc, 20 cc of strength 4.

Dosage: 750–3,000 million bacteria at 3–5 day intervals; larger doses in chronic cases.

Pneumococcus Vaccine **(Upjohn)**
Contains per cc
Pneumococcus I, II, III, IV.......... 1,000 million (250 million each)

Supply: Packages of six 1 cc ampules.

Dosage: Initial 1 cc.

3. PNEUMOCOCCUS COMBINED VACCINES

Pneumonia Bacterin **(Abbott)**

Contains per cc	
Pneumococcus Type I	2,000 million
Pneumococcus Type II	2,000 million
Pneumococcus Type III	2,000 million
Pneumococcus Group IV	2,000 million
Strept. hemolyticus	1,000 million
Strept. viridans	1,000 million

Supply: Bulk packages 5 cc, 20 cc.

Dosage: PROPHYLACTIC—initial 0.5 cc, then 2 doses of 1 cc each at 7–10 day intervals.
THERAPEUTIC—1 cc every 6–12 hr. during temperature of 101°; subsequently at 24 hr. intervals

Pneumococcus Combined Vaccine (Polyvalent) **(Lederle)**

Contains per cc	
Pneumococcus Types I, II, III	400 million
Strep. hemolyticus and viridans	200 million
Staph. albus and aureus	400 million

Supply: Vials 5 cc (dilution 4).

Dosage: ⅛, ¼, ½, 1 cc at intervals of 3–5 days.

Pneumo-Strep-Bacterin (Pneumococcic and Streptococcic Vaccine, Mixed) **(Mulford)**

Contains per cc	A	B	C	D
Pneumococcus Types I, II, III	50	100	200	400 million
Strept. hemolyticus, non-hemolyticus, viridans	100	200	400	800 million

Supply: Packages of 4 syringes of A, B, C, D strengths; Vials 5 cc of D strength.

Dosage: Initial one-fifth to full contents of syringe A.

Pneumo-Bacterin Mixed (Pneumococcic Vaccine Mixed) **(Mulford)**

Contains per cc

	A	B	C	D
Pneumococcus I, II, III	50	100	200	400 million
Strep. hemolyticus, non-hemolyticus, viridans	25	50	100	200 million
Staph. aureus	25	50	100	200 million
Staph. albus	25	50	100	200 million

Supply: Packages of 4 syringes of strengths A, B, C, D; Vials 5 cc of D strength.

Dosage: Initial—10–50 million bacteria.

Pneumo-Serobacterin Mixed (Pneumococcic Vaccine Mixed, Sensitized) **(Mulford)**

Contains per cc

	A	B	C	D
Pneumococcus I, II, III	250	500	1,000	2,000 million
Strep. hemolyticus, non-hemolyticus, viridans	250	500	1,000	2,000 million
Staph. aureus	250	500	1,000	2,000 million
Staph. albus	250	500	1,000	2,000 million

Supply: Packages of 4 syringes of strengths A, B, C, D; Vials 5 cc of strength D.

Dosage: Initial contents of syringe A.

Pneumococcus Combined Vaccine (Pneumo-Bacterin Mixed) **(National Drug)**

Contains per cc

Pneumococcus I, II, III, IV	2,000 million
Strep. hemolyticus, viridans	1,000 million
Bac. influenzae	1,000 million

Supply: Ampule-vials 5 cc, 15 cc, 30 cc.

Dosage: PROPHYLACTIC—¼, ½, 1 cc at 2–4 day intervals.
THERAPEUTIC—¼–½ cc increased by ¼–½ cc at 8–12 hr. intervals till temperature is reduced to 101°, then 1 cc daily.

Pneumonia Vaccine (Combined) **(Parke, Davis)**

Contains per cc

Pneumococcus I, II, III, IV	2,000 million
Bac. Friedlander	500 million
Strep. hemolyticus, non-hemolyticus	500 million

Supply: Vials 5 cc.

Dosage: THERAPEUTIC—initial 0.25–0.5 cc, increased by 0.25–0.5 cc up to 1 cc at 2–3 day intervals.

Pneumococcus Immunogen Combined **(Parke, Davis)**

An extract of diplococcus pneumoniae types I, II and III, and strep. hemolyticus and non-hemolyticus.

Supply: Vials 10 cc, rubber-diaphragm-capped.

Dosage: Initial 0.5 cc *intramuscularly* or 0.1–0.2 cc *subcutaneously;* gradually increased, avoiding severe reaction; daily or on alternate days; maximum dosage 2 cc or possibly 5 cc.

Pneumonia Phylacogen **(Parke, Davis)**

Culture filtrates of pneumococcus types I, II, III, IV (75%), and streptococci.

Supply: Vials 10 cc, rubber-diaphragm-capped.

Dosage: SUBCUTANEOUSLY—1 cc, increasing gradually to 10 cc; daily injections.
INTRAVENOUSLY—initial 2–4 m, increasing gradually to 5 cc; daily injections.

Pneumonia Vaccine **(Sherman)**

Contains per cc

Pneumococcus	100 million
Bac. influenzae	200 million
Streptococcus	100 million

Mic. catarrhalis	200 million
Staphylococcus	400 million

Supply: Bottles 5 cc, 12½ cc.

Dosage: 1–1½ cc every 6 hr. till temperature is 99°; continued with 1 cc at 12 hr. intervals, then at 24 hr. intervals.

Pneumococcus-Streptococcus Vaccine (Squibb)

Contains per cc	1	2	3	4
Pneumococcus	750	1,500	2,250	3,000 million
Streptococcus	250	500	750	1,000 million

Supply: Packages of 4 ampules of strengths 1, 2, 3, 4—Vials 5 cc, 20 cc of strength 4.

Dosage: THERAPEUTIC—0.3 cc increased.

POLIOMYELITIS SEROTHERAPY

Description: The sera available against poliomyelitis are concentrated antitoxins prepared from the blood of horses immunized in accordance with the Rosenow method with cultures of Pleomorphic Streptococci, believed to represent the globoid bodies and organisms of Flexner, the etiological factor of poliomyelitis; contain specific antibodies and are of considerable value in this disease.

Administration: Is administered *intramuscularly,* about 5 cc of serum for every 5 yr. of age of the child, every 12, 18 or 24 hr. in accordance with symptomatology and severity of epidemic.

PREPARATIONS

Antistreptococcic Serum Poliomyelitis (Concentrated Globulin) (Lilly)

Supply: Vials 20 cc.

Dosage: 5 cc for each 5 yr. of age, repeated in 12, 18 and 24 hr., *intramuscularly.*

Antistreptococcic Serum (Poliomyelitis, Rosenow) (Mulford)

Supply: Ampule-vials 20 cc.

Dosage: As above.

PUERPERAL FEVER SEROTHERAPY

Description: Antitoxic and antibacterial sera for the treatment of puerperal infections are prepared from the blood of horses, hyperimmunized to toxins and virulent cultures of a Streptococcus, isolated in pure culture from blood of sufferers from typical, severe, puerperal septicemia.

Administration: In prophylaxis or treatment, is administered in 10–20 cc dosage, as frequently as conditions demand.

PREPARATIONS

Antistreptococcic Serum (Concentrated, Globulin) (Lilly)

Supply: Syringes 20 cc.

Puerperal Septicemia Antistreptococcic Serum (Parke, Davis)

Supply: Syringes 10 cc with sterile needle.

Dosage: 10–20 cc.

PYORRHEA VACCINOTHERAPY

Description: Vaccines for use in pyorrhea alveolaris, in conjunction with topical, physical and surgical therapy, are prepared from the various organisms found to be the infective agents in this disease, principally the Streptococcus Hemolyticus, Non-hemolyticus and Viridans, but often also the Staphylococcus, Pneumococcus and Diphtheroids.

Administration: Several injections are given in strengths and at intervals as indicated in each preparation.

PREPARATIONS

Pyorrhea Serobacterin Mixed (Pyorrhea Vaccine Mixed, Sensitized) **(Mulford)**

Contains per cc	A	B	C	D
Strep. hemolyticus, non-hemolyticus, viridans	25	50	100	200 million
Staph. aureus	100	200	400	800 million
Staph. albus	100	200	400	800 million
Pneumococcus I, II, III	25	50	100	200 million
Mic. catarrhalis	25	50	100	200 million
Bac. influenzae	50	100	200	400 million
Bac. diphtheroid	50	100	200	400 million

Supply: Packages of 4 syringes—strengths A, B, C, D; Vials 5 cc—strength D.

Dosage: Initial—contents of syringe A; then continued in accordance with reactions.

RABIES VACCINOTHERAPY

Description: A sterile suspension of the brain and cord substance of rabbits inoculated with fixed rabies virus; is made non-virulent for humans by special treatment to decrease still further its infectivity and destroy its toxicity. The various methods employed, as drying (Pasteur), phenolizing (Semple), drying at freezing temperature (Harris), and dialization (Cummings) do not impair the antigenic or protective value of the vaccines. Are used to produce active immunity against rabies in those bitten by animals, suspected or proved to be rabid. As the incubation period of rabies is rather prolonged, it affords ample time for treatment either by the Semple method of 14 days' duration, or the Pasteur, 21 day method, if instituted immediately after injury is sustained.

Administration: Daily injections, *subcutaneously*, in interscapular region or anterior abdominal wall, late in the afternoons, 14 doses of the Semple strength or 21 doses of Pasteur preparations. In slight wounds of extremities, 14 injections may suffice; in extensive wounds, or those about the head, neck and shoulders, 21 treatments are more desirable.

Bibliography: *See Chap. XII.*

PREPARATIONS

Rabies Vaccine (Semple) (C.A.) **(Cutter)**
Contains 5% of brain emulsion, phenol killed.

Supply: Packages of seven 25 cc syringes for 7 doses; Two 7-syringe packages for 14 doses; Three 7-syringe packages for 21 doses.

Dosage: 14 or 21 doses depending upon severity and location of bites; 1–2 doses daily, *subcutaneously.*

Rabies Vaccine (C.A.) **(Gilliland)**

Supply: Packages of 14 doses of phenolized rabies vaccine in individual syringes with sterile needles.

Dosage: 14 doses at approximately 24 hr. intervals (Semple method); 21 doses for administration in 3 injections (Pasteur method).

Pasteur Antirabic Vaccine (C.A.) **(Gilliland)**

Supply: Dried cord, emulsified in 0.6 cc of 60% glycerin containing 0.3% tricresol—for 21 doses.

Dosage: 21 daily administrations of supplied cord sections, diluted with physiologic saline in syringes; administered in serial order.

Rabies Vaccine (Semple Method) (C.A.) **(Hixon)**

Supply: Packages of 14 doses in aseptic syringes with sterile needles for 1 complete treatment; Packages of 14 doses in individual vials with glass syringe needles for 1 complete treatment; Packages of 7 vials without syringe.

Dosage: 14 injections at 1 day intervals.

Rabies Vaccine (Semple) (C.A.) **(Jensen-Salsbery)**

Contains brain substance 2%; phenol 0.5%.

Supply: Packages of 14 vials or syringes; Packages of 21 vials or syringes.

Dosage: Vials 1 and 2 given 4–6 hr. apart, first day; then 1 vial daily; light injuries—14 doses; severe injuries—21 doses; given *subcutaneously* or *intramuscularly*.

Rabies Vaccine (Semple Method) (C.A.) **(Lederle)**

Supply: Packages of fourteen 2 cc syringes of phenolized rabies virus; a 4% saline solution of fixed virus.

Dosage: 14 injections at 1 day intervals.

Rabies Vaccine (C.A.) **(Lilly)**

Prepared by Harris modification of the Pasteur method.

Supply: Packages of fourteen 1 cc syringes, serially numbered.

Dosage: Daily *subcutaneous* injections.

Antirabic Vaccine (C.A.) **(Medical Arts)**

Contains a sterile suspension in distilled water of the brain and cord substance of rabbits injected with fixed rabies virus (Semple).

Supply: Packages of 14 ampules for 1 course.

Dosage: 2 cc for 14 daily, in the late afternoon, given *subcutaneously*.

Rabies Vaccine (C.A.) **(Mulford)**

Supply: Packages of 14 syringes of equal strength, for 1 complete treatment.

Dosage: Daily injections.

Rabies Vaccine—Human (Semple Method) (C.A.) **(National Drug)**

Contains phenolized virus of brain, medulla and spinal cord.

Supply: Packages of four 2 cc ampules for first 4 doses; Packages of ten 2 cc ampules for next 10 doses; Packages of fourteen 2 cc ampule-vials for complete immunization.

Dosage: Daily injections.

Rabies Vaccine (Harris) (C.A.) **(National Pathological)**

Supply: Packages of 10 tubes of vaccine and 10 vials of normal saline.

Dosage: 1 dose daily for 10 days.

Rabies Vaccine (Cumming) (C.A.) **(Parke, Davis)**

Supply: Packages of fourteen or twenty-one 2 cc syringes for complete treatments

Dosage: Daily injections; children under 4—1 cc.

Antirabic Virus (Semple) (C.A.) **(Pasteur Institute)**

Supply: Packages of fourteen 2 cc ampules.

Dosage: 1 ampule daily.

Pasteur Rabies Vaccine **(Squibb)**

Supply: Packages of 21 numbered syringes and ampules for 1 complete treatment.

Dosage: First 2 days—2 doses daily, then 1 dose daily.

Rabies Vaccine Semple (C.A.) **(Squibb)**

Supply: Packages of 14 doses in ampules for complete immunizing treatment.

Dosage: 1 syringe daily; children under 2 years—half dosage.

Rabies Vaccine (Phenolized) (C.A.) **(Terrell)**

Supply: Packages of fourteen 3 cc vials; Packages of twenty-one 3 cc vials.

Dosage: Daily injections.

Rabies Vaccine (Semple) (C.A.) **(U. S. Standard Products)**

Supply: Packages of fourteen 2 cc syringes; of 7 and 21 vials.

Dosage: 1 syringe daily.

SCARLET FEVER BIOTHERAPY

1. DIAGNOSTIC

Dick Test: For the diagnosis of susceptibility to scarlet fever the Dick Test is used; $\frac{1}{10}$ cc of the diluted toxin is introduced *intradermally* on the anterior surface of the arm after proper antiseptic cleansing. Observation is made after 18–24 hr.: positive reaction indicating the absence of immunity against scarlet fever is shown by the appearance of an area of redness, 1 cm wide, remaining for about 4 days. Non-specific serum reactions must not be confused with positive specific reactions. Children between the ages of 6 mo. and 6 yr., not being susceptible to scarlet fever, need not be tested by the Dick Test; older children and adults should be tested before being immunized.

Schultz-Carlton Test: Is used to establish the diagnosis of scarlet fever in doubtful scarlatiniform rashes. 0.1–0.2 cc of antitoxin injected *intradermally* will produce in a true scarlet fever case, by neutralization of tissue toxin with injected antitoxin, a blanching at the site of injection. Observation is made in 14–20 hours, in bright daylight and at a distance.

Bibliography: *See Chap. XII.*

DIAGNOSTIC PREPARATIONS

Scarlet Fever Streptococcus Toxin (For the *Dick* Test) **(Gilliland)**

Supply: Vial packages for 10 tests or 100 tests.

Scarlet Fever Streptococcus Toxin (C.A.) (For the *Dick* Test) **(Parke, Davis)**

Supply: Vials 1 cc of diluted toxin for 10 tests.

Scarlet Fever Streptococcus Toxin (For the *Dick* Test) **(Mulford)**

Supply: Packages of 1 cc vial of diluted toxin for 10 tests.

Scarlet Fever Streptococcus Antitoxin (For the *Schultz-Carlton* Reaction) **(National Drug)**

Supply: Ampules 1 cc for 5 tests.

Dosage: 0.1–0.2 cc *intradermally.*

Scarlet Fever Streptococcus Toxin (C.A.) (For the *Dick* Test) **(National Drug)**

Supply: Ampules 1 cc for 10 tests.

Dosage: 0.1 cc *intradermally.*

Scarlet Fever Streptococcus Antitoxin (For the *Schultz-Carlton* Test) **(Squibb)**

Supply: Vials 1 cc for 10 blanching tests.

Dosage: 0.1–0.2 cc *intradermally.*

Scarlet Fever Streptococcus Toxin (C.A.) (For the *Dick* Test) **(Squibb)**
Supply: Packages—Vials for 10 tests or 100 tests.
Dosage: 0.1 cc *intradermally.*

---

2. IMMUNIZATION

For immunization against scarlatinal infection, several *subcutaneous* injections of increasing strengths as measured in neutralizing units are given about every 5–7 days; usually 5 doses suffice. Two weeks after the last injection the Dick Test is repeated; if not completely negative, a sixth dose, of the higher concentration, is injected. Where antitoxic serum is used for immunization, 2,000 units are generally employed.

IMMUNIZATION PREPARATIONS

Scarlet Fever Streptococcus Toxin (For Prophylactic Immunization) **(Mulford)**

Contains per cc	1	2	3	4	5
Skin test doses	500	2,000	8,000	25,000	80,000–100,000

Supply: Packages of 5 ampule-vials of above strengths for 1 complete treatment; Packages of six 10 cc vials—1 each of strengths 1, 2, 3, 4, and 2 of strength 5.
Dosage: Four 1 cc doses and one 2 cc dose, at 5–7 day intervals.

Scarlet Fever Streptococcus Toxin (C.A.) **(National Drug)**

Contains per cc	1	2	3	4	5
Skin test doses	500	2,000	8,000	25,000	80,000

Supply: Packages of five 5 cc ampule-vials—strengths 1, 2, 3, 4, 5 for 1 immunization; Packages of fifty 5 cc ampule-vials—for 10 immunizations; Ampule-vials 100,000 skin test doses for sixth dose testing.

Scarlet Fever Streptococcus Toxin (C.A.) (For Immunization) **(Parke, Davis)**
Supply: Packages of 5 vials containing 500, 200, 800, 2,500, 80,000 skin tests—for individual immunization courses; Packages of six 10 cc rubber diaphragm-capped vials, numbered—500, 2,000, 8,000, 25,000, 40,000, 40,000 million—for 10 immunization courses.
Dosage: IMMUNIZATION—Injections at 5–7 day intervals, of graded dilutions.

Scarlet Fever Vaccine **(Sherman)**
Contains per cc

Streptococcus	100 million
Pneumococcus	100 million
Staphylococcus	400 million

Supply: Vials 5 cc, 12½ cc.
Dosage: 1 cc every 12 hr., until fever abates; continued 1 cc at 24–48 hr. intervals.

Scarlet Fever Streptococcus Toxin (C.A.) **(Squibb)**
(For Active Immunization)
Supply: Packages of five ampules for 1 complete immunization—500, 2,000, 8,000, 25,000, 80,000 skin test doses; Packages of six 10 cc vials for 10 complete immunizations.
Dosage: 5 injections of above strengths at 5–7 day intervals. Children under 1 yr.—half dosage.

---

3. THERAPEUTIC

Description: For treatment of scarlet fever, antitoxins are used; these are refined and concentrated sera prepared from the blood of horses inoculated with gradually increasing doses of the toxins of Streptococcus Hemolyticus Scarlatinae. The effect of antitoxin is antigenic, exciting the development of antibodies and neutralizing toxins circulating in the system, establishing immunity.

Administration: Is administered in dosages as indicated with each preparation. *intramuscularly* or *intravenously;* the former, though slower in action, has the advantage of being free from the disagreeable by-effects of serum rashes at times attending intravenous injections. The serum is administered usually in 1 day, at most in 2 days, relief being obtained usually within 24 hr. after injection.

ANTITOXIN PREPARATIONS

Scarlet Fever Streptococcus Antitoxin (Refined and Concentrated) **(Gilliland)** (C.A.)

Supply: Syringe packages for prophylactic or therapeutic doses.

Scarlet Fever Streptococcus Antitoxin (Concentrated) (C.A.) **(Mulford)**

Supply: Packages of 1 or 2 syringes containing 6,000 units, sufficient to neutralize at least 300,000 skin test doses (therapeutic)—Packages of 1 syringe of 2,000 units, sufficient to neutralize 100,000 skin tests (prophylactic).

Scarlet Fever Streptococcus Antitoxin (Refined and Concentrated) **(National Drug)** (C.A.)

Supply: Perfected serum syringe with adaptor-needle containing 6,000 U. S. Standard Units or 300,000 neutralizing units.

Scarlet Fever Streptococcus Antitoxin (C.A.) (Parke, Davis)

Supply: Therapeutic dose syringe containing 6,000 units, with sterile needle; Prophylactic dose syringe containing 2,000 units, with sterile needle; Bulbs 1 cc (3 tests), for Schultz-Charlton test.

Scarlet Fever Antitoxin (C.A.) N.I.H. **(Squibb)**

Supply: Therapeutic Dose—one 10 cc syringe containing 6,000 units.
Prophylactic Dose—1 syringe containing 2,000 units; Vial, 1 cc, Diagnostic Blanching test (10 tests).

Dosage: In severe cases and in Puerperal Scarlet Fever—2 therapeutic doses, or 12,000 units, repeated in 18–24 hr., as indicated. Mild and moderate cases—1 therapeutic dose (6,000 neutralizing units). Prophylaxis—2,000 neutralizing units. Diagnostic—in doubtful rashes, 0.2 cc intradermally where rash is brightest.

SMALLPOX VACCINOTHERAPY

Description: Smallpox vaccine is a glycerin-water suspension of killed virus, for immunization against smallpox; is used for the production of immunity against the disease through development of antibodies.

Administration: After thorough cleansing of outer surface of the arm below deltoid insertion, or of inner surface of the leg below the knee, where such vaccination is desired, vaccine virus is applied by the *scratch method* or *multiple puncture method* and lightly rubbed in. After 4 days a papule with zone of redness appears; after 6 days—a vesicle and umbilicated area which enlarges to the eighth day; then it dries completely and forms a scab at about the fourteenth day.

Bibliography: *See Chap. XII.*

PREPARATIONS

Smallpox Vaccine (Vaccine Virus) **(Cutter)**

Supply: Cases of 1, 5 or 10 capillary tubes of glycerinated virus—each tube for individual vaccination.

Vaccine Virus (Smallpox Vaccine) (C.A.) **(Gilliland)**

Supply: Packages of 1, 2, 5 or 10 capillary tubes—each tube for individual vaccination by multiple puncture method.

Vaccine Virus (Smallpox Vaccine) **(Lederle)**

Supply: Packages of 1, 5 or 10 capillary tubes for 1, 5 and 10 vaccinations.

Vaccine Virus (Green) **(Lederle)**

Cured with brilliant green.
Supply: Packages of 1, 5 or 10 capillary tubes for 1, 5 and 10 vaccinations.

Smallpox Vaccine Virus (C.A.) **(Lilly)**

Supply: Packages of 1 or 5 capillary tubes with scarifiers, for 1 and 5 vaccinations.

Smallpox Vaccine **(Mulford)**

Supply: Packages of 10 capillary tubes with 10 glass encased needles and 1 bulb, for 10 vaccinations; Packages of 1 or 10 improved tube points and 1 bulb, for use especially in the multiple pressure method—for 1 or 10 vaccinations.

Vaccine Virus **(National Drug)**

Supply: Packages of 1, 5 or 10 capillary tubes with sterile needles and bulbs, for 1, 5 and 10 vaccinations.

Smallpox Vaccine **(Parke, Davis)**

Supply: Packages of 1 or 5 capillary glass tubes, for 1 and 5 vaccinations.

Smallpox Vaccine (C.A.) **(Squibb)**

Supply: Packages of 1, 5 or 10 capillary glass tubes with bulbs and needles, for 1, 5 and 10 vaccinations.

STAPHYLOCOCCUS VACCINOTHERAPY

Description: Staphylococcus Vaccines are available in various strains of Staphylococcus Pyogenes Aureus, or of Aureus and Albus combined, or of these with Citreus; in strengths from 250 million to 2,000 million per cc. Are used for the production of immunity in minor staphylococcus infections, as furunculosis, carbunculosis, stye, sycosis, impetigo contagiosa; also in those susceptible to infection, and to prevent relapse.

Administration: In accordance with strength of vaccine, beginning with 0.1–0.2 cc *subcutaneously*, every 2–3 days, gradually increased, avoiding undue reaction; continued for several weeks.

PREPARATIONS

Staphylococcus Vaccine (Staphylococcic Bacterin) (C.A.) **(Cutter)**

Contains per cc
Staph. albus and aureus .... 2,000 million

Supply: Bottles of 5 cc.

Dosage: Initial 0.05 cc, *subcutaneously* or *intracutaneously*, increasing every 5–7 days, till 1 cc is reached.

Staphylococcic Vaccine (C.A.) **(Gilliland)**

Contains per cc	1	2	3	4
Staph. albus and aureus	250	500	1,000	2,000 million

Supply: Packages of four 1 cc vials of strengths 1, 2, 3, 4; Vials 5 cc, 10 cc of strength 4.

Dosage: Initial 50–250 million bacteria increased at 2–5 day intervals.

Staphylococcic Vaccine (C.A.) **(Hollister-Stier)**
Contains per cc
Staph. albus.......... 500 million
Staph. aureus.......... 500 million

Supply: Bottles 5 cc, 20 cc.

Dosage: Initial 0.1 cc.

Staphylococcus Vaccine (Polyvalent) (C.A.) **(Lederle)**
Staph. albus.......... 800 million
Staph. aureus.......... 800 million
Staph. citreus.......... 400 million

Supply: Vials 5 cc (Dilution 4).

Dosage: 1/8, 1/4, 1/2, 1 cc at intervals of 3–5 days.

Staphylococcus Albus Vaccine (C.A.) **(Lederle)**
Contains per cc
Staph. albus.......... 2,000 million

Supply: Vials 5 cc, 20 cc.

Dosage: Initial—0.05 cc.

Staphylococcus Aureus Vaccine (C.A.) (Furunculosis Vaccine, Polyvalent) **(Lederle)**
Contains per cc
Staph. aureus.......... 2,000 million

Supply: Vials 5 cc.

Dosage: 1/8, 1/4, 1/2, 1 cc at intervals of 3–5 days.

Staphylococcus Vaccine (Staphylococcus Combined) (C.A.) **(Lilly)**
Contains per cc
Staph. aureus.......... 2,000 million
Staph. albus.......... 2,000 million

Supply: Bottles of 5 cc, 20 cc.

Dosage: Initial 2–4 m.

Staphylococcus Aureus Vaccine (Staphylo-Aureus) (C.A.) **(Lilly)**
Contains per cc
Staph. aureus.......... 2,000 million

Supply: Vials 5 cc, 20 cc.

Dosage: Initial 2–4 m.

Staphylo-Serobacterin (Staphylococcic Vaccine, Sensitized) (C.A.) **(Mulford)**

Contains per cc	A	B	C	D
Staph. aureus..........	250	500	1,000	2,000
Staph. albus..........	250	500	1,000	2,000

Supply: Packages of 4 syringes of strengths A, B, C, D; Vials 5 cc of strength D.

Dosage: Initial—contents of syringe A.

Staphylococcus Vaccine (Staphylo-Bacterin) (C.A.) **(National Drug)**
Contains per cc
Staph. aureus.......... 1,000 million
Staph. albus.......... 1,000 million

Supply: Ampule-vials 5 cc, 15 cc, 30 cc.

Dosage: Initial—1/8–1/4 cc, increased to 1 cc at 2–3 day intervals.

Staphylococcus Vaccine (Combined) (C.A.) **(Parke, Davis)**
Contains per cc
Staph. aureus.......... 1,000 million
Staph. albus.......... 1,000 million

Supply: Packages of four 1 cc bulbs; Vials 5 cc, 20 cc.

Dosage: Initial 0.1–0.2 cc, increased at 3–5 day intervals.

Staphylococcus Immunogen (Parke, Davis)
An extract of staph. albus and aureus.

Supply: Vials 10 cc, rubber-diaphragm-capped.

Dosage: Initial 0.5 cc *intramuscularly* or 0.1–0.2 cc *subcutaneously*, gradually increased, avoiding severe reaction; daily or on alternate days; maximum dosage 2 cc or possibly 5 cc.

Staphylococcus Vaccine (Bacterial Vaccine) (C.A.) (Squibb)

Contains per cc	1	2	3	4
Staph. aureus and albus each	250	500	750	1000

Supply: Packages of 4 ampules of strengths 1, 2, 3, 4; Vials 5 cc, 20 cc of strength 5,000 million per cc.

Dosage: Initial 250 million, increased to 500, 1,000 and more at intervals of 3–5 days; after acute stage has passed, 0.5–1.0 cc weekly for several weeks.

Staphylococcus Mixed Vaccine (Upjohn)
Contains per cc

Staph. albus	1,000 million
Staph. aureus	1,000 million

Supply: Packages of six 1 cc ampules—Vials 5 cc, 20 cc.

Dosage: Initial 0.1–0.2 cc increased at 3–5 day intervals.

STREPTOCOCCUS BIOTHERAPY

1. STREPTOCOCCUS VACCINES

Description: Streptococcus vaccines are prepared from the various strains of Streptococcus Viridans, Streptococcus Hemolyticus and Non-hemolyticus, in concentrations of 500 million to 2,000 million per cc. *Used* for immunization in streptococcus disease, generally subacute or chronic: in tonsillitis, otitis media, mastoiditis, meningitis, rheumatic fever, endocarditis, pleurisy, synovitis, osteomyelitis, empyema.

Administration: Usually 3 or 4 injections, *subcutaneously* and *intravenously*, are given at intervals of 3–5 days, in dosages as specified and in accordance with directions for individual preparations. Some vaccines are recommended also for therapy.

PREPARATIONS

Streptococcus Vaccine (Streptococcus Bacterin) (Cutter)
Contains per cc

Strep. hemolyticus and non-hemolyticus	500 million

Supply: Bottles of 5 cc.

Dosage: 0.2–0.6 cc, increased.

Streptococcic Vaccine (Gilliland)

Contains per cc in proportions:	1	2	3	4
Strep. hemolyticus 50%, non-hemolyticus 10%, viridans 40%	125	250	500	1,000 million

Supply: Packages of four 1 cc vials of strengths 1, 2, 3, 4; Vials 5 cc, 10 cc of strength 4.

Dosage: Initial—50–100 million bacteria, increased at 5–7 day intervals.

Streptococcus Vaccine (Lederle)
Contains per cc

Strep. hemolyticus and viridans	400 million

Supply: Vials 5 cc (dilution 4).

Dosage: ⅛, ¼, ½, 1 cc at 3–5 day intervals.

Streptococcus Vaccine (Lilly)
Contains per cc
Streptococcus.. 500 million

Supply: Vials 5 cc, 20 cc.

Dosage: Initial—2–4 m.

Strepto-Serobacterin (Streptococcic Vaccine, Sensitized) (Mulford)

Contains per cc	A	B	C	D
Streptococcus.....................	250	500	1,000	2,000 million

Supply: Packages of 4 syringes of strengths A, B, C, D; Vials 5 cc of strength D.

Dosage: Initial—contents of syringe A.

Streptococcus Vaccine (Strepto-Bacterin) (National Drug)
Strept. hemolyticus and viridans...................... 2,000 million

Supply: Ampule-vials 5 cc, 15 cc, 30 cc.

Dosage: Initial ⅛–¼ cc, increased to 1 cc at 1–3 day intervals.

Streptococcus Vaccine (Parke, Davis)
Strep. hemolyticus and non-hemolyticus................. 500 million

Supply: Packages of four 1 cc bulbs; Vials 5 cc, 20 cc.

Dosage: 0.1–0.2 cc, gradually increased at 2–3 day intervals.

Streptococcus Immunogen (Parke, Davis)
An extract of strep. hemolyticus and non-hemolyticus.

Supply: Vials 10 cc, rubber-diaphragm-capped.

Dosage: Initial 0.5 cc *intramuscularly* or 0.1–0.2 cc *subcutaneously*, gradually increased, avoiding severe reaction; daily or on alternate days; maximum dosage 2 cc or possibly 5 cc.

Streptococcus Vaccine (Squibb)

Contains per cc	1	2	3	4
Streptococcus......................	250	500	750	1,000 million

Supply: Packages of 4 ampules of strengths 1, 2, 3, 4—Vials 5 cc, and 20 cc of strength 4.

Dosage: THERAPEUTIC—250 million, increased to 1,000 million at 3–5 day intervals.
PROPHYLAXIS—0.5, 1, 1 cc *subcutaneously*, at 3–5 day intervals.

Streptococcus Vaccine (Upjohn)
Contains per cc
Strep. hemolyticus...................................... 250 million
Strep. viridans.. 250 million

Supply: Packages of six 1 cc ampules.

Dosage: 0.5 cc increased.

2. ANTISTREPTOCOCCUS SERA

Description: The sera are most helpful in therapeusis of streptococcus infections; they are prepared from the serum of horses injected with various strains of streptococci; are tested and standardized. *Indicated* in acute streptococcus disease, endocarditis, rheumatism, alveolar abscess, periostitis, osteomyelitis.

Administration: Are most frequently administered *intravenously*, but also used *intramuscularly*, in dosages in accordance with preparation.

PREPARATIONS

Antistreptococcus Serum, Polyvalent (Concentrated) (Cutter)

Supply: Syringe container—10 cc, equivalent to 50 cc of unconcentrated serum.

Dosage: PROPHYLACTIC—2–10 cc.
THERAPEUTIC—10–20 cc or more.

Antistreptococcus Serum, Polyvalent (Unconcentrated) **(Cutter)**

Supply: Bottles 20 cc. Gravity package for intravenous use—50 cc.

Dosage: PROPHYLACTIC—10–50 cc.
THERAPEUTIC—50–100 cc or more.

Antistreptococcic Serum (Gilliland)

Supply: Syringes of 10 cc or 20 cc—Vials 50 cc with gravity injecting outfit.

Dosage: IMMUNIZING—10–20 cc *subcutaneously.*
THERAPEUTIC—Initial 50–100 cc *intravenously,* repeated according to results obtained.

Antistreptococcic Serum (Hemolytic and Viridans Strains) (Lederle)

Supply: Packages of one 10 cc syringe; Packages of one 50 cc syringe with intravenous outfit.

Dosage: PROPHYLACTIC—10–50 cc.
THERAPEUTIC—Initial 200 cc—adults; 50–100 cc—children; repeated at 4–6 hr. intervals where required.

Antistreptococcic Serum **(Lilly)**

Supply: Syringes of 10 or 20 cc.

Dosage: 10–20 cc; severe cases 50–100 cc.

Antistreptococcic Serum Purified (Concentrated) **(Lilly)**
Four to five times potency of Unconcentrated.

Supply: Syringes 10 cc—Vials 10 cc.

Dosage: 3–5 cc; severe cases 10–20 cc.

Antistreptococcic Serum (Polyvalent) **(Mulford)**

Supply: Packages of 1 syringe—20 cc; Packages of 1 double-end vial 50 cc with intravenous injection outfit.

Antistreptococcic Serum (Concentrated) **(Mulford)**
Is refined and concentrated to a high antibody potency.

Supply: Packages of one 10 cc syringe.

Dosage: 10–20 cc *intramuscularly* or *intravenously.*

Antistreptococcic Serum Hemolytic **(Mulford)**

Supply: Packages of 1 double end vial 50 cc with intravenous injection outfit.

Antistreptococcic Serum Viridans **(Mulford)**

Supply: Packages of one double end vial 50 cc with intravenous injection outfit.

Antistreptococcic Serum, (Polyvalent) (National Drug)

Supply: Packages of two 10 cc syringes—Packages of 50 cc or 100 cc intravenous outfits.

Dosage: 50–100 cc *intravenously,* repeated at 6–8 hr. intervals in severe infections.

Antistreptococcic Serum (Polyvalent) (Parke, Davis)

Supply: Packages of one 10 cc syringe or 20 cc syringe with sterile double pointed needle.

Dosage: 10–100 cc subcutaneously, intramuscularly or intravenously.

Antistreptococcic Serum, Concentrated (Polyvalent, Refined and Concentrated) (Parke, Davis)

Supply: Packages of one 10 cc syringe with sterile double pointed needle.

Dosage: 10–20 cc intramuscularly.

Antistreptococcic Serum (Polyvalent) **(Squibb)**

Supply: Packages of one or two 10 cc syringes; Vials 20 cc, 50 cc; Packages of 50 cc gravity container.

Dosage: Subcutaneously—20–100 cc daily, repeated in 8–24 hr.
Intravenously—50–100 cc daily, repeated in 8–24 hr.
Intramuscularly—10–20 cc simultaneously.

MIXED STAPHYLOCOCCUS-STREPTOCOCCUS VACCINOTHERAPY

Description: Vaccines for use in mixed infections are prepared in the usual manner from Staphylococcus Albus et Aureus and various strains of Streptococcus Hemolyticus and Viridans. Are used to stimulate antibody formation and immunity in various pyogenic infections caused by above organisms: sinusitis, conjunctivitis, bacteriocystitis, otitis media, pyorrhea alveolaris, adenitis; also in empyema, pleurisy, chronic appendicitis, cholecystitis, ischiorectal abscess.

Administration: Immunization—*subcutaneously*, every 2–3 days for 10–12 injections, in gradually increasing dosage and in accordance with the individual preparation.

Bibliography: *See Chap. XII.*

PREPARATIONS

Strepto-Pneumo-Staph. Bacterin **(Abbott)**

Contains per cc

Strept. pyogenes	200 million
Pneumococcus	100 million
Staph. aureus	300 million
Staph. albus	300 million

Supply: Bulk packages 6 cc, 20 cc.

Dosage: 3–15 m at 1–3 day intervals.

Staph-Strep Vaccine **(Cutter)**

Contains per cc

Staphylococci	500 million
Streptococci	50 million

Supply: Bottles of 5 cc.

Dosage: Initial 0.1–0.2 cc.

Staphylococcus-Streptococcus Vaccine **(Hollister-Stier)**

Contains per cc

Staph. albus	1,000 million
Staph. aureus	1,000 million
Streptococci	200 million

Supply: Bottles 5 cc, 20 cc.

Dosage: Initial 0.05–0.1 cc.

Staphylococcus Combined Vaccine (Polyvalent) **(Lederle)**
Dilution 4

Contains per cc

Staph. albus, aureus and citreus	800 million
Strept. hemolyticus and viridans	200 million
B. coli	400 million

Supply: Packages of 4 vials, graduated doses; Vials 5 cc, Dilution 4.

Dosage: 1/8, 1/4, 1/2, 1 cc at 3–5 day intervals.

Staphylococcus-Streptococcus Vaccine (Polyvalent) **(Lederle)**
Dilution 4

Contains per cc

Staph. albus and aureus	800 million
Strep. hemolyticus and viridans	200 million

Supply: Packages of 4 vials, graduated doses; Vials 5 cc Dilution 4.

Dosage: ⅛ cc, ¼ cc, ½ cc, 1 cc of Dilution 4 at 3–5 day intervals.

Streptococcus-Staphylococcus Vaccine (Staph-Strep.) (Lilly)

Contains per cc	1	2	3	4
Streptococci	25	50	100	200 million
Staph. aureus	125	250	500	1,000 million
Staph. albus	125	250	500	1,000 million

Supply: Packages of four 1 cc vials of strengths 1, 2, 3, 4; Vials 5 cc, 20 cc of strength 4.

Dosage: Initial—2–4 m of strength 4 or contents of Vial 1.

Staphylo-Strepto-Bacterin Mixed (Staphylo-Streptococcic Vaccine Mixed) **(Mulford)**

Contains per cc	A	B	C	D
Staph. aureus	25	50	100	200 million
Staph. albus	25	50	100	200 million
Strept. hemolyticus, non-hemolyticus, viridans	25	50	100	200 million

Supply: Packages of four syringes of strengths A, B, C, D; Vials 5 cc of strength D.

Dosage: Initial—one-fifth to entire contents of strength A.

Staphylo-Strepto-Serobacterin Mixed (Sensitized Staphylococcic and Streptococcic Vaccine, Mixed) **(Mulford)**

Contains per cc	A	B	C	D
Staph. aureus	125	250	500	1,000 million
Staph. albus	125	250	500	1,000 million
Strep. hemolyticus, non-hemolyticus, viridans	250	500	1,000	2,000 million

Supply: Packages of 4 syringes of strengths A, B, C, D; Vials 5 cc, 20 cc of strength D.

Dosage: Initial—contents of syringe A.

Strepto-Staphylo Combined (Strepto-Staphylo Mixed Bacterin, Polyvalent) **(National Drug)**

Contains per cc	
Strep. hemolyticus and viridans	1,000 million
Staph. albus	500 million
Staph. aureus	500 million

Supply: Ampule-vials 5 cc, 15 cc, 30 cc.

Dosage: Initial, ⅛–¼ cc, increased at 2–4 day intervals until 1 cc is given.

Streptococcus and Staphylococcus Vaccine (Combined) **(Parke, Davis)**

Contains per cc	
Strep. hemolyticus and non-hemolyticus	250 million
Staph. albus	500 million
Staph. aureus	500 million

Supply: Packages of four 1 cc bulbs; Vials 5 cc, 20 cc.

Dosage: 0.1–0.2 cc increased by 0.1 cc to 1 cc at intervals of 3–5 days.

Streptococcus Immunogen Combined **(Parke, Davis)**

An extract of strep. hemolyticus and non-hemolyticus, staph. albus and aureus.

Supply: Vials 10 cc, rubber-diaphragm-capped.

Dosage: Initial 0.5 cc *intramuscularly,* or 0.1–0.2 cc *subcutaneously,* gradually increased, avoiding severe reaction; daily or on alternate days; maximum dosage 2 cc or possibly 5 cc.

Exo-Sepsis Vaccine **(Sherman)**

Contains per cc	
Streptococcus	120 million
Staph. aureus	300 million
Staph. albus	300 million

Supply: Vials 5 cc, 12½ cc.

Dosage: Acute conditions—1 cc every 6–12 hr. until fever abates; continued with 1 cc every 24–48 hr.

Staphylococcus-Streptococcus Vaccine **(Squibb)**

Contains per cc

	1	2	3	4
Staph. albus	250	500	750	1,000 million
Staph. aureus	250	500	750	1,000 million
Streptococcus	250	500	750	1,000 million

Supply: Packages of 4 ampules of strengths 1, 2, 3, 4; Vials 5 cc, 20 cc of strength 4.

Dosage: THERAPEUTIC—0.3 cc, according to reaction; increased every 2–3 days for 10–12 injections.

Staphylococcus Vaccine Combined **(Squibb)**

Contains per cc

	1	2	3	4
Pneumococcus	125	250	375	500 million
Streptococcus	125	250	375	500 million
Staph. albus	125	250	375	500 million
Staph. aureus	125	250	385	500 million

Supply: Packages of 4 ampules—strengths 1, 2, 3, 4; Vials 5 cc, 20 cc—strength 4.

Dosage: THERAPEUTIC—0.3 cc, increased by 0.25 cc, for 6–8 injections, *subcutaneously.*

Streptococcus Mixed Vaccine **(Upjohn)**

Contains per cc

Strep. hemolyticus	100 million
Strep. viridans	100 million
Staph. albus	500 million
Staph. aureus	500 million

Supply: Packages of six 1 cc ampules; Vials 5 cc, 20 cc.

Dosage: 0.1–0.2 cc increased by 0.1–1 cc at intervals of 3–5 days.

TETANUS SEROTHERAPY

Description: Tetanus Antitoxins are highly concentrated and refined globulins obtained from the serum of horses hyperimmunized by injection of toxins of Tetanus Bacillus and accurately standardized. Are effective in neutralizing free toxins circulating in the blood, but not those toxins bound to the central nervous tissue, for which reason their administration soon after the injury is obligatory. *Used* as a specific prophylactic agent in wounds of a nature which are apt to be followed by tetanus infection.

Administration: *Prophylactic*—1,500 or more units, administered *intramuscularly* or *subcutaneously*, once weekly; continued until the wound is healed; is injected slowly and without massaging site of injection.

Therapeutic—given in large dosage, 10–20 thousand units and over, *intravenously;* from 5–10 thousand *intraspinally,* and in some cases about 10 thousand units injected in the vicinity of the wound after its thorough cleansing; injections are given daily for 4 days.

Caution: In those subject to asthma and other anaphylactic disturbances, or suspected of serum sensitivity, 1 or 2 drops of a 1 in 10 saline dilution of the serum is first injected intradermally as a test; in case of reaction—desensitization, if possible with small doses of the serum, gradually increased, should first be accomplished. Adrenalin chloride 1:1,000 may be required to combat urticaria and serum sickness where present.

PREPARATIONS

Tetanus Antitoxin—Human (Concentrated Globulin) (C.A.) **(Cutter)**

Supply: Syringes of 1,500, 5,000, 10,000 or 20,000 units; Vials 1,500 units.

Dosage: Prophylactic—1,500–5,000 units *subcutaneously*, once weekly for 2–3 weeks or until wound heals; children—same dosage.

Therapeutic—35,000–140,000 units, some *intraspinally*, some *intravenously* and some *subcutaneously*.

Tetanus Antitoxin (Concentrated and Refined) (C.A.) **(Gilliland)**

Supply: Syringe packages of 1,500, 5,000, 10,000 or 20,000 units; Vial packages of 1,500, 5,000 or 10,000 units.

Dosage: Immunizing—1,500 units repeated within 3 days.

Therapeutic—10,000 units repeated or increased at 6–8 hr. intervals for as long as necessary; *subcutaneously*, *intramuscularly*, *intravenously* or *intraspinally*.

Tetanus Antitoxin (C.A.) **(Hixson)**

Supply: Syringe packages of 1,500, 5,000, 10,000 or 20,000 units; Sheep Antitoxin—Syringes of 1,500 units; Vial packages upon request.

Dosage: Immunizing—1,500 units.

Therapeutic—5,000–20,000 units every 8 hr. where necessary.

Tetanus Antitoxin (Refined and Concentrated) (C.A.) **(Lederle)**

Supply: Prophylactic—Vials 1,500 units; Syringes 1,500 or 3,000 units; Packages of 10 syringes of 1,500 units each.

Therapeutic—Syringes of 5,000, 10,000 or 20,000 units; Syringes of 10,000 units for intraspinal use.

Dosage: Immunizing—1,500–3,000 units in accordance.

Therapeutic—10,000 units *intraspinally* and 20,000 units *intravenously*, repeated in 8 hr., then every 12–18 hr. until 4 or 5 treatments are given, with 10,000 units *subcutaneously* on fourth or fifth day after last treatment.

Tetanus Antitoxin (Purified, Concentrated) (C.A.) **(Lilly)**

Supply: Vials 1,500 units; Syringes of 1,500, 5,000, 10,000 or 20,000 units.

Dosage: Prophylactic—1,500 units, repeated if necessary once or twice at 5–7 day intervals.

Therapeutic—10,000–20,000 units *intravenously*, and 5,000 units *intraspinally*.

Tetanus Antitoxin (Superconcentrated) (C.A.) **(Mulford)**

Supply: Prophylactic—Vials or syringes of 1,500 units.

Therapeutic—Packages or vials of 5,000 units; Syringes of 10,000 units; Packages of 20,000 units.

Tetanus Antitoxin (Bovine) (C.A.) **(Mulford)**

Supply: Syringes of 1,500 units.

Tetanus Antitoxin (Extra Concentrated and Refined) **(National Drug)**

Supply: Ampule-vials of 1,500, 5,000, 10,000 or 20,000 units; Perfected syringes of 1,500, 5,000, 10,000 or 20,000 units.

Dosage: Immunizing—1,500–5,000 units.

Therapeutic—full dosage 20,000–50,000 units, best *intravenously*, repeated every 6–12 hr.; also *intraspinally*, *intracisternally* and around wound.

Tetanus Antitoxin (Refined and Concentrated) (C.A.) **(Parke, Davis)**

Supply: Bulbs 1,500 units; Syringes 1,500, 5,000, 10,000 or 20,000 units.

Dosage: Prophylactic—1,500 units, repeated in 1 week.

THERAPEUTIC—10,000–20,000 units or more, in vicinity of wound; then 10,000–20,000 units *intraspinally* and *intramuscularly* and *intravenously*—5,000–10,000 units every 6–12 hr., till recovery is assured.

Tetanus Antitoxin (C.A.) (Squibb)

Supply: PROPHYLACTIC—Packages of 1,500 or 3,000 units—vials of 1,500 units.
THERAPEUTIC—Packages of 5,000, 10,000 or 20,000 units.

Dosage: PROPHYLACTIC—1,500–3,000 units, *intramuscularly*.
THERAPEUTIC—10,000–20,000 units *intravenously*, 5,000–10,000 intraspinally, first and second day; then third and fourth day—5,000 *intramuscularly* every 12 hr. to 10,000 units, also *intraspinally*.

TETANUS-GAS GANGRENE SEROTHERAPY

Description: Prepared from serum of horses immunized against the toxins of Bacillus Welchi, Vibrion Septique, Bacillus Edematiens, Bacillus Sordelli and Bacillus Tetanus; neutralizes the toxins of the principle gas-gangrene producing bacterial species and prevents development of tetanus. *Is used* in conditions where gas-gangrene is threatening or probable: in deep, lacerated wounds with extensive tissue destruction, interference of blood supply and particularly where contaminated with soil; in crushed wounds, compound fractures, gunshot injuries.

Administration: *Prophylactic*—1 or more prophylactic doses, repeated at weekly intervals until the wound is healed.
Therapeutic—1 therapeutic dose repeated in 6, 12, 24 hr. and longer intervals, as demanded; administered *intramuscularly*, in some cases *intravenously*.

PREPARATIONS

Polyanaerobic Antitoxin (Tetanus—Gas Gangrene Antitoxin) (C.A.) **(Cutter)**

Supply: Packages of 1 prophylactic syringe or therapeutic dose syringe.

Dosage: Contents of 1 syringe at weekly intervals—prophylactic. Contents of 1 syringe every 6–12 hr.—therapeutic.

Tetanus-Gas Gangrene Antitoxin (Refined and Concentrated) (C.A.) **(Lederle)**

Supply: Packages of 1 syringe for prophylactic dose, containing tetanus antitoxin 1,500 units, perfringens antitoxin 1,000 units, vibrion septique antitoxin 1,000 units.

Dosage: 1 syringe *intramuscularly;* repeated in 5–7 days.

Tetanus-Gas Gangrene Antitoxin, Combined (C.A.) **(Lilly)**

Supply: Packages of 1 syringe containing tetanus antitoxin 1,500 units, perfringens antitoxin 1,000 units, vibrion septique antitoxin 1,000 units.

Dosage: *Intramuscularly*—1 syringe; repeated in 5–7 days.

Tetanus-Gas Gangrene Antitoxin **(Mulford)**

Supply: Packages of 1 syringe of prophylactic dosage containing Tetanus antitoxin 1,500 units, perfringens antitoxin 10 units, vibrion septique 10 units.

Tetanus-Perfringens Antitoxin (Tetanus—Gas Gangrene Antitoxin (C.A.) **(National Drug)**

Supply: Packages of 1 syringe or ampule-vial for prophylaxis, containing tetanus antitoxin 1,500 units, perfringens antitoxin 1,000 units.

Dosage: 1 syringeful, repeated in 1 week; 2 injections.

Tetanus-Gas Gangrene Antitoxin Combined (Refined and Concentrated) (C.A.) **(Parke, Davis)**

Supply: Packages of 1 syringe containing tetanus antitoxin 1,500 units, perfringens antitoxin 1,000 units, vibrion septique 1,000 units.

Dosage: 1 syringeful, repeated in 1 week—2 injections.

TUBERCULIN BIOTHERAPY

Tuberculins are products of the Tubercle Bacillus, introduced as aids in diagnosis, prophylaxis and treatment of tuberculosis. The following tuberculins are in common use:

Old Tuberculin (O.T.), Tuberculinum Koch.
New Tuberculin, Tuberculin Residue (T.R.) Tuberculin Rückstand, Koch.
New Tuberculin, Bacilli Emulsion (B.E.) Bacillen Emulsion, Koch.
Tuberculin Denys, Bouillon Filtrate Tuberculin, Bacillen Filtrat (B.F.).

Description: Old Tuberculin (O.T.), Tuberculinum Koch; is prepared after months of cultivation in glycerinated broth of strains of Bacillus Tuberculosis (human type), sterilization and evaporation to one-tenth the original volume and otherwise so treated as to contain no bacillary bodies, but only the products of their growth and metabolism; is a brown clear fluid of characteristic odor, and is used for diagnostic and therapeutic purposes.

Tuberculin Residue (T.R.) is an almost colorless, slightly opalescent fluid prepared from living and dried tubercle bacilli which are subjected to repeated grinding, suspension in water, centrifugation, and mixing with 20% glycerin; is finally standardized to represent 10 mg of dried tubercle bacilli to each cc of residue; is used by some clinicians in tuberculosis therapy.

Bacilli Emulsion (B.E.) is practically a 1/20% suspension of dead bacilli; is prepared from pulverized tubercle bacilli suspended in equal parts of water and glycerin, and after other processes in manufacture is standardized to contain 5 mg of tubercle bacilli per cc of emulsion; a colorless, slightly opalescent fluid; is used extensively in tuberculosis therapy.

Bacillen Filtrate (B.F.) is a glycerin broth culture of tubercle bacilli containing all soluble products of growth and metabolism of the tubercle bacillus; is used in tuberculosis therapy.

---

1. TUBERCULIN DIAGNOSTIC TESTS

Description: The tests in which Tuberculin products are used in diagnosis of tuberculosis are the Von Pirquet, Mantoux, Moro, and Calmette.

Administration: **Von Pirquet Test—Cutaneous.** *Technic*—2 superficial scarifications, at least 2 in. apart, are made by needle or scarifier; to one the content of a test capillary or a drop of Old Tuberculin (O.T.) is applied and gently rubbed into the scarified area by chisel or toothpick; the other scarification is treated in the same manner with a tuberculin-free control. Both vaccinations are allowed to remain for 10 minutes, then carefully dried, care being taken that no tuberculin is permitted to contaminate the control scarification. The areas are examined at the end of 24 and 48 hours. Positive reaction is shown by an area of reddening and infiltration at the site of tuberculin application, extending for about half inch or more; a negative reaction is accompanied by similar appearance as that of the control. The test is especially useful in children under six.

Mantoux Test—Intradermal. *Technic*—consists of 3 injections of dilute tuberculin, 3 days apart; careful observation is made for local, focal and general reaction symptoms. After careful cleansing of the skin, first dosage of 0.0002 cc is injected *intradermally;* if no reaction occurs, the second and third, 0.001 cc and 0.005 cc are given. In case of slightest reaction previous dosage is repeated but not increased. In the feeble and children, is administered in half doses and cautiously; in those with fever is not to be employed at all. Positive reactions are shown by rise of temperature, of at least 1°, and other symptoms as malaise, headache, pains in the limbs, palpitation; nausea and vomiting are occasionally present. Focal symptoms like increased rales, cough and sputum in pulmonary cases, or a visible flaring up of inflammation in the affected tubercular area are additional manifestations pointing to a positive reaction. The test is used more frequently in adults.

Moro Test—Percutaneous. *Technic*—after cleansing skin of some hairless part of body with alcohol and drying with ether, tuberculin ointment, 50%, is gently rubbed into the skin, for 1 minute; observation made 24 hours after. Positive reaction is shown by papulo-vesicular eruption.

Calmette Test—Ophthalmo-Reaction. *Technic*—after inspecting the eyes and excluding disease, with both conjunctivae of same appearance, 1 drop of freshly prepared sterile 1:100 saline solution Old Tuberculin (O.T.) is instilled with dropper at the medial canthus of one eye, and retained; observation made 24 hours later. Mild reaction—redness of the caruncle and inner surface of the lower lid; medium reaction—redness also of the ocular conjunctiva; violent reaction—purulent conjunctivitis. In doubtful reactions a drop placed in the other eye; resulting reaction will assist in definite conclusion.

DIAGNOSTIC PREPARATIONS

Diagnostic Tuberculin (C.A.) **(Cutter)**

Supply: Packages for 3 Von Pirquet cutaneous tests.

Tuberculin Solution O.T. (C.A.) (For Von Pirquet Test) **(Gilliland)**

Supply: Packages of 1, 5 or 10 capillary tubes; Vials 1 cc, 3 cc.

Von Pirquet Test (Tuberculin O.T.) (C.A.) **(Lederle)**

Supply: Packages with scarifiers for 3 or 10 tests.

Tuberculin (C.A.) (For Von Pirquet Test) **(Lilly)**

Supply: Packages of 3 capillary tubes for 3 tests.

Von Pirquet Test (C.A.) **(Mulford)**

Supply: Tuberculin Old, Human Type—Packages of 1, 3 or 10 capillary tubes with 1, 3, or 10 controls respectively for 1, 3 or 10 tests.

Tuberculin Old, Bovinn Type (C.A.)—Packages of 1, 3 or 10 capillary tubes with 1, 3 or 10 controls, respectively for 1, 3 or 10 tests.

Tuberculin O-T (C.A.) (For Von Pirquet Test) **(National Drug)**

Supply: Packages for 1, 3 or 10 tests, containing for each test 1 tube of tuberculin and 1 tube of concentrated glycerin bouillon for control.

Tuberculin Old (C.A.) (For Von Pirquet Test) **(Parke, Davis)**

Supply: Packages containing 3 sealed glass tubes of Old Tuberculin for 3 tests, and 3 tubes for control.

Dilute Tuberculin (C.A.) (For the Mantoux Test) **(Gilliland)**

Supply: Packages for 10 tests.

Intracutaneous Tuberculin (C.A.) (Test of Mantoux) **(Lederle)**

Supply: Packages for 10 tests, 1 vial 0.1 cc O.T., 1 vial 0.9 cc diluent.

Dosage: 0.1 cc *intracutaneously.*

Tuberculin Old, Concentrated (C.A.) **(Lilly)**

Supply: Vials 1 cc for subcutaneous tuberculin test (Mantoux), containing 1 Gm tuberculin, with 1 vial diluent.

Tuberculin, Intracutaneous (Tuberculin "O.T." Human Type) (C.A.) (For the Mantoux or Mendel Test) **(Mulford)**

Supply: Packages of intradermal syringes for 1 or 5 tests.

Dosage: 1/20 cc (0.2 mg).

Tuberculin, Intracutaneous (Tuberculin "O.T." Bovine Type) (C.A.) (For the Mantoux or Mendel Test) **(Mulford)**

Supply: Packages of intradermal syringes for 1 or 5 tests.

Dosage: 1/20 cc (0.2 mg).

Tuberculin Intracutaneous (O-T) (C.A.) **(National Drug)**
(For Mantoux Test)

Supply: Packages for Single Test—1 intradermal syringe and needle containing 1/10 cc of 1:1,000 dilution equivalent to 0.001 Gm O-T with glycerin bouillon for control; Packages for Double Test—2 intradermal syringes, 1 as above, 2 ten times strength of 1; Packages of one 1 cc ampule-vial for 10 single tests, each 1/10 cc containing 0.0001 Gm O-T with glycerin bouillon for control; Packages of two 1 cc ampule-vials for 10 double tests, Vial 1 as above, Vial 2 ten times strength of Vial 1; Packages of one 5 cc ampule-vial for 50 single tests, each 1/10 cc containing 0.001 Gm O-T with glycerin bouillon for control; Packages of one 5 cc ampule-vial for 50 single tests, ten times strength of above.

Tuberculin Old (C.A.) (For Mantoux Test) **(Parke, Davis)**

Supply: Packages of one 10 cc vial containing 0.01 cc Old Tuberculin, and one 10 cc vial of diluent—for 100 tests.

Tuberculin Ointment (C.A.) (For the Moro Test) **(Gilliland)**

Supply: Packages of 1 or 5 capsules, one for each test

Tuberculin Ointment (C.A.) (For Moro Test) **(Lilly)**

Supply: Collapsible tubes 2 Gm, containing equal parts of O.T. and anhydrous wool fat.

Tuberculin (C.A.) (For Ophthalmo-reaction) **(Parke, Davis)**

Supply: Tubes of 12 Disks, each 3.3 mg.

---

2. TUBERCULIN THERAPY

Description: The use of tuberculins in the treatment of tuberculosis demands thorough familiarity, good clinical judgment and accurate observation of the individual treated. Early tubercular cases are most favorable for tuberculins, but those moderately advanced with fever or positive sputum need not necessarily be excluded.

Administration: Initial dosage must be extremely minute; subsequent injections are tenfold, increased gradually; treatments given at intervals of sufficient length to allow the reaction after each injection to subside before the next dose is given.
To assure continuous increase in tolerance, injections are best made during height of the secondary rise of the middle phase, usually on fourth or fifth day after previous treatment, with intervals lengthened as dosage is increased. Slight reactions, as mild fever, malaise, mild active focal symptoms are to be anticipated; severe reactions must be avoided.
Tuberculin syringes only are to be used; dilutions must be made fresh and very accurately. Dosages are graded in each case as per specified schedules available with each preparation.

THERAPEUTIC PREPARATIONS

Concentrated Tuberculins O.T. (C.A.) **(Cutter)**

Supply: Packages, Tuberculin O.T. Human 1 cc, concentrated; Packages, Tuberculin O.T. Bovine 1 cc, concentrated.

Tuberculin Dilutions O.T. (C.A.) **(Cutter)**
(Also for intradermal test)

Supply: In bottles of about 7 cc.

No.	Per cc	Dilution
1	0.01 mg	1:100,000
2	0.1 mg	1:10,000
3	1. mg	1:1,000
4	10. mg	1:100
5	100. mg	1:10

Tuberculin Original (Old Tuberculin) **O.T.** (C.A.) **(Gilliland)**

Supply: Vials 1 cc, 3 cc with 10 cc diluent.

Tuberculin O.T. (Koch's Old Tuberculin) (C.A.) **(Lederle)**

Supply: Packages of 1 vial each of Concentrated 1.0 cc, "A" 0.1 cc, "B" 0.01 cc, "C" 0.001 cc, "D" 0.0001 cc, "E" 0.00001 cc, "F" 0.000001 cc. Each with 1 vial of diluent to make specified dilution.

Tuberculins Therapeutic (Human Strain) (C.A.) **(Lilly)**

Supply: Tuberculin Old, Concentrated—Vials 1 cc containing 1 Gm tuberculin. Tuberculin Old, Serial Dilutions—2 vials, of tuberculin and diluent, to make A. 0.1 cc, B. 0.01 cc, C. 0.001 cc, D. 0.0001 cc, E. 0.00001 cc, F. 0.000001 cc dilutions.

Tuberculin Concentrates (Undiluted) (C.A.) **(Mulford)**

Supply: Tuberculin Old "O.T." (Human Type)—Vials 1 Gm Tuberculin Old "O.T." (Bovine Type)—Vials 1 Gm.

Tuberculin Dilutions O.T. (Human Type) (C.A.) **(Mulford)**

Supply: Vials 8 cc, each 2 m containing:

Dilution 1	1–1,000 mg
Dilution 2	1–100 mg
Dilution 3	1–10 mg
Dilution 4	1 mg
Dilution 5	10 mg

Dosage: 2 m progressively increased by 2 m until 20 m are injected at 1 dose, after which the next stronger dilution is used in similar manner.

Tuberculin Old O.T. (Human Type) (C.A.) **(National Drug)**

Supply: Vials 1 cc, concentrated (representing 1 Gm undiluted tuberculin).

Tuberculin O.T. Serial Dilutions (C.A.) **(National Drug)**

Supply: Ampule-vials 10 cc, each 2 m containing:

Dilution 1	1/1,000 mg
Dilution 2	1/100 mg
Dilution 3	1/10 mg
Dilution 4	1 mg
Dilution 5	each minim equal to 10 mg.

Tuberculin Old O.T. (C.A.) **(National Drug)**

Supply: Vials 1 cc representing 1 Gm tuberculin; Vials 4 cc representing 0.25 Gm tuberculin per cc.

Tuberculin Old O.T. (C.A.) **(Parke, Davis)**

Supply: Packages of one 1 cc glass bulb, rubber diaphragm capped.

Tuberculin Bacillen Emulsion B.E. (C.A.) **(Gilliland)**

Supply: Vials 1 cc, 3 cc.

Tuberculin "B.E." (Bacillary Emulsion) (C.A.) **(Lederle)**

"F" 0.000001 cc; Each with 1 vial of diluent to make specified dilution; also vials 1 cc.

Tuberculin Concentrates (Undiluted) (C.A.) **(Mulford)**

Supply: Tuberculin Bacillen Emulsion "B.E." (Human Type)—Vials 1 Gm.

Tuberculin Dilutions, Tuberculin Bacillen Emulsion, B.E. (Human Type) (C.A.) **(Mulford)**

Supply: Vials, each 2 m containing:

Dilution 1	1–10,000 mg
Dilution 2	1–1,000 mg
Dilution 3	1–100 mg
Dilution 4	1–10 mg
Dilution 5	1 mg
Dilution 6	10 mg

Dosage: 2 m progressively increased by 2 m until 20 m are injected at 1 dose, after which the next stronger dilution is used in similar manner.

Tuberculin, Bacillen Emulsion B.E. (C.A.) (Parke, Davis)

Supply: Packages of one 1 cc glass bulb, rubber diaphragm capped, containing 1 mg tubercle solids.

Tuberculin, Bacillen Emulsion B.E. (C.A.) (Parke, Davis)

Supply: Tablets in vials of 10 each:

Vial 1	0.0001 mg
Vial 2	0.001 mg
Vial 3	0.01 mg
Vial 4	0.1 mg
Vial 5	1 mg

Tuberculin Dilutions, Tuberculin "T.R." (Human Type) (C.A.) **(Mulford)**

Supply: Vials each 2 m containing:

Dilution 1	1–10,000 mg
Dilution 2	1–1,000 mg
Dilution 3	1–100 mg
Dilution 4	1–10 mg
Dilution 5	1 mg
Dilution 6	10 mg

Dosage: 2 m progressively increased by 2 m until 20 m are injected at 1 dose, after which the next stronger dilution is used in similar manner.

Tuberculin Residue T.R. (C.A.) (Parke, Davis)

Supply: Concentrated—Packages of one 1 cc glass bulb, rubber diaphragm capped, containing 1 mg tubercle solids. Diluted—Packages of six 1 cc glass bulbs, rubber diaphragm capped, each containing 0.001 mg tubercle solids.

Tuberculin Residue T.R. (C.A.) (Parke, Davis)

Supply: Tablets in Vials of 10 each:

Vial 1	0.0001 mg
Vial 2	0.001 mg
Vial 3	0.01 mg
Vial 4	0.1 mg
Vial 5	1 mg

Concentrated Tuberculins (C.A.) (Cutter)

Supply: Packages, Tuberculin B.F. 1 cc, concentrated.

Tuberculin Bouillon Filtrate B.F. (C.A.) **(Cutter)**

Supply: Vials 1 cc.

Tuberculin Bouillon Filtrate B.F. (C.A.) **(Gilliland)**

Supply: Vials 1 cc, 3 cc, and in packages for dilutions.

Tuberculin B.F. Bouillon Filtrate (C.A.) **(Lederle)**

Supply: Vials 1 cc, and in packages for dilutions.

Tuberculosis Vaccine **(Sherman)**

Contains avirulent B. tuberculosis.

Supply: Vials 5 cc, 12½ cc—500 million bacteria per cc; Vials 5 cc, 12½ cc—1,000 million bacteria per cc.

Dosage: Initial 100 million bacteria, increased by 100 million at weekly intervals until 1,000 million is reached—controlled in accordance with reactions.

TYPHOID VACCINOTHERAPY

Description: Typhoid Vaccines are preparations of killed Bacillus Typhosus in physiologic saline suspension. Are used in vaccination against typhoid fever and the acquisition of an immunity lasting 2½–3 yr.; are also frequently used in non-specific protein therapy of other diseases.

Administration: Administered in 3 doses, at weekly intervals, *subcutaneously*, best late in the afternoon; in women, not during or near menstrual periods. Dosages in accordance with strength of individual preparations, generally 500, 1,000 and 1,000 million bacteria; in women and children dosage reduced according to weight.

PREPARATIONS

Typhoid Bacterin (C.A.) **(Abbott)**

Contains per cc

B. typhosus.................................... 1,000 million

Supply: Bulk packages of 6 cc, 20 cc.

Dosage: 0.5–1 cc at 7–10 day intervals.

Typhoid Vaccine (Typhoid Bacterin) (C.A.) **(Cutter)**

Contains per cc

B. typhosus.................................... 500 million

Supply: Bottles of 5 cc.

Dosage: 0.02–0.1 cc as initial dose, continuing with 0.1 cc at 3–7 day intervals.

Typhoid Prophylactic (C.A.) **(Cutter)**

Supply: Packages of 3 ambots (1 complete immunizing treatment); Syringe with 3 needles (1 complete immunizing treatment).

Dosage: 500 million, 1,000, 1,000 million bacteria at 5–7 day intervals.

Typhoid Vaccine (C.A.) **(Gilliland)**

Contains per cc	1	2	3
B. typhosus..............................	500	1,000	1,000 million

Supply: Packages of three 1 cc syringes or vials of strengths 1, 2 and 3; Vials 1 cc of strengths 1, 2 and 3—in packages of 30; Vials 5 cc, 10 cc, 20 cc of strength 3.

Dosage: PROPHYLAXIS—500, 1,000, 1,000 million bacteria at 7 day intervals.

Typhoid Vaccine (C.A.) **(Lederle)**

Contains per cc	1	2	3
B. typhosus..............................	500	1,000	1,000 million

Supply: Vials 5 cc.

Dosage: PROPHYLACTIC—3 injections—strengths 1, 2 and 3 or 1/8, 1/4 and 1/4 cc from vial, at intervals of 2–3 days.

Typhoid Vaccine, Prophylactic and Therapeutic (C.A.) **(Lilly)**
Contains per cc
B. typhosus.. 1,000 million

Supply: Single immunization package of three 1 cc vials 500, 1,000, 1,000 million bacteria; Packages of ten vials for 10 complete immunizations.

Typho-Bacterin (Typhoid Vaccine) (C.A.) **(Mulford)**

Supply: Packages of 3 syringes of 500, 1,000, 1,000 million bacteria—1 complete immunization; Packages of 30 vials for 10 complete immunizations.

Dosage: PROPHYLACTIC and THERAPEUTIC—Initial 50–125 million bacteria.

Typho-Serobacterin (Typhoid Vaccines, Sensitized) (C.A.) **(Mulford)**

Contains per cc	1	2	3
B. typhosus...........................	1,000	2,000	2,000 million

Supply: Packages of 3 syringes—strengths 1, 2, 3; Vials 5 cc of strength 2.

Dosage: Initial—contents of syringe 1.

Typhoid Vaccine (Typho-Bacterin) (C.A.) **(National Drug)**
Contains per cc
B. typhosus.. 1,500 million

Supply: Ampule-vials 5 cc, 15 cc, 30 cc.

Dosage: PROPHYLACTIC—0.5, 1, 1 cc at 7–10 day intervals.
THERAPEUTIC—0.25–0.5 cc increased by 0.25 cc at 8–24 hr. intervals.

Typhoid Vaccine (Prophylactic) (C.A.) **(Parke, Davis)**

Supply: Packages of 3 bulbs containing 500, 1,000 and 1,000 B. typhosus; Packages of ten 2.5 cc vials for 10 immunizations; Vials 20 cc, rubber diaphragm capped.

Dosage: 500, 1,000 and 1,000 million bacteria at intervals of 7–10 days; children according to weight.

Typhoid Vaccine **(Sherman)**
Contains per cc
B. typhosus.. 1,000 million

Supply: Vials 5 cc, 12½ cc.

Dosage: 0.5, 1, 1 cc at intervals of 7 days.

Typhoid Vaccine Immunizing (C.A.) **(Squibb)**

Contains per cc	1	2	3
B. typhosus..............................	500	1,000	1,000 million

Supply: Packages of 3 ampules—strengths 1, 2, 3; Packages of 30 ampules—10 each of strengths 1, 2, 3; Vials 5 cc, 20 cc of strength 3.

Dosage: Men—500, 1,000, 1,000 million bacteria at 7–10 day intervals. Women and children—in proportion to weight.

Typhoid Vaccine **(Upjohn)**

Contains per cc	1	2	3
B. typhosus..............................	500	1,000	1,000 million

Supply: Packages of three 1 cc ampules—strengths 1, 2, 3.

Typhoid Vaccine (C.A.) **(U. S. Standard Products)**

Contains per cc	1	2	3
B. typhosus..............................	500	1,000	1,000 million

Supply: Packages of three 1 cc vials; strengths 1, 2, 3; Vials 5 cc, 20 cc of strength 3.

Dosage: 500, 1,000 and 1,000 million bacteria at intervals of 7–10 days.

TYPHOID-PARATYPHOID VACCINOTHERAPY

Description: The Typhoid-Paratyphoid Vaccines are suspensions of killed Bacillus Typhosus, Bacillus Paratyphosus A and B, in physiologic saline solution; *are used* for the production of active immunity to typhoid and paratyphoid infections, the immunity lasting for about 3 yr., the first year being most active; also used frequently in non-specific protein therapy of other diseases.

Administration: Administered in 3 injections at weekly intervals, *subcutaneously;* best given late in the afternoon; in women, not during or near menstrual periods. Dosage in accordance with individual preparations, generally 1,000, 2,000, 2,000 million bacteria; in women and children dosage reduced according to weight.

PREPARATIONS

Typhoid-Paratyphoid Bacterin (Prophylactic) (C.A.) **(Abbott)**

Contains per cc	1	2	3
B. typhosus	500	1,000	1,000 million
B. paratyphosus A	375	750	750 million
B. paratyphosus B	375	750	750 million

Supply: Packages of three 1 cc vials—strengths 1, 2 and 3; Packages of 36 ampules, containing both strengths; Vials 6 cc, 20 cc of strength 3.

Dosage: 3 injections (strengths 1, 2 and 3) injected at 10 day intervals.

Typhoid-Paratyphoid Prophylactic (C.A.) **(Cutter)**

Contains	
B. typhosus	50%
B. paratyphosus A	25%
B. paratyphosus B	25%

Supply: Packages of 3 ambots (1 complete immunizing treatment) and 30 ambots (10 complete immunizing treatments); Bottles of 20 cc (8 full treatments); Syringe with 3 needles (1 complete immunizing treatment).

Dosage: 1,000, 2,000 and 2,000 million bacteria injected at 5–7 day intervals.

Typhoid-Paratyphoid Vaccine (Triple Typhoid Vaccine) (C.A.) **(Gilliland)**

Contains per cc	1	2	3
B. typhosus	500	1,000	1,000 million
B. paratyphosus A	250	500	500 million
B. paratyphosus B	250	500	500 million

Supply: Packages of three 1 cc syringes or vials of strengths 1, 2, 3 (1 immunization); Packages of thirty 1 cc vials of strengths 1, 2, 3. (10 immunizations); Vials 5 cc of strength 3 (2 immunizations); Vials 10 cc of strength 3 (4 immunizations)—Vials 20 cc of strength 3 (8 immunizations).

Typhoid Combined Vaccine (Typhoid-Paratyphoid Prophylactic) (C.A.) **(Lederle)**

Contains per cc	1	2	3
B. typhosus	500	1,000	1,000 million
B. paratyphosus A	250	500	500 million
B. paratyphosus B	250	500	500 million

Supply: Packages of 3 syringes or 3 vials—strengths 1, 2, 3, for 1 immunization; Packages of 30 vials for 10 immunizations; Vials 5 cc for 2 immunizations.

Dosage: 3 injections—strengths 1, 2 and 3, at intervals of 7 days.

Triple Typhoid Vaccine **(Lederle)**

Contains per cc	
B. typhosus	50%
B. paratyphosus A	25%
B. paratyphosus B	25%

Supply: Vials 5 cc—50 million bacteria per cc; Vials 5 cc; 100 million bacteria per cc.

Dosage: *For use* in non-specific intravenous therapy—initial dose 12½ million; second 25 million, third 50 million, fourth 75 million bacteria, at intervals of 3–4 days.

Typhoid Mixed Vaccine, Prophylactic and Therapeutic (Triple Typhoid T.A.B.) (C.A.) (Lilly)

Contains per cc	1	2
B. paratyphosus A	250	500 million
B. paratyphosus B	250	500 million
B. typhosus	500	1,000 million

Supply: Packages of three 1 cc vials—strengths 1, 2 and 2; Packages of 10 vials (10 complete immunizations); Vials 5 cc, 20 cc of strength 2.

Dosage: Initial—strength 1, followed at 5, 7 or 10 day intervals with strength 2 for 2 doses; from bulk packages—initial dose 0.5 cc, second and third doses 1 cc.

Typho-Bacterin Mixed (C.A.) (Mulford)

Contains	A	B	C	D
B. typhosus	125	250	500	1,000 million
B. paratyphosus A	62.5	125	250	500 million
B. paratyphosus B	62.5	125	250	500 million

Supply: Packages of 4 syringes—strengths A, B, C, D; Vials 5 cc and 20 cc of strength D; Packages of 30 vials (10 complete immunizations); Packages of 3 syringes or vials—strengths 1, 2 and 3 as follows:

	1	2	3
B. typhosus	500	1,000	1,000 million
B. paratyphosus A	250	500	500 million
B. paratyphosus B	250	500	500 million

Dosage: 3 injections of 1 cc each at intervals of 1 week or longer.

Typho-Serobacterin Mixed (Sensitized Typhoid Vaccine Mixed) (C.A.) (Mulford)

Contains	A	B	C	D
B. typhosus	250	500	1,000	2,000 million
B. paratyphosus A	125	250	500	1,000 million
B. paratyphosus B	125	250	500	1,000 million

Supply: Packages of four syringes—strengths A, B, C, D; Packages of 30 vials—10 complete immunizations (first, second and third doses)—Vials 5 cc of strength D; Packages of 3 immunizing syringes or 1 cc vials—first, second and third doses; Syringes and vials of immunizing packages contain as follows:

	First dose	Second dose	Third dose	
B. typhosus	1,000	2,000	2,000	million
B. paratyphosus A	500	1,000	1,000	million
B. paratyphosus B	500	1,000	1,000	million

Dosage: 3 injections of 1 cc each at intervals of 1 week.

Typhoid-Paratyphoid Mixed Vaccine (Typho-Bacterin Mixed) (C.A.) (National Drug)

Contains per cc	
B. typhosus	1,000 million
B. paratyphosus A	500 million
B. paratyphosus B	500 million

Supply: Ampule-vials 5 cc, 15 cc, 30 cc; Packages of three 1 cc ampule-vials (1 immunization); Packages of thirty 1 cc ampule-vials (10 immunizations).

Dosage: Prophylactic—0.5 cc, 1 cc, 1 cc at intervals of 7–10 days.
Therapeutic—0.25–0.5 cc, increased by 0.25 cc at 8–24 hr. intervals.

Typhoid-Paratyphoid (A) Vaccine (Typhoid-Paratyphoid (A) Bacterin) (C.A.) (National Drug)

Contains per cc	
B. typhosus	750 million
B. paratyphosus A	250 million

Supply: Ampule-vials 5 cc, 15 cc, 30 cc; Packages of three 1 cc ampule-vials (1 immunization); Packages of thirty 1 cc ampule-vials (10 immunizations).

Dosage: 1 cc at intervals of 7–10 days, for 3 doses.

Typhoid-Paratyphoid Vaccine (C.A.) (Parke, Davis)

Contains per cc

B. typhosus	1,000 million
B. paratyphosus A	750 million
B. paratyphosus B	750 million

Supply: Packages of 3 bulbs—0.5 cc, 1 cc and 1 cc; Packages of ten 2.5 cc vials; Vials 20 cc.

Dosage: 0.5 cc, 1 cc and 1 cc at 7–10 day intervals; children according to weight.

Typhoid Phylacogen (Parke, Davis)

Culture filtrates of bac. typhosus (50%), bac. paratyphosus A (25%) and bac. paratyphosus B (25%).

Supply: Vials 10 cc, rubber-diaphragm-capped.

Dosage: SUBCUTANEOUSLY—1 cc, increasing gradually to 10 cc; daily injections.
INTRAVENOUSLY—initial 2–4 m, increasing gradually to 5 cc; daily injections.

Typhoid Vaccine (Sherman)

Contains per cc

B. typhosus	1,000 million
B. paratyphosus A	750 million
B. paratyphosus B	750 million

Supply: Vials 5 cc, 12½ cc.

Dosage: PROPHYLACTIC—initial 0.5 cc, increased to 1 cc at 7 day intervals for 3 doses.
THERAPEUTIC—0.5 cc, increased by 0.1 cc at 24 hr. intervals until 1 cc is reached and continued at 24–48 hr.

Typhoid Vaccine Combined Immunizing (C.A.) (Squibb)

Contains per cc	1	2	3
B. typhosus	500	1,000	1,000 million
B. paratyphosus A	375	750	750 million
B. paratyphosus B	375	750	750 million

Supply: Packages of 3 and 30 ampules of strengths 1, 2, 3—Vials 5 cc, 20 cc of strength 3.

Dosage: Strengths 1, 2 and 3 at 7–10 day intervals; women and children in proportion to weight.

Typhoid Paratyphoid Mixed Vaccine (Upjohn)

Contains per cc	1	2	3
B. typhosus	500	1,000	1,000 million
B. paratyphosus A	375	750	750 million
B. paratyphosus B	375	750	750 million

Supply: Packages of three 1 cc ampules; Vials 5 cc, 20 cc of strength 3.

Dosage: PROPHYLACTIC—strengths 1, 2 and 3 at 7–10 day intervals.

Typhoid-Paratyphoid Vaccine Combined (C.A.) (U. S. Standard Products)

Contains per cc	1	2	3
B. typhosus	500	1,000	1,000 million
B. paratyphosus A	375	750	750 million
B. paratyphosus B	375	750	750 million

Supply: Packages of three 1 cc vials—strengths 1, 2, 3; Vials 5 cc, 20 cc of strength 3.

Dosage: 3 injections (strengths 1, 2 and 3) at 10 day intervals.

ULCERATIVE COLITIS BIOTHERAPY

Description: The sera are prepared in accordance with the method presented by Bargen, by immunization of horses with suspensions of living cultures of a Non-Hemolytic Streptococcus, isolated from typical, uncomplicated cases of chronic ulcerative colitis; the vaccines are prepared in the usual manner from the Diplo-streptococcus of Bargen.

Administration: To be employed only after exact diagnosis with the isolation and identification of the Bargen organism; given *intramuscularly* and *intravenously*, in repeated small doses over a considerably extended period.

SERUM PREPARATIONS

Streptococcus Antibody Globulin (Bargen Serum) (Mulford)

Supply: Ampule-vials 10 cc containing 20,000 units.

Ulcerative Colitis Antistreptococcic Serum (Parke, Davis)

Supply: Bottles rubber-diaphragm capped 20 cc.

Dosage: Initial 1–2 cc gradually increased to 5 cc daily or every other day.

VACCINE PREPARATIONS

Ulcerative Colitis-Streptococcus Vaccine (Bargen) (Cutter)

Contains per cc

Streptococci obtained from chronic ulcerative colitis..... 2,000 million

Supply: Vials 5 cc.

Dosage: Initial 0.2 cc, increasing by 0.1 cc every third day to maximum dose of 1–1.5 cc, then given weekly.

Bacterial Vaccine (Hollister-Stier)

Contains per cc

Diplo-streptococcus of Bargen........................ 2,000 million

Supply: Bottles of 5 cc, 20 cc.

Dosage: INTRADERMALLY—0.5–0.1 cc, rapidly increased to 1 cc.

Ulcerative Colitis Vaccine (Sherman)

Contains per cc

Diplo-streptococcus of Bargen..........1,000 million

Supply: Vials 5 cc, 12½ cc.

Dosage: Initial 0.2 cc, increased by 0.1 or 0.2 cc until 1 cc is reached, at intervals of 1–3 days, *subcutaneously*.

UNDULANT FEVER THERAPY

Description: The serum and vaccines available for treatment of undulant fever, or Malta, Mediterranean or rock fever, are prepared from cultures of Brucella Abortus and Brucella Melitensis and thus contain the antibodies of the two infecting agents; *are used* to raise the natural immunity against these brucellae in the treatment of undulant fever.

Administration: *Prophylaxis*—3 injections, at 7 day intervals, are usually given. *Therapy*—about 7 inoculations at 3 day intervals.

Bibliography: *See Chap. XII.*

PREPARATIONS

Undulant Fever Bacterin (Abbott)

Contains per cc

Brucella abortus................................ 2,000 million

Supply: Bulk packages 6 cc, 20 cc.

Dosage: 0.25–1 cc at 3 day intervals.

Undulant Fever Bacterial Vaccine (C.A.) **(Jensen-Salsbery)**
Contains per cc
Brucella melitensis abortus (bovine) 75%
Brucella melitensis suis (porcine) 25%
Killed organisms—5,950, suspended in saline.

Supply: Packages of six 2 cc vials.

Dosage: THERAPEUTIC—0.25 cc daily, *intramuscularly*, increased by 0.25 cc till 1 cc is reached; maximum number of doses—7; rest period of 2–3 weeks, then repeated.
PROPHYLACTIC—3 doses at 7–10 day intervals.

Brucella Melitensis Vaccine (C.A.) **(Lederle)**
Contains per cc
Brucella abortus .... 2,000 million

Supply: Vials 5 cc.

Dosage: 0.25–1 cc at 3 day intervals.

Abortion Test Antigen **(Lederle)**

For use in agglutination test in diagnosis of undulant fever.

Supply: Vials 20 cc, for 200 tests.

Antimelitensis Serum **(Mulford)**
A polyvalent serum containing antibodies for both melitensis and abortus groups of brucella organisms.

Supply: Packages of 1 double end 50 cc vial with intravenous injection outfit.

Dosage: 50–100 cc *intravenously*, repeated in 12–24 hr.

Undulant Fever Vaccine (Malta Fever, Abortus Vaccine) (C.A.) **(National Drug)**
Contains per cc
Brucella melitensis (Br. abortus) .... 1,000 million
Brucella abortus (bovine and porcine) .... 1,000 million

Supply: Ampule-vials 5 cc, 15 cc, 30 cc.

Dosage: PROPHYLACTIC—¼, ½, 1 cc at 7–10 day intervals.
THERAPEUTIC—¼ cc for 3 injections, ½ cc for 3 injections, 1 cc for 3 injections—at 3 day intervals.

Undulant "Malta" Fever Vaccine **(Sherman)**
Contains per cc
Brucella abortus .... 2,000 million

Supply: Vials 5 cc, 12½ cc.

Dosage: 0.1–0.2 cc increased by 0.2–0.5 cc until 1 or 1.5 cc is reached, at 1–3 day intervals.

VAN COTT'S VACCINOTHERAPY

Description: Polyvalent Vaccines are prepared from organisms most commonly associated with ordinary infections; *used* for the production of immunity in infections of bladder, kidneys, colon, sinuses; in otitis media, cellulitis, osteomyelitis, puerperal and other septic conditions, and in rheumatic affections.

Administration: Initial dosage small; continued in ascending doses to point of tolerance, guided by reactions, course of disease and the particular product used. Injections given every 2–3 days—6–8 or more per course.

PREPARATIONS

Sepsis Bacterin (Van Cott's Modified) **(Abbott)**

Contains per cc

Streptococcus	100 million
Pneumococcus	200 million
Bac. coli	500 million
Staph. aureus	250 million
Staph. albus	250 million

Supply: Bulk packages of 6 cc, 20 cc.

Dosage: Initial 3–5 m increased to 1 cc every 3–5 days.

Van Cott's Combination **(Cutter)**

Contains per cc

Staph. albus and aureus	500 million
Streptococcus	50 million
Bac. coli	100 million
Pneumococcus	100 million

Supply: Bottles of 5 cc.

Dosage: Initial 0.1–0.3 cc.

Staph-Strep-Coli-Pneumo Vaccine (Van Cott's Combination) **(Hollister-Stier)**

Contains per cc

Streptococcus	50 million
Staph. aureus	400 million
Staph. albus	400 million
Bac. coli	100 million
Pneumococci	100 million

Supply: Bottles 5 cc, 20 cc.

Dosage: Initial 0.25 cc.

Combined Bacterial Vaccine (Van Cott) **(Lederle)**

Contains per cc

Bac. coli	200 million
Pneumococcus I, II, III	200 million
Strep. hemolyticus, viridans	100 million
Staph. albus	400 million
Staph. aureus	400 million
Staph. citreus	200 million

Supply: Vials 5 cc.

Dosage: ⅛, ¼, ½, 1 cc at 3–7 day intervals.

Coli Combined Vaccine (Van Cott) **(Lilly)**

Contains per cc

Bac. coli	200 million
Staph. aureus	500 million
Staph. albus	500 million
Streptococcus	100 million
Pneumococcus	200 million

Supply: Vials of 5 cc, 20 cc.

Dosage: Initial 2–4 m.

Combined Vaccine (Van Cott) **(National Drug)**
(Pneumo-Strept. Bacterin)

Contains per cc

Pneumococcus Types I, II, III, IV	250 million
Strept. hemolyticus and viridans	500 million
Staph. albus and aureus	500 million
Bac. coli	250 million

Supply: Ampule-vials 5 cc, 15 cc, 30 cc.

Dosage: Initial 0.25 cc, increased by 0.25 cc every 1–3 days.

Combined Bacterial Vaccine (Van Cott) (Parke, Davis)

Contains per cc

Strept. hemolyticus and non-hemolyticus	100 million
Staph. albus	500 million
Staph. aureus	500 million
Bac. coli	200 million
Pneumococcus 4 types	200 million

Supply: Packages of four 1 cc bulbs; Vials of 5 cc, 20 cc.

Dosage: Initial 0.25 cc, increased to 1 cc at 3–5 day intervals.

Combined Immunogen (Van Cott) (Parke, Davis)

An extract of pneumococci types I, II, III, staph. albus and aureus, strep. hemolyticus and non-hemolyticus, bac. coli.

Supply: Vials 10 cc, rubber-diaphragm-capped.

Dosage: Initial 0.5 cc *intramuscularly* or 0.1–0.2 cc *subcutaneously*, gradually increased, avoiding severe reaction; daily or on alternate days; maximum dosage 2 cc or possibly 5 cc.

Mixed Infection Phylacogen (Parke, Davis)

Culture filtrates of staph. albus and aureus, strep. hemolyticus and non-hemolyticus, pneumococci types I, II, III, IV, bac. coli communis.

Supply: Vials 10 cc, rubber-diaphragm-capped.

Dosage: SUBCUTANEOUSLY—1 cc, increasing gradually to 10 cc; daily injections.
INTRAVENOUSLY—Initial 2–4 m, increasing gradually to 5 cc; daily injections.

Endo-Sepsis Vaccine (Improved Van Cott) (Sherman)

Contains per cc

Streptococcus	100 million
Pneumococcus	100 million
Bac. coli	200 million
Staphylococcus	600 million

Supply: Vials 5 cc, 12½ cc.

Dosage: PROPHYLACTIC—Initial 0.3 cc increased by 0.3 cc every 24 hr. for 2–3 injections.
PHYLACTIC—Increased to 1 cc dosage, three times weekly.

Van Cott's Vaccine (Squibb)

Contains per cc

	1	2	3	4
Strep. pyogenes	75	150	225	300 million
Staph. albus	125	250	375	500 million
Staph. aureus	125	250	375	500 million
Bac. coli	125	250	375	500 million
Pneumococcus	50	100	150	200 million

Supply: Packages of 4 ampules of 1, 2, 3, 4 strengths; Vials 5 cc, 20 cc of strength 4.

Dosage: 0.3 cc increased according to reaction, every 2–3 days, for 6–8 injections.

Colon Streptococcus Mixed Vaccine (Van Cott) (Upjohn)

Contains per cc

Bac. coli	200 million
Streptococcus	100 million
Pneumococcus	200 million
Staph. albus	500 million
Staph. aureus	500 million

Supply: Packages of six 1 cc ampules; Vials of 5 cc, 20 cc.

Dosage: Initial 0.25 cc, increased to 1 cc at 3–5 day intervals.

MISCELLANEOUS BIOLOGICALS

Bothrops Antitoxin (C.A.) **(Mulford)**
A serum prepared by immunization of horses against venom of American serpents, genus Bothrops, especially fer-de-lance; standardized on pigeons.

For use: In snake bites of the Bothrops group.

Supply: Syringes 10 cc.

Dosage: Intramuscularly or subcutaneously, 10 cc as early as possible following bite; in severe cases, intravenously.

Crotalus Antitoxin (C.A.) **(Mulford)**
A serum prepared by immunization of horses against venom of Crotalus snakes (Nearctic Crotalidae), of North American species; contains rattle snake 75%, copperhead 12½%, water moccasin 12½%.

For Use: In snake bites of above species.

Supply: Syringes 10 cc.

Dosage: Intramuscularly or subcutaneously, 50 cc.

Coley Toxins **(Parke, Davis)**
A mixed bacterial vaccine prepared from various strains of streptococcus pyogenes erysipelatis and bacillus prodigiosus.

For Use: In operable sarcoma.

Supply: Bulbs 1 cc, packages of 5—Bulbs 15 cc, packages of 1.

Dosage: 0.05–0.5 cc (1–8 m) hypodermically, partly into the tumor or adjoining tissues, and partly at a distance, this to secure local and systemic effect. Injections are given at intervals in accordance with reactions, which consist of chill and fever, and are continued until tolerance is established.

BACTERIOPHAGES

Description: Bacteriophage preparations are obtained from live bacterial cultures by the lytic action of undefined principles, specific for each bacterial organism. These lytic substances or phages are thought to be minute, inframicroscopic, living organisms, physically existing as corpuscles which penetrate presumably into the interior of the living microbes, colonize and multiply there, destroy the host and liberate a crop of young corpuscles endowed with similar and continued function. Such lysis of living bacteria by phages occurs in vitro as well as in vivo. The phages contain antigens, stimulate phagocytosis, are nontoxic, non damaging, harmless to tissue cells but are inhibited by antiseptics.

Bacteriophages are used in numerous infections; only phages specific to the particular microbe are to be employed in each case. May be administered topically, orally, subcutaneously and intravenously, in dosages in accordance with preparation and character of infection. Clinical experience must determine the frequency and method of administration as well as dosage in each case. Where injections are employed, like vaccines may be made at any desirable site; children are given smaller dosage.

PREPARATIONS

Bacteriophage-Staphylococcus Vials 30 cc; Ampule-vials 5 cc—Boxes of 6 **(Abbott)**

For use in boils, carbuncles, acne, cellulitis, osteomyelitis.

Administration—As dressing, two to three times daily; injections—0.2–0.5 cc topically.

Bacteriophage-Staphylococcus-Coli Vials 30 cc; Ampule-vials 5 cc—Boxes of 6 **(Abbott)**

For use in bed sores, abdominal surgical wounds, traumatic wounds, appendical abscess, fecal fistula.

Administration—As local wash, covered with cotton, oiled silk bandages; injected topically.

Bacte-Dysenteri-Phage Ampules 2 cc—Boxes of 10 and 50 **(Anglo-French)**
Containing in sterile broth suspension and bacterial substance.

Bacilli dysentery phage	10 billion
Bacilli para-dysentery phage	10 billion

For use in various types of acute bacillary dysentery.

Administration—Contents of 1 ampule in half glassful of cold water; every 4 hr. for 10 doses.

Bacte-Intesti-Phage Ampules 2 cc—Boxes of 10 and 50 **(Anglo-French)**
Containing in sterile broth suspension and bacterial substance.

Bacilli dysenteriae-phages	2,500 million
Para dysenteriae-phages	2,500 million
Bacilli proteus-phages	2,500 million
Enterococcus-phages	250 million
Bacilli pyocyaneous-phages	250 million
Bacilli coli-phages	250 million
Streptococcus-phages	250 million
Staphylococcus-phages	250 million

For use in various intestinal infections.

Administration—*Infectious diarrheas*—contents of 1 ampule in 20 cc water, in morning on empty stomach, and at night; acute cases—1 cc in 50 cc water, every 4 hr. *Infantile diarrhea*—1 ampule in 50 cc vichy or water, given 1 tablespoonful every hour; in gastric intolerance, 1 ampule in 40 cc water as enema.

Bacte-Coli-Phage Ampules 1 cc—Boxes of 50; Ampules 2 cc—Boxes of 10—Ampules 10 cc—Boxes of 5 **(Anglo-French)**
Each 2 cc ampule containing 1,000 million anti-coli and anti-paracoli bacteriophages with dissolved substance of 200 million bacillus coli and paracoli.

For use as specific for coli infections, especially of genitourinary tract.

Administration—*Cystitis*—bladder instillation of 10–20 cc diluted in 50 cc saline; retained as long as possible; repeated twice. *Pyelonephritis*—5 cc pure or mixed with Bacte-Staphy-phage, instilled into renal pelvis, accompanied by bladder instillation as for cystitis; repeated after 4 or 5 days. *Prostatitis*—slow intravenous injection of 10 cc diluted in 500 cc sterile saline, together with bladder instillation for 4 consecutive days; orally, 2 cc diluted in half glass water, mornings on empty stomach, for 20 days.

Bacte-Pyo-Phage Polyvalent Ampules 2 cc—Boxes of 10; Ampules 50 cc—Boxes of 1 and 10 **(Anglo-French)**
Each 2 cc ampule containing in sterile broth suspension with bacterial substance.

Staphylococcus-phages	3,000 million
Streptococcus-phages	500 million
Bacilli proteus-phages	500 million
Bacilli pyocyaneus-phages	250 million
Bacilli coli-phages	150 million
Para-coli-phages	150 million
Pneumo-bacillus-phages	150 million
Enterococcus-phages	100 million

For use in destroying various bacteria of pyogenic infections.

Administration—*Pustular acne*—applied locally as wet dressing. *Suppurations, Peritonitis, Osteomyelitis, Infected Wounds*—under local anesthesia pus cavity is aspirated and washed out with Bacte-Pyo-Phage. *Dental Phlegmon, Pyorrhea*—subcutaneous injection of 2 cc, combined with injection into infected tissues.

Bacte-Staphy-Phage Ampules 2 cc—Boxes of 10; Ampules 50 cc —Boxes of 1 and 50. **(Anglo-French)**

Each 2 cc ampule containing in sterile broth suspension and bacterial substance 250 million staphylococci-phages and 10,000 billion phages of selected strains active against staphylococcus aureus, citreus, albus.

For use in various staphylococcus infections.

Administration—Furunculosis—0.5–3 cc, twice, at 24–48 hr. intervals; local application as wet dressing. *Carbuncle*—several injections directly into lesion, with local application as wet dressings. *Tonsillar Phlegmon*—2 cc injected 1–2 cm from lesion; followed immediately with autohemotherapy, gluteal injections of 10 cc of patient's whole blood; may be repeated in 24 hr. with another autohemotransfusion. *Septicemia*—slow intravenous injection of 10 cc diluted in 500 cc saline.

Bacte-Rhino-Phage Ampules 2 cc—Boxes of 10 and 50 **(Anglo-French)**

Containing in sterile broth suspension and bacterial substance.

Streptococcus-phages	1,000 million
Staphylococcus-phages	1,000 million
Pneumo bacillus-phages	1,000 million
Proteus-phages	500 million
Para-coli-phages	500 million
Bacilli pyocyaneus-phages	100 million

For use against above bacteria.

Administration—Coryza, Bronchitis—sprayed into nose and throat.

Ento-Jel Tubes ½ oz., nasal tipped **(Lilly)**

Contains mixed lysates of micrococcus catarrhalis, staphylococcus aureus, streptococcus and pneumococcus—incorporated in water soluble, jelly base, with merthiolate 1:5,000.

For use in nasopharyngeal infections of above bacterial origin, by sniffing intranasally or by tampons two or three times daily.

Ento-Lysate Vials 5 cc, 20 cc **(Lilly)**

A sterile solution of the mixture of phage-lysed respiratory bacterial antigens, of micrococcus catarrhalis, staphylococcus aureus, streptococcus and pneumococcus.

For use in respiratory affections.

Administration—Locally by atomizer or dropper, three to five times daily, either pure or in 50% solution; hypodermically—injected 0.1–1 cc in accordance with extent of infection, to produce systemic immunity.

Staphylo-Jel Tubes of ½ oz. **(Lilly)**

Contains lysed staphylococcus aureus and albus principles, fortified with 25% of lysed streptococcus proteins and preserved with merthiolate prepared in the usual manner of bacteriophages, with water soluble jelly base.

For use in staphylococcus infections—boils, carbuncles, folliculitis, sycosis, impetigo, paronychia, abscesses, phlegmons, osteomyelitis, ulcer, styes, blepharitis, pustular acne.

Administration—Applied locally, being previously warmed; may also be injected into the infected area.

Staphylo-Lysate Vials 20 cc, rubber stoppered **(Lilly)**

A sterile solution of phage-lysed staphylococcus aureus and albus principles fortified with 25% of lysed streptococcus proteins and preserved with merthiolate; prepared in the usual manner of bacteriophages.

Uses as for Staphylo-Jel.

Administration—Locally, as wet dressing or tampon covered with silk; area cleaned before use; may also be injected into boils.

Strepto-Jel Tubes of ½ oz. (Lilly)
Contains mixed lysates of various strains of streptococcus pyogenes incorporated in water soluble jelly base, preserved with merthiolate, with lysed staphylococcus protein filtrate added.

For use in streptococcus infections of skin and mucous surfaces.

Administration—Applied locally, previous warmed and surface cleansed.

Strepto-Lysate Vials 20 cc, rubber stoppered (Lilly)
A sterile solution of phage-lysed streptococcus pyogenes of various strains, with sterile lysed staphylococcus protein filtrate, preserved with merthiolate.

For use in streptococcus infections of skin and mucosa.

Administration—Applied locally by tampon or wet dressings, area cleansed before use; injected locally where desired.

Colo-Jel (Combined) Tubes of 1½ oz. with metal pipe (Lilly)
Prepared from active cultures of bacillus coli, staphylococcus aureus, streptococcus and pneumococcus, lysed with their respective bacteriophages and incorporated in water soluble jelly base.

For use in mixed infections of abdomen, pelvis, perineum; rectal abscess, vaginitis, cervicitis and other coli infections.

Administration—Applied locally by tampon, as instillations through catheter, as lubricant for sounds and bougies; twice daily.

Bio-Cream Jars of ¼ oz., 1 oz. (Sherman)
An antivirus product obtained from autolyzed skin bacteria incorporated in creamy base.

For use in pustular rashes, pimples, boils, ulcerations, burns, acne.

Administration—Applied twice daily, gently rubbed in like a cream after cleansing parts with water and bland soap.

A-Vee 51 Preparation (Sherman)
Contains the antivirus principles of numerous strains of staphylococcus, incorporated in face cream.

For use in acne, boils, carbuncles, furuncles, sycosis.

Administration—Applied locally twice daily.

A-Vee 11 Preparation (Sherman)
Contains the antivirus principles of numerous strains of staphylococcus, in liquid form.

For use in above conditions.

Administration—Applied as wet packs or irrigation.

A-Vee 52 Preparation (Sherman)
Contains the antivirus principles of numerous strains of pyogenic organisms of mixed varieties, in creamy form.

For use in the treatment of suppurating wounds, bed sores, perineum infections, abscesses, phlegmons.

Administration—Applied locally after cleansing parts, two to three times daily.

A-Vee 12 Preparation (Sherman)
Contains the antivirus principles of numerous strains of pyogenic organisms of mixed varieties, in liquid form.

For use in the treatment of suppurating wounds, bed sores, perineum infections, abscesses, phlegmons.

Administration—Applied locally as wet dressing, tampon or irrigation two to three times daily.

Polyvalent Staphylococcus Bacteriophage Vials 20 cc, rubber-stoppered (Squibb) Contains broth culture of polyvalent staphylococcus aureus, specifically autolyzed by bacteriophage, and filtered.

For use in staphylococcus infections: carbuncles, furuncles, genitourinary infections, staphylococcus septicemia.

Administration—Topically by gauze dressings or saturated drains directly applied to lesion; injections into lesion—0.3–1 cc, repeated; *subcutaneously* 1 cc away from lesion, repeated following day; as instillations into bladder—10 cc diluted with saline to 40 cc; twice daily; *intravenously*, in emergencies and septicemia—1–3 cc.

Bibliography: *See Chap. XII.*

CHAPTER VII

ALLERGENS

This chapter presents 2223 Individual and 121 Group Protein Extracts for the diagnosis and therapeusis of allergic disturbances: hay fever, asthma, urticaria, eczema, angioneurotic edema, colitis and other similar disorders.

Description: The allergens of foods, bacteria, epidermals and furs here described are prepared from their respective substances and are available in the form of powdered extracts, as liquids and pastes, in various concentrations. Hay fever antigens are produced from mature, carefully and properly selected pollens; these are cleared from extraneous matter and either dried and pulverized, or extracted in saline, alcoholic or glycerol solutions; they are thus obtainable as powdered extracts, as buffered saline and glycerinated solutions or as pastes of glycerin-concentrated pollens mixed with glycerite of starch to a pasty consistency, with a minute quantity of antiseptic oil as preservative. Most allergens are standardized in nitrogen units, each unit being equivalent to 0.001 mg N-Protein; others are measured in pollen units, about ten times the potency of N-units. Allergens are used in diagnosis, immunization and therapeusis of allergic manifestations.

Diagnosis: Allergens for diagnosis are available as preparations of individual proteins, or of groups of several homologous substances: similar foods, epidermals, furs or seasonal and regional plants. The diagnostic tests are based on the phenomena of local hypersensitiveness and the reactions induced by foreign proteins.

Tests: The tests are performed by several methods:

Cutaneous, Percutaneous or Scratch Method—The flexor surface of forearm or arm is carefully cleansed (with water, saline, dilute alcohol or ether) and allowed to dry; scarifications, about ⅛–¼ in. long, 1–2 in. apart, in 2 rows if necessary are made with scalpel, needle or Von Pirquet scarifier, taking care not to penetrate epidermal layer and draw blood. The protein extracts in whatever form, are then applied to the abrasions, in definite order, so as to make their identification possible, and are carefully rubbed in, each with a fresh toothpick or other means; not more than 18–20 tests at each sitting, with one control of saline or other bland solution for comparison are to be given. Observation is made in 10–20 min.; reactions are compared with that of control and recorded; where *negative*, the reaction presents no particular difference from that of the control, no indurative or erythematous changes; a slight redness from irritation must not be interpreted as a positive reaction. Observation is to be repeated in 24 hr. for possible delayed reactions. Negative reactions are not exclusive and may have to be repeated for further corroboration. A *positive* reaction, if mild or moderate, is indicated by slight redness; where severe—by an urticarial, slightly raised wheal with pseudopodia, irregular in outline, surrounded by an erythema ½–1 in. in width; in *strongly positive* reactions, wheals and pseudopodia are markedly pronounced.

Intracutaneous, Intradermal Method—Is applied by injecting with extremely fine needle and syringe 1–2 drops (0.01–0.02 cc) of suitably diluted liquid allergens, *intradermally*, not subcutaneously. Observations made and results recorded in the same manner as in the scratch method. The intradermal method is more painful and presumably more dangerous than the scratch method; it is however the preferred method, as it is more sensitive, and lately is being more extensively used.

Ophthalmic Method—This test is infrequently applied; it is especially useful in the diagnosis of horse serum sensitivity. In this test a few drops of the fluid allergens are dropped into one eye, the other eye being used as control; where *positive*, a hyperemia of conjunctiva with itching or burning results; in severe reactions, a marked conjunctivitis.

Therapeusis: All protein antigens for immunization and treatment of allergic conditions are administered in ascending dosage, *subcutaneously*, at about 2–4 day intervals, beginning with the smallest, least provocative dose and continued in gradually increasing strengths until correct top dosage is established. In all instances it is also most essential that a correct diagnosis be first established before administering any specific protein; that the dosage and interval between injections be carefully graded; that severe reactions be avoided; and that the individuality also of the treated be taken into consideration.

In hay fever therapy consideration must also be given: 1. to the use of the correct extracts as indicated by the reactions to the diagnostic tests. 2. to the correct identification of the offending protein where a positive reaction is obtained by the group test, comprising several plants of the same genus. 3. to the limitation of treatment in combined injections to as few extracts as possible. 4. to the administration of allergens at the right time and season, in relation to symptoms and pollination period. 5. to the buoyancy of wind borne pollens and exclusion of insect pollinating plants. In those with spring and fall attacks, separate treatment should be administered preliminary to each season. Injections are to be continued well into the season, whether early or late summer or fall. In positive reactions to group combinations of 3–6 different protein extracts, tests for each individual constituent protein must be performed before desensitization is undertaken.

Immunization: In immunization against hay fever, treatment must begin early enough to permit the administration of the last injection before the time of expected attack. Fifteen doses are given preseasonally and 5–10 injections in slightly submaximal concentration are continued into the season; injections are made every 3–4 days. Three methods of immunization are used:

Intensive Preseasonal Method—Used in cases near the seasonal attack and too late for preseasonal therapy; treatment comprises 10–12 injections administered every 24 hr., the other injections of the series at longer intervals, but in dosages not as large as in preseasonal schedules.

Coseasonal Method—Used during seasonal period; here injections are given daily or even twice daily, but in much smaller dosage; they are very gradually increased and greater care is exercised to avoid severe reactions; where these occur treatment is discontinued for 1–2 weeks, then resumed.

Perennial Method—Now considered the most advisable and helpful method, here treatments are administered throughout the year, dosage increased gradually until the highest which is protective against an attack is reached; this is then continued bimonthly or even monthly. This method requires considerable skill and the use of a constant extract, but has the advantage of beginning treatment at any time of year and after first season may be carried out monthly.

Administration: Accurate dosage is essential; avoidance of injecting into vein is imperative. Allergic phenomena, local and constitutional, are to be avoided by careful dosage and cautious administration. Moderate local reactions are desirable; quantities above or below the maximum "top dose" producing undesirable reactions should be avoided. Dosages are governed in accordance with preparations; injections are given with fine needle and tuberculin syringe.

Constitutional Reactions: Reactions may appear soon after injection or within 24 hr.; they are shown, *locally*, by rapid spreading and elevation of a hot and itchy urticarial wheal, with surrounding erythema of about 4–5 in. and over. *Constitutionally*—reactions cause itching of palms, sneezing, coughing, swellings, dyspnea, coryza, asthmatic attacks and other symptoms. Reactions are treated by the subcutaneous injection of 0.5 cc epinephrin, which should always be on hand when allergens are administered, and repeated in a few minutes if necessary; a tight tourniquet around the arm where the extract has been injected, is helpful.

Bibliography: *See Chap. XII.*

Part I

Allergens*

I. Individual

Bacterials

(Arlington)

B. Coli Communis
Diphtheroid
Friedlander Bacillus
Micrococcus Tetragenus
Micrococcus Catarrhalis
Pneumococcus Type I
Pneumococcus Type II
Pneumococcus Type III
Staphylococcus Pyogenes Aureus
Staphylococcus Pyogenes Albus
Staphylococcus Pyogenes Citreus
Streptococcus Viridans
Streptococcus Haemolyticus
Streptococcus Non-haemolyticus

Supply: Diagnostic—Vials of 25 mg powdered extract—Packages of 1 or 6.
Therapeutic—Treatment sets for desensitization.

(Lederle)

Bacillus Coli
Micrococcus Catarrhalis
Pneumococcus Type I
Pneumococcus Type II
Staphylococcus Albus
Staphylococcus Aureus
Streptococcus Hemolyticus
Streptococcus Viridans

Supply: Vials 1 cc, for diagnosis and desensitization.

(Mulford)

Acne Bacillus
Coli (Polyvalent)
Diphtheroids (Polyvalent)
Diphtheroids (Polyvalent)
Dysentery (Shiga) Bacillus
Friedlander Bacillus
Gonococcus (Polyvalent)
Influenza Bacillus
Meningococcus (Gordon Types I, II, III, IV)
Micrococcus Catarrhalis
Paradysentery (Flexner, Strong, Y-Hiss, Sonne) Bacillus
Paratyphosus "A" Bacillus
Paratyphosus "B" Bacillus
Pertussis (Polyvalent) Bacillus
Pneumococcus (Types I, II, III, IV)
Staphylococcus (Albus and Aureus)
Streptococcus (Polyvalent)
Typhosus Bacillus

Supply: Diagnostic—Ampule-vials 1 cc (for 10 tests).

(Parke, Davis)

Colon Bacillus
Friedlander Bacillus
Gonococcus
Micrococcus Catarrhalis
Micrococcus Tetragenus
Pneumococcus Type I
Pneumococcus Type II
Pneumococcus Type III
Pseudodiphtheria Bacillus
Staphylococcus Albus
Staphylococcus Aureus
Staphylococcus Citreus
Streptococcus, Hemolyticus
Streptococcus, Non-hemolyticus
Typhoid Bacillus
Paratyphoid Bacillus A
Paratyphoid Bacillus B

Supply: Diagnostic—Collapsible tin tubes—glycerinated paste extract for about 50 tests.
Therapeutic—Supplied in graded dilutions.

(Squibb)

Bacillus Acne
Bacillus Coli
B. Friedlander
Bacillus Influenzae
Bacillus Pertussis
Bacillus Typhosus
Bacillus Diphtheroid
Gonococcus
Micrococcus Catarrhalis
Micrococcus Meningitis
Micrococcus Tetragenes
Pneumococcus I
Pneumococcus II
Pneumococcus III
Pneumococcus IV
Staphylococcus Aureus
Staphylococcus Albus
Staphylococcus Citreus
Streptococcus (Polyvalent)
Streptococcus Pyogenes
Streptococcus Viridans

* For simplicity the marking of C.A. preparations is omitted in this Chapter.

Supply: Diagnostic—Vials 25 mg—Cases containing 12, 24 or 50 individual allergen vials, assorted.

Epidermal Extracts **(Abbott)**

Chicken Feathers
Duck Feathers
Goose Feathers
Turkey Feathers
Cow Dander
Human Hair
Horse Dander
Cat Hair
Dog Hair
Hog Hair
Rabbit Hair
Wool

Supply: Diagnostic—Vials of 3 and 25 capillary tubes.

(Arlington)

Camel Hair
Canary Feather
Cat Hair
Cattle Hair
Chicken Feather
Deer Hair
Dog Hair
Dog Feather
Goat Hair
Goose Feathers
Guinea Pig Hair
Hog Hair
Horse Dander
Human Hair, White
Human Hair, Negro
Mouse Hair
Mule Dander
Ostrich Feather
Parrot Feather
Pigeon Feather
Rabbit Hair
Sheep Wool
Turkey Feather

Supply: Diagnostic—Vials 25 mg powdered extract, and 15 mg—Packages of 1 or 6 vials.

Therapeutic—Standardized treatment sets for desensitization.

(Hollister-Stier)

Angora Wool
Cat Hair
Cattle Hair
Deer Hair
Dog Hair
Chicken Feathers
Guinea Pig Hair
Horse Dander
Human Hair
Hungarian Stone
Hog Hair
Martin
Duck feathers
Mouse Hair
Rat Hair
Rabbit Hair
Sheep Wool
Goose Feathers

Supply: Diagnostic—Ampules 1 cc, with capillary tube (for 25 tests)—Packages of 1 or 6 assorted ampules.

Therapeutic—Sets of 5 vials each containing 1, 2 or more proteins, in concentrations of 1–10, 1–50, 1–100, 1–1,000, 1–5,000.

(Lederle)

Camel Dander
Cow Dander
Duck Feathers
Goose Feathers
Horse Dander
Muskrat Dander
Pigeon Feathers
Sheep Dander
Canary Feathers
Cat Dander
Fox Dander
Guinea Pig Dander
Mink Dander
Mule Dander
Opposum Dander
Rabbit Dander
Skunk Dander
Chicken Feathers
Dog Dander
Goat Dander
Hog Dander
Mouse Dander
Parrot Feathers
Raccoon Dander
Turkey Feathers

Supply: Diagnostic—Vials 6 cc, diluted fluid extract; Capillary tubes, glycerolated—Packages of 5 and 50.

Therapeutic—Vials 6 cc, fluid extract, undiluted; Concentrated extract with bottles of 4½ cc sterile diluting fluid.

(Mulford)

Cat Hair
Cattle Dander
Chicken Feathers
Dog Hair
Duck Feathers
Goose Feathers
Guinea Pig Hair
Horse Dander
Horse Serum
Rabbit Hair
Sheep Wool

Supply: Diagnostic—Tube—Vials 50 mg of dried powdered extract, for about 25 tests; Packages of 1 single cutaneous outfit for 1 test.

Therapeutic—Packages of one 5 cc vial, 500 protein units per cubic centimeter.

(National Drug)

Camel Hair
Canary Feathers
Cat Hair
Cattle Hair
Chicken Feathers
Dog Hair

Epidermal Extracts.—(*Continued*)

- Duck Feathers
- Goat Hair
- Goose Feathers
- Guinea Pig Hair
- Hog Hair
- Horse Dander
- Human Hair
- Monkey Hair
- Mouse Hair
- Ostrich Feathers
- Parrot Feathers
- Pigeon Feathers
- Rabbit Hair
- Sheep's Wool
- Turkey Feathers

Supply: DIAGNOSTIC (for scratch method)—Ampule-vials 1 cc.
THERAPEUTIC—Ampule-vials 5cc, in dilutions as requested.

(Parke, Davis)

- Chicken Feathers
- Duck Feathers
- Goose Feathers
- Hair of Cattle
- Hair of Cat
- Hair of Dog
- Hair of Goat
- Hair of Guinea Pig
- Hair of Horse
- Hair of Rabbit
- Human Hair
- Sheep's Wool

Supply: DIAGNOSTIC—Collapsible tin tubes of glycerinated paste extract for about 50 tests.
THERAPEUTIC—Supplied in graded dilutions, as ordered.

(Squibb)

- Burro Hair
- Burro Dander
- Cat Hair
- Cat Dander
- Chamois Skin
- Chicken Feathers
- Cow Hair
- Cow Dander
- Dog Hair
- Dog Dander
- Duck Feathers
- Goose Feathers
- Grouse Feathers
- Horse Hair
- Horse Dander
- Human Hair
- Human Dander
- Rabbit Hair
- Rabbit Dander
- Sheep's Wool

Supply: DIAGNOSTIC—Vials 25 mg of powdered extract—Boxes of 12, 24 or 50 individual allergen vials, assorted.

FOODS

(Abbott)

Sea Foods
- Clam
- Haddock
- Herring
- Lobster
- Oyster
- Salmon
- Shrimp
- Tuna Fish

Meat
- Beef
- Chicken
- Mutton
- Pork

Egg
- Egg Yolk
- Egg White
- Egg "Whole"

Milk
- Lactalbumin
- Milk

Cereals
- Barley
- Buckwheat
- Corn (Green)
- Corn Meal
- Oats (Rolled)
- Rice
- Rye Flour
- Wheat
- Wheat Flour

Nuts
- Almond
- English Walnut
- Pecan
- Walnut

Legumes
- Black-eye Pea
- Lima Bean
- Navy Bean
- Pea
- Peanut
- String Bean

Vegetables
- Beet
- Cabbage
- Carrot
- Cauliflower
- Celery
- Cucumber
- Lettuce
- Onion
- Potato
- Radish
- Spinach
- Sweet Potato

Fruits
- Apple
- Banana
- Blackberry
- Cantaloupe
- Grapefruit
- Orange
- Peach
- Pear
- Raspberry (Black)
- Raspberry (Red)
- Strawberry
- Tomato

Beverages
- Chocolate
- Coffee

Supply: DIAGNOSTIC—Vials of 3 or 25 capillary tubes.

Foods (Arlington)

Almond
Anchovy
Aniseed
Apple
Apricot
Artichoke
Asparagus
Avocado
Banana
Barley
Bass (Sea)
Bay Leaves
Bean
Beef
Beet
Blackberry
Black-eyed Pea
Black Walnut
Blueberry
Bluefish
Bran (Wheat)
Brazil Nut
Broccoli
Brussels Sprouts
Buckwheat
Butterfish
Cabbage
Calves' Brains
Cantaloupe
Caraway Seed
Carp
Carrot
Casaba
Casein
Cashew Nut
Castor Bean
Catfish
Cauliflower
Caviar
Celery
Cheeses:
- American
- Camembert
- Edam
- Cheddar
- Gjedeost
- Gorganzola
- Limburger
- Parmesan
- Roquefort
- Swiss

Cherry
Chehestnut
Chicken (Hen)
Chicken (Rooster)
Chicory
Chive
Cinnamon
Clam, hard
Clam, soft
Clove
Cocoa
Cocoanut
Codfish
Coffee
Corn
Crab
Cranberry
Crawfish
Cucumber
Currant, red
Dandelion
Date
Dill
Duck
Duckegg
Eel
Eggplant
Eggwhite (whole)
Eggwhite (Ovomucoid)
Eggwhole
Eggyolk (whole)
Eggyolk (Ovovitellin)
Endive
Escargot
Fig
Filbert (Hazelnut)
Flounder
Frogs' Legs
Garlic
Ginger
Goatmeat
Goose
Gooseberry
Goose Egg
Grape
Grapefruit
Guinea Hen
Haddock
Halibut
Hazelnut (Filbert)
Herring
Hickory
Honey Dew
Horse Radish
Jerusalem Artichoke
Kale
Kidney (Beef)
Kidney Bean
Kohlrabi
Lactalbumin
Lamb
Leek
Lemon
Lentil
Lettuce
Lima Bean
Liver (beef)
Lobster
Mackerel
Mango
Milk (Breast)
Milk (Cow)
Milk (Goat)
Mint
Mushroom
Mustard
Mutton
Mullet
Nutmeg
Oat
Okra
Olive
Onion
Orange
Oyster
Oyster Plant
Paprika
Parsley
Parsnip
Pea
Peach
Peanut
Pear
Pecan
Pepper (Red and Green)
Pepper (Black)
Perch
Pheasant
Pickerel
Pike
Pimiento
Pineapple
Pine Nut (Pignolia)
Pistachio Nut
Plum
Pompano
Poppy Seed
Pork
Potato
Prune
Pumpkin
Rabbit
Radish
Raisin
Raspberry
Redsnapper
Rhubarb
Rice
Rye
Salmon
Sage
Sardine
Scallops
Shad
Shad Roe
Shrimp
Smelts
Sole
Spinach
Squab
Squash
Strawberry
Sturgeon
String Bean
Sweet Bread
Sweet Potato
Swiss Chard
Swordfish
Tangerine
Tea
Terrapin
Tomato
Tripe
Trout (Lake)
Trout (Sea)
Tuna Fish
Turkey
Turnip
Turtle
Veal
Walnut (English)
Watercress
Watermelon
Weakfish
Wheat (Whole)
Wheat Gliadin
Wheat Globulin
Wheat Glutenin
Wheat Proteose
Wheat Leucosin
Whitefish (Lake)
Whiting

Supply: DIAGNOSTIC—Vials 50 mg powdered extract for 20 tests, and some tube 25 mg—Packages of 1 or 6,
THERAPEUTIC—Standardized treatment sets for desensitization.

(Hollister-Stier)

Beverages

Cocoa
Coffee
Tea

Cereals

Barley
Buckwheat
Corn
Oat
Rice
Rye
Sago
Tapioca
Wheat
Wheat (Glutenin)
Wheat Gliadin
Wheat Gluten

Condiments

Allspice
Black Pepper
Chili Powder
Cinnamon
Cloves
Dill
Garlic
Ginger
Green Pepper
Horse Radish
Mace
Mustard
Nutmeg
Okra
Paprika
Red Pepper
Sage
Thyme
Turmeric
Vanilla

Egg

Egg (All proteins)
Egg Yolk
Egg White

Sea Foods

Clam
Crab
Halibut
Haddock
Ling Cod
Lobster
Mackerel
Oyster (Eastern)
Oyster (Olympia)
Pickerel
Pike
Red Snapper
Rock-cod
Sabel Fish
Salmon
Sea Bass
Shrimp
Smelt
Sole
Trout
Tuna Fish
White Fish

Fruits

Apple
Apricot
Banana
Blackberry
Black Cap
Cantaloupe
Cherry
Cranberry
Currant
Date
Fig
Gooseberry
Grape
Grapefruit
Ground Cherry
Huckleberry
Lemon
Lime
Loganberry
Olive
Orange
Peach
Pear
Pineapple
Plum
Pomegranate
Prune
Quince
Raisin
Raspberry
Rhubarb
Strawberry
Watermelon

Meats

Beef
Beef Heart
Beef Tongue
Calves' Liver
Chicken
Duck
Goose
Lamb
Mutton
Pork
Rabbit
Turkey
Veal
Venison

Nuts

Almond
Black Walnut
Brazil Nut
Cashew Nut
Chestnut
Cocoanut
English Walnut
Filbert
Hickory Nut
Peanut
Pecan
Pistachio

Milk

Cheese
Cow's Milk
Cow's Milk (Albumin)
Cow's Milk (Casein)
Goat's Milk

Vegetables

Artichoke
Asparagus
Beet
Brussels Sprouts
Cabbage
Carrot
Casaba
Cauliflower
Celery
Cucumber
Curly Kale
Eggplant
Endive
Lentil
Lettuce
Lima Bean
Mushroom
Navy Bean
Onion
Parsely
Parsnip
Pea
Pimento
Potato
Pumpkin
Radish
Rutabaga
Soy Bean
Spinach
Squash
String Bean
Sweet Potato
Swiss Chard
Tomato
Turnip
Watercress
Wax Bean
Yam

Supply: Diagnostic—Ampules 1 cc with capillary tube for 25 tests; Packages of 1 or 6 assorted ampules.

Therapeutic—Sets of 5 vials, of 1, 2 or more proteins, in concentrations of 1–10, 1–50, 1–100, 1–1,000, 1–5,000.

Foods (Lederle)

Alligator Pear
Allspice
Almond
Anchovies
Anise Seed
Apple
Apricot
Artichoke
Asparagus
Banana
Barley
Bass
Coffee Bean
Kidney Bean
Lima Bean
Navy Bean
Soy Bean
String Bean
Beef
Beet
Blackberry
Black-eyed Pea
Black Pepper
Black Walnut
Blueberry
Bluefish
Brazil Nut
Broccoli
Brussels Sprouts
Buckwheat
Butterfish
Cabbage
Canary Seed
Cantaloupe
Caraway Seed
Carp
Carrot
Cashew Nut
Castor Bean
Catfish
Cauliflower
Caviar
Celery
Cherry
Chestnut
  (Spanish)
Chicken Meat
Chicory
Chive
Chocolate (Cocoa)
Cinnamon
Citron
Clam
Clove
Cocoanut
Codfish
Coffee Bean
Corn Meal
Corn, Sweet
Cow's Milk
Crab Meat
Cranberry
Cucumber
Currant, Red
Dandelion
Date
Dill Leaves
Duck Meat
Eel
Egg Plant
Egg White
Endive
English Walnut
Fig
Filbert
Flounder
Frog's Legs
Garlic
Ginger
Goat's Milk
Gooseberry
Goose Meat
Grape
Grapefruit Juice
Grapefruit Peel
Green Pea
Green Pepper
Guinea Hen Meat
Haddock
Halibut
Hazelnut
Herring
Hickory Nut
Honey Dew Melon
Hops
Horse Meat
Horse Radish
Huckleberry
Jerusalem
  Artichoke
Juniper Berry
Kale
Kidney Bean
Lake Trout
Lamb
Leek
Lemon Juice
Lemon Peel
Lentil
Lettuce
Lima Bean
Lima Juice
Lobster
Mace
Mackerel
Meal, Corn
Melon, Honey Dew
Milk (Cow's)
Milk (Goat's)
Mushroom
Mustard
Navy Bean
Nut:
  Black Walnut
  Cashew
  Chestnut
    (Spanish)
  Filbert
  Hickory
  Peanut
  Pecan
  Pignolia
  Pistachio
Nutmeg
Oat (Oatmeal)
Okra
Olive
Onion
Orange Juice
Oyster
Oyster Plant
Paprika
Parsley
Parsnip
Peach
Peach Skin
Peanut
Pear
Pecan
Pepper (Black)
Peppermint
Pepper (Green)
Pepper, Red
Perch
Pickerel
Pignolia Nut
Pike
Pineapple
Pistachio Nut
Plum
Pomegranate
Pompano
Poppy Seed
Pork
Potato, Sweet
Potato, White
Prune
Pumpkin
Quince
Radish
Radish, Horse
Raisin
Raspberry, Red
Red Currant
Red Pepper
Rhubarb
Rice
Rye
Sage
Salmon
Sardine
Scallion
Scallop
Sea Trout
Seed:
  Anise
  Caraway
  Poppy
Shad
Shad Roe
Shrimp
Smelt
Sole
Soy Bean
Spinach
Sprouts, Brussels
Squab
Squash
Squid
Starch, Corn
Strawberry
String Bean
Sugar Cane
Sweet Corn
Swiss Chard
Tangerine
Tapioca
Tea Leaf
Terrapin
Thyme
Tomato
Tuna Fish
Trout, Lake
Trout, Sea
Turkey Meat
Turnip
Vanilla
Walnut, English
Watercress
Watermelon
Weakfish
Wheat (Whole)
White Fish
White Potato
Whiting

Supply: DIAGNOSTIC—Special sets of 40 capillary tubes of individual allergens for 40 tests, by pressure, puncture or scratch method; Vials of 6 cc, diluted fluid extract; Capillary tubes, glycerolated—Packages of 5 and 50.

THERAPEUTIC—Vials of 6 cc, fluid extract, undiluted; Concentrated extract with bottles of 4½ cc sterile diluting fluid.

Foods **(Mulford)**

Almond
Apple
Apricot
Artichoke
Asparagus
Banana
Barley
Bean (Kidney)
Bean (Lima)
Bean (Navy)
Bean (String)
Beef
Beet
Blackberry
Buckwheat
Butternut
Cabbage
Cantaloupe
Carrot
Cauliflower
Celery
Cheese
Cherry
Chesnut
Chicken
Cinnamon
Clam
Cocoa
Cocoanut
Codfish
Coffee
Corn
Cottonseed
Crab
Cucumber
Duck
Eggplant
Egg Yolk
Egg White
Egg, Whole
Garlic
Ginger
Goose
Grape
Grapefruit
Haddock
Halibut
Herring
Hickory Nut
Lactalbumen
Lamb
Lemon
Lentil
Lettuce
Lobster
Mackerel
Milk (Casein), Cow
Mushroom
Mustard
Nutmeg
Oat
Okra
Onion
Orange
Oyster
Parsley
Parsnip
Paprika
Pea
Peach
Peanut
Pear
Pecan
Pepper (Black)
Pepper (Red)
Pepper (Sweet)
Pineapple
Plum
Pork
Potato
Prune
Pumpkin
Radish
Raisin
Raspberry
Rhubarb
Rice
Rye
Salmon
Shrimp
Sole
Soy Bean
Squash
Spinach
Strawberry
Sweet Potato
Swiss Chard
Tea
Tomato
Tuna Fish
Turnip
Veal
Walnut (English)
Walnut (Black)
Watermelon
Wheat

Supply: DIAGNOSTIC—Dried powder form, in Tube-vials 50 mg for about 25 tests; Packages of 1 single cutaneous outfit for 1 test.

THERAPEUTIC—Packages of one 5 cc vial, 500 protein units per cubic centimeter.

(National Drug)

Beverages

Cocoa
Coffee
Tea

Cereals

Barley
Buckwheat
Bran (Wheat)
Corn
Oatmeal
Rice
Rye
Wheat (Whole)

Cheese

American
Limburger
Roquefort
Swiss

Egg and Milk

Chicken Egg White
Chicken Egg Whole
Chicken Egg Yolk
Duck Egg
Milk (Cow)

Fruit

Apple
Apricot
Banana
Blackberry
Blueberry
Cantaloupe
Cherry
Cocoanut
Cranberry
Currant, red
Date
Elderberry
Fig
Grape
Grapefruit
Honey Ball
Honey-dew Melon
Huckleberry
Lemon
Lime
Olive
Orange
Peach
Pear
Pineapple
Plum
Prune
Raisin
Raspberry
Strawberry
Watermelon

Meats

Beef	Liver (Beef)
Calves' Brains	Pork
Chicken	Rabbit
Duck	Squab
Goose	Sweet Bread
Guinea Hen	Turkey
Kidney (Beef)	Veal
Lamb	

Nuts

Almond	Hickory
Brazil Nut	Peanut
Butternut	Pecan
Cashew Nut	Walnut (Black)
Chestnut	Walnut (English)
Filbert (Hazelnut)	

Sea Food

Anchovy	Halibut	Shrimp
Bass (Sea)	Herring	Smelts
Blue Fish	Lobster	Sole
Butterfish	Mackerel	Sturgeon
Carp	Oyster	Trout (Lake)
Caviar	Perch	Trout (Sea)
Clam	Porgies	Tuna Fish
Codfish	Salmon	Weakfish
Crab	Scallops	Whitefish
Flounder	Shad	
Haddock	Shadroe	

Spices

Aniseed	Paprika
Caraway Seed	Pepper (Black)
Cinnamon	Pepper (Red)
Clove	Poppy Seed
Ginger	Pimento (Allspice)
Mustard	Sage
Nutmeg	

Vegetables

Artichoke (Jerusalem)	Celery	Leek	Pepper (Green)
Asparagus	Chicory	Lentil	Potato (Sweet)
Bean (Kidney)	Chive	Lettuce	Potato (White)
Bean (Lima)	Cucumber	Mint	Pumpkin
Bean (Navy)	Dandelion	Mushroom	Radish
Bean (String)	Dill	Okra	Rhubarb
Beet	Egg Plant	Onion	Spinach
Broccoli	Garlic	Parsley	Squash
Cabbage	Horse Radish	Parsnip	Swiss Chard
Carrot	Kale	Pea (Black-eyed)	Tomato
Cauliflower	Kohlrabi	Pea (Green)	Turnip
			Watercress

Supply: DIAGNOSTIC (for scratch method)—Ampule-vials 1 cc.
THERAPEUTIC—Ampule-vials 5 cc, in dilutions as requested.

Foods **(Parke, Davis)**

Almond	Cantaloupe	Eggplant	Milk, Human
Apple	Carrot	English Walnut	Mutton
Apricot	Cauliflower	Fig	Oatmeal
Artichoke	Celery	Filbert	Onion
Asparagus	Cheese	Garlic	Orange
Banana	Cherry	Goose	Oyster
Barley	Chestnut	Grape	Parsley
Bean, Kidney	Chicken	Grapefruit	Parsnip
Bean, Lima	Chicory	Guinea Hen	Pea
Bean, Navy	Clam	Hazelnut	Peach
Bean, String	Cocoa	Hickory Nut	Peanut
Beef	Coffee	Hops	Pear
Beet	Corn	Kale	Pecan
Blackberry	Cottonseed	Lamb	Peppers, Sweet
Black Walnut	Crab	Lemon	Pineapple
Brazil Nut	Cucumber	Lentil	Plum
Brussels Sprouts	Duck	Lettuce	Pork
Buckwheat	Egg (all proteins)	Lobster	Prune
Butternut	Egg White	Milk, Cow's (all	Potato, Sweet
Cabbage	Egg Yolk	proteins)	Potato, White

Foods.—(*Continued*)

Pumpkin	Rutabaga	Squab	Turkey
Radish	Rye	Squash	Turnip
Raspberry	Scallop	Strawberry	Veal
Rhubarb	Shrimp	Tea	Watermelon
Rice	Spinach	Tomato	Wheat

Supply: DIAGNOSTIC—In glycerinated paste form, in collapsible tin tubes, for about fifty tests.

THERAPEUTIC—Supplied in graded dilutions, as ordered.

(Squibb)

Cereals		Milk	Egg
Barley	Rye	Cow's Milk (all proteins)	Egg (all proteins)
Buckwheat	Wheat	Cow's Milk Albumin	Egg Albumin
Corn	Wheat Gliadin	Cow's Milk Casein	Egg Yolk (all proteins)
Oats	Wheat Glutenin	Goat's Milk	Egg Yolk Globulins
Rice		Human Milk	Egg White (all proteins)

Sea Foods		Meat		Condiments
Bluefish	Pickerel	Beef	Lamb	Black Pepper
Butterfish	Salmon	Chicken	Mutton	Green Pepper
Clam	Scallops	Duck	Pheasant	Red Pepper
Codfish	Sea Bass	Frog's Legs	Pork	Ginger
Crab	Shad	Goat	Rabbit	Mustard
Haddock	Shad Roe	Goose	Sweetbreads	Paprika
Halibut	Shrimp	Guinea Hen	Turkey	Vanilla
Lobster	Smelt	Horse	Veal	
Mackerel	Sole			
Oyster	Whiting			

Fruits		Nuts	Vegetables	
Apple	Lemon	Almonds	Artichoke	Okra
Apricot	Olive (ripe)	Black Walnut	Asparagus	Onion
Banana	Orange	Brazil Nut	Beet	Parsnip
Blackberry	Peach	Butternut	Cabbage	Pea
Cantaloupe	Pear	Chestnut	Carrot	Potato (Sweet)
Cherry	Pineapple	English Walnut	Cauliflower	Potato (White)
Date	Plum	Filbert	Celery	Pumpkin
Fig	Prune	Hazel Nut	Cucumber	Radish
Grape	Raspberry	Hickory Nut	Egg Plant	Rhubarb
Grapefruit	Strawberry	Peanut	Kidney Bean	Spinach
Huckleberry	Watermelon	Pecan	Lentil	Squash
			Lettuce	String Bean
			Lima Bean	Swiss Chard
			Mushroom	Tomato
			Navy Bean	Turnip

Beverages

Cocoa
Coffee
Tea

Supply: DIAGNOSTIC—Fruits, beverages, condiments—Vials of 25 mg of powdered extract. All other foods—Vials of 50 mg.

THERAPEUTIC—Diagnostic cases containing 12, 24 or 50 individual allergen vials, assorted.

FURS

(Arlington)

Alaska Seal	Caracul	Monkey	Raccoon
Russian Hare	Chinese Dog	Muskrat (Hudson Seal)	Skunk
Australian Opposum	Fox	Nutria	Squirrel
Badger	Kolinsky	Opposum, American	Wolf
Bear	Leopard	Opposum, Ringtail	
Beaver	Marmot	Otter	

Supply: DIAGNOSTIC—Vials 15 mg powdered extract—Packages of 1 or 6.
THERAPEUTIC—Standardized treatment sets for desensitization.

(Hollister-Stier)

Beaver	Mink	Opossum (American)	Seal (Alaska)
Chamois Skin	Mole	Opossum (Australian)	Skunk
Fox	Muskrat	Raccoon	Squirrel

Supply: DIAGNOSTIC—Ampules 1 cc with capillary tubes for 25 tests; Packages of 1 or 6 assorted ampules.
TREATMENT—Sets of 5 vials of 1, 2 or more proteins, in concentrations of 1–10, 1–50, 1–100, 1–1,000, 1–5,000.

(National Drug)

Beaver	Lamb (Persian)	Muskrat	Raccoon
Caracul	Leopard	Nutria	Seal (Alaskan)
Chinese	Marmot	Opossum	Seal (Hudson)
Fox	Mink	Pony	Skunk
Kolinsky	Mole	Rabbit	Squirrel

Supply: DIAGNOSTIC (for scratch method)—Ampule-vials 1 cc.
THERAPEUTIC—Ampule-vials 5 cc, in dilutions as requested..

(Squibb)

Beaver	Kolinsky	Mole	Raccoon
Caracul	Lamb (Persian)	Opossum	Squirrel
Civet Cat	Leopard	Pony	Skunk
Fitch	Mink	Persian Cat (Angora)	Seal (Alaskan)
Fox	Muskrat	Rabbit Fur	Seal (Hudson)

Supply: DIAGNOSTIC—Vials 25 mg of powdered extract—Boxes of 12, 24 or 50 assorted vials.

POLLENS

(Abbott)

Ragweed Group		Carelessweed Group	Goosefoot Group
Short Ragweed	Marsh Elder	Pigweed (Redroot)	Lamb's Quarters
Giant Ragweed	Burweed Marsh Elder	Spiny Amaranth	Burning Bush
Western Ragweed	False Ragweed	Palmer's Amaranth	Russian Thistle
Southern Ragweed	Slender False Ragweed	Water Hemp	
Cocklebur			

Wormwood Group	Grass Group		Others	
Annual Sage	Bluegrass	Bermuda Grass	Red Sorrel	Oak
Biennial Sage	Timothy	Johnson Grass	English Plantain	Sycamore
Prairie Sage	Orchard Grass	Sweet Vernal Grass	Hemp	Ash
Sagebrush	Redtop		Yellow Dock	Hickory
			Cottonwood	Walnut
			Box Elder	Corn

Supply: DIAGNOSTIC—Vials of 3 or 25 capillary tubes of each pollen.

Graminae

(Arlington)

Timothy	Meadow Fescue	Western Wheat Grass
June Grass	Rough Stalked Meadow Grass	Tall Oat Grass
Orchard Grass		Velvet Grass (Mesquite Grass)
Red Top	Bermuda Grass	Indian Rice
Sweet Vernal Grass	Johnson Grass	Rye
Rye Grass (Ray Grass)	Sudan Grass	Wheat
Quack Grass	Sorghum	Oat
Red Fescue	Western June Grass	Corn

Chenopodiaceae

Burning Bush
Goosefoot
Mexican Tea
Shad Scale
Orach
Greasewood
Burroweed
Winter Fat
Sea Blite
Russian Thistle

Amaranthaceae

Pigweed
Carelessweed
Spiny Amaranth
Western Water Hemp

Leguminosae

Alfalfa
Clover
Sweet Clover

Compositae

Ambrosiaceae

Ragweed Short or Common
Ragweed Giant
Ragweed Western
Ragweed Western Giant
Slender Ragweed
Bur Ragweed
Prairie Ragweed
Poverty Weed
Marsh Elder (Iva ciliata "Wild")
Marsh Elder (Iva oraria "Bartlett")
Cocklebur

Carduaceae

Sage Brush (Artemisia tridentata "Nutt")
Sage Brush (Artemisia bigelovii)
Hill Sage
Carpet Sage
Prairie Sage
California Mugwort (California Sage)
Mugwort
Indian Wormwood
Silvery Wormwood
Sunflower
Goldenglow
Dahlia
Aster
Aster, China
Daisy Ox-eye
Yellow Daisy
Thistle
Fleabane
Goldenrod
Cosmos

Cichoriaceae

Dandelion

Trees **(Arlington)**

Pinaceae

Pine
Pine, Bull (Rock Pine)
Pine, Knob-cone
Mountain Cedar

Salicaceae

Willow
Willow, Pussy
Poplar (Cottonwood) (Populus deltoides)
Cottonwood Arizona
Poplar (Cottonwood) (Populus Eugeni)
Cottonwood, California
Cottonwood, Narrow-leaved
Cottonwood, Western

Juglandaceae

Hickory
Pecan
Black Walnut
Arizona Walnut
Walnut, California Black
Walnut, English
Butternut

Betulaceae

Birch, White
Birch, Black
Hazelnut Corylus (americana)
Hazelnut Corylus (avellana)
Blue Beach (Hornbeam)
Alder (alnus incana)
Alder (alnus sinuata)

Fagaceae

Oak, White
Live Oak
Oak, Mesa
Oak, Red
Oak, Scrub
Oak, Black

Ulmaceae

Elm

Platanaceae

Sycamore (Platanus racemosa "Nutt")
Sycamore (Platanus occidentalis)

Rosaceae

Apple

Leguminosae

Locust
Acacia (Acacia florabunda)
Acacia (Acacia scapulaformis)
Acacia (Acacia longifolia)

Simarubiaceae

Tree of Heaven

Aceraceae

Maple
Oregon Maple
Box Elder (Ash-leaved Maple)

Oleaceae

White Ash
Arizona Ash
Ash
Olive

Hippocastanceae

Horse Chestnut

Tilliaceae

Linden (Basswood)

Other Plants

Cat-tail Flag
Sweet Gale
Hemp
Dock
Dock, Curly or Yellow
Mesquite Prosopis
Ginkgo
Sweet Gum
Knotweed
California Poppy
Joe-pye Weed
Rose
Wild Carrot
Privet
English Plantain
Hackberry

Supply: Diagnostic—Capillary tubes of each pollen, in concentrated solution—Vials 1 cc (for about 15 tests).

Therapeutic—Standardized single pollen treatment sets for desensitization.

Pollens: **(Cutter)**

Alkali Weed
All Scale
Annual Saltbrush
Ash
Bermuda Grass
Black Walnut
Box Elder
Burning Bush or Mexican Firebush
Canary Grass
Careless Weed
Cocklebur
Corn
Cottonwood
Foxtail or Squirrel Tail
Johnson Grass
June Grass
Lambs Quarter
Marsh Elder
Mountain Cedar
Mugwort or Wormwood
Oak
Olive
Orchard Grass
Pigweed, Red Root
Plantain
Ragweed, Common
Ragweed, False
Ragweed, Giant
Ragweed, Western
Red Top
Rye Grass
Russian Thistle
Sage, Coast
Sagebrush, Mountain
Shad Scale
Timothy Grass
Tumbleweed
Velvet Grass
Western Water Hemp
Wild Oat Grass

Supply: Diagnostic—Separate capillary tubes of each extract.

Therapeutic—Single pollen treatment sets containing over 60,000 pollen units; Combined pollens—where requested.

Bottles 5 cc of dilutions: 1–10,000, 1–1,000, 1–100 or 1–33⅓ of single or combined pollens.

Grasses **(Hollister-Stier)**

Timothy
Red Top
Koeler's Grass
Orchard Grass
Kentucky Blue Grass
Sandberg's June Grass
Smooth Brome Grass
Cheat
Quack Grass
Corn
Perennial Rye Grass
Bermuda Grass
Sweet Vernal Grass
Tall Oat Grass
Velvet Grass
Annual June Grass
Canada Blue Grass
Soft Cheat
Giant Rye Grass
Blue Bunch Grass
Wheat
Squirrel Tail
Italian Rye Grass
Alkali Rye Grass
Crab Grass
Sudan Grass
Mediterranean Canary Grass
Dallis Grass
Cultivated Barley
Wild Oat
Slender Wild Oat
Needle or Thread Grass
Rye
Sheep's Fescue
Western Rye Grass
Small Flowered Melica
Ripgut Grass
Barnyard Grass
Wall Barley
Nodding Stipa
Darnell Grass
Johnson Grass
California Brome Grass

Trees **(Hollister-Stier)**

Yellow Pine
Hazelnut
Spring Birch
Aspen
Carolina Poplar
Black Cottonwood
Willow
Alder
Box Elder
Garry's Oak
California Black Oak
Ash
English Walnut
Black Walnut
Red Fir
Tamarack
Eucalyptus
California Sycamore
Acacia
Live Oak
Sycamore
Cedar
Juniper
Olive

Weeds **(Hollister-Stier)**

Nettle
Sheep Sorrel
Yellow Dock
Green Dock
Cocklebur
Atriplex
Silvery Atriplex
Greasewood
Lamb's Quarters
Russian Thistle
Bract-scale
Dandelion
Eastern Ragweed
Giant Ragweed
False Western Ragweed
Western Ragweed
Giant Poverty Weed
Small Poverty Weed
Common Sagebrush
Green Sagebrush
Mugwort
White Sagebrush
Mexican Tea
English Plantain
Redroot Pigweed
Tumbleweed Pigweed
Prostrate Pigweed
Careless Weed

Miscellaneous **(Hollister-Stier)**

Goldenrod
Sugar Beet
Castor Bean
Rose
Sunflower
Alfalfa
Red Clover
Sweet Clover
Scotch Brome

Supply: Diagnostic—Ampules ½ cc with capillary tube—in test sets for each district.

Therapeutic—Treatment Sets of 1 or more pollens comprising 20 prophylactic preseasonal graduated doses and 10 maximum seasonal doses; Treatment Sets comprising 5 vials of 1 or more pollens in concentrations of 20, 100, 1,000, 5,000 and 1,000 units per cubic centimeter; Mixed Pollen Treatment Sets for individual districts.

Pollens **(Lederle)**

Annual Saltbush
Arizona Ash
Arizona Walnut
Bermuda Grass
Black Walnut
Careless Weed
Cocklebur
Cottonwood
Giant Ragweed
Green Sage
Johnson Grass
June Grass
Lamb's Quarters
Marsh Elder
Mountain Cedar
Mugwort
Oak
Olive
Orchard Grass
Pasture Sage
Pecan
Perennial Rye Grass
Plantain
Prostrate Pigweed
Rabbit Bush
Ragweed
Ragweed, Giant
Ragweed, Slender
Ragweed, Southwestern
Ragweed, Western
Redroot Pigweed
Redtop
Russian Thistle
Sage Brush
Sage, Green
Sage, Pasture
Shad Scale
Sheep Sorrel
Slender Ragweed
Southwestern Ragweed
Spiny Amaranth
Summer Cypress
Sweet Vernal Grass
Timothy
Walnut, Arizona
Walnut, Black
Western Ragweed
Western Water Hemp
Yellow Dock

Supply: Diagnostic—Vial for 3 tests, with scarifier.

Therapeutic—Sets containing vials of antigen and of diluent as follows:

Complete treatment set—Doses 1–15: Series A—Doses 1–5; Series B—Doses 6–10; Series C—Doses 11–15; Series D—5 Doses of 15.

(Mulford)

Alder
Alfalfa
Apple
Ash
Ash, Arizona
Aster
Barnyard Grass
Bermuda Grass
Birch
Blue Beech
Boneset
Box Elder
Brome Grass
Burning Bush
Burweed Marsh Elder
Buttercup
Canary Grass
Careless Weed
Cedar
Cedar, Mountain
Chrysanthemum
Clover, Red
Clover, Sweet
Cocklebur
Corn
Cosmos
Cottonwood
Crab Grass
Dahlia
Daisy
Dandelion
Dock
Elm
Fescue Grass
Goldenglow
Goldenrod
Hickory
Johnson Grass
June Grass (Blue Grass)

Lamb's Quarters
Maple
Marsh
Mesquite
Milo Maize
Mexican Tea
Mock Orange
Mugwort
Mugwort, California
Oak
Oats
Oats, Wild
Olive
Orchard Grass
Pawpaw
Peach
Pecan
Pine
Plantain, Common
Plantain, English
Poverty Weed
Privet
Quack Grass
Rabbit Brush
Ragweed
Ragweed, False
Ragweed, High
Ragweed, Low
Ragweed, Slender
Ragweed, Western
Ragweed, Western Giant
Redtop
Redroot-Pigweed
Rose
Russian Thistle
Rye
Rye Perennial
Sage, Annual
Sage, Coast
Sage, Dragon
Sage, Pasture
Sage, Prairie
Sagebrush
Sagewort
Salt Bush
Saw Grass
Shad Scale
Sheep Sorrel
Spring Amaranth
Sudan Grass
Sugar Beet
Sunflower
Sweet Vernal
Sycamore
Timothy
Velvet Grass
Walnut, Arizona
Walnut, Black
Walnut, English
Water Hemp
Wheat
Willow
Winter Grass
Wormwood
Yellow Foxtail Grass

Supply: DIAGNOSTIC—Tube-vials, 50 mg of dried substance, for 25 tests—Packages of 1 or 12;
Packages of single cutaneous outfit for 1 test.
Packages of 3 tube-points of concentrated extract for 3 tests.
THERAPEUTIC—Vials 5 cc of 2,000 or 20,000 units of pollen extract per cubic centimeter.

Some of the pollen extracts are available as follows:
15 syringe or vial treatment (5 to 5,000 pollen units).
Series 1—5 syringes or vials, first 5 doses (5–60 pollen units).
Series 2—5 syringes or vials, second 5 doses (100–1,000 pollen units).
Series 3—5 syringes or vials, third 5 doses (1,500–5,000 pollen units).
Series 4—5 syringes or vials, fourth 5 doses (supplementary treatment, 6,000–10,000 pollen units).

{Spring hay fever group—sweet vernal, June or Kentucky blue grass, orchard, timothy, red top and rye grasses.
Fall hay fever group—giant and dwarf ragweeds.}

{Birch, Black Walnut}

{Cottonwood, Elder}

{Maple, Oak}

{Poplar, Willow}

{White Ash, Yellow Pine}

{Daisy, Primrose}

{Rose, Burning Bush}

{Johnson Grass, Golden Rod}

{June Grass, Timothy}

{Orchard Grass, Rye}

{Sweet Clover, Field Corn}

{Pigweed (Redroot), False Ragweed (Bur Ragweed)}

{Red Top, Wormwood} (National Drug)

{Pasture Sage (Carpet Sage), Green Sage}

{Sheep Sorrel, Sweet Vernal}

{Russian Thistle, Yellow Dock}

{Black Ash, Privet}

{Aster, Cosmos}

{Beech, Shagbark Hickory}

Cocklebur Lamb's Quarters	Plantain, large or giant Plantain, dwarf or small	Apple Cedar
Sycamore Scrub Oak	Prairie Ragweed Western Ragweed	Cultivated Rye Alfalfa
English Oak Pin Oak	Bermuda Grass Pigweed	Gama Grass Flat Cat Tail
Austrian Pine Elm	Winter Fat Fescue Grass	

Supply: DIAGNOSTIC—Packages of 2 tubes (for 2 tests of pollens, grouped as above). Packages of 10 tubes (10 tests of 1 pollen).

THERAPEUTIC—Series "AA" Ampule-vials 5 cc or 15 cc, 25 N-units per cubic centimeter.

Series "A" Ampule-vials 5 cc or 15 cc, 50 N-units per cubic centimeter.

Series "B" Ampule-vials 5 cc or 15 cc, 100 N-units per cubic centimeter.

Pollen Allergens, Glycerinated Pastes **(Parke, Davis)**

Alfalfa
Aster
Barnyard Grass
Bermuda Grass
Burweed
Chestnut
Clover, White
Cocklebur
Corn
Cosmos
Crab Grass
Dahlia
Daisy, Ox-eye
Daisy, Yellow
Dandelion
Goldenrod
Goose-foot, White
Halberd-leaved Orache
Indian Hair Tonic
Johnson Grass
June Grass
Juniper
Maple
Marigold
Mugwort (wormwood)
Oak
Oats
Orchard Grass
Pine
Plantain
Poplar, Lombarde
Prairie Sage
Ragweed, Common
Ragweed, Giant
Ragweed, Western
Rose
Rough Marsh Elder
Russian Thistle
Rye
Sagebrush
Sunflower
Sweet Vernal Grass
Timothy
Waterhemp, Western
Wheat
Willow
Wormwood (Mugwort)
Wormwood Sage
Yarrow
Yellow Dock

Supply: DIAGNOSTIC—Collapsible tin tubes for about 50 tests.

THERAPEUTIC—Supplied in graded dilutions, as ordered.

Pollen Allergens, Soluble Powder Extracts **(Squibb)**

Ash (White)
Black Walnut
Corn
Goldenrod
Hickory
Johnson Grass
June Grass
Oak (White)
Orchard Grass
Pine (White)
Poplar
Ragweed, Giant
Ragweed, Dwarf (Common)
Ragweed Mixed (Giant and Dwarf)
Rye
Timothy

Supply: DIAGNOSTIC—Vials of 25 mg—Cases of 12, 24 or 50 assorted vials.

Pollen Allergen Solutions, Glycerol Form **(Squibb)**

Early Spring

Ash (White Ash)
Ash (Oregon)
Black Walnut
California Black Walnut
Dandelion
Oak (White Oak)
Cottonwood
  Necklace Poplar

Summer

Annual Salt Bush (Orach)
Bermuda Grass (Scutch or Scotch Grass)
Corn (Maize, Indian Corn)
English Plantain (Buckthorn, Rib Grass)

Grasses Combined (equal parts of Bermuda Grass, June Grass, Orchard Grass, Red Top, Timothy)
Johnson Grass (Guinea Grass)
June Grass (Blue Grass, Kentucky Blue Grass)
Orchard Grass
Perennial Rye Grass
Red Top (Silk Grass)
Sweet Vernal Grass (Sweet Scented Vernal Grass)
Timothy (Cat Tail, Herd's Grass)

Autumn

Cocklebur (Clotbur)
Goldenrod
Marsh Elder
Mugwort (Sagewort)
Ragweed, Giant and Dwarf combined)
Ragweed, Giant
Ragweed, Dwarf
Russian Thistle
Sage Brush (Black Sage, Wormwood)
Slender Ragweed
Western Weeds Combined (equal parts of Marsh Elder, Mugwort, Sagebush, Slender Ragweed and Western Ragweed)

Supply: DIAGNOSTIC—Packages of 2 tubes, of any single pollen. Packages of 6 vials of 2 tubes each, assorted pollens. Vaccine syringes 1 cc, graduation 1–100 cc.
THERAPEUTIC—Vials 5 cc, containing 0.025 mg pollen-N per cubic centimeter.

(Terrell)

Alfalfa
Bermuda Grass
Box Elder
Cocklebur
Cottonwood
Dahlia
English Plantain
Goldenrod
June Grass
Marsh Elder
Mountain Cedar
Oak (Mixed)
Oriental Sycamore
Pasture Sage
Rabbit Bush
Rose
Russian Thistle
Shad Scale
Short Ragweed
Spiny Amaranth
Sudan Grass
Sweet Vernal Grass
Velvet Grass
Western Water Hemp
Yellow Dock
Annual Salt Bush
Black Walnut
Careless Weed
Corn
Crab Grass
Elm
Ralse Ragweed
Johnson Grass
Lamb's Quarters
Mesquite
Mugwort
Orchard Grass
Orris Root
Perennial Rye Grass
Red Top Grass
Rough Pigweed
Sage Brush
Sheep Sorrel
Slender Ragweed
Southern Ragweed
Sunflower
Timothy Grass
Western Ragweed
Willow

Supply: Single extracts only for treatment. Individual orders, in dilutions of 1:100, to 1:40,000; In bulk of 5 cc and upwards; In dropping bottles of 1 cc.

Miscellaneous Substances

(Abbott)

Cigarette Smoke
Corn Silk
Corn Smit (spores)
Cotton
Cottonseed
Flaxseed
Henna Leaves
Kapok
Orris Root
Pyrethrum
Silk
Tobacco

Supply: DIAGNOSTIC—Vial of 3 capillary tubes; Vial of 25 capillary tubes.

(Arlington)

Beef Serum
Boxwood
Cotton
Cotton Seed
Dust
Flaxseed
Gelatin
Glue
Henna
Hops
Horse Serum
Horse Meat
Jack Bean
Juniper
Kapok
Lycopodium
Orris Root
Pyrethrum
Red Cedar
Senna
Silk
Soy Bean
Tobacco
Vanilla
Yeast (Fleischmann)

Supply: DIAGNOSTIC—Powder form, in glass vials 50 mg (some in tubes of 25 mg, henna in tubes of 10 mg)—Packages of 1 or 6.

THERAPEUTIC—Standardized treatment sets for desensitization.

(Hollister-Stier)

Arrow Root	Hemp	Pyrethrum
Binding Twine	Henna	Rayon
Cedar	Jute	Silk
Cocoanut fibre	Kapok	Tamarack
Cotton	Orris Root	Tobacco
Cottonseed	Poison Ivy	White Pine
Flaxseed	Poison Oak	Yellow Pine
Fir	Primrose	

Supply: DIAGNOSTIC—Ampule 1 cc, with capillary tube (for 25 tests); Packages of 1 or 6 assorted; Complete test sets.

THERAPEUTIC—Sets of 5 vials (each containing 1, 2 or more proteins), of following concentrations—1:10, 1:50, 1:100, 1:1,000, 1:5,000.

(Lederle)

Alfalfa	Henna	Pyrethrum
Cotton Seed	Horse Serum	Tobacco
Dust, House	Kapok Seed	Wool
Flax Seed	Lycopodium	Control Tests
Glue (Fish)	Orris	Silk (silk worm)

Supply: DIAGNOSTIC—Capillary tubes of glycerolated extract—Packages of 5 and 50; Vials 6 cc of glycerolated extract, diluted.

THERAPEUTIC—Vials 6 cc of glycerolated extract, undiluted; Concentrated extracts with bottles of 4½ cc sterile dilution.

(Mulford)

Dust	Rice Powder (Polish)	Pyrethrum
Flaxseed	Silk (Extract only)	Tobacco
Orris Root	Kapok Seed	

Supply: DIAGNOSTIC—Tube—Vials 50 mg powdered extract, for about 25 tests. Packages of single cutaneous outfit, for 1 test.

(National Drug)

Beef Serum	Henna	Rayon
Cotton Seed	Hops	Rice Powder (Polishings)
Dust (House)	Horse Serum	Silk
Flaxseed	Kapok	Soy Bean
Gelatin	Lycopodium	Tobacco
Glue (Animal)	Orris Root	Vanilla
Glue (Fish)	Pyrethrum	Yeast (Fleischmann)

Supply: DIAGNOSTIC—Ampule-vials 1 cc (for scratch method).

THERAPEUTIC—Ampule-vials 5 cc, in dilutions, as requested.

(Parke, Davis)

Black Pepper	Orris Root	Serum, Beef
Cotton	Paprika	Serum, Horse
Ginger	Peptone	Silk
Kapok	Red Pepper	Tobacco
Mustard	Sage	

Supply: DIAGNOSTIC—Collapsible tin tubes, in glycerinated paste form, for about 50 tests.

THERAPEUTIC—Supplied in graded dilutions.

(Squibb)

Cheese	Flaxseed (Linseed)	Serum Horse
Cocoanut	Glue (Le Page)	Silk
Cotton Seed	Hay (Alfalfa)	Tobacco
Dust (House)	Orris Root	Yeast (all proteins)
Dust (Street)	Serum Beef	

Supply: DIAGNOSTIC—Vials 25 mg of powdered extract; Diagnostic cases containing 12, 24 or 50 individual allergen vials, assorted.

Part II

Allergens

Groups

Bacterials **(Parke, Davis)**

Group XX
- Bac. coli.
- Gonococcus
- Staph. aureus
- Staph. albus
- Staph. citreus

Group XXI
- Bac. Friedlander
- Mic. catarrhalis
- Mic. tetragenus
- Pseudodiphtheria

Group XXII
- Pneumococcus, I, II, III
- Strept. hemolyticus
- Strept. non-hemolyticus

Group XXIII
- B. Typhosus
- B. Paratyphosus "A"
- B. Paratyphosus "B"

Supply: Diagnostic—Collapsible tin tubes of glycerinated paste extract for about 50 tests, 1 tube for each numbered group.

(Squibb)

Group XXV
- B. Coli
- B. Diphtheroid
- B. Gonococcus
- B. Influenzae
- B. Pertussis
- B. Typhosus

Group XXVI
- Micrococcus catarrhalis
- Pneumococcus I
- Pneumococcus II
- Pneumococcus III
- Pneumococcus IV

Group XXVII
- Staph. aureus
- Staph. albus
- Staph. citreus
- Streptococcus (polyvalent)
- Strep. pyogenes
- Strep. viridans

Supply: Diagnostic—Vials of 25 mg of powdered extract, 1 for each numbered group; Cases of 12, 24 or 50 assorted vials.

Epidermals (Parke, Davis)

Group XXIV
- Cat Hair
- Cattle Hair
- Dog Hair
- Horse Hair

Group XXV
- Goat Hair
- Guinea-pig Hair
- Rabbit Hair
- Sheep Wool

Group XXVI
- Chicken Feathers
- Duck Feathers
- Goose Feathers

Supply: Diagnostic—Collapsible tin tubes of glycerinated paste extract, for about 50 tests, 1 tube for each numbered group.

Hair and Dander **(Squibb)**

Group XXI
- Cat
- Cow
- Dog
- Horse
- Rabbit

Supply: Diagnostic—Vials of 25 mg of powdered extract; Cases of 12, 24 or 50 vials.

Feathers **(Squibb)**

Group XXII
- Chicken
- Duck
- Goose

Supply: Diagnostic—Vials of 25 mg of powdered extract; Cases of 12, 24 or 50 vials.

Furs (Squibb)

Group XXVIII	*Group XXIX*	*Group XXX*
Beaver	Civet Cat	Kolinsky
Mole	Fox	Pony
Muskrat	Leopard	Raccoon
Opposum	Mink	Seal (Alaska)
Squirrel	Persian Cat (Angora)	Seal (Hudson)
		Skunk

Supply: DIAGNOSTIC—Vials of 25 mg of powdered extract, 1 for each numbered group;
Cases of 12, 24 or 50 assorted vials.

Inhalants (Lederle)

Series I

House Dust	Dog Dander	Cat Dander
Kapok	Cow Dander	Camel Dander
Rabbit Dander	Horse Dander	Tobacco
Feathers	Goat Dander	Horse Serum
Orris Root	Fish Glue	Pyrethrum
Cotton Seed	Flaxseed	Sheep Dander (Wool)

Supply: DIAGNOSTIC—Vials 6 cc packages of 18, in strengths for intracutaneous testing.

Foods (Lederle)

Series II

Egg White	Chicken Meat	Pork
Milk	Corn Meal	Rice
Wheat	Rye	Green Pea
Beef	Lima Bean	Spinach
Lamb	Orange	Chocolate (Cocoa)
White Potato	Mustard	Almond

Series III

English Walnut	Oyster	Celery
Cherry	Oat	Tomato
Peanut	Barley	String Bean
Crab	Buckwheat	Banana
Cod	Carrot	Grape Fruit
Flounder	Cabbage	Peach

Supply: DIAGNOSTIC—Vials 6 cc of each series, in packages of 18, in strengths for intracutaneous testing.

(Parke, Davis)

Meats:	**Egg and Milk:**	**Fowl:**	**Shell Fish:**
Group I	*Group II*	*Group V*	*Group VI*
Beef	Milk of Cow (all proteins)	Chicken	Clam
Lamb	Egg (all proteins)	Duck	Oyster
Pork	Cheese	Goose	Shrimp
Veal	Human Milk	Turkey	Scallop
Mutton		Squab	Lobster
		Guinea-Hen	Crab

Vegetables:

Group VII	*Group VIII*	*Group IX*	*Group X*
White Potato	Kidney Bean	Beet	Cabbage
Sweet Potato	Lima Bean	Asparagus	Cauliflower
Eggplant	Navy Bean	Onion	Radish
Tomato	String Bean	Spinach	Rutabaga
Sweet Pepper	Peas	Garlic	Turnip
	Lentil		

Group XI	Group XIV	Group XXXIII	**Seasonings:** Group XXVII
Pumpkin	Artichoke	Carrot	Black Pepper
Squash	Chicory	Celery	Mustard
Cucumber	Lettuce	Parsnip	Ginger
Cantaloupe	Buckwheat	Parsley	Red Pepper
Watermelon	Rhubarb		Paprika
			Sage

Fruits:

Group XVI	Group XVII	Group XVIII	**Beverages:** Group XIX
Apple	Apricot	Orange	Coffee
Pear	Plum	Lemon	Tea
Strawberry	Peach	Grapefruit	Cocoa
Blackberry	Prune	Banana	
Raspberry	Cherry	Pineapple	
Fig		Grape	

Nuts:

Group XII	Group XIII	**Cereals:** Group XV
Chestnut	Black Walnut	Wheat
Peanut	English Walnut	Rye
Brazil Nut	Hickory Nut	Barley
Almond	Butternut	Corn
Filbert	Pecan	Oatmeal
Hazelnut		Rice

Supply: Diagnostic—Collapsible tin tubes of glycerinated extract for about 50 tests, 1 for each numbered group.

(Squibb)

Vegetables:

Group I	Group II	Group III
Beet	Cabbage	Artichoke
Carrot	Celery	Asparagus
Parsnip	Lettuce	Cauliflower
Radish	Onion	Rhubarb
Turnip	Spinach	String Bean

Group IV	Group V	Group Va
Cucumber	Kidney Bean	Mushroom
Egg Plant	Lentil	Okra
Pumpkin	Lima Bean	Potato (Sweet)
Squash	Navy Bean	Potato (White)
Tomato	Pea	Swiss Chard

Fruits:

Group VI	Group VII	Group VIII	Group VIIIa
Apricot	Cantaloupe	Apple	Blackberry
Cherry	Grapefruit	Banana	Grape
Peach	Lemon	Fig	Huckleberry
Plum	Orange	Pear	Raspberry
Prune	Watermelon	Pineapple	Strawberry

Nuts:

Group IX		Group X	
Almond	Hazel Nut	Black Walnut	Hickory Nut
Chestnut	Peanut	Brazil Nut	Pecan
Filbert		English Walnut	

Cereals:

Group XI

Barley
Buckwheat
Corn
Oats
Rice
Wheat

Meats:

Group XII

Beef
Goat
Horse
Mutton
Pork

Group XIII

Frog Legs
Lamb
Sweetbread
Rabbit
Veal

Fowl:

Group XIV

Chicken
Duck
Goose
Guinea Hen
Turkey

Fish:

Group XV

Bluefish
Codfish
Haddock
Halibut
Mackerel

Group XVI

Butterfish
Salmon
Sea Bass
Sole
Whiting

Mollusks:

Group XVII

Clam
Crab
Lobster
Oyster
Scallops
Shrimp

Condiments:

Group XVIII

Black Pepper
Ginger
Mustard
Paprika
Vanilla

Beverages:

Group XIX

Cocoa
Coffee
Tea

Egg and Milk:

Group XX

Egg (all proteins)
Cow's Milk (all proteins)
Goat's Milk (all proteins)

Supply: DIAGNOSTIC—Vials 25 mg, each representing 1 numbered group; Diagnostic cases of 12, 24 or 50 assorted vials.

POLLENS

Ragweed Pollen Extract: **(Abbott)**

Containing 50 % Short and 50 % Giant Ragweed, in isotonic dextrose solution, a stable painless menstruum; for the prevention and treatment of Fall hay-fever (August and September).

Supply: Standardized Treatment Sets, for direct injection, 16 doses, each in rubber-stoppered vial, with vial of three ⅜ gr capsules of ephedrine hydrochloride in each set.

Dosages:

No. 1— 5 units	No. 6— 100 units	No. 11—1,500 units
No. 2—10 units	No. 7— 200 units	No. 12—2,000 units
No. 3—20 units	No. 8— 400 units	No. 13—3,000 units
No. 4—40 units	No. 9— 700 units	No. 14—3,500 units
No. 5—70 units	No. 10—1,000 units	No. 15—4,000 units
Packages of 1 Extra Dose.		Extra Dose—4,000 units

Mixed Grass Pollen Extract: **(Abbott)**

Containing equal quantities of extracts of timothy, bluegrass, orchard grass, redtop and sweet vernal grass, in isotonic dextrose solution; for the prevention and treatment of grass hay fever (May to July).

Supply: Standardized Treatment Sets, as above 16 doses; Packages of 1 Extra Dose (4,000 units).

Skin Test Sets, Diagnostic: (Abbott)

Assortment A (for Central and Northeastern States)—contains elm, oak, bluegrass, timothy, redtop, short and giant ragweed.
Assortment B (for Rocky Mountain States)—contains bluegrass, timothy, Russian thistle, burweed, marsh elder, short and giant ragweed, sagebrush.
Assortment C (for Southeastern States)—contains mountain cedar, elm, oak, Bermuda grass, Johnson grass, short and giant ragweed.
Assortment D (for Southwestern States)—contains cottonwood, ash, Bermuda grass, Palmer's amaranth, Russian thistle, giant ragweed, western ragweed.

Supply: Sets of 7 vials of 3 capillary tubes each.

Prescription Sets, Therapeutic: (Abbott)

Containing any single pollen or combination of pollens.

Supply: Sets of one 2 cc vial of 3% concentrated extract (single variety or mixed as prescribed) and 4 vials of diluent for making 4 decimal dilutions.

Pollen Mixtures: (Arlington)

Grass Mixture: June grass, orchard grass, timothy and red top.
Grass Mixture: June grass, orchard grass, timothy, red top and sweet vernal grass.
Grass Mixture: Bermuda grass and Johnson grass.
Ragweed Mixture: ragweed dwarf and ragweed giant.
Ragweed Mixture with cocklebur.
Ragweed Mixture with goldenrod.
Ragweed Mixture plus burweed marsh elder.
Triple Ragweeds: Ragweed dwarf, ragweed giant and western ragweed.
Ambrosia Mixture: Ragweed short, ragweed giant, western ragweed, burweed marsh elder, cocklebur.
Rocky Mountain Mixture: Western ragweed, bur ragweed, prairie ragweed, sage brush, carpet sage and prairie sage.
California Mixture: California mugwort, hill sage, poverty weed, indian wormwood, bur ragweed and western ragweed.
Artemisia Mixture: Sage brush, prairie sage, carpet sage and indian wormwood.

Tree Mixtures:

Alder Mixture
Birch Mixture
Cottonwood-Poplar Mixture
Hazelnut Mixture
Hickory Mixture
Hickory-Pecan Mixture
Maple Mixture
Oak Mixture
Pine Mixture
Walnut Butternut Mixture

Supply: Standardized treatment sets of each mixture, for desensitization.

Spring Mixed (Cutter)

Bermuda Grass
Black Walnut
Cottonwood
Johnson Grass
June Grass
Velvet Grass
Wild Oats
Orchard Grass
Red Top Grass
Rye Grass
Timothy

Fall Mixed (Cutter)

Annual Salt Bush
Careless Weed
Cocklebur
Lamb's Quarter
Mugwort
Red Root Pigweed
Ragweed Common
Ragweed False
Ragweed Giant
Ragweed Western
Russian Thistle
Mountain Sagebrush

California Spring Mixed

Black Walnut
June Grass
Bermuda Grass
Orchard Grass

California Fall Mixed

Mugwort
Sagebrush Coast
Ragweed Western

Northwest and Mountain Special

Mountain Sage
Russian Thistle

Ragweed Combined

Ragweed Common 50%
Ragweed Giant 50%

South San Joaquin Valley Mixed

All Scale — Russian Thistle

Supply: DIAGNOSTIC—In capillary tubes for each group.

THERAPEUTIC—Stock mixture treatment sets containing over 60,000 pollen units; Bottles of 5 cc of concentrated extract, dilutions of 1–10,000, 1–1,000, 1–100, 1–33⅓.

(Lederle)

Zone 1 (*New England, Eastern and Central States, Ontario and Maritime Provinces*)
- Sweet Vernal Grass
- Orchard Grass
- June Grass
- Timothy
- Redtop
- Ragweed
- Giant Ragweed

Zone 2 (*Southern States*)
- June Grass
- Bermuda Grass
- Timothy
- Redtop
- Johnson Grass
- Ragweed
- Giant Ragweed

Zone 3 (*Middle Western States, Manitoba*)
- Sweet Vernal Grass
- Orchard Grass
- June Grass
- Timothy
- Redtop
- Ragweed
- Giant Ragweed

Zone 4 (*Rocky Mountain States, Alberta, Saskatchewan*)
- Cottonwood
- Sweet Vernal Grass
- Orchard Grass
- June Grass
- Timothy
- Lamb's Quarters
- Annual Saltbush
- Redroot Pigweed
- Sage Brush
- Russian Thistle
- Summer Cypress
- Pasture Sage
- Western Ragweed

Zone 5 (*Southwestern States*)
- Cottonwood
- Shad Scale
- Rabbit Bush
- June Grass
- Bermuda Grass
- Johnson Grass
- Annual Saltbush
- Redroot Pigweed
- Sage Brush
- Russian Thistle
- Careless Weed
- Slender Ragweed
- Southwestern Ragweed

Zone 6 (*Pacific States, British Columbia*)
- Black Walnut
- Orchard Grass
- Perennial Rye Grass
- June Grass
- Bermuda Grass
- Timothy
- Redtop
- Johnson Grass
- Redroot Pigweed
- Sage Brush
- Russian Thistle
- Mugwort
- Careless Weed

Supply: DIAGNOSTIC—Packages for each zone comprising 3 capillary tubes and scarifying needle for each of the contained pollens.

(Lederle)

Spring Type Antigen
- June Grass
- Orchard Grass
- Sweet Vernal Grass
- Red Top
- Timothy

Ragweed Combined Antigen
- Common Ragweed
- Giant Ragweed
- (equal parts)

Supply: THERAPEUTIC—Each of above 2 antigens in packages containing syringes or vials, as follows:

Complete Treatment Set—(Doses 1 to 15).

Series A—(Doses 1 to 5).
Series B—(Doses 6 to 10).
Series C—(Doses 11 to 15).
Series D—(Dose 15).
Series E—(Dose 20).
Series F—(Doses 16 to 20).

(Lederle)

Rocky Mountain Antigen
- Russian Thistle
- Sage Brush
- Pasture Sage
- Summer Cypress
- Western Ragweed

Southern Formula Antigen
- Bermuda Grass
- Johnson Grass
- Common Ragweed
- Giant Ragweed

Combined Antigen

Sweet Vernal Grass
June Grass
Red Top
Orchard Grass
Timothy
Yellow Dock Rye
Wheat Corn
Ragweed
Sage Brush

Supply: THERAPEUTIC—Each of above 3 antigens in packages of vials, as follows:
Complete Treatment Set—(Doses 1 to 15).

Series A—(Doses 1 to 5).
Series B—(Doses 6 to 10).
Series C—(Doses 11 to 15).
Series D—(Dose 15).

(Mulford)

Zone I (*Appalachian and Great Lakes Region*)
Sweet Vernal
Orchard Grass
June Grass
Red Top
Timothy
Cocklebur
Lamb's Quarters
Plantain (English)
Redroot (Pigweed)
Ragweed (High and Low)

Zone III (*Rocky Mountain Areas*)
Box Elder
Orchard Grass
Timothy
Lamb's Quarters
Ragweed, False
Ragweed, Western
Russian Thistle
Sagebrush
Marsh Elder
June Grass

Zone V (*Southeastern Area*)
Marsh Elder
Bermuda Grass
Johnson Grass
June Grass
Timothy
Cocklebur
Lamb's Quarters
Redroot (Pigweed)
Ragweed
Spiny Amaranth

Zone II (*Plains Area*)
Cottonwood
Corn
June Grass
Orchard Grass
Timothy
Sage, Prairie
Ragweed
Russian Thistle
Redroot (Pigweed)
Cocklebur

Zone IV (*Pacific Coast Areas*)
Box Elder
June Grass
Velvet Grass
Mugwort, California
Orchard Grass
Ragweed, Western
Rye, Perennial
Redroot (Pigweed)
Coast Sage
Timothy

Zone VI (*Southwestern Area*)
Cedar, Mountain
Bermuda Grass
Johnson Grass
Ragweed, False
Mugwort
Russian Thistle
Salt Bush
Ragweed, Western
Cottonwood
June Grass

Supply: DIAGNOSTIC—Pollen Zone Test Packages—10 vials, each containing 3 capillary tube points of concentrated pollen extract.

Pollens: **(Mulford)**

Timothy Ragweed Grass Mixture; Grass Mixture—Southwestern.

Supply: Each supplied as all Mulford pollens; also as:
Packages of three 5 cc vials—100, 2,000, 20,000 pollen units respectively, offering equivalent of 15 dose and 20 dose syringe or vial treatment.

Spring Hay Fever Antigen: **(National Drug)**

Contains the antigens of the pollens of spring grasses. Standardized in nitrogen protein units; for treatment.

Supply: Treatment No. 1 Complete (24 doses)—in 5 cc ampule-vials, comprising:
Series "AA," 125 units (8 doses).
Series "A," 250 units (8 doses).
Series "B," 500 units (8 doses).
Treatment No. 2 (16 doses)—in 5 cc ampule-vials, comprising:
Series "A," 250 units (8 doses).
Series "B," 500 units (8 doses).
Single 5 cc Ampule-vials comprising:

Series "AA," 125 units (8 doses).
Series "A," 250 units (8 doses).
Series "B," 500 units (8 doses).
Special Series "C," 1,250 units.
Syringe Treatment Sets comprising:
Packages of sixteen 1 cc syringes marked from first to sixteenth dose, units graduated from 2½ to 100.
Packages of four syringes, 150 units each.

Timothy Antigen:

Supply: Complete Treatment No. 1 (24 doses)—as above.
Single 5 cc Ampule-vials—as above.
Syringe Treatment Sets—as above.

Ragweed Antigen (Fall Hay Fever Antigen):

Contains giant and dwarf ragweed.

Supply: Complete Treatment No. 1 (24 doses)—as above.
Treatment No. 2 (16 doses)—as above.
Syringe Treatment Sets—as above.

(Parke, Davis)

Gramineae:

Group XXVIII
Timothy
Johnson Grass
Orchard Grass
Bermuda Grass
Red Top

Chenopodiaceae and Related Families:

Group XXIX
Russian Thistle
White Goosefoot
Yellow Dock
Western Waterhemp
Halberd-leaved Orache

Ambrosiaciae:

Group XXX
Common Ragweed
Giant Ragweed
Western Ragweed
Rough Marsh Elder
Burweed Marsh Elder
Cocklebur

Artemisiae:

Group XXXI
Wormwood Sage
Mugwort
Prairie Sage
Sagebrush
Indian Hair Tonic

Supply: DIAGNOSTIC—Collapsible tin tubes of glycerinated extract for about 50 tests—Packages of 1, or 4 assorted.
THERAPEUTIC—Packages of 3 vials, 4 cc, rubber-diaphragm capped, of glycerinated extract.

Diagnostic Assortment Sets, Pollen Allergen Solutions, Glycerol Form: **(Squibb)**

New England and Eastern States

Spring—Oak
Summer—Orchard Grass
Timothy
June Grass
Fall—Ragweed (Giant and Dwarf)
Cocklebur

Central States

Spring—Oak
Poplar
Summer—June Grass
Timothy
Fall—Ragweed (Giant and Dwarf)
Marsh Elder

Southern States

Spring—Oak
Summer—Bermuda Grass
Johnson Grass
Timothy
Fall—Ragweed (Giant and Dwarf)
Marsh Elder

Middle Western States

Spring—Oak
Summer—June Grass
Timothy
Brome Grass
Fall—Ragweed (Giant and Dwarf)
Western Ragweed

Southwestern States
- Spring—Cottonwood
- Summer—Bermuda Grass
  - Johnson Grass
- Fall—Sagebrush
  - Slender Ragweed
  - Western Ragweed

Rocky Mountain States
- Spring—Black Walnut
- Summer—Brome Grass
  - June Grass
- Fall—Mugwort
  - Sagebrush
  - Western Ragweed

Pacific Coast States
- Spring—California Black Walnut
- Summer—June Grass
  - Timothy
- Fall—Sagebrush
  - Western Ragweed (Giant and Dwarf)

Pacific Coast States
- Spring—Cottonwood
- Summer—Perennial Rye
  - Bermuda Grass
  - Orchard Grass
- Fall—Russian Thistle
  - Mugwort

Supply: Packages of 6 vials of 2 capillary tubes with rubber bulbs and needles.

Treatment Sets, Pollen Allergen Solutions, Glycerol Form: **(Squibb)**

Grasses Combined (*Late Spring and Summer*)
- Equal parts of—
- Bermuda Grass
- June Grass
- Orchard Grass
- Red Top
- Timothy

Timothy (*Late Spring and Summer*)
- Cat-Tail
- Herd's Grass

Ragweed (*Fall*)
- Dwarf Ragweed
- Giant Ragweed

Supply: THERAPEUTIC—Treatment Set A, Complete, Doses 1–10 with diluent, and 1 tube Diagnostic Pollen Allergen Solution.
Treatment Set B, Complete, Doses 1–5, with diluent, and 1 tube Diagnostic Pollen Allergen Solution.
Treatment Set C, Complete, Doses 6–10, with diluent.
Treatment Set D, Complete, five doses of Dose 10 with diluent.

Grasses Combined
- Equal parts of—
- Bermuda Grass
- June Grass
- Orchard Grass
- Red Top
- Timothy

Timothy

Ragweed Combined
- Equal parts of—
- Ragweed Giant and Dwarf

Western Weeds Combined
- Equal parts of—
- Marsh Elder
- Mugwort
- Sagebrush
- Slender Ragweed
- Western Ragweed

Supply: THERAPEUTIC—Packages of 3 vials containing solutions of strengths for use without further dilution.

Sets; Pollen Allergens, Soluble Powder Extract:

Early Spring
- Ash
- Black Walnut
- Oak
- Poplar

Summer
- June Grass
- Johnson Grass
- Orchard Grass
- Rye
- Timothy

Fall
- Corn
- Goldenrod
- Dwarf Ragweed
- Giant Ragweed

Supply: DIAGNOSTIC—Vials 25 mg—Cases of 12, 24 or 50 assorted vials.

COMBINATION SETS

40 Test Set (Lederle)

Banana	Chocolate	Almond	Cotton Seed
Beef	Codfish	Buckwheat	Cow Dander
Chicken Meat	Corn Meal	Cat Dander	Crab Meat

40 Test Set.—*(Continued)*

Egg White	Peanut	Dog Dander	Kapok
Green Pea	Pork	Feathers	Orris
Lamb	Rice	Fish Glue	Pyrethrum
Lima Bean	Rye	Flax Seed	Rabbit Dander
Milk	Spinach	Goat Dander	Sheep Dander (Wool)
Mustard	Wheat	Horse Dander	Tobacco
Orange	White Potato	Horse Serum	000 Control
		House Dust	

Supply: Packages of 40 tests, glycerinated extract—each in separate tube.

Pocket Case Assortment **(Mulford)**

Bean (Navy)	Milk Casein (Cow)	Wheat	Horse Dander
Beef	Onion	Cat Hair	Horse Serum
Beet	Oyster	Cattle Dander	Lamb's Quarters
Cabbage	Pork	Chicken Feathers	Orris Root
Celery	Prune	Dog Hair	Ragweed
Egg, whole	Salmon	Duck Feathers	Timothy
Lamb	Strawberry	Goose Feathers	Wormwood
Lettuce	Tomato		

Supply: Powdered extract—Pocket case of 30 cutaneous outfits for 30 tests.

Diagnostic Test Case:

Pollens Dried

Bermuda Grass	Lamb's Quarters	Sage Brush
Box Elder	Marsh Elder	Sweet Vernal Grass
Careless Weed	Mountain Cedar	Timothy
Cocklebur	Mugwort	Walnut
Cottonwood	Orchard Grass	Water Hemp
False Ragweed	Plantain	Western Ragweed
Goldenrod	Ragweed (Common)	Wormwood
Johnson Grass	Redroot-Pigweed	Yellow Dock
June Grass	Russian Thistle	

Food Extracts Dried

Apple	Celery	Egg Yolk	Orange	Rye
Bean (Lima)	Chicken	Lamb	Oyster	Salmon
Bean (Navy)	Cocoa	Lettuce	Pea	Strawberry
Beef	Codfish	Milk Casein (Cow)	Pork	Sweet Potato
Beet	Coffee		Potato	Tomato
Cabbage	Corn	Oat	Prune	Walnut
Carrot	Egg White	Onion	Rice	Wheat

Epidermal and Miscellaneous Extracts Dried

Cat Hair	Dog Hair	Horse Dander	Rabbit Hair
Cattle Dander	Duck Feathers	Horse Serum	Rice Powder
Chicken Feathers	Goose Feathers	Orris Root	Sheep Wool

Supply: Case containing 50 mg vials, each vial sufficient for 25 tests.

CHAPTER VIII

FOODS AND BEVERAGES

209 Foods in 443 forms, classified into groups and presented alphabetically.

Description: The foods and beverages here described are chosen for their medical interest; they represent a variety of nutritional values and are adapted for the preparation of numerous infants' formulae and the dietetic regulation of systemic disorders. The infant foods are grouped in accordance with their intended function, into Milk Products, Milk Modifiers, Powdered Milk, etc.; the other food products, comprising Flours, Cereals, Vegetables, Soups, and others, are grouped together, to facilitate their ready selection in the preparation of dietaries.

Uses: The infant foods are used for various types of feeding of infants and children, under normal and abnormal conditions, as the premature, marasmic, anemic, those with alimentary disorders and numerous other disturbances; the food products for adults are indicated in the dietetic treatment of diabetes, obesity, nephritis, cardiorenal disease and undernutrition. The caloric value of the preparations may readily be computed from the analyses and tables accompanying descriptions; the preparation of individual dishes is omitted, as recipes for these usually accompany the marketed products or are obtainable from distributors.

1. BREADS

(Loeb)

Aerated Gluten Bread: A very light bread, a loaf 9 in. long weighing 1 oz.; *For use* in diabetes and carbohydrate restricted diets.

Analysis:

Carbohydrates	21 %	Fat	12 %
Protein	50 %		

Caloric value: per loaf 117 calories.

Supply: Carton of 12 loaves.

(Loeb)

Aerated Gluten Rolls: Light, crisp and nourishing breakfast rolls; *For use* in diabetes and carbohydrate restricted diets.

Analysis:

Carbohydrates	36 %	Fat	9 %
Protein	33 %		

Caloric value: per package 181 calories.

Supply: Carton of 6 rolls.

(Energen)

Energen Breads: Accurately standardized, of invariable composition of food elements, palatable, digestible and crisp, *For use* in diabetes, obesity and indigestion. Supplied as follows:

	Carbohydrate	Protein	Butter, Oz.	Weight per Gm	Calories	Supply, Tins of
Batons (large)	14¼	11½	1	32	345	8
Batonettes (small)	7	5½	½	15½	170	18
Rolls	2	1½	⅓	4½	90	40
Rusks (4)	4¼	3½	⅓	9½	115	96
Whole wheat batons	19½	14½	1	37½	370	8

(Loeb)

Genuine Gluten Bread: Prepared from standard gluten flour; is of fine texture and palatable; *for use* in diabetes and carbohydrate restricted diets.

Analysis:

Carbohydrates............ 25% Fat...................... 4%
Protein.................. 33%

Caloric value: per loaf 643 calories.

Supply: Individual loaves.

Sliced and toasted loaves (14 or more slices).

Gluten Bread: Made from 100% pure gluten flour: **(Dietetic Food)**

Analysis:

Protein.................. 43.15% Crude Fiber........... 1.52%
Carbohydrate............. 35.80% Ash................... 1.46%
Fat...................... 2.90% Moisture.............. 5.77%
Non-hydrolyzing carbohydrate 9.40%

Supply: Loaves of 8 oz.

2. BREADSTUFFS

(Energen)

Agar Bran Biscuits: Palatable, digestible and crisp; *For use* in diabetes, obesity and indigestion.

Analysis:

Carbohydrate............ ¼% Butter.................. ——
Protein.................. ——

Food value: per ounce 1 calorie.

Supply: Tins of 11.

(Loeb)

Assortment Package of 15 Varieties: Lady fingers, macaroons, bread, chocolate bars, wafers, croutons.

(Dietetic Foods)

Bran Cookies: Starch, sugar and salt-free; flavored.

Supply: Boxes of 8 oz.

Breadstuffs, Cakes, Cookies, Wafers **(Curdolac)**

Used for variation of diabetes and obesity diets.

Food Value	Protein, Gm	Fat, Gm	Carbohydrate, Gm	Supply
Cream cookie	0.7	1.2	0.1	Boxes of 12
Tea cake	2.7	2.8	0.5	Boxes of 12
Lady finger	0.8	1.7	0.4	Boxes of 12
Jumble	1.9	2.8	1.3	Boxes of 12
Chip	1.1	0.5	0.4	Boxes of 12
Pretzel	0.7	0.5	0.01	Packages of 24
Doughnut	5.2	3.5	0.9	Boxes of 12
Cocoa cake	2.5	2.5	0.9	Boxes of 12
Spice cake	2.1	2.0	0.0	Boxes of 12
Gold cake	2.1	2.0	0.0	Boxes of 12
Fruit cake (slice)	2.0	2.2	2.4	Package 6 servings
Favorite (slice)	2.0	2.0	0.85	Package 6 servings
Birthday cake	7.2	8.2	0.4	Packages of 2 layers
Diabetic crackers				
Wheat-soya crackers	3.0	3.2	1.6	Boxes of 24
Jay See crackers	4.7	3.2	1.7	Boxes of 24
Malted bran wafers no food value	...	...	....	Boxes of 12
Diabetic cookies:				
Vanilla square	1.6	1.3	1.8	Boxes of 18
Soyettes	1.6	2.9	0.6	Boxes of 18
Brownies	1.5	1.4	0.9	Boxes of 18
Ginger cookies	1.0	1.0	0.4	Boxes of 18
Spicynut cookies	1.3	2.8	0.6	Boxes of 18
Caramelettes	2.2	2.3	0.2	Boxes of 18
Fruit cookies	2.0	2.8	2.2	Boxes of 18
Cheese straws	1.0	0.4	0.6	Boxes of 24

Breadstuffs—Crackers, Wafers **(National Biscuit)**

Food Value	Moisture, %	Mineral, %	Protein, %	Fat, %	Carbohydrates, %	Calories, %	Packages, Pound
Shredded wheat	4.05	1.80	10.96	1.56	81.63	1,744	1
Uneeda biscuit	4.66	2.02	11.05	10.50	71.77	1,983	1
Holland rusk	6.42	1.24	12.62	5.97	73.75	1,850	1
Premium sodas { unsalted	3.40	1.91	10.57	9.93	74.19	1,957	1
Premium sodas { salted	3.40	3.08	10.38	9.91	73.26	1,974	1
Triscuit	4.40	1.79	10.52	1.55	81.74	1,747	1
Wheatsworth cereal crackers	8.07	1.66	11.68	1.80	76.79	1,721	1
Graham crackers	3.36	2.85	8.74	9.30	75.75	1,964	1

(Dietetic Foods)

Casein Lady Fingers: Starch, sugar and salt-free.
Supply: Packages of 24.

(Dietetic Foods)

Casein Sponge Cookies: Starch, sugar and salt-free.
Supply: Packages of 24.

(Loeb)

Dietetic Almond Macaroons: Prepared from casein flour, free from carbohydrates, sugar, salt.

Analysis:

Carbohydrate............. 0% Fat...................... 46%
Protein.................. 30%

Food value: per package 467 calories.
Supply: Packages—Sweetened and Unsweetened.

(Loeb)

Dietetic Gluten Breadsticks:

Analysis:

	Plain, Per cent	Almond, Per cent
Carbohydrate	35	31
Protein	42	39
Fat	4	12

Food value: per package 204 calories (Plain) and 226 calories (Almond).
Supply: Sealed packages—Plain and Almond.

(Loeb)

Dietetic Gluten Crackers: Palatable, crisp and tasteful.

Analysis:

Carbohydrate............. 31% Fat...................... 20%
Protein.................. 35%

Food value: per package 386 calories.
Supply: In sealed packages.

(Loeb)

Dietetic Gluten Zwieback: Palatable, crisp and nourishing; *For use* in diabetics, invalids and in restricted diets.

Analysis:

	Plain, Per cent	Almond, Per cent
Carbohydrate	36	33
Protein	43	41
Fat	3	8

Food value: per package 199 calories and 213 calories.
Supply: In sealed packages—Plain and Almond.

(Loeb)

Dietetic Lady Fingers:

Analysis:

Carbohydrate............. 2% Fat...................... 34%
Protein.................. 48%

Food value: per package 147 calories.
Supply: Packages of 24, Sweetened and Unsweetened.

(Loeb)

Dietetic Sponge Cookies: A pleasant, slightly sweetened cookie.

Analysis:

Carbohydrate............ 2% Fat..................... 34%
Protein.................. 50%

Food value: per package 148 calories.

Supply: Packages.

(Energen)

4 Digestive Biscuits: Palatable, digestible and crisp; *For use* in diabetes, obesity and indigestion.

Analysis:

Carbohydrate........... 13 % Butter.................... 7%
Protein.................. 6¾%

Food value: per ounce 146 calories.

Supply: Tins of ½ lb.

(Energen)

Endo Bran Biscuits: Palatable, digestible and crisp; *For use* in diabetes, obesity and indigestion.

Analysis:

Carbohydrate........... 5½% Butter.................. 8½%
Protein.................. 3½%

Food value: per ounce 115 calories.

Supply: Tins of 4.

(Loeb)

Genuine Gluten Croutons: *For use* in soups or as breakfast cereal.

Analysis:

Carbohydrate............ 35% Fat...................... 4%
Protein.................. 42%

Food value: per package 123 calories.

Supply: Packages.

(Loeb)

Gluten Butter Cookies: As substitute for pastries and cookies.

Analysis:

Carbohydrate............ 31% Fat...................... 12%
Protein.................. 37%

Food value: per package 330 calories.

Supply: Sealed packages—Sweetened (with saccharin) and Unsweetened.

(Loeb)

Gluten Cheese Tid-Bits: Crisp little crackers, salt free.

Analysis:

Carbohydrate............ 17% Fat..................... 38%
Protein.................. 34%

Food value: per package 240 calories.

Supply: Packages.

(Dietetic Foods)

Gluten Cookies: Low carbohydrate content; flavored.

Supply: Cartons of 7 oz.

(Dietetic Foods)

Golden Gluten Breadsticks: Crispy breadsticks for light meals.

Analysis:

Proteins.................. 41.10% Crude Fiber............ 1.00%
Carbohydrate............. 37.93% Ash.................... 1.60%
Fat...................... 4.03% Moisture............... 6.11%
Non-hydrolyzing Carbohydrate 9.40%

Supply: Packages of 10 sticks.

(Loeb)

Karlsbader Biscotten: High in caloric value and low in carbohydrates. *Used* as change from bread.

Analysis:

Carbohydrate	18%	Fat	40%
Protein	32%		

Food value: per package 508 calories.

Supply: In packages.

(Battle Creek)

Laxa Biscuit: A food laxative, prepared from 2 forms of cellulose, ceylon moss (agar-agar) and cooked bran; is palatable, nutritious, rich in vitamins; contains protein, phosphates and vitamins; eaten dry like toast or with butter; served in soup or juices.

Supply: Laxa Biscuit, Sweet and Unsweetened—Packages of 6 per can.

(Dietetic Foods)

Low Calory Cookies: Prepared from bran and low calory flour; palatable, easily digested and flavored.

Analysis:

Protein	8.12%	Hemicellulose	40.95%
Carbohydrate	0.00%	Ash	2.25%
Fat	0.70%	Moisture	3.84%
Cellulose	32.39%	Mineral oil	11.75%

Supply: Boxes of 8 oz.

(Ralston)

Rye Krisp (C.A.): A rye wafer prepared from whole rye grains; contains the whole germ and all the bran; *For use* in wheat sensitized patients, obesity, constipation.

Analysis:

Protein	13.1%	Dextrines	19.5%
Fat	2.0%	Minerals	4.1%
Carbohydrate	73.9%	NaCl	2.9%
Pentosans	9.8%	Phosphorus	0.3850
Fiber	2.2%	Iron	0.0039
Starch	42.4%	Moisture	6.8%

Food value: Wafer 6.1 Gm—20 calories; Disc 20 Gm—64 calories.

Supply: In packages.

(Dietetic Foods)

Snaps: Starch, sugar-free; flavors—ginger, anise, lemon, vanilla, almond, assorted.

Food value: practically none.

Supply: Boxes of 24.

(Loeb)

Starch-Free Bran Wafers: Rich in iron, phosphorus, vitamins, salt-free; *For use* in constipation and indigestion.

Analysis:

Carbohydrate	2%	Fat	19%
Protein	26%		

Food value: per package 328 calories.

Supply: Packages.

3. BREAKFAST FOODS

(Chicago Dietetic)

Bran Breakfast Food: A combination of washed bran and cellulose with flavoring; makes a palatable cereal substitute, without food value.

Supply: Packages 1 lb.—Cases of 10.

(Loeb)

Bran and Gluten Cereal: Has a carbohydrate content and food value lower than Loeb's Gluten Breakfast Cereal; is unsweetened, contains starch-free bran and is mildly laxative.

Supply: Sealed packages.

(Chicago Dietetic)

Bran Special Wafers: Prepared from fine bran; flavors—chocolate, almond and cheese.

Supply: Packages 1 lb.—Cases of 10.

(Chicago Dietetic)

Bran Wafers: Prepared from washed bran and Cellu Flour; *For use* as bread substitute; no food value.

Supply: Bran Wafers—Packages 1 lb.—Cases of 10.

(Curdolac)

Breakfast Food (C.A.): Prepared from starch-free bran and soy beans, with leavening, flavoring and traces of gluside; *For use* as breakfast food or as per recipes on packages.

Analysis:

Protein	15.19%	Nitrogen-free extract	50.39%
Carbohydrate	1.3%	Fibre	17.8%
Fat	5.26%	Moisture	2.0%

Food value: per 100 Gm—113 calories.

Supply: Packages of 24 oz.

(Dietetic Food)

Breakfast Food: Is starch and sugar-free. *For use* either dry or served with milk or cream as breakfast food as per recipe.

Analysis:

Protein	4.09%	Fat	2.69%
Carbohydrate	0.0 %	Ash	2.24%
Cellulose	64.46%	Moisture	5.55%
Hemicellulose	20.97%		

Supply: Boxes of 8 oz. for 15 servings.

(Loeb)

Gluten Breakfast Cereal: A wholesome, nutritious and palatable food *for use* as breakfast cereal; already cooked and sweetened.

Analysis:

Carbohydrate	26%	Fat	19%
Protein	32%		

Food value: per package—701 calories.

Supply: Sealed packages—Sweetened and Unsweetened.

(Dietetic Food)

Gluto-Lax Breakfast Food: *For use* at breakfast, dry or with milk or cream.

Analysis:

Protein	33.63%	Hemicellulose	22.02%
Carbohydrate	19.34%	Ash	2.09%
Fat	3.25%	Moisture	9.04%
Cellulose	10.63%		

Supply: Cans of 8 oz.

(Lister)

Starchless Breakfast Food: Contains ready cooked palm nut flakes, starch free bran and vegetable gums; *For use* as diabetic breakfast food; in soups—as substitute for noodle flakes and barley.

Analysis:

Moisture	7.3%	Protein	8.7%
Ash	2.5%	Sugar	0.0%
Fat	1.5%	Hemicellulose-cellulose	80.0%

Supply: Cartons of 1 lb.
Special recipes in carton.

4. CEREALS

(Ralston)

Baby Ralston (C.A.): A cereal food prepared from the 2 fractions of wheat—the endosperm and embryo.

Analysis: Each 30 Gm represents

Fat	0.60 Gm	Iron	0.00085 Gm
Protein	4.23 Gm	Calcium	0.037 Gm
Carbohydrate	20.10 Gm	Phosphorus	0.08 Gm
Ash	0.29 Gm		

Food value: per 30 gm—103 calories.
Nutritious cereal rich in vitamin B; *For use* in infant feeding; also in smooth diets of adults; cooked thoroughly for 10 min. and served.

Supply: In Tins.

Bibliography: *See Chap. XII.*

(Energen)

Bismeal: A low-starch breakfast food, containing per Gm:

Analysis:

Carbohydrate	13½%	Butter	1 oz.
Protein	10%		

Supply: Tins of 8 oz.

(Curdolac)

Breakfast Cereal (C.A.): Also called Vitabran, a carbohydrate poor brown cereal, prepared from soy beans, blended with wheat products, including starch-free bran.

Analysis:

Protein	25.9%	Fibre	8.68%
Carbohydrate	14.9%	Ash	12.40%
Fat	10.0%	Moisture	3.94%
Nitrogen-free extract	24.04%		

Food value: per 100 Gm—260 calories.
½ cupful of Vitabran mixed with cupful of boiling water, cooked in double boiler for ½ hr. makes 2 servings, each containing protein 8.8 Gm, carbohydrate 5 Gm, fat 3.3 Gm; caloric value about 85.

Supply: Packages of 1 lb.

(General Mills)

Embo (C.A.): A purified wheat embryo (germ), freed from bran and other impurities; contains vitamins A, B, E and G.

Analysis:

Protein	25–30%	Moisture	11–15%
Carbohydrates	50–37.5%	Ash	3.5–4.5%
Fat	9–12%	Crude fiber	1.5–2%

Food Value: per ounce: 108 calories.
Uses: Supplies essential vitamins in dietary, and thus improves appetite and assists growth; *used* to prepare bread, biscuits, or porridge. 2 tablespoonfuls daily, mixed with fruit juices, vegetable juices, or sprinkled over cooked fruits or cereals.

Supply: Cans hermetically sealed.

Bibliography: *See Chap. XII.*

(Gerber)

Gerber's Strained Cereal, Milk Cooked (C.A.): A cooked cereal consisting of a mixture of whole wheat and oats, strained to a fine consistency, of minimum roughage, with wheat germ added; cooked in whole fresh milk without sugar or salt.

Analysis:

Moisture	83.1%	Reducing sugars after inversion as lactose	3.6%
Total solids (vacuum, 4″ mercury 70C)	16.9%	Crude fiber	0.2%
Ash	0.7%	Carbohydrates other than crudefiber (by difference)	10.0
Fat (Rose Gottlieb method)	2.8%	Iron (Fe)	0.001
Protein (N × 6.25)	3.4%	Calcium (Ca)	0.09
Reducing sugars before inversion as lactose	3.4%	Phosphorus (P)	0.05

Food value: Calories: 0.8 per gram; 23 per ounce. A starting cereal for infants and for invalids; also for soft diets; is high in vitamins A, B, E and G and in calcium, phosphorus and iron.

Supply: Cans 10¼ oz.

(Pure Gluten)

Gluten-Bran Flakes "Hoyt": A cereal, half gluten and half bran, from which most of the starch has been removed; furnishes bulk, roughage and is laxative; ready to serve with fruit juices or skimmed milk for the obese; served with cream for diabetics; *used* in dietaries of restricted carbohydrates for weight reduction.

Supply: Packages 14 oz.

(Campbell)

Malto-Meal (C.A.): A wheat cereal flavored with barley malt; a breakfast food of individual flavor, well adapted for use by children.

Analysis:

	Per Cent		Per Cent
Moisture	11.47	Malt sugar	1.59
Ash (mineral)	.50	Soluble carbohydrate	1.96
Protein	10.93	Starch	71.55
Fat	1.15	Total carbohydrate	79.95
Fiber	.85	Calories per pound	17.91

Supply: Packages of 1 lb.

(Mead Johnson)

Mead's Cereal (C.A.): A cereal enriched with mineral and vitamin containing foods; contains calcium, iron, phosphorus, copper and other essential minerals and vitamins A, B, E and G.

Composition:

	Per Cent		Per Cent
Farina	53.0	Edible bonemeal (especially prepared for human use)	2.0
Wheat germ	15.0	Brewers' yeast	1.0
Oatmeal	18.0		
Cornmeal	10.0		
Alfalfa	1.0		

Analysis:

Fat	3.0	Minerals (ash)	3.2
Protein	15.0	Moisture	7.0
Carbohydrates	71.8		

Mineral Content:

Calcium	0.78	Magnesium	0.13
Phosphorus	0.62	Sulphur	0.015
Iron	0.024	Silicon	0.015
Copper	0.001	Manganese	0.00035
Chlorine	0.677	Zinc	0.00015
Sodium	0.458	Other minerals	traces
Potassium	0.396		
		Total approximately	3.2%

Food value per ounce: 106 calories. (4 level tablespoonfuls are equal to 1 oz.)

Supply: Packages of 1 and 4 lb.

Administration: 1 day's supply for average infant is thinned with milk and fed in number of tablespoonfuls prescribed. Other recipes are similar to those used for farina.

(Ralston)

Ralston Wheat Cereal (C.A.): A wheat cereal containing the proteins of wheat embryo, phosphates, bran; is rich in vitamins A, B_1, B_2, E and minerals—calcium, phosphorus, potassium, magnesium, sulphur, sodium, chlorine, iron; is growth promoting, stimulates appetite; *For use* in infant feeding; is mildly laxative in constipation.

Analysis:

Protein	14.15%	Ash	1.54
Fat	2.10	Carbohydrate	71.80
Fibre	1.24	Moisture	9.17

Food value per 30 Gm:

	Grams	Calories
Fat	0.63	5.67
Protein	4.24	16.96
Carbohydrates	21.54	86.56
Total calories		109

Supply: Packages of 16 oz.

Bibliography: *See Chapter XII.* Cereal.

5. CONCENTRATED MILK PRODUCTS

CONCENTRATED LIQUID SKIM MILK (S. M. A.)

Description: An evaporated, almost fat-free, skim milk; the milk is first pasteurized and then almost wholly defatted by centrifugal method and later concentrated until 68% of the water has been drawn off; sterilized.

Uses: For infant feeding; may be used whenever "Fat free" milk is indicated; also in reducing the fat content of the whole milk or evaporated milk.

Analysis:

Moisture	80.0%	Fat (ether extract)	0.3%
Total solids	20.0%	Protein (N × 6.38)	7.3%
Ash	2.0%	Lactose (by difference)	10.4%

Food Value: 0.8 calories per cubic centimeter; 23—per fluid ounce.

Supply: **CONCENTRATED LIQUID SKIM MILK** (C.A.)—Cans of 6.2 and 16½ oz.

Administration: According to formula desired.

LACTOGEN (Nestle)

Description: A dried mixture of fat-enriched cow's milk and lactose, in proportions to simulate human milk in percentage composition; provides a food of natural nutritive milk constituents only, the water alone having been extracted; contains Vitamins A, B, C, D.

Action and Uses: A modified milk powder for the feeding of normal infants.

Analysis:

Fat	25%	Mineral Salts	3.5%
Protein	16.2%	Water	2.0%
Carbohydrate (Lactose only)	53.3%		

Food Value: 156 calories per ounce; 39 calories per tablespoonful.

Supply: LACTOGEN (C.A.)—Cans of 1 lb.

Administration: According to formula desired.

PET MILK (Pet Milk)

Description: An evaporated, whole cow's milk; concentrated, homogenized and sterilized, evaporation abstracting about 60% of the water; is uniform in composition, standardized to a definite content of fat and non-fat solids and free from harmful microorganisms.

Action and Uses: Is readily digested, forming soft flocculent curds easily penetrated by the digestive juices. *Indicated* for the feeding of infants with acute alimentary disorders and diarrhea; in difficult feeding as in children, premature and marasmic, and in pyloric stenosis.

Analysis:

Fat	7.8–7.9%	Salts	1.5–1.6%
Sugar	9.5–10%	Water	74.2–73%
Protein	7–7.5%	Total Solids	25.8–27%

Food Value: 43 calories per ounce.

Supply: PET MILK (C.A.)—Cans of 6 oz., 13 oz.

Administration: According to formula desired.

6. FLOURS

CASEIN COMPOUND (Curdolac)

Description: A carbohydrate-free flour, well adapted for making low calory bread, shortcakes, muffins, drop cakes. *For use* in diabetic and obesity diets.

Contains:

Protein	42.7%	Fibre	3.36%
Carbohydrate	none	Ash	5.60%
Fat	0.75%	Moisture	5.23%
Nitrogen-free ext	42.35%		

Food Value: Per gram 100–182 calories.

Supply: CASEIN-COMPOUND (C.A.)—Cans of 1 lb.

CELLU FLOUR (Chicago Dietetic)

Description: A carbohydrate-free flour consisting of commercially pure cellulose; is of white or grayish-white color, odorless, tasteless; prepared from wood pulp, straw pulp and cotton fibre, specially treated.

Action and Uses. Has almost no nutritive value; supplies roughage and bulk and thus somewhat laxative. *For use* in diabetes, obesity and other conditions where carbohydrates are best excluded.

Supply: CELLU FLOUR (C.A.)—Packages of 2 and 5 lb.

Administration: Preparation of Cellu Flour Bread: Is made by separating the whites from 4 yolks of eggs, beaten until stiff; yolks are then beaten into thick spongy consistency; to this are added 2 tablespoonfuls of water, ½ gr saccharine, all of which are combined into a mixture to which ½ cupful of Cellu Flour, a teaspoonful of salt and a tablespoonful of mineral oil are added; is placed in baking pan and baked in moderate oven for about 40 min.

Food Value: Of 1 loaf—312 calories, containing protein 24 Gm, fat 24 Gm, carbohydrate none.

DIETETIC CASEIN FLOUR (Dietetic Food)

Description: A self-rising flour prepared from refined casein and Tagua palm nut; is starch and sugar-free but high in mineral salts; *For use* in making bread, pancakes, cakes, muffins, etc.

Analysis:

Protein	48.50%	Fat	0.53%
Carbohydrate	0.00%	Ash	8.78%
Cellulose	34.83%	Moisture	7.36%
Hemicellulose	0.00%		

Supply: DIETETIC CASEIN FLOUR—Cartons of 15 and 30—Boxes for 2 and 4 weeks' supply.

DIETETIC FLOUR (Lister)

Composition: A blend of caseins, cascinate, palm nut flour with leavening incorporated; is starch-free and self-rising.

Analysis:

Moisture	7%	Protein	56.9%
Ash	6.6%	Starch	0.0
Fat	0.5%	Sugar	0.0
Leavening, Fibre	28.9%		

Food Value: Per ounce—64.98 calories.

Action and Uses: In diabetic and obesity diets; is easily made into starch-free bread, muffins and other foods.

Supply: DIETETIC FLOUR—Cartons—large size (enough for 30 bakings).
DIETETIC FLOUR—Cartons—small size (enough for 15 bakings).
Booklet of recipes in each carton..

ENERGEN NUTRIENT FLOUR (Energen)

Description: Prepared from wheat and gluten; is free from baking powder, raising material and bleaching substances.

Uses: *For use* either alone or mixed with ordinary flours for the making of bread, biscuits and other foods.

Supply: ENERGEN NUTRIENT FLOUR—Packages of 1 lb.

EQUALIZED FLOUR (Lister)

Composition: A low carbohydrate, self-rising flour; a blend of starch-free bran, number 1 Miller's bran, and vegetable gums incorporated with leavening.

Analysis: Each carton of flour, sufficient for baking six large muffins or of any of the other recipes, contains 12 Gm carbohydrate, no protein, no fat; when combined with 2 eggs, gives a food containing 12 Gm carbohydrates, 12 Gm fat and 12 Gm protein.

Food Value: 204 calories, per carton.

Action and Uses: *For use* in more liberal carbohydrate diets with low and equal amounts of protein, fat and carbohydrate.

Supply: EQUALIZED FLOUR—Cartons—large size (30 day supply).
EQUALIZED FLOUR—Cartons—small size (15 days supply).
Booklet of recipes in each carton.

GLUTEN CRACKER MEAL (Loeb)

Description: A preparation made from gluten flour for breading chops, cutlets, sea foods.

Analysis:

Carbohydrate	31 %	Fat	11 %
Protein	40 %		

Food Value: Per package 335 calories.

Supply: GLUTEN CRACKER MEAL—Sealed packages—unsweetened.

GLUTEN FLOUR (Battle Creek)

Description: A flour containing 44.81 % of gluten, about 3 times the amount of iron present in meat; is poor in starch, having only ½ that of ordinary flour

Analysis:

Moisture	0 %	Crude fiber	0.49 %
Ash	.77 %	Actual starch	43.33 %
Protein	44.81 %	Other carbohydrates	8.80 %
Fat	1.80 %		

Composition: One ounce gluten bread contains—protein 7 Gm, carbohydrates 3.5 Gm, Fat—0.

Food Value: Of gluten bread—42 calories per ounce.

Action and Uses: *For use* in reduction therapy of the obese; in the diabetic and the anemic.

Supply: GLUTEN FLOUR—Bags of 5 lb.

Administration: As per accompanying recipes in each bag.

GLUTEN FLOUR (MacDowell)

Analysis:

Protein	44.17 %	Moisture	9.37 %
Starch	32.56 %	Fat	.97 %
N-Free Extract, undetermined	12.06 %	Ash	.49 %
		Fibre	.38 %

Action and Uses: For preparing bread, rolls, muffins, bread sticks, etc. in diabetic and reduction diets.

Supply: GLUTEN FLOUR—Sacks 5 lb.

GLUTEN SPECIAL FLOUR "HOYT" (Pure Gluten)

Composition: Average

		Calories
Protein	83.10	328
Fat	2.31	9
Carbohydrate	2.51	25

Food Value: 362 calories per 100 Gm

Description: A carbohydrate-poor flour prepared from gluten, free from bitter taste; is high in protein, non-fattening, and serves to overcome excess of carbohydrates in diet.

Uses: *Used* in diabetes mellitus and reduction dietaries with restricted carbohydrates; as gruel, flatcakes or bread.

Supply: GLUTEN SPECIAL FLOUR (C.A.)—Bags of 3 lb.

Combinations: 1. GLUTEN MUFFIN AND PANCAKE FLOUR "HOYT"—For biscuits, muffins, waffles, cakes and dumplings (recipes accompanying).

2. SPECIAL GUM GLUTEN FLOUR "HOYT"—For bread, rolls, flat cakes as addition to other foods (recipes accompanying).

3. GLUTEN BREAD FLOUR "HOYT"—For Government Standard Gluten Bread (recipes accompanying).

IMPROVED FLOUR (Curdolac)

Description: A flour of low carbohydrate value but less palatable than wheat soya flour; is prepared from casein, soy bean, carbohydrate-free bran with leavening and flavoring.

Analysis:

Protein	41.4 %	Nitrogen-free ext.	36.99 %
Carbohydrate	4.6 %	Fibre	6.53 %
Fat	12.0 %	Moisture	4.98 %

Food Value: Per 100 Gm—257 calories.

Supply: IMPROVED FLOUR (C.A.)—Packages of 5 lb.

JOHNNY CAKE FLOUR (Curdolac)

Description: A flour prepared from cereal products, soy bean, leavening and flavoring; tastes and looks like corn meal; *used* for making muffins, pancakes and waffles.

Analysis:

Protein	35.2 %	Fibre	6.22 %
Carbohydrate	20 %	Ash	5.13 %
Fat	16.3 %	Moisture	6.58 %
Nitrogen-free extract	10.52 %		

Food Value: Per 100 Gm—380 calories.

Supply: JOHNNY CAKE FLOUR (C.A.)—Packages 1 and 5 lb.

LOW CALORY FLOUR (Dietetic Food)

Description: A self-rising, refined flour prepared from tropical palm nut; composed chiefly of unassimilable carbohydrates; is sugar and starch-free.

Analysis:

Protein	3.37 %	Cellulose	40.58 %
Fat	0.56 %	Moisture	9.13 %
Carbohydrate	0.0 %	Ash	2.08 %
Hemicellulose	44.28 %		

Food Value: Almost none.

Supply: LOW CALORY FLOUR—Cartons of 15 boxes (2 week's supply).

Administration: *For use* in preparing low calory foods.

NEUTRALIZED FLOUR (Dietetic Food)

Description: A self-rising mixture of low calory flour and casein; is sugar and starch-free.

Analysis:

Protein	23.40 %	Hemicellulose	30.45 %
Fat	0.42 %	Ash	8.15 %
Carbohydrate	0.0 %	Moisture	6.14 %
Cellulose	31.44 %		

Supply: NEUTRALIZED FLOUR—Cartons 15 boxes (2 weeks' supply).

Administration: *For use* in preparing low calory food.

NUTRIVOID FLOUR (Nutrivoid)

Description: A white flour composed of unassimilable carbohydrates, mannas, salts; has a slight but palatable taste and odor.

Action and Uses: *Useful* in preparing foods of low nutritive value in cases of obesity, diabetes; in constipation for its roughage effect.

Analysis:

Glucose	none	Fat	0.92%
Cane Sugar	none	Protein	4.31%
Starch	none	Ash	1.17%
Dextrin	none	Moisture	8.23%
Non-utilizable Carbohydrates			85.37%

Supply: NUTRIVOID FLOUR (C.A.)—Cans of 1, 2, 5 lb.

Administration: In form of imitation bread, biscuits, muffins, cookies, etc. mixed with bran, eggs, baking powder and other auxiliaries; in quantities of similar ordinary food products.

PREPARED SOY BEAN FLOUR (WITH GLUTEN) (Loeb)

Description: A self-rising flour, for use in making muffins, pancakes, etc.

Supply: PREPARED SOY BEAN FLOUR (WITH GLUTEN)—Packages of 12 oz.

PURE GLUTEN FLOUR (Dietetic Food)

Description: Consists of 100% pure gluten, for use in preparing bread, pancakes, muffins, cookies, etc.

Analysis:

Protein	41.00%	Hemicellulose	16.58%
Carbohydrate	39.86%	Ash	1.74%
Fat	1.64%	Moisture	0.00%
Celluose	17.10%		

Supply: PURE GLUTEN FLOUR—Boxes 1 lb.—Bags 3 lb.

GENUINE GLUTEN FLOUR (Loeb)

Analysis:

Carbohydrate	37%	Fat	2%
Protein	42%		

Food Value: Per package of 1 lb. 1,550 calories.

Supply: GENUINE GLUTEN FLOUR—Packages of 1, 3 and 5 lb.

SELF-RISING GLUTEN FLOUR (Loeb)

Description: Contains all flour ingredients; makes batter with water only; palatable, self-rising.

Action and Uses: *For use* in making muffins, pancakes.

Supply: SELF-RISING GLUTEN FLOUR—Packages of 1 lb.

SOY BEAN FLOUR (Chicago Dietetic)

Description: A flour prepared from soy bean and defatted; contains about 45.5% protein, 25.5% carbohydrate, 8.5% fat, 6% ash, 4.7% fiber, 9.5% water; only about half of the carbohydrate is converted into utilizable sugar.

Action and Uses: Is *used* in conditions where low carbohydrate diet is desired; in diabetes, obesity, flatulence, amylaceous dyspepsia.

Food Value: 186 protein calories, 104 carbohydrate calories, 78 fat calories per 100 Gm.

Supply: SOY BEAN FLOUR (C.A.)—Packages 2 and 5 lb.

Combinations: CELLU SOY CRISP (C.A.)—Prepared from cooked soy beans; contains approximately protein 45.6%, carbohydrate 16.1%, fat 20.8%, ash 6.7%, fiber 6.8%, water 4%. *Used* as leguminous breakfast food, agreeably flavored.

Supply: Sealed packages.

CELLU SOY BEANS IN TOMATO SAUCE—Contains protein 11.4%, carbohydrate 2.0%, fat 3.0%.

Supply: Cans of 6 oz.

SOY BEAN FLOUR (MacDowell)

Description: Prepared from pulverized soy beans with part of the oil extracted; is starch free.

Supply: SOY BEAN FLOUR—Cartons 2 lb.

Administration: For preparing muffins, cookies, wafers, bread, gems, hermits. *For use* in diabetes and carbohydrate restricted diets.

Analysis:

Protein (N. × 6.25)	42.30%	Ash	4.60%
Starch and Sugar	0 %	Fibre	4.70%
Undetermined	19.03%	Water	4.40%
Fat	18.20%		

Recipes accompany each carton.

SOYA BRAN FLOUR (Curdolac)

Description: A low starch flour for preparing bread, muffins, pancakes for diabetics; is easily digestible and slightly laxative.

Contains approximately:

Protein	27.3%	Fibre	8.92%
Carbohydrate	7%	Ash	12.7%
Fat	15.7%	Moisture	4.61%
Nitrogen-free extract	23.68%		

Food Value: Per 100 Gm—239 calories.

Supply: SOYA BRAN FLOUR (C.A.)—Packages of 1 and 5 lb.

SOYA FLOUR (Curdolac)

Description: A carbohydrate-poor flour with a nutty and palatable flavor; is prepared from soya bean. *Used* for making muffins, bread, etc.

Contains:

Protein	42%	Fibre	7.86%
Carbohydrate	8%	Ash	4.10%
Fat	18%	Moisture	6%
Nitrogen-free extract	22.04%		

Food Value: Per 100 Gm—342 calories.

Supply: SOYA FLOUR (C.A.)—Packages of 1 and 5 lb.

STARCH-FREE BRAN (Dietetic Food)

Description: A flour prepared from selected bran, freed from starch by the diastase process; is sugar and starch free and somewhat laxative; *For use* in foods, alone or mixed with other flours, for bulk.

Analysis:

Protein	15.75%	Fibre	22.0%
Carbohydrate	0.0%	Moisture	5.0%
Fat	7.5%		
Hemicellulose and phosphorus compounds	49.75%		

Supply: STARCH-FREE BRAN—Cartons of 1 lb.

Administration: *For use* in preparing low calory food.

STARCH FREE BRAN (Lister)

Description: Bran rendered starch-free by the diastase method.

Food Value: None.

Supply: LISTER'S STARCH FREE BRAN—Cartons of 2 lb.

STARCH-FREE BRAN (Loeb)

Description: A cereal starch free-bran, containing iron, phosphates and vitamins.

Analysis:

Carbohydrate	3%	Fat	8%
Protein	18%		

Food Value: Per package 724 calories.

Action and Uses: For preparing biscuits, crackers; is slightly laxative.

Supply: Packages.

STARCH FREE BRAN (MacDowell)

Description: Prepared from wheat bran; washed, dried and toasted.

Analysis:

Moisture	9.65%	Dextrose	3.97%
Ash	5.92%	Fat	3.96%
Protein (N. × 6.25)	10.81%	Undetermined-non-utilizable	53.02
Fibre	12.67%		
Starch	(trace)		

Food Value: None.

Supply: STARCH FREE BRAN—Cartons 1 lb.

Administration: In diabetic and reduction diets.

WASHED BRAN (Chicago Dietetic)

Description: A starchless flour prepared for starch-restricted diets and bread substitutes of low food value; used alone or in combination with other flours to add bulk.

Food Value: Practically none.

Supply: WASHED BRAN—Cartons of 1 lb.

Combinations: PULVERIZED WASHED BRAN—Is pulverized to produce a finer bran product for those who find ordinary washed bran too coarse; is easily combined with eggs and other substances to make muffins, etc.

Food Value: Negligible.

Supply: Cartons of 2 lb.

ONE-TWO-THREE FLOUR—A pulverized washed bran with India gum, vegetable fat and salt, for muffins; contains protein 2%, carbohydrate 1%, fat 2%—per muffin.

Supply: Envelopes for 6 muffins—Cartons of 10.

WHEAT-NUT-CASEIN FLOUR (MacDowell)

Description: Prepared from wheat, nuts, casein and leavening, consisting of potassium bitartrate and sodium bicarbonate, and flavored with sodium chloride; a palatable flour for making bread, muffins, pancakes, etc.; also called Diaban Flour.

Action and Uses: In dietetic treatment of diabetes; in carbohydrate restricted diets; is made into muffins and bread.

Analysis:

Protein	28.67 %	Pentosans	5.26 %
Starch	27.77 %	Fibre	2.33 %
Fat	18.69 %	Sucrose	0.60 %
Water	8.49 %	Dextrose	0.25 %
Ash	5.64 %	Dextrin	0.06 %

Food Value: Per 500 Gm—2,190 calories; protein 588, fat 906 and carbohydrate 696 calories.

Supply: **DIETETIC FLOUR (C.A.)**—Tins of 6 oz.—Cans of 5 and 10 lb.

Combinations: **DIETETIC WAFERS**—Made from MacDowell's Dietetic Flour; *For use* in diabetic diet.

Analysis:

Protein (N × 6.25)	25 %	Ash	5.66 %
Carbohydrates	27.75 %	Water	3.60 %
Undetermined	19.10 %	Pentosans, Hemicelluloses	95.58 %
Fat	14.47 %		

Food Value: 100 Gm = 389 calories.

Supply: Plain, chocolate and ginger flavors—Cartons 8 oz.

WHEAT SOYA FLOUR (Curdolac)

Description: A low protein and low carbohydrate flour, palatable and slightly laxative; is prepared from starch-free bran, soy bean, small amount of wheat with leavening and flavoring. *Used* for making tasty bread, waffles, cakes, muffins etc.

Analysis:

Protein	23 %	Fibre	6.02 %
Carbohydrate	20.5 %	Ash	11.8 %
Fat	9.3 %	Moisture	5.52 %
Nitrogen-free extract	23.86 %		

Food Value: Per 100 Gr—264 calories.

Supply: **WHEAT SOYA FLOUR (C.A.)**—Packages of 1 and 5 lb.

7. FOOD ACCESSORIES

A. Confections (Loeb)

Chewing Gum: Sweet, peppermint flavored, of no food value.

Supply: Packages of 12.

(Dietetic Food)

Dietetic Candy: A flavored vegetable product; is starch, sugar, protein and fat free; of no food value.

Supply: Boxes of ½, 1 lb.

(Loeb)

Dietetic Chocolate Bars: Contains—

	Plain, Per Cent	Almond, Per Cent
Carbohydrate	7	5
Protein	15	15
Fat	52	53

Food value: 261 calories and 263 calories.

Supply: Packages, Sweetened and Unsweetened.

(Dietetic Food)

Dietetic Cocoa Bars: Contains moisture 3.82 %, ash (mineral matter) 2.37 %, protein (N × 6.25) 23.08 %, carbohydrates 20.14 %, fat (ether extract) 38.35 %, crude fibre 8.04 %, sugars 0.00 %, non-hydrolyzing carbohydrates, by difference, 4.20%.

For use as ordinary chocolate; or as beverage by dissolving ½ bar in cup of boiling water, with milk or cream.

Supply: Boxes of 10 bars.

(Lister)

Lister's Brittle: An imitation candy without sugar, starch or fat; protein only 2½ %; prepared from ceretonia gum, indian gum and gum acacia, sweetened with saccharin and dulcin 0.67 gr per oz. Food value: 100 Gm equals 10 calories.

Supply: Boxes of ½ lb.

(Loeb)

Unsweetened Chocolate: Prepared from cocoa beans; contains carbohydrates 13 %, protein 14 %, fat 52 %. Food value: 501 calories per package.

Supply: Packages.

B. Desserts (Chicago Dietetic)

Agar Dessert: A preparation of agar-agar, true fruit flavors, saccharin; is sugar-free; flavors—orange, lemon, raspberry, grape, cherry. Food value: not in excess of ½ %.

Supply: Boxes of 10 individual servings.

(Chicago Dietetic)

Cellu Agar Jelly: Flavors—raspberry, strawberry, cherry, grape, lemon, orange; of no food value.

Supply: Glasses of 6 oz.

(Chicago Dietetic)

Cellu Chili Sauce: Sugarless, but of carbohydrate content 6 %; palatable and well-seasoned.

Supply: Bottles of 8 oz.

(Curdolac)

Delecto Dessert Powder: Sugar free; flavors—lemon, orange, grape, cocoa.

Supply: Boxes of 8 individual servings.

(Loeb)

Dietetic Grape Jelly: Contains carbohydrate 5 %, protein—traces, fat—none. Food value: 21 calories per jar.

Supply: Jars.

(Dietetic Food)

Dietetic Pudding: Contains per serving protein 4.48 gr., fat 6 gr., carbohydrates 0.017 gr; flavors—chocolate, vanilla, lemon, butterscotch.

Supply: Boxes of 2 oz. for 4 servings.

(Chicago Dietetic)

D-Zerta: A powder for preparing sugar-free gelatin dessert; flavors—raspberry, lemon, orange. Food value per portion equivalent to 2.3 Gm gelatin.

Supply: Boxes of 20 servings.

(MacDowell)

D-Zerta: A sugar-free gelatin dessert; flavors—lemon, raspberry, orange; *For use* as dessert or pie filling.

Supply: Boxes of 20 envelopes for 20 servings.

(Chicago Dietetic)

Gelatin Dessert: Prepared from pure gelatin, artificial flavoring, certified colors and fruit acids; is unsweetened; flavors—raspberry, grape, cherry, orange, lemon. Food value: proteins 3 %, carbohydrates 5 %, fat—none.

Supply: Boxes of 20 envelopes for 20 servings.

(Hansen)

Junket Powder (C.A.): A concentrated rennin mixed with cane sugar and fruit flavors, cocoa or coffee; *For use* in preparing junket desserts; flavors—vanilla, orange, chocolate, lemon, raspberry, coffee. *Used*—by stirring directly in milk and cooling; one package per pint of milk.

Supply: Packages 1½ oz., cans 1 pound. **(Hansen)**

Junket Tablets (C.A.): A concentrated rennin mixed with pure table salt and standardized; added to milk, forms junket and palatable dessert; *For use* in children, convalescents, peptic ulcer, nephritis, obesity, tuberculosis, diabetes. *Used*—1 tablet to 1 pt. of milk, sweetened and flavored.

Supply: Tablets—Boxes of 10, with recipes.

(Knox)

Knox Jell: *For use* as base of desserts and salads.

Supply: Packages of 26 oz.

(Knox)

Sparkling Gelatine (C.A.): A gelatine preparation from hard bones of food animals, contains protein about 85%, fat 0.1%, carbohydrate none, moisture 13%; calcium phosphate 1–1.25%; *For use* in infant feeding, growing children, convalescence, gastric hemorrhage diet, diabetes, tuberculosis, constipation.

Supply: Plain and Sparkling, in boxes sufficient for 4 pt.

C. Dressings

(Chicago Dietetic)

Mayonnaise: Is high in fat, free from condiments; contains protein 0.9%, carbohydrate none, fat 87%.

Supply: Jars of 8, 16 oz.

(Curdolac)

Mayonnaise (C.A.): A delicious, carbohydrate free, low fat dressing.
Food value: protein 0.7%, carbohydrate none, fat 0.5%.

Supply: Jars of 6 oz.

(Loeb)

Mayonnaise, Dietetic: Prepared from mineral oil; is of low food value.

Supply: In jars.

(Chicago Dietetic)

Mineral Oil Dressing: Prepared from eggs, milk, oil, vinegar and salt; *For use* in obesity and laxative diets.
Food value: protein 1%, fat 1%, carbohydrate none.

Supply: Jars of 8, 16 oz.

(Curdolac)

Oil Dressing (C.A.): A mineral oil substitute for butter, lard and olive oil in solids; of no food value.

Supply: Bottles 1 pt., 1 qt.

D. Flavorings

(Dietetic Food)

Beverage Compounds (C.A.): Flavorings of ginger ale, root beer, strawberry, sarsaparilla, cherry, currant, raspberry, loganberry, orangeade; of no food value and sugar-free; *For use* with water, plain or carbonated.

Supply: Bottles of 4 and 8 oz.

(Winthrop)

Curtasal: Contains calcium, magnesium and sodium salts of aliphatic carbonic and oxycarbonic acids. A white crystalline powder easily soluble in water; is inert and excreted almost completely unchanged. *Used* as salt substitute for seasoning of food in cardiorenal disease, hypertension, arteriosclerosis, epilepsy, tuberculosis and renal complications of pregnancy; is added directly to food in amounts about twice as much as ordinary table salt.

Supply: Aluminum salt shakers—2 oz.; Bottles of 8 oz.

Citric Acid (C.A.): A vinegar substitute. **(Curdolac)**

Supply: Jars of 4½ oz.

(Loeb)

Dietetic Cocoa: Contains carbohydrates 11%, proteins 33%, fat 18%. Food value: per package—304 calories.

Supply: In tins.

(Loeb)

Dietetic Cocoa Shells: Has no food value; *used* for beverage purposes.

Supply: Packages.

(Abbott)

Hosal: A combination of aminoacids, low molecular fatty acids, with calcium and sodium. *Used* as salt substitute and flavoring agent, having the approximate taste of ordinary table salt, in conditions where salt-free diet is indicated: eclampsia, tuberculosis, arteriosclerosis, hypertension, cardiorenal disease, etc.; is added to food or incorporated with it.

Supply: Salt shakers ¾ oz.—Bottles of 8 oz.

(Loeb)

Imitation Maple Syrup: A sweetening agent.

Supply: Bottles of 1 pt.

(Lister)

Lister's Sugarless Sweetener: A blend of sodium caseinate, precipitated calcium carbonate, sweetened with saccharin and dulcin; *For use* in place of sugar in diabetic diets, in sweet sauces, icings, etc.

Supply: Sifter top cans, 2 oz.

(National Aniline)

Malic Acid F.F.: Chemical Formula—$CH_2(COOH)_2CH.OH$.
A white, crystalline substance, readily soluble in water and alcohol, of pleasant acid taste; occurs naturally in apples, peaches, plums and other stone fruits; combines readily with fruit flavors, essences or ginger into 1 single flavor; *used* in flavoring bottle beverages, jellies, confections, ice cream, desserts.

Supply: Cartons of 5 and 10 lb.

(Nutradiet)

Nutradiet-Honey: Strained—Jars of 16 oz.

(Burroughs Wellcome)

Saxin: A substitute for sugar, 600 times sweeter than cane sugar and without food value; *for use* as sweetening agent in diabetes.

Supply: Tabloids gr ¼ (0.016 Gm), representing 1 teaspoonful of cane sugar in sweetening value—Bottles of 100, 200 and 500.

(Chicago Dietetic)

Sugarless Syrup: Imitation syrup prepared from vegetable gum, artificial maple flavor, saccharin, certified color; of no food value.

Supply: Jugs of ½ pt.

(Frank Sons)

Tablets Chicory (C.A.): The white, milky roots of the plant Cichorium Intybus; a flavoring agent imparting color, body, aroma and pungency to coffee; is diuretic and tonic.

Analysis:

Moisture	3.5%	Crude fiber	7.9%
Ash	4.7%	Reducing sugar as invert	8.6%
Water soluble ash	2.9%	Sucrose	0.4%
Acid insoluble ash	0.4%	Total carbohydrate	73.0%
Fat	3.6%	Water extr	69.0%
Protein	7.3%		

Food value: 2.5 calories per Gm., 71 per ounce.

Supply: Boxes of 40; *Used*—1 tablet added to percolator of coffee.

E. Noodles

(Dietetic Food)

Gluten Noodles: Contains protein 36.95 %, carbohydrate 18.50 %, fat 2.84 %, cellulose 15.33 %, hemicellulose 14.93 %, ash 1.57 %, moisture 9.88 %.

Supply: Boxes of 8 oz. for 3 servings.

(Loeb)

Gluten Noodles: Contains carbohydrate 37 %, protein 41 %, fat 4 %; is salt-free. Food value per package: 303 calories.

Supply: Packages of fine and broad sizes.

(Chicago Dietetic)

Noodles: Prepared from cellu flour and eggs; is starch-free; contains protein 6 %, carbohydrate—none, fat 6 %.

Supply: Boxes of 5 oz.

(Curdolac)

Noodles (C.A.): Of low carbohydrate content; contains protein 22 %, carbohydrate 5 %, fat 14 %.

Supply: Packages of 10 oz.

(Energen)

Tapioca: (Starch-reduced) Contains carbohydrate 21½ Gm, protein 2¼ Gm; food value—97 calories per ounce.

Supply: Packages of 1 lb.

F. Miscellaneous

(Loeb)

Baking Powder, Starch-Free: Of no food value.

Supply: Tins.

(Chicago Dietetic)

Bouillon Cubes: An appetizer and stimulant; flavors—beef, vegetable, mushroom, tomato, chicken, liver.

Food value: 1 Gm of carbohydrates and proteins.

Supply: Jars of 12 cubes.

(Curdolac)

Bouillon Cubes (C.A.): Salt-free, *For use* by nephritics and cardiacs; flavors—beef, chicken.

Supply: Jars of 30 cubes.

(Curdolac)

Butter, Peanutless (C.A.): Has appearance and taste of peanut butter but contains no butter.

Food value: protein 20 %, carbohydrate 4 %, fat 12 %.

Supply: Packages of 10 oz.

(Loeb)

Dietetic Agar-agar: *For use* in thickening soups, gravies and sauces; of no food value.

Supply: Tins.

(Loeb)

Dietetic India Gum: For thickening soups, gravies; of no food value.

Supply: Tins.

(MacDowell)

India Gum Karaya: A selected grade of gum arabic.

Supply: Packages of 1 lb.

(Dietetic Food)

India Gum: A binder, to thicken soups, gravies or to replace corn starch.

Supply: Cans of 4 oz.

(Lister)

Lister's Golden Spread: A fat-free butter substitute, with appearance and taste of dairy butter; prepared from saturated hydrocarbons, emulsified with certified coloring, salt and a special culture to produce butter flavor; contains vitamin A and has no food value. *For use* in low fat diets for diabetics and the obese, in gall bladder disorders, food allergies; freely as butter on table and in kitchen.

Supply: Individual tubs of 1 lb. of butter.

(Lister)

Lister's Indian Gum: A vegetable product for use as binder and thickener.

Supply: Boxes of ¼ lb.

(Schieffelin)

Steero Cubes: *For use* as bouillon and to flavor soups and other foods; combines flavors of beef, vegetables, spices, seasoning.

Supply: Tins of 4, 12, 50 and 100; *Used*—1 cube in 1 cup boiling water.

8. FOOD CONCENTRATES

(H. H. Clapp)

Beef Broth (C. A.): Of value as an appetizer and as a meat stock for vegetable soup. The fat is removed.

Analysis: See page 855.

Supply: Jars 4 oz.; Cans 4½ oz.

(Armour)

Beef Peptone: A liquid food prepared from fresh, lean beef by a peptonizing process; contains in assimilable form, the entire nutritive content of fresh beef with extractives; 1 lb. of beef peptone is equivalent to 5½ lb. fresh lean beef. *For use* in malnutrition, as appetizer and gastric stimulant.

Supply: Containers—powder, containing 10% milk sugar, in 1, 5, 10 and 25 lb.

Administration: 1 tablespoonful three times daily.

(Valentine)

Valentine's Meat Juice (L.A.): An aqueous extract of lean meat, 1 oz. representing the water soluble extractives of 20 oz. of lean beef.

Analysis:

Water	57.64%	Total nitrogen	3.06%
Solids	42.36%	Total phosphoric acid	3.41%
Total meat bases	6.05%	Sodium chloride	1.77%
Total protein substance	5.63%	Ash	10.26%
Undetermined	15.02%		

For use as a gastric stimulant, appetizer and nutrient, in gastrointestinal disorders, acute infections, convalescence and after operation.

Supply: Flasks of 1⅗ oz.

Dosage: 1 teaspoonful three times daily in hot or cold water shortly before meals.

(Squibb)

Vitavose (C.A.): Fine golden yellow, very hygroscopic granules, of pleasant taste and soluble in water; compared with certified whole cow's milk contains no less than 100 times that of vitamin B_1 and 33 times that of vitamin B_2; has nutritive value of 3.9 calories per Gm; contains maltose 38%, maltodextrin 20%, dextrins, 20%, soluble proteins 8%, soluble amino acids and other nitrogen products 4% mineral salts, including iron in natural form 0.0125%, moisture 3%.

Supply: Tins of 1 lb.

Dosage: 1 tablespoonful one to three times daily with milk or water.

9. LACTIC ACID MILK PRODUCTS

(Mead Johnson)

Powdered Lactic Acid Milk: Plain (Non-Curdling)—A whole milk, acidified with U.S.P. lactic acid and spray-dried; prepared so that the desired carbohydrate additions may be made; can be reliquefied in water at any temperature; does not curdle when boiled. *For use* as complement in breast feeding, for marasmic infants and those intolerant of fat and sugar. Normal amount of Dextri-Maltose may be added.

Analysis:

Protein	26.0%	Minerals (ash)	6.0%
Lactose (by difference)	36.8%	Lactic acid	2.5%
Milk fat	27.2%	Moisture	1.5%

Food value: 141 calories per ounce (3½ packed level tablespoonfuls equal 1 oz.).

Supply: POWDERED LACTIC ACID MILK—Plain (C.A.)—Tins of 1 and 4 lb.

Administration: To reliquefy for normal dilution—1 packed level tablespoonful is added to 2 oz. water; containing then—

Protein	3.3%	Lactic acid	0.3%
Lactose (by difference)	4.6%	Moisture	87.6%
Milk fat	3.4%	pH	5.0%
Minerals (ash)	0.8%	Food value: 18 calories per ounce.	

Dosage: 5–15 level tablespoonfuls, with 3–8 level tablespoonfuls Dextri-Maltose, 10½–30 ounces water; 6–5 feedings of 2–7 oz. each in 24 hr.

Bibliography: *See Chap. XII.*

(Mead Johnson)

Powdered Lactic Acid Milk with Dextri-Maltose: (Non-Curdling)—A powdered, boilable lactic acid milk combined with 6% Dextri-Maltose; requires only dilution. *For use* as complement to breast feeding; for marasmic infants and those whose tolerance for fat and sugar is low.

Analysis:

Protein	18.3%	Milk fat	19.1%
Dextrins (by difference)	13.4%	Minerals (ash)	4.2%
Maltose (reducing sugars)	16.2%	Lactic acid	1.8%
Lactose (reducing sugars)	25.5%	Moisture	1.5%

Food value: 132 calories per ounce. (3 packed level tablespoonfuls equal 1 oz.)

Supply: POWDERED LACTIC ACID MILK WITH DEXTRI-MALTOSE (C.A.)—Tins of 20 oz. and 5 lb.

Administration: To reliquefy for normal dilution—1 packed level tablespoonful is added to 1½ oz. water; containing then—

Protein	3.3%	Moisture	82.1%
Carbohydrates	10.0%	Lactic acid	0.3%
Milk fat	3.5%	pH	4.6
Minerals (ash)	0.8%	Food value: 25 calories per ounce.	

Dosage: 10–20 packed level tablespoonfuls with 15–30 oz. water; 6–5 feedings of 3–7 oz. each in 24 hr.

Bibliography: *See Chap. XII.*

(Merrell-Soule)

Powdered Whole Lactic Acid Milk: A powdered milk for prematures, new-born, in milder diarrhea and for routine infant feeding.

Analysis:

Butterfat	28%	Free acidity	4.25%
Protein	26.5%	Total acidity	5.0%
Lactose	32.5%	Moisture	2.75%
Salts	6.0%		

Food value:

Calories per ounce	147	Calories per tablespoonful	41
Calories per gram	5.2		

Supply: POWDERED WHOLE LACTIC ACID MILK (C.A.)—Containers 1, 4, 25 and 50 lb. vacuum packed.

Administration: To prepare standard strength dilution: 4½ oz. or 16 tablespoonfuls are added to 1 qt. of water, making 35 oz. lactic acid milk; or 1 packed tablespoonful in 2 oz. water; dilution contains—butterfat 3.3%, protein 3.2%, lactose 3.9%, salts 0.7%, free lactic acid 0.5%, total acidity 0.6%, water 88.4%; pH = 4.6.

Food value: 18.5 calories per ounce, 0.64 per cubic centimeter.

Bibliography: *See Chap. XII.*

10. MILK MODIFIERS

ALERDEX (S. M. A.)

Description: A protein-free maltose and dextrins preparation; essentially a mixture of approximately equal parts of maltose and dextrins, rendered protein-free by special process and free from pathogenic organisms.

Composition:

Moisture	3.0%	Hydrolyzed proteins (N x 6.25)	0.5%
Ash	0.5%	Reducing sugars as maltose	50.0%
Fat (ether extract)	0.0%	Dextrins (by difference)	46.0%

Food Value: Calories: per gram 3.85; per ounce 109.

Uses: For the modification of the milk of infants requiring a protein-free or low protein milk, because of a state of sensitization.

Supply: ALERDEX (C.A.)—Tins.

Administration: As per formula desired.

BANANA POWDER (Merck)

Description: Spray dried ripe bananas in powder form, retaining their natural enzymes and vitamins; contains approximately vitamin A (100%), B (100%), C (20%) and G (100%) of bananas.

Uses: An easily assimilable and nourishing carbohydrate food; *useful* in modifying cow's milk and in supplementary infant feeding; as flavoring agent in foods, desserts.

Supply: BANANA POWDER (C.A.)—Cans, friction-plug, 10 and 22 oz.

Administration: For children and adults—1 tablespoonful or more to a glass of milk, or as substitute for sugar on cereals, desserts; as flavoring or sweetening agent.

Bibliography: *See Chap. XII.*

CASEC (Mead Johnson)

Calcium Caseinate

Description: A milk modifier, almost wholly a combination of protein with calcium.

Composition:

Protein	88.0%	Minerals (ash)	4.5%
Milk fat	2.0%	Calcium	1.8%
Moisture	5.5%	Phosphorus	0.6%

Food Value: 108 calories per ounce (12 packed level tablespoonfuls equal 1 oz.).

Action and Uses: Is growth promoting in non-thriving infants. *For use* as prophylactic against diarrhea during the onset of an infection; in colic and diarrhea of breast-fed infants; in fermentative diarrheas in the bottle-fed and older children.

Supply: CASEC (C.A.)—Tins of 3⅓ and 30 oz.

Preparation: ⅓ oz. added to 32 oz. of feeding mixture increases protein content 1%.

With Milk—Casec is mixed with enough cool, boiled water to make a thin paste; the balance of the water and milk is added and the mixture heated slowly, with constant stirring, until the Casec is dissolved. The mixture should not be heated to boiling.

With Water—The Casec is mixed with enough cool, boiled water to make a thin paste; the balance of the water is gradually added to the paste, with constant stirring to obtain a smooth mixture. The mixture is then placed in the refrigerator until ready to use.

Dosage: *With Water*—4 packed level tablespoonfuls.
3 to 10 oz. water.
With Milk—8 packed level tablespoonfuls.
16–20 oz. water.
10–16 oz. whole milk.
7–5 feedings of 2–9 oz. each in 24 hr.

Bibliography: *See Chap. XII.*

CITABS (Squibb)

Anhydrous Citric Acid

Description: Prepared from specially purified citric acid; readily soluble in warm water, very slowly soluble in milk.

Action: Forms a smooth homogeneous acid milk mixture, of uniform small curds, without large indigestible masses; gives the gastric contents of the infant a hydrogen ion concentration of 3.72, similar to that of the breast fed infant; has pleasant flavor, does not increase urine acidity, and is well tolerated.

Uses: For preparing acid-milk for artificially fed children, in very young infants with diarrhea caused by sugar fermentation and in intestinal disturbances common in summer.

Supply: CITABS (C.A.)—Tablets gr 7½ (0.5 Gm)—Bottles of 200.

Administration: 4 tablets for each pint of milk; after boiling and cooling of milk or feeding mixture, 4 tablets dissolved in 2–3 teaspoonfuls of water are added; the mixture is stirred before administering.

Bibliography: *See Chap. XII.*

CHOCOLATE FLAVORED VITAVOSE (Squibb)

Food Supplement

Composition: Contains Vitavose 30%, milk solids, cocoa and sugar, comprising carbohydrates 83%, proteins 10%, fats, 1.8%, ash, 3.3%; food value—115 calories per ounce.

Use and Administration: Makes a delicious, Vitamin B-rich drink in hot or cold milk, using about 2 teaspoonfuls to the glass; also *used* in preparation of fudge, ice cream, candies, and other articles of food.

Supply: CHOCOLATE-FLAVORED VITAVOSE—Cans of 1 lb.

DEXIN (Burroughs Wellcome)

Composition: Contains

Dextrins	75%	Ash	0.25%
Maltose	24%	Moisture	0.75%

Action and Uses: A high, non-fermentable dextrin carbohydrate for modifying cow's milk in infant feeding and for adult invalids; is easily assimilated, readily soluble in all proportions in cold fluids.

Supply: DEXIN—Tins of 12 oz.

Administration: Is added to the infant's feedings in accordance with age and weight; for adults, sprinkled on fruit or cereal or dissolved in milk, tea, coffee, etc.

Bibliography: *See Chap. XII.*

DEXTRI-MALTOSE 1 (Mead Johnson)

Description: A carbohydrate of high tolerance for modifying cow's milk and other infant feeding formulae.

Composition:

Maltose	51%	Sodium chloride	2%
Dextrins	42%	Moisture	5%

Food Value: 108 Calories per ounce (4 level tablespoonfuls are equal to 1 oz.).

Action and Uses: General infant feeding for carbohydrate modification of milk formulae.

Supply: DEXTRI-MALTOSE 1 (C.A.)—Tins of 1 and 5 lb.

DEXTRI-MALTOSE 2 (Mead Johnson)

Composition:

Maltose	52%	Moisture	5%
Dextrins	43%		

Food Value: 108 Calories per ounce. (4 level tablespoonfuls equal 1 oz.)

Action and Uses: Salt-free to permit freedom in salt modification; especially valuable as adjunct in diets of nursing mothers and invalids to increase caloric content of milk.

Supply: DEXTRI-MALTOSE 2 (C.A.)—Tins of 1 and 5 lb.

DEXTRI-MALTOSE 3 (Mead Johnson)

Composition:

Maltose	51%	Potassium bicarbonate	3%
Dextrins	41%	Moisture	5%

Food Value: 108 Calories per ounce (4 level tablespoonfuls are equal to 1 oz.).

Action and Uses: To counteract tendency toward constipation; promotes formation of soft, flocculent curds and soft stools; conserves alkali reserve.

Supply: DEXTRI-MALTOSE 3 (C.A.)—Tins of 1 and 5 lb.

Preparation: DEXTRI-MALTOSE 1, 2, and 3: Required amount of water is brought to a boil; required amount of milk is added and the mixture boiled for 3 min.; boiled water is added to replace that lost by evaporation; to this is added the required amount of Dextri-Maltose which is measured by means of a standard tablespoon and leveled with the aid of a table knife.

Dosage: DEXTRI-MALTOSE 1, 2 and 3: 3–6 level tablespoonfuls with 10–38 oz. whole milk and 2–11 oz. water; 7–5 feedings of 3–8 oz. each in 24 hr.

Bibliography: *See Chap. XII.*

DEXTRI-MALTOSE WITH VITAMIN B (Mead Johnson)

Description: Contains in addition to the carbohydrate value of Dextri-Maltose, also vitamin B complex (vitamins B and G) derived from yeast and wheat embryo.

Composition:

Maltose (Reducing sugars)	52.6%	Minerals (ash) including natural iron salts 0.012%	2.3%
Dextrins (By differences)	39.8%	Moisture	1.0%
Protein	4.3%		

Food Value: 112 calories per ounce (6 level tablespoonfuls equal 1 oz.).

Uses: For modifying milk formulae of infants exhibiting partial vitamin B deficiency; in anorexia, spasticity, irritability; for nursing mothers.

Supply: DEXTRI-MALTOSE WITH VITAMIN B (C.A.)—Tins of 12 oz. and 4 lb.

Preparation: Required amount of water is brought to a boil; required amount of milk is added and the mixture boiled for 3 min.; boiled water is added to replace that lost by evaporation; to this is added the required amount of Dextri-Maltose which is measured by means of a standard tablespoon and leveled with the aid of a table knife.

Dosage: 3½–9 level tablespoonfuls with 10–38 oz. whole milk, 2–11 oz. water; 7–5 feedings of 3–8 oz. each in 24 hr.

Bibliography: *See Chap. XII.*

DEXTROLAC (Upjohn)

Description: A lactic acid milk modifier for infant feeding, containing mixed carbohydrates including dextrin, maltose and detrose lactic acid, iron and potassium salts.

Action and Uses: Milk modifier in infant feeding; adjusts cow's milk to become easily digested like breast milk. *For use* in supplementary and complementary feeding of infants; in rickets; in the malnourished, infected, under weight child.

Supply: DEXTROLAC 1—Bottles 12 and 32 oz. Containing per fl. oz.—

Carbohydrates (dextrins, maltose, dextrose gr)		25.515 Gm
Iron lactate	0.033	0.002 Gm
Potassium lactate	4.136	0.268 Gm
Lactic Acid U.S.P.	m. 32.787	2.00 cc.

Food Value: 54 calories per tablespoonful.

DEXTROLAC 2—Same content as 1, except half the amount of lactic acid, only 1 %—Bottles 12 and 32 oz.

Administration: As per schedule and tables, obtainable from manufacturer.

DEXTRO-VITAVOSE (Squibb)

Description: Vitavose modified to supply a greater quantity of carbohydrates, especially of dextrose.

Composition:

Dextrose	65 %	Mineral salts	1½ %
Maltose	15 %	Moisture	1½ %
Dextrin	12 %	Iron	0.0004 %
Soluble proteins	5 %		

Contains about 30 times as much of the antineuritic Vitamin B factor as does fresh, raw, certified whole milk, and 10 times as much pellagra preventing Vitamin G; 3 tablespoonfuls are equal to a quart of milk and yield approximately 120 calories.

Uses: For modification of milk for very young infants, especially those suffering from gastro-intestinal disturbances.

Administration: The quantity to be used is first mixed into a paste with a little boiled but cooled water, and then added to the rest of the water, stirring constantly; this is then mixed with the milk and poured into nursing bottles.

Supply: DEXTRO-VITAVOSE (C.A.)—Tins-moisture proof, 1 lb.

Bibliography: *See Chap. XII.*

HYLAC (Nestle)

Description: A spray-dried, homogenized mixture of cow's milk, with milk fat, milk sugar, malted whole wheat extract (dextrins and maltose) and iron citrate.

Action and Uses: For the modification of cow's milk in infant feeding and for correct balancing of formulas, to closely simulate human milk.

Analysis:

Milk Fat	21.5 %	Dextrin	28 %
Carbohydrate	69.0 %	Protein	5.5 %
Lactose	17 %	Ash (iron 0.0036 %)	2.0 %
Maltose	24 %	Moisture	2.0 %

Food Value: 152 calories per ounce; 25 calories per tablespoonful.

Supply: HYLAC (C.A.)—Cans of 14 oz.

Administration: According to formula desired.

LAROSAN "STOELTZNER" (Roche)

Description: Calcium caseinate, containing 1.75% of calcium; is high in protein and low in carbohydrate and fat content; a white, light, powdery substance, odorless, tasteless and neutral in reaction; readily soluble in hot milk.

Uses: In the management of fermentative diarrheas and other nutritional disorders of infancy.

Supply: LAROSAN (C.A.)—Packages of ⅔ oz. each, 5 in carton.

Administration and Dosage: Is begun with 2 oz. of Larosan milk every 3 hr., prepared by mixing 1 pt. of milk and 1 pt. of water with a ⅔ oz. package of Larosan.

Bibliography: *See Chap. XII.*

MALT SUGAR (Borcherdt)

Analysis:

Maltose	87%	Dextrins	4.7%
Protein	4.4%	Mineral Salts, including calcium, sodium, potassium, magnesium, iron, sulphur, phosphorus	1.9%
Moisture	2%		

Food Value: 109.1 calories per ounce.

Action and Uses: Is biologically assayed for vitamin potency, B_1 and B_2 (G), 1 Gm being equivalent to 0.6 Gm dried yeast or 2.5 gr of moist yeast; is low in protein, easily digested and favorably affects intestinal flora; is not constipating. *Used* as sugar substitute in infant feeding.

Supply: MALT SUGAR (C.A.)—Tins of 1 lb.

Administration: In accordance with infant feeding formulae.

S. M. A. CONCENTRATED LIQUID FORM (S. M. A.)

Description: A homogenized mixture of skim milk, lactose, beef fat, cocoanut oil, cocoa butter, cod liver oil and potassium chloride; the chemical constants of the fat are similar to those of human milk fat.

Action: An antirachitic and antispasmophilic sterile food; when diluted according to directions, is essentially similar to human milk in percentages of protein, fat, carbohydrate and ash, in chemical constants of the fat and in many physical properties.

Analysis:

Moisture	72.9%	Protein (N × 6.38)	3.1%
Ash	0.7%	Lactose (by difference)	15.8%
Fat (ether extract)	7.5%		

Of dilution according to directions in each package:

Ash	0.2–0.3	Lactose (by difference)	7.3–7.5
Fat (ether extract)	3.5–3.6	pH	6.8–7.0
Protein (N × 6.38)	1.3–1.4		

Food Value: 1.4 calories per Gm, 40 calories per fluid ounce. After dilution 20 calories per fluid ounce.

Supply: S. M. A. CONCENTRATED LIQUID FORM (C.A.)—Cans of 6.2 and 16½ oz.

Administration: According to formula desired.

SMACO MALTOSE AND DEXTRINS (S. M. A.)

Description: Essentially a mixture of approximately equal parts of maltose and dextrins, spray-dried and bacteria free.

Composition:

Moisture	3.0%	Protein (N × 6.25)	0.5%
Ash	0.5%	Reducing sugars as maltose	50.0%
Fat (ether extract)	0.0%	Dextrins (by difference)	46.0%

Food Value: Per Gm 3.9 calories; per oz. 111 calories.

Uses: *For use* as a carbohydrate supplement for the modification of milk for infant feeding.

Supply: SMACO MALTOSE AND DEXTRINS (C.A.)—Tins, hermetically sealed.

11. POWDERED FOODS

BORDEN'S MALTED MILK (Borden)

Description: A powdered product of barley malt, whole milk and wheat flour, processed and evaporated to dryness; mixes readily with water, producing an even suspension.

Composition:

Fat	9.2%	Dextrin	20.2%
Protein	15.5%	Ash	3.8%
Lactose and Maltose	49.1%	Moisture	2.2%

Food Value: Calories per ounce 123.

Action: Is rich in enzymes and a source of vitamins A, B and G; adds flavor and digestibility to milk and assists digestion.

Uses: Valuable as a food for children, invalids, convalescents and the aged; also used as a carrier for barium in X-ray work.

Supply: BORDEN'S MALTED MILK (C.A.)—Tins of ½, 1, 5, 10 and 25 lb.

Bibliography: *See Chap. XII.*

MALTCAO (Merckens)

Composition: Contains cocoa, milk, malt, sugar and the organic phosphates of calcium and iron.

Action and Uses: A digestible, hematinic and tonic food and ready source of calcium; *used* in convalescence, for infants and nursing mothers.

Analysis:

Moisture	3.03%	Dextrin and carbohydrate	7.36%
Cocoa butter	4.42%	Mineral ash	3.99%
Butter fat	0.56%	Ash comprising	
Milk solids	10.09%	Sodium chloride	0.84%
Crude fiber	0.89%	Iron	0.09%
Cane sugar	45.07%	Calcium oxide	0.52%
Maltose	14.72%	Phosphate	1.41%
Total protein	9.87%		

Food Value: Per dram 35 calories; per pound 1,830 calories.

Supply: MALTCAO (C.A.)—Cans of 1 lb.

MALTED MILK (Horlick)

Description: A powdered food accessory prepared from whole cow's milk, extracts of wheat and malted barley.

Analysis:

Fat	8.78%	Total soluble carbohydrate	67.95%
Protein	16.35%	Minerals (ash)	3.86%
Dextrin	18.80%	Moisture	3.06–100.0%
Lactose and maltose	49.15%		

Ash Constituents:

Potassium oxide	31.3%	Chlorine	15.8%
Sodium oxide	16.7%	Phos. pentoxide	12.9%
Calcium oxide, Magnesium oxide, Ferric oxide	12.7%	Carbon dioxide	10.6–100.0%

Food Value: 121 calories per ounce, comprising

	Gm	Calories
Protein	4.65	19
Fat	2.49	23.1
Carbohydrate	19.26	78.9

Action and Uses: An easily digestible, palatable nutrient, *For use* in infant feeding, convalescence, peptic ulcer, constipation and in radiography.

Supply: MALTED MILK (C.A.)—Plain and Chocolate flavored—Tins of ½, 1 and 5 lb.

Administration: 1–2 tablespoonfuls mixed in 1 cup water or milk.

Bibliography: *See Chap. XII.*

MALTED NUTS (Battle Creek)

Description: A ground nut and malt sugar combination containing per ounce—

Carbohydrate	49.8 calories	Protein	26.9 calories
Fat	70.6 calories		

Action and Uses: *Useful* in infant feeding, especially for the child sensitized to milk, for growing children, nursing and expectant mothers, and in malnutrition.

Supply: MALTED NUTS—Jars of 7 and 14 oz. and 5 lb.

Administration: As food drink with milk and on cereals, salads, fruits, desserts.

NESTLE'S FOOD (Nestle)

Description: A powdered mixture of malted whole wheat, wheat malt (maltose, dextrins, starch, cereal protein and minerals), whole milk solids, sucrose, wheat flour tri-calcium and di-calcium phosphates, iron citrate and cod-liver oil extract with Vitamins A, B, D, and G.

Analysis:

Fat	1.3%	Ash	0.4%
Carbohydrate	9.5%	Moisture	86.8%
Protein	2.0%		

Food Value: 18 calories per ounce.

Action and Uses: For the feeding of infants who show limited tolerance to cow's milk, supplying its elements in easily digestible and non-irritating form.

Supply: NESTLE'S FOOD (C.A.)—Cans 1 lb.

Administration: According to formula desired.

SOBEE (Mead Johnson)

Description: A soy bean preparation free from milk proteins; contains soy bean flour 61.0%, sodium chloride 1.0%, arrowroot starch 9.0%, dextri-maltose 6.0%, dicalcium phosphate, pure 4.0%, olive oil 19.0%.

Analysis:

Fat	19.2%	Minerals (ash)	8.5%
Protein	32.0%	Moisture	2.4%
Carbohydrates	38.4%		

Food Value: 130 calories per ounce (6 level tablespoonfuls equal 1 oz.).

Action and Uses: For eczema and other diseases caused by milk-protein idiosyncrasy.

Supply: SOBEE (C.A.) Tins of 1 and 4 lb.

Preparation: To reliquefy for normal dilution—6 level tablespoonfuls are added to 7 oz. water; contains then—

Fat	2.4%	Minerals (ash)	1.0%
Protein	4.0%	Moisture 87.8%	pH 6.2
Carbohydrates	4.8%		

Food Value: 16 Calories per ounce.

Administration: Average feeding: 6 level tablespoonfuls Sobee, 7 oz. water with 1 level tablespoonful carbohydrate.

Bibliography: *See Chap. XII.*

STARCHLESS PORRIDGE POWDER (Lister)

Composition: Combines vegetable gums and palm nut flakes.

Analysis:

Moisture	10.9%	Starch	0.0%
Ash	6.1%	Sugar	0.0%
Fat	1.1%	Protein	2.7%
Cellulose, Hemicellulose	78.9%		

Food Value: A generous serving of porridge is made from ½ box of the powder. The food value of such a serving is:

Protein	0.8 Gm	Calories	6
Fat	0.3 Gm		

Uses: As cereal substitute.

Supply: **STARCHLESS PORRIDGE POWDER**—Carton 1 lb. Recipes in carton.

Administration: Prepared by stirring into boiling water.

THOMPSON'S DOUBLE MALTED MILK (Borden)

Description: A chocolate flavored, sweetened, powdered product of barley malt, wheat flour and whole milk evaporated to dryness, with sucrose and cocoa added; is a permanent, even suspension and an easily and quickly stirred food; is readily assimilated and of high flavor and aroma; is rich in Vitamins A, B and G.

Action: Converts cereal starches into malt sugars, prevents rancidity and aids digestion.

Uses: A valuable food for children and adults; an excellent carrier for barium in X-ray work.

Supply: **THOMPSON'S DOUBLE MALTED MILK** (C.A.)—Tins of ½, 1, 5, 10 and 25 lb.

Bibliography: *See Chap. XII.*

12. POWDERED MILK PRODUCTS

ALACTA (Mead Johnson)

Description: A powdered milk of low fat and low bacterial content.

Analysis:

Milk fat	12.0%	Minerals (ash)	7.0%
Lactose (by difference)	46.5%	Moisture	1.5%
Protein	33.0%		

Food Value: 121 calories per ounce (3½ packed level tablespoonfuls equal 1 oz.).

Uses: When milk of low fat is indicated.

Supply: **ALACTA** (C.A.)—Tins of 1 and 4 lb.

Preparation: To reliquefy for normal dilution—1 packed level tablespoonful is added to 2 oz. water; contains then—

Milk fat	1.5%	Minerals (ash)	0.9%
Protein	4.1%	Moisture	87.7%
Lactose (by difference)	5.8%		

Food Value: 15 calories per ounce.

Dosage: 7–17½ level tablespoonfuls Alacta, 3–5 level tablespoonfuls Dextri-Maltose, 20–36 oz. water; 7–5 feedings of 3–8 oz. each in 24 hr.

Bibliography: *See Chap. XII.*

DRYCO (Dry Milk)

Description: A powdered food prepared from fresh, liquid milk with part of butterfat removed; is irradiated by ultra-violet ray to increase Vitamin D content and dried by the "Just" Roller Process; is easily digested, nutritious, of small bulk; its protein forms a small flocculent precipitate and its fat is easily digestible.

Analysis:

Fat	12%	Mineral ash	7%
Lactose	46%	Moisture	3%
Protein	32%		

Food Value: Calories: per ounce 127; per level tablespoonful 16.

Action: Antirachitic, increasing mineral content of bones; is well tolerated, digested and assimilated often when other foods fail; always fresh, uniform, easily prepared, requires no refrigeration.

Uses: *Used* in infant feeding, rickets, eczema, gastrointestinal disturbances and diarrhea, vomiting; for the acutely ill and convalescent; for prematures.

Supply: DRYCO (C.A.)—Cans of 12 oz. and 3 lb.

Administration: 2½ level tablespoonfuls per day for each pound of infant body weight; dissolved in 1 or more ounces of water than there are tablespoonfuls of Dryco per feeding; made into a thick paste with hot water, stirred until smooth and diluted to proper quantity for each feeding.

Bibliography: *See Chap. XII.*

POWDERED PROTEIN MILK (Merrell-Soule)

Analysis:

Protein	37%	Free lactic acid	5%
Butterfat	27%	Moisture	3%
Lactose	23%	Total acidity	5.5%
Salts	5%		

Food Value: Calories: per ounce 146.7; per gram 5.2; per level tablespoonful 40.

Uses: For infant feeding in special cases; in alimentary intoxication, summer diarrhea, fermentative diarrhea, ileocolitis. celiac disease, prematurity, new-born babies.

Supply: POWDERED PROTEIN MILK (C.A.)—Containers 1 and 4 lb., vacuum packed.

Preparation: To prepare standard strength dilution: 10½ tablespoonfuls are *used* in 1 qt. of water; dilution contains—

Protein	3.0%	Salts	0.4%
Butterfat	2.2%	Free lactic acid	0.4%
Lactose	1.9%	Moisture	92.1%

Food Value: Calories: per ounce 12.1; per cubic centimeter 4.

Bibliography: *See Chap. XII.*

POWDERED PROTEIN MILK (Mead Johnson)

Description: A boilable protein milk prepared after the improved Finkelstein method, slightly modified to change casein content and assure a low bacterial count; is non-curdling.

Analysis:

Protein	39.0%	Minerals (ash)	6.0%
Lactose (by difference)	24.0%	Lactic acid	3.0%
Milk fat	26.5%	Moisture	1.5%

Food Value: 144 calories per ounce (3½ packed level tablespoonfuls equal 1 oz.)

Uses: In newborn infants, prematures, weight disturbances, decomposition (atrophy, marasmus); in fermentative (summer) diarrhea, alimentary intoxication (cholera infantum, ileocolitis), celiac disease.

Supply: **POWDERED PROTEIN MILK (C.A.)**—Tins of 1 and 4 lb.

Preparation: To reliquefy for normal dilution—1 oz. is added to 11 oz. water; dilution contains—

Protein	3.3%	Lactic acid	0.3%
Lactose (by difference)	2.0%	Moisture	91.8%
Milk fat	2.2%	pH	4.8
Minerals (ash)	0.5%	*Food Value:*	12 calories per ounce.

Dosage: 4 packed level tablespoonfuls Powdered Protein Milk, in 11 oz. water.

Bibliography: *See Chap. XII.*

RECOLAC (Mead Johnson)

Description: Contains soluble casein, lactalbumin, lactose, milk salts (all derived from fresh cow's milk), dextrins, maltose, minerals, extracts of yeast and wheat embryo, animal and vegetable fats and cod liver oil; the whole so proportioned as to meet almost all nutritional requirements of infants; contains vitamins A, B, D and G.

Analysis:

Protein	16.0%	Lactose (reducing sugars)	18.7%
Fats	27.0%	Minerals (ash)	3.3%
Dextrins (by difference)	16.2%	Moisture	1.4%
Maltose (reducing sugars)	17.4%		

Food Value: 148 calories per ounce (4 packed level tablespoonfuls equal 1 oz.).

Uses: An infant food for complementing breast feeding, for alternate feedings; where quality of fluid milk is questionable.

Supply: **RECOLAC (C.A.)**—Tins of 1 lb.

Preparation: To reliquefy for normal dilution—1 oz. is added to 7 oz. water; dilution contains—

Protein	2.0%	Minerals (ash)	0.4%
Fats	3.4%	pH	7.2
Carbohydrates	6.5%	*Food Value:*	19 calories per ounce.

Dosage: 1–4½ level tablespoonfuls Recolac in 2–7 oz. water.
7–5 feedings in 24 hr.

Bibliography: *See Chap. XII.*

SIMILAC (M and R Dietetic)

Description: A powdered milk, prepared from cow's milk for reliquefication to a composition similar to breast milk of uniform strength.

Action and Uses: A food for infants; meets the requirements for growth and nutrition in easily assimilable and digestible form and low curd-tension; for preparation of infant feeding formulae.

Supply: SIMILAC (C.A.)—Cans 1 lb.

Preparation: Reliquefication of 1 measureful in 2 oz. of water offers—

Protein	1.5%	Fat	3.4%
Sugar	6.8%	Salt	0.4%

Food Value: 19 calories per ounce of dilution.

S. M. A. POWDERED FORM (S. M. A.)

Composition: A dried, powdered homogenized mixture of skim milk, lactose, beef fat, cocoanut oil, cocoa butter, cod liver oil and potassium chloride. The chemical constants of the fat are similar to those of human milk fat; pathogenic microorganisms—none.

Description: A food for infants, prepared from tuberculin tested cows' milk, the fat of which is replaced by animal and vegetable fats, including biologically tested cod liver oil; milk sugar, potassium chloride and salts are added.

Action: The product contains sufficient cod liver oil to be antirachitic and antispasmophilic for the majority of babies; when prepared according to directions it approximates human milk in percentages of fat, protein, lactose and ash; the pH specific gravity and caloric value are also similar to those of human milk; the buffer value is low. Should be supplemented with orange juice or other adequate source of Vitamin C.

Analysis:

Moisture	1%	Protein (N × 6.38)	10%
Ash	2%	Lactose (by difference)	59%
Fat (ether extract)	28%		

Food Value: 5.3 calories per gram; 151—per ounce.

Preparation: Diluted with water according to directions, presents

Ash	0.2–0.3	Lactose (by difference)	7.3–7.5
Fat (ether extract)	3.5–3.6	pH	6.8–7.0
Protein (N × 6.38)	1.3–1.4	*Food Value:*	20 calories per fluidounce.

Uses: Is intended for infants of any age deprived of, or as a supplement to human milk; should be used when the infant is still well, or in the milder types of malnutrition.

Supply: S.M.A. POWDERED FORM (C.A.)—Tins 8 oz., 16 oz., with directions enclosed.

13. SKIMMED MILK PRODUCTS

(S. M. A.)

Hypo-Allergic Skim Milk: Sterilized, liquid, almost fat-free skim milk made hypo-allergic by prolonged processing. The milk is pasteurized and then almost completely defatted in centrifugal cream separator; is canned and processed under steam pressure for prolonged period; is immediately cooled and sterile. *For use* in individuals subject to allergic reactions from usual boiled skim milk or other skim milk preparations; may be used in regular feeding formulas.

Analysis:

Moisture	90.9%	Fat (ether extract)	0.1%
Total solids	9.1%	Protein (N × 6.38)	3.2%
Ash	0.7%	Lactose (by difference)	4.9%

Food Value: 0.35 calories per cc; 10 calories per fluid ounce.

Supply: HYPO-ALLERGIC SKIM MILK (C.A.)—Tins.

(S. M. A.)

Powdered Half-Skimmed Milk: A powdered, spray-dried, half-skimmed milk hermetically sealed in tins in an atmosphere of nitrogen and free from micro-organisms; for infant feeding wherever a partially skimmed milk is indicated.

Analysis:

Moisture	2.0%	Protein (N × 6.38)	31.0%
Ash	6.5%	Lactose (by difference)	45.0%
Fat (ether extract)	13.5%		

Preparation: Normal dilution, 5 level tablespoonfuls of powder to 8 fl. oz. of water; this contains—

Specific gravity 20/20 C	1.03	Protein (N × 6.38)	3.3
Total solids	10.6	Lactose (by difference)	4.9
Ash	0.7	pH	6.4
Fat (ether extract)	1.5		

Food Value: 4.3 calories per gram; 122—per ounce.

Supply: **POWDERED HALF-SKIMMED MILK** (C.A.)—Tins.

(S. M. A.)

Powdered Skim Milk: An almost fat free skim-milk powder, hermetically sealed in an atmosphere of nitrogen and bacteria free; the milk fat is almost entirely removed from pasteurized milk by centrifugal separation; the skim milk is dried by spraying under high pressure, the powder packed in vacuumized cans, filled with nitrogen gas to prevent oxidation of fats and vitamins, and hermetically sealed. Each 8 oz. can is equivalent to 2¼ qt. of normal strength liquid skim milk. Any desired concentration for infant feeding may be prepared; the pH of the dilution may be changed by the addition of lactic acid.

Analysis:

Moisture	2.0%	Protein (N × 6.38)	35.5%
Ash	8.0%	Lactose	51.0%
Fat (ether extracts)	2.0%		

Preparation: Normal dilution, 5 packed level tablespoonfuls to 6 fl. oz. of water; this contains—

Total solids	10.0	Protein (N × 6.38)	3.6
Ash	0.8	Lactose	5.2
Fat (ether extract)	0.2	pH	6.4

Food Value: 3.64 calories per gram; 103.4—per ounce.

Supply: **POWDERED SKIM MILK** (C.A.)—Cans of 8 oz.

(Merrell-Soule)

Powdered Skimmed Milk: For infant feeding where a fat-free milk is required.

Analysis:

Butterfat	1.0%	Salts	7.9%
Protein	36.5%	Moisture	2.8%
Lactose	51.8%		

Food Value: Calories per oz. 105.2; per gram 3.7; per level tablespoonful 30.

Supply: **POWDERED SKIMMED MILK** (C.A.)—Containers 1, 5, 25, and 50 lb., all vacuum packed.

Administration: To reliquefy to normal dilution or cow's skimmed milk—12 tablespoonfuls are added to 1 qt. of water, making 35 oz. skimmed milk, containing butter-fat 0.1%, protein 3.5%, lactose 4.9%, salts 0.7%, water 90.8%; food value 10.5 calories per ounce, .34 calories per cubic centimeter.

(Merrell-Soule)

Powdered Skimmed Lactic Acid Milk: For infant feeding; is similar to buttermilk.

Analysis:

Protein	36.0%	Free acidity	4.2%
Butterfat	1.0%	Total acidity	5.0%
Lactose	47.8%	Moisture	3.0%
Salts	8.0%		

Food value: Calories per ounce 105; per gram 3.5.

Supply: **POWDERED SKIMMED LACTIC ACID MILK** (C.A.)—Containers 1 and 5 lb. vacuum packed.

Administration: To reliquefy to normal dilution or standard buttermilk—12 tablespoonfuls are added to 1 qt. of water, making 35 oz. of buttermilk; or 3 packed level tablespoons in 8 oz. of water; dilution contains—butter fat 0.1%, protein 3.4%, lactose 4.5%, salts .7%, water 90.9%, free acidity 0.4%, total acidity 0.47%; pH 4.9.

Food value: 10.5 calories per fluid ounce, 3 calories per cubic centimeter.

Bibliography: *See Chap. XII.*

14. SOUPS

BABY SOUP (H. H. Clapp)

Composition: A combination of carrots, tomatoes, celery, cabbage, onions, potatoes, unpolished rice, whole grain barley, and beef juice.

Analysis: See page 855.

Supply: **BABY SOUP** (C.A.)—Strained (for infants)—Jars 4 oz., 14 oz,; Cans 4½ oz.
BABY SOUP (C.A.)—Unstrained (for older children)—Jars 14 oz.; Cans 4½ oz.

Administration: Served as is, or diluted 2 oz. to 1 oz. of milk, water or milk formula.

LIVER SOUP (H. H. Clapp)

Composition: Same as Baby Soup with the addition of calves' liver.

Analysis: See page 855.

Action and Uses: For use in nutritional anemia.

Supply: **LIVER SOUP** (C.A.)—Glass Jars 4 oz.

Administration: Served as is, or diluted 2 oz. to 1 oz. of milk, water or milk formula.

MALT SOUP EXTRACT (Borcherdt)

Composition: Contains: malt extract 100 Gm, potassium carbonate 1.1 Gm; vitamin B_1 and B_2 potency equivalent to 0.8 gr dried yeast or 3.2 gr moist yeast.

Food Value: 90 calories per ounce.

Administration: As Keller's malt soup: 4 tablespoonfuls of Malt Soup Extract are dissolved in 22 oz. water; is mixed with solution of 5½ level tablespoonfuls wheat flour in 11 oz. milk and mixture boiled for 5 min.; this contains—

Carbohydrates	12.1%	Protein	2%
Fat	1.2%		

Food Value: 1 oz. 23 calories; *For use* in malnourished, marasmic and atrophic infants; to relieve constipation is given 1 or 2 teaspoonfuls per feeding.

Supply: **MALT SOUP EXTRACT**—Bottles of 16 oz.

Combinations: **DRI-MALT SOUP EXTRACT** (C.A.)—A heavy semi-liquid malt soup extract, dried to a powder by a special drying process; it consists wholly of pure malt extract with potassium carbonate, combined in proportion of the original malt soup formula.

Dosage: 2–4 teaspoonfuls per feeding, in constipated infants.

Supply: Bottles of 16 oz.

MALT WITH SPLEEN MARROW—Contains in addition gr 10 spleenmarrow (Wilson) per ounce; for use in the treatment of malnutrition, anemia and convalescence; *administered* 1–2 teaspoonfuls three times daily after meals and at bedtime.

Supply: Bottles 8 and 16 oz.

VEGETABLE SOUP (H. H. Clapp)

Composition: Same as Baby Soup, except that wheat germ, a rich source of vitamin B, replaces beef juice.

Analysis: See page 855.

Supply: **VEGETABLE SOUP** (C.A.)—Jars 4 oz., 14 oz.; Cans 4½ oz.

Administration: Served as is, or diluted 2 oz. to 1 oz. of milk, water or milk formula.

WHEATHEART CEREAL SOUP (H. H. Clapp)

Composition: A well cooked combination of farina and wheat germ; a good source of vitamin B.

Analysis: See page 855.

Supply: **WHEATHEART CEREAL SOUP** (C.A.)—Glas Jars 4 oz., 14 oz.; Cans 4½ oz.

Administration: Served as is, or diluted 2 oz. to 1 oz. of milk, water or milk formula

15. WHOLE MILK PRODUCTS

(S. M. A.)

Concentrated Liquid Whole Milk: A canned evaporated high fat milk. The pasteurized milk is concentrated to ½ its original volume at 54–60°c and standardzed to conform with the United States Department of Agriculture standard for evaporated milk; is bacteria-free. *For use* exclusively for infant feeding; keeps indefinitely in the unopened can.

Approximate Analysis:

Total solids	25.9%	Protein (N × 6.38)	6.6%
Ash	1.5%	Lactose	9.5%
Fat (ether extract)	7.8%	pH	6.5%

Food Value: Calories 1.34 per gram; 38.1 per ounce.

Supply: **CONCENTRATED LIQUID WHOLE MILK** (C.A.)—Tins.

(S. M. A.)

Hypo-Allergic Whole Milk.—A sterilized whole milk made hypo-allergic by prolonged processing. Milk is pasteurized by the holding system, heated to a temperature of 61 to 65°c, is uniformly maintained at this temperature for 30 min. and cooled to 7°c or less; is then homogenized by forcing under high pressure through small apertures and canned. The canned milk is processed under steam pressure for a prolonged period, after which it is immediately cooled; is sterile. *For use* in individuals subject to allergic reactions from usual boiled milk or milk preparations; may be used in regular feeding formulas.

Analysis:

Moisture	87.6%	Fat (ether extract)	3.5%
Total solids	12.4	Protein (N × 6.38)	3.3
Ash	0.7	Lactose (by difference)	4.7

Food Value: Calories, 0.6 per cubic centimeter; 0.6 per Gram; 20 per fluid ounce.

Supply: **HYPO-ALLERGIC WHOLE MILK** (C.A.)—Tins.

(Merrell-Soule)

Klim Powdered Whole Milk: A powdered whole milk for infant and child feeding; wholesome, convenient, specially packed and containing all vitamins and other food elements of ordinary milk; is of uniform constitution and cream distribution; free from pathogenic bacteria, only 3,000 bacterial count per cubic centimeter, with easily digestible protein and fat. *Used* for normal infant feeding formulae and as a substitute for fluid milk; also in powder form in concentrated diets.

Analysis:

Butterfat	28.0%	Salts	5.8%
Protein	26.75%	Moisture	1.5%
Lactose	38.0%		

Food Value:

Calories per ounce	149	Calories per packed level tablespoonful	42
Calories per gram	5¼		

Supply: **KLIM POWDERED WHOLE MILK** (C.A.)—Containers 1, 2½, 5 and 50 lb., vacuum packed.

Administration: To reliquefy to normal dilution or cow's milk—1 packed level tablespoonful is used to 2 oz. of water or 4 oz. of powder to 29 oz. of water, making 1 qt. of cow's milk, containing butterfat 3.33%, protein 3.18%, lactose 4.53%, salts 0.69%, water 88.27%, of food value 20 calories per ounce, 0.64 calories per cubic centimeter. The milk is prepared by placing powder on top of warm or cold water, stirring, best with egg beater or whipper, until dissolved.

Bibliography: *See Chap. XII.*

(Mead Johnson)

Powdered Whole Milk: Fresh cow's milk from which the water has been removed, to be *used* as fluid cow's milk.

Analysis:

Milk fat	28.0%	Minerals (ash)	6.0%
Lactose (by difference)	37.7%	Moisture	1.5%
Protein	26.8%		

Food Value: 145 calories per ounce. 3½ packed level tablespoonfuls equal 1 oz.

Supply: **POWDERED WHOLE MILK** (C.A.)—Tins of 1 and 4 lb.

Administration: To reliquefy for normal dilution—1 packed level tablespoonful is added to 2 oz. water; dilution contains

Milk fat	3.5%	Protein	3.4%
Lactose (by difference	4.7%	Minerals (ash)	0.8%
Moisture	87.6%	Food value: 19 calories per ounce.	

Formula: 7–16 packed level tablespoonfuls powdered whole milk, 2–6 level tablespoonfuls Dextri-Maltose with 20–35 oz. water; 7–4 feedings of 3–8 oz. each in 24 hr.

Bibliography: *See Chap. XII.*

(S. M. A.)

Powdered Whole Milk: A powdered spray-dried whole milk, hermetically sealed in tins in an atmosphere of nitrogen. The pasteurized milk is homogenized to break up the fat particles, then passed through a centrifugal clarifier and spray-dried. The cans are vacuumized, filled with nitrogen gas to prevent oxidation of fats and vitamins, and hermetically sealed.

Analysis:

Moisture	2.0%	Protein (N × 6.38)	26.0%
Ash	6.0%	Lactose	37.5%
Fat (ether extract)	27.0%		

Normal dilution—2 packed level tablespoonfuls diluted to 3 fl. oz., presenting—

Specific gravity 20 C/20 C	1.03	Protein (N × 6.38)	3.3
Total solids	12.3	Lactose	4.7
Ash	0.7	pH	6.4
Fat (ether extract)	3.4	Food value: 4.97 calories per gram; 141.1—per ounce.	

Uses: Each 12 oz. can Powdered Whole Milk will make 2.8 qt. of liquid milk (normal strength) figuring 122 Gm per quart. The pH of the liquid mixture obtained by dilution according to directions is approximately 6.4. Should any other pH be required, proper adjustment can be made by addition of other Smaco specially acidified products.

Supply: **POWDERED WHOLE MILK (C.A.)**—Cans 12 oz.

(S. M. A.)

Whole Milk Sterilized: A canned sterilized homogenized whole milk; contains no foreign chemical substances or preservatives, no pathogenic bacteria, nor more than one million living bacteria per cubic centimeter before pasteurization; standardized and homogenized, canned and autoclaved.

Analysis:

Total solids	12.4%	Protein (N × 6.38)	3.3%
Ash	0.7%	Lactose (by difference)	4.9%
Fat (ether extract)	3.5%		

Food Value: Calories 0.64 per gram; 18.2 per ounce, 0.66 per cubic centimeter, 19.5 per fluid ounce.

Supply: **WHOLE MILK STERILIZED (C.A.)**—Cans.

Uses: Is recommended for all uses of whole milk and especially for infant feeding.

16. FRUITS

(Chicago Dietetic)

Canned Fruits: Fresh fruit packed in water without sugar; *For use* in diets restricted in carbohydrates; the more acid varieties marketed may be sweetened with saccharin and traces of baking soda.

Supply: 10% carbohydrate—grapefruit, peaches (sliced), pineapple (sliced) strawberries, 10% fruit salad combinations—Cans of 8 oz., 1 lb. Loganberries, pineapple (grated) pineapple juice—Cans of 1 lb.; 15% carbohydrate—apricots (halves), cherries (Royal Anne), pears (Bartlett)—Cans of 8 oz., 1 lb.; apple sauce, blueberries, cherries (red pitted) raspberries (black) raspberries (red)—Cans of 1 lb.

(H. H. Clapp)

Fruit Pulps (C. A.): Supply mineral salts, mild acid juices and roughage, all of which act as a stimulus to normal intestinal activity.

Analysis: *See page* 855.

Supply: Jars 4 oz.; Cans 4½ oz. Varieties—applesauce, apricots, prunes.

(Loeb)

Dietetic Canned Fruits: Containing carbohydrate 3–11%.

Supply: Cans of 8 oz. Varieties—peach, pear, pineapple, plum, apricot, cherry, strawberry, fruit salad.

(Nutradiet)

Nutradiet Fruits: Unsweetened; for carbohydrate restricted diets.

Analyses: Approximate, per 100 Gm portions:

	Protein	Carbo-hydrates	Fat	Water	Minerals	Fibre	Total Acidity
Apple sauce	0.21	11.44	0.04	87.12	0.18	0.50	0.51
Apricots	0.38	7.69	0.06	90.50	0.41	0.37	0.59
Blackberries	0.86	9.33	0.49	86.44	0.34	2.06	0.48
Cherries, R. A.	0.63	12.23	0.03	86.23	0.34	0.15	0.39
Figs, Delphia	0.41	10.42	0.16	88.10	0.31	0.52	0.08
Grapefruit	0.75	8.63	0.07	90.00	0.43	0.12	....
Peaches, sliced	0.30	5.77	0.07	93.06	0.23	0.23	0.34
Peaches, halves	0.43	5.83	0.08	92.81	0.24	0.25	0.36
Pears	0.22	8.42	0.07	90.31	0.16	0.64	0.18
Pineapple, sliced	0.34	11.80	0.06	87.30	0.33	0.18	....
Pineapple, tidbits	0.24	10.61	0.14	.....	....	....	....
Prunes	1.31	35.24	0.12	61.57	1.06	0.70	....
Youngberries	0.95	5.19	0.44	90.31	0.48	1.73	0.90

Supply: Cans of 1 lb. 4 oz.

(Nutradiet)

Nutradiet Berries:

Supply: Cans of 1 lb. 4 oz.

(Nutradiet)

Nutradiet Sun Dried Fruits:

Supply: Cans of 1 lb. 4 oz. Varieties—Figs, Black mission; figs—whole Calismyrna; prunes.

(Nutradiet)

Nutradiet Fruit Juices:

Analyses: Approximate, per 100 Gm portions:

	Protein	Carbo-hydrates	Fat	Water	Minerals	Fibre	Total Acidity
Grape juice	0.34	17.92	0.02	80.84	0.35	....	0.53
Grapefruit juice	0.63	9.44	0.06	87.73	0.40	0.03	1.71
Orange juice	1.04	9.46	0.07	87.72	0.68	0.02	1.01
Pineapple juice	0.29	12.44	0.27	.....	....	....	....
Tomato juice	1.11	4.25	0.07	93.32	0.49	0.19	0.57

Supply: Cans of 1 lb. 4 oz.

17. VEGETABLES

(Battle Creek)

Spinach Concentrate: A palatable concentrate prepared from fresh spinach, containing all its active elements: organic iron, calcium, phosphorus, copper, vitamins A and B; is rich in iron, has ten times the amount of calcium of fresh milk; hematinic, bone building, rich in vitamins; *For use* in infant feeding; to garnish foods, etc.

Analysis:

Iron	.094%	Vitamin A	(200 units per Gm)
Calcium	1.429%	Vitamin B (B and G)	7–8 units per Gm.
Phosphorus	.558%		

Supply: Cans of 1½ oz.

(Certifoods)

Sieved Vegetables: Fresh vegetables of standardized and guaranteed vitamin content; cooked and sieved, preserving the mineral salts, caloric value and soft roughage; no added seasoning or sugar; ready for use; *For use* in infant feeding; to promote growth and health; also of value to adults requiring special diets.

Supply: Cans, enamel lined 4½ and 10¼ oz. Varieties—carrots, tomatoes, spinach, green peas, green beans, vegetable puree. Is served warm.

(Chicago Dietetic)

Canned Vegetables: Fresh vegetables packed in water without salt or sugar. *For use* in diets limited in salt and as supply of fresh vegetables at all seasons.

Supply: Cans of 1 lb. 3 oz., except mushrooms—Cans of 4 oz. Varieties—5% carbohydrate—asparagus tips, asparagus (green cut) beans (green stringless) beans (yellow string), cauliflower, rhubarb, spinach, tomatoes, mushrooms, 5% vegetable salad combinations; 10% carbohydrate—beets, carrots (quartered) peas. 15% carbohydrate—corn.

(Clapp)

Strained Vegetables (C.A.): Presents maximum contents of mineral salts and vitamins.

Analysis: *See page* 855.

Supply: Jars 4 oz.; Cans 4½ oz. Varieties—asparagus, beets, carrots, peas, spinach, tomatoes, wax beans.

(Gerber)

Gerber's Strained Vegetables (C.A.): Presents a smooth strained vegetable with minimum roughage and most of the vitamins retained; *For use* in infant feeding and as supplementary diet; for invalids, soft diets, etc.

Supply: Cans 4¼ oz. Varieties—carrots, green beans, peas, prunes, spinach, tomatoes, beets, vegetable soup (consists of rice, barley, carrots, peas, beef, celery, spinach and tomatoes).

(Nutradiet)

Nutradiet Vegetables: Unsalted:

Analyses: Approximate, per 100 Gm portions:

	Protein	Carbo-hydrate	Fat	Water	Minerals	Fibre	Sodium Chloride
Asparagus, nat. green	2.75	2.70	0.15	93.33	0.44	0.63	0.06
Beans, stringless	1.36	2.17	0.10	95.58	0.37	0.42	0.02
Beets, whole	0.67	16.59	0.08	81.74	0.46	0.46	0.01
Carrots	0.41	6.88	0.11	91.69	0.29	0.62	0.01
Celery hearts	1.06	2.98	0.15	94.66	0.58	0.57	0.16
Corn, Dainty Pearl	2.48	12.38	0.66	83.33	0.35	0.80	0.01
Lima beans, green	3.50	8.68	0.21	85.84	0.73	1.04	0.11
Peas, green	3.21	6.20	0.51	88.62	0.34	1.12	0.11
Spinach	3.24	2.65	0.44	92.06	0.71	0.90	0.035
Sprouts, Brussels	2.13	3.36	0.08	93.20	0.58	0.65	0.004
Tomatoes	1.20	4.63	0.26	92.63	0.45	0.83	0.09

Supply: Cans of 1 lb. 4 oz.

18. BEVERAGES

(Hires)

Hires' Root Beer Extract: Prepared from juices of roots, herbs, barks, berries; free from synthetic or coal tar derivatives; a palatable drink, flavored.

Supply: **ROOT BEER (C.A.)**—Cans 1, 5, 10, 35 gal. Root Beer, Fountain Concentrate—Bottles of 1 qt., 1 gal. Root Beer Extract—Bottles of 1 pt; Also Ginger Beer, Birch Beer flavors.

Administration: 8 oz. extract mixed with 5¾ lb. sugar and dissolved in 2 qt. water makes 1 gal. finished syrup. 1 oz. finished syrup with 6 oz. carbonated water makes 1 glass or stein Hires' Root Beer.

(MacDowell)

Sugar Free Beverages: Prepared from carbonated water, saccharin and flavored. Ginger ale, orange, lime, grape, root beer.

Supply: Bottles of 12 oz.

(Squibb)

Beverage Acidophilus: Contains lactose 4.75% and more than 200 million acidophilus bacteria per cubic centimeter, and up to 6 weeks after manufacture, at least 100 million organisms; fruit flavored, carbonated. *For use* where acidophilus therapy is indicated—in intestinal toxemia, indigestion, flatulence, putrefaction, diarrheas, constipation, mucous colitis.

Supply: Bottles 7 fl. oz. (210 cc); expiration day dated.

Administration: 1 bottle daily for 3–4 days each week, at or between meals; must be preserved cold.

Analyses of Clapp's Strained Foods

	Total Solids	Ash	Fat	Protein	Carbo-hydrate	Crude Fiber	Calories per Oz.
Wheatheart Cereal Soup	13.44	0.88	0.39	2.11	9.90	0.16	14
Baby soup strained	11.39	1.43	0.08	1.05	8.61	0.22	11
Vegetable soup	14.07	1.74	0.18	1.95	9.86	0.34	14
Liver soup	13.19	1.39	0.45	3.26	7.90	0.20	14
Asparagus	5.88	1.20	0.24	1.40	2.59	0.45	6
Beets	11.35	0.51	0.26	1.07	6.62	2.41	10
Carrots	8.20	0.79	0.18	0.52	5.81	0.64	8
Peas	15.11	0.58	0.44	3.87	8.90	0.93	15
Spinach	6.41	1.21	0.30	1.71	1.95	0.63	4
Tomatoes	6.41	0.83	0.27	0.88	4.19	0.24	6
Wax beans	7.49	1.18	0.09	1.22	4.20	0.79	6
Applesauce	14.16	0.38	0.68	0.14	10.86	2.10	14
Apricots	15.39	1.10	0.52	0.69	10.73	2.35	14
Prunes	30.05	0.72	1.46	1.08	27.32	2.41	31
Beef broth	2.34	1.13	....	1.02	0.17	....	

CHAPTER IX

BOTTLED MINERAL WATERS

In this chapter are described 129 of the most popular bottled mineral waters and mineral salts, used in the United States, natural and artificial, domestic and imported.

Description: Mineral waters are complex inorganic bodies dominated in their properties by their physiochemical constitutions. They represent a perfectly balanced association of ions and molecules of specific chemical properties; they contain numerous elements, some waters as many as 50, in ionic state and continuous association and dissociation.

Natural waters are obtained directly from springs and are bottled without modification; the artificial are prepared in accordance with definite formulae of the chemical composition of the springs they represent. Many waters are also radioactive and thus possess additional properties because of such radioactivity; some waters are of the still type, others effervescing.

Analysis: Most analyses of the *natural* mineral waters here presented are complete; in a few instances only are they approximate, offering nevertheless sufficient information for practical use. The classification as alkaline, saline, chalybeate, etc. from the standpoint of chemical content, and as weak, medium, strong in accordance with their total solid content, follows the Fitch* standardization. The *artificial* waters closely simulate in composition the natural springs they represent; they serve in many instances as satisfactory substitutes.

Action: The action of mineral waters is dependent upon their chemical saturation, the extent of radioactivity, colloidal content and other physical and chemical features. They affect the organism; first, by virtue of the water itself, which is a universal solvent influencing cell activity, osmosis, metabolism and similar functions; second, through their chemical constituents, which variously affect every organ in the system, this depending upon the mineral components and the method of administration; the effect may be laxative, purgative, cholagogue or diuretic, uricolytic, hematinic and other.

Uses: Mineral waters are used quite extensively; while not a panacea for all derangements, they are decidedly helpful in many, provided the appropriate water is prescribed. Their employment in chronic cases must be prolonged, persistent and from time to time regulated. Spa treatment is for many reasons more successful, but home administration of waters is quite satisfactory in a majority of cases.

Administration: Dosage is in accordance with the type of water used, its concentration, the condition of the individual treated and object sought to be attained; it varies from a wineglassful to one or more quarts a day, taken cold or hot, and accompanied by regulation of diet, exercise and mode of living.

* Fitch, William Edward; Mineral Waters of the United States and American Spas; Lea and Febiger, Philadelphia, 1927.

Part I

Natural Mineral Waters

Domestic and Imported

ABILENA WELLS, Kansas (Hahn and Wessel)

Description: A strongly sulphated, very highly mineralized, sodic, potassic and saline water.

Analysis:

	Per Million Parts
Sodium chloride	588.3
Sodium sulphate	68,747.3
Potassium sulphate	1,797.0
Potassium nitrate	6.4
Magnesium sulphate	1,498.5
Calcium sulphate	817.8
Sodium bicarbonate	354.8
Calcium bicarbonate	1,047.9
Ferric bicarbonate	10.0
Silica	15.7
TOTAL SOLIDS	74,883.7

Action and Uses: Laxative, cathartic, purgative without causing griping. *Indicated* in gastrointestinal diseases, hepatic disturbances, hypertension and similar conditions.

Supply: Bottles, large—Cases of 12, 24.
Bottles, small—Cases of 12, 50.

ALQUA WATER, Shasta Springs, California (Hahn and Wessel)

Description: A moderately mineralized, clear alkaline water, rich in salts naturally present in the human body; sparkling and still.

Analysis: Glacier water from Shasta Springs contains calcium chloride, sodium phosphate, sodium chloride, sodium bicarbonate.

Action and Uses: *For use* to overcome acidosis and maintain alkali reserve in diabetes, uremia, nephritis, pyelonephritis, hypertension; in hepatic cirrhosis, diarrhea of infants, gastrointestinal disorders, vomiting, intoxication by drugs and burns; in wasting diseases, obesity, after narcosis, rheumatic affections.

Supply: Bottles 1 qt.—Boxes of 12.

APENTA, Hungary (Apollinaris Co.)

Description: Highly mineralized; magnesic, sodic, calcic; sulphated, carbonated.

Analysis:

	Per 1,000 Gm.
Magnesium sulphate	23.430
Sodium sulphate	15.530
Calcium sulphate	2.580
Potassium sulphate	0.096
Sodium chloride	1.716
Sodium carbonate	1.011
Silica	0.032
Oxide of iron	0.046
Alumina	0.121
Ammonia	traces
Bromine	traces
Fluorine	traces
Boron	traces
Lithia, Thallium } Presence ascertained by spectral rays.	

Action and Uses: A natural strong purgative spring water, rich in sodium and magnesium sulphates; of constant composition. *For use* as aperient in habitual constipation; in congestive inflammatory conditions of the respiratory and circulatory systems; in biliary and hepatic stasis; in obesity.

Supply: Bottles—Cases of 50.

Administration: Wineglassful dosage, one to two times daily; larger quantities where necessary.

APOLLINARIS, Germany (Apollinaris Co.)

Description: Moderately mineralized; sodic, calcic, magnesic, chloric; bicarbonated and carbonated water.

Analysis:

	Per 1,000 Gm
Potassium chloride	0.06902
Sodium chloride	0.36208
Sodium sulphate	0.26569
Sodium hydrocarbonate	2.035977
Calcium hydrocarbonate	0.42872
Magnesium hydrocarbonate	0.77727
Ferro hydrocarbonate	0.00483
Silicic acid	0.02808
	3.971667
Free carbonic acid	3.10

Action and Uses: A pleasant refreshing table water promoting normal digestion. *For use,* in catarrhal affections of upper respiratory tract; as diuretic in genitourinary disturbances and as tonic in gastric and intestinal affections.

Supply: Bottles of 1 pt. and 1 qt.—Cases of 50 and 100.

ARROWHEAD HOT SPRINGS, California (Arrowhead)

Description: PENYUGAL SPRINGS—Moderately mineralized, weak sulphated and thermic; sodic, saline; arsenated, sulphated, sulphuretted.

GRANITE AND PALM SPRINGS—Moderately mineralized, alkaline, saline; sodic, muriated, sulphated; calcic, bicarbonated, arsenated.

Analysis:

	Per Million Parts		
	Penyugal Springs	Granite Springs	Palm Springs
Ammonium chloride	0.150	0.110	0.135
Lithium chloride	trace	trace	trace
Potassium chloride	31.800	25.300	24.500
Sodium chloride	97.500	102.600	89.500
Sodium sulphate	782.000	737.100	644.000
Sodium metaborate	41.400	36.500	26.400
Disodium arsenate	0.744	0.496	0.595
Magnesium sulphate	4.400	2.000	3.900
Calcium phosphate	trace	trace	trace
Calcium bicarbonate	112.600	104.500	116.500
Mangano-manganic oxide	trace	trace	trace
Ferric oxide and alumina	1.500	0.080	2.000
Calcium silicate	9.600	1.750	
Silica	93.000	102.350	100.500
TOTAL SOLIDS	1,174.694	1,111.886	1,008.030
Gases at °c and 760 mm pressure:			
Hydrogen sulphide cc per liter	0.55	0.22	none
Free carbon dioxide cc per liter	none	none	none
Carbon dioxide on evaporation cc per liter	17.7	14.4	15.9

Action and Uses: Diuretic, antacid, laxative and alterative; *For use* in diseases of gastrointestinal tract, liver and kidney; in disorders of metabolism with general debility and anemia; in skin disorders, endocrine and lymphatic glandular affections.

Supply: Bottles—quart—Cases of 50—Cartons of 12.
Bottles—pint—Cases of 90—Cartons of 24.
Bottles—splits—Cases of 120—Cartons of 36.

BASSIN DE VICHY, France (Morris and Schrader) (Hahn and Wessel)

Description: Highly mineralized; sodic, potassic, calcic; bicarbonated, carbonated.

Analysis:

Bicarbonate of soda	4.980
Bicarbonate of potassium	0.275
Bicarbonate of calcium	0.308
Bicarbonate of magnesium	0.080
Bicarbonate of iron	0.020
Sulphate soda	0.262
Chloride sodium	0.509
Silica	0.025
Arsenic acid, phosphoric acid; Strontium, lithium, manganese; Alumina	Traces
Free carbonic acid gas	Abundant
TOTAL	6.459

Action and Uses: A pleasant palatable alkaline table water; assists digestion, relieves indigestion and hyperacidity. Is *used* in functional and organic disorders of digestive and genitourinary tracts.

Supply: Bottles of 1 qt.—Cases of 50.

BEAR LITHIA SPRINGS, West Virginia (Great Bear)

Description: Lightly mineralized, alkaline, slightly carbon-dioxated; calcic, magnesic, bicarbonated.

Analysis:

	Parts per Million
Ammonium chloride	0.063
Lithium chloride	trace
Potassium chloride	3.100
Sodium chloride	1.200
Potassium iodide	trace
Sodium sulphate	4.300
Sodium nitrate	1.220
Sodium nitrite	trace
Sodium bicarbonate	11.00
Magnesium bicarbonate	62.00
Calcium bicarbonate	73.700
Ferric oxide and alumina	0.200
Silica	15.500
TOTAL SOLIDS	172.283
Temperature °c	11.1
Gases, cc per liter:	
CO_2 free	6.8
CO_2 on evaporation	21.2

Action and Uses: Diuretic, tonic, alterative. *For use* in disorders of genito-urinary organs (bladder and kidneys); in gastric hyperacidity.

Supply: Sparkling—Bottles 1 pt.—Cases of 100.
Bottles 1 qt.—Cases of 50.
Splits—Cases of 100.

BEDFORD SPRINGS, Pennsylvania (Hahn and Wessel)

Description: Comprise about 12 individual springs of which the following waters are utilized medicinally:

MAGNESIA SPRING WATER—the most important; is moderately mineralized; calcic, sulphated, bicarbonated, saline, carbon-dioxated. Is *used* for its eliminative power in metabolic disorders; as intestinal cleanser in constipation, autointoxication, diabetes, obesity; as eliminator in renal and vesical disorders, gout, liver and gall-bladder affections, gastro-intestinal disorders; also as diuretic and tonic.

LIMESTONE SPRING WATER—Same composition; is antacid and tonic.

SULPHUR SPRING WATER—Moderately mineralized; calcic, magnesic, sulphated, bicarbonated, alkaline-saline, sulphuretted. *Used* as antacid, diuretic, alterative in rheumatism, gout, and gastro-intestinal catarrh.

SWEET SPRING WATER—Slightly mineralized; calcic, bicarbonated, alkaline, carbon-dioxated; diuretic in genito-urinary affections.

Analysis:

	Per Million Parts			
	Magnesia Spring	Limestone Spring	Sulphur Spring	Sweet Spring
Ammonium chloride	0.6	......	0.11	
Lithium chloride	trace		trace	trace
Potassium chloride	3.6	......	2.81	
Sodium chloride	4.4	2.93	4.12	0.8
Potassium sulphate	....	4.61		
Sodium sulphate	13.7	......	8.00	
Strontium sulphate	....	1.36		
Magnesium sulphate	70.3	4.96	324.20	3.1
Calcium sulphate	1,650.0	9.93	456.20	
Calcium phosphate	....	trace		
Magnesium bicarbonate	....	52.11	....	0.6
Calcium bicarbonate	267.3	196.52	544.40	13.3
Ferrous bicarbonate	....	1.10	....	1.6
Ferrous oxide	1.4	......	1.00	
Aluminum oxide	1.6	......	1.00	
Calcium silicate	45.7	......	25.20	
Silica	....	8.04	9.20	8.0
TOTAL SOLIDS	2,058.6	281.56	1,377.14	27.4

Gases: (MAGNESIA SPRING)
Carbon dioxide (free) cc per liter 8.9
Carbon dioxide, evaporated to dryness 36.7

Supply: **BEDFORD SPRING MINERAL (MAGNESIA) WATER**—Bottles ½ gal.—Cases of 12.

BEDFORD SPRINGS TABLE WATER (STILL)—Bottles ½ gal.—Cases of 12.

BEDFORD SPRINGS SPARKLING TABLE WATER—Bottles of 1 pt.—Cases of 24.

BERRY HILL MINERAL SPRINGS, Virginia **(Bleacho)**

Description: Moderately highly mineralized; calcic, saline water; sulphated, bicarbonated.

Analysis:

	Per Million Parts
Ammonium chloride	0.157
Lithium chloride	trace
Potassium chloride	6.500
Sodium chloride	37.600
Potassium bromide	trace
Potassium iodide	trace
Sodium sulphate	459.600
Magnesium sulphate	291.500
Calcium sulphate	1,618.700
Sodium metaborate	heavy trace
Sodium nitrate	trace
Sodium nitrite	0.014
Calcium bicarbonate	197.000
Ferrous bicarbonate	4.500
Mangano-manganic oxide	trace
Silica	27.600
TOTAL SOLIDS	2,643.171
Gases, cc per liter:	
Carbon dioxide, free	1.4
Carbon dioxide, set free on evaporation	27.7

Action and Uses: Diuretic, laxative, tonic, alterative. *For use* in gastro-intestinal disorders, hepatic and genitourinary affections.

Supply: Bottles of 5 gal.

BETHESDA MINERAL SPRING, Wisconsin **(Hahn and Wessel)**

Description: A moderately mineralized, weak alkaline, calcic, magnesic, 70% bicarbonated water.

Analysis:

	Per Million Parts
Sodium chloride	37.6
Potassium chloride	6.8
Calcium chloride	3.9
Calcium nitrate	34.9
Magnesium sulphate	96.5
Calcium bicarbonate	324.0
Magnesium bicarbonate	132.9
Iron bicarbonate	0.4
Lithium bicarbonate	trace
Silica	14.9
Aluminum	0.2
TOTAL SOLIDS	652.1

Action and Uses: Antacid and diuretic; *For use* in gastric hyperacidity and genitourinary affections.

Supply: Still—Bottles ½ gal.—Cases of 12.
Carbonated—Bottles 1 qt.—Cases of 50.
Bottles 1 pt.—Cases of 100.

BILINER SAUERBRUNN, Czecho-Slovakia **(Hahn and Wessel)**
(Morris and Schrader)

Description: A moderately mineralized, strongly alkaline, carbon-dioxated water.

Analysis:

	Per 1,000 Parts
Sodium Bicarbonate about	4.467
Lithium bicarbonate	0.033
Total solids	8.978

Action and Uses: Corrects gastric hyperacidity and digestion; relieves flatulence, intestinal fermentation and auto-intoxication; stimulates liver function, bile secretion and thus affects stone formation; improves renal function and vesical inflammation. *Useful* in acidosis, uric acid diathesis and other abnormal blood states; in gastric ulcer, diabetes and gastro-intestinal catarrh with hypersecretion.

Supply: Bottles of 1 qt.

Administration: 2 wineglassfuls after meals three to four times daily.

BIRMO, Switzerland **(Morris and Schrader)**
(Hahn and Wessel)

Description: A strongly mineralized, sodic, magnesic, calcic, sulphated, bicarbonated water.

Analysis:

	Per 1,000 Parts
Sulphate of potash	0.85552
Sulphate of soda	16.56464
Sulphate of calcium	0.31639
Sulphate of magnesium	12.04312
Chloride of magnesium	0.39219
Bicarbonate of calcium	1.23340
Bicarbonate of iron	0.00693
Aluminia	trace
Silicia	trace
TOTAL	31.41219

Action and Uses: A mild bitter cholagogue water; *For use* in jaundice, hepatic disease, habitual constipation with hemorrhoids.

Supply: Bottles 1 pt.—Cases of 50.

Administration: 1 wineglassful before breakfast, best taken hot.

BOGNANCO, Italy (Morris and Schrader)

Description: A highly carbonated, alkaline water obtained from Ansonia and San Lorenzo Springs; the former contains 1.21% mineral content and 1,514 free carbon dioxide per litre; the latter 4.22 solid residue and 1,700 free carbon dioxide per litre; contains also lithium carbonate and magnesia.

Action and Uses: A palatable table water *for use* in digestive disturbances; is slightly laxative and uricolytic.

Supply: Bottles of 1 qt.

Administration: 1 wineglassful four to six times daily.

BORJOM, Caucasia (Amtorg)

Description: A natural alkaline mineral water; sodic, calcic, bicarbonated, chlorated, iodated.

Analysis:

	Per Liter
Sodium bicarbonate	5.2162 Gm
Sodium chloride	0.6687 Gm
Basic ferric oxide bicarbonate	0.618 Gm
Magnesium bicarbonate	0.1233 Gm
Calcium bicarbonate	0.3659 Gm
Strontium bicarbonate	0.009 Gm
Sodium iodide	0.0006 Gm
Sodium bromide	0.0005 Gm
Potassium chloride	0.0428 Gm
Silica	0.003 Gm
Free carbonic acid	434 cc

Action and Uses: Mucus solvent and eliminant, gastric stimulant, slightly diuretic and uricolytic. *For use* as table water in nephrolithiasis, pyelitis, cholecystitis, gastric hyperacidity, acidosis.

Supply: Bottles of 1 pt.—Cartons of 10–30.

BRAUN MINERAL SPRINGS, Hot Springs, South Dakota (Hahn and Wessel)

Description: BRAUN SPRING—Moderately mineralized, thermic; calcic, sodic, magnesic, bicarbonated, sulphated, sulphuretted; an alkaline, saline diuretic and tonic water.

MINNEKAHTA SPRING—Moderately highly mineralized; predominantly potassic; otherwise of above composition.

KIDNEY SPRING—Moderately mineralized; has above constitution in addition to being muriated.

Analysis:

	Per Million Parts		
	Braun Spring	Minnekahta Spring	Kidney Spring
Sodium chloride	210.84	235.81	242.60
Potassium chloride	....	....	68.44
Magnesium chloride	....	....	118.00
Sodium sulphate	295.49	277.80	
Magnesium sulphate	184.68	73.87	
Potassium sulphate	....	333.62	
Lithium sulphate	....	....	15.21
Calcium sulphate	....	279.24	703.99
Calcium bicarbonate	539.84		
Calcium phosphate	....	....	2.76
Ferric oxide and alumina	1.03	trace	trace
Silica	5.64	42.04	23.64
TOTAL SOLIDS	1,237.52	1,242.38	1,174.64

Uses: In rheumatism, gout, neuralgia; in chronic diseases of the liver and digestive organs; in affections of kidney, bladder and skin; in malaria, tuberculosis, bronchial disease and neurasthenia.

Supply: Bottles, large and small.

BUCKHEAD SPRING NATURAL WATERS, Virginia **(Buckhead)**

Description: Lightly mineralized; magnesic, sodic; muriated, nitrated, silicated, bicarbonated alkaline water.

Analysis:

	Per Million Parts
Lithium chloride	0.016
Potassium chloride	3.610
Sodium chloride	1.140
Magnesium chloride	10.510
Calcium chloride	1.570
Potassium sulphate	1.260
Sodium nitrate	11.570
Sodium phosphate	0.017
Sodium arsenate	trace
Magnesium bicarbonate	0.570
Calcium bicarbonate	5.030
Manganese bicarbonate	0.020
Barium bicarbonate	0.040
Ferrous bicarbonate	0.360
Aluminum oxide	1.000
Silica	7.480
TOTAL SOLIDS	44.193
Gases:	
Carbon dioxide, free	6.4

Action and Uses: Diuretic. *For use* in gout, rheumatism, gastrointestinal disorders.

Supply: Bottles ½ gal.—Cases of 12.
Bottles 1 qt.—Cases of 24.
Bottles 1 pt.—Cases of 48.

BUCKHORN LITHIA SPRINGS, North Carolina **(Hahn and Wessel)**

Description: Lightly mineralized; calcic, lithic, bicarbonated, alkaline.

Analysis:

	Per Million Parts
Potassium chloride	1.02
Sodium chloride	10.43
Sodium sulphate	5.81
Sodium bicarbonate	6.50
Lithium bicarbonate	80.58
Magnesium bicarbonate	43.96
Calcium bicarbonate	165.96
Ferric oxide and alumina	3.08
Silica	27.37
TOTAL SOLIDS	343.71
Temperature °c	12.2

Action and Uses: Antacid, antilithic, diuretic, tonic. *For use* in gastric hyperacidity, anemia, chlorosis, genitourinary affections with renal and vesical calculi.

Supply: Bottles of ½ gal.—Cases of 12.

BUFFALO LITHIA SPRINGS, Virginia **(Hahn and Wessel)**

Description: SPRING 1 (BYRD)—Moderately mineralized; calcic, sulphated, bicarbonated, alkaline, carbon-dioxated. *For use* as diuretic, antacid, tonic.

SPRING 2 (GOODE)—Moderately mineralized; calcic, sodic, sulphated, bicarbonated, alkaline. *For use* as diuretic, antacid.

SPRING 3 (SOEKAHATTE)—Lightly mineralized; calcic, potassic bicarbonated, ferruginous (aluminic), carbon dioxated. *For use* as tonic, alterative.

SPRING 4 (POOLE WELL)—Moderately mineralized; potassic, sodic, magnesic, calcic; muriated, bicarbonated, alkaline-saline. *For use* as aperient, diuretic.

SPRING 5 (VIRGINIA CLUB)—Lightly mineralized; light calcic, alkaline, saline (silicious), ferruginous. *For use* as tonic, alterative.

SPRING 6 (MECKLENBURG)—Lightly mineralized; calcic, magnesic, bicarbonated, alkaline. *For use* as antacid, diuretic.

SPRING 8 (FORTUNA)—Lightly mineralized; sodic, magnesic, calcic; bicarbonated, silicated, alkaline. *For use* as antacid, diuretic.

BUFFALO MINERAL SPRINGS

	Per Million Parts						
	Spring 1	Spring 2	Spring 3	Spring 4	Spring 5	Spring 6	Spring 8
Ammonium chloride	0.05	......	......	0.07	0.03	......	0.025
Lithium chloride	0.45	0.29	trace	......	......	......	trace
Potassium chloride	0.39	9.90	......	10.80	2.80	......	4.060
Sodium chloride	......	6.74	3.80	125.80	10.90	14.6	2.890
Magnesium chloride	......	......	......	158.20			
Sodium iodide	......	......	trace				
Sodium sulphate	66.80	53.60	......	......	3.20	......	3.500
Potassium sulphate	6.40						
Aluminum sulphate	......	......	52.41				
Magnesium sulphate	26.40	41.29	2.59	48.30			
Calcium sulphate	397.40	459.72	40.52	......	......	15.6	trace
Calcium phosphate	2.30	1.19	trace	48.20	trace		
Sodium nitrate	trace	4.85	......	trace	4.30	......	1.350
Sodium nitrite	......	trace	......	trace			
Sodium metaborate							
Sodium bicarbonate	......	......	......	......	4.10	......	9.400
Magnesium bicarbonate	......	......	trace	24.10	8.40	22.0	
Potassium bicarbonate	......	......	51.67				
Calcium bicarbonate	253.80	93.54	43.45	255.20	37.30	70.6	
Ferrous bicarbonate	......	......	65.00				
Ferric oxide / Aluminum oxide	1.00	1.80	......	1.80	1.40	1.6	2.000
Sodium silicate	......	......	......	......	......	......	6.840
Magnesium silicate	......	......	......	......	......	......	11.540
Calcium silicate	......	66.55	......	66.80	0.90	......	19.370
Silica	44.70	1.46	9.85	2.00	37.90	52.8	24.850
TOTAL SOLIDS	799.69	740.93	269.29	741.27	111.23	172.2	95.705
Gases:							
Carbon dioxide (free) cc per liter	14.8	......	5.4	......	......	3.2	
Flow in gallons per day	1,500	1,900	2,448	10,000	30,100	200,000	5,000

Action and Uses: Antacid, diuretic, antilithic, aperient and tonic; are markedly radioactive; energize body enzymes; stimulate to greater activity the proteolytic and diastatic ferments; increase autolytic, glycolytic, uricolytic, pancreatic and peptic functions. *For use* in gastric hyperacidity, intestinal catarrh and retarded bowel action; in renal, vesical and hepatic calculi; in nephritis and albuminuria of pregnancy; in neurasthenia and other irritable nervous conditions; in anemia, chlorosis, debility, rheumatism, gout, uric acid diathesis; in menstrual and menopausal disorders.

Supply: Bottles of ½ gal.—Cartons of 6.
Bottles of 26 oz.—Cartons of 12.

CAPON SPRINGS, West Virginia **(Hahn and Wessel)**

Description: Lightly mineralized; calcic, lithic, magnesic bicarbonated; alkaline water.

Analysis:

	Per Million Parts
Sodium chloride	0.800
Potassium sulphate	2.420
Calcium sulphate	8.470
Strontium sulphate	trace

	Per Million Parts
Calcium phosphate	0.028
Calcium fluoride	trace
Sodium nitrate	trace
Sodium iodide	trace
Sodium bromide	trace
Lithium bicarbonate	45.960
Sodium bicarbonate	13.490
Magnesium bicarbonate	35.760
Calcium bicarbonate	192.640
Manganous bicarbonate	trace
Ferrous bicarbonate	0.890
Aluminum oxide	0.250
Silica	10.100
TOTAL SOLIDS	310.828
Temperature, °c	17.8
Gases, cc per liter:	
Oxygen	0.58
Nitrogen	1.28

Action and Uses: Antacid, diuretic, tonic, alterative. *For use* in acidosis of rheumatism, gout, uric acid diathesis; in gastrointestinal and liver disorders; in genitourinary diseases—renal and vesical calculi, renal catarrh.

Supply: Bottles ½ gal.—Cases of 12.
Demijohn 5 gal.

CARABANA, Spain **(Hahn and Wessel)**

Description: Very highly mineralized; sodic, magnesic, calcic; sulphated, chlorated, phosphated.

Analysis:

	Per 1,000 Parts of Water	
	Natural	American Concentrated
Sodium sulphate	100.111	50.005
Sodium sulphite	0.0499	
Magnesium sulphate	3.0711	30.971
Sodium chloride	1.6	2.503
Magnesium chloride	0.4774	
Calcium chloride	0.1967	
Sodium phosphate	0.021	
Alumina	0.0005	
Iron oxide and alumina	....	.016
Silica	....	.005
Calcium sulphate	....	2.817
Magnesium carbonate	....	.352
TOTAL SOLIDS	106.0826	86.669

Action and Uses: Purgative, alterative, antiseptic, detergent. *Useful* as cholagogue, hepatic stimulant, diuretic, intestinal sedative; in diseases with liver-stasis, autotoxemia, intestinal fermentation, constipation; in renal and bladder disorders; in malnutrition, anemia, rheumatism, gout, diabetes and diseases of children.

Supply: Bottles of 1 qt.

Administration: 1 wineglassful several times daily, then reduced as elimination is normally established.

CLOVERDALE LITHIA SPRINGS, Pennsylvania **(Cloverdale)**

Description: Lightly mineralized; calcic, magnesic, bicarbonated, alkaline water.

Analysis:

	Per Million Parts
Ammonium chloride	0.3
Lithium chloride	trace
Potassium chloride	1.7
Potassium sulphate	0.7
Sodium nitrate	trace
Sodium sulphate	26.6
Magnesium sulphate	2.5
Magnesium bicarbonate	48.1

	Per Million Parts
Calcium bicarbonate	98.6
Ferric oxide	0.4
Silica	15.9
TOTAL SOLIDS	194.8
Gases:	
Carbonic acid	1.070
Oxygen	1.109
Nitrogen	6.013
TOTAL GASES	8.910

Action and Uses: A clear sparkling, antacid, aperient, diuretic water. *Used* in gastric hyperacidity, gastric ulcer, intestinal stasis; in genito-urinary affections.

Supply: Sparkling—Cases of 12.

CONTREXEVILLE, France (Hahn and Wessel) (Morris and Schrader)

Description: A moderately highly mineralized radioactive water bottled from Pavillon Spring; calcic, magnesic, lithic, sodic; sulphated, bicarbonated, silicated.

Analysis: PAVILLON SPRING WATER.

	Per 1,000 Parts
Carbonic acid, free	0.080
Calcium sulphate	1.565
Magnesium sulphate	0.236
Sodium sulphate	0.030
Bicarbonate of calcium	0.402
Bicarbonate of magnesium	0.035
Bicarbonate of iron	0.007
Bicarbonate of lithium	0.004
Potassium chloride	0.006
Sodium chloride	0.004
Silicon	0.015
Arsenic	traces
Fluoride of calcium	traces
TOTAL	2.384

Action and Uses: A palatable, astringent, neutral water. *For use* as uricolytic, laxative, detoxicant in gout, rheumatism, arthritis, biliary calculi; in genito-urinary affections, diabetes, arteriosclerosis, obesity, anemia.

Supply: Bottles 1 qt.—Case of 50.

Administration: 1 bottle daily before breakfast.

CRAZY MINERAL WELLS, Palo Pinto County, Texas (Crazy Well)

Description: Comprise 4 springs; weak alkaline, weak saline; sulphated, moderately highly mineralized, muriated, bicarbonated, nitrated.

Analysis:

	Per Million Parts			
	Spring 1	Spring 2	Spring 3	Spring 4
Ammonium chloride	trace	trace	trace	trace
Potassium chloride	97.66	262.07	66.84	88.85
Sodium chloride	472.74	986.55	190.27	414.02
Sodium sulphate	1,015.20	1,887.08	3,326.76	4,573.32
Magnesium sulphate	682.00	579.55	752.00	123.33
Sodium nitrate	57.73	349.43	3.59	4.98
Sodium bicarbonate	20.69	35.85	89.17	66.29
Magnesium bicarbonate	164.76	322.42	10.87	223.08
Calcium bicarbonate	620.65	848.22	599.93	329.08
Ferric oxide and alumina	7.25	81.74	58.84	3.98
Silica	9.94	22.93	22.93	19.93
TOTAL SOLIDS	3,148.62	5,375.84	5,121.20	5,846.86

Action and Uses: Antacid, diuretic, laxative, tonic. *For use* in gastrointestinal disorders, constipation, autointoxication, intestinal and hepatic stasis.

Supply: In form of Crazy Water Crystals (*See* p. 891).

CROCKETT ARSENIC LITHIA SPRINGS, Shawsville, Virginia (Wilson)

Description: Moderately mineralized; calcic, magnesic, sodic; bicarbonated, sulphated, alkaline-saline (arsenated).

Analysis:

	Per Million Parts
Ammonium chloride	0.030
Lithium chloride	0.120
Potassium chloride	10.530
Potassium iodide	trace
Potassium sulphate	2.900
Sodium sulphate	53.300
Magnesium sulphate	79.200
Sodium metaborate	trace
Disodium arsenate	0.322
Sodium nitrate	0.300
Sodium nitrite	trace
Magnesium bicarbonate	30.000
Calcium bicarbonate	232.100
Ferric oxide and alumina	1.000
Calcium silicate	9.000
Silica	43.510
TOTAL SOLIDS	462.312

Action and Uses: Diuretic, antacid, alterative. *For use* in chronic skin disorders with scaly eruptions.

Supply: Bottles, large and small.

DUERKHEIM, Germany (Spa Products)

Description: Highly mineralized; sodic, calcic, potassic, magnesic; arsenic-sulphated, hydrocarbonated.

Analysis: **MAX SPRING** of Bad Duerkheim.

	Gm per 1,000 Parts
Potassium	0.1575
Sodium	5.462
Lithium	0.0158
Rubidium	0.00099
Caesium	0.00148
Calcium	1.121
Strontium	0.047
Magnesium	0.8
Iron	0.00255
Aluminum	0.00066
Strontium sulphate	0.0734
Magnesium chloride	0.255
Magnesium hydrocarbonate	0.879
Ferro-hydrocarbonate	0.00812
Aluminum oxide	0.00125
Arsenic tri-oxide	0.01735
Silicic acid	0.0141
TOTAL SOLIDS	17.79

Action and Uses: A natural non-irritating arsenical water, free from iron; does not establish arsenical tolerance; stimulating hematinic, aperient; improves gastro-intestinal motility, appetite, digestion and assimilation; increases hemoglobin and red blood cells. *For use* in primary and secondary anemia, functional neuroses, hysteria, neurasthenia; in menstrual disorders, malarial cachexia; also in syphilis, eczema, psoriasis, furunculosis, scrofula, arthritis and rheumatic affections.

Supply: Bottles 1 qt.

Administration: 30–50 cc increased daily by 10–25 cc until 300 cc are taken; continued 2–3 weeks and decreased. Children: 30–60 cc daily.

EMS, Bad Ems, Germany (Von der Bruck)

Description: Comprises 6 thermal, muriated, alkaline springs; highly mineralized; sodic, calcic, magnesic; bicarbonated, sulphated water.

Analysis: "Kraenchen" Spring.

	Per 1,000 Parts
Sodium bicarbonate	1,955,414
Lithium bicarbonate	0,003,732
Ammonium bicarbonate	0,001,883
Sodium sulphate	0,023,890
Sodium chloride	1,026,032
Sodium bromide	0,000,487
Sodium iodide	0,000,020
Sodium phosphate	0,001,353
Potassium sulphate	0,047,326
Calcium bicarbonate	0,234,073
Strontium bicarbonate	0,002,050
Barium bicarbonate	0,001,059
Magnesium bicarbonate	0,207,920
Ferrous bicarbonate	0,003,633
Manganous bicarbonate	0,000,166
Silicic acid	0,047,299
TOTAL	3,556,337
Free carbonic acid	1,099,528
TOTAL CONSTITUENTS	4,655,865

Action and Uses: An alkaline, saline water *for use* in chronic catarrhal conditions of nose and throat, bronchitis, asthma, emphysema; in biliary affections, uric acid and gynecologic disorders.

Supply: Bottles 1½ pt.—Case of 50.

Administration: 2–3 glasses before breakfast, taken warm.

EVIAN-CACHAT, France (Morris and Schrader) (Hahn and Wessel)

Description: Weakly mineralized, aerated; potassic, sodic, calcic, magnesic; carbonated, sulphated, nitrated, silicated water.

Analysis:

	Per 1,000 Parts
Cations	
Potassium	0.0023
Sodium	0.0069
Ammonium	——
Calcium	0.0784
Magnesium	0.0237
Iron	0.0002
Aluminum	——
Manganese	——
Anions	
Carbonic	0.3568
Sulphuric	0.0085
Chlorine	0.0018
Nitric	0.0021
Phosphoric	0.0005
Iodine	trace
Acids	
Silica	0.0142
Carbonic anhydride	0.0105

Action and Uses: An alkaline, mineral table water, sterile and palatable. Diuretic, eliminative. *For use* in uric acid diathesis, rheumatic affections, urinary infections; in fevers, for dilution of infant's milk; in gastro-intestinal disorders and as table water.

Supply: Bottles of 1 qt.

Administration: 1 glass, ½ hr. before meals.

FACHINGEN, Germany (Morris and Schrader) (Hahn and Wessel)

Description: Sodic, calcic, magnesic, ferric; lithiated, bicarbonated, chlorated water.

Analysis:

	Per 1,000 Parts
Sodium bicarbonate	2.425
Calcium bicarbonate	0.56
Magnesium bicarbonate	0.43
Sodium chloride	0.295
Ferrum bicarbonate	0.011
Lithium bicarbonate	0.01

Action and Uses: A natural, clear, alkaline mineral water; palatable, effervescent; maintains alkali reserve, restores blood chlorides. *For use* in gastric hyperacidity; in uric acid diathesis, nephrolithiasis, nephritis; in liver disorders, cholelithiasis, intestinal catarrh; in gout, diabetes, eczema, furunculosis; also used as table water.

Supply: Bottles of 1 qt.

Administration: 1 bottle daily in 3 portions, 1 hr. before meals, for 4–6 weeks.

FRANZENSBAD, Germany **(Spa Products) (Hahn and Wessel)**

Description: Sodic, potassic, chloric; hydrocarbonated, ferruginous, sulphated.

Analysis:

	Per 1,000 Parts per Gm
Crystalline glauber salt	36.5
Sodium sulphate	16.1
Sodium chloride	4.002
Potassium chloride	0.503

Action and Uses: Stimulates and facilitates digestion, corrects constipation; also useful in hepatic and portal congestion, plethora, circulatory disorders.

Supply: Bottles of 1 qt.

Administration: Average—1½–4 oz. several times daily, taken slowly. In constipation—7 oz. on empty stomach.

FRENCH LICK SPRINGS, Orange County, Indiana **(Hahn and Wessel)**

Description: Waters are cool, variously mineralized and radio-active, 1 spring being highly activated. The 4 bottled waters are as follows:

PLUTO SPRING—Moderately highly mineralized; sodic, muriated, magnesic, calcic, saline; sulphated, carbondioxated, sulphuretted.

BOWLES SPRING—resembles Pluto; is in addition sodium sulphated.

PROSPERINE SPRING—similar to Pluto Spring.

PLUTO CONCENTRATED—strongly magnesium and sodium sulphated.

Analysis:

	Per Million Parts			
	Pluto Spring	Bowles Spring	Prosperine Spring	Pluto Concentrated
Ammonium chloride	31.2	26.8	32.7	17.1
Potassium chloride	31.5	28.6	16.2	33.5
Sodium chloride	1,688.5	1,285.9	1,539.8	2,054.2
Magnesium chloride	77.5	....	51.8	
Magnesium sulphate	1,051.5	877.5	1,032.2	34,536.4
Sodium sulphate	....	285.8	....	62,843.7
Calcium sulphate	1,388.9	921.1	1,379.6	1,507.1
Calcium bicarbonate	379.5	373.4	325.6	323.9
Ferric oxide and alumina	5.0	3.0	16.0	16.0
Silica	28.0	21.0	13.0	13.0
TOTAL SOLIDS	4,681.6	3,823.1	4,406.9	101,344.9
Gases:				
Carbon dioxide, free	131.0	110.0	102.0	
Hydrogen sulphide	30.5	20.3	18.0	
Radio-activity	1.35	4.45	1.96	

Action and Uses: Laxative, diuretic and antacid; stimulate oxidation, cell activity and elimination. *Used* as bath to stimulate nerve endings and exert a soothing, healing action on the skin. *Internally*—in gastro-intestinal diseases, liver dysfunction, gall-bladder and duct infections, autointoxication; in obesity, anemia, diabetes and skin disorders.

Supply: PLUTO NATURAL—Bottles—Case of 24—Splits—Case of 50.

PLUTO CONCENTRATED—Bottles 1 qt.—Cases 24—Bottles ½ pt.—Cases 50.

BOWLES SPRING—Case of 24.

FIUGGI, Italy **(Societa Anonima Fiuggi)**

Description: Highly mineralized radioactive water; sodic, calcic, silicic; carbonated, sulphated.

Analysis:

	Per 100,000 Parts
Chloride of sodium	1.208
Nitrate of potassium	0.727
Carbonate of potassium	0.093
Sulphate of calcium	0.555
Carbonate of calcium	1.159
Chloride of magnesium	0.114
Carbonate of magnesium	0.945
Silica anhydride	1.073
TOTAL SOLIDS	5.874

Action and Uses: A clear tasteless water; uricolytic, laxative; *Used*—in gout, genito-urinary calculi and infections.

Supply: Bottles of 1 qt.—Cases of 50.

Administration: 1–3 liters before breakfast and with meals.

HAMBY'S GENUINE DAWSON SPRINGS, Hopkins County, Kentucky **(Dawson Spring)**

Description: Weak alkaline; sulphated, calcic, magnesic, potassic, sodic, ferruginous, manganic.

Analysis:

	Per Million Parts
Sodium chloride	155.514
Potassium sulphate	113.757
Sodium sulphate	704.178
Magnesium sulphate	866.336
Calcium sulphate	964.922
Sodium bromide	trace
Calcium nitrate	5.157
Sodium phosphate	15.273
Calcium bicarbonate	195.482
Magnesium bicarbonate	742.362
Lithium bicarbonate	trace
Manganese bicarbonate	49.475
Ferrous bicarbonate	87.774
Aluminum oxide	3.173
Silica	28.167
TOTAL SOLIDS	3,971.370

Action and Uses: Constipation, gastrointestinal catarrh, liver and gall bladder disorders: tonic, alterative in anemia, chlorosis, leucocythemia, malnutrition.

Supply: Bottles, large and small.

KARLSBAD SPRINGS, Germany **(Carlsbad Products)** **(Hahn and Wessel)**

Description: A natural mineral water obtained principally from the Muehlbrunn and Sprudel Springs; moderately highly mineralized; sodic, magnesic, potassic; sulphated, carbonated, phosphated water.

Analysis:

	Gr per Gal. Muehlbrunn Spring	Gr per Gal. Sprudel Spring
Potassium sulphate	0.70965	0.833366
Sodium sulphate	8.938566	8.768638
Sodium chloride	3.899588	3.829896
Sodium fluoride	0.018522	0.01134
Sodium borate	0.014742	0.01134
Sodium bicarbonate	7.674912	7.560378
Lithium bicarbonate	0.095634	0.063126
Calcium phosphate	0.001512	0.001512
Calcium bicarbonate	2.029860	2.016630
Strontium bicarbonate	0.001512	0.001512
Magnesium bicarbonate	1.106406	1.067850
Manganese bicarbonate	0.001890	0.000756
Iron bicarbonate	0.019218	0.007804
Aluminium oxide	0.000756	0.001134
Silicic anhydride	0.274050	0.271782
Free carbonic acid gas	1.914192	2.577960

Action: Eliminant and chemical catalyst; increases intestinal peristalsis, bile fluidity and secretion; affects blood alkalinity, urinary secretion and promotes uric acid solution and elimination.

Uses: Liver and gall bladder diseases: cholelithiasis, alcoholic cirrhosis, degenerative and congestive hepatitis, enlargement of spleen. Gastrointestinal: gastric hyperacidity, peptic ulcer, chronic constipation, infantile diarrheas and ulceration. Renal: nephritis, urinary infections, prostatic disease. General: gout, uric acid diathesis, obesity, diabetes, tropical infections, skin diseases.

Supply: KARLSBAD SPRUDEL SPRINGS—Bottles of 1 qt.

KARLSBAD MUEHLBRUNN—Bottles of 1 qt.

Administration: ½–1 glassful two to three times daily on empty stomach, warmed, for 3–6 weeks.

KISSINGEN, Germany

(Hahn and Wessel)
(Morris and Schrader)
(Spa Products)

Description: Strongly mineralized; potassic, sodic, magnesic, calcic; chlorated, sulphated, carbonated, ferrated.

Analysis:

	Per 1,000 Gm
Chloride of potassium	0.28640
Chloride of sodium	5.82205
Chloride of lithium	0.02002
Chloride of magnesia	0.30379
Bromine of sodium	0.00838
Sulphite of magnesia	0.58839
Sulphite of lime	0.38937
Nitrate of soda	0.00931
Phosphate of lime	0.00561
Carbonate of magnesia	0.01704
Carbonate of lime	1.06096
Carbonate of oxide of iron	0.63158
Silicic acid	0.01290
Ammonia	0.00091
TOTAL	8.55721
Free carbonic acid	1,305.5

Action and Uses: An alkaline, sulphated, radio-active, effervescent spring water bottled from Rakoczy Spring; promotes stomach secretion; is gastric sedative, intestinal laxative and bile stimulant. *For use* in gastrointestinal disorders; in cholelithiasis, cholecystitis, cholangitis, cirrhosis, and functional cardiovascular disorders.

Supply: Bottles 1 pt., 9 oz.—Boxes of 50.

Administration: ½–4 glasses daily, cold or warm on empty stomach; in liver affections, used in greater quantities.

LEVICO, Italy **(Hahn and Wessel)** **(Morris and Schrader)**

Description: A very strongly chalybeate mineralized water, containing iron and arsenic in soluble assimilable form.

Analysis:

	Per 10,000 Gr Levico Strong	Levico Mild
Anhydride of arsenic acid	0.060	0.020
Sulphate of manganese	0.145	0.072
Protosulphate of iron	46.027	18.154
Sulphuric acid, free	16.660	5.278
TOTAL DISSOLVED CONSTITUENTS	78.577	

Action and Uses: Hematinic, roborant and reconstructive. *For use* in anemia, debility, convalescence; in endocrine disturbances, chlorosis, dermatoses, nervous diseases, neuralgia and gynecologic disturbances.

Supply: Bottles 7½ oz.—Cases of 100.

Administration: 4 Tablespoonfuls daily.

MAN-A-CEA, Preston County, West Virginia **(Hahn and Wessel)**

Description: Obtained from Irondale Spring; moderately mineralized; calcic, sodic, potassic, sulphated.

Analysis:

	Per Million Parts
Ammonium chlorid	0.023
Potassium chlorid	3.536
Potassium sulphate	19.74
Sodium sulphate	12.19
Magnesium sulphate	16.425
Calcium sulphate	276.694
Sodium nitrate	16.51
Sodium nitrite	trace
Calcium bicarbonate	14.063
Calcium silicate	22.629
Iron oxid and alumina	1.50
Mangano-manganic oxid	1.20
Silica	0.47
TOTAL	384.980

Action and Uses: A soft palatable natural mineral water, slightly laxative, diuretic, tonic. *For use* in various gastro-intestinal disturbances, catarrh, dysentery, diarrhea, anemia.

Supply: Bottles of quarts, pints and splits.

MANITOU SPRINGS, El Paso County, Colorado **(Hahn and Wessel)**

Description: Highly radio-active and energizing.

MANITOU SPRING—Moderately highly mineralized; sodic, calcic; bicarbonated, muriated, carbon-dioxated, sulphuretted; alkaline.

NAVAJO SPRING—Moderately highly mineralized; sodic, calcic, magnesic; alkaline.

CHEYENNE SPRING—Moderately highly mineralized; sodic, calcic; bicarbonated, muriated, carbon-dioxated; alkaline.

SHOSHOWE SPRING—Moderately highly mineralized; calcic; bicarbonated, carbon-dioxated; alkaline and highly radio-activated.

Analysis:

	Manitou Spring	Navajo Spring	Cheyenne Spring	Shoshowe Spring
	Per Million Parts			
Ammonium chloride	0.15			
Lithium chloride	1.38	trace	trace	none
Potassium chloride	136.10	137.7	213.95	trace
Calcium chloride	....	....	....	17.31
Sodium chloride	303.20	309.8	242.76	60.25
Sodium sulphate	324.20	343.7	316.20	
Calcium sulphate	....	....	....	318.19
Sodium bicarbonate	1,193.20	1,056.7	1,218.50	298.14
Magnesium bicarbonate	476.80	437.5	381.20	298.14
Calcium bicarbonate	1,854.50	1,877.6	1,756.50	3,725.80
Ferrous bicarbonate	5.70	15.6	12.25	11.14
Mangano-manganic oxide	2.40			
Silica	47.20	49.0	42.50	58.10
TOTAL SOLIDS	4,344.83	4,227.8	4,183.86	4,489.64

Action and Uses: Stimulate cell activity, promote absorption and glandular function; contain considerable carbonic acid gas. *For use* in functional gastric disorders with hyperacidity, fermentation, motor insufficiency; in gastric ulcerations and dilatation; in chronic Bright's, uricacidemia, vesical disorders; in arthritis, rheumatism, lumbago, sciatica, neuritis, gout, obesity and chronic skin disorders.

Supply: Bottles—Boxes of 50.
Half bottles and Splits—Cases of 100.

MARIENBAD, Czecho-Slovakia (Hahn and Wessel) (Spa Products)

Description: Clear, strongly sulphated, alkaline spring water, bottled from Kreuzbrunnen and Ferdinandsbrunnen; strongly mineralized; potassic, sodic, magnesic; ammoniated, sulphated, hydro-carbonated; ferruginous.

Analysis:

	Kreuzbrunnen	Ferdinandsbrunnen
	Per 1,000 Parts	
Cations		
Potassium	0.2484	0.02212
Sodium	2.612	2.772
Lithium	0.00117	0.003143
Ammonium	....	0.001709
Calcium	0.2273	0.1759
Strontium	0.00051	
Barium	0.00026	
Magnesium	0.1142	0.1200
Ferrum	0.0144	0.02316
Manganese	0.0040	0.005704
Aluminum	0.00342	0.001002
Anions		
Nitrate	....	0.008912
Chloride	1.042	1.095
Sulfate	3.458	3.224
Hydrocarbonate	2.430	2.612
Hydrophosphate	0.00094	0.005328
Silicic acid	0.0563	0.1008
Free carbon dioxide	2.212	3.179
TOTAL	12.42	13.35

Action and Uses: Laxative, diuretic and tonic. *For use* in metabolic disorders, gastro-intestinal disturbances and obesity.

Supply: Bottles 1 qt.—Cases of 50.

Administration: 2 glasses warmed, mornings before breakfast.

MATTONI "GIESSHUBLER," Czecho-Slovakia (Hahn and Wessel) (Muller)

Description: Strongly mineralized; sodic, calcic, potassic, lithic, magnesic; bicarbonated, borated, hydrophosphated, silicated.

Analysis:

	Per 10,000 Gm
Potassium fluoride	0.0232
Potassium nitrate	0.0023
Potassium chloride	0.3070
Potassium bicarbonate	1.1952
Potassium sulphate	0.3180
Sodium bicarbonate	13.5892
Lithium bicarbonate	0.0233
Calcium hydrophosphate	0.0017
Calcium bicarbonate	3.5535
Strontium bicarbonate	0.0055
Magnesium bicarbonate	2.3052
Iron bicarbonate	0.0958
Manganese bicarbonate	0.0090
Aluminum sulphate	0.0038
Meta boric acid	0.0285
Meta silicic acid	0.8279
TOTAL	22.2891
Free carbonic acid	27.1747
	49.4638

Action and Uses: An acidulated water *used* in respiratory affections, colds, pleurisy, bronchitis, laryngitis, pneumonic infections; in gastric hyperacidity, catarrh, anorexia, nausea and constipation; in gout, arteriosclerosis, diabetes, renal and vesical disorders.

Supply: Bottles—Boxes of 50.
Half Bottles—Boxes of 100.

Administration: May be taken in milk and fruit juices.

MERGENTHEIM, Germany (Hahn and Wessel) (Spa Products)

Description: Strongly mineralized; sodic, potassic, calcic, magnesic; carbonated, chlorinated, sulphated, bicarbonated; ferruginous.

Analysis:

Karl Spring	Per 1,000 Parts
Sodium chloride	16.644124
Potassium chloride	0.376193
Lithium chloride	0.009046
Ammonium chloride	0.005664
Sodium bromide	0.008308
Sodium iodide	0.000373
Sodium sulphate	3.345013
Calcium sulphate	0.907396
Magnesium sulphate	2.262723
Strontium sulphate	0.078762
Barium sulphate	0.000988
Calcium bicarbonate	1.645187
Ferrous bicarbonate	0.014655
Manganous bicarbonate	0.001156
Calcium borate	0.006521
Calcium phosphate	0.000144
Silicic acid	0.026110
TOTAL	20.332363
Carbonic acid, completely free	1.053048
TOTAL OF ALL CONSTITUENTS	21.385411

Action and Uses: A cold alkaline saline spring water from Karl Spring, containing in abundance Glauber and Epsom salts; is laxative, cholagogue. *For use* in cholelithiasis, cholecystitis, chronic constipation, intestinal disorders; also *used* in diabetes.

Supply: Bottles of 1 qt.—Cases of 50.

MOUNTAIN VALLEY SPRINGS, Garland County, Arkansas (Hahn and Wessel)

Description: Moderately mineralized; calcic, magnesic; alkaline, bicarbonated.

Analysis:

	Per Million Parts
Sodium chloride	7.36
Sodium sulphate	10.95
Potassium sulphate	1.03
Magnesium sulphate	12.66
Aluminum sulphate	7.59
Ferrous sulphate	0.34
Magnesium bicarbonate	52.66
Calcium bicarbonate	315.43
Silica	15.57
TOTAL SOLIDS	423.59

Action and Uses: Antacid, diuretic and tonic. *Useful* in renal and vesical disorders, in diabetes and other conditions.

Supply: Bottles—Cases of 50, ½ Gal.—Cases of 12. Carbonated—Bottles 1 pt.—Cases of 50.

MOUNT CLEMENS MINERAL SPRINGS, Mount Clemens, Mich. (Mount Clemens)

Description: Highly mineralized; sodic, calcic, magnesic (lithic, bromidic, iodic); muriated saline, sulphuretted.

Analysis:

	Per Million Parts
Lithium chloride	105.9
Potassium chloride	1,707.1
Sodium chloride	76,108.8
Magnesium chloride	14,948.8
Calcium chloride	34,039.9
Potassium bromide	725.0
Potassium iodide	3.0
Calcium sulphate	777.6
Sodium metaborate	trace
Ferric oxide and alumina	4.2
Silica	11.0
TOTAL SOLIDS	128,648.8
Gases:	
Hydrogen sulphide	14.3

Action and Uses: Laxative, tonic, diuretic and alterative. *Used* in scrofulus disorders of the skin, bone and skin diseases, luetic manifestations; in sciatica, neuritis, gout, uric acid diathesis, renal and vesical affections; in constipation and neurasthenia.

Supply: Bottles of 1 pt.

NARZAN, Caucasia (Amtorg)

Description: A lightly mineralized, natural carbonic water; magnesic, calcic, sodic; bicarbonated, sulphated, chlorated.

Analysis:

	Gm per Liter
Sodium sulphate	0.1342
Magnesium sulphate	0.4183
Calcium bicarbonate	0.4204
Ferri bicarbonate	0.00105
Lithium chloride	0.000286
Sodium chloride	0.1591
Potassium chloride	0.02535
Free carbonic acid (CO_2)	1.8871

Action and Uses: A refreshing table water, slightly appetizing and mildly laxative. For use in various conditions.

Supply: Bottles of 1 pt.—Cartons of 20–100.

NEUENAHR, Germany

(Hahn and Wessel)
(Spa Products)

Description: A Rhineland natural mineral water obtained from the Grosse Sprudel and the Willibrordus thermal alkaline springs; potassic, sodic, calcic, magnesic; chlorated, sulphated, carbonated.

Analysis:

	Per 1,000 Parts
Cations	
Potassium	0.02566
Sodium	0.3553
Lithium	0.000523
Ammonium	0.001085
Calcium	0.08444
Magnesium	0.09566
Ferrum	0.006639
Manganese	0.000293
Chloride	0.06590
Bromide	0.000188
Iodide	0.000003
Sulfate	0.06165
Anions	
Hydrophosphate	0.000594
Hydroarsenate	0.000203
Hydrocarbonate	1.547
	2.245
Boric acid (meta)	0.001498
Silicic acid (meta)	0.02756
	2.274
Free carbonic acid	1.150
	3.424

Action and Uses: Cholagogue, laxative, diuretic and tonic. *For use* in hepatic disorders with or without jaundice, cholelithiasis, gastric hypoacidity, intestinal disorders, peptic ulcer and diabetes.

Supply: Bottles of 1 qt.—Boxes of 50.

Administration: 3–7 oz., three times daily, before meals; sipped slowly and taken cold or lukewarm.

PANACEA SPRINGS, Littleton, N. C.

Description: Lightly mineralized; sodic, magnesic, calcic, manganese-ferruginous chlorated, bicarbonated, carbon-dioxated.

Analysis:

	Per Million Parts
Potassium chloride	5.66
Sodium chloride	1.11
Sodium sulphate	3.33
Potassium sulphate	
Sodium bicarbonate	54.78
Magnesium bicarbonate	33.86
Calcium bicarbonate	48.58
Ferrous bicarbonate	50.16
Manganese bicarbonate	12.22
Aluminum oxide	0.99
Silica	18.35
TOTAL SOLIDS	229.00

Action and Uses: Tonic, alterative, reconstructive, hematinic. *Used* in hyperacid gastric states, anorexia; as diuretic in renal and vesical catarrh; in chronic skin disorders, rheumatism, debility, anemia, chlorosis.

Supply: Bottles—large and small.

POLAND SPRINGS, South Poland, Me. **(Hahn and Wessel)**

Description: Lightly mineralized; calcic, magnesic; bicarbonated, carbon-dioxated and radioactivated.

Analysis:

	Per Million Parts
Ammonium chloride	0.03
Potassium chloride	2.31
Sodium chloride	2.06
Magnesium chloride	0.54
Magnesium sulphate	1.86
Sodium nitrate	7.27
Magnesium bicarbonate	13.02
Calcium bicarbonate	34.24
Ferric oxide and alumina	trace
Silica	19.26
TOTAL SOLIDS	80.59
Gases:	
Carbon dioxide (free)	2.1
Carbon dioxide (free on evaporation)	10.2

Action and Uses: An alkaline, antacid and diuretic water, mildly depurative. *For use* in renal disturbances—nephritis, albuminuria of pregnancy, after kidney operations, renal calculi and their prevention; in some gastro-intestinal and gall bladder disturbances and in rheumatism.

Supply: Bottles ½ gal.—Cases of 24.
Bottles—Aerated—Cases of 50.
Half Bottles—Cases of 50.

RHENS, Germany **(Hahn and Wessel)** **(Von der Bruck)**

Description: A natural highly mineralized water; sodic, magnesic, calcic, chloric; carbonated, carbon-dioxated; is iron-free.

Analysis:

	Per 1,000 Parts
Sodium bicarbonate	0.889005
Lithium bicarbonate	0.010177
Ammonium bicarbonate	0.009722
Calcium bicarbonate	0.462290
Strontium bicarbonate	0.000319
Magnesium bicarbonate	0.343774
Ferrous bicarbonate	0.022935
Manganous bicarbonate	0.001474
Sodium chloride	1.253636
Sodium bromide	0.001457
Sodium iodide	0.000017
Potassium sulphate	0.042666
Sodium sulphate	0.760467
Sodium phosphate	0.000986
Sodium arsenate	0.000149
Sodium biborate	0.005719
Silicic acid	0.016994
TOTAL	3.821727
Free carbonic acid	3.108049

Action and Uses: A palatable table water; is slightly diuretic, mildly laxative and tonic.

Supply: Bottles large (24 oz. each)—Case of 50
Bottles small (12 oz. each)—Case of 100
Bottles split (8 oz. each)—Case of 100

ROCKBRIDGE ALUM SPRINGS, Virginia **(Rockbridge)**

Description: Moderately mineralized; aluminic, sulphated (ferruginous).

Analysis:

	Per Million Parts
Ammonium chloride	0.514
Lithium chloride	trace
Potassium chloride	2.900
Sodium chloride	1.200
Potassium iodide	trace
Sodium sulphate	18.200
Magnesium sulphate	33.700
Calcium sulphate	13.900
Manganous sulphate	0.400
Aluminum sulphate	336.900
Ferrous sulphate	9.200
Sodium nitrate	1.820
Ferric oxide	0.400
Silica	46.800
TOTAL SOLIDS	459.934

Action and Uses: Styptic, tonic, alterative. *For use* in scrofula, ulcers, diarrhea, chronic colitis and dysentery.

Supply: Bottles ½ gal.—Cases of 12.

RUBINAT-LLORACH, Spain (Hahn and Wessel) (Ingold)

Description: Moderately mineralized; sodic, potassic, calcic, magnesic, chloric and sulphated; bacteria-free water.

Analysis: Approximate:

	Per 1,000 Parts
Sulphate of soda	99.024
Sulphate of potash	.236
Sulphate of magnesia	3.353
Sulphate of lime	1.995
Chloride of sodium	2.114
Silica, alumina / Ferric oxide (traces)	.030
TOTAL	106.752

Action and Uses: Aperient, purgative, uricolytic, diuretic. *For use* in gastro-intestinal disorders, constipation, flatulence, colic, intestinal intoxication; in acute infections, gout, rheumatism, anemia, dermatoses; in hepatic, cardiac and renal disease.

Supply: Bottles ½ pt.—Cases of 50.

Administration: 1 wineglassful on empty stomach; repeated one to two times daily.

SAINT-GALMIER BADOIT, France (Hahn and Wessel)

Description: Contains sodium bicarbonate, calcium bicarbonate, azotates.

Action and Uses: A pleasant table water and diuretic. For table use and in urinary disorders.

Supply: Bottles—Large—Cases of 12 and 50.
Bottles—Half size—Cases of 12 and 100.

SALVATOR WATER, Hungary (Hahn and Wessel)

Description: Moderately highly mineralized; sodic, calcic, magnesic, chloric; carbonated, sulphated.

Analysis:

	Per 10,000 Parts
Bicarbonate of	
Sodium	3.0536
Magnesium	9.1708
Lithium	0.2282
Calcium	16.9452
Sodium of borate	0.9689
Sulphate of sodium	1.4804

	Per 10,000 Parts
Potassium sulphate	0.7476
Sodium chloride	1.7405
Sodium bromide	0.0092
Sodium iodide	0.0028
Earthy salts	0.0840
Silicic acid	0.3340
TOTAL SOLID CONTENTS	34.7652
TOTAL CARBONIC ACID	40.0365
Free Carbonic acid	23.5571

Action and Uses: Dietetic, eliminative, metabolic stimulant, diuretic. *For use* in renal and vesical affections, gout, rheumatism, chronic metallic poisoning, gastrointestinal disorders; in upper respiratory diseases, diabetes, uric-acid diathesis.

Supply: Bottles—Cases of 50.

Administration: 1 Glass to 1 liter daily.

SAN PELLEGRINO (FONTI NUOVE), Bergaino, Italy (Hahn and Wessel)

Description: Lightly mineralized, radioactive, alkaline; lithic, sodic, potassic, calcic, magnesic, silicic; ferrated, sulphated, chlorated, nitrated and carbonated water.

Analysis:

	Per 1,000 Parts
Sodium	0.02876
Lithium	0.00030
Calcium	0.06090
Magnesium	0.2696
Sulphuric	0.0748
Chlorine	0.00461
Monocarbonic	0.29646
Silica	0.01118
Iron	traces
Nitric	traces

Action and Uses: Diuretic, uricolytic. *For use* in uricacidemia, gout, arthritis, arteriosclerosis; in affections of the genitourinary, gastrointestinal tract; in nephritis.

Supply: Bottles—Boxes of 50.

Administration: 1 pt. daily for 15–20 days; repeated after 3–4 weeks.

SARATOGA SPRINGS WATER, New York (State of New York)

Description: Of the numerous naturally carbonized springs the waters bottled are:

GEYSER SPRING—Alkaline, highly mineralized; strong sodic, potassic, magnesic; muriated, bicarbonated, carbon-dioxated.

HATHORN 2 SPRING—Alkaline-saline, highly mineralized; sodic, potassic, magnesic; muriated, bicarbonated, carbon-dioxated.

COESA SPRING—Alkaline, saline, moderately mineralized; sodic, potassic, calcic; muriated, bicarbonated, carbon-dioxated.

Analysis:

	Per Milligram		
	Geyser Spring	Hathorn 2 Spring	Coesa Spring
Ammonium chloride	61.17	53.54	34.42
Lithium chloride	27.00	65.26	27.00
Potassium chloride	233.81	723.97	437.58
Sodium chloride	2,511.61	11,290.17	5,967.45
Potassium bromide	32.00	120.00	31.50
Potassium iodide	1.60	1.60	1.75
Sodium sulphate	trace	trace	trace
Sodium metaborate	trace	trace	trace
Sodium nitrate	trace	trace	trace
Sodium nitrite	trace	trace	trace
Sodium bicarbonate	2,206.54	241.23	512.07
Calcium bicarbonate	1,877.09	3,962.24	3,467.52

	Per Milligram		
	Geyser Spring	Hathorn 2 Spring	Coesa Spring
Barium bicarbonate	trace	46.83	27.22
Strontium bicarbonate	trace	trace	trace
Ferrous bicarbonate	23.15	9.38	13.40
Magnesium bicarbonate	874.71	2,837.48	2,047.44
Alumina	1.59	15.80	24.00
Silica	6.60	9.20	10.00
TOTAL SOLIDS	7,856.87	19,376.70	12,601.35

Action and Uses: HATHORN 2 WATER—cathartic, mildly purgative. *For use* in constipation.

COESA WATER—Mildly laxative, antacid, diuretic. *For use* in gastro-intestinal catarrh, liver and gall bladder diseases.

GEYSER WATER—Antacid, uricolytic, hematinic. *For use* in gastric acidity and dyspepsia, arthritis, rheumatism, anemia, general sclerosis.

Supply: HATHORN 2—Bottles of 1 pt.—Boxes of 24.

COESA—Bottles of 1 pt.—Boxes of 24.

GEYSER—Bottles of 1 pt.—Boxes of 24.

Administration: HATHORN 2—1 pt. mornings, warmed or at room temperature.

COESA—After meals; in gall bladder disease—in the morning before breakfast.

GEYSER—With or after meals.

SILOAM SPRINGS, Howell County, Mo. (Excelsior)

Description: Weak, alkaline, saline water; moderately mineralized; calcic, magnesic, alkaline; bicarbonated, nitrated, carbon-dioxated, sulphuretted.

Analysis:

	Per Million Parts
Sodium chloride	17.3
Magnesium chloride	10.1
Magnesium sulphate	6.4
Magnesium nitrate	44.6
Magnesium bicarbonate	211.4
Calcium bicarbonate	305.8
Ferric oxide and alumina	trace
Silica	5.0
TOTAL SOLIDS	600.6

Action and Uses: Antacid and diuretic. *For use* in gout, rheumatism, uric-acid diathesis; in gastric hyperacidity, hepatic disease, renal and vesical catarrh.

Supply: Bottles—Cases of 50.
Bottles—half size—Cases of 100.

STAFFORD MINERAL SPRINGS WATER, Vossburg, Miss. (Stafford Springs)

Description: A calcic, magnesic, bicarbonated, radioactive water.

Analysis:

	Parts per Million
Ammonium chloride	0.091
Potassium chloride	1.353
Sodium chloride	8.150
Potassium iodide	.017
Sodium sulphate	5.170
Magnesium sulphate	1.200
Calcium sulphate	6.400
Calcium phosphate	.108
Magnesium bicarbonate	17.060
Calcium bicarbonate	234.050
Ferrous bicarbonate	4.490
Alumina	.110
Silica	29.500
TOTAL	309.017

Action and Uses: Stimulates kidney function. *Used* in renal dysfunction as diuretic.

Supply: Bottles of ½ gal.—Cases of 12.

Administration: Mild cases—1 glassful every hour, beginning 2 hr. before breakfast and continuing until 3 or 4 o'clock in the afternoon; after that hour, taken only when thirsty; treatment continued until urine is free from casts and albumin. Severe Cases—1 wineglassful every 30 min. during day, and occasionally during night; daily dosage ½ gal., gradually increased to 1 gal.

SUWANEE SULPHUR SPRINGS, Suwanee County, Florida **(Kalish)**

Description: Lightly mineralized; calcic, magnesic; bicarbonated, sulphuretted.

Analysis:

	Per Million Parts
Sodium chloride	11.00
Potassium chloride	1.10
Sodium sulphate	4.00
Magnesium sulphate	30.00
Magnesium bicarbonate	35.00
Calcium bicarbonate	211.00
Ferrous bicarbonate	0.51
Silica	14.00
TOTAL SOLIDS	220.00

Gas: Sulphuretted hydrogen, abundant.

Action and Uses: Hematinic and alkaline water of sulphur odor. *For use* in gastro-intestinal disorders, rheumatism, nervous disorders, liver diseases and anemia.

Supply: Bottles of ½ gal.—Cases of 12.

VADE MECUM SPRINGS, Stokes County, N. C. **(Tise)**

Description: Moderately highly mineralized; alkaline, saline; calcic, sodic, potassic; sulphated, carbon-dioxated.

Analysis:

	Per Million Parts
Sodium chloride	11.09
Potassium sulphate	15.00
Sodium sulphate	177.40
Calcium sulphate	1,512.00
Magnesium bicarbonate	219.80
Calcium bicarbonate	97.75
Silica	13.20
TOTAL SOLIDS	2,046.15

Action and Uses: Diuretic and laxative. *For use* in intestinal stasis and for diuresis.

Supply: Bottles ½ gal.—Cases of 12.

VERONICA SPRINGS, Santa Barbara County, California **(Hahn and Wessel)**

Description: Highly mineralized; sodic, magnesic; sulphated, muriated, saline.

Analysis:

	Per Million Parts
Ammonium chloride	0.24
Potassium chloride	169.50
Sodium chloride	3,170.00
Magnesium chloride	
Potassium iodide	trace
Sodium sulphate	802.70
Magnesium sulphate	14,151.40
Calcium sulphate	744.30
Magnesium nitrate	
Calcium phosphate	trace
Sodium nitrate	2,384.90
Potassium bicarbonate	
Calcium bicarbonate	1,397.80
Ferric oxide and alumina	3.70
Silica	18.10
TOTAL SOLIDS	22,842.64

Action and Uses: Diuretic, purgative and cholagogue. *For use* in constipation, digestive insufficiency, chronic dyspepsia.

Supply: Bottles 1 qt.—Cases of 12.

VICHY, France (American Agency)

Description: Of 14 springs of Vichy, 4 are the most popular: Celestins, Grande Grille, Hopital and Chomel; waters contain about 41 elements, principally bicarbonates of sodium, potassium, calcium with chlorides, sulphate of sodium and free carbonic acid.

Analysis:

	Per 1,000 Parts			
	Celestins Spring	Grande Grille Spring	Hopital Spring	Chomel Spring
Sodium bicarbonate	3.3090	5.5830	5.5852	5.6120
Potassium bicarbonate	0.2490	0.3502	0.4407	0.3521
Lithium bicarbonate	0.0281	0.0350	0.0418	0.0418
Calcium bicarbonate	0.7400	0.3641	0.5445	0.3612
Magnesium bicarbonate	0.1016	0.0736	0.0795	0.0709
Ferrous bicarbonate	0.0012	0.0038	0.0038	0.0012
Sodium chloride	0.3830	0.5737	0.5675	0.5751
Sodium sulphate	0.2430	0.2795	0.2667	0.2757
Silica	0.0300	0.0652	0.0620	0.0640
Sodium arseniate, phosphate and nitrate	present	trace	trace	trace
Carbon dioxide	2.1750	0.8494	1.1770	0.9729

Action and Uses: CELESTINS—Cholagogue, antacid, diuretic; stimulates secretions, encourages elimination. *Used* in functional and organic disorders of digestive and genitourinary tracts; in diseases of spleen and skin; in uterine affections, metabolic disorders, diabetes, gout, rheumatism and arthritis.

GRANDE GRILLE—Specially indicated in liver and gastrointestinal disorders.

HOPITAL —Used mostly as analgesic in gastrointestinal disorders.

CHOMEL—Indicated in respiratory disorders.

Supply: VICHY CELESTINS—Bottles—large—Cases of 12 and 50.
Bottles—small—Cases of 12 and 100.
Bottles—splits—Cases of 12 and 100.

GRANDE GRILLE—Bottles—large—Cases of 12 and 50.

HOPITAL—Bottles—large—Cases of 12 and 50.

VILLACABRAS, Spain (Hahn and Wessel)

Description: Strongly mineralized; sodic, magnesic, sulphated.

Analysis:

	Gm per Liter
Sodium sulphate	122.05
Magnesium sulphate	0.984

Action: A natural, palatable, laxative water of salty taste; filtered by the Pasteur system and free from sulphurous smell.

Uses: Laxative in constipation.

Supply: Bottles 1 qt.—Cases of 50.

Administration: ⅓–½ glassful before breakfast.

VITTEL, France (Hahn and Wessel) (Morris and Schrader)

Description: Slightly mineralized; calcic, magnesic, lithic. Bottled from 2 springs, Grande Source, which is less mineralized and strongly diuretic and Source Hepar, the more magnesic.

Supply: Bottles ½ pt.—Cases of 50.
Bottles, large—Cases of 24.

WHITE SULPHUR SPRINGS, West Virginia (Hahn and Wessel) (Morris and Schrader)

Description: Obtained from 4 springs of the following qualities.

WHITE SULPHUR SPRING—Moderately highly mineralized; calcic, magnesic, saline; sulphuretted, bicarbonated; sulphated; has considerable free carbonic acid and hydrogen sulphide.

RADIO-CHALYBEATE SPRING—Lightly mineralized; calcic, ferric, alkaline; sulphated and strongly radioactive.

ALUM SPRING—Moderately mineralized; aluminic, magnesic, calcic, sulphated.

ALVON SPRING—Lightly mineralized; sodic, calcic, carbondioxated.

Analysis:

	Per Million Parts			
	White Sulphur Spring	Radio-chalybeate Spring	Alum Spring	Alvon Spring
Ammonium chloride	....	....	....	0.05
Lithium chloride	0.20	trace	....	trace
Sodium chloride	30.62	5.830	16.260	2.76
Potassium chloride	....	....	....	1.86
Sodium iodide	....	0.008	0.003	
Potassium iodide	....	....	....	trace
Potassium sulphate	8.98	1.090	11.970	.
Sodium sulphate	31.92	2.830	2.980	7.50
Magnesium sulphate	515.72	2.460	583.110	0.56
Calcium sulphate	1,303.77	45.540	198.500	2.67
Manganous sulphate	....	16.960	51.370	
Aluminum sulphate	....	....	298.120	
Strontium sulphate	....	1.500		
Cobalt sulphate	....	....	trace	
Lithium sulphate	....	....	trace	
Cupric sulphate	....	....	trace	
Nickel sulphate	....	....	15.95	
Calcium phosphate	0.07			
Sodium phosphate	....	0.990	0.630	
Sodium nitrate	trace	....	3.590	trace
Sodium nitrite	....	....	....	none
Sodium bicarbonate	trace			
Magnesium bicarbonate	60.55	6.880	....	17.87
Calcium bicarbonate	156.50	20.180	....	93.48
Strontium bicarbonate	2.83			
Ferrous bicarbonate	2.98			
Ferric sulphate	....	22.770		
Ferric persulphate	....	....	11.29	
Ferrix oxide and alumina	....	....	....	1.49
Manganum bicarbonate	trace			
Aluminum oxide	0.92	1.990		
Silica	9.97	22.940	30.44	7.78
Sulphuric acid	....	....	38.90	
TOTAL SOLIDS	2,125.03	151.968	1,268.013	136.02
Gases:				
Carbon dioxide (free) / Hydrogen sulphide (free) / Radio-activity	....	2 4		

WILDUNGEN, Germany (Von der Bruck) (Morris and Schrader)

Description: Is obtained principally from Helenen-Quelle and George-Victor Spring, and of 2 other springs, Koenigsquelle and Stahlquelle.

Analysis:

	Per 1,000 Parts Helenen Spring	George Victor Spring
Potassium chloride	0.03856	
Sodium chloride	1.035	0.007581
Sodium bromide	0.000536	
Sodium iodide	0.000032	
Sulphuric acid	0.03819	0.068602
Calcium sulphide	——	——
Potassium sulphide	——	0.00928
Sodium bicarbonate	0.9471	0.065213
Lithium bicarbonate	0.009021	0.000770
Ammonium bicarbonate	——	0.000439
Ammonium chloride	0.002032	
Calcium phosphate	0.000159	
Calcium arsenate	0.001053	
Calcium bicarbonate	1.437	0.731939
Magnesium bicarbonate	1.554	0.553820
Strontium bicarbonate	0.02914	
Barium bicarbonate	0.000677	0.000016
Iron protoxide bicarbonate	0.02641	0.029949
Manganous protoxide bicarbonate	0.001724	0.002180
Aluminium phosphate	——	0.000065
Alumina	——	0.000102
Silica	0.03280	0.021677
Free carbonic acid	2.529	2.550242
TOTAL CONSTITUENTS	7.681514	4.041939

Action and Uses: HELENEN SPRING WATER is sodic, chloric, calcic, magnesic; bicarbonated, muriated, alkaline, acidulous; GEORGE VICTOR WATER—of same composition with abundance of free carbonic acid. *For use* in uric acid diathesis, gout, renal calculi, nephritis, pyelitis, cystitis and hematuria.

Supply: Bottles 24 oz.—Cases of 12 and 50.

Administration: 1–2 glasses three times daily before meals for 4–8 weeks.

WYRICK MINERAL SPRINGS, Crockett, Va.

Description: Lightly mineralized and radio-active alkaline water; calcic, magnestic sodic; bicarbonated.

Analysis:

	Per Million Parts
Lithium chloride	trace
Sodium chloride	1.8
Potassium sulphate	6.0
Sodium bicarbonate	35.4
Magnesium bicarbonate	32.7
Calcium bicarbonate	97.2
Ferric oxide and alumina	4.2
Silica	8.4
TOTAL SOLIDS	185.7

Action and Uses: Diuretic, antacid and tonic. *Used* in gastric hyperacidity, dyspepsia, gastritis nervousness; in rheumatism, uric acid diathesis, in renal and vesical affections, Bright's disease; in diabetes, hepatic calculi; for its radio-active stimulation in psoriasis, eczema, scrofula, gland disorders.

Supply: Bottles, large and small.

PART II

ARTIFICIAL MINERAL WATERS

ALKA WATER (Schultz)

Description: A pleasantly carbonated, palatable, artificial water containing per 100,000 parts: lithium bicarbonate 20, calcium bicarbonate 90, potassium bicarbonate 70, sodium bicarbonate 586, sodium chloride 82, sodium phosphate 70 parts. (Each 6 oz. contains 36 gr of minerals.)

Action and Uses: Diuretic, uricolytic, antacid, cholagogue. *For use* in uric acid diathesis, gout, rheumatoid arthritis, constipation, gastro-intestinal affections.

Supply: Bottles 25 oz.—Boxes of 12.
Bottles 12 oz.—Boxes of 24.

BILIN (Schultz)

Description: An alkaline mineral water, artificially prepared to chemically approximate natural Bilin (Josephsquelle) water; contains among others per 100,000 parts of water: sodium bicarbonate 467.67, sodium sulphate 82.68, calcium bicarbonate 65.16, sodium chloride 38.22 parts (Each 6 oz. represents 19.40 gr minerals).

Action and Uses: Diuretic and uricolytic. *For use* in genito-urinary affections, with or without calculi; in gout, biliary disease, diabetes.

Supply: Bottles 25 oz.—Boxes of 12.
Bottles 12 oz.—Boxes of 24.

CARLSBAD (Schultz)

Description: A moderately mineralized, alkaline, sulphated water; bottled in 2 strengths, double and quadruple the strength of normal Carlsbad Sprudel water; contains among others per 100,000 parts of water—sodium sulphate 240.49, sodium bicarbonate 208.43, sodium chloride 102.23, calcium bicarbonate 52.18, potassium sulphate 18.62 parts. (Each water glass (6 oz.) represents 18.1 gr of mineral ingredients.)

Action and Uses: Laxative, antacid and diuretic. *For use* in gastric hyperacidity, peptic ulcer, hepatic and biliary affections, constipation and other gastrointestinal disorders; also in gout, diabetes and obesity.

Supply: Bottles 25 oz.—Boxes of 12.
Bottles 12 oz.—Boxes of 24.

GLEICHENBERG (Schultz)

Description: A lightly mineralized, alkaline saline water, resembling in its chemical constitution, Constantinquelle Spring in Styria, with a saline strength about one-half its alkalinity; contains among others per 100,000 parts of water: sodium chloride 225.15, sodium bicarbonate 126.94, magnesium bicarbonate 45.19, calcium bicarbonate 39.41 parts; (Glass of 6 oz. contains 20.47 gr minerals).

Action and Uses: Soothing in respiratory catarrhal affections, effective in scrofulosis, in cardiac affections and in mild catarrhal jaundice.

Supply: Bottles 25 oz.—Boxes of 12.
Bottles 12 oz.—Boxes of 24.

HOMBURG (Schultz)

Description: A moderately mineralized saline water, resembling in chemical constitution Elizabethbrunnen water, in Hesse-Nassau; contains among others per 100,000 parts of water: sodium chloride 985.79, calcium bicarbonate 250.36, magnesium chloride 76.27, calcium chloride 65.05 parts. (Glass of 6 oz. represents 39.07 gr minerals.)

Action and Uses: *For use* as antacid, diuretic, uricolytic in hyperacidity, gout, anemia.

Supply: Bottles 25 oz.—Boxes of 12.
Bottles 12 oz.—Boxes of 24.

HUNYADI (Schultz)

Description: A moderately, highly mineralized sulphated water, similar in its chemical constitution to the Janos spring in Hungary; contains among others per 100,-

000 parts of water: sodium sulphate 1,966.21, magnesium sulphate 1,949.42, sodium chloride 142.41, calcium bicarbonate 141.4 parts. (Glass of 6 oz. represents 115.6 gr minerals.)

Action and Uses: Strongly purgative. *For use* in conditions where purgation is indicated, as in cerebral hyperemia, edema, ascites.

Supply: Bottles 25 oz.—Boxes of 12.
Bottles 12 oz.—Boxes of 24.

KALAK (Kalak)

Description: Highly mineralized; sodic, potassic, calcic, magnesic, chloric; carbonated, phosphated, alkaline water; colorless, odorless, of saline taste, palatable. Contains per 100,000 parts: sodium carbonate 3655, sodium chloride 606, potassium chloride 117, calcium carbonate 475, sodium phosphate 122, magnesium carbonate 58 parts.

Action and Uses: Alkalizer for use in acidosis, rheumatism, gout, arthritis; in fevers, rickets and tetany.

Supply: Bottles of 1 qt.—Cases of 50.
Splits—Cases of 100.

KISSINGEN (Schultz)

Description: A lightly mineralized saline water, chemically resembling the Rakoczy spring in Bavaria; contains per 100,000 parts of water: sodium chloride, 581.57, calcium bicarbonate 175.42, magnesium sulphate 37.69, calcium sulphate 36.72, potassium sulphate 33.52 and other mineral parts. (Glass of 6 oz. represents 25.32 gr minerals.)

Action and Uses: Antacid, diuretic and uricolytic. *For use* in gastric hyperacidity, gastric atony, urinary affections with or without calculi, gout, rheumatism and secondary anemias.

Supply: Bottles of 25 oz.—Boxes of 12.
Bottles of 12 oz.—Boxes of 24.

KISSINGEN BITTER WATER (Schultz)

Description: A highly mineralized sulphated bitter water; resembles chemically, the Bitterquelle in Bavaria; contains among other minerals per 100,000 parts of water: sodium chloride 1,280.12, magnesium sulphate 1093.29, calcium bicarbonate 102.63, potassium sulphate 19.83 and sodium bromide 12.75 parts. (Glass of 6 oz. represents 70.2 gr minerals.)

Action and Uses: Laxative, purgative. *For use* in habitual constipation, intestinal toxemia, dyschezia, arterial hypertension and edema.

Supply: Bottles of 25 oz.—Boxes of 12.
Bottles of 12 oz.—Boxes of 24.

LITHIA WATERS (Schultz)

Description: Artificial mineral waters with the addition of Lithium salts.

LITHIA CARLSBAD—Contains minerals corresponding to single Carlsbad water, with the addition of lithium 60 parts to 100,000 parts of water: sodium sulphate 240.49, sodium bicarbonate 208.43, sodium chloride 102.23, lithium bicarbonate 60.73, calcium bicarbonate 52.18 parts. Glass of 6 oz. represents 1.66 gr of lithium bicarbonate and 18.03 gr Carlsbad minerals.

LITHIA SELTERS—Contains minerals corresponding to Selters water, with the addition of lithium 58 parts to 100,000 parts of water: sodium chloride 112.57, sodium bicarbonate 63.47, lithium bicarbonate 30.00, calcium bicarbonate 19.70 parts; Glass of 6 oz. represents 0.8 gr of lithium bicarbonate and 6.17 gr of minerals of Selters, one-half strength.

LITHIA VICHY—Contains minerals corresponding to Vichy water, with the addition of Lithium 58 parts to 100,000 of water: sodium bicarbonate 602.25, lithium bicarbonate 58.48, sodium chloride 57.87, calcium bicarbonate 40.50, potassium sulphate 20.40 parts. Glass of 6 oz. contains 1.6 gr of lithium bicarbonate and 20.45 gr of minerals of Vichy.

LITHIA WATER—Contains per 100,000 parts lithium bicarbonate 146.1 and sodium chloride 125.66 parts. Glass of 6 oz. represents 4 gr of lithium bicarbonate; bottled Sparkling and Still.

Action and Uses: Diuretic, uricolytic and somewhat laxative; offer in addition characteristics of the mineral waters they represent without the lithia; *For use* in rheumatism, gout, gastro-intestinal catarrh and similar instances.

Supply: Bottles of 25 oz.—Boxes of 12.
Bottles of 12 oz.—Boxes of 24.

MARIENBAD (Schultz)

Description: A lightly mineralized alkaline sulphated water, of the chemical constitution of Kreuzbrunnen in Bohemia; contains among other minerals per 100,000 parts of water: sodium sulphate 472.25, sodium bicarbonate 180.68, sodium chloride 145.39, calcium bicarbonate 97.12, magnesium bicarbonate 79.92 parts. (Glass of 6 oz. represents 27.4 gr minerals.)

Action and Uses: Laxative and aperient in habitual constipation, plethoric obesity.

Supply: Bottles, 25 oz.—Boxes of 12.
Bottles 12 oz.—Boxes of 24.

OBERSALZBRUNN (Schultz)

Description: An alkaline mineral water, prepared to resemble in its chemical constitution the natural spring in Prussian Silesia; contains among other minerals per 100,000 parts of water: sodium bicarbonate 209.08, magnesium bicarbonate 46.69, sodium sulphate 43.59, calcium bicarbonate 43.49 parts. (Glass of 6 oz. represents 10.14 gr minerals.)

Action and Uses: Uricolytic and intestinal corrective; *for use* in intestinal acid fermentation and urinary calculi; and as diluent for milk and whey.

Supply: Bottles, 25 oz.—Boxes of 12.
Bottles 12 oz.—Boxes of 24.

PIPERAZINE (Hahn and Wessel)

Description: Each quart bottle of carbonated water is stated to contain 15 gr of Piperazine.

Action and Uses: An artificial, alkaline, uricolytic mineral water *for use* in arthritis, gout, rheumatism, acidosis and uric acid diathesis.

Supply: Bottles of 1 qt.—Boxes of 12.

Dosage: 1 bottle daily in divided doses, warmed, on empty stomach.

PUELLNA (Schultz)

Description: A moderately highly mineralized sulphated water, prepared to represent in its chemical constitution the Bitterwasser springs in Bohemia; contains among other minerals per 100,000 parts of water: magnesium sulphate 1516.31, sodium sulphate 1287.29, sodium chloride 267.29, magnesium bicarbonate 108.55, potassium sulphate 62.50, calcium bicarbonate 56.63 parts.

Action and Uses: *For use* as purgative in acute and severe constipation.

Supply: Bottles, 25 oz. Boxes of 12.
Bottles 12 oz. Boxes of 24.

PURGOS (Hahn and Wessel) (American Agency)

Description: A French artificial mineral water comprising a mixture of salts with French Vichy; alkaline, magnesic, sodic; contains per 1,000 parts: carbonic acid (free) 0.1082, calcium bicarbonate 0.0293, iron bicarbonate 0.0040, lithia bicarbonate traces, magnesium bicarbonate 0.0052, potassium bicarbonate 0.0135, soda bicarbonate 8.000 parts.

Action and Uses: Digestive stimulant, laxative, diuretic, purgative. *For use* in gastrointestinal disturbances, atony, catarrh, constipation, hepatic congestion, obesity.

Supply: Bottles of 14 oz.—Boxes of 12 and 50.

Administration: 1 wineglassful in the morning before breakfast; as purgative, 1 tumblerful mornings; children, ½ dosage.

PYRMONT **(Schultz)**

Description: A lightly mineralized chalybeate water, prepared to resemble in its chemical constitution the Neubrunnen, in Waldeck-Pyrmont; contains among other minerals per 100,000 parts of water: calcium bicarbonate 162.23, sodium chloride 115.98, magnesium sulphate 41.04, sodium sulphate 28.90 parts. (6 oz. represents 10.55 gr minerals.)

Action and Uses: Antacid, chalybeate, hematinic in anemia.

Supply: Bottles, 25 oz. Boxes of 12.
Bottles 12 oz. Boxes of 24.

SARATOGA VICHY **(Hahn and Wessel)**

Description: An artificially carbonated and lithiated water for table use.

Supply: Bottles, large—Boxes of 50.
Bottles, 1 pt.—Boxes of 100.
Splits—Boxes of 100.

SCHWALBACH **(Schultz)**

Description: A lightly mineralized chalybeate water, prepared to represent in its chemical constitution the Strahlbrunnen in Hesse-Nassau; containing among other minerals per 100,000 parts of water: calcium bicarbonate 24.90, magnesium bicarbonate 24.20, ferrous bicarbonate 9.32 parts. (6 oz. contains 1.86 gr minerals.)

Action and Uses: *For use* as antacid, chalybeate, hematinic in anemia, neuralgia, hypochondriasis.

Supply: Bottles, 25 oz. Boxes of 12.
Bottles 12 oz. Boxes of 24.

SELTERS **(Schultz)**

Description: A mineralized alkaline popular table water, resembling in its chemical constitution the Selters spring in Hesse-Nassau; contains per 100,000 parts of water: sodium chloride 225.15, sodium bicarbonate 126.94, magnesium bicarbonate 45.19, calcium bicarbonate 39.41 and others. (Each 6 oz. contains 12.35 gr minerals.)

Action and Uses: Antacid, mucolytic, diuretic; For use in gastrointestinal, respiratory and genito-urinary affections; in bronchial catarrh, urinary calculi, intestinal disturbances.

Supply: Cases of 10 Siphons.

VICHY **(Schultz)**

Description: A strong alkaline water, similar in its chemical constitution to the Grande Grille Spring in France; contains per 100,000 parts of water among others: sodium bicarbonate 602.25, sodium chloride 57.87, calcium bicarbonate 40.50, potassium sulphate 20.40 parts. (Each 6 oz. represents 20.45 gr of minerals.)

Action and Uses: Antacid, diuretic, uricolytic; *For use* in affections of the genito-urinary and respiratory tracts; in hyperacidity, gout, biliary and urinary calculi; in arthritis, rheumatism, acidosis, vomiting.

Supply: Bottled both Sparkling and Still.
Cases of 10 Siphons.

WILDUNGEN **(Schultz)**

Description: A lightly mineralized alkali-earthy water, prepared to represent in its chemical constitution the Helenenquelle, in Waldeck; contains among other minerals per 100,000 parts of water: magnesium bicarbonate 155.51, calcium bicarbonate 142.86, sodium chloride 103.75, sodium bicarbonate 95.62 parts. (6 oz. contains 13.90 gr minerals.)

Action and Uses: *For use* as antacid, diuretic, uricolytic in hyperacidity, urinary calculi, etc.

Supply: Bottles, 25 oz. Boxes of 12.
Bottles of 12 oz. Boxes of 24.

Part III

Mineral Water Salts

CRAZY WATER CRYSTALS **(Crazy Well)**

Description: A pure product of evaporation of the natural waters of Crazy Mineral Wells; when diluted for use, 1 level teaspoonful to 1 pt. of water, it presents per million parts: calcium bicarbonate 3.5, magnesium bicarbonate 7.2, magnesium sulphate 1.0, sodium sulphate 3695.8, sodium chloride 69.4, sodium nitrate 0.1, potassium chloride 42.9, total solids 3819.9, total alkalinity in terms of sodium bicarbonate 11.80.

Action and Uses: Diuretic, laxative and antacid; *Uses* as for the natural Crazy Mineral Water—in gastrointestinal disorders, constipation, autointoxication, intestinal and hepatic stasis.

Supply: Packages of 1 lb.

Administration: 1 glassful of above mentioned dilution four times daily, before breakfast and between meals, cold for diuresis and hot as laxative.

EMS MINERAL SPRING SALT **(Von der Bruck)**

Description: A product of evaporation of the natural waters of Ems Thermal Springs, containing their ingredients in concentration.

Action and Uses: Alkaline and saline; *For external use* in catarrhal affections of the upper respiratory tract, conjunctivitis and as mouth wash; internally—in the conditions as for natural Ems products.

Supply: Bottles of 2 oz.

Administration: ½ teaspoonful of Salt to tumblerful of water, as required.

FRANZENSBAD NATURAL MUD SALT **(Spa Products)**

Description: A product of evaporation from Franzensbad Mineral Mud deposits; contains per 100 parts: ferrous oxide 24.83, ferric oxide 0.50, aluminum oxide 1.18, manganese oxide 0.25, calcium oxide 0.58, magnesium oxide 0.18, potassium oxide 1.16, sodium oxide 1.66, ammonia 0.43, sulphuric anhydrid 32.50, phosphoric anhydrid 0.03, chlorine 0.01.

Action and Uses: Stimulates circulation, is astringent and disinfectant; *For use* in gynecologic disturbances, rheumatic affections and neuralgias.

Supply: Packages of 2½ lbs.

Administration: For irrigation—1–2 tablespoonfuls to 1 qt. of water; for full bath—contents of 1 package, for sitz or foot bath—½ package. Bath should not exceed ½ hr., and be followed by plain water bath.

Caution: Tub should be thoroughly scoured to prevent mineral particles injuring enamel.

KARLSBAD BATH SALT (Carlsbad Products)

Description: Concentrated extract from the waters of Karlsbad Sprudel, containing approximately equal parts of sodium chloride and sodium carbonate.

Action and Uses: For bathing, in rheumatism or gout and other diseases where strong brine baths are indicated.

Supply: Packages of 2½ lbs.

Administration: 1–2 kg. added to bathtub of water, warm or hot.

KARLSBAD SPRUDEL SALT (Carlsbad Products)

Description: A powder obtained by evaporation of the water of Karlsbad Sprudel; contains per package: potassium sulphate 3.41, lithium carbonate 0.19, sodium hydrocarbonate 34.04, sodium carbonate 1.77, sodium sulphate 42.10, sodium chloride 18.14, sodium tetraborate 0.01, ferric oxide 0.002, silicic acid 0.002, sodium iodide 0.00046, water 0.32, calcium and magnesium traces.

Action and Uses: As for natural Karlsbad Sprudel Water; is recommended in gastric hyperacidity, acute gastritis, gastric ulcer, chronic constipation and other intestinal and biliary disorders; also in genitourinary and metabolic affections.

Supply: Bottles of ⅛ lb.
Packages of 5 Gm in boxes of 10.

Administration: In hyperacid states—5–10 Gm in ½ pt. of water, warm, taken mornings on an empty stomach; in hypoacid states—1–3 Gm in carbonated water; in obesity—10–15 Gm, in other conditions—5 Gm to 1 litre of warm water three to four times daily, in 200–250 cc doses.

MARIENBAD NATURAL SPRING SALT (Spa Products)

Description: A product of evaporation from the water of Ferdinandsbrunnen; contains per 100 parts: potassium sulfate 0.66, sodium sulfate 54.38, sodium chloride 20.40, sodium carbonate 23.81, lithium carbonate 0.08, water 0.67, with traces of sodium biborate, sodium nitrate, sodium bromide, silicic acid, ferric oxide; 15 gr of the Salt are equivalent to about 3½ oz. of the natural water.

Action and Uses: Increases elimination, stimulates secretory function of digestive organs and is diuretic; *Uses* as for the natural waters.

Supply: Bottles of 3½ oz.

Administration: 1 teaspoonful to 1 pt. of water, warmed, taken mornings and evenings.

MONTECATINI SALTS (Banfi)

Description: A product of extraction from the mineral waters of Montecatini; contains per 100 parts: **Plain**—sodium sulphate 44.715, sodium chloride 1.250, sodium carbonate 0.035, water of crystallization 54.000, with traces of potassium, lithium, bromine and manganese; **Iodated**—above contents plus 0.20% of iodine.

Action and Uses: For use in stomach, liver and biliary diseases and dysfunction, in constipation and intestinal diseases; in metabolic disorders and arthritic disease.

Supply: **MONTECATINI IODATED SALTS**—Bottles of 115 Gm.
MONTECATINI PLAIN SALTS—Bottles of 115 Gm.

Administration: 1 teaspoonful in 8 oz. of hot water, ½ hour before breakfast; half or full dosage repeated ½ hour before evening meal, if necessary. The Iodated Salts to be used in those diseases in which the additional administration of iodine is indicated.

Caution. [illegible]

KARLSBAD BATH SALT [illegible]

Description. [illegible]

Action and Uses. [illegible]

Supply. [illegible]

Administration. [illegible]

KARLSBAD SPRUDEL SALT [illegible]

Description. A powder [illegible]

Supply. [illegible]

Administration. [illegible]

KARLSBAD [illegible]

Description. [illegible]

Action and Uses. [illegible]

Supply. [illegible]

Administration. [illegible]

MONTE [illegible]

Description. [illegible]

Action and Uses. [illegible]

[illegible]

Administration. [illegible]

Pharmaceutical Drug *and* Drugs Products

(With their description, medicinal preparations, administrations and therapeutic uses)

Pharmaceutical Drug *and* Drugs Products

(With their description, medicinal preparations, administrations and therapeutic uses)

A presentation of 8160 modern, non-pharmacopeal, medicinal preparations, comprising: 1878 drugs and chemicals, 535 biologicals, 860 endocrines, 1563 ampule medicaments, 209 medicinal foods, 129 mineral waters, 2344 individual and group allergens and 642 miscellaneous products.

By :
JACOB GUTMAN, M.D., Phar.D., F.A.C.P.
WILLIAM E. FITCH
Consulting Physician, Manhattan General Hospital, New York; the Riverdale, Shore Road, Williamsburg Maternity and Borough Park General Hospitals of Brooklyn; Director, Brooklyn Diagnostic Institute. Formerly Professor of Materia Medica College of Dentistry, University of State of New Jersey; Professor Clinical Chemistry Jersey City College of Pharmacy; Instructor of Medicine, New York Post Graduate Medical School and Hospital; Attending Physician Wyckoff Heights and Unity Hospitals.

Volume 3

SHREE PUBLISHERS & DISTRIBUTORS
NEW DELHI-110 002

Edition : 2008

Published by :
SHREE PUBLISHERS AND DISTRIBUTORS
20, Ansari Road, Daryaganj
New Delhi-110 002

3 Volumes Set

ISBN : 978-81-8329-255-9

Printed by :
Ruchika Printers
Delhi-110032

PREFACE

This treatise is designed to meet the demand of the progressive physician for information concerning the most modern therapeutic agencies placed at his command by Research Laboratories. It presents without bias or comment all the popular non-pharmacopeal preparations and other remedies found useful in the treatment of disease.

The pharmaceutical concerns of America spend millions of dollars yearly for the discovery and preparation of medicinal agents of high merit. Medicine is indeed indebted to these organizations for the many epoch-making discoveries and invaluable additions to modern therapeusis made during the past few decades; most of the curative sera, vaccines, allergens, potent drugs and endocrines are the result of their researches. The physician, however, has at present no adequate means of keeping informed on all the newer additions to his armamentarium; commercial descriptions of these reach him at inopportune times and usually find their way into the waste basket, thus seldom being on hand when wanted; and except for the official publication of only Council-Accepted products, there are no authoritative sources of information embracing all the modern preparations. To provide such source is the purpose of this work.

An endeavor is here made to present without favoritism or discrimination all the non-official products-proprietary, patented, Council Accepted and others, that are popular with the medical profession. Descriptions, statements, analyses and all other data are offered without change or comment, but as found available in the numerous standard works and references consulted, or as obtained from the producers and distributors of the respective products. Every effort has been made to present the information accurately yet concisely, excluding elaborate discussions, quotations, theories and other time consuming topics of but little practical value to the clinician. The embodiment in three volumes of such a mass of material necessitated the use of phraseology as brief as was found consistent with the complete description of every important feature.

To insure ease in locating a desired preparation and to afford equal consideration to all products and producers, the arrangement throughout the book is alphabetical, by drug or distributor. Separate chapters are devoted to preparations of similar character; in each chapter like products are grouped, and preceded in each instance by a brief description with suggestions for their practical application; for each drug its various methods of administration, with dosages in the metric and U. S. systems, are presented. Incompatibilities, contraindications, strengths of solutions and methods of their preparation are given where deemed serviceable; where emphasis is desirable, italics or capitals are employed; verbiage is avoided throughout the book.

The Therapeutic Guide is intended to provide for the clinician, whether general practitioner or specialist, a wide choice of preparations of use in the numerous pathologic conditions encountered in his daily service to the sick; also to assist him in the selection of a remedy for a particular purpose. The comprehensive Index is arranged into three sections-Distributors', Drug and Therapeutic, this to assure convenience and rapidity in locating a desired drug, disease or other topic.

GLOSSARY

Definitions of the Newer Trade Terms

Alkpule: A specially treated glass vial containing chemically pure, normal 4% sodium hydroxide solution, in the exact quantity necessary to alkalize the corresponding dose of the accompanying drug.

Ambot: An ampule-bottle containing a solution for hypodermic use.

Ampacoid: A sterile, isotonic solution containing a physiologically standardized hormone of high concentration and purity.

Ampule-vial: A vial containing a sterile solution for hypodermic injection.

Aspirol: A trade name for Ampule-vial.

Bacterin: A bacterial vaccine; a suspension of killed bacteria for use in immunization.

Billet: A small tablet.

C.A.: Council or Committee Accepted (accepted by the Council on Pharmacy and Chemistry or Committee on Foods of the A.M.A., 1933).

Carpule: A glass cartridge-ampule containing in sterile solution a medicament, in definite dosage and strength.

Collosol: A suspensoid colloid with the active ingredient in the disperse phase; non-dialysable, slowly diffusible and disintegrating; is electrically charged and affected by electrolytes.

Crinogen: A preparation of glandular substance, protein and alcohol-free, in concentrated solution.

Dragee: A sugar coated pill or medicated confection.

Elixoid: A fluid preparation favorably flavored.

Emplet: An endocrine product with a protective, inert, salol-free enteric coating, insoluble in stomach but soluble in duodenal and intestinal secretions.

Enteric Coated: Specially coated to traverse the stomach intact without causing irritation, and disintegrating only in the intestines.

Enterocap: A capsule devised to protect its contents against gastric action.

Enterosol Coated: So coated as to be insoluble in gastric secretion.

Enule: A rectal suppository wrapped individually in tin foil.

Glaseptic Ampule: An ampule made of an alkali-free, non-soluble glass, assuring stability of contents.

Hypoloid: An ampule containing a solution for hypodermic injection.

Immunogen: Extraction from living bacterial culture, principally ectoplasm, free from toxic autolysates, bacterial substances, with only 1/10% of the protein content of ordinary vaccines.

Isopule: An ampule containing a measured dose of a medicament.

Kapseal: A special gelatine capsule with joints hermetically sealed to keep contents airtight and prevent deterioration.

Kerakote: A keratin-composition acid resisting, coating, for carrying into the intestines medicinal products which may be impaired or destroyed in the stomach.

Keratin Coated: Coated with acid-resistant keratin, enabling contained medication to pass through the stomach unimpaired.

L.A.: Laity Advertised; popular preparations advertised to the public.

Phylacogen: A bacterial culture filtrate free from organisms.

Pulvule: A dry powdered preparation enclosed in thin walled, quickly soluble capsule of a special gelatin, assuring stability of medication.

Sanitablet: A tablet mechanically packed in cellophane to prevent contamination from handling.

Serobacterin: A bacterin or vaccine sensitized with its corresponding immune serum and of use in smaller dosage.

Soloid: A tablet of soluble ingredients for the making of solutions.

Sucret: A preparation with sucrose.

Swab-Seal: An Ampule-vial mechanically sealed for preservation of contents in sterile state.

Tabloid: A form of medicinal tablet or lozenge.

TABLE OF CONTENTS

CHAPTER V

HYPODERMIC MEDICAMENTS

CHAPTER VI

BIOLOGICALS

CHAPTER VII

ALLERGENS

CHAPTER VIII

FOODS AND BEVERAGES

CHAPTER IX

BOTTLED MINERAL WATERS

CHAPTER X

MISCELLANEOUS PRODUCTS

CHAPTER XI

THERAPEUTIC GUIDE

CHAPTER XII

CHAPTER XIII

CHAPTER XIV

CHAPTER XV

CHAPTER X

MISCELLANEOUS PRODUCTS

In this chapter are assembled 642 preparations for topical application, comprising—

32 Buccal Preparations	172 Ophthalmic Ointments
30 Dusting Powders	46 Rectal Suppositories
4 Ear Drops	7 Styptics
37 Liquid Antiseptics	10 Soaps, Medicated
14 Lotions and Emollients	8 Urethral Bougies and Pencils
19 Lozenges and Troches	45 Vaginal Antiseptics
69 Nasal Preparations	5 Miscellaneous Preparations
144 Ointments	

Brief descriptions of practical interest accompany each preparation; those marked *"See Chap."* will be found more fully described in previous chapters; the arrangement is alphabetical, by product.

---

1. BUCCAL PREPARATIONS

A. Anesthetics

A.L.A. Ampules 2 cc; Packages of 6. Bottles of 30 cc and 500 cc **(Sutliff and Case)**
Contains

Para-amino-benzoic acid ethyl ester	3.0%
Phenmethylol	5.0%
Ether	10.0%
Olive oil	82.0%

For use topically as dental anesthetic in painful manipulations of the mouth. Must *not* be injected intravenously. *See Chap. II.*

Apothesine Tablets (C.A.) Tubes of 20; Packages of 5 tubes **(Parke, Davis)**
Contains

	Gr	Gm
Apothesine	1/3	(0.02)
Adrenalin	1/2500	(0.00002)

For use in infiltration anesthesia in dental operations. One tablet dissolved in 1 cc normal saline makes a 2% solution. *See Chap. I.*

Beta Euçaine Hydrochloride Bottles 1/8 oz. **(Schering and Glatz)**
Contains trimethylbenzoxypiperidine hydrochloride; *for use* as dental anesthetic in 2–3% solution; for infiltration anesthesia—4–5% solution. *See Chap. I.*

Beta Eucaine Lactate Bottles 1/2 oz. **(Schering and Glatz)**
Contains betacaine; *for use* in infiltration anesthesia in 0.12% solution. *See Chap. I.*

Borocaine Tablets, Tubes 20, Bottles 100. **(Sharp and Dohme)**
Contains ethocaine borate; *for use* in infiltration anesthesia (1/2–1% solution) in root canal work. *See Chap. I.*

Butyn Solution (C.A.) Bottles 1 oz. **(Abbott)**
Contains p-aminobenzoyl-gamma-dinormalbutylamino-propanolsulphate. *For use* in infiltration anesthesia in 2% solution, in painful dental operations. *See Chap. I.*

Dentaline Vials 2 dr. **(Smith-Dorsey)**
Contains per oz.

	Gr	Gm
Phenol	24	1.55
Benzocaine	12	0.78
Chloroform and oil of cloves	q.s.	

For use as toothache drops; *applied* by packing dental cavity with pledget saturated in solution or by rubbing on the gums.

Neurocaine Billets, Vials of 100. **(Schieffelin)**
Contains cocaine hydrochloride gr 1/12. *For use* in pressure anesthesia for marginal cavity and pulp chamber work, cavity preparation and pulp removal; *applied* by inserting into cavity or directly into pulp chamber.

Tooth Ache Drops Bottles ¼ oz. **(McKesson and Robbins)**
Contains oil of cloves, phenol and glycerine. *For use* in relief of dental pain; *applied* by inserting pellet saturated in solution, directly into dental cavity.

B. Antiseptics

Chloro-Camphene Bottles ½ oz. **(McNeil)**
Contains para-mono-chlor-phenol; *for use* as dental antiseptic for infected root canals; *applied* locally by cotton pledget inserted directly into canal.

Chloroseptine Aromatic Powder Bottles 2 oz., 1 lb. **(Strasenburgh)**
Contains chloroseptine 5% with sodium bicarbonate, sodium chloride, saccharin and eucalyptol, equal parts. For use as gargle or spray in oral and nasal affections; *Administration*—as gargle, ½ teaspoonful in ½ glass of warm water; as nasal douche, ¼ strength.

Collosol Chlor Carvacrol Bottles 1 oz. **(Crookes)**
For use as dental antiseptic and mouth wash in oral hygiene; *applied* twice daily with tooth brush or as gargle. *See Chap. I.*

Dentinol Bottles 1 and 2 oz. **(Dentinol)**
Contains cresol, oils of eucalyptus, birch, sassafras, camphor, capsicum, turpentine, alcohol and ether. *For use* as oral germicide in infected dental sockets, pyorrhea, and after extractions; *applied* full strength as mouth wash or gargle.

Lavoris (L.A.) Bottles 8, 16 oz. **(Lavoris)**
Contains zinc chloride. *For use* as liquid antiseptic and astringent in throat and tonsillar irritation; also as mouth wash; *Applied*—full strength or diluted with equal parts of warm water.

Noviform Powder Bottles 1 oz. **(Heyden)**
For use as dental antiseptic for tamponing abscesses and after extraction; *applied* in powder form or mixed with talcum. *See Chap. I.*

Phenandyne Individual bottles, Cartons 12. **(Schieffelin)**
Contains acetic acid-ester of phenol. *For use* as dental antiseptic in treatment of cavities, pulpitis, pericementitis, alveolar abscess and pyorrhea; is especially adapted for "Buckley Treatment"; *applied* full strength by inserting pledget directly into cavity.

Sodiphene Bottles 3, 7, 16 oz. **(Sodiphene)**
An alkaline germicide with local anesthetic effect; is pleasant, non-caustic; *for use* in oral manipulations to prevent gagging, in pyorrhea, Vincent's infections and post extraction. *Applied* topically, full strength, three or four times daily; as gargle, diluted in 3 parts of warm water. *See Chap. III.*

C. Astringents

Red Gum Tabloids, Bottles of 100 **(Burroughs Wellcome)**
For use as astringent in treatment of relaxed fauces; *applied* by dissolving 1 tablet slowly in the mouth, several times daily.

Root Canal Filling Individual bottles. **(Burnham)**
Contains—Powder 1—free iodine, bismuth subnitrate and calcium phosphate; liquid 2—free iodine solution in oil. *For use* as dental filling in root canals to keep the periapical area sterile and to stimulate regrowth of healthy tissue in this region; *applied* by mixing #1 and #2 to form a smooth paste for use as root canal filling. *See Chap. XII.*

D. Hemostatics

Hemarestors Boxes of 20 **(McNeil)**
Aseptic medicated discs in a gelatin glycerin base. *For use* as styptic in arresting hemorrhage or secondary oozing following extractions or other oral operations.

Thromboplastin (C.A.) Individual vials **(Squibb)**
A hemostatic serum for treatment of persistent bleeding following dental operations; *applied* by subcutaneous injection, preferably preoperatively as prophylactic. *See Chap. I.*

E. Tooth Pastes

Collosol Argentum Dentifrice Individual tubes, packages 12 **(Crookes)**
Contains collosol argentum; *for use* as dental antiseptic, and as dentifrice. *See Chap. I.*

Dental Magnesia Individual tubes—large and small **(Phillips)**
Contains milk of magnesia 75 %. *For use* as dentifrice; *applied* twice daily with tooth brush.

Detoxol Paste Individual tubes **(Merrell)**
Contains soricin 2 % (sodium ricinoleate). *For use* as dentifrice for the care of teeth, gums and mouth; *applied* twice daily with tooth brush.

Hexyl Resorcinol Tooth Paste Tubes 2 oz. **(Sharp and Dohme)**
Contains hexyl resorcinol 1:1,000. *For use* as dentifrice and oral antiseptic; *applied* twice daily with tooth brush. *See Chap. I.*

Iodent Tooth Paste (L.A.) Individual tubes **(Iodent)**
Contains

	1	2
Calcium carbonate precipitated	55 Gm	30.14 Gm
Soap	6 Gm	7.23 Gm
Glycerin	34 Gm	28.9 Gm
Petrolatum	1.25 Gm	1.51 Gm
Saccharin	0.25 Gm	0.30 Gm
Oil of peppermint	1.0 Gm	1.20 Gm
Water	2.26 Gm	0.30 Gm
Iodides (Ca and K)	0.24 Gm	0.24 Gm

For use as dentifrice in oral hygiene; *applied* twice daily with tooth brush.

Ipana Tooth Paste (L.A.) Individual tubes—large and small **(Bristol-Myers)**
Contains soap, calcium carbonate ziratol and flavoring oils. *For use* as dentifrice and in oral hygiene; *applied* by massaging into gums twice daily with finger or tooth brush.

Pepsodent Tooth Paste (L.A.) Individual tubes. **(Pepsodent)**
Contains

Special calcium phosphate	59.400 %
Benzoic acid	0.100 %
Tragacanth gum	0.600 %

Karaya gum	1.200 %
Calcium chloride	0.237 %
Glycerin, water, flavor	38.463 %

For use as dentifrice, *applied* twice daily with tooth brush.

Pycopé Tooth Powder (L.A.) Cans, 2 oz. (Pycopé)

Contains	Per Cent
Sodium chloride	59.471273
Bicarbonate of soda	19.823757
Magnesium carbonate	4.944939
Sodium perborate	14.867818
Oil of cloves	.293463
Methyl salicylate	.587738
	99.999988

For use as dentifrice; *applied* twice daily with tooth brush.

Pyrozide Tooth Powder (L.A.) Individual boxes (Dentinol)
Contains dentinol, (composed of cresol, oils of birch, camphor, capsicum, eucalpytus, sassafras, turpentine with alcohol, ether) with sodium perborate, magnesia, cinchona bark and effective cleansing agents. *For use* twice daily as dentifrice.

Pyrozone (L.A.) Individual tubes. (McKesson and Robbins)
Contains hydrogen peroxide 25% solution. *For use* as tooth bleach; *applied* to discolored teeth with tooth brush twice daily.

---

2. DUSTING POWDERS

Anazyme Dusting Powder Boxes of 1 oz. (Maltbie)
Contains boric acid, phenol, bismuth salts, thymol iodide, zinc sulphocarbolate, alum, menthol, eucalyptol, thymol, zinc stearate. *For use* as antiseptic dry dressing in wounds, burns, ulcers and certain skin diseases; *applied* locally. *See Chap. III.*

Antiseptic Borated Talcum Cans 4⅛ oz. (Mennen)
For use as an antiseptic dusting powder on babies' skin; *applied* locally.

Aristol Powder (C.A.) Bottles 1 oz. (Winthrop)
Contains thymol iodide. *For use* as surface antiseptic and anesthetic in skin affections; *applied* locally, freely. *See Chap. I.*

B. F. I. Powder Cans, large and small (Sharpe and Dohme)
Contains bismuth-formic-iodide gr 70, acetanilid gr 30, zinc sulphocarbolate gr 10, bismuth subgallate gr 20, powdered alum gr 3, boric acid gr 128 per ounce; *applied* locally, freely as antiseptic and astringent. *See Chap. II.*

Bismuth Thymol Iodide Cans 5½ oz., 2 oz. bottles (Strasenburg)
Contains bismuth oxyiodide, thymol iodide, boric acid. *For use* as surgical dressing; *applied* locally. *See Chap. II.*

Camphaseptic Powder Individual cans, sifter top. (Irwin, Neissler)
Contains acetanilid, bismuth subnitrate, boric acid, camphor, phenol. *For use* as antiseptic dusting powder, locally. *See Chap. III.*

Chlomine Powder Cans 4 oz. (Columbus)
Contains chlorbutanol 1%, boric acid, sodium borate, thiosulphate and aromatics. *For use* as fungicide and deodorant in parasitic skin affections. *See Chap. III.*

Chloramine Powder (C.A.) Bottles 1 and 5 lb. (Squibb)
For use as dry Dakin antiseptic in suppurative wounds; *applied* freely. *See Chap. I.*

Chlorazene Surgical Powder (C.A.) Cans, sprinkler top, 1 oz. (Abbott)
Contains active chlorine 11.5–13 %; *For use* as antiseptic and deodorant in infected wounds. *See Chap. I.*

Dermalgen Powder Cans 2 oz. (National Drug)
Contains alum, bismuth, iodine, acetanilid, phenol, boric acid, antiseptic oils. *For use* as antiseptic, analgesic and deodorant in ulcerations; *applied* by dusting freely. *See Chap. III.*

Dimazon Powder (C.A.) Boxes of 1 oz. (Heilcraft)
Contains diacetylamidoazotoluene 5 % in talcum 95 %. *For use* as cell proliferant and dry dressing. *See Chap. I.*

Drosine Metal containers, sprinkler top. (National Drug)
Contains magnesium peroxide, zinc sulphocarbolate, salicylic acid, boric acid, Italian talc, antiseptic aromatic oils. *For use* as soothing, antiseptic, astringent, deodorant to relieve chafing, irritation, burns and prickly heat and to neutralize body odors; as foot powder for the relief of tired sweating feet; on sanitary napkins; *applied* locally to axillae, perineum, feet or dusted into shoes.

Golden Powder Jars 4 oz. (Columbus)
Contains magnesium sulphate, boric acid, berberine, eucalyptol, menthol, thymol and phenol. *For use* as antiseptic deodorant and styptic in minor surgical affections, burns, pruritus.
Applied locally as dusting powder; as mouth wash—½–1 teaspoonful to glass of water; as vaginal douche and for rectal irrigation—1–2 teaspoonfuls to pint of water.

Iodine-Boric Acid Dusting Powder "Sulzberger" Powders 1 % and 2 %— (Pilling) bottles of 1 oz.
Contains iodine and boric acid in intimate association, as a fine impalpable powder; penetrating, antiseptic and deodorant, its iodine vapor affecting surrounding tissues. *For use* in suppurative otitis media; *applied* by daily insufflation as long as necessary; irrigations are best avoided.

Iodoformal Powder Bottles of 2 oz., 1 lb. (Warner)
Contains per 100 Gm

Thymol iodide..........	equivalent to 0.156 Gm thymol
Bismuth subiodide......	equivalent to 2.0 Gm bismuth subnitrate
Cinchonine periodide....	equivalent to 4.92 Gm cinchonine sulphate
Formaldehyde-Gelatine..	equivalent to 1.25 Gm 40 % formaldehyde sol.
Acetanilid..............	20.0 Gm
Phenol..................	0.5 Gm
Phenyl salicylate........	1.0 Gm
Boric acid..............	67.39 Gm

For use as antiseptic surgical dressing, astringent and analgesic; for local application.

Inoton Powder Carton 125 Gm. (Fougera)
Contains sulfo-schistol 0.01 Gm, lithol 0.03 Gm extract hamamelis 0.2 Gm, sod. borate 0.08 Gm, zinc oxide 0.4 Gm, calcium carb. 1.6 Gm, magnesia silicate 36 Gm. *For use* as antiseptic, antipruritic dry dressing. *See Chap. II.*

Lorate Containers of 8 oz. (Lorate)
Contains sodium perborate, monosodium carbonate, sodium chloride and menthol. *For use* as non-astringent, antiseptic deodorant in endocervicitis, gonorrheal vaginitis, leukorrhea; *applied* as vaginal douche—2 teaspoonfuls to the quart of warm water.

Noviform Powder Bottles 1 oz. (Heyden)
Contains bismuth tetrabrompyrocatechin. *For use* as antiseptic, astringent dry dressing in various infections. *See Chap. I.*

Orphol Powder (C.A.) Bottles 1 oz.; 1 lb. (Schering and Glatz)
Contains bismuth betanaphthol. *For use* as astringent, antiseptic on wounds and ulcers; *applied* topically. *See Chap. I.*

Orthoform (C.A.) Bottles 1 oz.; vials 5 Gm. **(Metz)**
Contains methylamino paraoxy-benzoate. *For use* as surface anesthetic and antiseptic in burns, varicose ulcers; *applied* topically. *See Chap. I.*

Protonuclein Powder Bottles 1 oz. and 8 oz. **(Reed and Carnrick)**
Contains mixed gland substance and boric acid. *For use* to stimulate granulations; *applied* locally. *See Chap. II.*

Quinothesine Powder Individual cans **(McNeil)**
Contains orthesin 5%, quinosol salicylate 1/10%, soda hyposulphite and boric acid q.s. *For use* as antiseptic, analgesic and parasiticide in burns, scalds, ringworm, psoriasis. *See Chap. II.*

Salamene-X Bottles 4 oz. **(Tailby-Nason)**
A chlorinated powder. *For use* as non-caustic deodorant in pelvic affections; *Administered* as vaginal douche, 1 teaspoonful to the quart of warm water.

Surgical Powder Bottles of 4, 8, 16 oz. **(Boericke and Tafel)**
Contains boric acid, calendula, hydrastis, acetanilid, thymol. *For use* as anesthetic stimulating powder in various skin and minor surgical affections; *applied* as local dusting powder.

Surgical Powder Cans, sprinkler top, large and small sizes **(Wyeth)**
Contains

Bismuth oxyiodide	5%
Bismuth subgallate	5%
Phenol, thymol, menthol, eucalyptol	1%
Acetanilid	7%
Absorbent base	82%

For use as astringent, analgesic, antiseptic and hemostatic dry dressing in wounds, ulcerations and herpes zoster; *applied* by dusting.

Tinapo Cans, sifter top. **(Irwin, Neisler)**
Contains sodium thiosulphate, oxyquinoline sulphate, thymol, powdered boric acid. *For use* as parasiticide in ringworm, epidermophytosis, dermatitis; *applied* as dusting powder.

Vioform Powder (C.A.) Cans, sprinkler top; Bottles ½ oz., and 1 lb. **(Ciba)**
Contains iodochloroxyquinolin; *For use* as antiseptic and styptic in infected wounds, ulcers, burns. *See Chap. I.*

Vulnerine Tins 1 oz.; Bottles ¼ lb., 1 lb. **(Rorer)**
Contains

Boric acid	50%
Bismuth subgallate	30%
Zinc stearate, camphor, phenol	q.s.

For use as surgical dressing in infections, burns and wounds; *applied* by dusting, locally.

Xeroform Powder (C.A.) Bottles 1 oz., 1 lb. **(Schering and Glatz)**
Contains bismuth tribromphenate. *For use* as astringent and antiseptic dry surgical dressing; *applied externally. See Chap. I.*

---

3. EAR DROPS

An-Gly-Flav Bottles of ½ oz. **(Angly Lab)**
Contains antipyrine, neutral acriflavine hydrochloride in heavy glycerine, with 2% adrenaline chloride, 1:1,000 sol. *For use* to relieve inflammation and pain in otitis media; *applied* by local instillation into affected ear.

Auralgan Bottles ½ oz. (Doho)
Contains 5% Pyrazolon phenyl-dimethyl in solution in high specific gravity glycerin;
For use in acute otitis media before suppuration;
Administration—by medicine dropper. *See Chap. II.*

Auraline Drop bottles ½ oz.—cartons of 12 (Smith-Dorsey)

Contains	Gr	Gm
Phenol	24	1.55
Menthol	12	0.78
Benzocaine	12	0.78
Oil base		

For use as analgesic in earache; *applied*—2–3 drops, warmed, by instillation into affected ear.

Otalgyne Bottles of 1 pt. (Irwin, Neisler)
Contains phenol, menthol, chloral hydrate, benzocaine, in glycerine base. *For use* as analgesic and antiseptic in earache; *applied*—2–3 drops, warmed, by instillation into affected ear.

---

4. LIQUID ANTISEPTICS

Absorbine Jr. (L.A.) Bottles 4, 12 oz. (Young)
A compound of vegetable extracts and essential oils. *For use* as antiseptic, germicide and analgesic in athlete's foot, insect bites, abrasions, infections, burns, bruises; also as gargle and local application in muscle soreness and sprains;
Administration—for massage, full strength, without bandaging; if bandaged, only 10% solution; for inhalation, a few drops in bowl of steaming water; for ringworm, 10–30% solution.

Alkalol Bottles of 6, 8, 16 oz. (Alkalol)
An alkaline, saline, non-irritating liquid antiseptic. *For use* to dissolve mucus and pus, in irrigation of nasal cavities; also as gargle for singers, smokers, speakers; locally on itching areas, burns, stings and bites;
Administration—full strength or diluted with equal parts of water.

Alpha-Naphthol Camphor Oil Bottles of 1¼ and 3 oz. (Carel)
Contains alpha-naphthol 0.5 Gm, a colorless or faintly gray crystalline powder of faint phenolic odor and pungent taste, readily soluble in alcohol, ether, chloroform, benzene and watery alkaline solutions; slightly soluble in water; is mixed with camphor, 0.5 Gm, cottonseed oil 12 Gm, liquid petrolatum q.s. 100 Gm. *For use* as local antiseptic in 0.1–1% solution; as gargle, vaginal douche or irrigation—in 0.05–0.5% solution.

Analka Bottles 3, 8, 16 oz. (Bristol-Myers)
Contains ziratol, alcohol 22%, in alkaline saline menstruum. *For use* as salivary stimulant, astringent and cleansing agent; as mouth wash, gargle, for gum massage and dental hygiene; as spray in nasal affections and as wet dressing in skin irritations, chafing, insect bits, rashes and abrasions;
Administration—full strength or diluted one-half.

An-Nu-Tol Bottles 1 pt. (Columbus)
Contains camphor, menthol, resorcin, eucalyptol, phenol, thymol iodide, balsam of Peru in neutral oil base. *For use* as emollient and antiseptic dressing in burns and minor surgical affections; *applied* one to two times daily, as necessary.

Antiseptic Gargle Bottles 4, 12 oz., 1 gal. (Fraser)
Contains pheno-glycerite of tannin and mint. *For use* to remove infective discharges, check minor oozing, promote granulation in inflammatory conditions of mouth, gums, throat and in colds;
Administration—full strength as gargle when necessary.

Antiseptic Solution 59 Bottles 16 oz. **(McKesson and Robbins)**
Contains oil of pine, fluid ext. baptesia, methyl salicylate, eucalyptol, thymol, menthol, boric and benzoic acids, in 25% alcoholic solution. *For use* as antiseptic mouth wash, spray and gargle.

Bensolyptus Bottles 1 pt., 1 gal. **(Schieffelin)**
Contains formaldehyde 0.1%, boric, salicylic and benzoic acids, methyl salicylate, alcohol 26%. *For use* as antiseptic deodorant and mucolytic, as mouth wash and dentifrice;
Administration—locally as gargle, full strength.

Bon-Sol Bottles 3, 6, 16 oz. **(Wampole)**
Contains menthol, eucalyptol, thymol, methyl salicylate, aromatic oils, glycerine, boric acid, benzoic acid, alcohol 15%. *For use* as antiseptic, deodorant, mouth wash, gargle, spray or lotion;
Administration—full strength.

Boro-Cap-Tol Bottles 1, 5 gal. **(Boericke and Runyon)**
For use as antiseptic (alcohol 30%), moist dressing, gargle, mouth wash, nasal spray and deodorant;
Administration—externally in full strength; oral cavity—diluted with equal parts of water.

Borolyptol Bottles 3, 6, 12 oz. **(Arlington)**
For use as antiseptic and mucolytic, for spongy gums and soreness; as gargle, mouth wash and as wet dressing for minor surgical affections;
Administration—full strength, where necessary.

Borolyptol Cans 1 gal. **(Irwin, Neisler)**
Contains benzoic acid, boracic acid, thymol, eucalyptol, oil of peppermint, oil of wintergreen, oil of thyme. *For use* as antiseptic mouth wash in stomatitis, gingivitis. aphthae;
Administration—full strength as mouth wash and gargle.

Chloroseptine Tablets gr 4.6; Bottles of 500 and 1000. **(Strasenbergh)**
Contains chloramine-T. *For use* as antiseptic gargle or spray in nose and throat affections;
Administration—in 2% solution, or 2 tablets dissolved in 1 oz. of water.

Chlorothol Compound Tablets—bottles of 100, 500, 1,000 **(Stoddard)**
Contains beta-naphthol, eucalyptol, camphor, menthol, sodium salts. *For use* as antacid, detergent; as douche, spray or gargle after dental extraction.
Administration—as solution, 1–2 tablets in half glass hot water as often as required.

Dermalene Cans 1 qt., 1 gal. **(Ohio Chemical)**
For use as fat solvent, to remove preoperatively grease and foreign matter from the skin, and to remove adhesive tape;
Administration—by scrubbing surface where solution is to be used.

Eau De Botot Bottles 50 cc, 125 cc, 200 cc, 500 cc, 1,000 cc **(Gane-Ingram)**
For use as astringent, detergent and antiseptic mouth wash, for irrigation of dental cavities, and for pyorrhea alveolaris;
Administration—by direct application to the gums with swab or brush, followed by rinsing mouth.

Eucalyptus-Thymol Compound Bottles 1 pt., 1 qt. **(Smith-Dorsey)**
Contains sodium benzo-borate, baptisia, glyceryl borate, thymol, eucalyptol, menthol, methyl salicylate, alcohol 12%. *For use* as nasal douche, gargle and mouth wash as necessary.

Formula L-F Bottles 7 oz. **(Lehn and Fink)**
Contains 6-chloro-3-hydroxy-1-methyl-benzene 2%. *For use* as germicide for surgical instruments and for wet dressings; *applied* in 2–3% solution for 15 min.

Iodex Liquid Bottles of 2 oz. (Menley and James)
A non-irritating, non-corrosive, elemental iodine preparation combined with absorbent mixed fatty acids. *For use* in sprains, ulcers, wounds, skin diseases, burns and scalds; *applied* locally, freely, to affected area.

Irrigol Packages of 6, 16 oz. (Alkalol)
An alkaline, saline, non-irritating astringent solution. *For use* in dissolving mucus and pus in pelvic affections—vaginitis, cervicitis;
Administration—1 heaping teaspoonful per quart of warm water for douching.

Lagarg Bottles 4, 16 oz. (McKesson and Robbins)
Contains synthetized phenols in alcohol-aqueous solution. *For use* as antiseptic deodorant; *applied* externally in full strength; as gargle diluted with 2 parts of water.

Lavoris (L.A.) Bottles 3½, 8, 20 oz. (Lavoris)
Contains zinc chloride and aromatics. *For use* as antiseptic, deodorant, astringent and cleansing agent in catarrhal conditions of the mouth; as vaginal douche in vaginitis, endocervicitis and erosions, in pruritus and other skin affections; *applied* as lotion or douche in 10–50% strength; as instillation or tampon 50% or full strength; in oral cavity—full strength.

Metoso Bottles 5 oz. (Abbott)
Contains in aqueous solution metaphen 1:2,000, alcohol 14%, sodium chloride and essential oils. *For use* as mouth and dental antiseptic in infections of the mouth, teeth and throat; *applied* as gargle or spray when desired.

Myodine Bottles 4 oz. (Eimer and Amend)
Contains vegetized iodine in aqueous solution. *For use* as oral and dental antiseptic in affections of mouth, throat, gums and teeth, and as gargle for singers; *applied* as gargle or spray, 1 teaspoonful to the half ounce of water; in dentistry, after extraction —same strength; for exposed nerve—topically, full strength.

Nuzon Bottles 1 pt., 1 gal. (Schieffelin)
For use as general disinfectant and deodorizer; *applied* full strength as necessary.

Obtundia Bottles 1 oz., 4 oz., 1 pt., 1 qt. (Otis Clapp)
For use as non-irritating antiseptic and antipruritic in minor surgical affections, burns and boils; *applied* locally as necessary.

Orazin Bottles 1 pt. (Schieffelin)
Contains zinc chloride, oil of cinnamon, oil of cloves, menthol, formaldehyde. *For use* as astringent, mouth wash and deodorant; *applied* as gargle full strength, as necessary.

Pepsodent Antiseptic (L.A.) Bottles 3, 7, 16 oz. (Pepsodent)
Contains

Chlor-thymol	0.07%
Benzoic acid	0.20%
Tartaric acid	0.10%
Citric acid	0.10%
Boric acid	1.00%
Flavoring	0.0687%
Coloring	0.0015%
Solvents	98.4598%

For use as antiseptic gargle and mouth wash; *applied* as frequently as necessary.

Petrogen Products Bottles 2, 7 oz. (Wyeth)
Contains the active medicament in a modified mineral oil.
Combinations:

- Petrogen Camphor 20%
- Petrogen Guaiacol 20%
- Petrogen Ichthyol 10%
- Petrogen 5% and 10%
- Petrogen Methyl Salicylate 20%

For use as analgesic, antiseptic dressings for wounds, ulcers and dermatoses; *applied* locally by dropper or inunction as necessary.

Phenandyne Small bottles—Cartons of 12 (Schieffelin)
Contains acetic acid-ester of phenol. *For use* as oral antiseptic and analgesic in the treatment of dental cavities, pulpitis, pericementitis, alveolar abscess, pyorrhea; especially suitable for the "Buckley Treatment"; *applied* full strength on cotton pledget and inserted into cavity.

Pixalbol Bottles 1, 8 oz. (Bilhuber-Knoll)
A preparation of tar. *For use* as antiparasitic, antipruritic and to promote epithelia-zation, in eczema, urticaria, alopecia, hyperhidrosis;
Administration—as paint, ointment, or as alcoholic solution.

S. A. S. Bottles ¼, 1 pt. (Schieffelin)
Contains thymol, eucalyptol, menthol, methyl salicylate, boric acid, benzoic acid, alcohol 25%. *For use* as antiseptic gargle and mouth wash, for douching and as wet dressing in minor surgical affections; also as shampoo in dandruff; *applied* in full strength or diluted as desired, when necessary.

Sodiphene Bottles 3, 7, 16 oz. (Sodiphene)
An alkaline germicide with local sedative effect; is pleasant and non-escharotic. *For use* particularly in dentistry, to prevent gagging during oral manipulation, in pyorrhea alveolaris, Vincent's disease; also in various minor skin affections, in antral disease and for vaginal douching;
Administration—full strength, topically; for cavity irrigations—25%; in minor surgery, small burns and dandruff—full strength; for vaginal douching, 1 oz. per quart of warm water. *See Chap. III.*

Stannoxyl Glycerin (Anglo-French)
Contains metallic tin and tin oxide in glycerine. *For use* as staphylocide in boils, pustular acne, suppurating wounds, chronic osteomyelitis, mastitis, mixed infections; *Administration*—by local application. *See Chap. I.*

Stomaseptine Glass jars 6, 14¾ oz. (Stomaseptine)
Contains menthol, thymol, eucalyptus, methyl salicylate, sodium boro salicylate, sodium chloride, sodium bicarbonate, sodium perborate. *For use* as alkaline antiseptic and deodorant in trichomonas vaginalis; as douche in leukorrhea and pelvic affections; also as mouth wash and nasal irrigation. *Applied:* 1–2 tablespoonfuls to quart of warm water, as douche and for oral use.

Sy-Lac (L.A.) Individual bottles. (Anacin)
Contains sodium perborate. *For use* as mouth wash and for gum massage in oral affections; *applied* twice daily as necessary.

Zemacide Bottles 4, 16 oz. (Tilden)
Contains zinc oxide, zinc carbonate, liquor calcis and phenol. *For use* as antipruritic in eczema, pruritus, excoriations, sunburn and poison ivy; *applied* locally as necessary.

---

5. LOTIONS, EMOLLIENTS

Albatum Bottles 2 oz., 4 oz. (McKesson and Robbins)
Contains menthol, camphor, eucalyptol and essential oils. *For use* as rubefacient in colds, congestions, chilblains and neuralgia; *applied* by rubbing thoroughly into parts affected.

Antiseptic Oil (L.A.) Bottles 5 oz. (Mennen)
An antiseptic medicated blend of oils for the protection of infant's skin, preventing pemphigus, intertrigo, thrush, erythema, chafing, excoriation and diaper rashes; also in impetigo, pemphigus neonatorum and scaly scalps; *applied* by anointing the infant's skin.

Chloretone Emollient Bottles 16 oz. 1 gal. (Parke, Davis)
Contains chloretone, gr 5 (0.324 Gm) per fluid ounce of liquid petrolatum, with camphor, menthol. *For use* as dressing in burns and wounds. *See Chap. I.*

Collosol Calamine Lotion Bottles 3, 6, 12, 80 oz. **(Crookes)**
Is a 10% suspension of calamine. *For use* in localized affections; *applied* locally with sponge and allowed to dry. *See Chap. I.*

Collosol Scalp Lotion, Oily and Non-Oily Bottles 6 oz., 16 oz., 80 oz. **(Crookes)**
Contains collosol hydrargyrum and collosol sulphur, with or without oil. *For use* in alopecia, seborrhea and as hair dressing; *applied* by vigorous scalp massage night and morning. *See Chap. I.*

Collyrium Bottles of 4 and 7 oz. with eye-cup. **(Wyeth)**
Contains sodium borate and boric acid in 0.4% antipyrine solution. *For use* as mild astringent and eye wash in conjunctival inflammations; *applied* as eye bath.

I-Bath Bottles 6 oz. with aluminum eye cup. **(McKesson and Robbins)**
Contains boric acid, sodium chloride, hydrastine hydrochloride, camphor. *For use* as antiseptic astringent eye wash in catarrh and irritations of the eye; *applied* as lotion with cup or by medicine dropper.

Larkspur Lotion Bottles 2 oz., 6 oz. **(McKesson and Robbins)**
Contains alcoholic solution of larkspur, stavesacre and aromatic oils. *For use* as scalp wash to destroy lice, nits and itch mites; *applied*—locally.

Lotion Cormatal Bottles 3 oz., 1 gal. **(McNeil)**
Contains resorcin, zinc oxide in boroglycerinated vehicle. *For use* as prophylactic in impetigo; *applied* without bandaging, by atomizer or tampon.

Painol Bottles 4 oz., 16 oz., 1 gal. **(Boericke and Runyon)**
Contains menthol, methyl salicylate, arnica, capsicum and calendula in absorbent base. *For use* as analgesic and anodyne in neuralgia, rheumatism, sciatica, lumbago, sprains, bruises, etc.; *applied* by rubbing freely into painful part as often as required.

Pinotol Bottles 3 oz., 16 oz. **(McKesson and Robbins)**
Contains pine oil 90% in sulphonated vegetable oil. *For use* as disinfectant and deodorant; *applied* by sprinkling locally.

Poison Ivy Lotion Bottles 2 oz., 6 oz. **(McKesson and Robbins)**
Contains an alcoholic solution of poison ivy concentrate, menthol, cedar leaf, essential oils. *For use* as antigen in poison ivy and oak dermatitis; *applied* locally on affected areas.

Sunburn Lotion Bottles 2 oz. **(McKesson and Robbins)**
Contains magnesium sulphate, zinc oxide and glycerine. *For use* as soothing emollient in sun- and wind-burn, for local application.

White Liniment Bottles 4 oz. **(Columbus)**
Contains camphor, spirit of turpentine, ammonia water, ammonium chloride, soap. *For use* as stimulating rubefacient, anodyne liniment in sprains, bruises, congestions; *applied* by rubbing locally, plain or diluted, two or three times daily.

---

6. LOZENGES AND TROCHES

Anesthesin-Calcidin Troches Bottles of 100, 1,000; Boxes of 12, 24. **(Abbott)**
Contains, anesthesin, ¼ gr (0.016 Gm); calcidin, ⅓ gr (0.021 Gm); licorice and aromatics. *For use* in throat irritations;
Administered—dissolved in mouth as necessary. *See Chap. I.*

Angier's Throat Tablets Boxes of 50. **(Angier)**
Contains purified petroleum, pure elm bark and excipients; *used* by dissolving in mouth, as necessary.

Caloxidine Compound Throat Tablets Bottles of 500, 1,000. **(Strasenburgh)**
For use in the relief of tonsillitis and pharyngitis;
Administered—1 dissolved in mouth as necessary.

Cocoanilid Lozenges Tube-vials of 24 **(Hancock)**
Contains acetanilid gr 2 (0.130 Gm) per lozenge. *For use* as anesthetic and analgesic in dysphagia and throat irritations, in tonsillitis, after tonsillectomy, in laryngitis, pharyngitis;
Administered—1 dissolved in mouth as necessary.

Euphagin Boxes of 25; Bottles of 100, 500 **(American Bio-Chem)**
Contains amido-benzoic ethyl-ester with sodium borate and menthol. *For use* as analgesic and anesthetic in painful conditions of the mouth and throat, in peroral endoscopy, electrocoagulation of tonsils, after tonsillectomy; in pharyngitis, stomatitis, laryngeal tuberculosis, dysphagia, intra-oral cancer.
Administered—1 lozenge dissolved in mouth as required.

Glucal Lozenges Bottles 1 and 5 lb. **(McNeil)**
Contains per lozenge gr 15 calcium gluconate. *For use* as alterative and tonic in calcium deficiencies. *See Chap. III.*

Guai-Ammon Lozenges Tube vials of 24 **(Hancock)**
Contains per lozenge ammoniated guaiacum gr 2 (0.130 Gm). *For use* as tonic in relaxed throats, for cough with expectoration, in voice strain by singers, public speakers and in hoarseness;
Administered—1 dissolved in mouth as necessary.

Guaiatan Lozenges Tube-vials of 24. **(Hancock)**
Contains guaiacum and colloidally iodized tannic acid. *For use* as astringent and alterative in relaxed throat, tonsillitis, pharyngitis.
Administration—1 dissolved in mouth as necessary.

Hexyl-Resorcinol Sucrets Boxes of 24 **(Sharpe and Dohme)**
Contains per lozenge, 2½ mg of hexylresorcinol. *For use* as oral antiseptic. *See Chap. I.*

Iodithesin Lozenges Packages of 1 lb., 5 lb. **(Searle)**
Contains

	Gr	Gm
Anesthesin	1/4	0.016
Iodicalcium	1/3	0.02
Powd. ipecac	1/40	0.0016
Creosote	1/10	0.006
Guaiacol	1/20	0.003
F. E. senega	1/6	0.012
Ext. squills	1/4	0.016
Aromatics	q.s.	

For use as respiratory tract antiseptic and stimulating expectorant, to allay irritation in obstinate cough;
Administration—1 dissolved in mouth, as required.

Lozenges Benzocaine Comp. Bottles of 100, 500, 1,000 **(Stoddard)**
Contains benzocaine gr 1/10 (0.006 Gm), powdered sugar, powdered elm bark, oil of orange. *For use* as demulcent and local palliative in laryngitis, hoarseness and throat irritation with cough;
Administration—1 dissolved in mouth as required.

Neutral Acriflavine Throat Troches (C.A.) Boxes of 30—Cartons of 12 **(National Aniline)**
Contains per troche neutral acriflavine 0.006 Gm.
Administered—1 dissolved in mouth as required. *See Chap. I.*

Orthesine-Epinephrine Compound Bottles of 100, 500, 1,000, 5,000 **(McNeil)**
Contains

	Gr
Orthesine	1/25
Epinephrine hydrochloride	1/1000
Powdered ipecac	1/50
Benzoic acid	1/40
Aromatics	q.s.

For use as surface anesthetic and antiseptic in throat irritations with cough;
Administration—1 lozenge dissolved in mouth as required.

Orthesine-Iodine Troches Bottles of 100, 500, 1,000, 5,000 **(McNeil)**
Contains

	Gr
Orthesine	1/6
Iodized calcium	1/3
Aromatics	q.s.

For use as surface anesthetic and antiseptic in throat affections;
Administration—1 dissolved in mouth as required.

Orthesine-Quinosal Lozenges Bottles of 100, 500, 1,000, 5,000 **(McNeil)**
Contains

	Gr
Orthesine (anesthesine)	1/4
Quinosal (oxyquinoline sulphate)	1/100
Aromatics	q.s.

For use as surface anesthetic and antiseptic in painful conditions of the throat;
Administration—1 dissolved in mouth as required.

Ortho-Troches Bottles of 100 **(Metz)**
Contains per troche orthoform gr 1/4 or 1/2.
For use as surface anesthetic in throat irritations;
Administered—1 dissolved in mouth as required. *See Chap. I.*

Para-Troches Bottles of 100 **(Metz)**
Contains parathesin gr 1. *For use* as surface anesthetic in painful conditions of the throat;
Administration—1 dissolved in mouth as required.

Pastilles Tins of 2 oz. **(Crookes)**
Contains iodine and black currant gr 1/10, in hard base. *For use* as iodine therapy in glandular disorders. *See Chap. I.*

Thantis Lozenges Tubes of 12, boxes of 2 tubes **(Hynson, Westcott and Dunning)**
Contains per lozenge merodicein gr 1/8 (0.008 Gm), saligenin gr 1 (0.0064 Gm). *For use* as oral antiseptic. 1 tablet dissolved in mouth as often as required. *See Chap. I.*

---

7. NASAL PREPARATIONS

Adrenalin Inhalant (C.A.) Bottles of 1 oz. **(Parke, Davis)**
Contains adrenalin 1:1,000 in aromatized bland oil, with chloretone 3%. *For use* in nasal affections;
Administered by dropper, as necessary. *See Chap. I.*

Adrephine Inhalant Bottles 1 oz. **(Parke, Davis)**
Contains adrenalin 1:10,000, ephedrine hydrochloride 1%, benzocaine 1%, chloretone 0.5%, alcohol 12%, glycerine q.s. *For use* in nasal congestion;
Administered by dropper, as necessary. *See Chap. I.*

Albomist Bottles 1 oz. with dropper. **(McKesson and Robbins)**
Contains ephedrine alkaloid, menthol, thymol, eucalyptol, in light mineral oil with camphor. *For use* as sedative and analgesic decongestive in affections of the nose and throat;
Administered by spray or dropper as necessary.

Anespray Bottles 4 oz., 1 pt. **(Abbott)**
Contains anesthesin 2%, camphor, menthol, thymol, thymol iodide and methyl salicylate. *For use* in catarrhal affections of the nose and throat;
Administered by spray or dropper. *See Chap. I.*

Alpha-Naphco Jelly Nasal Capsules Boxes of 6 and 80. **(Carel)**
Contains alpha-naphthol. *For use* as protective and antiseptic in nasal affections. *See Chap. II.*

Alpha-Naphco Nasal Ointment (C.A.) Tubes 2 oz. **(Carel)**
Contains alpha-naphthol in suitable base. *For use* as nasal antiseptic in upper respiratory affections;
Administration by local application, as necessary.

Benzedrine Inhaler (C.A.) Tubes 0.30 Gm **(Smith, Kline and French)**
Contains benzyl methyl carbinamine as volatile salt. *For use* as vasoconstrictor in allergic states, vasomotor rhinitis, hay fever, asthma; for relief of nasal congestion, to shrink the turbinates and in sinusitis;
Administered by insertion into the nostril, closing the other with the finger; deep and slow inhalations are made through the tube, twice only for each nostril; repeated in 1 hr. *See Chap. XII.*

Blandine Compound Bottles 1 pt., 1 gal. **(Sharpe and Dohme)**
Contains per fluid ounce camphor gr 1⅓, menthol gr ⅕, thymol gr ⅕, eucalyptol m ⅖, methyl salicylate m 1½, hydrastine gr 1/40, liq, petrolatum q.s. *For use* as protective in colds, catarrhs and nasopharyngeal affections. *Applied* by spray or swab. *See Chap. II.*

Camolus Spray and Camolus Spray with Ephedrine 0.5% Bottles 2 oz. **(Wyeth)**
Contains camphor, menthol, eucalyptol, in bland mineral oil. *For use* as soothing antiseptic spray in rhinitis, grippe, hay fever and asthma;
Administration by atomizer or dropper, as necessary.

Camphaseptic Bottles 1 pt., 1 gal. **(Irwin, Neisler)**
Contains camphor, phenol, in a suitable base. *For use* as non-irritating decongestive in nasal affections;
Administered by dropper, as necessary.

Camphaseptic Nasal Balm Individual tubes—cartons of 12 **(Irwin, Neisler)**
Contains camphaseptic, ephedrine 1%, benzocaine 1%. *For use* as decongestive and anesthetic in colds, nasal catarrh and hay fever;
Administration by local application, as necessary.

Camphaseptic Nasal Oil Bottles ½ oz., 1 pt. **(Irwin, Neisler)**
Contains camphaseptic, ephedrine alkaloid 1%, benzocaine 1%. *For use* as anesthetic decongestive in nasal and nasopharyngeal affections;
Administration by dropper, as necessary.

Carbolic Acid and Benzoinol Ointment Individual tubes **(Manhattan)**
Contains

Carbolic acid	0.5%
Benzoinol	20.0%
Petrolatum	q.s. 100%

For use as decongestive in nasal affections; *applied* one to two times daily as necessary.

Chloretone Inhalant (C.A.). Bottles 2, 4, 16 oz. and 1 gal. **(Parke, Davis)**
Contains per 100 Gm, chloretone 1.0 Gm, camphor 2.5 Gm, menthol 2.5 Gm, oil cinnamon 0.25 Gm, refined liquid petrolatum 93.75 Gm. *For use* as antiseptic and emollient in rhinitis, laryngitis, pharyngitis, bronchitis. *Applied* by spray, as necessary. *See Chap. I.*

Compound Camphor and Menthol Ointment Individual tubes **(Manhattan)**
Contains camphor 2%, menthol 2%, benzoinol 20%, petrolatum 76%. Uses and application as above.

Compound Eucalyptol and Gaultheria Ointment Individual tubes **(Manhattan)**
Contains menthol 0.25%, oil pinus pumilio 1%, oil gaultheria 0.5%, oil eucalyptol 0.5%, petrolatum q.s. 100%. *For use* as nasal decongestive; *applied* one to two times daily.

Compound Iodine and Glycerine Ointment Individual tubes **(Manhattan)**
Contains iodine 1%, potassium iodide 2%, glycerine 25%, petrolatum q.s. 100%. *For use* as emollient antiseptic in nasal affections; *applied* one to two times daily as necessary.

Cresatin Spray (C.A.) Bottles 4 oz. **(Sharp and Dohme)**
Contains metacresyl acetate 5%, methyl salicylate 2%, camphor ½%, menthol 1% in oil base. *For use* as analgesic and antiseptic in nasopharyngeal affections. *Applied* by sponge, as necessary. *See Chap. I.*

Emoleo Plain, Emoleo Iodized, Emoleo with Camphor and Menthol All in bottles 1 oz., 16 oz. **(McKesson and Robbins)**
Contain benzoin, zinc oxide, camphor, iodine and menthol. *For use* as decongestive in irritations of the nose and throat;
Administration by dropper as necessary.

Ephedol Bottles 1 pt. **(Irwin, Neisler)**
Contains parts of ephedrine 10, thymol 2, menthol 8, camphor 16, eucalyptol 8, oil gaultheria 4, petrolatum oil q.s. 1,000. *For use* as decongestive in colds, coryza, sinusitis;
Administration as spray, when necessary.

Ephedrine Butesin Jelly (C.A.) Tubes ½ oz. **(Abbott)**
Contains butesin 0.66%, ephedrine 1%, in a jelly base. *For use* as anesthetic decongestive in hay fever and coryza;
Administration locally as necessary. *See Chap. I.*

Ephedrine Butesin Spray (C.A.) Bottles 1, 4, 16 oz. **(Abbott)**
Contains butesin 1% with ephedrine. *For use* as anesthetic decongestive in hay fever, rhinitis and asthma;
Administration as spray when necessary. *See Chap. I.*

Ephedrine Compound (C.A.) Tubes ½ oz. **(Lilly)**
Contains ephedrine 1%, menthol 0.65%, camphor 0.65%, oil of thyme 0.375%, in petroleum base. *For use* as nasal decongestive in asthma, hay fever, rhinitis, bronchitis, pertussis;
Administration by local application as necessary. *See Chap. I.*

Ephedrine Compound Inhalant 30 (C.A.) Bottles 1 oz., 1 pt. **(Lilly)**
Contains ephedrine 1%, merthiolate 1:500 with menthol, camphor and oil of thyme. *For use* as antiseptic decongestive for the relief of swollen turbinates;
Administration by local application or inhalation. *See Chap. I.*

Ephedrine HCl Inhalant (1%) (C.A.) Bottles ½ oz. **(Abbott)**
Prepared in light mineral oil. *For use* as vasoconstrictor and analgesic in nasopharyngeal affections; *applied* by spray or dropper, as necessary. *See Chap. I.*

Ephedrine Inhalant (1%) (C.A.) Bottles 1 oz. **(Lederle)**
Prepared in light mineral oil, tinted and perfumed with oil of roses. *For use* as vasoconstrictor and analgesic in nasopharyngeal affections. *Applied* by spray or dropper, as necessary. *See Chap. I.*

Ephedrine Inhalant 66 (C.A.) Bottles ½ oz. with atomizer **(Abbott)**
Contains ephedrine 1% in mineral oil, perfumed with oil of rose. *For use* to promote ventilation and drainage in colds, coryza, hay fever. *Applied* by spray or dropper. *See Chap. I.*

Ephedrine Inhalant Compound (1%) (C.A.) Bottles of 1, 4 oz., 1 pt. **(Fraser)**
Contains ephedrine alkaloid 1%, gum camphor 1%, menthol 1%, oil of thyme ½%, in liquid petrolatum; action and uses as above. *See Chap. I.*

Ephedrine Inhalant Compound (1%) (C.A.) Bottles of 1 oz. and 1 pt. **(Lilly)**
Contains per 100 cc ephedrine 1 Gm, menthol 0.66 Gm; camphor 0.66 Gm; oil of thyme 0.31 cc; in paraffin oil q.s. *For use* as vasoconstrictor and analgesic in nasopharyngeal affections. *Applied* by spray or dropper, as necessary. *See Chap. I.*

Ephedrine Inhalant Compound (C.A.) Bottles 1, 16 oz. **(Parke, Davis)**
Contains ephedrine 1%; menthol 0.6%; camphor 0.6%; geraniol 0.32% in liquid petrolatum base. *For use* as vasoconstrictor and analgesic in nasopharyngeal affections. *Applied* by spray or dropper, as necessary. *See Chap. I.*

Ephedrine Inhalant Compound Individual bottles (Schieffelin)
Contains ephedrine 1%, menthol, camphor, eucalyptol, ethyl salicylate, liquid petrolatum. *For use* as vasoconstrictor, antiseptic, analgesic and astringent; in nasal catarrh, pharyngitis, tonsillitis, hay fever;
Administration by swab or dropper as necessary. *See Chap. I.*

Ephedrine Inhalant Compound Bottles 1 oz., 1 pt. (Smith-Dorsey)
Contains ephedrine alkaloid 1%, camphor, oil of thyme, menthol, paraffin oil. *For use* as decongestive in nasal affections and sinusitis;
Administration by dropper.

Ephedrine Inhalant Plain (1%) (C.A.) Bottles 1, 4 oz., 1 pt. (Fraser)
A solution of 1% ephedrine alkaloid in liquid petrolatum. *For use* as vasoconstrictor and analgesic in nasopharyngeal affections. *Applied* by spray or dropper, as necessary. *See Chap. I.*

Ephedrine Inhalant Plain (1%) (C.A.) Bottles 1 oz., 1 pt. (Lilly)
Contains per 100 cc ephedrine 1 Gm, combined with cinnamic aldehyde and benzaldehyde in aromatized paraffin. *For use* as vasoconstrictor and analgesic in nasopharyngeal affections. *Applied* by spray or dropper, as necessary. *See Chap. I.*

Ephedrine Inhalant Plain (1%) (C.A.) Bottles 1, 16 oz. (Parke, Davis)
Prepared in liquid petroleum base. *For use* as vasoconstrictor and analgesic in nasopharyngeal affections. *Applied* by spray or dropper, as necessary. *See Chap I.*

Ephedrine Jelly Individual tubes (Schieffelin)
Contains ephedrine inhalant, white pine and boric acid. *For use* in nasal congestions; *applied* locally as necessary. *See Chap. I.*

Ephedrine Nasal Jelly (C.A.) Tubes ¼ oz. and ½ oz. (Maltbie)
Contains ephedrine sulphate 1%, sodium benzoate 0.5%. *For use* as decongestive in nasal affections; *applied* locally, as necessary. *See Chap. I.*

Ephedrine Sulphate Jelly (1%) (C.A.) Tubes ½ oz. (Lilly)
Contains ephedrine sulphate 1%; eucalyptol 0.1% with aromatics, in water soluble base. *For use* as vasoconstrictor and analgesic in nasopharyngeal affections. *Applied* by spray or dropper, as necessary. *See Chap. I.*

Ephedrinol Bottles ½ oz., 1 oz., 1 pt. (Smith-Dorsey)
Contains ephedrine alkaloid 1%, oil of thyme, menthol, camphor, anesthesin. *For use* as anesthetic decongestive in nasal affections; *applied* locally by dropper.

Epinine Nasal Jelly Individual Tubes (Burroughs Wellcome)
Contains epinine 0.5%; camphor 1%; menthol 1%, in water soluble base. *For use* as vasoconstrictor and analgesic in nasopharyngeal affections. *Applied* by spray or dropper as necessary. *See Chap. I.*

Eucalyptol and Benzoinol Ointment Individual tubes (Manhattan)
Contains eucalyptol 3%, benzoinol 20%, wool fat, petrolatum aa q.s. 100%. Uses and application as above.

Iodosyl Nasal Suppositories Boxes 30, 144 (Nelson-Baker)
Contains iodosyl 56 parts, sodium chlorate 112 parts, sodium borate 56 parts, eucalyptol 9 parts. *Used* as antiseptic, alterative and analgesic in nasopharyngeal affections. *See Chap. I.*

Metaphedrin Inhalant Bottles 4, 16 oz., 1 gal. (Abbott)
For use as antiseptic decongestive in hay fever, sinus infections; *applied* locally by dropper. *See Chap. I.*

Metaphedrin Inhalant 99 Bottles 1, 4, 16 oz. (Abbott)
Contains metaphen 1:2,500, ephedrin 1% in mineral oil. *For use* as vasoconstrictor and analgesic in nasopharyngeal affections. *Applied* by spray or dropper, as necessary. *See Chap. I.*

Nasal Cream Tubes ¼, ½ oz.; jars 1 lb. (Maltbie)
Contains benzocaine and menthol each 1 %, thymol 0.3 %, phenol 0.3 %, camphor 1 %, eucalyptol 0.5 %, sodium bicarbonate 2 %, lanolin and petrolatum q.s. *For use* as anesthetic, decongestive in coryza, rhinitis and catarrh; *applied* locally as necessary.

Nasal Cream Tubes ½ oz. (Noyes)
Contains phenol, boric acid, bismuth subnitrate, menthol, eucalyptol, thymol, lanolin. *For use* as anesthetic astringent in hay fever, ozena, colds, influenza; *applied* locally two to three times daily and at night.

Nasal Cream with Ephedrine (1 %) Tubes ¼ oz. (Noyes)
Uses as above.

Nasal Cream with Procaine (1 %) Tubes ½ oz. (Noyes)
Uses as above.

Nasal Jelly Individual tubes (McKesson and Robbins)
Contains phenol, menthol, geronial, oil of rose, geranium, petroleum, white petrolatum. *For use* as decongestive in irritations of the nose and throat; *applied* locally as necessary.

Nasedra Aplikol Individual tubes (Buffington)
Contains ephedrine hydrochloride 1 %, menthol 1 % with camphor, eucalyptus, pinus compound. *For use* as decongestive in colds, coryza, hay fever, sinusitis, nasopharyngitis; *applied* locally as necessary.

Obtundia Ephedrine Inhalant Bottles 1 oz., 4 oz., 1 pt., 1 qt. (Otis Clapp)
Contains obtundia and ephedrine 1 % in light mineral oil. *For use* as nasal spray in sinusitis;
Administration—as necessary.

Obtundia Inhalant Bottles 1 oz., 4 oz., 1 pt., 1 qt. (Otis Clapp)
Contains obtundia in light mineral oil. *For use* as decongestive in nasal affections by inhalation.

Obtundia Nasal Cream Tubes ¼ oz., ½ oz. (Otis Clapp)
For use as decongestive in nasal affections; *applied* locally as necessary.

Paroleine Spray Compound Bottles 1, 16 oz. (Burroughs Wellcome)
Contains menthol gr 5 (0.324 Gm), chlorbutol gr 6 (0.389 Gm), eucalyptia m 5 (0.9 cc), paroleine q.s. 29.5 cc. *For use* as vasoconstrictor and analgesic in nasopharyngeal affections. *Applied* by spray or dropper, as necessary. *See Chap. I.*

Phedrolene Inhalant Bottles 1, 4 oz., 1 pt. (Zemmer)
Contains ephedrine alkaloid 1 % in light oil base. *For use* as decongestive in colds, coryza, nasal affections;
Administration—locally by dropper.

Pineoleum Liquid Bottles 100 cc. Dropper bottles 30 cc, and (Pineoleum)

Pineoleum Outfit, with Nebulizer and Oil
Contains camphor, menthol, eucalyptus globulus, pine needle oil, oil of cassia, aromatics in liquid petrolatum. *For use* as emollient and decongestive in coryza, pharyngitis, laryngitis, hay fever; *applied* locally by spray or dropper.

Resorcinol Ointment Individual tubes (Manhattan)
Contains resorcinol 10 % and petrolatum 90 %. *For use* as decongestive and antiseptic in nasal affections; *applied* one to two times daily.

Rubrol with Ephedrine Bottles of 2 oz. (Rubrol)
Jelly—tubes of 1 oz.
Contains ephedrine, menthol, eucalyptol, thymol and pinus pumilio; a non-staining, non-irritating nasal decongestive; is antiseptic, crust solvent and capillary constrictor *For use* in nasal congestion and softening of nasal crusts;
Administered by spray or dropper, as often as required.

Solution Ephedrine Hydrochloride (3 %) Bottles 1, 4 oz., 1 pt. (Zemmer)
For use as decongestive in nasal affections; *applied* by spray or dropper.

Suprarenalin Ointment (C.A.) Tubes ⅝ oz. **(Armour)**
Contains suprarenalin 1:1,000 in petrolatum base. *For use* as decongestive in catarrhal affections of the nasopharynx, asthma, urticaria; *applied* locally as necessary. *See Chap. I.*

Terpoflor Capsules—boxes of 20. **(Fougera)**
Contains cedrene 1 %, pinene 1 %, terpinol 0.4 %, sesquiterpenes 3.5 %, anethol 1.2 %, camphoric aldehyde 1 %, cineol 0.8 %, orthoquido-benzoate of methyl 0.7 %, acetate of linalyl 0.4 %, in paraffin oil. *For use* as antiseptic decongestive in nasal congestion and catarrhal affections of upper respiratory tract;
Administration by cutting off tip of capsule, allowing fluid to drain directly onto nasal mucous membrane, several times daily; children—½ capsule.

Vem Tubes ⅘ oz. **(Schoonmaker)**
Contains eucalyptus, menthol, in heavy petrolatum base. *For use* as emollient in nasal affections, coryza, rhinitis, hay fever; *applied* directly into the nostrils with injector.

Vem with Boric Acid Tubes ⅘ oz. **(Schoonmaker)**
Contains oil of eucalyptus m 15, boric acid ½ dr.

Vem with Camphor Tubes ⅘ oz. **(Schoonmaker)**
Contains camphor m 15, oil of eucalyptus m 15

Vem with Ichthyol Tubes ⅘ oz. **(Schoonmaker)**
Contains ichthyol gr 10, menthol gr 1, oil of eucalyptus m 15.

Zyl Tubes ⅘ oz. **(Schoonmaker)**
Contains oil of eucalyptus m 15, menthol gr 1/10, ephedrine ½ %.

---

8. OINTMENTS

Acriflavine Neutral Ointment (C.A.) Tubes 2½ oz., Jars 1 lb. **(Abbott)**
Contains acriflavine neutral 1:1,000 in Karaya gum jelly. *For use* as antiseptic and germicide; *applied* locally as necessary. *See Chap. I.*

Acriflavine Neutral Ointment (C.A.) Tubes 2 oz. **(National Aniline)**
Contains 1 % acriflavine neutral. *For use* as antiseptic in various surface infections; *applied* directly. *See Chap. I.*

Adrenalin Ointment (C.A.) Tubes ½ oz. **(Parke, Davis)**
Contains adrenalin 1:1,000 in oleagenous base. *For use* as local astringent; *applied* as necessary. *See Chap. I.*

Adrephine Ointment Tubes ½ oz. **(Parke, Davis)**
Contains adrenalin 1:5,000, ephedrine hydrochloride 2 %. *For use* as local astringent, as necessary. *See Chap. I.*

Albolene Solid Jars ½ lb., 1 lb., 5 lb., 25 lb. **(McKesson and Robbins)**
For use as ointment base, skin cleanser and massage cream; *applied* locally, as necessary.

Alpha-Naphco Ointment (C.A.) Jars 1, 2, 6½, 16 oz. **(Carel)**
Contains alpha naphthol. *For use* as antiseptic ointment in various surface infections. *Applied* directly. *See Chap. II.*

Amertan Tubes 1, 5 oz., Jars 1, 5 lb. **(Lilly)**
Contains tannic acid 5 %, merthiolate 1:5,000. *For use* as soothing antiseptic in extensive burns and scalds; *applied* liberally ½ in. thick until tanning occurs. *See Chap. II.*

Analgesic Balm Tubes, large and small sizes. **(McKesson and Robbins)**

Analgesic Balm Tubes ½ oz., Jars 1 oz., 1 lb. **(Maltbie)**
Contains menthol, methyl salicylate, camphor, lanolin. *For use* as analgesic in neuralgias, congestions, headache; *applied* locally when necessary.

Anazyme Ointment Boxes 1 oz., Packages 1, 5 lb. (Maltbie)
Contains anazyme (phenol and boric acid), zinc oxide, balsam of Peru. *For use* as anesthetic and emollient in skin diseases and ulcers; *applied* locally as necessary.

Aneskreme (C.A.) Tubes ½, 1 oz., Jars 1 lb. (Abbott)
Contains anesthesin 1%, sodium borate, menthol, thymol, camphor, methyl salicylate. *For use* as anesthetic and antipruritic in pruritus, hay fever and rhinitis; *applied* as necessary. *See Chap. I.*

Anesthone Cream Tubes ½ oz. (Parke, Davis)
Contains adrenalin 1:5,000, ephedrine hydrochloride, benzocaine 10%. *For use* as anesthetic and astringent; *applied* locally where necessary. *See Chap. I.*

Antiphlogistine Tins 5½, 10½, 17½, 34½, oz.; 5 lb. (Denver Chemical)
Contains dehydrated silicate of aluminum, glycerine, compounds of iodine, minute quantities of boric and salicylic acids, oils of peppermint, gaultheria, and eucalyptus. *For use* as analgesic poultice in painful affections, sprains, infections. *Applied* in thick layer, warmed. *See Chap. III.*

Aquadine Ointment Jars 2 oz., 1 lb. (Govett)
For use as analgesic and antiseptic in ringworm and congestions; *applied* locally as necessary.

Aquafor Tins 1, 5 lb. (Duke)
For use in chapped skin and rosacea and as ointment base; *applied* as necessary.

Argentiform Ointment (0.2% and 1%) Individual tubes—boxes of 12 (Nelson-Baker)
For use as antiseptic in the urethra; *applied* locally as necessary.

Argocol Ointment (10%) Tubes ½ oz.—packages of 12 (Mulford Colloid)
For use as local antiseptic in eczema, ringworm and ulcers; *applied* topically.

Argolaval Ointment Packages 1 oz.; ½ lb. (Doho)
Contains silver hexamethylene tetramine nitrate (equivalent to 1% solution nitric acid) *For use* as astringent antiseptic in surface infections; *applied* locally. *See Chap. I.*

Anemollient Individual tubes, Jars 1, 5 lb. (Searle)
Contains benzocaine 1%, alum, zinc oxide, camphor, oil of thyme. *For use* as anesthetic and protective dressing in burns and skin affections; *applied* locally as necessary.

Atomidine Ointment Tubes 1 oz. (Schieffelin)
Contains iodine 1%. *For use* as antiseptic and absorbent in burns, scalds and glandular enlargements; *applied* locally, two and three times daily. *See Chap. II.*

Azinol Tubes 1 oz., Jars 1 lb. (Schieffelin)
Contains alum, zinc oxide, phenol. *For use* as antipruritic and antiseptic in minor surgical affections, boils and burns.

Balmogen Tubes 1¼ oz. (40 Gm) (Balmogen)
Contains extr. belladonna 3%, camphor 5%, menthol 4%, methyl salicylate 5%, oleum sinapis 0.5%, adeps lanae hydrosus 67% with petrolatum 15.5%. *For use* as analgesic in myalgia, torticollis, neuralgia, lumbago; *applied* locally by rubbing into affected part after hot towelling for 5 min.

Baume Bengué Tubes 1 oz. (Leeming)
Contains menthol, methyl salicylate and lanolin. *For use* as analgesic and counterirritant in bruises, myalgia, colds and influenza; *applied* topically by rubbing into affected area; by inhalation—for 20 min., ¼ teaspoonful dissolved in steaming water; internally 1 teaspoonful with white vaseline dissolved in the mouth, at bedtime.

Benzalba Jars 1 oz., 1 lb. (Columbus)
Contains benzoic acid, salicylic acid, chloral hydrate, phenyl salicylate and thymol in white petrolatum. *For use* as emollient antiseptic in parasitic and fungus infections; *applied* locally as necessary.

Benzocomp Ointment Tubes 1 oz., Jars 1, 5 lb. **(Maltbie)**
Contains benzocaine 1%, phenol 1%, zinc oxide 5%, aromatics q.s. *For use* as antiseptic and analgesic in burns, wounds and ulcers; *applied* locally as required.

B. F. I. Ointment Tubes 1 oz.; jars 1, 5 lb. **(Sharp and Dohme)**
Contains bismuth-formic-iodide comp. powder gr 42, balsam peru 7 m, diachylon ointment gr 60, petrolatum q.s. 1 oz. *For use* as astringent, antiseptic, surgical dressing in minor surgical affections. *See Chap. II.*

Bismolan Individual tubes **(Cavendish)**
Contains bismuth oxychlorate 0.1 Gm, zinc oxide 0.15 Gm, solution suprarenin 1:1,000 0.05 Gm, eucaine hydrochloride 0.05 Gm, menthol, lanolin 0.05 Gm, vaseline solid 2.0 Gm. *For use* as astringent and hemostatic in fissures, ulcerations, and proctitis; *applied* to rectum as necessary.

Bismuth Violet Ointment (1%) Jars 1 oz., 4 oz., 1 lb. **(Table Rock)**
For use as antiseptic in impetigo, ringworm and burns; *applied* locally as necessary. *See Chap. II.*

Bis-Thiodide Ointment Individual tubes, Jars 1 lb. **(Strasenburgh)**
Contains bismuth oxy-iodide, thymol iodide, boric acid. *For use* as dressing in minor surgical affections; *applied* locally as necessary.

Borofax Individual tubes, Jars 16 oz. **(Burroughs Wellcome)**
Contains boric acid 10% in suitable base. *For use* as sedative and emollient antiseptic where necessary.

Burn Ointment 2 Tubes 2 oz., Jars 1 lb. **(McNeil)**
Contains orthesin 1%, quinosal 0.1%, sodium bicarbonate 3%, white petrolatum q.s. *For use* as sedative antiseptic in burns; *applied* locally, freely.

Burn Ointment 3 Tubes 2 oz., Jars 1 lb. **(McNeil)**
Contains orthesin benzoate 1%, picric acid 0.25%, sodium borate 0.50%, white petrolatum, lanum and white wax q.s. *For use* as soothing antiseptic in burns; *applied* freely where necessary.

Burntone Individual tubes **(McKesson and Robbins)**
For use as emollient antiseptic in minor surgical affections, burns and insect bites; *applied* locally where necessary.

Butesin Picrate Ointment (C.A.) Jars 1, 2 oz., 1, 5 lb. **(Abbott)**
Contains butesin picrate 1%, sodium borate, petroleum, paraffin, water, white wax. *For use* as soothing antiseptic in burns and ulcers; *applied* locally as necessary. *See Chap. I.*

Calamoin Tubes 1½ oz.—cartons of 12 **(Upjohn)**
Contains calamine and zinc oxide 10%, camphor-phenol 1%. *For use* as antipruritic and antiseptic in skin irritations; *applied* locally as necessary.

Calmitol Tubes 1 oz. **(Leeming)**
Contains solution chlorcamphoric aldehyde, organic iodine 0.5%, menthol, laevo-hyoscine oleinate, ether-alcohol-chloroform base. *For use* as antipruritic and antiseptic in acne, tinea trichophyton, eczema, pruritus ani et vulvae and rectal irritation; *applied* locally as necessary.

Calomelol Ointment (C.A.) Tubes 2 oz. **(Heyden)**
Contains calomel with colloidal aluminate (soluble mercury 28%, insoluble 2%). *For use* as antiluetic by inunction 1.5 dr. daily for 30 days. *See Chap. I.*

Cal-Zo Jars 1, 5 lb. **(Ulmer)**
Contains calamine and zinc oxide. *For use* as astringent and antiseptic dressing in the ambulant treatment of varicose ulcers; *applied* thickly directly to the lesions, applying constant pressure or support to the extremity.

Camiofen Ointment (C.A.) Tubes ½ oz. **(Schering and Glatz)**
Contains iocamfen 50% with lard, wax and oleum theobromatis. *For use* as antiseptic dressing in itching dermatoses; *applied* freely to affected area, one to two times daily, avoiding mercurial applications. *See Chap. I.*

Camphaseptic Ointment Individual tubes **(Irwin, Neisler)**
Contains camphaseptic, boracic acid, zinc oxide, mercury nitrate. *For use* as protective dressing; *applied* locally one to two times daily.

Colloidal Sulphur Compound Tubes 1 oz. **(National Drug)**
Contains menthol, camphor and phenol aa gr 8, anesthesin gr 16, sulphocol gr 40, boric acid gr 60, cold cream q.s. 1 oz. *For use* as antipruritic and antiseptic in eczema, dermatitis, epidermophytosis; *applied* locally twice daily.

Colloplasma Tins 8, 16, 32, 64 oz. **(Crookes)**
Contains collosol kaolin, boric acid, glycerol, collosol iodine, aromatic essential oils. *For use* as poultice in inflammations and congestions; *applied* well warmed on cotton wool for various conditions as required.

Collosol Hydrargyrum Cream Jars 1, 3, 16 oz. **(Crookes)**
Contains colloidal mercury 5% cream for antiluetic inunctions; *applied* as necessary. *See Chap. I.*

Collosol Ichthyol with Resorcin Jars 1, 3, 8, 16 oz. **(Crookes)**
For use as antiseptic ointment in surface infections. *See Chap. I.*

Collosol Ichthyol with Resorcin and Chrysarobin Jars 1, 3, 8, 16 oz. **(Crookes)**
For use as antiseptic ointment in surface infections. *See Chap. I.*

Collosol Iodine Paste Jars 1, 3 oz. **(Crookes)**
For use in iodine therapy. *Applied* by inunction. *See Chap. I.*

Collosol Sulphur Cream Jars 1, 3, 16 oz. **(Crookes)**
Contains collosol sulphur. *For use* in skin affections. *Applied* locally. *See Chap. I.*

Collosol Zinc Cream Tubes 1 oz.; jars 1, 18 oz. **(Crookes)**
Contains 5% zinc stearate in sodium stearate base. *For use* in skin affections; *applied* locally.

Compound Ichthyol Ointment Tubes 1, 2 oz., Jars 1 oz., 5 lb. **(Noyes)**
Contains ichthyol, bismuth subnitrate, phenol, lanolin. *For use* as anesthetic and antiseptic dressing in burns, eczema and dermatoses; *applied* locally twice daily.

Crutar Ointments "Grossman" Tubes 2 oz., Jars 1 lb. **(Tailby-Nason)**

Contains	1	2	3
Crude coal tar	20%	10%	5%
Zinc oxide	4%	4%	4%
Powdered starch	4%	4%	4%
Petrolatum	q.s.		

For use in infantile eczema; *applied* twice daily, reducing strength of ointment as improvement occurs.

Danish Ointment Jars 2 oz., 1 lb. **(Tilden)**
Contains sublimed sulphur, potassium hydroxide, zinc sulphate, sodium hydroxide, petrolatum, lanolin, with oil of bitter almonds. *For use* in scabies; *applied* by general body inunction after hot bath; followed by hot bath in 24 hr.

Dermalin Jars 1, 5 lb. **(Fraser)**
Contains diacetylamidoazotoluol 2% in suitable base. *For use* in minor surgical affections, decubitus ulcer, eczema; *applied* freely twice daily and covered.

Derma-Medicone Tubes 1 oz. **(Medicone)**
Contains anesthesin 5%, oxyquinoline sulphate 3%, ephedrine muriate 0.1%, oleo cadinum-ichthyol comp. 1%, non-oxidizable base q.s. *For use* as antipruritic, antiparasitic, vasoconstrictor dressing in eczema, pruritus, minor surgical affections; *applied* twice daily.

Dimazon Ointment (C.A.) Tubes 1 oz. **(Heilkraft)**
Contains 2% ointment in petrolatum 98%. *For use* in varicose ulcers, non-granulating wounds, burns, and dermatoses; *applied* as daily dressing. *See Chap. I.*

Eczol Jars 1, 8 oz., Cans 5 lb. **(C. D. Smith)**
Contains sodium soziodolate, sodium hyposulphite, ichthyol, salicylic acid, oil of ruse, zinc oxide, ammoniated mercury, echinacea. *For use* as antipruritic and antiseptic in eczema, impetigo, pruritus, psoriasis, minor surgical affections; *applied* locally as necessary.

Espinol Jars 50 Gm **(Spicer)**
Contains synthetic chrysarobin, starch, zinc oxide and vaseline. *For use* as stimulating antiseptic in psoriasis, eczema, pityriasis rosea, lichen planus; *applied* nightly by rubbing into involved area, repeated as necessary.

Eupinol Ointment Jars 2, 16 oz. **(Tilden)**
For use as soothing antiseptic in burns, ulcers, insect bites and minor surgical affections; *applied* locally as necessary.

Glandoid Compound "Lowenthal" Tubes 2 oz. **(American Organotherapy)**
Contains thyroid, orchitic substance, resorcin, menthol, camphor, sulphur, phenol 5%. *For use* as metabolic stimulant in skin affections—eczema, acne, psoriasis; in glandular disorders and rheumatism; *applied* locally twice daily. *See Chap. IV.*

Guaia-Camph Compound Individual tubes, Jars 1, 5 lb. **(Smith-Dorsey)**
Contains guaiacol, menthol, methyl salicylate, camphor, oil of pine needles. *For use* as counter-irritant in pulmonary congestion and as inhalant; *applied* by inhalation, ½ teaspoonful in cup of boiling water, externally by inunction.

Hazeline Cream Jars 1 lb., Individual tubes **(Burroughs Wellcome)**
For use as stimulating dressing in dermatoses; *applied* locally where necessary.

Hazeline Snow Jars 1 lb. **(Burroughs Wellcome)**
For use as vanishing cream where necessary.

Hemodal Tubes ½ oz. **(Maltbie)**
Contains benzocaine, extr. hamamelis, ichthynat, zinc oxide, alum, phenol, eucalyptol. *For use* as antipruritic in rectal irritations; *applied* locally where necessary.

Hydrosal Jars ½, 2 oz. **(Hydrosal)**
Contains colloidal aluminum acetate. *For use* as astringent dressing in furunculosis, burns and for infantile skin affections; *applied* freely ⅛ in. thick, directly to affected parts and covered with wax paper. *See Chap. III.*

Hydrosal Compound Tubes 1 oz. **(Hydrosal)**
Contains colloidal aluminum acetate, belladonna, tannic acid, in lanolin-petrolatum base. Uses and application as above. *See Chap. III.*

Ichthorcin Tubes 1 oz., Jars 1 lb. **(Sharp and Dohme)**
Contains ichthyol, resorcin and mercury in suitable neutral base. *For use* as antipruritic and anodyne in eczema, herpes, plant dermatitis and pruritus; *applied* twice daily without rubbing.

Ichthorgin Tubes 1 oz. **(Sharp and Dohme)**
For use as antipruritic and antiseptic in itching dermatoses; *applied* twice daily without rubbing.

Ichthylate Ointment Jars 1 lb. **(Westerfield)**
Contains ammonium ichthylate 20%, resorcinol 4%, boric acid 4%, eucalyptol 2%, lanum and petrolatum q.s. *For use* as stimulating dressing in wounds, ulcers and eczema; *applied* locally twice daily.

Ichthymall Tubes 1 oz., ¼ lb. **(Mallinckrodt)**
For use as astringent antiseptic in acne, eczema and dermatitis; *applied* locally as necessary. *See Chap. I.*

Ichthyol Bottles 1 oz. ¼ lb.; tubes 1 oz., ¼ lb. (Crookes)
Contains ammonium sulphoichthyolate. *For use* in 5–50% ointment in various surface affections; locally *applied*. *See Chap. I.*

Inoton Ointment "Debat" Tubes 1½ oz., 1 lb. (Fougera)
Contains per 50 Gm, lithol 0.5 Gm, ammonium ichthyol sulphonate 0.25 Gm, extract of witch hazel 0.5 Gm, titanium oxide 2.5 Gm, hydroxide ortho-titanique colloidal 0.5 Gm, zinc oxide 7.5 Gm, sodium borate 0.05 Gm, non-oxidizable base 39.0 Gm; *For use* as astringent and antiseptic in acne, eczema, impetigo, pruritus, psoriasis, varicose ulcers, burns; *applied* locally when necessary.

Iodahl Ointment Jars ½, 1 oz., 1 lb. (Maltbie)
Contains iodine 4% in suitable base. *For use* as counter-irritant and antiseptic in myalgia, glandular swelling and skin affections; *applied* locally twice daily.

Iodex Ointment Tubes ½ oz., Jars 1 oz. (Menley and James)
Contains elemental iodine combined with absorbent mixed fatty acids and suspended in petroleum base. *For use* in arthritis, burns, glandular enlargements, pruritus, sprains, hemorrhoids; *applied* locally by inunction, freely. *See Chap. III.*

Iodine Ointment Jars 1, 16 oz. (Burnham)
Contains free iodine with anesthesin. *For use* as anesthetic antiseptic in infected wounds, glandular enlargements, bruises, parasitic infections; *applied* by rubbing into affected parts, covered lightly.

Iodoformal Ointment (10%) Jars 1 oz., 1 lb. (Warner)
Contains iodoformal powder 10% in petrolatum, benzoinated lard, cera flava. *For use* as analgesic, astringent and antiseptic; *applied* locally as necessary.

Iodostan Jars 1 oz., 1 lb. (Strasenburgh)
Contains free iodine 5%, methyl salicylate 5%. *For use* as analgesic and antiseptic; *applied* by rubbing freely and completely into affected part, without covering.

Iodosyl Ointment (6%) Individual tubes, large, small and medium sizes—Tins 1 lb. (Nelson, Baker)
For use as local anesthetic; *applied* locally, as necessary.

J & J Analgesic Balm Individual tubes. (Johnson and Johnson)
Contains K-Y lubricating jelly, camphor, menthol, methyl salicylate. *For use* as analgesic in muscular congestions and rheumatism; *applied* locally after hot towelling.

Joncolia Burn Ointment Individual tubes, Tins of 1 lb. (Johnson and Johnson)
Contains zinc oxide, phenol, menthol, thyme in petrolatum base. *For use* as sedative antiseptic in burns, blisters; *applied* locally as necessary.

Kerolysin Jars ¾, 2 oz. (Upjohn)
Contains benzoic acid 12%, salicylic acid 6%, chlorthymol 0.25% in suitable base q.s. *For use* as antipruritic and keratolytic in eczema and epidermophytosis; *applied* locally, daily or every other day, after previous cleansing.

K-Y Lubricating Jelly Tubes 2, 8 oz. (Johnson and Johnson)
Contains boric acid and gelatinous vegetable products in jelly form. *For use* as surgical lubricant for gloves and instruments, as surface dressing in wounds; *applied* locally where necessary.

Lenigallol Zinc Ointment (6%) (C.A.) Tubes ½ oz. (Bilhuber-Knoll)
Contains lenigallol, zinc oxide in suitable base. *For use* as antiseptic and keratolytic in eczema, psoriasis and dermatoses; *applied* locally as necessary. *See Chap. II.*

Liantral Casein Ointment (5%) Tubes 50 Gm. (Duke)
Contains liantral (a tar product) in suitable casein ointment base. *For use* as astringent antiseptic in seborrhea of the scalp; *applied* locally as necessary.

Lubafax Tubes 2 oz. (Burroughs Wellcome)
For use as surgical lubricant for instruments and gloves; *applied* as necessary.

Lubricant Individual tubes (McNeil)
Contains glycerinated jelly. *For use* as surgical lubricant; *applied* as necessary.

Mazon Ointment Jars 1, 2, 4 oz. (Belmont)
For use as antipruritic and antiseptic in parasitic skin affections, eczema, psoriasis, sycosis; *applied* by rubbing into affected area, without covering.

Merciol Ointment (5%) Tubes ½ oz. (Mulford Colloid)
Contains colloidal mercuric iodide; *For use*—as antiluetic in all stages of syphilis. *See Chap. I.*

Mercurettes (C.A.) Packages of 6, 50, 100 (Parke, Davis)
Oblong cakes of cacao butter, each containing gr 50 (3.25 Gm) metallic mercury. *For use* as antiluetic; *applied* by inunction two to three times weekly. *See Chap. I.*

Mercurocol Ointment (10%) Tubes ½ oz. (Mulford Colloid)
Contains suspension of metallic mercury. *For use* as antiluetic; *applied* locally. *See Chap. I.*

Mersalv Jars 4 oz. (Anglo-French)
Contains metallic mercury 10% in suitable ointment base. *For use* as antiluetic; *applied* by inunction, 1 dr. nightly.

Merthiolate Ointment (C.A.) Tubes 1 oz.; Jars 1 lb. (Lilly)
Contains merthiolate 1:2,000. *For use* as antiseptic in surface infections. *Applied* locally. *See Chap. I.*

Metaphedrin Ointment 1:5,000 Tubes of 2 oz. (Abbott)
Contains 1:5,000 metaphedrin. *For use* as parasiticide in scabies, pediculosis, sycosis and similar infections; *applied* externally. *See Chap. I.*

Metaphen Ointment (C.A.) Individual Tubes (Abbott)
Contains metaphen 1:5,000. *For use* as antiseptic in parasitic skin infections. *Applied* locally as necessary. *See Chap. I.*

Molan Individual tubes, Jars 1 lb. (Irwin, Neissler)
Contains ichthymall, zinc oxide, phenol, alum compound, antiseptic oils, lanum and petrolatum. *For use* as astringent antiseptic in burns; *applied* locally as necessary.

Mustarx Bottles 1, 4 oz. (McKesson and Robbins)
Contains mustard in ointment form. *For use* as mustard plaster; *applied* where necessary.

Mycozol Ointment Tubes 1 oz.; packages 12 (Parke, Davis)
Contains chloretone 5%, salicylic acid 4%, mercury salicylate 48%, aromatics and base q.s. *For use* as fungicide in dermatoses; *applied* locally, as necessary. *See Chap. II.*

Neo-Silvol Ointment (C.A.) Individual tubes (Parke, Davis)
Contains neosilvol 5%. *For use* as antiseptic in surface infections; *applied* locally. *See Chap. I.*

Neutral Acriflavine Ointment (C.A.) Tubes 2 oz. (National Aniline)
For use as a general antiseptic in numerous external affections. *See Chap. I.*

Nupercaine (C.A.) Tubes 1 oz., Jars 1 lb. (Ciba)
Contains nupercaine 1% in neutral ointment base. *For use* as anesthetic ointment in burns, eczema, ulcers, pruritus ani, rectal irritations; *applied* as necessary, several times daily. *See Chap. I.*

Ointment Antiseptinol Individual tubes, Jars 1 lb. (McNeil)
Contains ichthyonate, boric acid, phenol, alum, zinc oxide, thymol iodide, aromatic oils, lanum and petrolatum. *For use* as soothing antiseptic in burns and minor surgical affections; *applied* daily and covered.

Ointment Chlorung Individual jars, large and small (McNeil)
Contains chloramin T, U.S.P., 1% in vanishing cream base. *For use* as antiseptic and emollient dressing for wounds and burns; *applied* locally in thick layer and covered.

Panthesine Ointment Tubes 10, 20, 100 Gm (Sandoz)
Contains panthesine 5%, in vegetable emollient base. *For use* as surface anesthetic and antipruritic in itching dermatoses. *Applied* locally two to four times daily. *See Chap. I.*

Paraffin Compound Packages 2½ lb. (Sharp and Dohme)
Contains beta naphthol 0.25%, olive oil 5%, oil eucalyptus 2%, paraffin ointment 25%, paraffin 67.75%. *For use* as emollient antiseptic in extensive burns; *applied* by nebulizer or fine brush, and covered.

Parresine (C.A.) Cakes ½ lb. (Abbott)
Contains paraffin 94–96%, gum elemi 0.2–0.25%, japan wax 0.4–0.5%, asphalt 0.2–0.25%; eucalyptol 2%; alkannin 0.5–1% gentian violet q.s.; analgesic and healing ointment for burns; *applied* in thin layer by spray, covered thinly with cotton, resprayed and bandaged. *See Chap. II.*

Phenofax Individual tubes, Glass jars (Burroughs Wellcome)
Contains carbolic acid 3% in suitable base. *For use* as antiseptic and antipruritic dressing in minor surgical affections; *applied* locally as necessary.

Picratol Tubes 1 oz. (Wyeth)
Contains silver trinitrophenolate 30%. *For use* as styptic and antiseptic in burns, hemorrhoids and infections; *applied* locally twice daily.

Picro-Benzyl Tubes 2 oz., Jars 1, 5 lb. (Ulmer)
Contains phenyl carbinol, phenol and picric acid. *For use* as antiseptic and astringent dressing in minor surgical affections and burns; *applied* locally daily, and covered.

Poison Ivy Balm Tubes 1 oz. (Squibb)
Contains zinc oxide, methyl salicylate, phenol, with vegetable solvent of poison ivy toxins. *For use* in plant dermatitis of various types, insect bites; *applied* to involved skin and washed off after 15 min. with hot suds and running water; reapplied in 1 hr.; skin must not be rubbed.

Posterisan "Kade" Individual tubes (Beisner)
For use as antiseptic ointment in Bac. coli infections and rectal irritations; *applied* freely two to three times daily.

Pronusin Tubes 1 oz. (Bischoff)
Contains ethyl-aminobenzoate and zinc oxide. *For use* as local anesthetic and astringent in hemorrhoids, eczema and ulcers; *applied* freely on affected area several times daily.

Protonuclein Ointment Jars 1 oz. (Reed and Carnrick)
Contains protonuclein special powder 19% and balsam peru 12%. *For use* as stimulating dressing in skin affections. *See Chap. II.*

Pyridium Ointment Jars 25 Gm. (Merck)
Contains pyridium 10%. *For use* as antiseptic, for local application. *See Chap. I.*

Quinothesin Ointment Tubes 1, 12 oz.; jars 1, 5 lb. (McNeil)
Contains orthesin 1%; quinosol 1/10%, sodium bicarbonate and white petrolatum, q.s. *For use* as antiseptic and stimulating dressing in dermatoses. *Applied* locally, as necessary. *See Chap. II.*

Rectal Ointment (Keno) Individual tubes. (McKesson and Robbins)
Contains carbolic acid, powdered camphor and bismuth subgallate. *For use* as antipruritic and astringent in rectal irritations; *applied* locally several times daily.

Reso-Lanae Ointment Tins 1 oz., Jars 1, 5 lb. (Maltbie)
Contains resorcin, zinc oxide, oil of cade, balsam peru, bismuth subnitrate, lanolin and petrolatum. *For use* as antiseptic and analgesic in eczema, herpes and pruritus; *applied* locally twice daily.

Res-Unguentum Tubes 1 oz., Jars 1 lb. (Sharp and Dohme)
Contains resorcin, zinc oxide, bismuth subnitrate, oil of cade and phenol, in neutral base. *For use* as antipruritic and antiseptic in itching dermatoses and plant poisoning; *applied* several times daily without rubbing.

Salit Cream Individual tubes (Heyden)
Contains borneol salicylate. *For use* as analgesic in rheumatic and gouty affections. *Applied* by inunction, two times daily. *See Chap. I.*

Scabiola Tins 4 oz., 1, 5 lb. (Norwich)
Contains per ounce precipitated sulphur gr 30, balsam peru gr 15, beta-naphthol gr 4, oil of cade gr 6 in petrox base. *For use* as antiparasitic in scabies and ringworm; *applied* externally one to two times daily.

Scarlet Red Ointment (C.A.) A—Tubes 1 oz.; B—Jars ½ lb. (Parke, Davis)
Scarlet red ointment (A) contains scarlet red sulphonate 5 %, petrolatum and wax 95 %; scarlet red ointment (B) contains scarlet red sulphonate 10 %, petrolatum and wax 90 %. *For use* as stimulating ointment and epithelial proliferant in dermatoses. *Applied* locally as necessary. *See Chap. I.*

Scarlet Red Salve "Biebrich" (C.A.) Jars 1 oz. (Heilkraft)
Contains scarlet red 8 %, eucalyptol 2 %, petrolatum 90 %. *For use* as local antiseptic in burns, ulcers, minor surgical affections; *applied* locally twice daily. *See Chap. I.*

Sherman A-Vee 51 Individual tubes. (Sherman)
Contains staphylococcus antivirus cream of mixed strain. *For use* as vaccine in acne, boils, carbuncles, furuncles, sycosis; *applied* once or twice daily. *See Chap. VI.*

Sherman A-Vee 52 Individual tubes. (Sherman)
Contains mixed virus cream. *For use* as vaccine in mixed suppurating wounds, bed sores and abscesses; *applied* locally one to two times daily. *See Chap. VI.*

Sherman Bio-Cream Jars ¼, 1 oz. (Sherman)
Contains autolyzed skin bacteria in creamy base. *For use* in pustular rashes, acne, boils, pimples; *applied* as cold cream, twice daily. *See Chap. VI.*

Siocol Ointment Tubes ½ oz.; packages of 12 (Mulford)
Contains colloidal silver iodide 10 %. *For use* as fungicide and antiseptic where indicated. *Applied* locally, freely, as necessary. *See Chap. I.*

Sketofax Individual tubes (Burroughs Wellcome)
Contains a combination of aromatic essential oils *for use* as deterrent against insects; *applied* by smearing lightly on the skin.

Stannoxyl Ointment Individual tubes (Anglo-French)
Contains metallic tin and tin oxide in suitable base. *For use* as staphylocide in boils, styes, pustular acne, suppurating wounds, mixed infections; *applied* locally two to three times daily. *See Chap. I.*

Storaxin Individual tubes, Jars 1 lb. (Smith-Dorsey)
Contains resorcin, storax, menthol, camphor, carbolic acid, lac sulphur. *For use* as antipruritic and antiparasitic in ringworm, insect bites and pruritus; *applied* locally twice daily.

Sulophen Ointment 1 Jars 2 oz. (McNeil)
Contains para-thio-cresol 0.25 % in anhydrous lanum. *For use* as antiseptic and epithelializer in wounds and ulcers; *applied* full strength three times weekly. *See Chap. II.*

Sulophen Ointment 2 Jars 2 oz. (McNeil)
Contains para-thio-cresol 0.25 % in vanishing cream base; uses and application as above. *See Chap. II.*

Sulphocol Ointment Tubes ½ oz.; packages of 12. (Mulford Colloid)
Contains colloidal sulphur 10 %. *For use* in metabolic and arthritic affections. *Applied* locally, as necessary. *See Chap. I.*

Sunex Individual tubes. (Abbott)
Contains butesin and metaphen. *For use* as analgesic antiseptic in sun and wind burn, insect bites and poison ivy; *applied* locally one to two times daily.

Surgical Lubricant Individual tubes, Jars 1 lb. (Parke, Davis)
Contains mucilage of tragacanth, chondrus, glycerin and boric acid with aromatics. *For use* as emollient dressing and as surgical lubricant; *applied* when necessary.

Taroxide Tubes 1 oz., Jars 1, 5 lb. (Abbott)
Contains coal tar distillate 5 parts, zinc oxide 50 parts, starch and petrolatum 120 parts. *For use* in chronic infantile moist eczema, poison ivy; *applied* locally, daily for 1 week; rest period several days and repeated. *See Chap. XII.*

Tricocide Ointment Tubes ½, 1 oz. (Maltbie)
Contains cresol, beta-naphthol, benzocaine, zinc oxide. *For use* as antiseptic in ringworm and fungus infections; *applied* locally twice daily.

Tricotox Jars 2 oz. (Stearns)
Contains salicylic acid, benzoic acid, chlorthymol, lanolin. *For use* as parasiticide in epidermophytosis; *applied* twice daily after washing parts; when desquamation occurs bland ointment is used.

Unguentine Tubes large and small, Tins 1, 5 lb. (Norwich)
Contains alum compound, phenol, ammonium sulfoichthyolate, zinc oxide, parahydrecin, aromatic oils, petrolatum, purified animal fats. *For use* as astringent and antiseptic in burns, minor surgical skin affections; *applied* locally twice daily.

Vaseline Preparations Individual tubes, Jars 1, 5 lb. (Chesebrough)
Contains semisolid mixture of hydro-carbons obtained from petrolatum. *For use* as antiseptic and anesthetic in minor surgical affections, chafing, sunburn, bruises, dermatoses.
Combinations:
"Vaseline" Borated Jelly; "Vaseline" Carbolated Jelly; "Vaseline" Mentholated Jelly; "Vaseline" Camphor Ice; "Vaseline" Eucalyptol Jelly.

Vulnerine Tubes ½ oz., Jars 2, 4 oz., 1 lb. (Rorer)
Contains boric acid 50%, bismuth subgallate 30%, zinc stearate, camphor, phenol q.s. *For use* as surgical dressing in infections, burns and wounds.

---

9. OPHTHALMIC OINTMENTS

Ammoniated Mercury Tubes ⅛ oz.; Boxes of 12 (Abbott)
Contains ammoniated mercury 3%, white petrolatum 97%. *For use* as stimulating antiseptic in eczema of lids, blepharitis, catarrhal or trachomatous conjunctivitis. *Applied* locally to the lid margins several times daily.

Ammoniated Mercury Ointment Tubes 1 dr.; Boxes of 12. (Lilly)
Contains ammoniated mercury ½%, 3%.

Argenol Ointment Tubes ⅛ oz.; Boxes of 12. (Wyeth)
Contains mild silver protein 5%, in bland base.

Argental Tubes ⅛ oz. Boxes of 12 (Abbott)
Contains mild silver protein 20%, (colloidal) 10%, ophthalmic ointment base 90%. *For use* as astringent antiseptic in inflammatory conditions of the lids and conjunctivae, in corneal ulcer, styes, marginal blepharitis. *Applied* locally several times daily.

Argentiform Ointment Tubes 1 dr.; Boxes of 12. (Nelson, Baker)
Contains argentiform 1% or argentiform 1:500.

Argolaval Ointment Bottles of 5 and 10 Gm; Bottles of 3 oz. (Doho)
Contains equivalent to 1% silver nitrate.

Argyrol Ointment Tubes 1 dr.; Cartons of 12. (Manhattan)
Contains argyrol (Barnes) 10%; wool fat 25% in petrolatum. *See Chap. I.*

Argyrol Ointment Tubes ⅛ oz.; Boxes of 12. (Smith-Dorsey)
Contains argyrol 10% in special base.

Atropine Alkaloid Ointment (1%) Tubes 1 dr.; Cartons of 12. (Manhattan)

Atropine and Bichloride Ointment Tubes 1 dr.; Cartons of 12. (Manhattan)
Contains atropine sulphate 1%; mercury bichloride 1/30% in petrolatum.

Atropine and Iodosyl, 1 (Regular) Ointment Tubes 1 dr.; Boxes of 12. (Nelson, Baker)
Contains atropine 1%; iodosyl 2%.

Atropine and Iodosyl, 3 (Special) Ointment Tubes 1 dr.; Boxes of 12. (Nelson, Baker)
Contains atropine 0.5%; iodosyl 6%.

Atropine Ointment Tubes 1 dr.; Cartons of 12. (Manhattan)
Contains atropine alkaloid ½%; olive oil 20% in petrolatum.

Atropine Ointment Tubes 1 dr.; Cartons of 12. (Manhattan)
Contains atropine sulphate 2%; wool fat 10% in petrolatum.

Atropine Sulphate (1%) Tubes ⅛ oz; Boxes of 12 (Abbott)
Contains atropine sulphate 1%, ophthalmic ointment base 99%. *For use* as mydriatic of prolonged action. *Applied* locally as necessary.

Atropine Sulphate (2%) Tubes ⅛ oz; Boxes of 12 (Abbott)
Contains atropine sulphate 2%, boric acid 5%, ophthalmic ointment base 93%. *For use* as powerful mydriatic. *Applied* as necessary.

Atropine Sulphate Ointment Tubes 1 dr.; Boxes of 12. (Lilly)
Contains atropine sulphate 1%.

Atropine Sulphate Ointment Tubes ⅛ oz.; Boxes of 12. (Sharp and Dohme)
Contains atropine sulphate 1%.

Atropine Sulphate Ointment Tubes ⅛ oz.; Boxes of 12. (Smith-Dorsey)
Contains atropine sulphate 1% in special base.

Bichloride Ointment Tubes 1 dr.; Cartons of 12. (Manhattan)
Contains mercury bichloride 1–5,000 in petrolatum.

Bichloride Ointment (White) Tubes 1 dr.; Cartons of 12. (Manhattan)
Contains mercury bichloride 1–3,000 in petrolatum.

Boric Acid (10%) Tubes ⅛ oz. Boxes of 12 (Abbott)
Contains boric acid 10%, white petrolatum 90%. *For use* as sedative to relieve pain and reduce inflammation. *Applied* locally several times daily.

Boric Acid Eye tubes ⅛ oz. (Maltbie)
Contains boric acid 5%.

Boric Acid Compound Tubes ⅛ oz. Boxes of 12 (Abbott)
Contains boric acid 5%, carbolic acid 1%, white petrolatum 94%. *For use* as sedative antiseptic, *Applied* locally as necessary.

Boric Acid Ointment Tubes ⅛ oz.; Boxes of 12. (Sharp and Dohme)
Contains boric acid 5%.

Boric Acid Ointment Tubes ⅛ oz.; Boxes of 12. (Smith-Dorsey)
Contains boric acid 5% in special base.

Boric Acid Ointment Tubes 1 dr.; Boxes of 12. (Lilly)
Contains boric acid 5%.

Boric Acid Ointment Tubes 1 dr.; Boxes of 12. (Upjohn)
Contains boric acid 10%.

Boric Acid Ointment Tubes 1/8 oz.; Boxes of 12. (Wyeth)
Contains boric acid 5 %.

Boric Acid and Phenol Ointment Tubes 1/8 oz.; Boxes of 12. (Smith-Dorsey)
Contains boric acid 5 % and phenol 1 %, in special base.

Butesin Picrate (1 %) (C.A.) Individual tubes 1/8 oz. Boxes 12. (Abbott)
Contains butesin picrate 1 % in petrolatum base. *For use* as antiseptic and anesthetic in corneal burns, ulcers and inflammations. *Applied* locally several times daily. *See Chap. I.*

Butyn (2 %) (C.A.) Tubes 1/8 oz. Boxes 12. (Abbott)
Contains butyn 2%, metaphen 1:10,000, ophthalmic ointment base q.s. *For use* as antiseptic and anesthetic of long duration. *Applied* locally post-operatively, as necessary. *See Chap. I.*

Butyn Ointment (1 %) (C.A.) Tubes 1 dr.; Cartons of 12. *See Chap. I.* (Manhattan)

Butyn and Bichloride Ointment Tubes 1 dr.; Cartons of 12. (Manhattan)
Contains butyn (Abbott) 1/2 %; bichloride ointment 1–3,000.

Butyn and Bichloride Ointment Tubes 1 dr.; Cartons of 12. (Manhattan)
Contains butyn (Abbott) 1 %; bichloride ointment 1–3,000.

Calomel Ointment (5 %) Tubes 1 dr.; Cartons of 12. (Manhattan)

Cocaine Hydrochloride Ointment Tubes 1/8 oz.; Boxes of 12. (Smith-Dorsey)
Contains cocaine hydrochloride 2 % in special base.

Colloidal Silver Salts Ointment Tubes 1/8 oz.; Boxes of 12. (Smith-Dorsey)
Contains colloidal silver salts 5 %, in special base.

Compound Mercury 14 Ointment Tubes 1/8 oz.; Boxes of 12. (Smith-Dorsey)
Contains yellow oxide of mercury 1 %; adrenalin chloride solution 1:2,000 5 %; phenol 1/6 %; menthol 1/25 %.

Compound Novocaine Ointment Tubes 1/8 oz.; Boxes of 12. (Smith-Dorsey)
Contains novocaine 1 %; adrenalin chloride solution 4 %; special base.

Compound Silver Iodide Ointment Tubes 1 dr.; Cartons of 12. (Manhattan)
Contains neo-silvol (P.D. Co.) 20 %; wool fat 10 % in petrolatum.

Compound Yellow Oxide Mercury and Adrenalin Oint. (C.A.) Tubes 1 dr.; Cartons of 12. (Manhattan)
Contains hydrarg. oxid. flav. 1 %; adrenalin chloride solution (P.D. Co.) 2 %; acid carbol. 1/5 %; menthol 1/25 %; wool fat 25 % in petrolatum.

Congestive Ointment Tubes 1/8 oz.; Boxes of 12. (Wyeth)
Contains yellow mercuric oxide 4 parts; epinephrine 1 part; boric acid 2 parts; ointment base q.s. 1,000 parts.

Conjunctivitis Ointment Tubes 1/8 oz.; Boxes of 12. Tubes 1/4 oz.; Boxes of 12. (Sharp and Dohme)
Contains Epinephrine 1 part; Yellow mercuric oxide 4 parts; Ointment Boroglyceride 240 parts; Ointment Base q.s. 1,000 parts.

Copper Citrate Ointment Tubes 1 dr.; Boxes of 12. (Lilly)
Contains copper citrate 5 %.

Copper Citrate Ointment (C.A.) Tubes 1 dr.; Cartons of 12. (Manhattan)
Contains copper citrate 5 % in petrolatum.

Copper Citrate Ointment (C.A.) Tubes 1 dr.; Cartons of 12. (Manhattan)
Contains copper citrate 10 % in petrolatum.

Copper Citrate Ointment Tubes 1/8 oz.; Boxes of 12. Tubes 1/4 oz.; Boxes of 12. (Sharp and Dohme)
Contains copper citrate 5 %.

Copper Citrate Ointment Tubes ⅛ oz.; Boxes of 12 **(Sharp and Dohme)**
Contains copper citrate 10%.

Copper Citrate Ointment Tubes ⅛ oz.; Boxes of 12. **(Smith-Dorsey)**
Contains copper citrate 5% or 10% in special base.

Copper Sulphate Ointment (½%) Tubes 1 dr.; Cartons of 12. **(Manhattan)**

Dionin Ointment Tubes of ⅛ oz.; Boxes of 12. **(Smith-Dorsey)**
Contains dionin 2½% or 5% in special base.

Eserine Alkaloid Ointment Tubes ⅛ oz.; Boxes of 12. **(Smith-Dorsey)**
Contains eserine alkaloid ¼% in special base.

Eserine (¼%) Tubes ⅛ oz. Boxes 12. **(Abbott)**
Contains eserine alkaloid ¼%, ophthalmic ointment base q.s. 100%. *For use* to contract the pupil, to diminish intra-ocular tension and in the treatment of adhesions of the iris, photophobia, glaucoma, keratitis; is antagonistic to atropine. *Applied* locally as necessary.

Eserine Ointment Tubes 1 dr.; Cartons of 12. **(Manhattan)**
Contains eserine alk. 1%; olive oil 20% in petrolatum.

Holocain and Adrenalin Ointment (C.A.) Tubes 1 dr.; Cartons of 12. **(Manhattan)**
Contains holocain (Metz) 1%; adrenalin chloride sol. (P.D.) 2%; wool fat 10% in petrolatum. *See Chap. I.*

Holocain and Bichloride Ointment Tubes 1 dr.; Cartons of 12. **(Manhattan)**
Contains holocain (Metz) 1%; bichloride of mercury 1/30%, in petrolatum.

Holocain and Bichloride Ointment Tubes 1 dr.; Cartons of 12. **(Manhattan)**
Contains holocain (Metz) 2%; bichloride of mercury 1/30%, in petrolatum.

Holocaine and Epinephrine (C.A.) Tubes ⅛ oz. Boxes 12. **(Abbott)**
Contains holocaine 1%, epinephrine hydrochloride solution 4%, ophthalmic ointment base 95%. *For use* as anesthetic and astringent; does not dilate the pupil, reduces inflammation and congestion, shrinks engorged capillaries and relieves pain. *Applied* three to five times daily as required.

Holocaine Hydrochloride Ointment (C.A.) Tubes 1 dr.; Boxes of 12. **(Lilly)**
Contains holocaine hydrochloride 2%.

Holocaine Hydrochloride Ointment Tubes ⅛ oz.; Boxes of 12. **(Smith-Dorsey)**
Contains holocaine hydrochloride 2% in special base.

Holocaine Hydrochloride and Mercury Yellow Oxide Ointment **(Smith-Dorsey)**
Tubes ⅛ oz.; Boxes of 12.
Contains holocaine hydrochloride 2% and mercury yellow oxide 1%.

Holocain Ointment (1%) (C.A.) Tubes 1 dr.; Cartons of 12. **(Manhattan)**
See Chap. I.

Hyzin Tubes ⅛ oz. Boxes 12. **(Abbott)**
Contains hydrastine white alkaloid 1:1,500, zinc sulphate gr 6/10, boric acid gr 18, camphor gr 6/10, petrolatum q.s. 1 oz. *For use* as astringent antiseptic to reduce inflammation. *Applied* locally as necessary.

Ichthyol Ointment Tubes ⅛ oz.; Boxes of 12. **(Sharp and Dohme)**
Contains ichthyol 5%.

Ichthyol Ointment Tubes ⅛ oz.; Boxes of 12. **(Smith-Dorsey)**
Contains ichthyol 5% in special base.

Iodoform Ointment Tubes 1 dr.; Boxes of 12. **(Lilly)**
Contains iodoform 2%. *See Chap. I.*

Iodoform Ointment, Sterile Tubes 1 dr.; Cartons of 12. **(Manhattan)**
Contains iodoform 10%; wool fat 20% in petrolatum.

Iodosyl Ointment Tubes 1 dr.; Boxes of 12. Tubes 6 dr.; Boxes of 12. **(Nelson, Baker)**
Contains iodosyl 2%, or iodosyl 6%.

Mercuric Chloride (Corrosive) Ointment Tubes ⅛ oz.; Boxes of 12. **(Wyeth)**
Contains mercuric chloride, corrosive 1:5,000.

Mercuric Chloride Corrosive Ointment Tubes ⅛ oz.; Boxes of 12. **(Sharp and Dohme)**
Contains mercuric chloride, corrosive 1:5,000.

Mercuric Oxide and Atropine, 1 Ointment Tubes 1 dr.; Boxes of 12. **(Lilly)**
Contains mercuric oxide, yellow 1%; atropine sulphate 1%.

Mercuric Oxide Yellow with Atropine Ointment Tubes ⅛ oz.; Boxes of 12. **(Sharp and Dohme)**
Contains mercuric oxide, yellow gr 4; atropine gr 1; petrolatum q.s. oz. 1.

Mercuric Oxide and Ephedrine Ointment Tubes 1 dr.; Boxes of 12. **(Lilly)**
Contains ephedrine sulphate 0.1%; mercuric oxide yellow 1.0%.

Mercuric Oxide Yellow (½%) Tubes ⅛ oz. Boxes 12. **(Abbott)**
Contains mercuric oxide yellow ½% in white petrolatum. *For use* as stimulating antiseptic dressing in infections of the lids. *Applied* locally two to three times daily.

Mercuric Oxide Yellow (1%) Tubes ⅛ oz. Boxes 12. **(Abbott)**
Contains mercuric oxide yellow 1% in white petrolatum. *For use* as above.

Mercuric Oxide Yellow (2%) Tubes ⅛ oz. Boxes 12. **(Abbott)**
Contains yellow mercuric oxide 2% in white petrolatum. *For use* as above.

Mercuric Oxide Yellow Compound Tubes ⅛ oz. Boxes 12. **(Abbott)**
Contains mercuric oxide yellow 4 parts, ointment boroglyceride 24 parts, solution epinephrine hydrochloride 50 parts, ophthalmic ointment base q.s. 1,000 parts. *For use* as stimulating antiseptic for congested eyelids and to constrict the small blood vessels, relieving inflammatory conditions. *Applied* locally several times daily.

Mercuric Oxide Yellow Ointment Tubes 1 dr.; Boxes of 12. **(Lilly)**
Contains mercuric oxide yellow ½%.

Mercuric Oxide Yellow Ointment Tubes 2 dr.; Boxes of 12. **(Lilly)**
Contains mercuric oxide yellow 1%, or mercuric oxide yellow 2%.

Mercuric Oxide Yellow Ointment Tubes 1 dr.; Boxes of 12. **(Nelson, Baker)**
Contains mercuric oxide, yellow ¾%, or 1%, or 2%.

Mercuric Oxide, Yellow Ointment Tubes ⅛ oz.; Boxes of 12; Tubes ¼ oz.; Boxes of 12. **(Sharp and Dohme)**
Contains mercuric oxide, yellow 1% or 2%.

Mercuric Oxide Yellow Ointment Tubes ⅛ oz.; Boxes of 12; Tubes ¼ oz.; Boxes of 12. **(Wyeth)**
Contains yellow mercuric oxide, 1%, or 2%.

Mercuriform Ointment Tubes 1 dr.; Boxes of 12. **(Nelson, Baker)**
Contains mercuriform 1:3,000.

Mercurochrome Ointment Tubes 1 dr.; Cartons of 12. **(Manhattan)**
Contains mercurochrome (H.W.D.) 1%; wool fat 10% in petrolatum.

Mercurochrome Ointment Tubes 1 dr.; Cartons of 12. *See Chap. I.* **(Manhattan)**
Contains mercurochrome (H.W.D.) 2%; wool fat 10% in petrolatum.

Mercurochrome Ointment Tubes ⅛ oz.; Boxes of 12. **(Smith-Dorsey)**
Contains mercurochrome 1% or 2% in special base.

Mercury, Ammoniated Ointment Tubes ⅛ oz.; Boxes of 12. **(Sharp and Dohme)**
Contains ammoniated mercury, 3%.

Mercury, Ammoniated Ointment Tubes ⅛ oz.; Boxes of 12. **(Smith-Dorsey)**
Contains ammoniated mercury 3% in special base.

Mercury Bichloride 1:3,000 Tubes ⅛ oz. Boxes 12. **(Abbott)**
Contains mercury bichloride 1:3,000, ophthalmic ointment base q.s. *For use* as stimulating germicide. *Applied* locally when required.

Mercury Bichloride 1:5,000 Tubes ⅛ oz. Boxes 12. **(Abbott)**
Contains mercury bichloride 1:5,000, ophthalmic ointment base q.s. *For use* as lid dressing in purulent infections; *applied* locally two or three times daily, to prevent adhering of lids.

Mercury Bichloride Ointment Tubes 1 dr.; Boxes of 12. **(Lilly)**
Contains mercury bichloride 1:3,000, or 1:5,000.

Mercury Bichloride Ointment Tubes ⅛ oz.; Boxes of 12. **(Smith-Dorsey)**
Contains mercury bichloride 1:3,000 in special base.

Mercury Bichloride Ointment Tubes of 1 dr.; Boxes of 12. **(Upjohn)**
Contains mercury bichloride 1:3,000.

Mercury Bichloride and Sodium Chloride Ointment Tubes ⅛ oz.; Boxes of 12. **(Smith-Dorsey)**
Contains mercury bichloride 1:3,000; sodium chloride 5:3,000.

Mercury Compound 18 Ointment Tubes ⅛ oz.; Boxes of 12. **(Smith-Dorsey)**
Contains adrenalin chloride solution 1:2,000; yellow oxide mercury, 1%; ointment boroglyceride 20%; special base.

Mercury Oxide, Yellow Ointment Tubes ⅛ oz.; Boxes of 12. **(Smith-Dorsey)**
Contains mercury oxide, yellow 1% in special base, or 2%.

Mercury Oxide Ointment Tubes of 1 dr.; Boxes of 12. **(Upjohn)**
Contains yellow oxide mercury, 1 or 2%.

Mercury Yellow Oxide Compound Eye tubes ¼ oz., ⅛ oz. **(Maltbie)**
Contains mercury yellow oxide 1%; benzocaine ½%.

Mercury Yellow Oxide Compound Ointment Tubes of 1 dr.; Boxes of 12. **(Upjohn)**
Contains yellow oxide mercury gr 3½; zinc oxide gr 3½.

Mercury Yellow Oxide Ointment Eye tubes ⅛ oz., ¼ oz. **(Maltbie)**
Contains mercury yellow oxide 1%.

Mercury, Yellow Oxide and Atropine Sulphate Ointment Tubes ⅛ oz.; Boxes of 12. **(Smith-Dorsey)**
Contains yellow oxide mercury, 1% and atropine sulphate ½% in special base.

Merthiolate Ointment Tubes 1 dr.; Boxes of 12. **(Lilly)**
Contains merthiolate 1:5,000. *See Chap. I.*

Metaphen Ophthalmic Ointment 1:3,000 (C.A.) Tubes ⅛ oz. Boxes 12. **(Abbott)**
For use as non-irritating, penetrating antiseptic and dressing, pre- and post-operatively as prophylactic and for the treatment of ulcers and infections. *Applied* locally two to three times daily. *See Chap. I.*

Novocaine Ointment Tubes ⅛ oz.; Boxes of 12. **(Smith-Dorsey)**
Contains novocaine 1% in special base.

Ointment 38 Tubes 1 dr.; Cartons of 12. **(Manhattan)**
Contains atropine sulph. 1%; hydrarg. oxid. flav. 1% in petrolatum.

Ointment 39 Tubes 1 dr.; Cartons of 12. **(Manhattan)**
Contains orthoform (Metz) 5%; balsam Peru 1%; novocain 1% in petrolatum.

Ophthalmic Cream Tubes ⅛ oz. (Maltbie)
Contains—Solution epinephrine 1:20,000, boric acid gr 12 (0.77 Gm), zinc sulphocarbolate gr 3 (0.19 Gm).

Ophthalmic Ointment Acid Boric Small tubes; Boxes of 12. (McNeil)
Contains boric acid 5%.

Ophthalmic Ointment Adrenal Comp. Small tubes; Boxes of 12. (McNeil)
Contains ext. suprarenal gland 2.5%; mercuric oxide, yellow 1.0%; menthol 0.04%; phenol 0.2%.

Ophthalmic Ointment Atropine Small tubes; Boxes of 12. (McNeil)
Contains atropine 1%.

Ophthalmic Ointment Copper Citrate Small tubes; Boxes of 12. (McNeil)
Contains copper citrate 5%.

Ophthalmic Ointment Mercuric Chloride, Corrosive Small tubes; Boxes of 12. (McNeil)
Contains corrosive mercuric chloride, 1:3,000.

Ophthalmic Ointment Mercuric Chloride with Procaine Small tubes; Boxes of 12. (McNeil)
Contains corrosive mercuric chloride, 1:3,000; procaine (base) ½%.

Ophthalmic Ointment Mercuric Oxide, Yellow Small tubes; Boxes of 12; Jars 1 lb. (McNeil)
Contains mercuric oxide yellow, 1% and 2%.

Ophthalmic Ointment Mercuric Oxide Yellow with Ephedrine Small tubes; Boxes of 12. (McNeil)
Contains mercuric oxide, yellow 1%; Ephedrine sulphate 1/10%.

Ophthalmic Ointment Procaine with Epinephrine (C.A.) Small tubes; Boxes of 12. (McNeil)
Contains procaine (Base) 1%; epinephrine 0.02%.

Ophthalmic Ointment Quinosol Small tubes; Boxes of 12. (McNeil)
Contains quinosol 1:3,000.

Ophthalmic Ointment Silver Albuminate Small tubes; Boxes of 12. (McNeil)
Contains silver albuminate 5%, or 10%.

Orthoform Ointment Tubes ⅛ oz.; Boxes of 12. (Smith-Dorsey)
Contains orthoform 1% in special base.

Petrolatum, Sterile Ointment Tubes 1 dr.; Boxes of 12. Tubes 1 oz.; Boxes of 12. (Lilly)
Contains sterile petrolatum.

Petrolatum (White) Sterile Ointment Tubes, prescription size; Cartons of 12. (Manhattan)

Petrolatum (White) Sterile Ointment Carbolated 1%. Tubes, prescription size; Cartons of 12. (Manhattan)

Phenacaine and Epinephrine Ointment Tubes 1 dr.; Boxes of 12. (Upjohn)
Contains phenacaine 1%; epinephrine hydrochloride (1:1,000) 4%.

Pilocarpine Muriate Ointment Tubes ⅛ oz.; Boxes of 12. (Smith-Dorsey)
Contains pilocarpine muriate 1% in special base.

Scarlet Red Ointment Tubes 1 dr.; Cartons of 12. *See Chap. I.* (Manhattan)
Contains scarlet red (Biebrich) 5% in petrolatum.

Silloid Ointment Tubes 1 dr.; Boxes of 12. (Upjohn)
Contains colloidal silver salt (Upjohn), 5% or 10%.

Silver Nitrate Ointment (1%) Tubes 1 dr.; Cartons of 12. (Manhattan)

Silvol Ointment Dispensing packages; Boxes of 12. Large tubes; Boxes of 12. **(Parke, Davis)**
Contains colloidal silver 5%.

Thiosinamine Ointment Tubes 1 dr.; Cartons of 12. **(Manhattan)**
Contains thiosinamine 10% in petrolatum.

Thiosinamine Ointment Tubes 1/8 oz.; Boxes of 12. **(Smith-Dorsey)**
Contains thiosinamine 10% in special base.

Unguentum Acidum Boricum Ointment Tubes 1/8 oz.; Boxes of 12. **(Zemmer)**
Contains acid boric 5%; Petrolatum (white) q.s.

Unguentum Acidum Boricum Compound Ointment Tubes 1/8 oz.; Boxes of 12. **(Zemmer)**
Contains acid boric 5%; acid carbolic 1/4%.

Unguentum Argentum Ointment Tubes 1/8 oz.; Boxes of 12. **(Zemmer)**
Contains argyrol gr 48; lanolin and petrolatum aa q.s. 1 oz.

Unguentum Atropine Sulphate Ointment Tubes 1/8 oz.; Boxes of 12. **(Zemmer)**
Contains atropine sulphate 1/2%.

Unguentum Atropine Sulphate Ointment Tubes 1/8 oz.; Boxes of 12. **(Zemmer)**
Contains atropine sulphate 1 or 2%.

Unguentum Butyn Ointment Tubes 1/8 oz.; Boxes of 12. **(Zemmer)**
Contains butyn 1%.

Unguentum Cocaine Hydrochloride Ointment Tubes 1/8 oz.; Boxes of 12. **(Zemmer)**
Contains cocaine hydrochloride 2%.

Unguentum Cupric Citrate Ointment Tubes 1/8 oz.; Boxes of 12. **(Zemmer)**
Contains cupric citrate gr 24 or gr 48; lanolin and petrolatum (white) aa q.s. 1 oz.

Unguentum Cupric Sulphate Ointment Tubes 1/8 oz.; Boxes of 12. **(Zemmer)**
Contains cupric sulphate 1/2%.

Unguentum Dionin Ointment Tubes 1/8 oz.; Boxes of 12. **(Zemmer)**
Contains dionin 2 1/2% or 5%.

Unguentum Eserine Salicylate Ointment Tubes 1/8 oz.; Boxes of 12. **(Zemmer)**
Contains eserine salicylate 1/4%.

Unguentum Holocaine et Adrenalin Ointment Tubes 1/8 oz.; Boxes of 12. **(Zemmer)**
Contains holocaine gr 4; adrenalin (1/3,000) m 20; lanolin anhydrous and white petrolatum q.s. 1 oz.

Unguentum Hydrargyri Chloridi Corrosivum Ointment Tubes 1/8 oz.; Boxes of 12; Tubes 1/4 oz.; Boxes of 12. **(Zemmer)**
Contains hydrarg. chlor. corros. 1:3,000; sodium chloride q.s.; lanolin and petrolatum (white) aa q.s. 1 oz.

Unguentum Hydrargyri Oxidum Flavum Ointment Tubes 1/8 oz.; Boxes of 12. Tubes 1/4 oz.; Boxes of 12. **(Zemmer)**
Contains hydrarg. oxid. flav. gr 4; ointment base q.s. 1 oz.

Unguentum Hydrargyri Oxidum Flavum Ointment Tubes 1/8 oz.; Boxes of 12. **(Zemmer)**
Contains hydrarg. oxid. flav. gr 8; ointment base 1 oz.

Unguentum Hydrargyri Oxidum Flavum et Atropine Ointment Tubes 1/8 oz.; Boxes of 12. **(Zemmer)**
Contains hydrarg. oxid. flav. gr 4; atropine sulphate gr 1; petrolatum album q.s. 1 oz.

Unguentum Hydrargyri Oxidum Flavum et Adrenalin Comp. Ointment Tubes 1/8 oz.; Boxes of 12. **(Zemmer)**

Contains hydrarg. oxid. flav. gr 4; adrenalin chloride 1:1,000 25 gtt.; menthol gr 1/10; acid carbolic gr 1; lanolin 1/2 oz.; petrolatum album q.s. 1 oz.

Unguentum Ichthyol (5%) Ointment Tubes 1/8 oz.; Boxes of 12. (Zemmer)

Unguentum Lunosol (10%) Ointment Tubes 1/8 oz.; Boxes of 12. (Zemmer)

Unguentum Mercurochrome (1%) Tubes 1/8 oz.; Boxes of 12. Tubes 1/4 oz.; Boxes of 12. (Zemmer)
In special ointment base.

Unguentum Mercurochrome (2%) Tubes 1/8 oz.; Boxes of 12. Tubes 1/4 oz.; Boxes of 12. (Zemmer)
In special ointment base.

Unguentum Optochin Hydrochloride (1%) Tubes 1/8 oz.; Boxes of 12. (Zemmer)

Unguentum Optochin Hydrochloride (2%) Tubes 1/8 oz.; Boxes of 12. (Zemmer)

Unguentum Orthoform (1%) Tubes 1/8 oz.; Boxes of 12. (Zemmer)

Unguentum Orthoform (2%) Tubes 1/8 oz.; Boxes of 12. (Zemmer)

Unguentum Pilocarpine Muriate (1%) Tubes 1/8 oz.; Boxes of 12. (Zemmer)

Unguentum Thiosinamine (10%) Tubes 1/8 oz.; Boxes of 12. (Zemmer)
In lanolin and petrolatum base.

Unguentum Zinci Acetas Tubes 1/8 oz.; Boxes of 12. (Zemmer)
Contains zinc acetate gr 1/2; lanolin and petrolatum aa q.s. 1 oz.

Unguentum Zinc Sulphate (1/2%) Tubes 1/8 oz.; Boxes of 12.

Unguentum Zinc-Ichthyol Tubes 1/8 oz.; Boxes of 12. (Zemmer)
Contains zinc sulphate gr 1/2; ichthyol ointment 5% q.s. 1 oz.

White's Ointment Tubes 1/8 oz. Boxes 12. (Abbott)
Contains mercury bichloride 1:3,000, sodium chloride 5:3,000 in ophthalmic ointment base q.s. *For use* as pre-operative dressing in ocular infections. *Applied* locally as necessary.

White's Ointment Tubes 1 dr.; Boxes of 12. (Lilly)
Contains mercury bichloride 1:3,000; sodium chloride 5-3,000.

Yellow Oxide of Mercury Ointments Dispensing packages (small); Boxes of 12. Tubes 1/4 lb.; Boxes of 12. (Parke, Davis)
Contains yellow oxide of mercury 1 or 2%.

Yellow Oxide Mercury and Atropine Ointment Tubes 1 dr.; Cartons of 12. (Manhattan)
Contains hydrarg. oxid. flav. 1%; atropine sulph. 1/2% in petrolatum.

Zinc Acetate Ointment Tubes 1/8 oz.; Boxes of 12. (Smith-Dorsey)
Contains zinc acetate 1:1,000 in special base.

Zincol Ointment Tubes 1/2 oz. 10% (Mulford)
An astringent and antiseptic preparation. *For use* in ophthalmic affections.

Zinc Oxide Ointment (10%) Tubes 1 dr.; Cartons of 12. (Manhattan)

Zinc Sulphate Ointment (1/2%) Tubes 1/8 oz. Boxes 12. (Abbott)
Contains zinc sulphate 1/2% in ophthalmic ointment base. *For use* as astringent dressing in inflammatory conditions.

Zinc Sulphate Ointment Tubes 1 dr.; Boxes of 12. (Lilly)
Contains Zinc sulphate 1/2%.

Zinc Sulphate Ointment Tubes 1 dr.; Cartons of 12. (Manhattan)
Contains zinc sulphate 1/2%; wool fat 5% in petrolatum.

Zinc Sulphate Ointment Tubes 1/8 oz.; Boxes of 12. (Smith-Dorsey)
Contains zinc sulphate 1/2% in special base.

10. RECTAL SUPPOSITORIES

Adrenalin Suppositories (C.A.) Boxes of 12 **(Parke, Davis)**
Contains adrenalin 1:1,000 in oil of theobroma; also containing adrenalin gr 3/200, chloretone gr 3; astringent and hemostatic in hemmorrhoids, fissures. *See Chap. I.*

Adrenalin Compound Suppositories (C.A.) Boxes of 12 **(Parke, Davis)**
Contains adrenalin gr 1/300, apothesin gr 1/2, formidine gr 1, extr. hamamelis gr 1; action and uses as above. *See Chap. I.*

Adrephine Suppositories Boxes of 12 **(Parke, Davis)**
Contains adrenalin gr 1/300, ephedrine hydrochloride gr 1/6, benzocaine gr 4/5, chloretone gr 1/2; action and uses as above. *See Chap. I.*

Alpha-Naphco Suppositories (C.A.) Boxes of 12 **(Carel)**
Contains alpha naphthol; antiseptic, for rectal application. *See Chap. II.*

Anusol Suppositories Boxes of 6 **(Schering and Glatz)**
Contains bismuth iodoresorcinol-sulphonate, zinc oxide, balsam of peru. *For use* as antiseptic and analgesic in hemorrhoids, fistulae and fissures; *applied* twice daily.

Aesculol Suppositories Boxes of 12 **(C. D. Smith)**
Contains aesculus gr 1½, collinsonia gr 1½, hamamelis gr 1½, benzocaine gr ¼; *For use* as antipruritic and astringent in hemorrhoids and pruritus; *applied* once or twice daily.

Aminophyllin Suppositories Tubes of 12 **(Pharmedic)**
Contains gr 5 aminophylline. *For use* as diuretic, cardiotonic in hypertension, coronary disease; *applied* intrarectally twice daily. *See Chap. I.*

Anuform Suppositories Cartons of 12 **(Irwin, Neisler)**
Contains ephedrine alkaloid gr 1/2, benzocaine gr 1, oxyquinoline sulphate gr 1½, bismuth thymol-iodide gr 4; *For use* as anesthetic, astringent and antiseptic rectal suppository; *applied* once or twice daily.

Bismolan Suppositories Boxes of 12 **(Cavendish)**
Contains bismuth oxychlorate 0.1 Gm, zinc oxydate 0.15 Gm, solution suprarenin 1:1,000 0.05 Gm, eucaine hydrochloride 0.05 Gm, menthol 0.05 Gm, lanolin and solid vaseline q.s. 2.0 Gm. *For use* as anesthetic and astringent in rectal fissure, ulceration and proctitis; *applied* at night before retiring, after enema.

Butesin Compound Suppositories **(Abbott)**
Contains butesin gr 2½, extr. hydrastis gr 1/3, ext. hamamelis gr 1. *For use* as local anesthetic and astringent. *See Chap. I.*

Calmitol Suppositories Boxes of 12 **(Leeming)**
Contains chlorocamphoric aldehyde, iodine 0.5% (organic), menthol, laevo-hyoscine oleinate. *For use* as anesthetic, antiseptic and antipruritic in hemorrhoids, rectal irritation and pruritus ani and vulvae.

Collosol Cuprum Suppositories Boxes of 12 **(Crookes)**
Contains colloidal copper; *For use* as astringent for rectal disorders. *See Chap. I.*

Collosol Ichthyol Suppositories Boxes of 12. *See Chap. I.* **(Crookes)**

Collosol Iodine Suppositories Boxes of 12. *See Chap. I.* **(Crookes)**

Collosol Sulphur Suppositories Boxes of 6. *See Chap. I.* **(Crookes)**

Cresatin Suppositories Rectal. *See Chap. I.* **(Sharp and Dohme)**

Dilaudid Suppositories Boxes of 6 **(Bilhuber-Knoll)**
Contains dihydromorphinone HCl gr 1/24 (0.0025 Gm) in oleum theobromatis. *For use* where narcotics are indicated. *See Chap. I.*

Euphydigtal Suppositories Boxes of 6, 12 **(Hurst)**
Each contains 0.2 Gm metaphyllin, 0.15 Gm fol. digitalis. *For use* as diuretic and cardiotonic; *applied* two or three times daily. *See Chap. II.*

Glycerine Suppositories Boxes of 12, adult and infant sizes. **(McKesson and Robbins)**
Contains glycerine, stearic acid and sodium bicarbonate. *For use* in rectal stasis and constipation; *applied* as necessary, inserted into rectum.

Hazeline Suppositories Boxes of 12 **(Burroughs Wellcome)**
Contains volatile principles of hamamelis virginiana. *For use* as astringent and hemostatic. *See Chap. III.*

Iodosyl Compound Suppositories Boxes of 12, 48 **(Nelson-Baker)**
Contains iodosyl 50 parts, tannin 50 parts, alum 25 parts, atropine sulphate ¼ part, cacao butter 874¾ parts. *For use* as astringent antiseptic. *See Chap. I.*

Hemodal Suppositories Boxes of 12 **(Maltbie)**
Contains benzocaine, extr. hamamelis, ichthynat, zinc oxide, alum, phenol, eucalyptol. *For use* as antipruritic in hemorrhoids, pruritus ani; *applied* as necessary.

Ichthyol Suppositories. *See Chap. I.* **(Crookes)**

Iodine Suppositories Boxes of 12 **(Burnham)**
Contains free iodine, resorcinol 1%, anesthesin. *For use* as astringent, antiseptic, in rectal affections; *applied* as necessary.

Iodoformal Suppositories Boxes of 12 **(Warner)**
Contains iodoformal gr 5, acetanilid gr 1, cocoa butter q.s. *For use* as antiseptic astringent in rectal affections; *applied* as necessary.

Medinal Suppositories Boxes of 6 **(Schering and Glatz)**
Contains barbital-sodium gr 10 (0.643 Gm). *For use* as sedative, hypnotic. *See Chap. I.*

Medicated Suppositories Cartons of 12 **(Micajah)**
Contains sodium borate, alumen, ichthyol, balsam peru, belladonna leaves., ol. theobromatis. *For use* as astringent antiseptic and anesthetic in hemorrhoids and rectal infections, pruritus ani, fissure, proctitis; *applied* as necessary.

Metaphyllin Suppositories Boxes of 10 **(Hurst)**
Contains aminophyllin 0.36 Gm. *For use* as diuretic and cardiotonic; *Administered* two to four times daily. *See Chap. I.*

Metaphyllin with Calcium Suppositories Boxes of 10 **(Hurst)**
Uses as above. *See Chap. I.*

Metaphyllin with Calcium and Iodine Suppositories Boxes of 10 **(Hurst)**
Uses as above. *See Chap. I.*

Neo-Silvol Suppositories (C.A.) Boxes of 12 **(Parke, Davis)**
Contains neo-silvol 5% in glycero-gelatin base. *For use* as local antiseptic; *applied* as necessary.

Obtundobulbs Boxes of 12 **(Otis Clapp)**
Contains obtundia, hamamelis and aesculus. *For use* as astringent in rectal irritations; *applied* as necessary.

Phedrocaine Suppositories Boxes of 12, each gr ½ (0.32 Gm) **(Colwell)**
Contains ephedrine, ethyl aminobenzoate, para-aminobenzoyl-diethylaminoethanol. *For use* as astringent anesthetic in rectal affections; *applied* as necessary.

Picratol Suppositories Boxes of 20 **(Wyeth)**
Contains silver picrate 30% (silver trinitrophenolate). *For use* as antiseptic anesthetic in rectal affections; *applied* as necessary.

Posterisan "Kade" Suppositories Boxes of 10. **(Beisner)**
For use as rectal antiseptic in coli infections; *applied* once to twice daily, inserted into rectum.

Pronusin Suppositories Boxes of 12 **(Bischoff)**
Contains ethyl-aminobenzoate and zinc oxide. *For use* as astringent, anesthetic and antipruritic in rectal affections; *applied* twice daily after enema.

Quassin Suppositories Boxes of 12 **(Burroughs Wellcome)**
Contains the bitter principle of quassia wood, each gr ½ (0.032 Gm). *For use* as anthelmintic suppository for thread worms; *applied* rectally, once each night for several nights.

Rectal Suppositories Hemastin Boxes of 12, 50. **(McNeil)**
Contains suprarenal gland, creosote, tannic acid, lead oxide, zinc oxide, extr. stramonium. *For use* as astringent, hemostatic and antiseptic in rectal affections; *applied* locally as necessary.

Rectal Suppositories Quinosal Orthesine Boxes of 12, 50 **(McNeil)**
Contains quinosal and orthesine. *For use* as anesthetic and antiseptic in rectal affections; *applied* as necessary.

Rectal Medicone Boxes of 12 **(Medicone)**
Contains anesthesin gr 2, ephedrine hydrochloride gr 1/16, oxyquinolin sulfate gr ¼, bismuth subgallate gr 1, balsam peru gr 1, oleum theobromatis q.s. *For use* as anesthetic, antiseptic and decongestive in inflamed, thrombotic and bleeding hemorrhoids; *applied* three times daily, inserted into rectum.

Silver Sal Suppositories Boxes of 12 **(Smith-Dorsey)**
Contains mild protein 5% in glyco-gelatine base. *For use* as antiseptic in rectal gonorrheal affections. *See Chap. III.*

Supposidines Boxes of 12 **(Loeser)**
Contains iodine in suitable base. *For use* as antiseptic in rectal affections; *applied* as necessary.

Suppositories "Erge" Boxes of 12 **(Anglo-French)**
Contains grey oil (0.04 Gm mercury) and saponifiable fat base. *For use* as antiluetic; inserted into rectum at night.

Supsalvs Boxes of 6 **(Anglo-French)**
Contains salvarsan 0.10 gr (0.006 Gm) for adult, 0.08 gr (0.005 Gm) for infant. *For use* as antiluetic; *applied* every 2 days, inserted into rectum, for 24 doses; rest period 2 weeks, and course repeated. *See Chap. XII.*

Tannichthol Suppositories Boxes of 12 **(Sharp and Dohme)**
Contains phenol gr ¾, tannic acid gr 2½, ichthyol gr 1, extr. stramonium gr ¼, extr. belladonna gr ¼, extr. witch hazel gr ¼; *For use* as anesthetic, antiphlogistic, hemostatic in hemorrhoids, fissures, fistula, proctitis; *applied* locally, inserted into rectum as necessary.

Thephyldin Suppositories Boxes of 12 **(Kretschmar)**
Contain theophyllin ethylene diamine 0.36 Gm. *For use* as diuretic, cardiotonic; *Administered* two to four times daily. *See Chap. I.*

11. STYPTICS

Arzol Silver Nitrate Applicators **(Sklar)**
Wooden sticks 6 in. long, tipped at 1 end with a fused mass of silver nitrate 75% and potassium nitrate 25%. *For use* as astringent, hemostatic and escharotic, in various sores, ulcerations, oozing and erosions; *applied* directly to diseased area.
Supply—Boxes of 100.

Arzol Mercurochrome Applicators **(Sklar)**
Wooden sticks 6 in. long, tipped at 1 end with mercurochrome 10% in solid but soluble form. *For use* as local antiseptic in various surface diseases; *applied* directly.
Supply—Boxes of 10 folders, each 20 applicators.

Causticks (C.A.) (Tappan Zee)
Fused silver nitrate mounted like match head on wood applicator; contains silver nitrate 75%, potassium nitrate 25%. *For use* as antiseptic and escharotic in the healing of sore navel and nipples, in controlling secondary hemorrhage with erosion of cervix and verumontanum; *applied* by touching diseased area as with ordinary silver caustic pencil; to be used once and discarded.
Supply—Glass tubes of 100, sizes 1½, 6, 12 in.

Cupricsticks (C.A.) (Tappan Zee)
Fused copper nitrate mounted like match head on wood applicator; contains copper sulphate 25%, potassium sulphate 25%, alum 25%. *For use* as antiseptic and escharotic in trachoma, cervical erosions and other granular surfaces; *applied* by touching diseased area as with ordinary copper caustic; to be used once and discarded.
Supply—Glass tubes of 100, sizes 1½, 6, 12 in.

Hemarestors (McNeil)
Rounded cones or thin flexible sheets of a styptic in gelatin-glycerin base. *For use* in arresting hemorrhage or secondary bleeding after tonsillectomy, epistaxis, dental extraction; *applied* locally as styptic.
Supply—Boxes of 12, for tonsil and nasal use. Boxes of 20, for dental use.

Mercurosticks (Tappan Zee)
Solidified mercurochrome mounted like match head, on wood applicator. *For use* as first aid antiseptic in abrasions and similar injuries; *applied* by touching diseased area as with ordinary caustic pencil; to be used once and discarded.
Supply—Glass tubes of 100, sizes 1½, 6, 12 in.

Stypsticks (C.A.) (Tappan Zee)
Fused alum mounted like match head, on wood applicator; contains alum 75%, potassium nitrate 25%. *For use* as astringent in all superficial skin affections and mucous abrasions; *applied* by touching diseased area as with ordinary styptic pencil; to be used once and discarded.
Supply—Glass tubes of 100, sizes 1½, 6, 12 in.

12. SOAPS, MEDICATED

Antiseptic Soaps Individual bars (Schieffelin)
Contains

1. Benzoin 5%
2. Boric acid 5%
3. Ichthyol 5%
4. Ichthyol 10%
5. Ichthyol 3%, Tar 3%
6. Resorcin 5%
7. Resorcin 3%, Salicylic acid 3%, Sulphur 10%
8. Sublimate 0.5%
9. Sulphur 10%
10. Sulphur 5%, Camphor 5%, Balsam of Peru 3%

For use as detergent and antiseptic for the hands, and pre-operatively for surface sterilization.

Collosol Soap Boxes of 3 tablets. *See Chap. I.* (Crookes)

Collosol Ichthyol Soap Boxes of 3 tablets. *See Chap. I.* (Crookes)

Hazeline Soap *See Chap. III.* (Burroughs Wellcome)

Iodex Soap Individual cakes, packages of 3. (Menley and James)
Non-irritative, non-corrosive, medicated soap.

Metaphen Liquid Soap 1:1,000 Bottles of 4 oz. (Abbott)

Metaphen Antiseptic Bar Soap 1:500 Individual bars (Abbott)

Mazon Soap Individual cakes. (Belmont)
For use as shampoo in dandruff and for preparing the skin preliminary to application of Mazon Ointment.

Stearnize Tubes, collapsible, 4 oz. **(Stearns)**
Contains mercuric iodide, chlorthymol, glycerine, and a neutral base prepared from vegetable oils. *For use* as germicidal detergent and for the surgical sterilization of hands and operative areas;
Administered by rubbing in, like cold cream, for 1 min. on the dry skin, then rinsing off.

Mosquitone Sticks, in glass vials. **(McKesson and Robbins)**
An alcoholic soap stick containing mosquito-repelling essential oils. *For use* in keeping away mosquitoes and other insects, by rubbing on skin.

13. URETHRAL BOUGIES AND PENCILS

Argentiform Urethral Pencils Boxes of 14, 30, 72—packages of 12 **(Nelson, Baker)**
Contains argentiform gr ¼ (0.016 Gm). *For use* as local antiseptic and astringent in urethral affections;
Administration—1 inserted into urethra, as indicated.

Cargentos Urethral Bougies (C.A.) Boxes of 12 **(Sharp and Dohme)**
Contains colloidal silver gr 2 and a modified casein preparation. *For use* as local antiseptic in urethral affections;
Administration—1 inserted into urethra, as indicated.

Collosol Argentum Bougies *See Chap. I.* **(Crookes)**

Iodosyl Urethral Pencils Boxes of 14, 30, 72 **(Nelson, Baker)**
Contain iodosyl 50 parts, sod. borate 12½ parts, alum 12½ parts, zinc phenolsulphonate 5 parts, mercuric oleate 2½ parts, cacao butter 917½ parts. *See Chap. I.* *For use* in urethral disease.

Iodosyl Pencils (Milder) Boxes of 14, 30, 72 **(Nelson, Baker)**
Contains same formula as above except ½ of zinc phenolsulphonate and mercuric-oleate. *See Chap. I.*

Picratol Urethral Bougies Boxes of 2 **(Wyeth)**
Contains silver picrate gr ½ and 1. *See Chap. II.*

Silvol Bougies *See Chap. I.* **(Parke, Davis)**

Stylolactin Rods Boxes of 6 **(Hurst)**
For use as urethral bougie; *applied* as necessary.

14. VAGINAL ANTISEPTICS

Argentiform Cones Boxes of 12 **(Nelson, Baker)**
Contains a combination of silver and hexamethylenamine, each cone gr 3 (0.16 Gm). *For use* as antiseptic and germicide. *Applied* directly. *See Chap. I.*

Acriflavine Neutral Suppositories 1:2,000 (C.A.) Boxes of 12 **(Abbott)**
For use as vaginal antiseptic in pelvic infections; *applied* as necessary.

Alpha-Naphco Suppositories (C.A.) Boxes of 7 and 16 **(Carel)**
Contains alpha-naphthol. *For use* as antiseptic and germicide. *Applied* directly. *See Chap. II.*

Alquinco Suppositories Tablets—Bottles of 100 and 1 lb. **(McNeil)**
Contains powdered alum 12½ gr; copper sulphate 12½ gr, quinisal and oil of rose. *For use* as antiseptic and astringent douche, 1 tablet dissolved in 1 pt. of water. *See Chap. II.*

Asepticaps Boxes of 12 and 24 **(Wyeth)**
Contains boric acid 82%, alum 8%, zinc sulphate 6.5%, zinc phenolsulphonate 2.5%, sodium salicylate 2.5%, phenol 1%, aromatics q.s. *For use* as astringent, deodorant and antiseptic in vaginal affections; *applied* as vaginal douche—1 capsule dissolved in quart of warm water.

Aseptovols Boxes of 20 **(Sharp and Dohme)**
Contains acetanilid gr 2, sodium borate gr 5, zinc borate gr ½, benzothymol benzoate dr. 1, hydrastine m 15, boroglycerine base q.s; *For use* as alkaline antiseptic and astringent; *applied* once or twice daily as required.

Boro-Glyceride with Neo-Silvol Boxes of 12 **(Noyes)**
Contains neo-silvol 3%, boroglyceride base 5%. *For use* as vaginal antiseptic; *applied* as necessary.

Cargentos Suppositories Boxes of 12 **(Sharp and Dohme)**
Each contains gr 5 mild silver protein. *For use* as antiseptic and germicide in vaginal affections; *applied* locally. *See Chap. I.*

Cavosept Tubes of 12 **(Cavendish)**
Contains dichlorylsulfamid benzoate. *For use* as vaginal antiseptic in pelvic affections; *applied* 1 tablet intravaginally as necessary.

Collosol Argentum Boxes of 6 and 12 **(Crookes)**
Each contains 0.25% colloidal metallic silver; *For use* as vaginal antiseptic and astringent; *applied* locally. *See Chap. I.*

Collosol Hydrargyrum *See Chap. I.* **(Crookes)**

Collosol Iodine Pessaries Box of 6 **(Crookes)**
Contains 1% iodine in glyco-gelatin base. *For use* as vaginal antiseptic and germicide. *Applied* locally. *See Chap. I.*

Collosol Iodine Suppositories Box of 12 **(Crookes)**
Contains 1% iodine in glyco-gelatin base. *For use* as iodine therapy and for local action in pelvic affections. *See Chap. I.*

Collosol Sulphur Pessaries Box of 6 **(Crookes)**
Contains 0.1% colloidal sulphur solution. *For use* as parasiticide and antiseptic; *applied* topically. *See Chap. I.*

Cresatin Suppositories (10%) Box of 20 **(Sharp and Dohme)**
Contains metacresyl acetate. *For use* as antiseptic in pelvic affections; *applied* locally. *See Chap. I.*

Douchal Jars 2 oz. **(Irwin-Neisler)**
Contains oxyquinoline sulphate, magnesium sulphate, boric acid, alum, menthol. *For use* as vaginal antiseptic and deodorant in pelvic affections; *applied* as vaginal douche, when necessary.

Duo-Ban Tubes—boxes of 12 **(Irwin-Neisler)**
Contains oxyquinoline sulphate 1:500, lactic acid 20%, salicylic acid, boric acid, glycerine. *For use* as vaginal antiseptic jelly; *applied* as necessary.

Duofoam Tubes of 4 or 12, in 2 sections **(Burchard)**
Contains karacoll, sodium bicarbonate and boric acid, placed in 2 separated compartments. *For use* as vaginal antiseptic and prophylactic; *applied* intravaginally by mixing contents of each tube, when necessary.

Fomos Tablets Tubes of 10 **(Fomos)**
Contains quinol oxyquinoline sulphate, boric acid, tartaric acid and sodium bicarbonate; each tablet 1¼ Gm. *For use* as antiseptic, deodorant, and contraceptive. 1 tablet inserted intravaginally two times daily, or before exposure. *See Chap. III.*

Globulactin Pellets Box of 12 **(Hurst)**
Contains lactinium in a mixture of gelatin and glycerine. *For use* as antiseptic and astringent in pelvic affections. *See Chap. III.*

Hyva Sani-Tablets Vials of 10—packages of 12 **(Holland-Rantos)**
For use as vaginal antiseptic and prophylactic; *applied*—1 tablet dissolved in quart of warm water as vaginal douche.

Ichthyol Pessaries Box of 6 (Crookes)
Contains colloidal ichthyol. *For use* as antiphlogistic and antiseptic in vaginal affections. *See Chap. I.*

Koromex Individual tubes, Jars of 8 oz. (Holland-Rantos)
For use as vaginal prophylactic and antiseptic, deodorizer; *applied* intravaginally as necessary; often in connection with H-R Vaginal Diaphragm, in sizes 50–105 mm.

Lygel Individual tubes. Contains a combination of halogen and alkyl phenol derivatives as active principle. (Lehn and Fink)
For use as vaginal prophylactic; *applied* as necessary.

Marvosan Tubes 2½ oz. (Tablax)
Contains oxyquinoline sulfate, lactic acid, starch-glycerite base. *For use* as vaginal prophylactic and antiseptic; *applied* as necessary, using one-quarter turn of key.

Medicated Wafers Cartons of 25 (Micajah)
Contains sodium borate, alumen. *For use* as astringent and antiseptic in leucorrhea, cervicitis and other vaginal infections; applied as douche, 1 tablet in 4 oz. of water, or inserted high in vaginal canal after cleansing douche.

Mercurochrome Suppositories (C.A.) Boxes of 12, each 100 gr (6.48 Gm) (Aces)
Contains mercurochrome 2% solution, phenol 1/12%, thymol 1/12%, eucalyptol 1/12%, menthol 1/12%, in hydro-glycero-gelatin base. *For use* as vaginal antiseptic in pelvic affections; *applied* as necessary.

Mercurochrome Pessaries (C.A.) Box of 6 (Crookes)
Contains colloidal mercury. *For use* as antiseptic and germicide for vaginal application. *See Chap. I.*

Neo-Silvol Suppositories (C.A.) Boxes of 12 (Parke, Davis)
Contains neo-silvol 5% in glycero-gelatin base. *For use* as vaginal prophylactic in gonorrheal infections; *applied* as necessary.

Normolactol Tablets Boxes of 20 and 50 (Bischoff)
Contains calcium-sodium lactate. *For use* in leucorrhea. *Applied* intravaginally, 1 tablet each evening, for 3 days, followed by douche of normolactol solution on fourth day.

Norwich Douche Powder Cartons of 1 lb. (Norwich)
Contains boric acid 81.25%, salicylic acid 2.0%, zinc sulphate 15.5%, phenol 0.5%, menthol, eucalyptol, thymol q.s.; *For use* as vaginal astringent and prophylactic; *applied* as douche, 1 tablespoonful in quart of warm water, as necessary.

Obtundia Vagiobulbs Boxes of 12. (Otis Clapp)
Contains obtundia in glyco-boron or cocoa butter base. *For use* as vaginal antiseptic; *applied* as necessary.

Ortho-Gynol Tubes 2½ oz.—packages A, B, C, D, E. (Johnson and Johnson)
Contains oxyquinoline sulphate in gum base. *For use* as vaginal antiseptic and prophylactic; *applied* as necessary.

Oxyquinolin Suppositories Boxes of 12. (Noyes)
Contains oxyquinoline sulphate gr 1, salicylic acid gr 2, boric acid gr 10, quinine alkaloid gr 1; *For use* as vaginal antiseptic and prophylactic; *applied* as necessary.

Picratol Suppositories Box of 20 (Wyeth)
Contains silver picrate in boroglyceride and gelatin, sizes gr 1, gr 2. *For use* as astringent and antiseptic in vaginal infections. *See Chap. II.*

Progene Individual vials. (Holland-Rantos)
Contains glycocoll in saline vehicle. *For use* as an aid to conception; *applied* as necessary, 1 vial dissolved in 1 qt. warm water as vaginal douche. *See Chap. XII.*

Quinseptikons Boxes of 12 (Tablax)
Contains oxyquinolin-sulphate in suitable base. *For use* as vaginal antiseptic and prophylactic; *applied* as necessary.

Ramses Vaginal Jelly Collapsible tubes 2¼ oz., with or without Hycoloid applicator—cartons of 12. (Schmid)
Contains non-toxic ingredients in non-irritating easily distributable base, providing an antiseptic protective coating over vaginal wall and arresting motility of spermatozoa; is odorless, colorless, painless. *For use* as vaginal antiseptic in catarrhal infections; as contraceptive in connection with Ramses Velvet Finish Diaphragm and followed by douching.

Silver Sal Suppositories Boxes of 12. (Smith-Dorsey)
Contains colloidal silver 5% in suitable base. *For use* as vaginal antiseptic; *applied* as necessary.

Silvol Suppositories Boxes of 12. (Parke, Davis)
Contains mild silver protein 20%. *For use* as vaginal antiseptic; *applied* as necessary.

Sulfax Suppositories Box of 12 (Boericke and Tafel)
Contains oxyquinoline sulphate. *For use* as antiseptic in vaginal infections; *applied* locally. *See Chap. I.*

Suppository-Vaginal Boxes of 6. (Medicone)
Contains lactic acid jelly in cocoa-butter capsule. *For use* as vaginal antiseptic and prophylactic; *applied* as necessary.

Suppository 8 Boxes of 12, 36. (Smith-Dorsey)
Contains silver sal (colloidal) 5% in glycero-gelatine base. *For use* as vaginal antiseptic; *applied* as necessary.

Vaginettes Boxes of 12. (Buffington)
Contains mercurochrome 2.16%. *For use* as vaginal antiseptic in pelvic affections and gonorrhea; *applied* nightly for 2 weeks.

Vagitories Boxes of 12. (Hance)
Contains boric acid, quinine alkaloids, salicylic acid, red iodide of mercury in cocoa butter base. *For use* as vaginal antiseptic and prophylactic; *applied* as necessary.

15. MISCELLANEOUS

Saf-T-Top (C.A.) (Bernhard)
Glass ampules filled with one of the following solutions and covered with removable cap:
Mercurochrome 2%; Mercurochrome 2% in 25% glycerine; Iodine 3½%; Metaphen (1:200 Tincture); Ferric chloride (for poison ivy); Isopropyl alcohol (for creosote burns).
For use as local antiseptics in various external conditions; *applied* by sprinkling like fountain pen or painting with ampule after slipping off cap.
Supply—Ampules 2 cc, 15 cc—Packages of 6.

Saf-Fast (Bernhard)
A sterile liquid adhesive, resisting water, oil and gasoline; when dried is smooth and keeps bandage clean and fastened. *For use* in fastening bandages by spreading over ends of bandages.
Supply—Tubes, Cans of 1 gal.

Paraco Gauze (McNeil)
A sterilized paraffined gauze netting, 6 in. wide, permitting cutting regardless of meshes and free from loose threads. *For use* as initial dressing to prevent adherence to granulations and permit free drainage.
Supply—Cartons of 1 and 5 yd.

Stannoxyl Gauze (Anglo-French)
Sterile gauze impregnated with Stannoxyl, a compound of tin and tin oxide. *For use* as dressing in boils, styes, pustular acne, suppurating wounds of bones, breasts, tubercular infections.
Supply—In packages

Gelatin Compound Phenolized (C.A.) **(Sharp and Dohme)**
Contains gelatin 625 parts, zinc oxide 250 parts, glycerin and water each 1,900 parts, phenol 1½%; an antiseptic dressing for the preparation of bandages for chronic ulcers and burns; also as special bandage for varicose veins, medically treated. *Administered* by warming the liquid and applying with brush; is covered with bandage and reapplied; repeated for 3–4 layers.

CHAPTER XI

THERAPEUTIC GUIDE

The Therapeutic Guide is designed to assist the practitioner in the ready choice of a desirable remedy for a particular purpose.

In Part I all previously described products are classified: (1) *Chemically*—as all arsenical, iodine, silver, bismuth, sulphur preparations, etc. and (2) *Pharmacologically*—presenting all preparations of similar function or purpose, as antacids, antiluetics, laxatives, parasiticides, uricolytics.

Part II presents many preparations popular in each Specialty with brief descriptions for their use.

Part III enumerates diseases with the preparations found serviceable in their treatment.

PART I

CLASSIFICATION*

Chemical and Pharmacologic

Acidophilus Preparations

Acados
Acidophilus Blocks
Bacid Culture
B. Acidophilus Milk
B. A. Culture
B. A. Lactose-Dextrin Mixture
B. A. Liquid
Condensed Acidophilus
Lactobacillus
Lactobacillus Culture
Neo Acidophilus
Neocultol

Bacillus Bulgaricus

Virilus

Agar Preparations

Agar
Agar Agar
Agarol
Albagar
Analax
Kasagra
Petrolagar
Regulin

Allergens

Bacterials
Epidermals
Feathers
Foods
Furs
Inhalants
Pollens

Alteratives

Alterative Compound
Armervenol
Armicol
Aurocol
Aurol
Cali-Chlorides
Chionacea
Collosol Iodine
Delbiase
Ecthol
Elarson
Elixir Arsylene Compound
Elixir Iodo-Bromide of Calcium Comp.
Gray's Glycerine Tonic Compound
Guaiacose
Hagee's Original Cordial Comp.
Iodia
Metatone
Neo-Riodine
Optarson
Orargol
Solarson
Syr. Hypophosphite of Sodium
Vito Lecithin

* For Complete Descriptions of the Following Drugs See Previous Chapters

Amebacides

Acetarsone
Anayodin
Carbarsone
Chiniofon
Paroxyl
Quinoxyl
Stovarsol
Vioform

Analgesics, Systemic

Acetidine
Acetonyl
Allonal
Alphebin
Amarbital
Amatin
Amifeine
Amphenal
Ampydin
Anacin
Analgine
Aspirofein
Aspiro-lithine
Barbenzal
Barmidon Tablets
Barmiphen Capsules
Butyl Chloral Hydrate
Calcium Benziodoxyl
Cannabine Tannate
Cibalgine
Cinchophen
Colchicum Comp.
Combinal
Compral
Darol
Guphen
Gynalgos
Ichthamol
Magnespirin
Melubrin
Mesotan
Methenos
Neomagnephen
Optalidon
Panalgyn
Peralga
Phenacetin
Pheno-Bromate
Pyramidon
Pyraminal
Salcetol
Sal-Ethyl Carbonate
Salipyrin
Salophen
Salysal
Silosan
Spirosal
Tolysin
Tongaline
Valital

Analgesics, Local

Amphenal
Analgesic Balm
Anesthesin
Anesthone Cream Improved
Apothesine
Auralgan (ear)
Benacol Solution
Butesin Picrate
Butesin
Camphro-Salyl Amp.
Coryfin
Ethyl Salicylate
Ichthamol
Mentholic Comp.
Menthol-Y
Numotizine
Orthoform
Panthesin Ointment
Poison Ivy Balm
Sal-Ethyl
Trichlorethylene

Anesthetics

1. *Local*

Adrocaine
A-L-A
Alypin
Anesthesin
Antidolorin
Apothesine
Benzyl Alcohol
Benacol
Benzoinol
Beta-Eucaine Hydrochloride
Beta-Eucaine Lactate
Borocaine
Butesin
Butesin Picrate
Butyn
Chlorbutanol
Chloretone
Holocain
Kelene
Larocaine
Metycaine
Neocaine
Novocaine
Nupercaine
Oleothesine
Pantocain
Parathesin
Phedrocaine
Phenol-Procaine
Procaine
Procaine-Borate and Epinephrin
Quinine and Urea Hydrochloride
Trichlorethylene

2. *Spinal*

Apothesine
Gravocain
Novocaine
Nupercaine
Pantocain
Spinocain
Tutocain

3. *Rectal*

Avertin
Barb-Eth-Oil (Obstetrical)
Barb-Eth-Oil (Surgical)
Rectal Analgesia (Gwathmey)

4. *General*

Carbon Dioxide-Oxygen Mixtures
Kelene
Lennox-Ethylene

5. *Preoperative*

Pantopon
Pentobarbital Sodium
Phenobarbital Sodium
Pernoston
Sodium Amytal
Veronal-Sodium

Anhidrotics

Betanaphthol
Salvysate
Syr. Histosan

Antacids, Gastric

Alcaroid
Alkacarb
Alucol
Bicarbonate of Soda
Bisodol
Bismutose
Bisurated Magnesia
Cal-Bis-Ma
Calcium Bismuth Compound
Calcium Peroxide
Calcol
Calmoxide
Carbovescent
Cerogen
Citro-Sodine
Combined Carbonates
Compound
Cremo-Carbonates
Entacarb
Gastro-Gallate
Gingament
Lac Bismo
Magnesium Peroxide
Neogestin
Neutralizing Cordial
Neutralon
Oxinol
Oxycaine
Peroxoids
Pulvis Alkantis
Soda Mint Tablets
Soda Mint and Pepsin
Sodinco

Antacids, Systemic

Alcaroid
Alka-Carb
Alvesen
Bisurated Magnesia
Calsoma
Cal-so-mag
Collosol Lactalumina
Collosol Lactomagnesia
Cremo Carbonates
Diskets Alkaline
Entacarb
Macarbo
Magnesium Peroxide
Magnesium Phosphate Tribasic
Milk of Magnesia
Neutralon
Peroxoids
Sodinco
Thialion

Antiarthritics

1. *Resolvents*

Alycin
Amiodoxyl Benzoate
Ami-Salox
Ampule "Reipar"
Befsal
Calcium Benziodoxyl
Diskets Sodium Salicylate Comp.
Farastan
Oxyl-Iodide
Oxo-ate
Oxo-ate B
Phytosalicyl
Panalgyn

2. *Vaccines*

See chapter on Vaccines

3. *Systemic*

Activin
Amp "Repiar"
Colsul
Omnadin
Proteolac
Selencol
Synodal

4. *Symptomatic*

Alycin
Anacin
Analeptine
Atophan
Atoquinol
Chloroxyl
Cincho-Iodide
Cinchophen
Colchi-Sal
Diskets-Sodium Salicylate Comp.
Guphen
Iodoxyl
Manakali
Mesotan
Natural Salicylate
Neocinchophen
Neomagnephen
Nopirine
Novaspirin
Panalgin
Piperazine
Salicin
Salicionyl
Salicylic Acid and Colchicine Comp
Salit
Salophen
Silosan
Spiroform
Tartar-Lithine

Antiluetics

1. *Arsenicals*

Acetarsone
Arsphenamine
Diarsenol
Neoarsphenamine
Neodiarsenol
Neosalvarsan
Sodium Diarsenol
Tryparsamide

2. *Bismuth Preparations*

Bicreol
Biliposol
Bi-Na-Gluconate
Bisempco Cream
Bismarsen
Bismodide
Bismogenol
Bismocymol
Bismoid
Bismol
Bismosol
Bismuthoidol
Bismuth Salicylate
Bisocol
Bi-Sod-Tartrate
Metallic Bismuth
Iodobismitol
Iodobismuth of Quinine
Iodobismuthate of Quinine
Oleo-Bi
Potassium Bismuth Tartrate with Butyn
Potassium Mercuric Iodide
Sol-Bi

3. *Mercurials*

Calomelol
Collosol Hydrargyrum
Flumerin-H
Merciol
Mercurials
Mercurocol
Mercury Benzoate
Mercury Oxycyanide
Mercury Salicylate
Mercurettes
Mercurosal
Mercurol
Mercury Succinimide
Mergal
Mesurol

4. *Iodides*

Collosol Iodine
Iodo-Alboid
Katolox
Naiodine
Neo-Riodine
Quiniobine
Tartro-Quiniobine

5. *Mixed Therapy*

Bismarsen
Iodobismitol
Mesurol
Red Mercuric Iodide
Silver Salvarsan
Sulfarsphenamine

Antimony Preparations

Anticol
Antimony Thioglycollamide
Antimony and Potassium Tartrate
Collosol Antimony
Neostam
Sodium Antimony Thioglycocholate

Antiphlogistics

Alkanite
Antiphlogistine
Ichthamol
Ichthynat
Icthyol
Inoton
Mazon
Thigenol

Antipruritics

Benzyl Alcohol
Calmitol
Dermocaine
Eczemol
Ekzebrol
Gynergen
Ichthymall
Ichthynat
Ichthyol
Inoton
Isarol
Mazon
Mycozol
Panthesin
Sarcoptal
Thigenol
Thiol
Tricotox

Antipyretics

Amatin
Amifeine
Amosol
Ampydin
Antifebrin
Barmiphen
Camphor Compound
Cibalgine
Coco-quinine
Colchicum Compound
Cryogenine
Darol
Elixir Aspiral
Empirin
Euquinine
Magnespirin
Melubrin
Phenacetin
Pyramidon
Quinine Camphor Compound
Quinisal
Saladin
Salysal
Salipyrin
Tolysin

Antiseptics

Acecolex
Acriflavine
Acriflavine Neutral
Acriviolet
Alkanite
Alquinco
Argyn
Aristol
Alpha-Naphco
Argentiform
Argocol
Argolaval
Argyrol
Benzosol
B. F. I. Powder

Antiseptics.—(*Continued*)

Bismuth Thymol Iodide
Bismuth Violet
Borolyptol
Cali-chlorides
Causticks
Calcium Peroxide
Camphenal
Chlomine
Chloramine
Chlorine Gas
Chlorazene
Collene
Collargol
Collosol Ichthyol
Collosol Argentum
Collosol Chlor-Carvacrol
Collosol Palladium
Collosol Trimine
Cupristicks
Camphenal
Dermalgen
Dermalin
Dibromin
Dihydranol
Dioxogen
Eupinol
Euresol
Formalin
Formin
Germicidal Discs
Gentian Violet
Hegonon
Hexylresorcinol
Hychlorite
Hydrosal
Ichthyol
Ichthorcin
Ichthymall
Ichtholdine
Inoton
Iodosyl
Isarol
Iodomuth
Kalmerid Germicidal Tablets
Lenigallol
Lar-Io-Ben
Liantral
Lunosol
Lysol
Mangacol
Mebluco
Meroxyl
Metabol
Metaphen
Mercurophen
Merthiolate
Mercurosticks
Mercurochrome 220
Neorobin
Neo-Reargon
Neo Silvol
Noviform
Orphol
Physillin
Pixalbol
Proflavine
Protargol
P-Thiocresol
Pyrozone
Quicamphol
Reargon
Resorcinol
Rivanol
Saf-T-Top Antiseptics
Silvogon
Sodium Perborate
Sodium Peroxide
Solargentum
Silver Nitrate
Strontium Peroxide
Silvol
Stypsticks
Sulphocol
Sulfidal
Sublamine
Thigenol
Tricotox
Vioform
Vivargin
Xeroform

Antispasmodics

Alepsal
Allisatin
Antiasthmatic
Asthmolysin
Aubromid
Belladenal
Bellafoline
Benzyl Aromatic
Benzene Medicinal
Benzyl Benzoate
Benzyl Fumarate
Benzyl Succinate
Bromsalizol
Bulbocapnine Hydrochloride
Camphogen
Compral
Cypress Oil
Dial
Diatussin
Dioviburnia Compound
Dysco
Elixir Ma Huang
Ephcaben
Ephetal
Ephedrine
Epinephrine
Epinine
Esterol
Felsol
Glyco-Cypress
Luminal
Lumodrin
Mentholic Compound
Neonal
Novatropine
Nurobromyds
Orthoben
Papaverine Hydrochloride
Pertussin
Somnos
Spasmolysin
Suxiphen
Theominal

Aphrodisiacs

Aphrodin Tablets
Cannabin Compound
Forto-Testin
Orchaton
Remogland
Testogan
Thelygan
Yohimboid
Yohimbin

Arsenicals

Acetarsone
Arsenocol
Arsenoferratose
Arsphenamine
Carbarsone
Collosol Arsenic
Diarsenol
Elarson
Elixir Arsylen Compound

Arsenicals.—(*Continued*)

Neoarsphenamine
Neodiarsenol
Neosalvarsan
Neosalvarsan-Glucose
Optarson
Sodium Diarsenol
Solarson
Sulpharsphenamine
Tryparsamide

Astringents

1. *Gastric*

Adsorgan
Alumnol
Bismolan
Bismuth and Anesthesin Compound
Bismuth Hydrate Compound
Collosol Kaolin
Collosol Lactalumina
Gallo-Bismuth Compound
Nepenthe
Gastric Mucin
Gastrosan
Mucin
Silver Lactate
Silver Nitrate-Anesthesin Compound

2. *Intestinal*

Bismogen
Bismutose
Calomel Camphor Compound
Eldoform
Enteri-drastis
Protan
Tannalbin
Tanichthol
Tannigen
Tannismut

3. *Surface*

Amertan
Blenol
Collosol Calamine Lotion
Collosol Lacto-Calamine
Collosol Zinc Cream
Hazeline
Hydrosal
Iodomuth
Lunosol
Red Gum
Silargel
Sulphodine
Tannic Acid Spray
Thiol
Zincol
Zinc Perborate
Zinc Permanganate
Zinc Peroxide

4. *Ophthalmic*

Collosol Zinc
Estivin

Bacteriophages

Bacteriophage-Staphylococcus
Bacteriophage-Staphylococcus-Coli
Bacte-Dysenteri-Phage
Bacte-Intesti-Phage
Bacte-Coli-Phage
Bacte-Pyo-Phage Polyvalent
Bacte-Staphy-Phage
Bacte-Rhino-Phage
Ento-Jel
Ento-Lysate
Staphylo-Jel
Staphylo-Lysate
Strepto-Jel
Strepto-Lysate
Colo-Jel (Combined)
Bio-Cream
A-Vee 51 Preparation
A-Vee 11 Preparation
A-Vee 52 Preparation
A-Vee 12 Preparation
Polyvalent Staphylococcus Bacteriophage

Bismuth Preparations

Bicreol
Biliposol
Bi-na-gluconate
Bisempco Cream
Bismarsen
Bismo-Cymol
Bismodide
Bismogenol
Bismoid
Bismol
Bismosol
Bismuth Anesthesin Compound
Bismuth Hydrate Compound
Bismuthoidol
Bismuth Salicylate
Bismuth Sodium Tartrate
Bismuth Violet
Bismutose
Bisocol
Bi-Thymol Iodide
Iodo-Bismitol
Iodo-Bismutholate of Quinine
Iodo-Bismuth of Quinine
Iodomuth
Kaomin
Metallic Bismuth
Mesurol
Oleo-Bi
Potassium Bismuth Tartrate
Quiniobine
Sol-Bi
Thio-Bismol
Tartro Quiniobine
Vivargen

Bromine Preparations

Aubromid
Brometone
Bromhosal
Bromidia
Bromidonna Elixir
Bromiphen Elixir
Bromionyl
Bromipin 10 %
Bromo-adonis

Bromine Preparations.—(*Continued*)

Bromocol
Bromo-Mangan
Brosedan
Collosol Bromide
Collosol Bromoform Compound
Diskets Bromides
Diskets Sodium Bromide Compound
Elixir Bromo-valerianate Compound
Neurobromyds
Peacock's Bromides
Pentabromides
Sedobrol
Sabromine
Solmides

Calcium Preparations

Afenil
Calcidin
Calcilact
Calcionates
Calciphos
Calcium Gluconate
Calcium Granular
Calcium Lactophosphate
Calcium Levulinate
Calcium Phosphate Tribasic
Calcol
Calglucon
Chloro Calcium
Collosol Calcium
D.C.P. 340
Elixir Neurogenic
Glucal
Gluco-Calcium
Iodicalcium
Neofosfan
Parathyroid with Calcium Lactate
Phytine
Syrup Hypophosphites of Calcium
Syrup Hypophosphites of Lime and Soda
Tetanol Collosol
Thyrocalx

Cell Proliferants

Acecolex
Amfetin
Dermalin
Dimazon
Enzymol
Neorobin
P-Thiocresol
Scarlet R Salve

Chaulmoogra Preparations

Chaulmestrol
Moogrol

Cholagogues

Ago-Cholan
Amisalox
Atophan
Betaphos
Bilein
Bile Salts
Bile Salts Compound
Bilina
Bilival
Bilox
Bisalco
By-Kem
Cascarine Compound
Cholaphen
Choleol
Cholphenolate
Chionacea
Colactol
Colalin
Decholin
Evacuant
Exicol
Felamine
Gallo-gogue
Glycotauro
Hepatone
Icterosan
Kolagog
Neocinchophen
Nuchol
Ovagal
Oxachol
Oxiphen
Pancrobilin
Phenobilin
Phenosagra
Phospho-Soda
Pthalox
Sodium Glycocholate Comp.
Taurocol
Taurophen
Thaleocolates
Tyloid
Veracolate
Zilatone

Cod Liver Oil and Concentrates

1. *Concentrates*

Accessorone
Adex Tablets
Cod Liver Oil Concentrate
Cod Liver Oil Concentrate "White"
Codamines
Cod Liver Oil and Concentrate
Vitamin Concentrate Cod Liver Oil

2. *Oils*

Cod Liver Oil with Viosterol 10D and 250D
Cod Liver Oil Emulsion
Cod Liver Oil, Norwegian
Cod Liver Oil
Emulsion Metagen and Cod Liver Oil
Gaduol Cordial
Irradol A
Kepler's Cod Liver Oil
Marinol
Morotol
Morrhuol Chapoteaut
Myeladol
Novatone
Oscodal
Super-D-Cod Liver Oil
Vitamexol

Contraceptives

Aseptovols
Chiniofon
Duofoam
Fomos
Lactin Preparations
Normolactol
Ortho-Gynol
Oxyquinoline Sulfate
Vaginal Suppository

Copper Preparations

Collosol Cuprum
Cupramin
Cuprico
Cuproglobin
Cupriferrum

Counterirritants

Absorbine, Jr.
Betulol
Balmogen
Colloplasma
Ethidol
Libradol
Mustarx
Numotizine
White Liniment

Creosote Preparations

Benzosol
Calcreose
Creosotal
Creosote Carbonate
Creosotide
Creo-Terpin
Creothyol
Duotal
Guaiacol Compound
Guaiacose
Guaiaphedra
Guaiaphon
Guaiatonic
Guphen
Neodyne
Proposote
Syrup Guaiacol Ammonium Comp.
Syrup Histosan
Thiocol

Detoxicants

Adsorgan
Kaylene
Merrillized Yeast
Occy-crystine
Silargel
Sodium Thiosulphate
Soricin
Sulfactol

Dextrose Preparations

Dextrose
See also Ampules
Dextrose-Ringer's Concentrate

Diagnostic Agents

Bromsulphalein
Ergamine
Fluorescein
Histamine
Phenolsulphonphthalein
Phenoltetrachlorphthalein
Phloridzin
Tetrabromphenolphthalein Sodium
Tetraiodophenolphthalein Sodium
Trichophytin Extract

Digestives

1. *Gastric*

Acidone
Alkarhein
Bisodol
Cagestol Elixir
Carminzym
Caroid Powder
Chymogen
Caripeptic Liquid
Elixir of Enzymes
Enzymol
Essence of Pepsin
Gastrogen Tablets
Gastron
Holadin
Pepsencia
Pepetal
Peptonizing Tubes
Pepana
Peptenzyme
Rennett

2. *Intestinal*

Alcaroid
Amylgestin
Boerenzyme
Cagestol Elixir
Cellasin
Diastase
Digestone Elixir
Diazyme Glycerole
Duodenin
Elixir Maltopepsin
Enzymatase
Extract Pancreatis
Enzymes Solution
Elixir Caricans
Glyco-Hydrastin
Liquor Diastos
Liquid Diastase
Liquenzyme
Luizyme
Lactopeptine
Panopsin
Panacoids
Pan-bis-cal
Pankreon
Panteric Preparations
Papain
Panpeptic Elixir
Pancreo-Bismuth and Pepsin
Peptogenic Powder
Protenzamyl
Taka-Diastase
Trypsin
Trypsogen
Secretogen

Digitalis Preparations

Cactus Compound
Cardysate
Digalen
Digicardalis
Digicardium
Digifoline
Digifortis
Digiglusin
Diginfuse
Diginutin
Digipit
Digipoten
Digitalin
Digitaline "Nativelle"
Digitalis
Digitalis and Duo-Test
Digitalis Leaves Powder
Digitaligen
Digitabs
Digitan
Digitora
Digitos
Digitoxin
Digismith
Digilutea
Elixir Digitalin Compound
Natibaine "Nativelle"
Pulv. Digitalis Folium
Pasanol
Syndrome Tablets

Dioxygen Products

Alphozone
Dioxogen
Manganese Dioxide
Magnesium Peroxide
Octozone
Peroxoids
Sodium Peroxide
Strontium Peroxide
Zinc Peroxide

Disinfectants. Deodorants

Alphozone
Antiformin
Camphenal
Chlomin
Chlorine Gas
Chlorine Soda Ampules
Creolin
Dermalgen
Dioxogen
Di-Phen
Eau-de-Botot
Formalin
Formin
Halazone
Hychlorite
Lysol
Me-Ox-Ol
Nonspi
Octozone
Phenoco
Sublamine
Vioform
Zonite

Diuretics

Agurin
Aminophyllin
Arbutin
Asparagus Comp.
Cymarin
Dialkalos
Diuretin
Diurol
Euphydigtal
Glycine
Hydragogin
Kidnoids
Lithiated Sorghum Comp.
Metaphyllin
Nacitra
Nephroson
Novasurol
Phyllicin
Salyrgan
Scillaren
Solurea
Theamin
Theocalcin
Theocin
Thephyldine
Urea
Uvursin

Dusting Powders

Anazyme Dusting Powder
Aristol
B.F.I. Powder
Bismuth Thymol Iodide
Borated Talcum
Camphaseptic Powder
Chlomine Powder
Chloramine Powder
Chlorazene Surgical Powder
Dermalgen Powder
Dimazon Powder
Drosine
Golden Powder
Iodoformal Powder
Inoton Powder
Kora Konia
Lorate
Noviform Powder
Orphol
Orthoform
Protonuclein Powder
Quinothesine Powder
Salamene-X
Surgical Powder
Tinapo
Vioform Powder
Vulnerine
Xeroform Powder

Ear Drops

An-Gly-Flav
Auralgan
Auraline
Otalgyne

Emollients

Amertan
Anemollient
Anesthone Cream
Antiseptic Baby Oil
Aquafor
Blandine Compound
Borofax
Chloretone Emollient
Emoleo
Gastric Mucin
Paraffine Comp.
Parresine
Sunburn Lotion

Endocrines

Endocrines Uniglandular
Endocrines Pluriglandular Groups 1–30

Ephedrine Preparations

Adrephine Compounds
Butyn-Ephedrine Sol.
Dysco Tablets
Elixir of Ephedrine
Ephedrin-Butesin Jelly
Ephedrin-Butesin Spray 1
Ephedrin-Butesin Spray 2
Ephedrine
Ephedrine and Amytal
Ephedrine Hydrochloride
Ephedrine Inhalant Comp.
Ephedrine Nasal Ointment
Ephetal Tablets
Ethyl-Morphine and Ephedrine Comp.
Metaphedrin Aqueous
Metaphedrin Inhalant

Ergot Preparations

Ergamin
Ergot Aseptic
Ergotoxine
Ernutin
Gynergen

Expectorants

Anastil
Angier's Emulsion
Bromoform Bronchial Anodyne Comp.
Bronchol
Calcreose
Caloxidine
Cerose
Cheracol with Codein
Creothyol
Chiquenia
Coci-Codein
Collosol Bromoform Comp.
Creo-Terpin
Di-Efrin
Ethyl Morphine and Ephedrine Comp.
Euphillana
Euphorbia Comp. Syrup
Expectorant
Glykeron
Glypectus
Guaiacol Comp.
Hyotole
Iocol
Kigo
Kresival
Linctus Comp.
Loingia
Maltine with Yerba Santa
Mar-Phedaco
Mobe
Neodyne
Orthoben
Pertussin
Pine and Somnos Cordial
Pinus-Codeia
Polygalysate
Sanguinaria Comp.
Sedaco
Sedatole
Suxiphen
Syr. Ammon. Hypophosphite
Syr. Ephedrine Hydrochloride
Syr. Guaiacol Ammonium Comp.
Syr. Histosan
Terpazone
Thiate
Thiocol
Toluphen
Tritussis
Yerba Santa-Creo Comp.
Yersanco

Foods

Beverages
Breads
Bread Stuffs
Breakfast Foods
Concentrated Milks
Crackers, Wafers, etc.
Flours
Food Accessories
Lactic Acid Milk
Milk Modifiers
Powdered Foods
Powdered Milks
Soups
Vegetables, Fruits
Whole Milks

Gastric Hydrochloric Acid Substitutes

Acidol
Acidol-Pepsin
Acidone
Acidulin
Betaine-Hydrochloride
Oxyntin

Gold Preparations

Allochrysine
Aubromid
Aurocol
Aurol
Collodaurum
Collosol Aurum
Gold Sodium Thiosulphate
Orargol
Triphal

Halibut Liver Preparations

Collosol Brand Halibut Liver Oil
Halibut Liver Oil Undiluted
Haliver Oil
Haliver Oil in Viosterol
Haliver Oil Plain
Haliver Oil with Viosterol 250D
Haliver Oil Plain and with Viosterol

Hematinics

Accessorone
Armicol
Arsenocol
Arsenoferratose
Bone Medulla
Cali-Chlorides
Cofron
Cofron Liver Extract
Collosol Arsenic
Collosol Cuprum
Collosol Ferro-Malt
Collosol F.C.V.D.
Collosol Ferro-Arsenicum and combinations
Collosol Ferro-Manganese Arsenic
Collosol Ferrum
Copfertabs
Copper Iron Comp.
Cupramin
Cupricol
Cupriferrum
Cuproglobin
Elarson
Elixir I.A.S.
Elixir Arsylene Comp.
Endomin Tablets
Extract Red Bone Marrow
Ferric Ammonium Citrate
Ferriquin
Ferro-Ca-Mang
Ferrocol
Ferro-Cop
Ferrodine
Ferro-Elarson
Ferro-Manganese Peptonated
Ferro-Mangan Peptonized
Ferrophytine
Ferruginous Comp.
Food Ferrin
Gastron with Iron
Haemobuminate
Hemaboloids
Hemaboloids Arseniated with Strychnia
Hemec Tablets
Hemogenin
Hemoglobin
Hemoglobin Comp.
Hemoquinine
Hemo-Nucleo-Spleen Comp.
Hemo-Vitol
Idozan
Iodo-Mangan
Iron Citrate Green
Iron Lactate
Maltine with Iron Iodide
Mancuhemin
Manganese Dioxide
Neobovinine 20
Neoferrum
Neurempco 3
Neurempco 4
Neurempco 8
Neurotrophol
Neusthenic "Fraisse"
Novatone
Optarson
Ovoferrin
Panopeptin Ferruginous
Pepto-Mangan
Pepto-Mangan "Gude"
Phos-hepatic Extract
Pulvules Lextron 55
Siderol
Solarson
Solbumin
Syr. Hypophosphites of Iron and Quinine
Syr. Hypophosphite of Manganese
Susto
Triglucon
Waterbury's Comp.

Hemopoietics

Cofron
Cofron Elixir
Concentrated Liver Extract
Concentrated Liver Extract with Iron
Erythgen Liver Extract
Extralin
Hemo-S
Hepati-Cole
Hepaticon
Hepatrat
Jeculin
Liver Extract
Liver Extract 29
Liver Extract 343
Liver Extract 55
Stomachon
Ventriculin
Liver Extract 95
Liver Extract A 5
Liver Extract 100 X
Liver Extract Plain
Liver Extract with Iron
Liver Extract Oral
Liver Extract Subcutaneous
Liver Meal

Hemostatics and Styptics

Adrenalin
Adrin
Calcilact
Calcium Gluconate
Ceanothyn
Chloro-Calcium
Coagulen
Fibrogen, Local, Oral and Subcutaneous
Hazeline
Hemagulen
Hemostatic Serum
Hydrastinin
Kephalin
Normal Horse Serum
Pitocin
Pituitary Solution
Pituitrin
Stypticin
Styptysate
Tenamin
Thromboplastin
Trillin

Hormone Extracts

Agomensin
Amniotin
Ampacoids
Anabolin
Anteri-Cole
Antophysin
Antuitrin-S
Eschatin
Follutein
Iodobesin
Nephritin
Ovarialhormone Folliculin
Parathormone
Paroidin
Pitocin
Pitressin
Pituitary Extract
Pituitrin

Hormone Extracts.—(*Continued*)

Plestrin
Progynon
Protonuclein
Sistomensin
Suprarenalin
Theelin
Theelol
Thelestrin
Thyracoids
Thyractin
Thyroxin
Thyroxin Synthetic

Hypnotic Preparations

Adalin
Adalin-Luminal
Alepsal
Allonal
Alphebin
Alurate
Amarbital
Amytal
Amytal and Sodium
Baramid
Barbromid
Brometone
Bromidia
Butyl-Chloral Hydrate
Chloretone
Combinal
Dial
Hypno-Bromic Comp.
Ipral
Lumalgin
Luminal
Luminal Sodium
Medinal
Neonal
Neuronidia
Neurosine
Nostal
Ortal Sodium
Pentobarbital Sodium
Pernoston
Phenobarbital Sodium
Phanodorn
Pyraminal
Recvalysate
Sandoptal
Somnos
Sulphonal
Trional
Veronal
Veronal Sodium

Hypotensives

Alepsal
Anabolin
Arsclero
Bromsalizol
Cucurbocitrin
Diasystol
Diciturin
Hepvisc
Hypotan
Hypotens "Fraisse"
Kacyan
Kathesina
Liver Extract
Nitrobar
Nitrocon
Nitrophen
Nitroscleran
Pulvoids Natrico
Thiocyan Elixir

Infants' Foods

1. *Baby Soups*

Baby Soup
Liver Soup
Dri-Malt Soup Extract
Malt Soup Extract

2. *Cereals*

Mead's Cereal
Ralston Wheat Cereal
Baby Ralston
Gerber's Strained Cereal

3. *Concentrated Milk*

Concentrated Liquid Skim Milk
Lactogen
Nestle's Food
Pet Milk
S.M.A. Concentrated Liquid Milk

4. *Lactic Acid Milk*

Powdered Lactic Acid Milk Plain
Powdered Lactic Acid Milk with Dextri-Maltose
Powdered Whole Lactic Acid Milk

5. *Milk Modifiers*

Alerdex
Casec
Citabs
Dexin
Dextri-Maltose 1, 2, 3
Dextri-Maltose with Vitamin B
Dextrolac
Dextro-Vitavose
Hylac
Larosan
Malt-Sugar
Protolac
Smaco, Maltose and Dextrins

6. *Powdered Milk*

Alacta
Dryco
Recolac
Powdered Protein Milk
Similac
S.M.A.

7. *Powdered Foods*

Maltcao
Malted Milk
Sobee

8. *Skimmed Milk*

Hypo-Allergic Skim Milk	Powdered Half Skimmed Milk	Powdered Skimmed Milk
	Powdered Skim Milk	Powdered Skimmed Lactic Acid Milk

9. *Vegetables*

Gerber's Strained Vegetables	Nutradiet Vegetables	Canned Vegetables
	Sieved Vegetables	Strained Vegetables
	Spinach Concentrate	

10. Whole Milk

Concentrated Liquid Whole Milk	Klim Powdered Whole Milk	Powdered Whole Milk
Hypo-Allergic Whole Milk		Whole Milk Sterilized

Insulin Preparations

Iletin		Insulin

Intestinal Antiseptics

Anayodin	Beta Naphthol	Ichthalbin
Benzyl Naphthol Benzoate Comp.	Dimol	Sulfax
	Gastrosan	Sulofen

Intestinal Stimulants

Duodenin	Prostigmin	Secretogen
Peristaltine		

Iodine Preparations

Alterative Comp.	Idocol	Miscidine
Anayodin	Iodalbin	Naiodine
Aquadine	Iodex	Neo-Riodine
Atomidine	Iodicalcium	Organidin
Bismodide	Iodine Ointment	Oridine
Calcidin	Iodia	Providin Tablets
Collosol Iodine	Iodicin	Riodine
Elixir Iodo-Bromide of Calcium Comp.	Iodo-Casein	Sajodin
	Iodostarine	Soluble Iodine
Ethidol	Iodo-Peptonoids	Sulfodine
Ethyl Iodide	Iodosyl	Stearodine
Fer-Iodine	Iodotone	Surgodine
Ferrodine	Iothion	Syr. Hydriodic Acid
Ferro-Sajodin	Katolox	Tiodine
Homiodin	Lipoiodine	

Laxatives

Agar	Flamin-Ol	Occy-Crystine
Agar Agar	Haley's M-O	Pamol
Agarol	Hepatic Saline	Para-Psyllium
Alaxa	Hepatone	Phospho-Soda
Albagar	Hygem	Psylla
Albolene	Isacen	Psyllium
Analax	Kaosyl	Petrobran
Baga	Kasagra	Petrolagar
Brandreth's Pills	Kelpamalt	Pheno-Sagra
Caroid Laxative	Kondremul	Paralax
Colactin	Lapactic Pill	Paroleine
Collosol Sulfur-Paraffin Emulsion	Laxamel	Peristaltine
	Maltine with Mineral Oil and Cascara	Pepule Eliminant
Coreine		Pthalox
Evacuant (Biliary)	Mineral Oil Emulsion	Regulin

Laxatives.—(*Continued*)

Rythmin
Saline Laxative
Saraka
Sennetal
Syl-Agg-Ol
Tasteless Castor Oil
Thiocyan Elixir

Lead Preparations

Collosol Lead
Plumbicol
Lead Selenide

Lotions

Collos. Calamine Lotion
Collosol Scalp Lotion—Oily
Collosol Scalp Lotion—Non-oily
Larkspur Lotion
Lotion Calmitol
Poison Ivy Lotion
Sunburn Lotion

Lozenges and Troches

Anesthesin-Calcidin Troches
Acriflavine Throat Troches
Angier's Throat Tablets
Creomint Lozenges
Caloxidine Compound Throat Tablets
Cocoanilid Lozenges
Euphagin
Glucal Lozenges
Guai-Ammon Lozenges
Guaiatan Lozenges
Hexyl Resorcinol Sucrates
Iodithesin Lozenges
Lozenges Benzocaine Comp.
Neutral Acriflavine Throat Troches
Ortho-Troches
Orthesine-Epinephrine Comp.
Orthesine-Iodine Troches
Orthesine-Quinosal Lozenges
Para-Troches
Pastilles
Thantis Lozenges

Lytics

Bichloracetic Acid
Fibrolysin
Iocamfen
Tiodine Cognet

Malt Preparations

A.B.D. Malt Extract with Cod Liver Oil and Viosterol 5D
Albomalt
Kepler's Malt Combinations
Malt Extract Plain
Maltine Plain
Maltine with Cascara
Maltine with Cod Liver Oil
Maltine with Cod Liver Oil and Iron Iodide
Maltine with Creosote
Maltine Ferrated
Maltine with Hypophosphites
Maltine with Iron, Quinine and Strychnine
Maltine with Mineral Oil and Cascara
Maltine with Yerba Santa
Marrow-Malt Comp.
Morotol

Manganese Preparations

Manganese Butyrate
Manganese Dioxide
Mangocol

Mercurials

Armervenol
Calomelol
Collosol Hydrargyrum
Collosol Lead
Colloidal Mercury Sulphide
Flumerin H
Mercurettes
Mercurochrome 222 Sol.
Merciol
Mercurials
Mercurocol
Mercurol
Mercurophen
Mercurosal
Mercury Benzoate
Mercury Cyanide
Mercury Salicylate
Mercury Succinimide
Mergal
Potassium Mercuric Iodide
Red Mercuric Iodide
Salyrgan
Sublamine
Sol Mercury

Mineralizers

Acido Sodium
Alkasal
Alkazane
Carbovescent
Citrocarbonate
Citrico
Citro Soda
Citro Sodine
D.C.P. 340
Delbiase
Diskets
Eupeptic Hypophosphites
Lecithol
Mineral Mixture Tablets 85
Mineralization Tablets
Minerasal
Neurotrophal
P.M.C.
Syr. Hypophosphite of Sodium
Tetra-Citrates
Vito Lecithine

Mineral Oils

Agarol
Albagar Plain
Albagar Compound
Albolene
Albomalt
Blandine Comp.

Mineral Oils.—(*Continued*)

Colactin
Collosol Sulphur Paraffin Emulsion
Fla-Min-Ol
Kaylene-Ol
Kondremul
Liquid Petrolatum with Agar
Maltine with M.O. and Cascara
Mineral Oil Emulsion
Pamol
Paralax
Para-Psyllium
Para-Psyllium with Phenolphthalein
Paroleine
Petrobran
Petrolagar
Petromul
Radolatum

Mineral Waters

Artificial
Domestic
Imported

Mineral Water Salts

Crazy Water Crystals
Ems Mineral Spring Salt
Franzensbad Natural Mud Salt
Karlsbad Bath Salt
Karlsbad Sprudel Salt
Marienbad Natural Spring Salt
Montecatini Iodated Salt
Montecatini Plain Salt

Mydriatics

Euphthalmine
Euphthalmine Hydrochloride
Homatropine Hydrochloride

Narcotics

Dilaudid
Dionin
Ethyl Morphine and Ephedrine Co.
Pantopon
Papaverine and its Hydrochloride
Papine

Nasal Preparations

Adrin Solution
Albomist
Alumnol
Alypin
Argyn
Aristol
Blandine Comp.
Bismuth Violet
Butyn Ephedrine Sol. 2%
Butyn Solution 2%
Cargentos
Chloramine
Chlorazene
Coagulin
Collosol Argentum
Coryfin
Cresatin
Ento-Jel
Ento-Lysate
Ephedrine Inhalant
Ephedrine Inhalant Comp.
Ephedrine Hydrochloride
Hexyl Resorcinol Solution
Larioben
Larocaine
Lunosol
Metaphedrin Inhalant
Metaphen in Oil-C
Neo-Silvol
Noviform
Novocaine
Parathesin
Paroleine Spray Comp.
Protargol
Rivanol
Scarlet Red Medicinal
Silvogon
Silvol
Solargentum
Terpoflor
Tutocaine

Non-specific Therapy Agents

Activin
Aolan
Caseosan
Citrosalven
Colsul
Endo-Mangalac
Hemoprotein "Brooks"
Lac-Proteinate
Lactigen
Lacto-Protein
Manganese Butyrate
Mervenol
Omnadin
Peptone Sol. 5%
Siliform
Spleen Liquid
Synodal
Terpichin
Yatren-Casein

Nucleotides

Adenine Sulphate
Colsul
Leucocyte Extract
Nuclein
Pentnucleotide

Nasal Ointments

Alpha-Naphco Nasal Jelly
Alpha-Naphco Nasal Ointment
Carbolic Acid and Benzoinol Ointment
Compound Camphor and Menthol Ointment
Compound Iodine and Glycerine Ointment
Compound Eucalyptol and Gaultheria Ointment
Ephedrine Jelly
Ephedrine Nasal Jelly
Ephedrine Butesin Jelly
Epinine Nasal Jelly
Ephedrine Sulphate Jelly
Eucalyptol and Benzoinol Ointment
Nasal Cream
Nasal Jelly
Obtundia Nasal Cream
Resorcinol Ointment
Vem

Oral Antiseptics

Absorbine, Jr.
Alphozone
Analka
Antiseptic Gargle
Antiseptic Solution 59
Bonsol
Borocaptol
Borolyptol
Chlorazine
Chloroseptine
Chlorothol Comp.
Collosol Chlor-Carvacrol
Collosol Lacto-Magnesia
Eau De Botot
Hychlorite
Lagarg
Larioben
Medicated Wafers
Me-Ox-Ol
Metoso
Pyrozone
Red Gum
Root Canal Filling
Salvarsan Glucose Solution
Stomaseptine
Tolamine

Oral Diabetic Drugs

Cellasin
Fer-iodine
Glycosuretics
Oralsulin
Pancrasin
Pancrepatine
Pancresal
Pansuline
Trypsogen
Uvursin

Parasiticides

Anticol
Carbon Tetrachloride
Chiniofon
Chinoplasmin
Coco-Quinine
Collosol Arsenic
Collosol Antimony
Collosol Chrysarobin
Euquinine
Iocamfen
Mycozol
Neorobin
Neostam
Plasmochin
Quicamfol
Quinarsin
Salvarsan-Glucose Solution
Soamin
Solvochin
Stovarsol
Trichophytin
Zymocide

Phosphorus Preparations

Eupeptic Hypofosfites
Fortossan
Lecibrin
Lecithin
Lecithin Glycerole
Lecithol
Neo-Fosfan
Neurophosphates "Eskay"
Phospho-Lecithin
Phosphorcin
Phospho-Vitamine B
Phostone
Phytine
Pursang
Robinol

Radiopaque Media

Brominol
Bromipin 33 %
Campiodol Solution
Chole-Cysto-Col
Iodeikon and Emulsion
Iodipin 40 %
Iodochlorol
Iso-Iodeikon
I-X-Barium Meal
Keraphen
Kerakote
Lipiodol
Lipoiodine Diagnostic
Neo-Iopax
Neosilvol
Neo-skiodan
Shadocol
Skiabaryt-Oral
Skiagenol
Skiodan
Solargentum
Tetrabromphenolphthalein Sodium
Tetradol Emulsion
Tetraiodophenolphthalein Sodium
Thorotrast
Umbrathor

Radium Preparations

Radium Salts
Radon

Sclerosing Agents

Episol
Lithium Salicylate 30 %
Quinine Hydrochloride and Urethane
Quinine and Urea Hydrochloride
Quinine and Urethane
Sodium Morrhuate 7 % Sol.
Sodium Morrhuate 5 % with Benzyl Alcohol
Solution Invert Sugar
Vari-Chlor-Ose
Varitose

Sedatives

Gastric

Aerophagyl
Belladenal
Bismuth and Anesthesin Comp.
Blenol
Chlorbutanol
Gastric Mucin
Kaomin
Mucin
Oxycaine
Silver-Nitrate Anesthesin Comp.

General

Abasin
Adalin
Allonal
Baramid
Barbromide
Barlupulin
Bismolate
Brometone
Bromhosal
Bromidia
Bromidonna Elix.
Bromiphen Elix.
Bromo-Adonis
Bromipin 10%
Bromocol
Bromomangan
Bromural
Brosedan
Brovalol
Bulbocapnine Phosphate
Butyl-Chloral Hydrate
Cafumal
Cannabin Tannate
Chamomilla Comp.
Collos. Bromide
Diskets Sodium Bromide Compound
Diskets Sodium Bromides
Elix. Barmival
Elix. Bromo-Valerianate
Elix. Neurogenic
Ephedrine and Amytal
Hypno-Bromic Compound
Ipral
Lecithin Glycerole
Muskola
Neo-Bornyval
Neonal
Nervinal
Neurempco
Neurilla
Neurinase
Neurobromyds
Neuro-Calm
Neuronidia
Neurosine
Optalidon
Ortal Sodium
Pantopon
Pascarnata
Passiflora Compound
Passiphen
Peacock's Bromides
Pentobarbital Sodium
Peralga
Pernoston
Phanodorn
Phenobarbital
Phenobarboid
Prokliman
Pyraminal
Recvalysate
Restophen
Sabromin
Sandoptal
Scopolamine
Sedobrol
Sedormid
Sodium Amytal
Solmides
Somnos
Sulphonal
Trional

Selenium Preparations

Collosol Selenium
Lead Selenide
Selencol Solution
Selenium

Silver Preparations

Argentiform
Argocol
Argolaval
Argyn
Argyrol
Cargentos
Collargol
Collene
Collosol Argentum
Choleval
Hegonon
Ichthargan
Lunosol
Neo-Silvol
Neo-Reargon
Orargol
Protargol
Reargon
Silargel
Silver Lactate
Silver Nitrate
Silver Sal
Silver Salvarsan
Silvogon
Silvol
Siocol
Solargentum
Targesin

Staphylocides

Collosol Manganese
Collosol Stannum
Mangacol
Manganese Butyrate
Man-Na-Gluconate
Stannoxyl
Stanno-Yeast
Stan-Protein
Tinox
Tinoxide
Tinpronate

Stimulants (Cardio-Respiratory)

Adrenalin
Alpha-Lobelin
Cactina Pillets
Cactus Comp.
Cadechol
Camphogen
Coramine
Cymarin
Elixir Digitalin Comp
Ephedrine
Homocamfin
Homo-Camphin
Metrazol
Myorgal
Myoston
Natibaine
Ouabain
Ouabaine "Arnaud"
Passanol
Quinicardine Nativelle
Quinidin
Syndrome Tablets
Verodigen

Sulphur Preparations

Colsul
Ichthymall
Ichthynat
Ichthyol
Sufrogel
Isarol
Sodium Thiosulphate
Sulfactol
Sulfidal
Sulphocol
Thigenol
Thiol
Tiodine

Suprarenal Preparations
See Adrenal Cortex
Medulla
Whole Gland
In Chap. IV, Uniglandular

Suppositories (Rectal)
See Chap. X

Suppositories (Vaginal)
See Chap. X, Vaginal Antiseptics

Tar Preparations

Liantral Casein Ointment
Liantral Ointment
Pixalbol

Tonics, General

A.B.D. Malt Extract
Adgene
Albomalt
Beef Peptone
Beta Lactose
C.C.C. Tonic
Chocolate Vitavose
Coco-Vitamine
Cofron Elixir
Collosol Ferro Malt
Dextrose
Dry Peptonoids
Elixir Arsylen Compound
Elixir Neurogenic
Enemose
Eupeptic Hypophosphites
Ferrophytine
Firolyptol
Gaduol Cordial
Glucose
Glycana
Glycerophan
Gray's Glycerine Tonic Comp.
Hagee's Original Cordial Comp.
Hema-Glycon
Hemol
Holadin
Kola
Liquid Peptonoids
Malt Extract Kepler
Malt Extract Plain
Malt Extract with Cod Liver Oil
Manola
Marrow Malt Comp.
Metatone
Morotol
Myeladol
Neo-Sevetol
Neurotrophol
Neurasthenic Ampule
Novatone
Pabutole
Panopepton
Peptonal
Phospho-Vitamin B
Phostone Elixir
Protonuclein
Robinol
Roboline
Seng
Siderol
Trophonine
Vitafood
Vitamexol
Vito-Lecithin
Wampole's Perfected Preparation

Trypanosomicides

Anticol
Antimony Thioglycollamide
Arsphenamine
Carbarsone
Collosol Arsenic
Formin
Germanin
Neoarsphenamine
Paroxyl
Quinarsen
Quinoxyl
Sodium Antimony Thioglycocholate

Uricolytics

Alkasal
Alvesen
Analeptine
Aspiro-lithine
Atoquinol
Befsal
Calculi-Sol
Carbovescent
Chloroxyl
Cinchophen
Citrico
Dialkalos
Neo-Cinchophen
Piperazine
Salithia
Spiroform
Tartarlithine
Tongaline
Urasal

Urinary Preparations

Acetylcholine Bromide
Acriflavine Neutral
Ambazin
Ammoform
Amylsal
Argolaval

Urinary Preparations.—(*Continued*)

Argyn
Arheol
Arhovin
Atrobutin
Benzoacetate
Benzosol
Buchuform
Caprokol
Coteremul
Chloramine
Chlorazene
Chlorhydrionic with Hexamethylene Tetramine
Clymocol
Collosol Argentum
Collosol Palladium
Collosol Trimine
Dibromin
Formohydrion
Formin
Gentian Violet
Gonosan
Hexalet
Hexarbutin
Helmitol
Hexylresorcinol Solution
Hychlorite
Hyoszea
Kalmerid Germicidal Tablets
Kavalactol
Liquor Santaiva
Lithiated Sorghum Comp.
Lunosol
Mallophene
Mebluco
Mercurochrome
Meroxyl
Metaphen 2500
Metaphen in Oil
Methenos
Methylets
Niazo
Nizin
Phospho Soda
Pyridium
Rivanol
Salihexin
Salysal
Sanmetto
Sanpaiba
Santyl
Serenium
Terogon
Tolamine
Uvalysate
Urasal
Uraseptine
Urethral Bougies and Pencils
  Argentiform Pencils
  Cargentos Bougies
  Collos. Argentum Bougies
  Iodosyl Pencils
  Iodosyl Pencils Mild
  Picratol Bougies
  Silvol Bougies
  Stylolactin Rods
  Unguentum Crede
Uriform
Urocedrol
Urotropin
Utros

Uterine Preparations

Dysmenatone
Emmenagogue
Ergoapiol
Ergot
Ergotoxine
Ernutin
Gynalgos
Gynergen
Genitone
Hayden's Viburnum Comp.
Hydrastinin
Hyperol
Infundin
Liquor Santaiva
Neo Ergot
Ovaritone
Pituitary Extract Solution or Liquid
Tenamin
Thymo Pitsin
Utros
Viburno

Vaccines and Sera

Acne Vaccines
Anthrax Sera
Arthritis Vaccines
Bothrops Antitoxin
Bubonic Plague Vaccines
Cholera Vaccines
Coley Toxins
Colon Vaccines
Crotalus Antitoxins
Diphtheria Toxins
Diphtheria Antitoxins
Diphtheria Toxoids
Diphtheria Tests
Erysipelas Antitoxins
Furunculosis Vaccines
Gas-Gangrene Vaccines and Sera
Gonococcus Vaccines
Influenza Vaccines
Meningococcus Sera
Pertussis Vaccines
Plant Poisoning Sera
Pneumonia Sera and Vaccines
Poliomyelitis Sera
Puerperal Fever Sera
Pyorrhea Vaccines
Rabies Vaccines
Scarlet Fever Sera and Vaccines
Smallpox Vaccines
Staphylococcus Pyogenes Vaccines
Staphylococcus and Streptococcus Mixed Vaccines
Streptococcus Vaccines and Sera
Tetanus Antitoxins
Tetanus-Gas Gangrene Antitoxins
Typhoid Vaccines
Typhoid Parathyroid Vaccines
Ulcerative Colitis Vaccines
Undulant Fever Vaccines
Van Cott's Vaccines

Vasoconstrictors

Adrenalin
Adrin Solution
Ephedrine
Ephedrine Hydrochloride
Ephedrine Salts
Ephedrine Sulphate
Epinephrine
Epinephrine Hydrochloride
Epinine
Infundin
Neo-Synephrine
Pituitary Extract

Pituitary Liquid
Pituitary Solution
Pituitrin
Suprarenalin
Suprarenin
Synephrine Tartrate
Tyramine

Vasodilators

Acecoline
Acetylcholine
Acetylcholine Bromide
Benzedrine Inhaler
Calcium Thiocyanate
Collosol Silica with Drosera Rutondifolia
Diuretin
Erythrol Tetranitrate
Euphydigtal
Haimased
Histamine
Padutin
Potassium Iodo-Theocalcin
Theamin
Theominal
Tissue Extract 568
Viscysate

Vehicles

Elixir Glyconda
Elixir of Enzymes
Elixir of Maltopepsin
Essence of Pepsin
Gastron
Lactopeptine
Liquenzyme
Panpeptic Elixir
Panopepton
Pepsencia
Peptenzyme

Vermifuges

Ascaridole
Benzene
Betanaphthol Benzoate
Butolan
Carbon Tetrachloride
Pelletierine Tannate
Quassin

Vitamines

A.B.D. Malt Extract
Alpha-Betamin
Bemax
B-Vitamines
Caritol
Coco-Vitamine
Crystalline Carotene
Natural Vitamine D
Savita
Tabl. Vitamines A and D
Vegex
Viosterol in Oil 250D
Viosterol
Vitafood
Vitamines A and D

Yeast Preparations

Brewers' Yeast
Brosedan
Cerevisine
Eldoform
Fermogen
Fleischmann's Yeast
Merrillized Yeast
Savita
Stanno Yeast
Vegex
Yeastamine
Yeast Bouillon Cubes
Yeast Capsules
Yeastone

Obesity Preparations

Dextrettes
Dinitrenal Capsules
Iodobesin
Lipolysin
Phytolacca Compound
Remolysin

Part II

Preparations Used in Specialties

Anesthesia

Preparations Used in Anesthesia

1. Spinal Anesthetics

Apothesine: A local anesthetic of the procaine type; used in 4–6% solution, 2 cc.

Gravocain: A 40% novocain solution with strychnine; is of higher specific gravity than spinal fluid; injected *intraspinally*, principally in obstetric cases, with patient in sitting or semi-recumbent position; dose 1 ampule.

Neocaine: A spinal anesthetic; used by dissolving the crystals in the spinal fluid which is permitted to flow directly into ampules; is then slowly injected, aspirated and reinjected.

Nupercaine: A local anesthetic; in caudal anesthesia, 30–35 cc of 1:1,000 solution, or 20–25 cc of 1:500 in physiologic saline.

Pantocain: A 1% solution for use as spinal anesthetic in surgery, urology, otolaryngology and ophthalmology; 1 to 2 cc of ampule preparation, administered in usual manner.

Spinocain: A 10% novocain solution with strychnine sulphate, in a solvent of specific gravity lower than the spinal fluid; 1 ampule *intraspinally*, according to specified technic.

Tutocain: A butamin anesthetic for use in general surgery, gynecology and urology; *intraspinally*, in ½–1% solution.

2. Rectal Anesthetics

Avertin: As basal anesthetic; after preoperative preparation on evening preceding operation, by cleansing enema, mild hypnotic, etc., a maximum dosage of 0.1 cc per kilogram of body weight, the total not to exceed 6–8 cc in the female, 9–10 cc in the male, and with consideration for the debilitated, cachectic and very obese; is administered as high retention enema.

Barb-Eth-Oil: For use in surgical and obstetrical cases, to eliminate fear and induce relaxation; given after cleansing soap-suds enemas and administration of 1 oz. of plain mineral or olive oil; in dosage of 4 oz. for 130 lb. of body weight or over, 3 oz. for 100 to 130 lb., 2 oz. for 100 lb. or less; instilled slowly, taking 20–30 min. for injection.

Rectal Anesthesia (Gwathmey): Is presented in 2 strengths; principally for use in obstetrics; instillation of medication is preceded by the mineral oil accompanying each ampule; is introduced by means of rectal analgesia set supplied with anesthetic.

3. Preoperative Sedatives

Luminal-Sodium: To eliminate fear and apprehension and induce restful sleep; 1 capsule on evening preceding operation; an additional capsule, with or without morphine and atropin ½–¾ hr. immediately before operation; in unusually nervous cases, as in thyroid disease—double dosage.

Ortal Sodium: To effect preoperative sedation; gr 3 four hours and gr 6 one hour before giving general anesthetic.

Pantopon: For preoperative sedation and for control of pain; is administered instead of morphine, ⅓ gr 45 min. before operation.

Pentobarbital-Sodium: Technic and dosage as for Luminal-Sodium.

Pernoston: For use in obstetrics, surgery and gynecology; 1 cc per 12½ kg. of body weight, 1 hr. preoperatively.

Phenobarbital Sodium: Technic and dosage as for Luminal-Sodium.

Sodium Amytal: Surgical cases—1 pulvule orally, at night, and 2–3 pulvules 2 hr. preoperatively; obstetrical—only when cervix is dilated 26 mm, 1 pulvule; a second after 1–4 hr.

Veronal Sodium: In surgical cases; technic as for Luminal-Sodium, but in dosages of 5–8 gr.

4. Inhalation Anesthetics

Carbon Dioxide-Oxygen Mixtures: For use during general anesthesia; administered by usual technic, with special inhalation apparatus.

Kelene: For inhalation anesthesia in minor surgical procedures of short duration; for induction preliminary to ether in major surgical procedures; administered by the open cone method.

Lennox-Ethylene: For induction of deep surgical anesthesia; administered by passing the gas into inhalation apparatus, in proportions by admixture with required amount of oxygen.

5. Local Anesthetics

Adrocain: For local and infiltration anesthesia, in minor surgery and dentistry; Tablets ℞ "A" in 2% solution, ℞ "B" in 1% solution.

A. L. A.: An oily solution used in dentistry for extraction and other painful operations; in medicine—in injection therapy; given intramuscularly or subcutaneously at 5–7 points within a 3 in. circle surrounding the painful area, 0.1–0.5 cc at each point or a total of 1 cc.

Alypin: As surface anesthetic; in cystoscopy 1–4 %, in ophthalmology 2–4 %, in rhinolaryngology 5–10 %.

Anesthesin: Principally for its analgesic effect; dusted on painful ulcers, postoperative wounds.

Antidolorin: For local refrigeration and general inhalation anesthesia in short surgical operations; applied by direct spray, locally; by inhalation mask, internally.

Apothesine: In nerve block and pressure anesthesia; subcutaneously, 0.5–2 % with adrenalin, in sterile water or physiologic saline.

Benacol Solution: In anal pruritus; *subcutaneously* or submucously, never into skin; 1 ampule, injected slowly in fan-shaped manner, repeated in 5 days.

Beta-Eucaine Hydrochloride: In minor surgery *subcutaneously,* 1 % solution; in sciatica injected perineurally.

Beta-Eucaine Lactate: In regional anesthesia. in 2–5 % solution; as infiltration anesthetic, in 0.12 % solution.

Borocaine: In dental root canal work, 1–2 cc of 2 % solution; in infiltration anesthesia, ½–1 %; in nerve block 1–2 %; in minor surgery ½–1 %; topically from 2–10 %, as required.

Butesin: As surface anesthetic in ulceration, sore throat, minor surgical and dental affections; applied freely as dusting powder.

Butesin Picrate: For use in abrasions, ulcers, extensive burns and other destructive surface injuries; applied as 5 % powder, 1 % ointment.

Butyn: For use in dentistry, genitourinary surgery, ophthalmology and rhinology; as infiltration anesthetic in general surgery; in the eye, in 2 % solution for topical use, in profound anesthesia 5 %; in nose and throat, 2 % solution; in infiltration anesthesia, ¼–1/10 %; in genitourinary work, in 1 % solution for topical uses.

Chlorbutanol: In dentistry, nose and throat disorders, hypodermically, in saturated aqueous solution; also as preanesthetic sedative—0.3–1.3 Gm, in capsules or dry.

Holocain: As ocular surface anesthetic in 1 % solution.

Kelene: As local refrigeration anesthetic, by spray.

Larocaine: As surface anesthetic; in ophthalmology, 2–5 % solution; in nose and throat work, 5–10 %; in urology, for vesical anesthesia, 30–50 cc, ¾–1 %; in general surgery, ½–1 %, occasionally ¼–2 % solution.

Metycaine: As local anesthetic on skin and mucous membranes; by instillation and infiltration, in 2–4 % solution.

Neocaine: In local and regional anesthesia in 1 % solution.

Novocain: In infiltration anesthesia ¼–½ %; for nerve block, 1 % solution; in nose and throat work, ½–1 % solution with suprarenin 1:1,000 in concentration of 3–5 m per ounce; in ophthalmology, conduction and infiltration, 2 % solution.

Nupercaine: For infiltration and nerve block in general, 1:2,000 to 1:1,000 solution, with epinephrine hydrochloride; in nose and throat conditions—as spray, 1:500–1:200, as anesthetic—1–2½ % solution; in ophthalmology—1:1,000–1:200; in genitourinary work—1:1,000 to 1:500 solution.

Pantocain: As surface anesthetic, ¼, ½, 1, 2 % solution, with or without suprarenin.

Parathesin: As surface anesthetic in the surgical treatment of wounds, burns, ulcers, bed sores and similar lesions 5–20 %, in oily solution or ointment; in rhinology as spray or swab 3–20 % in oily or alcoholic solution.

Procaine: In dentistry for conductive anesthesia 2 % (intra and extra nerve block); in medicine, for infiltration anesthesia—1–2 %; for contact and high pressure, infiltration, intraosseous, peridental, subperiosteal, for nerve block, direct and perineural ½–1 %; as urethral anesthetic 5 %.

Procaine Borate and Epinephrin: Same strength as Procaine; in medical and dental anesthesia.

Quinine and Urea Hydrochloride: For nerve blocking and infiltration, especially in pruritus ani or vulvae, ¼ % solution.

Trichlorethylene: As inhalation analgesic, in trigeminal neuralgia.

Cardiology

Preparations Used in Cardiac Disturbances*

Adrenalin and Adrin: In shock and collapse 5 drops 1:1,000 solution in 1 oz. normal saline *intravenously*, slowly; in severe cases—by centripetal transfusion; in suspended animation—0.5–1 cc intracardially.

Alpha Lobelin: As respiratory stimulant in anesthesia accidents and asphyxia neonatorum, ½–1 ampule, *intramuscularly* or *intravenously;* in surgical shock, collapse, deetherization, prostration, drug and morphine poisoning, 1 ampule or gr ¼ as required *intramuscularly* or *subcutaneously;* or gr 1/13–1/6 *intravenously.*

Arbutin: As diuretic in edema and anasarca, 1–2 tablets every 2 hr., or 15–23 gr several times daily.

Butyl-Chloral Hydrate: As sedative and analgesic in stenocardia, cardiac insomnia 1½–5 gr; as hypnotic 5–18 gr.

Cactus Compound: As cardiac stimulant and anodyne in angina pectoris, palpitation and similar symptoms; 1 tablet four to five times daily.

Cadechol: As cardiac tonic in myocardial insufficiency; 1–2 tablets four to five times daily.

Camphogen: As stimulant in syncope, acute infections, cardiovascular depression; *intramuscularly* 1–2 cc; *intravenously* in urgent cases only.

Cardysate: As cardiac stimulant and diuretic in most cardiac insufficiencies where digitalis is indicated; 5–15 m, as required.

Coramine: As cardio-respiratory stimulant in cardiac failure during acute infections, in poisoning by morphine, chloral, barbital, etc.; *orally* 15–30 m three to four times daily; *hypodermically* 1 or 2 ampules or more.

Cymarin: As cardiac tonic and diuretic in valvular and myocardial disease; 1–2 tablets daily; *intravenously* or *intramuscularly* 1–2 ampules only.

Digalen "Cloetta": In cases where digitalis therapy is indicated; 1–2 tablets; or 0.5–1 cc of liquid, or 1 ampule *hypodermically.*

Digicardalis: As for digitalis therapy.

Digicardium: As for digitalis therapy.

Digifoline: In cardiac disease as for digitalis therapy; *orally* 1 tablet or 1 cc of liquid four times daily until desired results are obtained; *hypodermically* 1 ampule 1–4 times daily, as indicated. Digitalization—initial dose 11 gr or 2 fl. dr. of liquid per 100 lb. of body weight; repeated every 6 hr. until desired effect or toxic symptoms occur, or until 22 gr of tablets or 4 dr. of liquid is reached. *Maintenance dose* 1½ gr daily in tablets, or 16 m of liquid.

Digifortis: Digitalization as for other digitalis preparations; *maintenance dose* 1 tablet or 1 kapseal daily.

Digiglusin: As for digitalis—same dosage.

Diginfuse: Same dosage as for infusion of digitalis.

Diginutin: As for digitalis—1 cc being equivalent to 1 cat unit.

Digipit: As for digitalis.

Digipoten: As for digitalis.

Digismith and Digilutea: Standardized in I.U.; liquids are 25% stronger than corresponding U.S.P. preparations, solids are twice as potent; dosage—one-twelfth of body weight represents about the number of international units for digitalization; given in capsule or liquid form in divided dose; *maintenance dose*—1–2 I.U.

Digitabs: 1 or more tablets as indicated.

Digitaligen: As for digitalis therapy.

Digitalin (Amorphous): *Hypodermically* 1–2 tabloids, maximum 3 tablets; *orally* 1–3 tabloids daily; *maximum dose* 1/60 gr.

Digitalin (Crystalline): A crystalline glucoside of digitoxin type; 1 ampule or 1 tabloid as required, given with great caution.

Digitaline "Nativelle": As cardiac stimulant in insufficiencies: mild—0.1 mg or 5 drops daily for 5 days of each 10 days; moderate—double dosage for first 5

***** *See also* **Parts I and III of this chapter for diseases and classified preparations pertaining to this specialty.**

days, theobromine salts during second 5 days; severe—0.2 mg or 10 drops daily for first 5 days, then 0.1 mg or 5 drops daily; supplemented if required by 1 ampule daily, for 3–4 days.

Digitalis: For digitalization; first day—$\frac{1}{4}$ of total calculated dose or 4 units, then 2 units at 6 hr. intervals or a total of 10 units during first 24 hr.; second day—2 units three times at 6 hr. intervals; third day, and subsequently—1 or 2 units in 1 dose as *maintenance dose;* providing no digitalis has been previously given; if so, or doubtful, 1 unit three to four times daily, watching for symptoms.

Digitalis "Duo-Test": Defatted and doubly standardized; dosage as for digitalis.

Digitan: As for digitalis therapy.

Digitora: As for digitalis therapy.

Digitos: *Intramuscularly* and *intravenously* only; 5–60 m at intervals of 24–48 hr.

Digitoxin: A powerful irritant glucoside; $\frac{1}{240}$–$\frac{1}{60}$ gr three times daily, *maximum single dose* $\frac{1}{30}$ gr; maximum daily, $\frac{1}{20}$ gr.

Diurol: As diuretic for relief of vesical or renal disturbances; 2–4 dr. three to four times daily.

Elixir Digitalin Compound: In shock and cardiac depression, 1 dr. orally.

Ephedrine: As vasoconstrictor in congestive states, in shock, anesthetic accidents; *orally*, tablets gr $\frac{1}{2}$ or 0.3% solution 5–15 m every 4–8 hr.; *hypodermically*, for rapid action if required, $\frac{1}{2}$–1 ampule daily.

Euphydigtal: As cardiac stimulant and diuretic, as vasodilator in coronary disease; 1–2 tablets three to four times daily, or 2–3 suppositories daily.

Glycine: As diuretic in hepatic disease with oliguria and stasis; 75 gr daily.

Homocamfin: As cardiorespiratory stimulant in cardiovascular failure during pneumonia, narcotic poisoning, myocarditis; *intramuscularly* 1$\frac{1}{2}$–2 cc; *intravenously* in emergencies only, 1 cc.

Hydragogin: As diuretic in cardiorenal edema, hepatic cirrhosis; from 3–15 drops every 3–4 hr. in water; in severe cases 15–24 drops every hour, for 24–36 hr.

Metaphyllin: As diuretic and cardiotonic in edema, myocardial insufficiency, coronary disease; 1–2 tablets three to four times daily; *hypodermically* 1–3 ampules daily.

Metrazol: As cardiotonic in acute heart failure, collapse or shock; *subcutaneously* 1 or 2 ampules several times daily; *orally* 1$\frac{1}{2}$–3 gr several times daily.

Natibaine "Nativelle": In auricular fibrillation, ventricular dilatation, myocardial insufficiency, hypertensive heart—10–25 drops daily; in emergencies 30–60 drops.

Neo-Riodine "Astier": As alterative in aortitis, vascular sclerosis, luetic heart disease; *intramuscularly* or *intravenously* 1 cc, increased up to 5 cc, three to four times weekly.

Nitrobar: As antispasmodic and vasodilator in angina and hypertension; 1–2 tablets three times daily.

Nitroscleran: As vasodilator in coronary sclerosis, angina pectoris, degenerative myocarditis—*subcutaneously* 0.04 Gm, slowly increased to 0.1 Gm for 8–15 injections; courses repeated every 4–6 weeks.

Novasurol: As effective diuretic in cardiac dropsy, cardiorenal edema; *intramuscularly* or *intravenously never subcutaneously;* tolerance dose 0.5 cc, injections 1–2 cc once or twice weekly, with simultaneous administration of ammonium chloride or nitrate, 90–150 gr daily.

Ouabain: As stimulant in cardiac emergencies, as acute dilatation, broken compensation, acute failure; *intravenously* $\frac{1}{2}$–1 ampule once in 24 hr.; *intramuscularly* 1 ampule daily; to be avoided where digitaline or strophanthine has been given within 24 hr.

Papaverine: As anodyne in angina pectoris, cardiac asthma, hypertensive heart; *orally* or *hypodermically*—$\frac{1}{2}$–1$\frac{1}{3}$ gr per dose; daily dose up to 7$\frac{1}{2}$ gr.

Papaverine Hydrochloride: As anodyne and antispasmodic in angina, arterial sclerosis, cerebral congestion; gr $\frac{3}{4}$–1$\frac{1}{3}$ single dosage, up to 4 gr daily; *intravenously* gr $\frac{1}{12}$–$\frac{1}{6}$ increased up to gr $\frac{2}{3}$.

Pasanol: As cardiac stimulant in functional disturbances; dosage 1 teaspoonful two to three times daily.

Phanodorn: As sedative and hypnotic in cardiac neuroses and similar disorders; 1 tablet, in obstinate cases 2 tablets at bedtime, with copious hot drinks.

Phyllicin: As diuretic, cardiac stimulant and analgesic in angin ous pains of coronary disease, congestive heart failure, and cardiac dyspnea; 1 tablet or 4 gr of powder two to four times daily after meals.

Potassium Iodo-Theocalcin: As vasodilator and diuretic in stenocardia and hypertensive heart; 1–2 tablets crushed, with water, at meals and at bedtime.

Pulvoids Digitalis Folium: In digitalis therapy; dosage as for digitalis.

Quinicardine "Nativelle": As rhythm normalizer in fibrillation, arrhythmia, tachycardia; first day—tolerance dose 1 tablet repeated in 2 hr.; second day if no susceptibility, 6–8 tablets, continued until tenth day and followed by digitalis therapy.

Quinidine: As rhythm regulator in auricular fibrillation, recent and paroxysmal; tolerance dose 3 gr; if not susceptible 3–6 gr four to five times daily until normal rhythm is established; *maintenance dose* in accordance with conditions.

Salyrgan: As powerful diuretic in cardiorenal edema, pericardial effusions; *intravenously* or *intramuscularly, never subcutaneously,* 0.5 cc; where tolerated, 1 ampule, in severe cases 2 ampules repeated every 3–4 days; with simultaneous administration of ammonium chloride or nitrate from 90–150 gr daily.

Scillaren: Cardiodiuretic in valvular disease, cardiac edema, chronic myocarditis, aortic insufficiency; 2 tablets or 40 drops of oral solution three to four times daily. In urgent cases *intravenously* Scillaren B, about 1 cc daily. *Maintenance dose* 1 tablet or 20 drops, two to three times daily.

Suprarenin: As vasoconstrictor, to raise blood pressure, to stimulate cardiac muscle in shock and heart failure; *subcutaneously* 10–15 m, *intravenously* 30 m to pint of saline or glucose, *intramuscularly* 5–15 m; *intracardially* up to 2 cc.

Syndrome Tablets: As general cardiac stimulant—1 tablet every 4 hr.

Theamin: As diuretic and vasodilator in edema of myocardial origin, chronic passive congestion, coronary thrombosis, angina; 3–5 pulvules three to five times daily for several days.

Theobromine: As diuretic and cardiac stimulant, in cardiorenal edema, pericardial effusion; 5–8 gr four times daily.

Theocalcin: As diuretic in congestive heart failure, cardiac asthma, angina and myocarditis; 1–3 tablets daily, after meals.

Theominal: As vasodilator and antispasmodic in angina pectoris and hypertensive heart; 1 tablet two to three times daily, as indicated.

Thephyldine: As diuretic and vasodilator in coronary sclerosis, cardiac asthma and angina pectoris; 1–2 tablets, or 2–4 suppositories, or 1–3 hypodermic injections daily.

Tissue Extract 568: As vasodilator in stenocardia and angiospasm; *hypodermically* 3–5 cc every few days for 5–10 weeks, then gradually reduced.

Tyramine: As vasoconstrictor and cardiac stimulant in shock and collapse; hypodermically ⅓–⅔ gr.

Verodigen: As cardiotonic where digitalis is indicated; 1 tablet three times daily, later dosage or frequency reduced.

Dentistry

Preparations of Use in Dental Practice*

Acriflavine: An antiseptic and bacteriostat in gingivitis and similar infections in 1:1,000 solution; as wet dressing or for irrigation of sinuses, in 1:5,000 to 1:10,000 solution.

Acriviolet: As antiseptic and germicide in Vincent's disease, leucoplakia and ulcerative stomatitis; in 1% solution, applied directly to diseased area.

Adrenalin and Cocaine Tablets: Containing cocaine hydrochloride gr ⅙ and adrenalin gr 1/1,300; for pressure anesthesia in extractions and other painful operations.

* *See also* "Buccal preparations," Chapter X and diseases of interest in Dentistry in Part III of this chapter.

A.L.A.: Containing para-amino-benzoic acid ethyl ester 3%, phenmethylol 5%, ether 10%, olive oil 82%; as dental anesthetic in painful manipulations of the mouth; *not* to be used intravenously.

Alphozone: As germicide for topical application in dentures; solution of 1:500 to 1:250.

Amarbital: As sedative, hypnotic and analgesic in preoperative and postoperative dentistry; 1–2 tablets 45 min. preoperatively; postoperatively as required.

Analka: As mouth wash, gargle and for gum massage; either full strength or one-half diluted, where desired.

Apothesine: As anesthetic in nerve block and pressure anesthesia; *subcutaneously,* 0.5–2% solution with adrenalin in sterile water or physiologic saline.

Benzolyptus: As mouth wash and gargle in oral infections; full strength.

Beta-Eucaine Hydrochloride: For local anesthesia in painful operations; in 2–3% solution; as infiltration anesthetic, in 4–5% solution.

Beta-Eucaine Lactate: As local anesthetic in dental manipulations; in 2–3% solutions.

Borocaine: As local anesthetic in root canal work; in 2% solution, 1–2 cc; for infiltration anesthesia, in ½–1% solutions; for nerve block, 1–2%; topically 2–10% strengths.

Butyl-Chloral Hydrate: As sedative for the relief of toothache; applied externally with equal parts of phenol.

Butyn, with or without Epinephrin: For all procedures demanding anesthesia; in infiltration, 1/10–¼% solutions; topically, 2%.

Butyn Solution: *For use* in infiltration anesthesia, in painful dental operations; in 2% solutions.

Caseosan: As non-specific therapy agent to increase leucocytosis and general resistance in root infections, severe gingivitis and in facial neuralgia; *intramuscularly* or *subcutaneously,* in graduated dosage from 0.5–5 cc; injections at 1–3 day intervals.

Chlorbutanol: As local anesthetic; in aqueous saturated solution, *hypodermically.*

Chloro-Camphene: As dental antiseptic in infected root canals; applied directly into canal, or locally by cotton pledget.

Chloroseptine Powder: As oral antiseptic and for oral hygiene; used as mouth wash or gargle, twice daily.

Chlorothol Compound: As local antiseptic for douching, spraying or gargle after dental extraction; 1 or 2 tablets in glass of hot water.

Cinchophen: As analgesic and uricolytic in infections as pyorrhea alveolaris, and in diseases of uratic diathesis; 1–2 tablets three to four times daily, with rest period of 3–5 days after each course; total dosage not to exceed 150 gr during 1 course

Collosol Argentum Dentifrice: As dental antiseptic for use as dentifrice.

Collosol Chlor-Carvacrol: As colloidal antiseptic for use in dental sepsis and decay, as gargle, spray or mouth wash; 5–10 drops in wineglassful of water.

Collosol Lactalumina: As astringent mouth wash and gargle; 1–2 teaspoonfuls in wineglassful of water several times daily.

Collosol Lactomagnesia: As alkaline mouth wash for oral hygiene; 2 teaspoonfuls in half glass of water, several times daily.

Dentaline: Containing phenol, benzocaine, chloroform and oil of cloves; as toothache drops; applied by packing dental cavity with saturated pledget or by rubbing solution on the gum.

Dental Magnesia: As alkaline dentifrice, containing milk of magnesia 75%; applied twice daily with tooth brush.

Dentinol: As oral germicide in infected dental sockets, in pyorrhea and after extractions, as mouth wash or gargle; in full strength.

Detoxol Paste: Containing 2% sodium ricinoleate (or soricin); applied as dentifrice twice daily with tooth brush.

Eau de Botot: As astringent, detergent and antiseptic; for use as mouth wash and in irrigation of dental cavities, pyorrhea; applied directly by swab or brush.

Eucalyptus-Thymol Compound: As antiseptic gargle and mouth wash; used in full strength.

Fibrogen (Local): As hemostatic in topical bleeding; applied by saturating cotton pledget well shaped before insertion and packed into tooth socket.

Hemarestors: As styptic to arrest hemorrhage or secondary oozing following extractions or other operations; applied directly into cavity.

Hexyl-Resorcinol Solution S.T. 37: In oral hygiene; used undiluted after brushing teeth.

Hexyl Resorcinol Tooth Paste: As dentifrice and oral antiseptic; applied twice daily with tooth brush.

Hyclorite: In oral hygiene, post-extraction therapy and pyorrhea; topically, one-half or full strength.

Iodent Tooth Paste: 1 and 2 as dentifrices in general hygiene; twice daily used with tooth brush.

Ipana Tooth Paste: As dentifrice in oral hygiene; applied by massaging into gums with finger or tooth brush, twice daily.

Katolox: As alterative; applied topically full strength on gums, dental sockets and other tissues.

Kelene: As local anesthetic and in inhalation anesthesia for short surgical procedures, extractions; local—by refrigeration, by spray from tube held 6–10 in. from treated area; in inhalation—by the open cone method.

Lagarg: As antiseptic gargle, mouth wash and deodorant; in full strength.

Lar-Io-Ben: As antiseptic and deodorant in dental and oral hygiene; in various dilutions up to 50%.

Lavoris: As antiseptic and astringent mouth wash in oral catarrh and hygiene; full strength or diluted.

Lumalgin: As sedative in preoperative dentistry; 1–3 tablets 45 min. preceding operation; also postoperatively.

Magnesium Peroxide: As antacid, antiseptic in the treatment of pyorrhea alveolaris and oral acidity; locally as dentifrice, internally 5–20 gr.

Mallophene: As local antiseptic in packing sockets after extraction, in marginal gingivitis and trench mouth; applied in form of paste mixed with glycerine.

Maradol: As general stimulant in dental caries; 2–4 teaspoonfuls three times daily.

Menthol Y: As analgesic and antiseptic; applied in pure crystal form into cavity.

Mercurochrome 220 Soluble: For sterilization of root canals, in gingivitis, stomatitis, aphthous disease; in 3–5% solution.

Metoso: As antiseptic mouth wash in dental affections; as spray or gargle in full strength.

Metycaine: As local anesthetic; hypodermically, in 2–4% solution.

Myodine: As antiseptic mouth wash and spray; in full strength.

Neo-Silvol: As colloidal antiseptic in dental caries; in 20% solution on cotton; in the treatment of erosions and exposed roots, in 50% solution; in pyorrhea, 10% solution.

Neurocaine: As pressure anesthetic in marginal cavity and pulp chamber work; also in cavity preparation and pulp removal; applied by inserting into cavity or directly into pulp chamber.

Noviform: As antiseptic, astringent and deodorant in tamponing abscesses, in post-extraction, ulcerated gums, osteomyelitis; applied in powder form, pure or mixed with talcum.

Optalidon: As anodyne and sedative in toothache; 1–2 tablets repeated as indicated.

Orazin: As antiseptic mouth wash and deodorant; used in full strength.

Pepsodent Antiseptic: As antiseptic mouth wash and gargle: used in full strength or 50% diluted.

Pepsodent Tooth Paste: As dentifrice; applied with tooth brush twice daily.

Peralga: As analgesic in toothache and neuralgia, also as preoperative sedative; 1 tablet or 5 gr of powder as indicated.

Phenandyne: As antiseptic and analgesic in pyorrhea, pulpitis and dental caries; for use in the Buckley treatment; applied full strength on pledget into cavity.

Procaine: As anesthetic in conductive anesthesia for intra- and extra-nerve block, 2%; in infiltration anesthesia, for contact and high pressure, intraosseous, peridental and subperiosteal, 1–2% solution.

Procaine Borate and Epinephrin: As anesthetic; used in conditions and strengths as procaine.

Pycopé Tooth Powder: As dentifrice; used twice daily with toothbrush.

Pyrozide: As tooth polish and cleanser and in oral hygiene; applied twice daily as dentifrice.

Pyrozone: As tooth bleach in discolored teeth; applied with toothbrush, twice daily.

Red Gum: As astringent in the treatment of relaxed fauces; used by dissolving 1 tablet slowly in mouth, several times daily.

Root Canal Filling: As dental filling in root canals to keep periapical areas sterile and to stimulate regrowth of healthy tissue; applied by mixing the 2 powders into smooth paste and inserting as filling.

Salvarsan Glucose Solution: As specific therapy in Vincent's angina and pyorrhea alveolaris of spirillae origin; applied locally. *See Chap. I* for systemic and local therapy.

S.A.S.: As antiseptic gargle and mouth wash; used full strength or diluted.

Silver Lactate: As astringent antiseptic in irrigating root abscesses; in 1:500 solution.

Sodiphene: As antiseptic and sedative in oral manipulations, and post-extraction; applied topically, full strength, several times daily; as gargle, diluted in 3 parts of warm water; for sinus irrigation, 25%.

Sodium Perborate: As oxidizer and antiseptic in dental surgery and Vincent's angina; used as mouth wash and toothpowder.

Sodium Peroxide: As bleaching agent for non-viable teeth, discolored pulps and in root canal disinfection; used in form of paste prepared with liquid paraffin.

Soluble Iodine: In root canal infections, periapical disease, gingivitis, Vincent's angina and for ionization; applied in full strength.

Strontium Peroxide: As antiseptic and deodorant in dentifrices; in full strength and diluted.

Stypticin: As hemostatic for local oozing, bleeding after extraction and other operations; applied pure or in strong solution, or as 30% on cotton or gauze; orally, ¼–4 gr four to five times daily as indicated.

Sy-Lac: As antiseptic mouth wash and for gum massage; used full strength twice daily.

Thromboplastin: As hemostatic in oral hemorrhages; 2 cc applied into site of bleeding, the remainder subcutaneously injected; locally, by direct pressure; as prophylactic, preoperatively, 1 cc hypodermically.

Toothache Drops: For relief of pain; applied by inserting pellet saturated in solution. directly into dental cavity.

Zonite: As antiseptic and deodorant; 3 teaspoonfuls to ¼–½ glass of water; for preserving artificial dentures overnight or when not in use—several drops in ½ glass of water.

Dermatology

Preparations of Use in Skin Diseases*

Acriflavine: As antiseptic and bacteriostat in furunculosis and eczema; as wet dressing 1:1,000 solution.

Acriflavine Neutral: In the treatment of burns, erysipelas and similar infections; in 1:100 to 1:500 solutions, as ointment 1:1,000; applied locally as often as necessary.

Acriviolet: As antiseptic and germicide in furunculosis and similar skin infections; pencilled in 1% solution once or twice daily.

Afenil: As non-specific therapy agent in toxic manifestations and arsenical dermatitis; hypodermically, 10 cc of 10% aqueous solution once or twice daily, or several times weekly as indicated in each case.

Alphozone: As antiseptic in abrasions, burns and other superficial skin injuries; in 1:500 to 1:250 solution; as dusting powder, mixed with talcum or boric acid, 1:20.

* *See also* "Ointments," "Vaccines," "Antiluetics," "Parasiticides," "Systemic Diseases" etc.

Alumnol: As astringent antiseptic for erosions, ulcerations, ulcus molle, abscesses, eczema, acne and sycosis; in pure powder form or 10% mixture with equal parts of French chalk and starch; also in 5% aqueous solution, 2½–10% alcoholic and as 2½–20% lanolin ointment.

Analka: As emollient dressing for chapped skin, insect bites, rashes and abrasions; full strength or half diluted.

Anesthesin: As topical analgesic and antipuritic in intertrigo, pruritus, eczema and similar affections; as dusting powder 10%, or as 4–10% ointment.

Anticol: As non-specific therapy agent in the treatment of boils, abscesses and impetigo; *hypodermically*, 0.25–3 cc every other day; *orally*, ½–5 gr per dose.

Aolan: As non-specific therapy agent in the treatment of various infections; *see Chap. I.*

Aquaphor: As ointment base and emollient cleanser in chapped skin, windburn; pure or mixed with other medicaments in any desired proportion.

Argocol: As antiseptic colloidal silver in ringworm, pustular eczema, septic ulceration; applied locally as ointment or in solution.

Atoquinol: In skin disorders with uratic basis; 4–8 tablets daily with plenty of water.

Benzene (Benzol) Medicinal: As parasiticide in scabies, pediculosis, pityriasis; applied pure or in ointment form.

Benzyl Benzoate: As antiparasitic in various skin infections; used in 25% solution in castor oil, or as ointment.

Betanaphthol Benzoate: As parasiticide and germicide in pediculosis, favus, prurigo, scabies, eczema, alopecia, hyperidrosis cutis, psoriasis; in 2–10% ointment.

B.F.I.: For chafing and other minor skin irritations; applied in powder form or in ointment.

Bicarbonate of Sodium: As antacid and antipruritic in eczema and other itching skin affections, in 2–5% solution; in superficial burns is mixed with water as paste.

Bichloracetic Acid: As keratolytic in corns, warts, calluses; applied locally at 3–4 day intervals, 1–4 applications.

Bismuth Violet: As antiseptic and germicide in impetigo, ringworm, scabies; applied in ointment form as often as required.

Bromipin 33%: As sedative to relieve irritation in frost bites; used with equal parts of castor oil.

Butesin Picrate: As protective and analgesic in extensive burns and other destructive skin lesions; used as 1% ointment or 5% powder with sodium stearate 95%.

Calamoin: As antipruritic and antiseptic in various skin irritations; applied locally as often as necessary.

Calcidin: As desiccating antiseptic for chronic ulcers and septic wounds; applied as dusting powder.

Calcium Gluconate and Calglucon: In itching and oozing dermatoses, in arsenical dermatitis, in psoriasis; *Intravenously* or *intramuscularly*, every 1–3 days, 10 cc or more; *orally*, 1 or 2 tablets three times daily, chewed before swallowing.

Calmitol: As antipruritic and antiseptic in tinea trichophyton, eczema, pruritus ani et vulvae, rectal irritation and acne; applied locally.

Calomelol: As antiluetic on syphilitic sores; applied in powder or ointment form.

Cal-Zo: As astringent and antiseptic dressing in ambulant treatment of varicose ulcers; applied thickly to lesions with steady pressure or support to the extremity.

Camiofen Ointment: As antiseptic dressing in itching dermatoses; applied freely to affected area once or twice daily.

Camphaseptic Ointment: As protective dressing; applied once or twice daily.

Cerevisine "Chapelle": As yeast therapy; 1 tablet every hour orally and as paste made with water, or as poultice—for local application to infected areas.

Chlorazene: As antiparasitic in epidermophytosis, eczema; applied as dusting powder or as 1% solution wet dressing, as frequently as required.

Collosol Argentum: As antiseptic in impetigo contagiosa, ringworm, tinea versicolor, pustular eczema, follicular impetigo; applied as ointment or wet dressing.

Collosol Aurum: In lupus, tuberculides, psoriasis; orally, 1 teaspoonful three times daily, well diluted in water; *intramuscularly*, 1 ampule every 2–4 days.

Collosol Calamine Lotion: As colloidal astringent and antiseptic in suppurative skin affections; applied locally with sponge and permitted to dry.

Collosol Chrysarobin: As colloidal parasiticide in various parasitic infections; applied topically as indicated.

Collosol Ferro-Manganese: As hematinic in anemia accompanying impetigo contagiosa, follicular impetigo, eczema; *intramuscularly,* 1–2 cc every 4 days; *orally,* 1 teaspoonful three times daily.

Collosol Hydrargyrum: As antiseptic on luetic ulcers; applied as often as necessary.

Collosol Ichthyol: As antiphlogistic and antiseptic in numerous inflammatory conditions; applied locally as ointment 5–40%, or as lotion, 10%.

Collosol Manganese: As colloidal bactericide and protective in acne suppurativa and vulgaris, in furuncles, boils, sycosis, impetigo and other coccogenic infections; *intramuscularly* from 0.5–1 cc every 2–3 days until 6–8 cc are administered; *orally,* 1 teaspoonful in water three times daily after meals.

Collosol Stannum: As colloidal antiphlogistic in furunculosis; 1 cc every 2–3 days *intramuscularly.*

Collosol Sulphur: As colloidal antiseptic in the form of sulphur baths, 4 oz. to 20 gal. warm water, immersion for 10–15 min.; topically, diluted ten to twenty times.

Collosol Zinc Cream: For infants, chapped skin, rough skin; as zinc stearate ointment massaged gently into affected area to leave a fine coating of zinc on the skin surface.

Coryfin: As antipruritic in itching dermatoses; applied locally as lotion.

Crutar Ointments "Grossman": As antiseptic in infantile eczema; applied twice daily as ointment, reducing strength.

Danish Ointment: As antiseptic in scabies; applied by inunction after hot bath, followed by second bath in 24 hr.

Dermalin: As epithelial proliferant in abrasions, burns, bed sores, erosions, ulcers; applied locally and covered with gauze.

Derma-Medicone: As antipruritic and antiseptic in eczema and pruritus; applied locally twice daily.

Dermocaine: As antipruritic and antiseptic in athlete's foot, eczema, impetigo; applied locally, three times daily.

Dimazon Ointment: As epithelial proliferant in indolent ulcers, sluggish wounds, ulcus cruris, erythroderma, eczema, intertrigo, severe burns; applied as ointment dressing; may be alternated with powder or other preparations.

Eczemol: As antipruritic in eczema; applied as wet dressing two to three times daily.

Eczol: As antiseptic and antipruritic in eczema, impetigo, pruritus, psoriasis; applied locally.

Espinol: As stimulating antiseptic in psoriasis, eczema, pityriasis rosea, lichen planus; applied nightly by rubbing into involved area and repeated as necessary.

Ethyl Iodide: In mycotic skin affections; applied locally by painting, two or three times daily.

Eupinol Ointment: As soothing antiseptic in burns, ulcers, insect bites; applied locally.

Euresol: As antiseptic and astringent in itching dermatoses, seborrhea, urticaria, sycosis, dandruff; applied as ointment 5–50%, every other day for 1–3 weeks; on scalp used as inunction, 2–5%, alcoholic solution; scalp dried and well rubbed with olive oil.

Ferrocol: As local bactericide in cellulitis and erysipelas; applied full strength as wet dressing.

Gold Sodium Thiosulphate: In lupus therapy, also in lichen scrofulosum; *intravenously* or *intramuscularly,* cautiously employed, gr 1/6; subsequent dosage increased by 0.01 Gm, at weekly intervals, with frequent rest periods; *maximum dose* for *male* 100 mg, *female* 75 mg.

Gynergen: In general prurigo of hepatic and renal origin; *intramuscularly,* 0.5–1 cc once or twice weekly; *orally,* 1 tablet three to four times daily for 3 days.

Hazeline Cream: As stimulating dressing in dermatoses; applied as necessary.

Hydrosal: As astringent dressing in burns, infantile skin affections and furunculosis; applied thickly on affected parts and covered with wax paper.

Ichthalbin: As local antiseptic in moist infantile eczema, scrofula, congestive dermatitis, seborrhoeic disorders, lichen strophulus; applied as dusting powder.

Ichthargan: As antiseptic in furunculosis; applied in ointment, 5–10%, twice daily.

Ichthorgin: As antiseptic in eczema, herpes; applied as ointment, twice daily.

Ichthymall: As antipruritic in acute dermatitis, erythema nodosum, eczema, chilblains; applied locally as ointment or by painting with solution as often as necessary.

Ichthyol: As antiphlogistic, mildly antiseptic in all inflammatory skin conditions, burns, scalds, chilblains, etc.—in 5–10% ointment; in scarlet fever 5–50% ointment.

Inoton "Debat": As analgesic in herpes zoster, pruritus, intertrigo, eczema, pityriasis; applied liberally and covered with 2 layers of gauze.

Iocamfen: As parasiticide in ringworm of the feet, body, scalp or nails; applied locally by swab or brush to dry surfaces only, after cleansing.

Iodine, Tincture: As antiseptic in athlete's foot; applied once or twice daily.

Iodomuth: As antiseptic and deodorant in burns, ulcers and varicose ulcerations; as dusting powder or as 40% ointment.

Iothion: As antiseptic in ringworm, sycosis barbae and other infections; used chiefly as Iothion Oil, undiluted or diluted with alcohol, olive oil and glycerin; in petrolatum ointment, 5–20%; applied area must not be too heavily painted or bandaged.

Isarol: As antipruritic in conditions where sulphur is indicated; in 5–50% ointment with lanolin, petrolatum, zinc oxide, castor oil or glycerin.

Joncolia: As emollient in burns; applied locally as often as required.

Kelene: As analgesic and parasiticide in herpes zoster, trichophyton, condylomatosis, lupus and skin transplantation; applied by spray.

Kerolysin: As keratolytic in epidermophytosis and eczema; applied daily or every other day after previous cleansing.

Lenigallol: As antiseptic in eczema, mycosis, dermophytosis, psoriasis; applied fresh as ointment 1–6%, once or twice daily; in mycosis, ¼–½%.

Lenigallol Zinc Ointment: As antiseptic and keratolytic in eczema, psoriasis and other dermatoses; applied locally.

Liantral: As antiseptic in lichen planus, lichenoid eczema, neurodermatitis; applied locally twice daily and dusted freely with corn starch.

Liantral Casein Ointment: As astringent antiseptic in seborrhea sicca; applied locally as necessary.

Mangacol: As germicide in boils, carbuncles, furuncles, folliculitis, impetigo, eczema; administered *intramuscularly* and *intravenously*, ¼–1 gr, also locally, full strength.

Mazon: As antiseptic in eczema, psoriasis, dandruff; rubbed thoroughly in form of ointment into area without covering, as often as necessary.

Mercurettes: As antiparasitic in various parasitic skin affections; applied by vigorous rubbing two or three times weekly.

Mercurophen: As mercurial germicide in parasitic skin infestation; in 1–1:1,000 solution, for 1 min.

Metaphen: As germicide in sycosis, ringworm, pediculosis, scabies; undiluted or as ointment, 1:5,000.

Molan: As astringent antiseptic in burns; applied locally.

Mycozol: As fungicide in epidermomycosis, athlete's foot, soft corns, fungi; after scrubbing affected area with antiseptic soap, washing with alcohol and drying, ointment is freely rubbed in, covered with bandage; repeated next night; between ointment applications boro-chloretone is dusted on.

Neorobin: As chrysarobin therapy in psoriasis, dermatitis seborrhoeica, pityriasis rosea, dandruff; applied externally in 1–5 gr per ounce of petrolatum.

Nizin: As astringent antiseptic in moist eczema and sluggish ulceration; applied topically in strength of 6 gr per ounce.

Noviform: As antiseptic and deodorant in condylomata, chancre, balanitis, intertrigo; used in powder form, pure or mixed with talcum.

Nupercaine: As anesthetic in burns, painful ulcers, cancerous lesions, prurigo; applied locally as often as required.

Omnadin: As non-specific protein therapy. *See Chap. I.*

Orthoform: As surface anesthetic in itching and painful dermatoses; dusted either plain or mixed with aristol, calomel, europhen and other drugs, and in ointment form.

Panthesine Ointment: As antipruritic and anesthetic in paronychia, herpes zoster, pruritus, sunburn, furuncles; rubbed in gently two to four times daily, or more frequently.

Parathesin: As antipruritic in eczema; applied locally as dusting powder or 5–20% ointment as often as required.

Paroleine: As emollient for burns and ulcerations; applied in full strength or in combination with other medicaments.

Petrogen: As analgesic antiseptic dressing in wounds, ulcers and dermatoses; applied externally.

Pixalbol: As antiseptic and antipruritic in eczema, urticaria, strophulus, alopecia; as ointment, paint or alcoholic solution.

Quinothesin: As antiseptic in burns, scalds, psoriasis, athlete's foot; in ointment or powder form.

Resorcinol Monoacetate: As antiseptic in sycosis, seborrhea, alopecia, acne; in 5–20% ointment or acetone solution; in alopecia, best—3–5% alcoholic solution.

Sarcoptol: As antipruritic, antiparasitic in scabies, is thoroughly rubbed in until absorbed; in dandruff, applied diluted with 4–5 parts of olive oil; in pediculosis, ringworm, prurigo, applied locally or painted with brush.

Scabiola: As antiparasitic in scabies and ringworm; applied once to twice daily.

Scarlet Red Salve "Biebrich": As antiseptic in soft chancre, lupus, ulcus cruris, skin suppurations; applied after previous cleansing and drying of wound, anointing with bland ointment skin surrounding wound, covering wound with the Scarlet Red Salve, then applying gauze; dressed every 1–2 days.

Stannoxyl: As staphylocide in boils, pustular acne, suppurative dermatitis and other coccogenic infections; orally, 4–8 tablets daily after meals, with water; as bath in generalized furunculosis.

Stanno-Yeast: As corrective in furunculosis; orally, 1–3 tablets every 3 hr.

Storaxin: As antiparasitic in ringworm and pruritus; applied twice daily.

Sufrogel: As non-specific therapy. *See Chap. I.*

Sulfactol: As non-specific therapy agent. *See Chap. I.*

Sulfidal: As non-specific therapy agent. *See Chap. I.*

Targesin: As astringent and antiseptic in pyodermia, intertrigo, impetigo, eczema; in 2–5% solution or 5% ointment.

Taroxide: As antiseptic in chronic infantile moist eczema, poison ivy; applied locally for 1 week and after several days' rest, repeated.

Thiol: As sulphur antiseptic and antiphlogistic in dermatitis, erythema, impetigo, intertrigo, sycosis, tinea tonsurans, pemphigus; in ointment, 10–25%, or powder form 5–10%.

Tin Oxide: As staphylocide in boils and furuncles; orally, 1 capsule every 3 hr.

Tinpronate: As staphylocide in acne and furunculosis; orally, 2 tablets every 3 hr.

Trichophytin-Extract: In trichophyton infections; *subcutaneously,* 0.05 cc diluted to 1 cc with sterile saline, injected every 4–5 days, in increased dosage; also given *intradermally.*

Tricocide Ointment: As antiseptic in ringworm and fungus disease; applied twice daily, locally.

Tricotox: As parasiticide in epidermophytosis; applied locally twice daily.

Triphal: As gold therapy in lupus erythematosus; *intravenously,* twice weekly. *See Chap. I.*

Xeroform: As antiseptic in weeping eczema and ulcus cruris; applied locally as dusting powder.

Yatren Casein: As non-specific therapy agent. *See Chap. I.*

Yeastone: As corrective in furunculosis and acne; 1 tablet four times daily.

Zincol: As astringent in insect bites and stings; topically as powder, diluted.

Zinc Peroxide: As antiseptic in plant dermatitis and eczema, and as skin protective; as dusting powder, pure or mixed with starch or tartaric acid; as ointment in 2–25% of paraffin.

Gastro-Enterology

For additional topics of interest in Gastro-Enterology, the reader is referred to "Internal Medicine" and to the following articles in Parts I and III of this chapter, the descriptions of which for brevity sake are here omitted:

Part I

Acidophilus Preparations
Agar Preparations
Amebacides
Antacids, Gastric
Astringents, Gastric
Cholagogues
Digestives
Foods
Gastric HCl Substitutes
Hematinics
Intestinal Antiseptics
Intestinal Stimulants
Laxatives
Mineral Oils
Mineral Waters
Non-specific Therapy
Sedatives, Gastric
Tonics, General
Vermifuges

Part III

Amebiasis
Biliary Derangements
Cancer
Colic
Colitis
Constipation
Gastric Disorders
Intestinal Disorders

Functional Tests

Bromsulphalein: For liver function diagnosis; *intravenous* injection of 0.002 Gm per kilogram of body weight, undiluted; determination is made from 4–5 cc of blood obtained from other arm; the serum is centrifuged and compared colorimetrically with established standards.

Ergamine: As secretory stimulant, in functional test for hydrochloric acid in gastric analyses; 1 tabloid gr 1/64 *subcutaneously* or *intramuscularly;* injection is followed by withdrawal of gastric contents at stated intervals, for determination of its hydrochloric acid concentration.

Histamine: As secretory stimulant, in functional test for hydrochloric acid in gastric analysis; *subcutaneously* and *intramuscularly,* 1 ampule; injection is followed by withdrawal of gastric contents at stated intervals, for determination of its hydrochloric acid concentration.

Iso-Iodeikon: As combination liver and gall bladder function test; 40 mg per kilogram of body weight, total not to exceed 2.5 Gm; solution is prepared by dissolving Iso-Iodeikon in 1 oz. of freshly distilled water, sterilized over boiling water bath for 15 min. and injected by gravity method, after dilution with about 150 cc of Ringer's or normal saline solution during a period of at least 15 min. Where the syringe method is used, concentration should not exceed 8% and the injection period not less than 15 min.; radiography 4, 8 and 12 hr. after administration; fatty meals where desired, given after 8 hr. observation and radiographed 1 or 2 hr. after; liver function test made ½–1 hr. after dye injection.

Phenoltetrachlorphthalein: For determination of liver function by the Rosenthal method; 5 mg per kilogram of body weight or 0.05–0.4 Gm of the disodium salt, administered *intravenously;* blood is colorimetrically examined 1 hr. after injection.

Gynecology

Preparations for Use in Diseases of Women*

Alphozone: As vaginal douche in cervicitis and vaginitis; 1:1,000–1:250 for irrigation twice daily.

Alumnol: As astringent and antiseptic for various pelvic inflammations with increase of discharge; as douche in 2–5% solution, pessaries 5%, gauze dressings 5%.

Argyn: As astringent and antiseptic in pelvic infections and cervical erosions; in 50–75% solution on tampons.

* *See also* "Vaginal Suppositories," "Liquid Antiseptics," "Anesthetics" and other drugs and diseases of gynecologic interest, in respective chapters.

Caseosan: As non-specific therapy agent in low grade pelvic infections, parametritis (*See Chap. I.*)

Causticks and Cupristicks: For cauterization of cervical erosions; applied directly to ulcerated area once daily.

Cerevisine "Chapelle": As yeast therapy and local germicide in vaginitis, cervical lesions, and leukorrhea; applied directly in form of paste mixed with water.

Chlorazene: In vaginitis and other pelvic infections; in 0.5–1 % solution as douche as frequently as necessary.

Clymocol: As germicidal douche in pelvic infections, in 0.5 % dilution.

Collargol: As silver antiseptic in gonorrheal cervicitis; painted twice daily with 0.02 %–1 % solution; as vaginal suppositories ¾ gr and as tampons.

Compral: As analgesic and antispasmodic for relief of pain in dysmenorrhea, postoperatively, postpartum and in climacteric discomfort; orally 1–2 tablets three to four times daily, as indicated.

Dibromin: As germicidal agent in vaginitis, cervicitis and endometritis; for douching 1:5,000 solution twice daily.

Dionin: As sedative and antispasmodic in pain and insomnia, gynecological operations, and prior to chloroform anesthesia; administered *orally* or *subcutaneously* ⅙–1 gr if necessary two to three times daily; as hypnotic ¼–½ gr.

Douchal: As vaginal antiseptic and deodorant in pelvic affections; for douching 1 tablespoonful to quart of warm water, as required.

Duoban: As vaginal antiseptic and contraceptive; 1 tablet introduced vaginally as required.

Duofoam: As vaginal antiseptic in pelvic affections and as contraceptive; applied as jelly as required.

Ergot Aseptic: As uterine contractor where ordinarily ergot is employed; 1 tabloid *subcutaneously* or *intramuscularly;* larger dosage to be given with caution.

Ergotoxine: As uterine stimulant in disturbances where ergot is employed; *subcutaneously* or *intramuscularly*, 1 or 2 tabloids, with or without strychnin.

Esterol: As antispasmodic in dysmenorrhea or excessive labor pain; orally 3–4 tablets, after 1 hr. 1–4 tablets if necessary; given in hot water.

Fomos: As vaginal antiseptic in pelvic affections and as contraceptive; used as required.

Germicidal Discs: As pelvic antiseptic for use in vaginal irrigation; in dilution of 1:20,000, preserved in closed vessels.

Gynergen: As uterine stimulant to induce contractions in postpartum hemorrhage, menorrhagia, metrorrhagia and after Cesarean operation; *orally* 1 tablet two to four times daily; *intramuscularly* 0.5 cc, maximum 1 cc, repeated if necessary in 20 min. only in emergencies.

Hydrastinin: Uterine hemostatic, for use in subinvolution, menorrhagia, menopausal hemorrhage; 20–40 drops or 1 tablet three to four times daily.

Ichthargan: As gonocide in female genitourinary infections; applied by tampon 1–100 to 1–20 in glycerin or as washes in 1:1,000 glycerin.

Ichtholdine: Antiphlogistic and antiseptic in pelvic affections; for local application with fine brush or cotton applicator and wool tampons.

Ichthynat: As emollient and antiseptic; applied by tampon or topical painting.

Ichthyol: Antiphlogistic and decongestive in pelvic affections; painted locally with 5–50 % solution; for douching 2 %, tampons 10–25 % in glycerin, suppositories 10 %.

Infundin: As oxytocic in uterine inertia and postpartum hemorrhage; 2 international units ante-partum, 10–15 units postpartum.

Iothion Oil: Antiseptic in vaginitis and cervicitis; applied by tampon or as 5–20 % ointment.

Isarol: Antiseptic in pelvic infections; used pure or in combination with other drugs on tampons.

Koromex: As vaginal prophylactic and antiseptic; applied as necessary.

Lavoris: As antiseptic in leucorrheal discharge, endocervicitis, erosion and pruritus vulvae; as tampon 50 % or full strength, as douche or lotion 10–50 %.

Lubafax: As lubricant in pelvic examinations; applied freely.

Lunosol: As vaginal antiseptic and astringent in gonorrheal infections; on tampon 10%, application to cervix 10%, as vaginal douche 0.25%.

Lygel: As vaginal antiseptic and prophylactic in pelvic affections, as required.

Lysol: As deodorizer in pelvic cellulitis and cervical discharges; for douching 0.5–1%.

Marvosan: As vaginal prophylactic and antiseptic; applied as required.

Medicated Wafers: As vaginal antiseptic in cervicitis, erosions and leukorrhea; inserted intravaginally once or twice daily.

Medicone Suppositories: As prophylactic and in vaginal infections; applied as required.

Me-Ox-Ol: As germicide and antiseptic; for douching 8–16 cc to quart of water once or twice daily.

Mercuristicks: For local application to cervical erosions; once daily.

Meroxyl: Antiseptic in vaginitis, cervicitis; douching 0.1% once or twice daily.

Neosilvol: As silver antiseptic in pelvic infections; as tampons 5–50%.

Nizin: As astringent and antiseptic douche; 1 teaspoonful to quart of warm water; in urethral injection 2 gr to ounce of water.

Normolactol: As antiseptic in leukorrhea; 1 tablet inserted intravaginally each evening for 3 days, followed on the fourth by cleansing therapy.

Norwich Douche Powder: As vaginal astringent and prophylactic; 1 tablespoonful in quart of warm water.

Ortho-Gynol: As vaginal antiseptic and prophylactic; applied as necessary.

Oxyquinolin Sulphate: As vaginal antiseptic and prophylactic; for irrigation 1:1,000–1:100 solution; as suppository applied when necessary.

Papaverine Hydrochloride: As antispasmodic in dysmenorrhea and other painful pelvic conditions; *orally* ¾–1⅓ gr, up to 4 gr daily, *subcutaneously* gr ¾ per dose, *intravenously* 1/12–⅙ gr.

Pernoston: As pre- and postoperative hypnotic, for reduction from 50–80% of inhalation anesthetic; 1 cc per 12½ kg of body weight, 1 hr. before operation.

Phenoco: As antiseptic in gynecologic and obstetric conditoins; for douching in 1–5% solution.

Plestrin Solution: For ovarian organic insufficiency, infantilism, maldeveloped uterus and appendages, in primary amenorrhea and sterility; *intramuscularly* 1 ampule every 1–2 days for several months, particularly during 10 days preceding menses, supplemented by 1–3 capsules one to three times daily.

Progene: As vaginal antiseptic and prophylactic; 1 vial dissolved in 1 qt. of warm water for douching.

Progynon: As placental sex hormone in ovarian organic deficiency, sterility, uterine maldevelopment, primary amenorrhea; 1 tablet three times daily or 1 ampule for 10 days prior to expected menstrual period; in menopausal disorders 1 tablet three times daily.

Prokliman: For climacteric disturbances and hypertension; 2 tablets two to three times daily after meals.

Protargol: As antiseptic and germicide in infections of genitalia, endometritis, vaginitis, and endocervicitis; applied in 2–10% solution.

Radon: As radium therapy in uterine hemorrhage, fibromyomata, to induce artificial menopause; applied topically by special technic.

Rectal Anesthesia "Gwathmey": For use principally in obstetrics, in 2 strengths; instillation of medication is preceded by mineral oil accompanying each ampule, and is introduced by means of rectal analgesia set supplied with anesthetic.

Santyl: As urinary sedative in gonorrheal and non-gonorrheal infections; 25–50 m three times daily after meals.

Silvogon: For gonorrheal infections; as irrigation 1:500.

Silvol: As mild silver protein antiseptic and astringent; vaginal suppositories 5%.

Sistomensin: As ovarian hormone therapy in menopausal disturbances, metrorrhagia, dysmenorrhea and hemorrhages of ovarian deficiency; *orally* 1–3 tablets three times daily, supplemented by *intramuscular* injections two to three times weekly.

Solargentum: As silver antiseptic and astringent in cervical and vaginal infections; as tampons 25% in glycerin.

Stomaseptine: As antiparasitic for vaginal douching in trichomona vaginalis vaginitis, and leukorrhea; 1–2 teaspoonfuls in quart of warm water.

Stypticin: As astringent and hemostatic in profuse menstruation, endometritis, climacteric hemorrhage; *orally* ½–4 gr, four to five times daily in gelatin capsules, *subcutaneously* in urgent cases gr 1½–4 of 10% solution.

Sublamine: As antiseptic and disinfectant; vaginal douche, 1:500 to 1:1,000 solution.

Sulfax: For antiseptic douching in 1:3,000 solution.

Surgical Lubricant: For direct application and examination.

Tanichthol: As antiseptic in vaginal infections, vaginitis; applied as necessary.

Targesin: As antiseptic in gonococcus infections; on tampons from 15–20% solution for vaginal use.

Thigenol: As antipruritic and antiseptic; on tampons saturated with 10–50% solution in glycerin or petrolatum; as suppositories 15–25% in cocoa butter.

Thiol: As antiseptic in cervical erosions; on tampon, diluted with water.

Trillin: As regulator of excessive menstruation; 2–5 tablets every 3–4 hr.

Yatren-Casein: As foreign protein therapy agent in pelvic septic infection. *See Chap. I.*

Zinc Permanganate: As astringent and antiseptic in vaginitis, cystitis; in 1:4,000 solution for local application.

Internal Medicine

Preparations of Special Interest to the Internist*

Acetidine: As analgesic for relief of headache, neuralgia, myalgia; as antipyretic in fevers; 1 tablet every 1–2 hr.

Adrenalin and Adrin Solution: As hemostatic in hematemesis, 1 dr. to 1 oz. orally; in hematuria, 1 oz., 1:5,000 or 1:10,000, instilled into bladder; as antispasmodic in asthma, 2–10 m *subcutaneously* or *intramuscularly*, repeated if necessary and site of injection massaged; in allergy to forestall reactions, 0.5 cc of 1:1,000 solution injected before specific medication is administered.

Coagulen: As hemostatic in gastric, intestinal, pulmonary and other hemorrhages; *intravenously*, 2–3 cc of ampule content several times daily; as prophylactic, 1.5–5 cc *subcutaneously* or *intramuscularly*.

Collosol Argentum: As colloidal antiseptic in general sepsis, septicemia, pyemia, meningitis following suppurative otitis media, and similar instances; administered *intravenously* or *intramuscularly*, 1 ampule every second day.

Collosol Aurum: As colloidal gold therapy in sepsis, septic bronchopneumonia, septic typhoid and similar infections; *intramuscularly* 1 ampule every 2–4 days; orally 1 teaspoonful three times daily, well diluted in water.

Collosol Ferro-Manganese: As hematinic, particularly in suppurative and infectious conditions, as erysipelas, cellulitis, lues and others; *intramuscularly*, 1–2 cc every 3–4 days; *orally* 1 teaspoonful three times daily.

Collosol Palladium: As antiinfective in various coccogenic infections, including gonorrhea, endocarditis, cellulitis, boils, gonorrheal arthritis; *intramuscularly*, 0.5–1 cc every second day; *orally*, 1 teaspoonful two to three times daily after meals, in water.

Diskets Alkaline: As alkalizer in general acidosis of infectious diseases, starvation, severe vomiting, exhaustive diarrheas, rheumatism, etc.; 1 disket in glass of water, repeated as often as necessary.

Diskets Sodium Bromide Compound: As sedative in mild migraine, gastric neuroses, menstrual disorders, hypertension and hyperthyroidism; 1 disket in half glass of water on empty stomach, repeated in 1 hr. and as necessary.

* *See also* Chapters on "Biologicals," "Endocrines," "Allergens," "Foods," "Mineral Waters" and Parts I and III of this chapter for special drugs and diseases.

Elixir Arsylen Compositum: As reconstructive, tonic and appetizer in anemia, convalescence, debility, malnutrition and chronic invalidism; 1 or 2 teaspoonfuls three times daily before meals.

Entacarb: As gastric and systemic alkalizer; in gastric hyperacidity and systemic acidosis; 2 or more tablets every 2–3 hr.

Ephedrin Products: As general stimulant in shock, Stokes-Adams' syndrome, hypoadrenia, myasthenia gravis; *orally*, ⅜–¾ gr two to three times daily; *hypodermically*, 1–2 ampules as indicated.

Ferro-Sajodin: As iodine therapy associated with anemia, in arteriosclerosis, syphilis, asthma, scrofula, arthritis, goitre; 1–3 tablets three times daily, chewed and crushed before swallowed.

Fibrogen: As hemostatic in concealed hemorrhages; *orally*, 3–6 cc in 6–8 oz. of ice water, in gastric hemorrhage; in other inaccessible hemorrhages—*subcutaneously*, never intravenously, 2–4 cc, repeated if necessary within 6 hr.

Formin: As systemic disinfectant in typhus, typhoid fever, infectious enteritis, encephalitis lethargica, meningitis; also in pneumonia, liver infections and bronchopneumonia; *intravenously*, 4–30 gr in 25% solution; *orally*, 5–15 gr several times daily.

Gentian Violet Improved Medicinal: As germicide in staphylococcic infections and septicemia; *intravenously*, 1–5 mg per kilogram of body weight, in 0.5% dilution, slowly and cautiously administered; in cyanosis during injection—cardiac stimulants.

Gynergen: As antipruritic in general prurigo of renal and hepatic origin; 1 tablet three to four times daily for 3 days or 1 ampule *intramuscularly* daily; in Graves' disease, same dosage, progressively diminished, for period of 2–3 weeks; course repeated after 1–3 weeks' intermission.

Helmitol: As urinary antiseptic in non-gonorrheal genitourinary disease—cystitis, prostatitis, pyelitis; as prophylactic against kidney involvement in scarlet fever, typhoid and other infections; 10–15 gr three to four times daily, dissolved in water.

Hemostatic Serum: As hemostatic in internal hemorrhages; prophylactically, 5 cc in fruit juice or other beverage, several times; in hemorrhage, *intravenously*, 2–5 cc, repeated as indicated.

Iodalbin: As alterative therapy in bronchial affections and in thyroidal disease; dosage 1 capsule after meals, as often as required.

Iodicin: As iodine therapy in replacement of potassium iodide; 1–3 tabloids three to four times daily; in simple goitre, as prophylactic—1 tabloid weekly, as treatment—2–3 tabloids weekly for 1 mo.

Iodostarine: As goitre therapy; preventive, 1 tablet weekly during school year, during pregnancy, 1–2 tablets throughout term; therapeutic, 2–3 tablets per week.

Iodotone: As alterative in arterial hypertension, arteriosclerosis, aneurysm, myocardial sclerosis, angina, rheumatism; 1–2 teaspoonfuls three to four times daily before meals.

Lipoiodine: As iodine therapy in lues, asthma, arteriosclerosis, plumbism and goitre; 2 tablets alternated with 1 tablet on each successive day; in goitre prophylaxis—2–4 tablets daily for 10 days during year; in hypothyroidism, 2–6 tablets daily as indicated.

Magnespirin: As general analgesic and antipyretic in colds, headaches, painful affections of the eyes, ears, nose, throat or joints; 2 tablets two to four times daily with water.

Melubrin: As antipyretic and analgesic in various fevers; 15–30 gr every 2–4 hr.; *maximum daily dosage* 150 gr.

Methylene Blue: As antidote in carbon monoxide and cyanide poisoning; 50–100 cc of 1% solution, *intravenously;* repeated if necessary.

Metrazol: As cardiac stimulant in shock, acute circulatory or respiratory failure, drug depression, asphyxia; *subcutaneously*, 1–2 ampules several times daily; *orally*, 1½–3 gr several times daily.

Normal Horse Serum: As hemostatic in pulmonary and other internal hemorrhages; *subcutaneously* or *intramuscularly*, 10–20 cc daily, repeated until 100 cc are given; orally, 30–100 cc repeated in 12–24 hr. if necessary.

Novatropin: For the decrease of secretions in ptyalism, hyperchlorhydria, hyperidrosis; orally, 1–2 tablets three times daily; or 10 drops of solution three to five times daily; *subcutaneously*, 1–3 ampules daily.

Nuclein: As leucocytosis stimulant in pneumonia, typhoid, tuberculosis; subcutaneously, 1 ampule daily or 1 or more tabloids after meals.

Optarson: As reconstructive and tonic in malarial, tubercular, neurologic and convalescent anemias; *subcutaneously* or *intramuscularly*, 1 ampule two to three times weekly.

Orargol: As alterative to raise resistance in pneumonia, influenza, sepsis, bronchopneumonia, typhoid; *intravenously* or *intramuscularly*, 5–20 cc every 1–2 days; orally (non-injectable), 20–100 drops daily as continuation to parenteral therapy.

Organidin: As iodine therapy in arterial hypertension, gout, asthma, thyroidal disease; 5–20 drops, diluted, three times daily before meals.

Otophen: As cholagogue in biliary stasis, catarrhal jaundice, constipation; 1 tablet, evenings, increased where necessary.

Pantopon: As injectable opium for use where morphine or codein is required; sedative dose, 1/24–1/12 gr; analgesic, 1/6–1/3 gr.

Papaverine Hydrochloride: As antispasmodic in biliary colic, uremic convulsions, whooping cough, bronchial asthma; as sedative in intestinal spasticity, sea sickness and hemoptysis; orally, 3/4–1 1/3 gr single dosage, up to 4 gr daily dosage; *subcutaneously*, 3/4–1 1/2 gr; *intravenously*, 1/12–1/6 gr per dose.

Para-Thor-Mone: As parathyroid therapy in delayed blood coagulability, chronic ulcerative colitis, radium poisoning, tuberculosis, nephrosis and to affect calcium metabolism; 28–60 units daily in spasmodic conditions; in hemorrhage 38–50 units; administered *hypodermically*.

Paroidin: As parathyroid therapy in above conditions; *subcutaneously* or *intramuscularly*, 0.2–0.4 cc (30–60 units) for 5–6 days; repeated if necessary after rest of 1 or 2 weeks.

Peroxoids: As systemic antacid in conditions with acidosis; 2–3 tablets or 1/2–1 teaspoonful in water, as often as required.

Phloridzin: In renal function test; for administration and interpretation *See Chap. I.*

Phytine: To stimulate calcium phosphorus metabolism in tuberculosis, convalescence, nervous diseases, and others; 1–4 tablets daily with meals.

Pitressin: As vasoconstrictor in hypotension, in shock during pneumonia, diphtheria and similar infectious diseases; in diabetes insipidus; *hypodermically*, 3–5 m; *intranasally*, by spray, or pledget.

Pituitrin: Indications and dosage as for Pitressin.

Proteolac: As non-specific protein agent in septicemia, thrombophlebitis, peptic ulcer and acute infections of various types; *intramuscularly*, 1–2 cc, rapidly increased to 5–10 cc, at intervals of 2–5 days; also given *intravenously* where quick and strong action is desired, every 2–5 days.

Pulvules Lextron 55: As hematinic and hematopoietic in secondary and primary anemias; 3 pulvules three times daily after meals.

Salyrgan: As powerful diuretic in hydrothorax, tubercular peritonitis, hepatic ascites and general anasarca; *intravenously* or *intramuscularly*, never subcutaneously, 0.5–1 cc every 3–4 days, in conjunction with ammonium chloride or ammonium nitrate, 90–150 gr daily, orally.

Solvochin: As quinine therapy in lobar pneumonia; *intramuscularly*, 2 cc for 3 successive days, given as early as possible; in malaria, 2 cc twice daily for 14 days, continued 1 cc for 14 additional days.

Sulphocol: As colloidal sulphur in sulphur metabolism deficiencies, liver impairment, intestinal toxemias; *hypodermically*, 0.25–5 cc, orally 1/2–3 gr, several times daily.

Stypticin: As hemostatic in hemoptysis, vesical and ureteral hemorrhages; orally, ½–4 gr four to five times daily if necessary; *subcutaneously* in urgent cases, 1½–4 gr in 10% solution.

Terpichin: As non-specific agent in the treatment of severe infections—sepsis, phlebitis, bronchial pneumonia, bronchiectasis, septic arthritis; *intramuscularly*, 1 cc every 2–3 days, increased to 2 cc.

Theobromine: As cardiac stimulant and diuretic in renal and hepatic edema, uremia, pleuritic effusions and aortitis; 3–8 gr four times daily.

Thromboplastin: As hemostatic in hemophilia, intestinal, gastric and pulmonary hemorrhage, bleeding of hepatic origin; *subcutaneously* or *intramuscularly*, never intravenously, 10–20 cc repeated as necessary.

Trillin: As hemostatic in intestinal and pulmonary hemorrhages; 3–5 tablets every 3 hr. as indicated.

Tyramine: As vasoconstrictor in shock, collapse, morphine poisoning; hypodermically, ⅓–⅔ gr.

Urotropin: As biliary and urinary antiseptic in gall bladder affections, in jaundice, ocular disease, sinusitis, meningitis; *intravenously*, 5 cc of 40% solution, also *intramuscularly* and *subcutaneously;* orally, 7½ gr two to four times daily.

Valital: As analgesic in painful affections—headache, irritable cough; 1–2 tablets every 4 hr.; in severe cases, larger doses more frequently.

Zilatone: As choleretic and cholagogue in biliary disease, constipation, atonic dyspepsia, hepatic insufficiency; 2 tablets with copious water intake twice daily; regulated as required.

Neuropsychiatry

Preparations Useful in Neurology and Psychiatry*

Abasin: To allay irritability and nervousness in menopausal neuroses, hysteria and mental disorders; 1–2 tablets three to four times daily.

Adalin and Adalin-Luminal: As sedative in neuroses and various mental disorders; sedative 5–10 gr two to three times daily; hypnotic 10–20 gr at bedtime or when indicated.

Alepsal: As sedative in various neuroses; 1–2 tablets as often as required.

Allonal: As analgesic and hypnotic in insomnia with or without pain; in mild cases, 1–2 tablets; in severe cases, a third table about 1 or 2 hr. after first dose.

Alurate: As hypnotic in milder forms of nervous excitation; in the more severe types of psychoses requiring hospitalization; in mild insomnia, 1 tablet at bedtime; in obstinate insomnia, 2–4 tablets or 2 teaspoonfuls of elixir; in severe cases, injectable ampule to be used.

Alphebine: As sedative in neuroses; 1–2 tablets as often as required.

Amarbital: As analgesic and hypnotic in many psychoses accompanied by pain and discomfort; 1–2 tablets as often as required.

Amatin: As analgesic in headache, various neuralgias; 1–3 tablets several times daily.

Am-Phen-Al: As analgesic and hypnotic in headache, neuritis and neuralgia; 1–2 tablets repeated in 1 hr. if necessary.

Amifeine: As sedative; 1–2 tablets or capsules as often as necessary.

Ampydin: As analgesic in neuralgia, neuritis, sciatica, migraine, headaches; 5 gr repeated as long as pain persists.

Amytal: As sedative and hypnotic in nervousness, insomnia of fatigue, neurasthenia and hyperthyroidism; sedative, ¾–1½ gr few times daily; hypnotic, 1–2 tablets at bedtime, taken in hot milk or water.

Analgine: As general nerve sedative; 1–2 tablets repeated in 2 hr. if necessary.

Antifebrin: As analgesic in neuralgia, migraine, sciatica, crises of locomotor ataxia; 1 tabloid every 1–2 hr., administered with caution.

* *See also* Parts I and III of this Chapter for additional drugs and diseases of interest in these specialties.

Arsenoferratose: As hematinic in neurasthenia, functional diseases, chorea minor; 1–3 teaspoonfuls three times daily.

Aspirofeine: As analgesic in various nervous disturbances; 1–2 tablets or capsules as often as indicated.

Atoquinol: As analgesic in neuralgia, myalgia, various painful neuritides; in moderate pain, 4–6 tablets in 24 hr.; in severe pain, up to 8 tablets every 3–4 hr. for 3 doses.

Aurol: As sedative in neuroses and neurasthenia; 15 m three times daily; *intravenously* or *intramuscularly*, 1–5 cc three times weekly.

Avertin: As rectal anesthetic and antispasmodic in violent and maniacal neuropsychiatric cases, in tetanus, epilepsy; 0.1 cc per kilogram of body weight, total dosage not to exceed in females 6–8 cc, in males 9–10 cc; the debilitated, cachectic, dehydrated and very obese must be given smaller doses.

Baramid: As sedative; 1–2 tablets or capsules as often as required.

Barbenzal: As analgesic in headache, ovarian neuralgia, neuritis; 1–2 tablets in warm fluid every 4–6 hr. until relieved.

Barbromide: As hypnotic; 1 capful at bedtime.

Barlupulin: As sedative in nervous disorders; 1–2 capsules as required.

Belladenal: As antispasmodic in epilepsy, Parkinsonism, nervous erethism, neurasthenia and psychoneuroses; 2–4 tablets daily or ¼ tablet every half hour.

Bellafoline: As antispasmodic in Parkinsonism; 1–2 tablets or 10–20 drops three times daily; as hypnotic, 0.5 cc when required.

Brometone: As sedative in epilepsy, severe headaches and various neurotic disturbances; 5 gr two to three times daily.

Bromionyl: As bromide therapy; 60–75 gr daily divided in 4 or 5 doses.

Bromiphen Elixir: As sedative in nervous disorders; 1–2 teaspoonfuls in water four or five times daily.

Bromipin 33%: As sedative in epilepsy, muscular twitchings, migraine, neurasthenia; 20 m increased to 40, up to 160 m; rectally, as enema, 4–10 dr.

Bromipin 10%: As sedative in neurasthenia, insomnia, twitchings, mild epilepsy; ½–2 tablespoonfuls three or four times daily.

Bromocol: As sedative in all conditions where bromides are indicated; 2–10 gr as often as required.

Bromural: As sedative in allaying hyperexcitation, irritability and restlessness. 1 tablet several times daily; as hypnotic, 2–4 tablets at bedtime.

Brovalol: As nerve sedative in hysteria, neurasthenia and various nervous excitation stages; 1–3 pearls several times daily.

Butyl-Chloral Hydrate: As analgesic in trigeminal neuralgia, also other neuralgias and tabetic pains; *maximum single dose* 30 gr; *maximum daily dose* 60 gr; average dose 1½–5 gr.

Cafumal: As sedative and hypnotic; 1–3 tablets daily.

Calcium Granular: For relief of vasomotor excitation in convulsive states; 2 teaspoonfuls before meals.

Camphro-Salyl: As analgesic in neuralgias; subcutaneously or intramuscularly into painful area; 1 ampule every 2–3 days for 5–6 injections.

Chamomilla Compound: As nerve stimulant in neurasthenia; 1 teaspoonful in hot water four times daily.

Chloretone: As sedative and hypnotic; 10 gr, repeated in half hour.

Chloroxyl: As analgesic in neuralgia, neuritis, lumbago and sciatica; 1–3 tablets repeated as indicated.

Cibalgine: As analgesic in cephalalgia, tabetic crises and other painful conditions; 1 tablet, 1 teaspoonful or 1 ampule every 3–6 hr.

Collosol Bromide: As sedative in epilepsy and similar states; 1–2 teaspoonfuls three times daily in water; or 2–4 teaspoonfuls at bedtime.

Collosol Palladium: In epilepsy; intramuscularly, 0.5–1 cc; orally, 1 teaspoonful in water two to three times daily after meals.

Colsul: For fever therapy in various mental disorders; *hypodermically*, 0.5 cc increased by 0.5 cc to *maximum dosage* of 5 cc until desired results are effected; if necessary, up to 10–12 cc.

Combinal: As analgesic in conditions accompanied by painful manifestations; sedative, 1 tablet three times daily; hypnotic, 2–3 tablets at bedtime.

Compral: As analgesic and antispasmodic in migraine, neuralgia, headaches; 1–2 tablets repeated as often as indicated.

Cryogenine: As analgesic in headache, migraine, neuralgia, sciatica, lumbago; 15–45 gr daily.

Decholin: As choleretic in melancholia, schizophrenia and biliary migraine; 1–2 tablets two to three times daily after meals, for 3–5 weeks, when dosage may be decreased; *intravenously*, 1 ampule of 20% solution, slowly injected on 3 successive days.

Dial: As sedative and hypnotic in migraine, chorea major, drug addiction, tetanus, strychnine poisoning; sedative, 1 tablet or ½ dr. of elixir one to four times daily; hypnotic, 1–3 tablets, 2–6 teaspoonfuls of elixir or 1–2 ampules 1 hr. before effect is desired.

Diskets Bromides: As sedative in insomnia, hysteria, nervous palpitation and epilepsy; 1 disket dissolved in water, repeated as necessary.

Elixir Bromo-Valerianate: As sedative in neurasthenia, hysteria, nervous irritability and functional disorders; 1 dr. three times daily.

Formin: As systemic antiseptic in meningitis, encephalitis, poliomyelitis; 5–15 gr two to three times daily; intravenously, 4–30 gr only, in 25% solution.

Gynergen: As liver detoxicant in migraine; as prophylactic, 1–2 tablets; during attack, *intramuscularly*, 0.5 cc–1 cc, repeated if necessary in 20 min.

Hypno-Bromic Compound: As hypnotic in insomnia, nervousness, hysteria; ½–1 teaspoonful in water at bedtime.

Ipral Calcium: As sedative and hypnotic in restlessness, irritability and sleeplessness; sedative 1–2 tablets followed by hot drink; hypnotic 2–3 tablets; repeated in 6–12 hr. if necessary.

Kola "Astier": As stimulating tonic in functional nervous disorders, neurasthenia and mental disturbances; 2 teaspoonfuls daily, plain or with fluids.

Lecithin Glycerole: As tonic in psychoses and neurasthenia; 1 teaspoonful in ice water or on cracked ice, as required.

Lumalgin: As hypnotic in nervousness, insomnia, migraine and various neuroses; 1–3 tablets in accordance with severity of condition.

Luminal-Sodium: For quick sedation in dementia, drug addiction, status epilepticus and cocaine intoxication; as enema or suppository, 3–6 gr; in emergency cases, hypodermically, gr 2.

Medinal: As hypnotic and sedative in insomnia, nervousness; orally, 5–15 gr, or elixir, 1–2 teaspoonfuls at bedtime; rectally, 5–10 gr as suppository.

Melubrin: As analgesic in neuralgia, neuritis, sciatica; 15–30 gr every 3–4 hr.; *maximum daily dose* 150 gr.

Naiodine "Logeais": As iodine therapy in trigeminal and intercostal neuralgia, sciatica, herpes zoster; *intramuscularly*, 20–40 cc two to three times daily; *maintenance dose*, 5–10 cc daily.

Narkogen: As hypnotic in manic states, nymphomania and nervous irritability; 1 or more teaspoonfuls as required.

Neo-Bornyval: As nerve sedative in hysteria, neuroses, morbid and emotional states, hypochondriasis, anaphrodisia; 1–3 pearls two to four times daily after meals.

Neomagnephen: As analgesic in neuritis and neuralgia; 2–3 tablets four times daily.

Nervinal: As nerve sedative in neurasthenia, hysteria and insomnia; 1–2 tablets three times daily, reduced with improvement.

Neuronidia: As sedative and hypnotic in insomnia, nervousness, neurasthenia, mild psychoses; sedative, 1 teaspoonful two to three times daily; hypnotic, 2 teaspoonfuls.

Neurosine: As hypnotic in migraine, neuralgia, neurasthenia; 1 dessertspoonful in water three or more times daily.

Neusthenic "Fraisse": As nerve tonic in neurasthenia, nerve exhaustion; *hypodermically*, 1 ampule daily for 12 days, followed by another series after 5 day interval; *orally*, 25 drops daily for 12 days; repeated after 5 day interval.

Nostal: As sedative and hypnotic in nervousness, neurasthenia, insomnia without pain; sedative, ½–1 tablet; hypnotic, double dosage; in severe cases, triple dosage; in hot water, milk or tea.

Ortal Sodium: As sedative and hypnotic in nervousness, insomnia, migraine, epilepsy, alcoholism and drug addiction; average dosage 1 to 2 capsules, in epilepsy 2 to 3 capsules daily; repeated as required.

Papaverine Hydrochloride: As anticonvulsive in epilepsy, chorea major, cerebral diseases; *subcutaneously*, ¾–1½ gr daily; *orally*, ¾ gr twice daily.

Passiflora Compound: As sedative in nervous irritability, hysteria and insomnia; 1–2 tablets several times daily after meals.

Pentobarbital-Sodium: As antispasmodic and sedative to control convulsions in tetany, strychnine poisoning and mania; rectally, 5–8 gr; orally, 1½–5 gr; intravenously, 1 ampule.

Peralga: As analgesic in painful affections—migraine, neuralgia, neuritis; 1 tablet as often as indicated.

Pernoston: As hypnotic and antispasmodic in psychiatric disturbances and drug addiction during withdrawal treatment of the habit forming drug; *intramuscularly* and *intravenously* by special technic; 1 cc per 27½ lb. of body weight. *See Chap. I.*

Phanodorn: As hypnotic in hysteria, psychoses, neurasthenia and nervous insomnia; 1 tablet, in obstinate cases 2 tablets, at bedtime, with copious hot drinks.

Phenobarbital-Sodium: As hypnotic in dementias, cocaine intoxication and other drug addictions; *hypodermically*, 20% solution, 1½–5 gr; rectally, in 20% solution.

Phospho-Lecithin: As nerve tonic in various disturbances; 2 teaspoonfuls four times daily before meals.

Pyramidon: As analgesic in neuralgia, headaches, migraine; 3–5 gr, repeated in 3–4 hr.

Pyraminal: As sedative in headache, migraine and neuralgias; 1 tablet repeated in ½–1 hr. if necessary; in severe cases, double dosage.

Sabromin: As sedative in nervousness, neurasthenia, insomnia and restlessness; 5–20 gr three to four times daily 1 hr. after meals.

Sandoptal: As sedative and hypnotic in mild nervous disturbances; 1 tablet, in obstinate cases 2–4 tablets, before retiring.

Scopolamine Stable: As cerebral sedative in acute mania, delirium tremens, drug addiction, tetanus, alcoholism and similar disturbances; hypodermically, 1 ampule as required.

Sedobrol: As sedative in neurasthenia, restlessness; 2 cubes dissolved in hot water, taken in evening.

Sedormid: As hypnotic in mild excitation, restlessness and insomnia; 1–2 tablets at bedtime; half dosage as sedative.

Sodium Amytal: As sedative, hypnotic and antispasmodic in convulsive diseases; 2–4 pulvules until convulsions are controlled; 1–2 pulvules every 6 hr. in other conditions.

Somnos: As sedative and soporific in delirium, mania, nocturnal epilepsy, hysteria; 1 teaspoonful every ½–1 hr.; double dosage at bedtime as hypnotic; rectally, in tetanus and strychnine poisoning, 2 oz. in 5% sodium bicarbonate as retention enema.

Sulfonal: As sedative and hypnotic in mental disturbances; 15–30 gr dissolved in hot fluid.

Trichlorethylene: As anodyne in trigeminal neuralgia; by inhalation, 6–7 breaths several times daily for several weeks.

Trional: As sedative and hypnotic in insomnias without pain; 10–15 gr or more half hour before retiring, in warm fluid.

Veronal and Veronal-Sodium: As hypnotic in epilepsy, morphinism, cocainism, delirium tremens and psychoses; 5–15 gr in hot drink; rectally and subcutaneously, 5–8 gr of the sodium salt dissolved in 5 cc of water.

Obstetrics

Preparations Useful in Obstetrical Practice*

Adrenalin and Adrin: In dystocia due to contraction ring spasm; 5 m of 1:1,000 solution *subcutaneously* or *intramuscularly*.

Avertin: As rectal anesthetic to ease delivery and in eclampsia; administered after cleansing enema and mild hypnotic, with or without morphine and atropine; is introduced into rectum; *maximum dosage* 1/10 cc per kilogram of body weight, total not to exceed 6–8 cc.

Calcium Gluconate and Calglucon: To allay irritability in preeclamptic stage; *intravenously* 1 ampule every 2 days; also administered intragluteally.

Chloretone: As analgesic in painful labor, 10–20 gr as required.

Colactol: As sedative in hyperemesis gravidarum, 2–4 teaspoonfuls three to four times daily after meals.

Dial: As sedative or to induce seminarcosis; 2–4 cc *intramuscularly*, or 2–4 tablets or equivalent of elixir *orally*, repeated in 2–3 hr.; *maximum dosage* 9 gr in 24 hr.

Dilaudid: As narcotic for relief of pain and preoperatively; oral initial dose 1/48 gr increased to 1/24 and 1/16 gr when required; hypodermically gr 1/32.

Dioviburnia: As antispasmodic in threatened abortion and in uterine subinvolution; 1 dessertspoonful three times daily in water after meals.

Ergotoxine: As uterine stimulant in relaxed uterus; 1 or 2 tabloids with or without strychnin, *subcutaneously* or *intramuscularly*.

Gravocain: As obstetric spinal anesthetic; administered in primiparae only after cervix is fully dilated, in multiparae—after 5–6 cm dilatation; injected *intraspinally* with patient in sitting position, or head and shoulders raised 15–20 degrees.

Gynergen: As uterine stimulant; orally 1 tablet two to four times daily, *intramuscularly*, 0.5 cc, maximum 1 cc; in emergencies repeated in 20 min.

Infundin: As uterine stimulant; *hypodermically* 2 m antepartum 10–15 m postpartum.

Luminal: As sedative in eclampsia and vomiting of pregnancy; gr ½–1½ every 4–6 hr. or 3–6 gr in individual doses, as required.

Luminal-Sodium: For conditions as above; *hypodermically* 1 ampule as often as demanded.

Neo-Ergot: As uterine stimulant and hemostatic; 15–30 m after labor, 30–60 m post partum hemorrhage.

Ortal Sodium: As preoperative sedative; gr 6 when active labor has begun, repeated in 3 hours if necessary.

Pantopon: As injectable opium in labor cases as sedative with or without scopolamine; dosage 1/24–1/12 gr, as analgesic 1/6–1/3 gr.

Pernoston: As antispasmodic and hypnotic for induction of twilight sleep and in postpartum eclampsia; 4–5 cc intravenously, slowly injected.

Pitocin: As uterine stimulant and hemostatic in uterine inertia, protracted labor without physical impediment, in pre-eclamptic and eclamptic states; *intramuscularly* 0.2–0.5 cc, repeated if necessary at intervals of 20–30 min.

Pituitary Extract: As vasoconstrictor and uterine stimulant; *intramuscularly* 2–4 units every 4 hr. for 3 doses, in first stage only in marginal placenta praevia with incomplete dilatation of cervix; in second stage, in secondary uterine inertia; in third stage, to prevent hemorrhage and to complete expulsion of placenta; in hemorrhage 5–10 units.

Pituitary Liquid: Uses and dosage as for pituitary extract; also in the Watson technic for induction of labor.

Pituitary Solution: As vasoconstrictor and uterine stimulant, and in obstetrical conditions; *subcutaneously* or *intramuscularly* 3–10 units, repeated if necessary.

* *See also* Parts I and III of this chapter for additional products of interest in this specialty.

Pituitrin: As uterine stimulant, for weak labor pains; 0.2–0.5 cc *hypodermically*, repeated if necessary in about ½ hr.; in postpartum hemorrhage from 0.5–0.8 cc.

Pyridium: As urinary antiseptic in pyelitis of pregnancy; 1 tablet or 1 dr. of solution four times daily.

Rectal Analgesia (Gwathmey): As analgesic for relief of pain in childbirth; rectally, after instillation of mineral oil and ether mixture.

Rivanol: As systemic antiseptic in puerperal sepsis; *intravenously* 1:1,000 solution in 1 part of drug to 2 parts of dextrose.

Scopolamine Stable: As preoperative sedative in obstetrics to produce twilight sleep; *hypodermically* gr 1/100 at 2 fingers' dilatation, repeated at intervals of 2 hr. as indicated; for optimal effect pantopon gr ⅓ is given with first injection but not repeated.

Sodium Amytal: For preoperative sedation and for the control of labor in obstetrics; orally 1 pulvule at 2 fingers' dilatation, repeated every 1–4 hr. as required; in eclampsia, 2–4 pulvules given orally at frequent intervals as required until convulsions are controlled.

Solvochin: In uterine inertia to induce labor; *intramuscularly* ½–1 cc at half hour intervals.

Tenamin: As uterine hemostatic to control postpartum hemorrhage and in metrorrhagia; orally 15–20 drops three to four times daily; *subcutaneously* and *intramuscularly*, 1 ampule repeated as necessary, *never intravenously.*

Thymo-Pitsin: In uterine inertia to induce labor and to control postpartum hemorrhage; *intramuscularly* 0.5 cc every hour for 3 doses.

Tyramine: As uterine stimulant and vasoconstrictor to control postpartum hemorrhage; *hypodermically* gr ⅓–gr ⅔, repeated as necessary.

Ophthalmology

Preparations Useful in Ophthalmologic Practice*

1. Anesthetics

Alypin: As local anesthetic in 2–4 % solution; must be freshly prepared, sterilized by boiling for several minutes in previously boiled distilled water.

Beta-Eucaine Lactate: As local anesthetic in 2–3 % solution.

Butyn: As local anesthetic for removal of foreign bodies, in corneal abrasions, all operations and painful affections; in 2 % solution for topical instillation, up to 5 %, for profound anesthesia; operation to begin not later than 10 min. after last instillation.

Holocain: As ocular surface anesthetic in keratitis, glaucoma, conjunctivitis; in 1 % solution, dropped into eye or applied to lids with cotton wrapped probe.

Larocaine: As local anesthetic in 2–5 % solution; is prepared from distilled water or saline, sterilized by boiling for 10 min.

Metycaine: As local anesthetic in 2 % solution.

Novocain: As local anesthetic 3–5 cc or 2 %, as indicated.

Nupercain: As local anesthetic 2–5 % solution, as indicated.

Orthoform: As surface anesthetic in tubercular and syphilitic lesions, corneal ulcers, conjunctivitis; applied as ointment or powder.

Panthesine Ointment: As local anesthetic and antipruritic, in blepharitis, corneal erosions and ulcers; applied in ointment form.

Pantocain: For surface and mucosa anesthesia; ¼, ½, 1 and 2 % solution, with or without suprarenin.

Tutocain: As local anesthetic for surface application 2–5 %; for infiltration ⅕–½ %.

2. Antiseptics

Argentiform: As ophthalmic antiseptic where silver therapy is indicated; applied topically, in form of ointment.

* *See in addition* "Ophthalmic Ointments" in this chapter, "Vitamines" and other preparations pertaining to this specially in respective chapters.

Argocol: As silver application in colloidal form in various eye affections, conjunctivitis, ophthalmia; applied as ointment or in solution.

Argolaval: As antiseptic and astringent; 5–50 %, pure or in combination with atropin, cocaine nitrate (not hydrochloride) and as ointment.

Argyn: As astringent in conjunctivitis, trachoma, corneal ulcers and ophthalmorrhea; in 10–25 % solution.

Argyrol: As gonocide and astringent in acute inflammatory conditions, in prophylaxis and treatment of ophthalmia neonatorum; 10–50 % for instillation; for prophylaxis 10–25 % solution.

Bismuth Violet: As germicide and analgesic; in 10 % aqueous glycerin solution.

Cargentos: As antiseptic and astringent in conjunctivitis in 25 % solution or 10 % ointment; in corneal ulcer 50 %; preoperatively and in prophylaxis of ophthalmia 25 %.

Chloramine: As Dakin antiseptic in 1⁄10 % solution in physiologic saline.

Chloroxyl: As analgesic and antipyretic in iritis, episcleritis and hemicrania; orally 1–3 tablets, repeated if necessary.

Collene: As colloidal antiseptic in eye affections; used full strength.

Collosol Argentum: As antiseptic for wounds, corneal ulcers, interstitial keratitis, blepharitis, dacryocystitis, gonorrheal ophthalmia; 2–3 drops of undiluted solution; for irrigation is diluted in 5–6 parts of warm saline; used as subconjunctival injections.

Collosol Hydrargyrum: As colloidal antiluetic in subconjunctival injections, in sympathetic ophthalmia, iritis, choroiditis, choroidoretinitis, retrobulbar neuritis.

Collosol Zinc: As astringent in 0.05 % or double strength, for local application.

Collyrium: As mild astringent eye wash in conjunctival inflammations; administered as eye bath.

Cupristicks: As astringent for topical application to the lids.

Dimazon Ointment: For local application in conjunctivitis, keratitis; applied daily by gentle massage over cornea with instillation of scopolamine.

I-Bath: As antiseptic and astringent eye wash for catarrhal conditions and irritations; applied with cup or by medicine dropper.

Iodosyl: An antiseptic where iodine is helpful; applied in 2–6 % ointment or with atropine 1 %.

Iothion-Oil: As iodine therapy in trachoma, pannus, blepharitis; used plain or diluted with olive oil.

Lunosol: As astringent antiseptic applied to granulated lids; plain or diluted.

Mercurochrome-220-Soluble: As antiseptic in ophthalmia; in 0.5–2½ % solution.

Mercurosticks: As antiseptic and astringent for granulated lids and marginal ulcers: applied topically.

Metaphen: As antiseptic eye wash and ointment, 1:3,000 dilution.

Merthiolate: As antiseptic eye wash, in 1:5,000 dilution.

Neo-Silvol: As colloidal antiseptic in purulent and simple conjunctivitis; in 10–50 % solution as indicated.

Noviform: As antiseptic in blepharitis and blenorrhagia; applied as ointment.

Palpebrine: As antiseptic eye wash in conjunctivitis, blepharitis and other external eye affections; applied by dropper three to four times daily.

Protargol: As antiseptic and astringent in prophylaxis of ophthalmia neonatorum; in 2 % solution; in conjunctivitis and blepharitis ½–2 %; in trachoma 20–25 %.

Rivanol: As antiseptic in acute conjunctivitis; 1–500 applied two to three times daily.

Solargentum: As silver antiseptic and gonocide in ophthalmia neonatorum; in 25 % solution.

Targesin: As gonocide and astringent in conjunctivitis, blepharitis and corneal ulcer; in 5 % solution or ointment.

Tolamine: As germicidal eye wash, postoperatively and for granular lids, for purulent ophthalmia; in 1⁄10 % solution.

Zincol: As astringent for instillation into conjunctival sac or topical application; 1–5 gr to the ounce of water.

3. Pupillary and Other Remedies

Cinchophen: As analgesic in iritis and episcleritis, 1–2 tablets three to four times daily, continued in acute cases for 2–5 days; in chronic, same dosage followed by rest period of several days.

Dionin: As analgesic and for chemosis in corneal affections, iritis, glaucoma, interstitial keratitis, conjunctival catarrh, opacities of vitreous humor; 1–2 drops of 5–10% solution or pure to produce chemosis; 2 drops of 0.5%–2% solution four times daily as analgesic.

Ephedrine: As local mydriatic; 1–2 drops of 3% solution.

Epinine: As mydriatic; 1 tabloid applied directly to conjunctiva there to be dissolved; or 1 tabloid in 10 m of water to form a 1:100 solution and applied.

Euphthalmine Hydrochloride: As mydriatic; 1 tabloid placed on conjunctiva, repeated in 20 min. if required; or 2–3 drops of 5–10% solution.

Fluorescein: As diagnostic aid in corneal ulcers and lesions; 1 tabloid placed on conjunctiva or solution instilled with dropper.

Neocinchophen: As uricolytic before intraocular operations; 7½–15 gr 3–4 times daily after meals, with copious draughts of water.

Novatropin: As mydiatic; in 2–5% solution.

Optochin Base and Optochin Hydrochloride: As próphylactic in cataract operation and treatment of serpiginous ulcers; see special technic, *Chap. I.*

Ovarialhormon Folliculin Menformon: Lately used in retinitis pigmentosa; *hypodermically* 1–2 ampules daily for 30 injections.

Oto-Rhino-Laryngology

Preparations Used in Otology, Rhinology and Laryngology*

Acriflavine: As antiseptic and bacteriostat in otitis media purulenta; as wet packing in 1:500 of 50% alcohol; for irrigation in this and other conditions 1:10,000 normal saline.

Acriflavine Neutral: As antiseptic in nose and throat infections, also in Ludwig's angina; as spray and gargle in 1:1,000 to 1:3,000 solution.

Acriviolet: As antiseptic spray and gargle in nose and throat affections in 1% solution every 3 hr.; in otitis media, auditory canal is filled with 1% solution while patient is directed to swallow; in sinusitis 4–6 cc of 1% solution injected several times.

Alumnol: As astringent and antiseptic in purulent otitis and in nasopharyngeal catarrh; for irrigation, gargling, douching in 0.5% solution; topically used in powder form or in ½–1% aqueous solution.

Alypin: As local anesthetic in rhinolaryngologic procedures; in 5–10% solutions.

Analka: As spray in nasal affections; full strength or 50% dilution.

Anesthesin: As topical analgesic in laryngitis, tubercular and syphilitic ulceration; as spray 3% in 1–2 parts of mucilage.

Antiseptic Sol 59: For mouth wash, gums, throat, colds; full strength.

Argocol: As colloidal silver application in nasal catarrh, tonsillitis, faucial inflammation; in pure solution or ointment form.

Argyn: As astringent in naso-pharyngitis, ozena, tonsillitis; in 5–10% solution, for nasal douching, gargling or direct application; for swabbing in 10–25% solution.

Argyrol: As astringent and antiseptic in acute nasal infections; as spray, gargle, tampon treatment 5–10% solution; topically, in 10–25% solution.

Auralgan: As analgesic for earache; by filling fully the auditory canal and retaining it there until relieved.

Beta-Eucaine Hydrochloride: As local anesthetic for various surgical manipulations; in 5–10% solution.

Beta-Eucaine Lactate: As local anesthetic in surgical manipulations; in 10–15% solution; in infiltration anesthesia 0.12% solution.

* *See also* "Nasal Preparations," "Vaccines," "Bacteriophages," "Buccal Preparations" and "Liquid Antiseptics" in this and other Chapters.

Bicarbonate of Soda: As solvent for impacted cerumen; by lavage of external canal with 5–10% solution.

Bismuth Violet: As germicide and analgesic in nasal and sinus infections; by local application in 10% aqueous solution.

Blandine Compound: For nasal affections as nose drops by swab or spray; full strength, when required.

Bon-Sol: As mouth wash and gargle, full strength or diluted one half.

Borocaine: As local anesthetic in various surgical procedures; in tonsillectomy ½–1%, nerve block 1–2%, topically 2–10%.

Borolyptol: As antiseptic and deodorant in stomatitis, gingivitis, aphthae; full strength or half diluted.

Butesin: As local anesthetic and decongestive in nasal affections, also hay fever, asthma and coryza; as jelly in bland base, or spray with ephedrine, ⅔–1%.

Butyn: As local anesthetic in submucous resection and other operations and examinations; in infiltration 1⁄10–¼%; topically in 2% solution.

Cargentos: Antiseptic, astringent; as spray 10–20%; for swabbing 25–50%.

Chloramine: As antiseptic in ½% solution for mouth, nose and throat.

Chlorbutanol: As local antiseptic in nose and throat disorders; hypodermically in aqueous solution.

Chlorazene: As Dakin antiseptic for gargle, spray or douching, in ¼% strength.

Chloretone: As antiseptic spray in rhinitis, laryngitis, pharyngitis, as inhalant with camphor, menthol and essential oils; applied by spray.

Chloroseptine: As antiseptic gargle or spray; in 2% solution, prepared by dissolving 2 tablets in 1 oz. of water.

Collene: As colloidal antiseptic in ear, nose and throat therapy; full strength.

Collosol Argentum: As silver antiseptic in otitis media suppurativa; pure or diluted with warm normal saline; as spray or gargle in nose and throat conditions, diluted with 2–4 parts of warm saline, also undiluted.

Coryfin: As local anodyne in nasal catarrh; is painted lightly on mucous membrane, full strength or sprayed in 30% solution with liquid petrolatum; in pharyngitis, also given 3–4 drops on lump of sugar, slowly dissolved in mouth; in laryngitis, by inhalation 10 drops to pint of boiling water.

Cresatin: As antiseptic and analgesic in purulent otitis media and auditory furunculosis; full strength or diluted with oil or alcohol; as spray by atomizer and nebulizer.

Ephedrine and Compounds: As decongestive to shrink swollen turbinates in hypertrophic rhinitis, sinusitis; by inhalation and topically by swab, dropper or spray.

Epinine: As vasoconstrictor to nasal passages for relief of congestion; applied in solution or nasal jelly.

Ferrocol: As local bactericide in nasopharyngeal catarrh and laryngitis; applied locally by dropper.

Fibrolysin: As fibrous tissue resolvent in middle ear deafness; *intramuscularly* also *subcutaneously*, 1 ampule or smaller dosage every second to third day, from 20–50 injections.

Formalin: As antiseptic and disinfectant in oral and pharyngeal infections; by spray in 2% solution, topically in 1½–2% solution; the latter also for irrigation of sinus cavities.

Homiodin: As absorptive in catarrhal otitis media; *subcutaneously* 1 cc twice weekly for 2–6 injections.

Kalmerid Germicidal Tablets: For sinus irrigation; in 1:5,000 to 1:20,000 solution.

Lar-Io-Ben: As antiseptic and deodorant gargle or spray; in dilutions up to 50%.

Larocaine: As local anesthetic in all surgical procedures; in 5–10% solutions.

Lunosol: As antiseptic and astringent in all nose, throat and ear infections; in 5% solution.

Mercury Cyanide: As germicide in diphtheria, croup and membranous rhinitis; 0.01% solution.

Metaphen: As antiseptic, for direct application, inhalation and irrigation; in 1:5,000 solution, or with ephedrine 1% added.

Metycaine: As local anesthetic; topically or hypodermically, 2% solution.

Neo-Silvol: As colloidal antiseptic in rhinitis, pharyngitis, sinusitis, post-tonsillectomy; in 10–50% solution, by swab 10%; for sinus irrigation 5%.

Neo-Synephrin: As decongestive in nasal congestion and in allergy; applied in ¼% aqueous solution or as emulsion.

Noviform: As antiseptic and astringent after removal of polyps, septum operation, turbinectomy; in powder form, pure or with talcum.

Novocain: As local anesthetic in all rhinolaryngologic procedures; in ½–1% with suprarenin 1:1,000 in concentration of 3–5 m per ounce.

Nupercaine: As local anesthetic, alone or in combination with ephedrine or epinephrin; as spray in 1:500 to 1:200 solution.

Orthoform: As surface analgesic, in tubercular or syphilitic lesions, in rhinitis and pharyngitis; as insufflation in powder form; in painful mouth and throat infections as troches dissolved on tongue.

Oxyquinolin Sulphate: As antiseptic in nasal and pharyngeal affections; for douching 1:3,000, as gargle 1:2,000.

Panthesine Ointment: As anesthetic in aphthous stomatitis and nasal affections; applied in small quantities as ointment, several times daily.

Parathesin: As surface anesthetic in ulcerative stomatitis, rhinitis and otalgia; in 3–20% oily or alcoholic solution, by swab or spray.

Phenoco: As antiseptic and disinfectant; in dilutions of 1:300 water for local application.

Protargol: As silver antiseptic in all infections of nose and throat; applied topically in ½–10% solution.

Quinothesin: As antiseptic in various catarrhal infections; as lozenges, ointment and powder for topical application.

Rivanol: As antiseptic in purulent rhinitis, as spray in 1:1,000 solution; in tonsillitis and pharyngitis in 1:2,000 solution.

Silver Lactate: As astringent and antiseptic in sore throat, tonsillitis, pharyngitis; as mouth wash and gargle in 1:100 to 1:2,000 solution.

Silvogon: As antiseptic and germicide in infections, wounds and ulcers of nose and throat; in 1:2,000 solution.

Sodium Perborate: As hemostatic in epistaxis, as antiseptic in other nose and throat affections; applied locally as dusting powder or wash.

Sublamine: As antiseptic, especially in luetic affections of nose and throat; as gargle and irrigation in 1:5,000 solution.

Sulfax: As antiseptic in nasal and oral hygiene and as gargle; in 1:2,000 solution.

Suprarenalin and Suprarenin: As decongestive and vasoconstrictor, applied locally in 1:5,000 to 1:1,000 solution.

Synephrin Tartrate: As vasoconstrictor and decongestive in sinusitis, hypertrophic rhinitis, allergy, hay fever; applied topically to mucous membranes.

Thantis Lozenges: As antiseptic and anesthetic; tablets dissolved in mouth as often as indicated.

Thiol: As sulphur antiseptic in angina, otitis media, rhino-pharyngitis, as 2% liquid solution; applied by painting or spraying.

Tiodine "Cognet": As fibrous tissue resolvent in otosclerosis; *intramuscularly* 1 ampule every other day; orally 2–5 pills daily.

Tolamine: As germicide in various affections of the nose and throat, in Vincent's angina, ozena, tonsillitis and pharyngitis, as 0.2% spray; for oral hygiene, in stomatitis, abrasions or pyorrhea, in 1% solution.

Tutocain: As local anesthetic for various surgical and examination procedures; surface application 2–5% solution; infiltration ⅕%; conduction anesthesia ½–1%.

Pediatrics

Preparations Useful in Diseases of Children*

1. Gastrointestinal

Allisatin: As sedative and antispasmodic in intestinal hyperperistalsis, colic, enterocolitis, flatulence, diarrhea; 1–2 tablets three times daily.

Beta Lactose "National": As milk modifier; 3–12% of formula, graded with child's development and dentition; as laxative in constipation, 1–4 teaspoonfuls in water, two to three times daily.

Bismuth Hydrate Compound: As intestinal astringent in diarrheas; ½–1 teaspoonful every ½ hr. for 6–8 doses.

Bismutose: As antacid and antiseptic in gastritis and gastric ulcer; 15–30 gr and over in gruel, milk or water, 1–3 times daily.

Butolan: As vermifuge; in children below age of 10—¼–½ tablet 3 times daily taken for 1 week, when a purgative as castor oil or calomel is given; in obstinate cases —a second course may be administered; during and after treatment, enemas are employed of 1 tablespoonful of liquor aluminis acetatis to quart of water or of limewater.

Calcium Peroxide: As antacid instead of milk of lime, in summer diarrheas of infants; 1–5 gr in water or with sodium bicarbonate, two to three times daily.

Citabs: As milk modifier; after boiling and cooling of pint of milk or feeding mixture, 4 tablets dissolved in 2–3 teaspoonfuls of water are added to mixture and stirred before use.

Collosol Lactomagnesia: As colloidal antacid and laxative in infantile disorders; ¼–1 teaspoonful in water two to three times daily; infants—1 teaspoonful to pint of milk, or ½ teaspoonful per bottle.

Coreine "Daniel-Brunet": As laxative in constipation, colitis and fermentative diarrheas; ½–1 dr. twice daily.

Dexin: As milk modifier in infant feeding; is added to food in accordance with age and weight of infant.

Diskets Alkaline: As alkalizer in cyclic vomiting and acid fermentation; 1 disket in glass of water, repeated as indicated.

Eldoform: As intestinal astringent in enterocolitis, dysentery, intestinal tuberculosis; 1–2 tablets several times daily, crushed and stirred in fluid.

Glycotauro: As cholagogue in various biliary disorders; 2½ gr three times daily for 8 days; dosage reduced during following 12 days.

Ichthalbin: As intestinal antiseptic in gastrointestinal catarrh, tubercular enteritis and peritonitis; 2–10 gr two to three times daily according to age; given in powdered form.

Kondremul: As laxative in constipation; 1 teaspoonful at night, best given with hot fluids.

Liquid Petrolatum with Agar: As intestinal lubricant and laxative in spastic constipation, diarrheas, impacted feces; 1–2 teaspoonfuls in water.

Magnesium Peroxide: As antiseptic and antacid in acid stomach and in diarrhea with acid stools; 2–4 gr, for older children in keratin coated capsules.

Orphol: As astringent and antiseptic in tubercular diarrhea, dysentery, gastrogenous diarrhea; 30–60 gr daily.

Paroleine: As intestinal lubricant in constipation and other intestinal conditions; ½–1 teaspoonful before meals.

Protan: As intestinal astringent in infantile diarrhea; 3 gr every 2–3 hr.; in chronic cases, double dosage.

Sodinco: As alkalizer in intestinal disorders of children, and in acidosis; ½–1 tablet every 2–3 hr.

Tannalbin: As intestinal astringent in summer complaint; infants—5 gr three times daily; children—larger dosage in accordance with age; continued 1–2 days after symptoms have subsided.

* *See also* "Foods," "Endocrines," "Biologicals," "Emollients," "Vitamines" and other items of interest in this specialty in respective chapters.

Tannigen: As intestinal astringent in children's diarrheas; 5–10 gr administered in water, food or with milk sugar.

Tannismut: As intestinal astringent in all intestinal diarrheas; children under 1 yr.—0.03–0.1 Gm; children over 1 yr.—0.1–0.5 Gm; given three to five times daily.

Xeroform: As intestinal antiseptic in dysentery, choleraic diarrheas, gastrointestinal catarrh; 2–5 gr daily.

2. Respiratory

Anastil: As antiseptic expectorant in various chronic bronchial infections; 0.5 cc *intramuscularly*, slowly injected, every few days, 6–25 injections.

Creosotal: As antiseptic in phthisis therapy and in intestinal tubercular infections; ¼–1 dr. daily, in emulsion, milk, with cod liver oil.

Creo-Terpin: As expectorant in bronchial affections; 10–15 drops every 2–3 hr.

Duotal: As phthisis therapy, in chronic bronchitis, pneumonic infections and tuberculosis; 2–8 gr several times daily.

Ethyl Morphine and Ephedrine Compound: As expectorant in spasmodic coughs; ¼–½ teaspoonful four to six times daily.

Felsol: As antispasmodic in asthma, croup and other disorders with spasm; ¼–½ of powder as marketed, older children larger dosage; given in sweetened warm water; in severe attacks is followed in 1 hr by another dose.

Ferro-Sajodin: As alterative in asthma, scrofula, cretinism, congenital syphilis; ½–1½ tablets once or twice daily.

Guaiacose: As expectorant and deodorant in chronic bronchitis, whooping cough, influenza and measles; ½ teaspoonful in milk, cocoa or other fluid, two to three times daily.

Guaiaphon: As expectorant in bronchial affections; ½–3 teaspoonfuls according to age.; the Guaiaphon Compound Syrup—double dosage.

Hyotole: As expectorant in bronchial affections; 1–3 mo.—10 drops, 4–12 mo.—20 drops, 1–3 yr.—30 drops, 4 yr. and upwards—½–1 teaspoonful.

Iodotone: As alterative in bronchitis, asthma, influenzal pneumonia, tuberculosis; ½ teaspoonful three times daily.

Kresival: As expectorant in acute and chronic bronchitis, laryngitis, cough in measles, whooping cough and pneumonia; 1 teaspoonful mixed with equal parts of water several times daily.

Lumodrin: As antispasmodic in whooping cough and asthma; ½–1 tablet in children above 5.

Optochin Hydrochloride: As irrigation in pneumococcus empyema of children; for application *see Chap. I.*

Orargol: To stimulate resistance in bronchopneumonia and other infectious fevers; *intramuscularly*, 1 cc for each year of age, every second day.

Pertussin: As antispasmodic and expectorant in whooping cough and similar spasmodic affections; ½–1 teaspoonful every 1–2 hr.

Proposote: As expectorant in chronic bronchitis and tuberculosis; 5 m three times daily.

Salophen: As analgesic in influenza, coryza and other acute infections; 3–8 gr, repeated if necessary.

Somnos: As sedative and soporific in whooping cough, spasmodic croup, convulsions; ½–1 teaspoonful two to three times daily, larger doses at bedtime; in spasmophilia as hypnotic; rectally, ½–1 oz. in 5% sodium bicarbonate solution.

Thiocol: As sedative expectorant in cough, colds, tuberculosis and other respiratory affections; ½–1 teaspoonful of syrup every 2–3 hr.

Tolyphen: As expectorant in acute respiratory infections; ½–2 teaspoonfuls according to age.

3. Deficiency Diseases

Adex Tablets 10D: To promote growth, stimulate immunity, raise calcium-phosphorus metabolism, in rickets; 2–4 tablets daily with water, milk or orange juice.

Calcium Phosphate Tribasic: To stimulate calcium and phosphorus metabolism; ¾–1½ gr for eacy year of age.
Caritol: In primary vitamin A therapy; 3–5 drops daily for infants and young children; larger doses in older children; given plain or with cod liver oil, halibut liver oil or viosterol.
Codamines Tablets: In vitamin A and D therapy; 1–3 tablets crushed in milk one to three times daily.
Cod Liver Oil with Viosterol 10D: As nutrient and vitamin D therapy; in infants' and young children 35–40 drops daily; in mild and moderate rickets ½–⅔ teaspoonful three times daily.
Cod Liver Oil with Viosterol 250D: As nutrient and vitamin therapy; prophylactic—5–15 drops twice daily; curative—10–20 drops twice daily.
Cod Liver Oils: Kepler, Newfoundland, Peter Moller's and others—As nutrient and vitamin therapy; ½–1½ teaspoonfuls twice daily, in accordance with age of infant or child.
D.C.P. 340: As calcium therapy in dental caries, rickets, developmental disturbances; ½–¾ teaspoonfuls daily with milk feedings.
Fortossan: As phosphorus therapy in rickets and other metabolic disorders; infants under 2 mo.—10 gr; 2–6 mo.—20 gr; 6–12 mo—30 gr; 1–2 yr.—40 gr; four times daily.
Haliver Oil Plain: In vitamin A therapy; 10 drops daily.
Haliver Oil with Viosterol 250D: In vitamin A and D therapy; normal infants—10 drops; premature and rapidly growing infants—15 drops; older children 10–20 drops; daily dosages.
Irradol A: In vitamin A therapy; infants ½–1 dr. three times daily; children 2 dr., three times daily.
Marinol: As nutritive and antirachitic; infants—drop doses several times daily; children—dram doses 3–4 times daily.
Myeladol: As hematinic and A, B, and D vitamin therapy; 1–2 teaspoonfuls three times daily.
Natural Vitamin D: In vitamin D therapy in rickets; prophylactic—10 drops daily; curative—15–30 drops daily, in accordance with severity of case.
Oscodal: In vitamin A and D therapy; 1–2 tablets three times daily.
Super D Cod Liver Oil: In vitamin A and D therapy; ¼–1 teaspoonful three times daily.
Super D Concentrate: In vitamin A and D therapy; 10–20 drops three times daily.
Undiluted Halibut Liver Oil: In vitamin A therapy; infants—30 drops; prematures and rapidly growing children—50 drops; older children—35–50 drops; daily.

4. Other Disorders

Alpha Lobelin: As respiratory stimulant in asphyxia neonatorum; ½ ampule *injected* directly into umbilical vein after clearing respiratory passages of mucus and keeping infant's head down; other half of ampule given *intramuscularly*.
Arsenoferratose: As hematinic in various anemias of children; 1 teaspoonful two to three times daily.
Aubromid: As antispasmodic in whooping cough; infants—½ tablet; children—1–2 tablets; given in water three times daily.
Bellafoline: As antispasmodic in enuresis; 1 drop of solution for each year of age; maximum 10 drops; given three times daily.
Bismo-Cymol: As antiluetic in congenital syphilis; *intramuscularly* 0.1–0.2 cc; older children, 2½–11 yr.—1 cc; given twice weekly for 12–16 injections.
Bismogenol: As antiluetic in congenital syphilis; *intramuscularly*, warmed, twice weekly for 30 injections, in following dosage: up to 2 yr.—0.1 cc, 2–4 yr.—0.4 cc, 4–6 yr.—0.6 cc, 6–8 yr.—0.8 cc, 8–10 yr.—1 cc; given in 5% suspension.
Bromhosal: As bromide therapy and salt substitute in epileptiform and nephritic cases; used from salt shaker as condiment on foods.
Bromipin 10%: As sedative in epilepsy; 2–4 teaspoonfuls per day in emulsion with peppermint water and syrup, or flavored; as enema—children under 1 yr., 15 m

for each month of age; from 1–4 yr., 3–4 dr.; over 4 yr., 4–5 dr.; older children 6–8 dr.; mixed with milk or flaxseed tea.

Bulbocapnine Phosphate: As sedative in behavior disorders of children; 1 tablet three times daily; *hypodermically* if necessary.

Cadechol: As sedative in enuresis; 1–2 tablets evenings.

Caprokol: As urinary antiseptic in pyelitis and other urinary disturbances of the kidneys; 1 teaspoonful every 4 hr., increased to 3 and 6 teaspoonfuls daily according to age; diuretics, citrates or bicarbonates are to be avoided.

Coramine: As cardiorespiratory stimulant in cases of poisoning, asphyxia, acute toxemias during infectious diseases; *subcutaneously* or *intramuscularly*, ½–1 ampule as required.

Cupriferrum: As hematinic in secondary anemia and nutritional diseases; ½–1 teaspoonful of syrup one to three times daily.

Cuproglobin: As hematinic in secondary and nutritional anemias; ½–2 teaspoonfuls three to four times daily.

Dimol: As antiarthritic in articular rheumatism with intestinal toxemia; infants, ½–1½ dr.; children, 1½–3 dr.; four to five times daily.

Euquinine: As antipyretic and antimalarial; 1–3 gr according to age; repeated as required.

Homocamfin: As cardiorespiratory stimulant in acute failure; *intravenously*, in emergencies only, 0.3–0.5 cc cautiously administered, to children from 2–12 yr.

Iodicalcium Tablets: As prophylactic in hypothyroidism and cretinism; ½ tablet one to two times daily.

Iodotone: In therapy of cretinism and myxedema; ½ teaspoonful three times daily.

Manola: As nutrient and tonic; ½–1 teaspoonful two to three times daily after meals.

Mesurol: As antiluetic in congenital syphilis; *intramuscular* injections once or twice weekly, beginning with 0.1 cc increased to 0.5 cc according to age; infants, from 0.05–0.1 cc.

Metatone: As nutrient in anemia, malnutrition and convalescence; ½–1 teaspoonful several times daily.

Miscidine: In prophylaxis of goitre and cretinism; 2–5 drops as required.

Neobovinine-20: As hematinic and dietary adjuvant in anemia and malnutrition; ½–1 teaspoonful several times daily.

Neosalvarsan: As antiluetic; *intramuscularly;* 3–9 mo.—0.1–0.15 Gm, 1–2 yr.—0.2 Gm, 2–3 yr.—0.25 Gm, 3–5 yr.—0.3 Gm; injections at weekly intervals.

Panopepton: As nutrient and vehicle; infants—few drops to half teaspoonful; older children, up to 1 teaspoonful; three times daily.

Para-Thor-Mone: As hormone therapy in tetany and hemorrhagic diathesis; infants—18–20 units; older children—in accordance with blood calcium.

Phytine: As calcium-phosphorus therapy in tetany, spasmophilia, urticaria and other allergic phenomena; 2–6 yr., 1–2 tablets; 6–10 yr., 2–3 tablets; daily.

Pitressin: In enuresis nocturna; *intranasally*, by dropper or tampon, 3–5 m; also hypodermically.

Pituitary Extract: As hormone therapy in diabetes insipidus; beginning with 1–2 units, increased daily until intestinal reaction is induced.

Pituitrin: In enuresis nocturna; 5–8 m *intranasally* by dropper or tampon; also *hypodermically*.

Plasmochin: As antimalarial; ½–1 tablet two to three times daily; Plasmochin Compound—1 tablet one to four times daily, infants—1 tablet daily; treatment continued for 2 weeks, then dosage reduced during the next 4 weeks.

Pyramidon: As antipyretic and analgesic in measles; also in colds, influenza and other febrile diseases; 1 gr per year of age; maximum, 5 gr every 4 hr.

Quiniobine: As antiluetic in congenital syphilis; infants—0.05–0.1 cc semi-weekly, increased by 0.05 cc until a total of 3 cc is administered; course is repeated after interval of 6 weeks.

Silver Nitrate Solution: As gonocide in ophthalmia prophylaxis; capsule is pierced with needle, solution expelled 1 drop at time, and few drops instilled in each eye.

Sulpharsphenamine: As antiluctic in congenital syphilis; *intramuscularly*, once or twice weekly; infants 3–8 weeks—0.05–0.75 Gm, 2–6 mo.—0.1 Gm, ½–1 yr.—0.15 Gm, 1–2 yr.—0.15–0.2 Gm.

Thyracoids: In enuresis, hypothyroidism and physical or mental underdevelopment; dosage graded according to conditions, age and sex.

Thyrocalx: In calcium deficiencies, spasmophilia, tetany; 1 tablet three times daily, reduced to 1 daily.

Proctology

Preparations of Service in Proctologic Practice*

A.L.A.: As local anesthetic in hemorrhoids or fissures; injected *intramuscularly* or *subcutaneously*, at 5–7 points within a 3 in. circle surrounding the painful area, from 0.1–0.5 cc at each point, a total of 1 cc.

Anesthone Cream: As analgesic in hemorrhoids and ano-rectal fissure; applied locally.

Argyn: As antiseptic for fissures, hemorrhoids and ulcerative colitis; in 1:100 to 1:500 solution.

Aristol: As antiseptic and analgesic in painful ulcerative anal disease; as suppository, 5–15 gr in cocoa butter.

Benacol Solution: For relief of intense itching and to relax sphincter spasm in anal fissure and pruritus; *subcutaneously* and *submucously* only, never into skin; 1 ampule injected in fan-shaped manner, repeated in 5 days.

Butesin: As local anesthetic in painful rectal affections; applied as suppository or solution.

Butyn: As local anesthetic for pruritus; in ½% solution injected around anus; in infiltration anesthesia, ⅒–¼%, maximum ½% solution.

Cargentos: As astringent and antiseptic; rectal irrigation, ⅒–1%; as suppository—same strength.

Collene: As colloidal antiseptic in colitis and proctitis; for irrigation in 25% dilution.

Isarol: As antiseptic in infections and inflammations of the rectum and perianal region; in 5–50% ointment, applied as often as necessary.

Nupercaine: As local anesthetic in pruritus ani, hemorrhoids, rectal ulcers and fissure; in 1:4,000–1:1,000 solution, and as 1% ointment.

Orthoform: As anesthetic antiseptic in hemorrhoids; applied as suppository or dusting powder.

Panthesine: As antipruritic in hemorrhoids; applied in ointment form two to three times daily.

Parathesin: As anesthetic in hemorrhoids, fissure and pruritus ani; applied in 5–20% ointment as often as necessary.

Protargol: As antiseptic and germicide in colitis and proctitis; for irrigation, 2%.

Quinine and Urea Hydrochloride: As infiltration therapy in pruritus ani; sufficient solution is injected until tissue is infiltrated.

Xeroform: As antiseptic anesthetic for painful fissure, irritation and ulceration; applied locally as dusting powder.

Radiology

Diagnostic Agents of Service to the Radiologist

Brominol: For visualization of respiratory tract, nasal sinuses, localization of spinal cord tumors and obstructions, the study of uterus, fallopian tubes and blood vessels; about 20 cc slowly injected by catheter or syringe.

Bromipin 33%: In bronchography; 2½–8 dr., warmed to body temperature before or during injection.

Campiodol Solution: For study of the respiratory tract, spinal canal, cerebral ventricles, nasal sinuses and uterine adnexae; quantity and method in accordance with part radiographed.

* *See also* "Rectal suppositories" and "Ointments" in Chapter X.

Chole-Cysto-Col: For cholecystography; 1 dose package administered in water or grape juice or ginger ale 12 hr. preceding examination, with special orders.

Iodeikon and Iodeikon Emulsion: For cholecystography; intravenous method, 55 mg per kilogram of body weight, total not to exceed 3½ Gm, dissolved in 1 oz. of distilled water, diluted with 200 cc Ringer's or normal saline and injected slowly; radiographs taken 4, 8 and 12 hr. after. Orally, 3½–4 Gm dissolved in 1 or 2 oz. of water and grape juice, taken 12 hr. preliminary to first radiograph.

Iodipin 40%: For x-ray diagnosis of bronchiectasis, pulmonary abscess, tumors, tuberculosis; also fistulae, stenosis, spinal cord affections; bronchography, 15–20 cc for each lung; myelography, 2 cc; pyelography and ureterography of both sides, 15–20 cc.

Iodochlorol: For radiography of uterine adnexae and sinuses; 5–15 cc, in accordance.

Iso-Iodeikon: For combined cholecystography and liver function test; 40 mg per kilogram of body weight, total not to exceed 2½ Gm, dissolved in 1 oz. distilled water, injected in combination with 150 cc Ringer's or normal saline solution; radiography 4, 8 and 12 hr. after administration; function test from blood ½–1 hr. after injection.

I-X Barium Meal: As radiopaque medium for gastrointestinal study; 1 measureful, 4–8 oz., in water, thoroughly mixed before using; usual technic.

Keraphen: For cholecystography; contents of 1 bottle dissolved in ¼ glass of water, stirred, mixed with lemonade, orange juice or grape juice; taken 12 hr. before cholecystography; radiography 12, 15, 18, 24 hr. after dye administration.

Lipoiodine: In bronchography, uterosalpingography, in sinus and ureteral study; from 5–20 cc, warmed, injected in accordance with area studied.

Lipiodol "Lafay": For study of cerebrospinal tumors, fistulae, sinuses, cysts and genitourinary tract affections, also in bronchography; in cerebral radiography 1–2 cc; in other studies 5–20 cc.

Neo-Iopax: As radiopaque medium for the visualization of structures in the genitourinary tract; *intravenously*, 20 cc; exposures made from 10–30 min. after injection; in retrograde method, injection made through ureteral catheters.

Neo-Silvol: As radiopaque medium in urography; administered *ureterally* in 20% solution.

Neoskiodan: As radiopaque medium for the study of the urinary tract; 1 ampule injected *intravenously*, films taken 10–20 min., in some cases 30 min. after injection.

Shadocol: As radiopaque medium in oral cholecystography; 1 oz. by the usual technic.

Skiabaryt-Oral: For study of the gastrointestinal tract; 5–6½ oz. administration and technic usual.

Skiagenol: In bronchography, uterosalpingography, sinuses, etc.; quantities and methods as for other radiopaque media.

Skiodan: For urography, retrograde pyelography, arteriography; intravenous urography, 50 cc of 40% solution; retrograde, in 10 and 15–20% concentrations.

Solargentum: As substitute for bismuth paste in the study of sinuses, fistulae and similar conditions; 200 gr is mixed with heavy petrolatum and lanolin to make a 4 oz. mixture of proper consistency.

Tetrabromphenolphthalein Sodium Salt: For cholecystography; quantity and method of administration—that of similar radiopaque media.

Tetradol Emulsion: For cholecystography; *oral*—1 dose of emulsion stirred in half to ¾ glass of cold water or fruit juice, taken 15 hr. preliminary to radiography; *intravenous*—50 mg of powder per kilogram of body weight, total not to exceed 3½ Gm; dissolved in distilled water, filtered, sterilized, diluted to 200 cc with Ringer's or saline solution, and slowly injected.

Thorotrast: In splenohepatography, arteriography, retrograde pyelography and cystography; hepato-lienography—20–25 cc *intravenously* every 1–2 days for 3 doses; radiographs taken 1–2 days after last injection; arteriography—peripheral, 10–12 cc into upper, 20–25 cc into lower extremity; cerebral arteriography —8–15 cc into common carotid; in retrograde pyelography—is diluted with equal parts of water or saline, in cystography—in 1–5 parts of water.

Umbrathor: For depiction of gastric, intestinal and bladder mucosa. (*See Chap. I.*)

Surgery

Preparations for Use in Surgical Conditions*

Acriflavine Neutral: Antiseptic and bacteriostat; for sterilization of the skin preoperatively, 5% solution with alcohol 50%, acetone 10%, water 40%; as wet dressing in surgical infections, 1:100–1:500 solution; in surgical sepsis, *intravenously* 10–50 cc, 0.5% of a freshly prepared warm saline solution; orally, gr 1–1½ daily in water.

Adrenalin and Adrin Solution: In surgical shock and collapse, 5 drops of 1:1,000 solution; 1 oz. in normal saline *intravenously*, slowly; in urgent cases 0.5–1 cc *intracardially*, or by *centripetal* transfusion.

Alpha Lobelin: As cardio-respiratory stimulant in suspended animation, surgical shock, collapse and de-etherization; *intramuscularly* or *subcutaneously* gr ¼, *intravenously* gr 1/13–⅙.

Alpha-Naphco: As antiseptic for wet surgical dressings.

Alphozone: In surgical infections; as wet dressing in 1:500–1:250 solution; as dusting powder mixed with talcum or boric acid 1–20.

Alumnol: As astringent antiseptic for wet dressings or irrigation of abscesses; in 0.5–3% solution.

Amertan: As emollient dressing for burns; applied locally, freely till tanning occurs.

Amfetin: As surgical prophylactic to stimulate serous surface defense in abdominal operations; 50–200 cc instilled at body temperature into the peritoneal cavity before closing of abdomen.

Ampule Glucose: As nutrient stimulant in acidosis, toxemia and postoperatively; *intravenously*, in calculated dosage as required in each case.

Anesthesin: As topical analgesic for painful wounds; applied externally as dusting powder 10% or ointment 4–10%.

An-Nu-Tol: As emollient dressing for burns; applied locally, freely as required.

Antiformin: As antiseptic wet dressing in surgical infections; 1–2% solutions.

Argolaval: As topical antiseptic and wet dressing in surgical infections; in 25% to full strength solutions.

Aristol: As desiccating antiseptic in surgical wounds; applied freely as dusting powder.

B.F.I. Powder: As local antiseptic, in surgical wounds; applied freely, as dusting powder.

Bismuth Thymol Iodide: As surface antiseptic and dry dressing in surgical affections; applied freely as dusting powder.

Bismuth Violet: As surface antiseptic following skin grafts, burns or wounds; applied locally in 10% aqueous-glycerin solution, as required.

Borocaine: As local anesthetic in minor surgical procedures; for nerve block in 1–2% solution; for mucous membrane anesthesia ½–1%.

Butesin: As local anesthetic in surgical wounds; applied freely as dusting powder.

Butesin Picrate: As anesthetic and antiseptic dressing for burns and surgical infections; applied locally as ointment, as 1% solution, or as dusting powder 5% with sodium stearate 95%.

Butyn: As local anesthetic in surgical procedures; by infiltration in 1/10–¼% solution; or combined with epinephrin for bloodless field work.

Caseosan: As non-specific protein agent in various infections, adenitis, periostitis, osteomyelitis and systemic infections; *intramuscularly* and *subcutaneously* 0.5, 2.0, 3.0 and 5.0 cc at 3 day intervals; *intravenously* 0.25–2 cc; *intracutaneous* 0.3–1 cc.

Chloramine: As Dakin antiseptic in various infections; as dry powder or 2% solution for irrigation.

Chlorazene: As Dakin antiseptic in various surgical infections; in powder form or in 1 or 2% solution as irrigation.

Chlorine-Soda: As antiseptic; uses as for chlorinated soda. (*See Chap. I.*)

* *See also* "Anesthetics," "Antiseptics," "Biologicals" and other topics of interest to Surgery, in respective chapters.

Clymocol: As germicide; for topical application, 2% solution; for instillation into body cavities 0.5% solution; for disinfection of instruments and operating room utensils 2–5%; for irrigations 2%.

Coagulen: As hemostatic for oozing wounds and bleeding after surgical operation; as preoperative prophylactic, *subcutaneously* or *intramuscularly* 1.5–5 cc postoperatively—up to 20 cc; *intravenously*—2–3 cc several times daily if necessary; orally—5–10 Gm dissolved in water and sipped slowly; topically—1 or 2 small ampules injected simultaneously with local anesthetic.

Collosol Calcium: To effect blood coagulability and control postoperative hemorrhage; 1 cc 12 and 6 hr. before operation, 1 cc immediately after operation and 6 hr. later; orally 1 dr. three times daily in water.

Dermalene: As detergent to prepare operating surface.

Dextrose: As nutrient stimulant in postoperative states, shock, toxemia; intravenously slowly administered, in quantities in accordance with demands of the individual case.

Dextrose-Ringer's Concentrate: As stimulant and nutrient in shock, sepsis and in hemorrhage; *intravenously* 500 cc of 5% solution per hour, diminished to 100 cc on improvement and continued for several days as necessary; in acute shock, 200 cc per hour.

Dibromin: As antiseptic in ulcers, wounds, abscesses and fistulae; for irrigation 1:1,250–1:2,500.

Dilaudid: As narcotic, anodyne and morphine substitute in all surgical conditions necessitating such therapy; hypodermically gr 1/32; orally 1/24, increased if necessary to gr 1/16.

Enzymol: As surgical solvent for destroying necrotic tissues, sloughs and stimulating ulcers and slow healing wounds; applied topically in ½–2% solution; in irrigation of abscess cavities and bone sinuses in 0.2% hydrochloric acid solution.

Ephedrine: As vasoconstrictor, preoperatively, in spinal anesthesia; ½–1 ampule as required.

Felamine: As choleretic after abdominal operations especially of gall bladder and biliary tract; 2–3 tablets two to three times daily.

Fibrogen (Local): As topical hemostatic in surgical surface bleeding; used on gauze or tampon or poured into wound undiluted, applying gentle pressure for 5 min.

Fibrolysin: As cicatrix resolvent for the softening and loosening of scars, adhesions, strictures and other fibrous tissues; *intramuscularly* also *subcutaneously*, 1 ampule every second to third day for 20–50 injections.

Formalin: As antiseptic and disinfectant in wounds, abscesses, in general and local sepsis; for irrigation and other uses; topically 1½–2% solution; for systemic infections *intravenously* 500–700 cc of 1–5,000 solution in normal saline.

Gentian Violet Improved Medicinal: As germicide and antiseptic in staphylococcus infections of joints, burns, pleural cavity; in dilution of 1:1,000.

Hemostatic Serum: As hemostatic in bone surgery and other operative procedures; prophylactic, orally—5 cc, 3–6 hr. prior to operation; in bad risks, several doses at 6 hr. intervals; *intravenously*—about 5 cc before and after operation, repeated if necessary.

Hexyl-Resorcinol Solution S.T. 37: As germicidal agent for topical use in abrasions, bruises, wounds, ulceration; applied full strength by swab or otherwise.

Homocamfin: As respiratory stimulant in surgical shock; in emergencies, *intravenously* 1 cc, cautiously increased if imperative; *intramuscularly* 1½–2 cc.

Hyclorite: As antiseptic and deodorant where Dakin solution is indicated; in osteomyelitis, chronic ulcers, empyema, abdominal infections, skin grafting and burns; in 1:200 solution as wet dressing.

Ichthynat: As antiphlogistic in early inflammatory conditions, in carbuncles, abscesses, mastitis, synovitis; in 5–50% ointment.

Infundin: As vasoconstrictor in surgical shock, in intestinal atony and paresis, in postoperative anuria; *intramuscularly* or *rectally*, in saline solution, 5–10 International units.

Ipral Calcium: For pre- and postoperative sedation; 1 or 2 tablets taken with hot drink the evening before operation; as sedative and hypnotic 2–3 tablets postoperatively.

Kalmerid Germicidal Tablets: For disinfection of skin, instruments, suture tubes hands, and as wet dressing; for skin 1–100 alcoholic solution; surgeon's hands 1:5,000; instruments 1:2,000 aqueous solution; wet dressings, 1:1,000 to 1:5,000 watery solution with sodium carbonate or bicarbonate.

Kelene: As anesthetic for minor surgical operations and preliminary to ether anesthesia; administered by spray, for topical effects and by open cone method in general anesthesia.

Kephalin: As hemostatic in local oozing; applied in 0.1–0.2 saline suspension on gauze sponges or directly to bleeding area.

Larocaine: As local anesthetic in all surgical procedures; in ¼–2% solutions, usually ½–1%, with or without epinephrin.

Mercurochrome-Collosol Brand and Mercurochrome 220 Soluble: *For use* as antiseptic in all infections, local and systemic; topically—0.5–5% solution, of stronger concentration in special cases; *intravenously*—in general sepsis, 1–5 mg per kilogram of body weight, freshly prepared and not boiled.

Mercurophen: As germicide for sterilization of instruments, catheters, gloves, in 1:5,000 solution; of excreta and utensils, 1:2,000 solution; as antiseptic in mucous membrane infections, in 1:5,000 to 1:15,000 solution.

Merthiolate: As antiseptic for skin disinfection, in 1:1,000 solution; for instruments 1:1,000; for septic infected wounds and irrigation 1:2,000 to 1:5,000 solution.

Metaphen: As antiseptic and germicide for sterilization of skin, instruments, gloves, the tincture 1:200; in systemic infections, 1 ampule *intravenously* repeated as necessary.

Neonal: As preoperative sedative; ¾–6 gr in divided doses.

Normal Horse Serum: As hemostatic in persistent bleeding wounds and accidental hemorrhage; topically, applied with cotton or gauze saturated with the serum; *subcutaneously* or *intramuscularly* 10–20 cc daily, repeated until 100 cc are used.

Noviform: As antiseptic in abscesses, carbuncles, tubercular fistulae and other infections; applied in powder form; as 10% oily solution for injection into tubercular joints.

Numotizine: As antiphlogistic in the earlier stages of abscesses, boils, carbuncles, sprains, bruises and mastitis; applied topically at body temperature, ⅛ in. thick on thin cloth, to remain until dry; repeated after skin cleansing.

Nupercaine: As local anesthetic in infiltration, nerve block, caudal and spinal anesthesia. *See Chap. I.*

Orphol: As antiseptic, astringent in wounds and ulcers; applied as dusting powder.

Orthoform: As anesthetic and antiseptic in superficial ulcers and sores; applied as dusting powder or as ointment.

Pantocain: As local anesthetic for surface and mucosa conditions; in ¼, ½, 1 and 2% solution, with or without suprarenin.

Pantopon: As anodyne in all conditions demanding morphine or its salts; ⅙–⅓ gr as required.

Paraffin Compound: As dressing for burns. *See Chap. II.*

Parathesin: As surface anesthetic in wounds, burns, ulcers, bed sores, cracked nipples, suppurating buboes; applied as dusting powder or in 5 to 20% oily solution or ointment.

Parresine: As emollient for burns and abrasions; applied in thin layer by spray, covered with cotton, resprayed and bandaged.

Peristaltine: As intestinal stimulant in postoperative stasis, in prophylaxis *hypodermically* 1 ampule; repeated in 12 hr. if passage of flatus or stool does not occur.

Phenoco: As antiseptic and disinfectant for various surgical purposes; in dilutions of 1–5%.

Picratol: As styptic and analgesic in burns and similar skin affections; applied as 2% ointment.

Pituitary Extracts and Solutions: As vasoconstrictor in surgical shock; given intravenously or intramuscularly in accordance with urgency, 10–20 units and repeated if necessary.

Potassium Mercuric Iodide: As disinfectant for instruments and excreta; in 1:100 to 1:1,000 solution; as irrigation in 0.9% saline solution.

Procaine: As infiltration anesthesia; for nerve block ½–1%; direct and perineural 1.5%; spinal 5–10% solution.

Prostigmin: As stimulant in postoperative intestinal paralysis or distention; 1 ampule subcutaneously and intramuscularly followed in 30 min. by glycerin enema, 150–200 cc; if no evacuation in 4–5 hr., injection is repeated.

Protargol: As antiseptic in ordinary wounds and ulcers; in 1–10% solution.

P-Thiocresol: As epithelial proliferant for the healing of wounds and abrasions: applied in 1:10,000 solution every 48 hr., with saline wet dressings between applications.

Quinine and Urea Hydrochloride: As local anesthetic and nerve block: *For use and preparation of solution see Chap. II.*

Rectal Analgesia (Gwathmey): As analgesic for the relief of pain in childbirth; administered rectally by instillation of the mineral oil and ether mixture.

Rivanol: An antiseptic and germicide in wounds, abscesses and similiar infections; in 1:1,000 to 1:500 solution; in purulent arthritis 10–15 cc of 1:1,000 to 1:500 is injected into joint; in pleural empyema after pus evacuation, 50–200 cc of a 1:500 solution is used; repeated if necessary three or four times.

Scarlet R Salve "Biebrich": For burns, skin grafts, decubitus ulcers, wounds; is applied after wound is first cleansed, surrounding skin anointed with bland ointment and covered with gauze; dressed every 1–2 days alternating with bland ointment.

Scopolamine Stable: As cerebral sedative, preliminary to anesthesia; *hypodermically,* 1/100 gr.

Silvogon: As antiseptic for wounds, ulcers and irrigation in 1:1,000 sol.; for wet dressings 1:10,000 sol.

Silvol: As silver antiseptic for external use; in 5% ointment or 10% solution.

Soricin Surgical 40%: In various infections, ulcers, burns; as wet dressings 2–4%; in abdominal infections in 2% saline solution.

Stannoxyl Glycerin: As staphylocide in boils, pustules, suppurating wounds, chronic osteomyelitis; by local application.

Strontium Peroxide: As mild antiseptic in minor surgical affections; applied as dusting powder or ointment.

Stypticin: As astringent and hemostatic in parenchymatous bleeding; applied pure, or in strong solution, or as 30% ointment, on cotton or gauze.

Suprarenalin and Suprarenin: As vasoconstrictor and hemostatic in shock and hemorrhage; *hypodermically* 1–15 m of 1:1,000 solution in pint of isotonic saline; *intramuscularly* 5–15 m; also injected locally with an anesthetic to intensify and prolong the effect.

Surgical Maggots: To digest necrotic tissue in osteomyelitis, suppurating wounds, decubitus, and tendon sloughs; applied locally with adhesive straps exposing wound to open end of maggot container; allowed to remain 5 days then flushed out with saline and re-applied fresh; repeated for 6–10 weeks.

Tannic Acid Spray: For burns; applied topically by spraying scalded area.

Thromboplastin: As hemostatic in bleeding after circumcision, tongue tie and similar operations; applied locally with cotton or gauze held firmly until clot is formed; for internal hemorrhages administered *subcutaneously* or *intramuscularly, never intravenously,* 10–20 cc., repeated if necessary.

Tolamine: As antiseptic for wounds, bed sores, ulcers, burns, abrasions; in 2% solution.

Trypsin: As proteolytic digestant in the treatment of diphtheritic membranes, purulent tuberculosis and cancerous ulcers. *For administration see Chap. I.*

Tutocain: As local anesthetic; for infiltration ¼%; conduction anesthesia ½–1%; spinal ½–1%.

Tyramine: As stimulant in shock and collapse; *hypodermically* ⅓–⅔ gr.

Vioform: As deodorating antiseptic in ulcers, wounds, burns, septic suppurations; applied by dusting or sprinkling of lesions.

Vivargin: As germicidal wet dressing; full strength.

Zinc Perborate: As local antiseptic in minor surgical affections; applied as dusting powder or ointment.

Zonite: As antiseptic in abrasions, wounds; 2 tablespoonfuls to quart of warm water for irrigation; 3 teaspoonfuls to ¼ glass of water for topical use.

Urology

Preparations for Use in Genito-Urinary Affections*

Acriflavine: As antiseptic and gonocide; urethral injections, 1:1,000 to 1:10,000 solutions; irrigations, 1:10,000 in normal saline.

Acriflavine Neutral: As urethral injection, 1:500, irrigation, 1:3,000; for vaginal swabbing and tampons, 1:500–1:1,000.

Activin: As non-specific therapy in infectious epididymitis, orchitis and prostatitis; *intramuscularly*, beginning with ½ cc, gradually increased in accordance with reaction; daily in acute cases, twice weekly in chronic conditions.

Ambazin: As urinary antiseptic in all infections; orally, 1 capsule three times daily.

Amylsol: As urinary antiseptic; orally, 1 capsule three times daily with meals, increased slowly to a maximum of 12 capsules daily.

Alypin: As local anesthetic in urologic manipulations; in 1–4% solution, topically.

Anastil: As non-specific therapy agent in infections, including pyelitis; *intramuscularly*, 1 cc every 2–3 days; *intravenously*, 1 cc in 3–5 cc saline, slowly injected every 2–3 days.

Aolan: As non-specific therapy agent; also as provocative in diagnosis of chronic gonorrheal infections; *intradermally*, 0.2–0.3 cc sufficient for 2 wheals; *intramuscularly*, 10 cc at 5–6 day intervals. As provocative, the intradermal method is employed, the suspected infected organs are examined and secretions searched for gonococci 10–24 hr. after injection.

Argentiform: As silver antiseptic and astringent; in form of urethral bougies, ointment or vaginal cones, for topical effect.

Argolaval: As local antiseptic and astringent in cystitis and pyelitis; for irrigations, 1% solution, increased to 10%.

Argyn: As antiseptic and gonocide in gynecologic infections, in 10–25% solutions; in venereal prophylaxis in 10% solution.

Argyrol: As gonocide; urethral injection, 3–10% solution; bladder irrigation, 1:500 solution; kidney pelvis lavage, 5% solution; vesiculitis, 5% solution; in venereal prophylaxis, 10% solution.

Arheol "Astier": As urinary sedative and antiseptic in dysuria and pollakiuria; 3–4 pearls orally three to four times daily with meals.

Arhovin: As antigonorrhoeic and uric acid eliminant; orally, 0.25 cc in capsules three times daily; locally by suppository, ¾ gr, by tampon or in 1–2% oily solution for vaginal application.

Atrobutin: As urinary antiseptic; 1 tablet four times daily.

Benzosol: As urinary antiseptic in cystitis and pyelitis; 3–10 gr in powder, pill or emulsion three to four times daily.

Benzyl Benzoate: As antispasmodic in ureteral colic, urolithiasis and vesical spasm: 5–7 m in gelatin capsules, or 3–6 globules or 1–2 teaspoonfuls of 20% solution; repeated in ½–1 hr. where relief is not obtained; ampule medication where rapid action is desired.

Beta-Eucaine Hydrochloride: As local anesthetic in cystoscopy; 0.2% solution.

Buchuform: As urinary antiseptic; 1 tablet four times daily with water.

Butyn: As local anesthetic in endourethral and endovesical examination; 4 cc of 1% solution, applied topically with cotton pledget for 3 min. immediately preceding examination.

Cadechol: In enuresis; 1–2 tablets on retiring.

Calcium Gluconate and Calglucon: To stimulate phagocytosis and increase systemic resistance; *intramuscularly* and *intravenously*, 10 cc every 1–3 days.

* *See also* "Biologicals," "Urethral Bougies," "Urinary Antiseptics" and diseases associated with this specialty, in respective chapters.

Caprokol: As urinary antiseptic and sedative; 2–4 capsules three times daily for several weeks until urine becomes bacteria-free.

Cargentos: As astringent and antiseptic; injections—acute urethritis, 3–10%, chronic—10–20%, for irrigation, 0.1%, urethral suppositories, 2 gr; in bladder irrigation, 5 cc of 20–50% solution or 30 cc of 10–25% solution.

Chloramine: For urethral injections; in ½–2% solutions.

Chlorazene: For irrigation of infected bladder, vagina, urethra; 0.1% solution, increased.

Chlorhydrionic with Hexamethylene Tetramine: As urinary antiseptic, 3–5 teaspoonfuls daily.

Choleval: As antigonorrhoeic; injection, 0.25% increased to 1.5% two to three times daily, then decreased; irrigation, 1:1,000 to 1:500.

Collene: As astringent and antiseptic in urethral and vaginal irrigation, half strength; for bladder irrigation, 30% solution.

Collosol Argentum: As astringent antiseptic; for injection is diluted in 2–4 parts of warm water, later increased to full strength; as pessaries and suppositories.

Collosol Hydrargyrum: In gonorrheal arthritis; *intramuscularly*, 3 cc three times weekly.

Collosol Manganese: As non-specific therapy agent in gonorrheal infections with septic bacteremia; *intramuscularly*, 0.5–1 cc every 2–3 days until 6–8 cc have been administered.

Collosol Palladium: In gonorrheal and other coccigenic infections; *intramuscularly*, 0.5–1 cc as required.

Collosol Trimine: As gonocide in septic gonorrheal infections; *intramuscularly*, 0.5–1.5 cc every 3 days until 6 cc have been injected.

Dibromin: As genitourinary antiseptic; for hand injections, 1:500 to 1:1,000; irrigations, 1:1,250 to 1:2,500; in gonorrheal vaginitis and cystitis, 1:5,000 solution.

Formin: As antiseptic, diuretic and uric acid solvent in pyelitis, cystitis, scarlatinal nephritis and postoperative anuria; 5–15 gr two to three times daily with large quantities of water, in conjunction with 15–20 gr sodium biphosphate to acidify urine.

Formohydrion: As antiseptic and acidifier; 1 heaping teaspoonful in 6 oz. of water five to eight times daily between meals.

Gentian Violet Improved Medicinal: As antiseptic; for irrigation, in 1:1,000 to 1:3,000 solution.

Gonosan: As urinary antiseptic and sedative; 2 capsules three times daily after meals.

Gono-Yatren: As non-specific therapy agent in acute affections; *intravenously*, 0.5–2.5 cc every 2–4 days; *intramuscularly*, 0.5–4 cc as frequently as reaction permits.

Hegonon: As antiseptic; injections, 0.25% solution; irrigations, 1:200–1:6,000 solution.

Helmitol: As urinary antiseptic; 10–15 gr dissolved in water, three to four times daily.

Hexalet: As antiseptic and uricolytic; 15 gr dissolved in water, three to six times daily after meals.

Hex-Arbutin: As urinary antiseptic; 1 tablet three times daily with meals.

Hexyl-Resorcinol Solution S.T. 37: As irrigation, diluted with 3–4 parts of water.

Hyclorite: As antiseptic and disinfectant; 1:2,000 to 1:200 solution for irrigation and injection.

Hyos-Zea: As urinary sedative in dysuria, vesicular and urethral irritation; 2 teaspoonfuls in water every 3 hr.

Ichthargan: As gonocide; hand injections, 1:1,000 solution; irrigations 1:3,000; as urethral bougie in chronic urethritis, 5–10%.

Iodosyl: As local antiseptic; in form of pencils and 6% ointment.

Kalmerid Germicidal Tablets: As antiseptic for genitourinary irrigation, 1:20,000.

Kephalin: As hemostatic for coating of catheters in catheterization after prostatectomy; in 0.1–0.2% saline solution.

Lactigen: As non-specific therapy agent; *intramuscularly*, beginning with 1 cc, increased to 10 cc; injections given every 3–5 days.

Larocaine: As local anesthetic in vesical surgery; 30–50 cc of a ¾–1% solution.

Liquor Santaiva: As genitourinary sedative; 1 dr. in wineglassful of water several times daily after meals.

Mallophene: As genitourinary antiseptic; orally, 2 tablets three times daily; for injection, 0.5%; preoperatively, 2 tablets, repeated in 3–4 hr.

Mercurochrome—220 Soluble: As antiseptic for ureteral catheterization; for kidney pelvis lavage 1%; for injection and irrigation, 1–2½%; in septic complications, *intravenously*, 0.4% freshly prepared, 1–5 mg per kilogram of body weight.

Mercurophen: As urinary antiseptic; for irrigation, 1:5,000 to 1:15,000.

Mercury Benzoate: As antiseptic in urethritis; for irrigation with equal parts of sodium chloride in 1:2,000 to 1:1,000 solution.

Merthiolate: For bladder irrigation; in 1:5,000 to 1:10,000 solution.

Metaphen: As antiseptic and bacteriostat; for irrigation, in 1:2,500 solution; for *intravenous* injection, in septic infections, prostatitis, cystitis 1:1,000 solution, 10 cc.

Methylets: As gonocide and sedative; 1–2 pearls three to four times daily.

Metycaine: As local anesthetic; topically or hypodermically, 2–4% solution.

Narcogen: As antispasmodic in priapism, chordee, vesical tenesmus; 1 or more teaspoonfuls orally as frequently as demanded.

Neo-Silvol: As colloidal antiseptic and astringent; in urethritis, injection or irrigation, 1–15%; in cystitis, 5–10 cc of 10% solution, or weaker dilutions in larger quantities; in vaginitis and cervicitis, 5–10% for irrigation or tamponade.

Niazo: As genitourinary antiseptic; 2 tablets three times daily for several weeks.

Nizin: As astringent and antiseptic; urethral injections, 2 gr to ounce; as vaginal douche, 1 teaspoonful to quart of warm water; topically, in concentrations of 6 gr per ounce.

Noviform: As antiseptic and deodorant in chancre, balanitis, intertrigo and condylomata; as dusting powder or ointment.

Novocain: As local anesthetic; for urethral anesthesia, 3%.

Numotizine: As antiphlogistic; for external application in orchitis, epididymitis and ovaritis; applied ⅛ in. thick at body temperature, on thin cloth; repeated as indicated, after skin cleansing.

Omnadin: As non-specific therapy agent; *intramuscularly*, 1 ampule once daily, repeated several times where necessary.

Orchaton: As aphrodisiac; 1 tablet three times daily.

Parathesin: As surface anesthetic in vesical tenesmus, cystitis and urethritis; in the form of bougies, 3–8 gr each.

Picratol: As antiseptic and styptic in suppurative genital infections; applied externally as required.

Pituitary Extract: In vesical atony with incontinence of urine; beginning with 10–20 units, gradually increased.

Procaine: As local anesthetic; in 5% solution for urethral application.

Protargol: As antiseptic and astringent; in acute urethritis, ½–1%, in chronic—2–5%; as prophylactic, 2%.

Proteolac: As non-specific therapy agent in gonorrheal complications; *intramuscularly*, 1–2 cc increased to 5–10 cc every 2–5 days.

Pyridium: As genitourinary antiseptic in colon, gonococcus and mixed infections; orally, 1–2 tablets three times daily; as urethral injection, 1:3,000–1:1,000; as bladder irrigation, 1:6,000–1:1,000; kidney lavage, 1:10,000 to 1:1,500.

Rivanol: As germicidal agent; urethral irrigations, 1:3,000 to 1:4,000; in cystitis, 30–50 cc of 1:5,000 to 1:1,000 solution; for pelvic lavage, 1:2,000.

Salihexin: As antiseptic; orally, 2 capsules every 3–4 hr.; *intravenously*, 1 ampule every 2 days or daily, for 15 doses.

Sanmetto: As urinary sedative and antiseptic; 1 teaspoonful four times daily.

Santyl: As urinary sedative and gonocide; 25–50 m three times daily after meals.

Salysal: As analgesic; 1–3 tablets three times daily, in water.

Sanpaiba: As urinary antiseptic; 2 capsules several times daily.

Serenium: As genitourinary antiseptic; 2 tablets three times daily for 4–5 days a week; continued for 2 weeks after symptoms have subsided.

Silvogon: For local application in vaginitis, 1:2,000; in cervicitis, 1:500; for irrigations, 1:1,000 to 1:5,000.

Silvol: As silver protein antiseptic; for topical application, in 5% bougies or vaginal suppositories.

Solargentum: As urinary antiseptic; in urethral injections, 10%; as irrigation, 1:1,000; for bladder instillation, 5 cc of 20–50% solution.

Solurea: As diuretic and uricolytic; 1–2 capsules or tablets with water, several times daily.

Targesin: As gonocide and astringent; urethral injections, 1–5%; bladder irrigation, 0.2%; in female urethritis and abortive therapy, 5–10% solution.

Terogon "Schiftan": As sedative and antiseptic in pain and strangury; 3–4 tablets three times daily.

Terpichin: As non-specific therapy agent; *intragluteally*, 1 cc twice weekly, increased to 2 cc.

Tolamine: As germicide for urethral, bladder and uterus irrigations; in 0.5% solutions.

Tutocain: As surface anesthetic in urethral manipulations; 1½–2% solution.

Uriform: As urinary antiseptic; 1–2 teaspoonfuls three times daily, with liberal use of water.

Urocedrol: As urinary antiseptic; in acute infections, 10 capsules daily, 5 before midday meal, 5 before evening meal; in chronic infections, 6 capsules daily, 2 before each meal.

Urotropin: As urinary antiseptic; orally, 7½ gr two to four times daily; *intravenously*, in general infections; *intramuscularly* or *subcutaneously*, 5 cc of 40% solution.

Yohimbin: As aphrodisiac in impotency and deficient libido; 1 tablet three times daily after meals; or ampules, given hypodermically.

Yohimboid "Lowenthal": As nerve stimulant in impotence, sexual neurasthenia and sterility; 1 tablet after meals and at bedtime.

Zinc Permanganate: As astringent; for urethral injection and irrigation; 1:4,000 solution.

Part III

Diseases and Preparations Indicated in Their Treatment

ACIDOSIS: *Systemic (Acute infections, Starvation, Vomiting, Cyclic vomiting, Pregnancy, Diabetes, Diarrheal diseases, Nephritis, Rheumatism)*

Alvesen—1–2 tablets in glassful of water as frequently as necessary.

Alka Carb—1 teaspoonful dissolved in glassful of water after meals.

Alka-Sal—1–3 teaspoonfuls daily, continued until urine is alkaline, then reduced.

Ampule Glucose—*intravenous* injections, slowly administered in quantities and frequency as demanded in each case.

Bicarbonate of Soda—in 4% solution as Murphy drip, quantities of 3–4 oz. or more.

Bisodol—1 teaspoonful in water three to four times daily or more frequently.

Bisurated Magnesia—1 teaspoonful in water three to four times daily.

Calcium Phosphate Tribasic—8–20 gr four times daily after meals; children ¾–1½ gr per year of age.

Diskets Alkaline—1 disket in glassful of water, repeated as frequently as necessary.

Magnesium Phosphate Tribasic—15–75 gr three to four times daily after meals.

Sodinco—1 teaspoonful between meals several times daily.

ACNE

Acriviolet—1% solution, pencilled twice daily after first drying surface.

Cerevisine—internally, 1 tablet every 1–2 hr.; topically, in form of paste made with water, or applied as poultice.

Collosol Argentum—in form of ointment or wet dressing.

Collosol Ichthyol—in form of ointment, soap, tampons and dressing; used topically.

Collosol Manganese—for *intramuscular* injections, 0.5–1 cc every 2–3 days till 6–8 cc are administered; also orally.

Collosol Stannum—for *intramuscular* injections, 1 cc every 2–3 days.

Ichthalbin—as dusting powder.

Ichthargan—as 5%–10% ointment.

Mangacol—for above purpose, *intramuscular* injections ¼–1 gr.

Manganese Butyrate—for above purpose, *intramuscular* injections 0.5–1 cc.

Man-Na-Gluconate—as non-specific therapy, *hypodermic* injections 1 cc every fourth day for 12 injections.

Resorcinol Monoacetate—in 5%–20% ointment or in acetone solution.

Stannoxyl—orally 4–8 tablets daily after meals; *intramuscularly* 1–2 ampules every second day; topically 1%–2% lotions; also general Stannoxyl baths.

Stanno-Yeast—as corrective, 1–3 tablets every 3 hr.

Stanprotein—as alterative, 6 gr every 3 hr. for 24 hr., then every 4 hr. for 24 hr., thereafter 3 gr every 3 hr.

Tinpronate—for non-specific therapy, 2 tablets every 3 hr. first day, every 4 hr. second day, thereafter 1 tablet every 3 hr.

Vaccines—*see* "Biologicals," "Acne Vaccinotherapy," *Chap. VI.*

ADDISON'S DISEASE: (*Also all cases of Severe Hypoadrenia*)

Adreno-Cortin—1–2 capsules two to three times daily, or 1 ampule of solution daily, *subcutaneously.*

Eschatin—*intravenously* 20 cc in extreme collapse; in moderate severity 1–5 cc *subcutaneously*, repeated as indicated; single dose generally 10 cc.

Suprarenal Cortex—1 ampule daily, *subcutaneously.*

ADENITIS: (*Glandular enlargements: Scrofulous, Infectious, Tubercular, Luetic, etc.*)

Atomidine—as alterative and absorbent; orally 5–10 drops in water two to three times daily; locally as ointment applied twice daily.

Collosol Iodine—as alterative and absorbent; orally 1–3 teaspoonfuls three times daily; locally as iodine oil or ointment by gentle massage, once or twice daily.

Creosotide—in tubercular adenitis 1 tablet three times daily, orally.

Ethidol—as alterative and absorbent; 0.5–1 cc injected intraglandularly on alternate days; locally—rubbed lightly until absorbed, or spread on applied dressing.

Iodotone—as alterative and absorbent; 1–2 teaspoonfuls three to four times daily.

Ointments—*See Chapter X* "Ointments."

Proteolac—as non-specific therapy, injected intradermally, 3 m every 5 days.

Soluble Iodine—as absorbent; locally—full strength for painting or injection; internally—8 m three times daily.

AMEBIASIS

Acetarsone—as amebacide; 2–3 tablets for 7–10 days, orally; *intravenously,* contents of 1 ampule dissolved in 9 cc of normal (4%) sodium hydroxide of accompanying alkpule and diluted with 11 cc of sterile distilled water; for 7–10 days.

Anayodin—as amaebicide; in acute amebiasis oral therapy only, 4 pills increased to 8 pills, three times daily before meals for 8 days; rest period of 10 days; course repeated until relieved; in chronic amebiasis, oral therapy is preferred and administered as in acute; in severe cases, enemas of 200–300 cc tepid 1½–3% solution of Anayodin, after cleansing enema, for 6–8 evenings; rest period of 6 days with 3 pills orally daily; course repeated where indicated. Hospitalized cases are given in addition, through Rehfuss tube, duodenal instillations of 1,000 cc warm hypertonic saline, followed after 30 min. by 200–300 cc of 1–2% warm Anayodin solution; given semiweekly for 4 weeks.

Bile Salts—as cholagogue in amebic dysentery, 1–4 tablets daily before meals; dosage reduced on improvement.

Carbarsone—as amebacide; 1 pulvule, twice daily after meals, for 10 days; after 10 days rest, second course; in severe cases, in addition—retention enemas (2 Gm dissolved in 200 cc of warm bicarbonate solution) slowly injected, preceded by alkaline cleansing enema; 5 injections, one every other night.

Chiniofon—as amebacide; on first day 1 tablet, three times daily after meals; on second to fifth day 2 tablets; then 3 tablets on sixth and seventh day, where tolerated; rectally, to prevent relapses and in the treatment of chronic cases. *See Chap. I.*

Paroxyl (Spirocid)—as amebacide; 1 tablet three times daily for 1 week, repeated after 10 days' interval, as indicated.

Quinoxyl—as amebacide; orally, 1–4 tabloids, three times daily; rectally, retention enemas of 200 cc of 2½% solution, administered daily.

Stovarsol—as amebacide; 1 tablet two to three times daily for 7 days; rest period and repeated as indicated. *See Chap. I.*

Vioform—as antiseptic, in amebic ulceration; orally, 8 gr three times daily for 10 days.

ANAPHYLACTIC SHOCK: *(In Intravenous protein, Sera, Vaccines, Antitoxins therapy; Intravenous Arsenicals and other drugs; Non-specific Protein Therapy)*

Adrenalin—prophylactic—0.5 cc, 1:1,000 solution administered before the specific medication; therapeutic—5 drops in 1 oz. saline, *intravenously*, slowly administered; *subcutaneously*, 10–15 min.

Ephedrin—*subcutaneously*—1–2 ampules as indicated; *intravenously* or *intramuscularly*, ½–1 ampule.

Epinephrin Hydrochloride—3–10 m *intramuscularly;* site massaged to aid absorption.

Epinine—1 hypoloid *intravenously* in 500 cc saline.

Suprarenalin—1–15 m of 1:1,000 *intravenously* in 1 pt. of saline solution.

Suprarenin—*intravenously*, 30 m to pint of normal saline or glucose; or 5–15 m *intramuscularly*.

ANASARCA: *(General, Ascites, Cardiorenal, Pleural effusion, Edema, Hepatic cirrhosis)*

Agurin—8–15 gr in capsule two to three times daily after meals.

Aminophyllin—1–2 tablets three to four times daily after meals; *hypodermically* 1–3 ampules daily; *rectally* 2–4 suppositories daily.

Arbutin—1–2 tablets every 2 hr. in water, or 15–23 gr three to four times daily.

See also—"Diuretics," "Purgatives," "Cardiac stimulants." *Chap. XI.*

ANEMIA: *(Secondary, Post-infectious, Post-hemorrhagic, Nutritional; Chlorosis)*

Accessorone—as vitamin source and hematinic; 1–4 dr. three to four times daily before meals.

Armicol—1–5 gr three times daily after meals.

Arsenocol—½–5 gr orally, ¼–3 cc *hypodermically.*

Arsenoferratose—1–3 teaspoonfuls three times daily orally.

Bone Medulla—1 or more tabloids after meals, with water.

Collosol Arsenic—in anemias accompanying spirillosis, orally—½–1 teaspoonful two to three times daily in water, increased if necessary; *intramuscularly*—1 cc twice weekly for 10 injections.

Collosol Cuprum—1 teaspoonful two to three times daily diluted in water.

Collosol Ferro-arsenicum—orally; 1 teaspoonful three times daily after meals, *hypodermically* 2 cc one or two times weekly.

Collosol Ferro-manganese—orally; 1 teaspoonful three times daily after meals, *hypodermically*, 0.5–1.5 cc one or two times weekly.

Collosol Ferrum—orally, 1 teaspoonful three times daily in water; *intramuscularly* 2 cc one or two times daily.

Cupricol—½–5 gr orally; *hypodermically* ½–3 cc.

Cupriferrum—1–2 tablets or 1–2 dr. of elixir or of syrup—one to three times daily after meals.

Elarson—2 tablets three to five times daily, increased if indicated.

Elixir I.A.S.—1 teaspoonful four times daily after meals.

Endomin—1–3 tablets three times daily.

Ferric Ammonium Citrate—2–4 capsules three times daily.

Ferri-Quin—1–2 capsules two to three times daily before meals.

Ferro-ca-mang—1–2 dr. or 2–4 pulvoids after meals, three times daily; hyposols *intravenously* or *intramuscularly* twice weekly.

Ferro-Cop—1–3 tablets three times daily.

Ferro-mangan Peptonized—1–2 dr. three times daily before or after meals.

Ferrophytine—1–2 pills three times daily after meals.

Ferruginous Compound—*hypodermically*, 1 ampule daily for 12 injections; orally 25 drops daily for 12 days.

Ferruginous Compound "Fraisse"—in convalescence and pregnancy; *subcutaneously* or *intramuscularly*, 1 ampule daily for 12 days, repeated after 5 day interval; orally, 25 drops daily for 12 days, repeated after 5 day interval.

Hemaboloids—1 tablespoonful or 2 tablets three to four times daily, increased if necessary.

Hemec—1–2 tablets three times daily after meals.

Hemoglobin—1 or more tabloids three times daily after meals.

Hemoglobin Compound—1–3 tablets at meals, in water.

Hepatrat—in anemias of metallic poisoning; *intramuscularly*—3 cc daily, in severe cases 6 cc; course of 6–8 weeks.

Iron Citrate, Green—*intramuscularly*, ¼–1½ gr, as indicated.

Iron Lactate—2–10 gr several times daily; average dose 5 gr.

Jeculin—2–4 teaspoonfuls three times daily after meals; also used in primary anemia.

Liver Extract with Iron 55—2–4 level teaspoonfuls with orange juice, grape fruit, lemonade, ginger ale—daily.

Liver Meal—2 heaping teaspoonfuls three times daily, in soups, milk, cereal, fruit juices, added to foods directly; also used in primary anemia.

Mancuhemin—1–2 tablets or half teaspoonful of elixir three to four times daily.

Manganese Dioxide—2–4 teaspoonfuls in water three times daily, half hour after meals.

Manola—1–2 teaspoonfuls four times daily after meals.

Neoferrum—1 tablespoonful three times daily, before or after meals.

Neobovinine—1 tablespoonful four times daily.

Neurempco—*intramuscularly*, two to three times weekly.

See also—"Hematinics," "Malt preparations," "Cod liver oil products," "Vitamines," *Chap. XI.*

ANGINA: (*Vincent's, Agranulocytic*)

Acriviolet—as spray; four times daily, 1% solution.

Adenine Sulphate—to stimulate polymorphnucleosis in Vincent's; 0.5 Gm in 20 cc normal saline solution, twice daily, *intravenously*.

Bisempco Solution—topically by swab, as frequently as necessary.

Collosol Argentum—as spray or gargle; undiluted or diluted with 2–4 parts of warm saline.

Pentnucleotide—10 cc *intramuscularly*, first twice, then once daily; in severe cases 20 cc twice daily for 4 days, then 10 cc.

Salvarsan Glucose Solution—applied topically daily, with cotton wrapped applicators and left in contact with tissues as long as possible; applications are made after previous cleansing with peroxide swabs, rinsing mouth with water, and drying of lesions.

ANGINA PECTORIS

Aminophyllin—as vasodilator and cardiostimulant, to relieve pain; orally 1–2 tablets three to four times daily after meals; *intramuscularly* or *intravenously* 1–3 ampules; rectally 2–4 suppositories daily.

Benzyl Succinate—for antispasmodic effect; 5–15 gr as frequently as indicated.

Diuretin—as cardiovascular dilator; 1 or 2 tablets three to four times daily after meals; in severe pain, 24–60 gr daily.

Erythrol Tetranitrate—as vasodilator, ¼–1 gr every 4–6 hr.

Ethyl Iodide Vaporole with Chloroform—1 vaporole crushed and contents inhaled until relief is obtained.

Felsol—as antispasmodic; 1–2 powders three times daily in water; in severe attack, repeated in half hour.

Metaphyllin—as cardiotonic; 1–2 tablets three to four times daily or 1–3 ampules *intramuscularly* or *intravenously;* or 2–4 suppositories.

Papaverine—as sedative, orally or *subcutaneously*, ½–1⅓ gr per dose, daily up to 7½ gr.

Papaverine Hydrochloride—as sedative, orally ¾–1½ gr per dose, up to 4 gr daily; *subcutaneously*, same dosage, as often as necessary; *intravenously*, 1/12–⅙ gr, daily up to ⅔ gr.

Theamin—as vasodilator; 3–5 pulvules three to five times daily for several days.

Theocalcin—as vasodilator; 1–3 tablets daily after meals, up to 60 gr daily, where necessary.

Theominal—as vasodilator; 1–2 tablets two to three times daily, as indicated.

Thephyldine—as vasodilator; 1–2 tablets three to four times daily after meals, *intravenously* or *intramuscularly* 1–3 ampules daily; rectally 2–4 suppositories daily.

Tissue Extract 568—*hypodermically*, 2–5 cc every 2–3 days for 5–10 weeks.

See Also—"Antispasmodics," "Vasodilators," "Narcotics," "Diuretics" and "Cardiology," *Chap. XI.*

ANGIONEUROTIC EDEMA: *See* "Allergy." *Chap. VII*

ANTHRAX: *See* "Biologicals"; "Anthrax Serotherapy," *Chap. VI.*

ANAPHRODISIA

Cannabin Compound—1–2 tablets four times daily.

Yohimbin—1 tablet three times daily after meals, orally; 1 cc ampule *hypodermatically* daily.

See also—"Endocrines, uniglandular, pluriglandular," "Aphrodisiacs," *Chap. IV.*

ARTERIAL DISEASE: (*Arteritis, Arterial spasm, Intermittent claudication, Endarteritis, Raynaud's disease; Senile, diabetic and amputation stump gangrene, Decubitus*)

Acecoline—as vasodilator, to relieve spasm and pain; *subcutaneously* or *intramuscularly*, never intravenously—1 ampule once or twice daily.

Acetylcholine and Acetylcholine Bromide—*intramuscularly* or *subcutaneously*. never intravenously—0.05–0.2 Gm daily, increased, as 5% solution.

Anespray—applied locally in discharging gangrene.

Anesthesin Powder—as dusting powder in decubitus ulcer.

Benzyl Fumarate—as antispasmodic; 1–4 tablets as often as indicated.

Calcium Thiocyanate—as vasodilator; 1 tablet three times daily after meals for 6–8 weeks; in severe cases, up to 4 tablets.

Erythrol Tetranitrate—as vasodilator; ¼–1 gr every 4–6 hours.

Hypotan—as hypotensive, 4–6 tablets daily.

Neo-Riodine "Astier"—as alterative; *intramuscularly* or *intravenously*, beginning with 1 cc, increased to 2, 3 and 5 cc three to four times weekly for 8–10 injections; repeated if necessary.

Organidine—as alterative, 5–20 drops three times daily before meals.

Oridine—as alterative; 1–2 tablets three times daily.

Padutin—as vasodilator; *intramuscularly*—½ ampule daily for 2 days, then 1 full ampule twice daily for 10–14 days; severe cases, 4 ampules daily.

Papaverine Hydrochloride—as anodyne; *intravenously* 1/12–1/6 gr, *subcutaneously* 3/4–1 1/2 gr as required.
Riodine "Astier"—as alterative; 2–6 capsules daily after meals.
Sajodin—as alterative; 5–15 gr three to four times daily, chewed before swallowing, after meals.
Tiodine "Cognet"—*intramuscularly*, 1 ampule every other day; orally, 2–5 pills daily, children 1–3 daily.
Tissue Extract 568—as vasodilator; *hypodermically* 2–5 cc every 2–3 days, gradually reduced; course of 5–10 weeks.
See Also—"Anodynes," "Narcotics," "Sedatives," "Hypnotics," "Vasodilators" and "Anti-spasmodics," *Chap. XI.*

ARTERIOSCLEROSIS: (*Hypertension, Coronary disease, Aneurysm, Aortitis*)
Allisatin—for relief of general symptoms; 2 tablets three times daily after meals, increased to 10–12 tablets.
Arsclero—for hypertension; 1–2 tablets two to three times daily.
Benzyl Benzoate—for arterial spasm; 5–7 m increased to 20 or 30 m as required; also 1–2 teaspoonfuls of solution or elixir; repeated as necessary.
Benzyl Fumarate—as antispasmodic; 1–4 tablets as frequently as required.
Bromural—for sedation and hypnosis; 1–2 tablets several times daily.
Diasystol—as vasodilator; 1 dr. three to four times daily.
Diuretin—as vasodilator; up to 24 gr daily.
Ferro-Sajodin—as alterative; 1–3 tablets three times daily.
Hepvisc—for cerebral spasm; 3–6 tablets daily.
Lipoiodine—as alterative in prolonged therapy; 1 or 2 tablets on alternate days.
Nitrocon—as hypotensive; 1–2 capsules or tablets three times daily.
Nitroscleran—as vasodilator and for relief of symptoms; *subcutaneously*, beginning with 0.04 Gm, slowly increased to 0.1 Gm for 8–15 injections; repeated at intervals of 4–6 weeks in intensive treatment.
Potassium-Iodo-Theocalcin—as vasodilator and diuretic; 1–2 tablets at meals.
Soluble Iodine—as alterative, average 8 m three times daily, well diluted.
Theominal—as vasodilator; 1 tablet two to three times daily.
Theamin—as vasodilator and diuretic; 3–5 pulvules three to five times daily for several days.
Theocin—as diuretic; 1–2 tablets two to three times daily, with abundance of fluid.
Thephyldine—as diuretic; orally 1–2 tablets three to four times daily after meals; *intramuscularly* or *intravenously* 1–3 ampules daily; rectally 2–4 suppositories daily.
Tiodine—as alterative; 1 ampule *intramuscularly* every other day; orally, 2–5 pills daily.
See Also—"Iodine preparations," "Vasodilators," "Alteratives," "Sedatives," *Chap. XI.*

ARTHRITIS: (*Infectious, Hypertrophic, Atrophic; Rheumatism, Gout, Uric acid diathesis, Uratic dermatoses, Lumbosacral disease, Fibrositis, Lumbago, Myositis*)
Activin—to stimulate defense mechanism; *intramuscularly*—initial dose 0.5 cc, gradually increased, twice weekly; larger doses in acute, smaller in chronic forms.
A.L.A.—as local anesthetic; injected *intramuscularly* or *subcutaneously* at 5–7 points within a 3 in. circle of painful area, in 0.1–0.5 cc at each point; total 1 cc.
Albatum—for rubefacient action; locally applied.
Amatin—as antipyretic and analgesic; 1–3 tablets three times daily.
Amiodoxyl Benzoate—as phagocytic and immunity stimulant, especially in hypertrophic and gonorrheal arthritis; *intravenously* 0.75–1 Gm in 100 cc sterile saline, slowly, followed by saline; twice weekly for 5–10 injections; orally, as its calcium salt, calciodoxyl benzoate, 1.5–3 Gm.
Ami-Salox—as analgesic and uric acid eliminant; 10–30 gr every 3–4 hr.
Ampule Reipar—as anesthetic; *hypodermically*, 1–10 cc at most painful points.

Anacin—as antiarthritic; 1–2 tablets in ½ glassful of water, repeated in 1 hr. if no relief is obtained.

Analgesic Balm—for local use; applied freely after hot towelling.

Antifebrine—antipyretic and analgesic; gr 3 as frequently as required.

Atophan—antiarthritic, uricolytic and analgesic; orally 1 tablet or 5–10 gr powder two to three times daily with large draughts of alkaline fluid, for 3–4 days; rest period of several days, then repeated; also *intravenously* and *intramuscularly*, as indicated.

Atoquinol—analgesic, uricolytic in acute and subacute cases; 4–8 tablets with liberal supply of water, in 24 hr.; in severe pain, 8 tablets every 3–4 hr. for 3 doses.

Balmogen—for external use; small amount is rubbed in gently, preceded by hot towelling; repeated as often as necessary.

Befsal—as uricolytic; 2–3 dr. daily, or 4–6 tablets four times daily.

Calcium Benziodoxyl—as antiarthritic; 1 capsule every 1–2 hr. with water, on empty stomach, three or four times daily; repeated every 3–4 days for 6 weeks; rest period of 2 weeks, then course repeated.

Calcium Thiocyanate—as vasodilator in gouty arthritis; 1 tablet three times daily after meals for 6–8 weeks; severe cases 4 tablets daily.

Camphro-salyl Ampules "Fraisse"—as analgesic; 1 ampule every 2–3 days, *subcutaneously* or *intramuscularly*, into painful areas; 5 or 6 injections.

Caseosan—as non-specific therapy agent; *intramuscularly* or *subcutaneously*, 0.5, 2.0, 3.0–5.0 cc at 1–3 day intervals; *intravenously* 0.25–3 cc; *intracutaneously*, 0.3–1 cc.

Chloroxyl—uricolytic, analgesic; 1–3 tablets repeated as indicated.

Cibalgine—as analgesic; 1–2 tablets or 1–2 dr. of elixir every 3–4 hr.

Cinchophen—analgesic, uricolytic; in acute cases 1–2 tablets three to four times daily for 2–5 days; chronic—same dosage, followed by rest period of 3–5 days, and repeated; total dosage not to exceed 150 gr during 1 course; tablets powdered before use.

Citrico—as alkalizer and uricolytic; 2 dr. in water before breakfast.

Colchicum Compound—as analgesic in gout; 1 tablespoonful every half hour for 6 doses, then every 1–2 hr.

Collosol Iodine—alterative; orally 1–3 teaspoonfuls three times daily after meals; *intramuscularly* 1 cc of 1% solution every fourth day; *intravenously*, from 5–100 cc in accordance with strength of solution; topically, ointment or oil for gentle massage.

Collosol Kaolin—as adsorptive in cases with intestinal toxemia; orally, 1 dessertspoonful in 1 oz. of water mornings and evenings; as colonic irrigation, 1 or 2 heaping tablespoonfuls to gallon of warm water.

Collosol Sulphur—in painful joints with intestinal toxemia; orally 1 teaspoonful three times daily in water; *intramuscularly* 1–2 cc twice weekly; externally as sulphur baths and as topical application diluted ten to twenty times.

Colsul—as pyretic to increase leucocytosis; *hypodermically*, initial dose 0.5 cc, increased by 0.5 cc to *maximum dose* of 5 cc; in larger dosage where necessary.

Combinal—as analgesic; 1–2 tablets as frequently as required; as hypnotic 2–3 tablets at bedtime.

Compral—as analgesic; 1–2 tablets three to four times daily or as indicated.

Dialkalos—as uric acid eliminant; 1 tablespoonful in water two to three times daily after meals.

Dimol—in cases with intestinal toxemia; 2–4 pulverettes with water after meals.

Diskets Sodium Salicylate Compound—as antiarthritic; 1–2 diskets in glass of warm water every 2–3 hr.

Empirin—as antipyretic and analgesic; 1–3 tabloids with water two to three times daily; as analgesic, 15 gr.

Ethidol—as alterative; used externally by rubbing lightly into affected part until absorbed, or spread on dressing.

Farastan—as analgesic and antiphlogistic in gout; 2 capsules three times daily after meals, with large amount of water.

Guphen—as analgesic and antipyretic, 1–2 tablets three or four times daily.

Ichthalbin—as detoxicant in cases with intestinal toxemia, 10–30 gr two to three times daily before meals.

Ichthyol—as antiphlogistic; as ointment from 5–50 %, applied twice daily.

Iodoxyl—as antiarthritic; 2 capsules three times daily after meals; larger doses in protracted cases.

Kaylene—as intestinal detoxicant; 1 tablespoonful in water before meals.

Lipoiodine—as alterative; 1–2 tablets on alternate days.

Magnesium Peroxide—as antacid and eliminant; gr 5–20 as often as required.

Magnespirin—as analgesic and antipyretic; 2 tablets three to four times daily with water.

Manakali—as analgesic and antiarthritic; ½–1 teaspoonful three times daily with water.

Mesotan—as analgesic and antiarthritic; 1 part to 2, 3 or 4 parts of olive or cottonseed oil, applied gently without rubbing; changed at intervals of 1–2 days.

Mustarx—as counterirritant; applied one or two times daily.

Naiodine "Logeais"—as alterative, 20–40 cc *intramuscularly* two to three times daily in intensive therapy; *maintenance dose* 5–10 cc daily.

Natural Salicylates—as antiarthritic and analgesic; initial therapy 1 gr per pound of body weight, then 15 gr daily, after first day's alkalization.

Neocinchophen—analgesic and uricolytic; 1–2 tablets three to four times daily after meals, with abundance of water; continued at intermittent periods of 3–4 days.

Neomagnephen—as analgesic; 2–3 tablets three to four times daily.

Neo-Riodine "Astier"—as alterative; *intramuscularly* or *intravenously;* initial dose 1 cc increased to 2 cc, 3 cc and 5 cc, three to four times weekly; 8–10 injections per course.

Novaspirin—as antiarthritic; 10–15 gr several times daily; severe cases increased to 30 gr.

Omnadin—as non-specific therapy agent; *intramuscularly,* 1 ampule once daily, and guided by local and general reactions.

Oxo-ate—as antiarthritic; *intravenously,* 1 Gm in 100 cc sterile solution, injected slowly, at body temperature; twice weekly for 8–10 doses; rectal retention enema, 1 Gm in 50 cc water twice weekly for 3–4 weeks.

Oxo-ate-B—antirheumatic; 1 tablet four times daily after meals.

Oxyl-Iodide—alterative and antiarthritic; 2 tablets after meals with plenty of water, as often as necessary.

Panalgin—as analgesic; 1–2 teaspoonfuls increased to 1 tablespoonful every 3–4 hr., followed by water or milk.

Panthesine Ointment—as analgesic, applied locally two to four times daily.

Phenacetine—as analgesic and antipyretic, 1–2 tablets every 4–6 hr.

Phytosalicyl—as antiarthritic, 1–2 teaspoonfuls in water five to six times daily.

Piperazine—as uricolytic, 15–20 gr daily, with abundance of alkaline drinks.

Proteolac—as non-specific therapy agent; *intramuscularly* 1–2 cc increased to 5–10 cc every 2–5 days.

Pyramidon—as analgesic; 3–5 gr every 3–4 hr.

Quinisal—as analgesic; 1–2 tablets every 2 hr., or less frequently.

Riodine "Astier"—as alterative; 2–6 capsules daily.

Rivanol—in purulent arthritis; injected into joint, 10–15 cc of 1:500 to 1:1,000 solution.

Sajodin and Ferro-Sajodin—as alteratives and tonics; 5–15 gr three to four times daily after meals.

Sal-Ethyl-Carbonate—as analgesic; 5–15 gr as often as required.

Salicin—as antipyretic and analgesic; 1–4 tablets after meals.

Salicionyl—antipyretic and antirheumatic; 1–6 oz. in water every 1–2 hr. until relieved, then at longer intervals.

Salipyrin—as analgesic and antipyretic; 7½–15 gr two to three times daily.

Salit—as rubefacient; rubbed in twice daily as cream or oil, after skin cleansing and drying.

Salophen—as analgesic; 15 gr three to four times daily.

Salysal—as analgesic; 1–3 tablets three times daily.
Selencol—as non-specific therapy agent; *hypodermically* 0.25–2 cc repeated according to reaction.
Silosan—as analgesic, 1–3 tablets repeated as necessary.
Silosan Compound—1–2 tablets with water at 3–4 hr. intervals.
Soluble Iodine—as alterative; average dose 8 m three times daily, well diluted, on empty stomach.
Spiroform—as intestinal antiseptic and antipyretic; 1–2 tablets three times daily.
Spirosal—as rubefacient; diluted in 2–3 parts of alcohol and olive oil, (1 dr. to the ounce), rubbed in thoroughly and covered.
Sufrogel—as non-specific therapy agent; *intramuscularly* 0.2–0.4 cc every 8 days for 6 doses.
Sulphocol—as non-specific therapy agent; orally ½–3 gr several times daily; *hypdermically*, 0.25–5 cc, repeated according to reaction.
Syrup of Hydriodic Acid—as alterative, ½ to 3 teaspoonfuls well diluted.
Thiol—as rubefacient; rubbed in as ointment several times daily.
Tiodine "Cognet"—as alterative and resolvent; 1 ampule *intramuscularly* every other day; orally, 2–5 pills daily.
Tolysin—as analgesic; 1–2 tablets every 3 hr., with frequent rest periods between courses.
Yatren-Casein—as non-specific therapy agent; *intramuscularly* 1 cc every 2–5 days, increased according to reaction.
See also—"Arthritis vaccinotherapy," *Chap. VI;* "Non-specific therapy agents," "Alteratives," *Chap. XI;* "Ointments," *Chap. X.*

ASCITES: *See* "Anasarca," *Chap. XI*]

ASTHMA

Adrenalin and Adrin Solution—as bronchial antispasmodic; *subcutaneously* or *intramuscularly* 2–10 m, massaging periodically site of injection; repeated as necessary.
Anti-asthmatic—½–1 ampule *subcutaneously* several times daily.
Atomidine—as alterative; 5–20 drops several times daily.
Belladenal—as antispasmodic; 2–4 tablets daily (¼ tablet every half hour).
Bellafoline—as antispasmodic; 1–2 tablets or 10–20 drops three times daily; hypodermically 0.5–2 cc daily.
Benzyl Benzoate—as antispasmodic; 5–8 m as required.
Benzyl Fumarate—as antispasmodic; 1–4 tablets as required.
Benzyl Succinate—as antispasmodic; 5–15 gr in capsules as required.
Ephedrine Preparations—as bronchial antispasmodics; *hypodermically* 1 ampule as required; orally, in accordance with preparation—tablets, syrups, elixirs, etc.
Ephetal Tablets—as antispasmodic; 1–2 tablets as frequently as required.
Esterol—as antispasmodic, 2–4 tablets three to four times daily (see contraindications).
Ethyl Iodide—as antispasmodic; for inhalation for 10 min. once or twice daily, 3 cc.
Papaverine Hydrochloride—in severe instances; *intravenously*, 1/12–½ gr, *subcutaneously* ¾–1½ gr, repeated if necessary.
Peptone Solution—as foreign protein therapy agent; *intramuscularly* 0.3 cc increased by 0.2 cc till 1.5 cc is reached; injections twice weekly.
Proteolac—as non-specific therapy agent; *intramuscularly*, initial dose 1–2 cc, rapidly increased to 5–10 cc; injections every 2–5 days; also *intravenously* where quick action is desired.
Sufrogel—as non-specific therapy agent; *intramuscularly*, 0.2–0.4 cc every 8 days for 6 doses; larger doses in certain instances; overdosage to be avoided.
Suprarenalin and Suprarenin—as antispasmodics; 5–10 m *intramuscularly;* in severe instances *intravenously.*
See Also—"Allergens," *Chap. VII*, "Antispasmodics," *Chap. XI*, "Nasal Preparations," *Chap. X.*

BACILLURIA: *See* "Urology" and "Urinary Antiseptics," *Chap. XI.*

BILIARY DERANGEMENTS: (*Cholangitis, Cholecystitis, Cholelithiasis, Hepatic diseases, Hepatic insufficiency, Jaundice*)

Afenil—as cholagogue; 1–3 tablets two to three times daily after meals.

Ago-Cholan—as cholagogue; 1–3 tablets two to three times daily.

Ami-Salox—as cholagogue laxative; 10–30 gr every 3–4 hr., avoiding alkaline medication.

Atophan—as choleretic and cholagogue; 1 tablet two to three times daily with copious alkaline drinks, for several days; after rest period of several days, may be repeated.

Bellafoline—as antispasmodic in biliary colic; 1–2 tablets or 10–20 drops three times daily; hypodermically 0.5–2 cc daily.

Benzyl Benzoate—as antispasmodic in biliary tract infections; 5–7 m in gelatine capsules, or 3–6 globules or 1–2 dr. of 20% solution; repeated in ½–1 hr. if necessary; *hypodermically* where rapid action is desired.

Benzyl Fumarate—as antispasmodic; 1–4 tablets as indicated.

Benzyl Succinate—as antispasmodic; 5–15 gr as often as indicated.

Betanaphthol Benzoate—as biliary and intestinal antiseptic; average dose 4–6 gr, *maximum single dose* 15 gr; daily dose 34 gr.

Bilein—as cholagogue and laxative; ¼–1 gr as often as indicated.

Bile Salts—as cholagogue and laxative, 1–4 tablets daily before meals, reduced where indicated.

Bile Salts Compound—as cholagogue and choleretic; 2 tablets night and morning in hot water.

Bilival—as cholagogue; acute infections—2–4 pills three times daily, reduced to 3 pills daily after meals; chronic conditions—1 pill three times daily, part of each month.

Bilox—as cholagogue, 1–2 tablets as required.

Bisalco—as cholagogue, 1–2 tablets once or twice daily.

By-Kem—in pre- and postoperative cases, as cholagogue; 2–6 tablets daily with meals.

Cascarine Compound—as cholagogue laxative; 1–2 tablets at night.

Chionacea—as cholagogue alterative; 1–2 dr. as often as required.

Cholaphen—as cholagogue; 1–2 tablets about 2 hr. after meals.

Choleol—as cholagogue laxative; 1 dr. every 3 hr.

Choleval—as bactericide in acute infections, including residual typhoid and hepatic abscess; *intravenously*, 1½ gr in 10 cc sterile water, daily if necessary; in severe cases, double dosage.

Cholphenolate—as cholagogue in liver stasis and catarrhal jaundice; 1–3 tablets four times daily.

Cibalgine—as antispasmodic to relieve biliary colic; *intramuscularly* 1 ampule every 4 hr.

Colactol—as cholagogue; 2–4 tablets three to four times daily after meals.

Decholin—as choleretic in insufficiency and hepatic cirrhosis; 1–2 tablets two to three times daily after meals for 3–5 weeks, then dosage decreased; *intravenously* 1 ampule or 5% or 20% solution on 3 successive days, in accordance with condition.

Diskets Sodium Salicylate Compound—as cholagogue, 1–2 diskets in warm water every 2–3 hr.

Felamine—as cholagogue and biliary antiseptic; in acute cases 2–3 tablets three times daily, chronic, 1–2 tablets for several weeks; several courses during year.

Formin—as biliary antiseptic; 5–15 gr two to three times daily with large quantities of water; in acute infections, *intravenously* 4–30 gr only, in 25% solution.

Gallo-Gogue—as cholagogue in cholelithiasis; 1–2 tablets four to five times daily.

Glycotauro—as cholagogue; 5 gr three times daily for 8 days, reduced to 2 doses daily for 12 days, and single dose for 24 days, with rest intervals before repeating course.

Hepatone—as cholagogue laxative in biliousness and jaundice; ½–1 tablespoonful well diluted in water, half hour before breakfast.

Icterosan—as cholagogue and choleretic; 1 ampule *intravenously*, warmed and slowly injected, daily; also *intramuscularly*.

Kolagog—as cholagogue; ½–2 teaspoonfuls after meals.

Nuchol Tablets—as cholagogue; 2 tablets at night and in morning.

Ovogal—as cholagogue; three capsules 2 times daily after meals, with water.

Oxachol—as cholagogue; 1–2 teaspoonfuls three times daily after meals.

Panteric Tablets and Capsules—as digestant; 1 or 2 tablets or capsules three times daily after meals.

Phenobilin—as cholagogue laxative; 1 or 2 tablets before meals.

Pthalox—as cholagogue laxative, 1 or 2 tablets at night.

Sal-Ethyl Carbonate—as cholagogue; 5–15 gr as often as indicated.

Sodium Glycocholate Compound—as cholagogue; 2–3 tablets 2–3 hr. after meals.

Taurocol—as cholagogue; 1–2 tablets before meals.

Tyloid "Lowenthal"—as cholagogue; 1 tablet after meals.

See also—"Powerful diuretics," "Hydrogogue cathartics," "Intestinal antiseptics," *Chap. XI.*

BLOOD DYSCRASIAS: (*Hemophilia, Hemorrhagic diseases of infancy, Leukemia, Hodgkin's disease, Polycythemia, Purpura hemorrhagica, Weil's disease, Hemorrhagic diathesis*)

Amniotin—as hemostatic; 1–2 cc *subcutaneously* on alternate days; orally 15 drops three times daily.

Benzene (Benzol) Medicinal—as leucocyticide in lymphatic leukemia and polycythemia; 2–10 m every 3 hr. in emulsion, on sugar or in capsules; or 8 m gelatine capsules as initial dose, slowly increased to 15 m, until 60–75 m are given daily; single *maximum dose* 45 m.

Calcilact—to increase blood coagulability; 1 capful three times daily in water before meals.

Calcium Gluconate—to increase blood coagulability; 1 dr. three times daily after meals; *intravenously* or *intragluteally*, 1 ampule every 1–2 days.

Calcium Granular—to increase blood coagulability; 2 teaspoonfuls in water during meals.

Calcium Levulinate—to increase blood coagulability; *intravenously* 10–20 cc warmed, slowly injected; *intramuscularly*, 2 cc as indicated.

Calcium Phosphate Tribasic—to increase blood coagulability; 8–10 gr, average dose 15 gr, as indicated.

Calcol—to increase blood coagulability; orally 2½–15 gr; *intravenously* 0.25–10 cc as indicated.

Calglucon—to increase blood coagulability; 1–2 tablets three times daily; *intramuscularly* and *intravenously*, 10 cc or more every 1–3 days.

Chloro-calcium—to increase blood coagulability; 1–2 dr. in water, as indicated.

Coagulen—as hemostatic; 5–10 Gm in ¼–1 glass of water, sipped slowly; *intravenously*, 2–3 cc several times daily.

Collosol Calcium—to increase blood coagulability; 1 dr. three times daily in water.

Hemostatic Serum—as hemostatic, principally in operations; orally 5 cc, 1 or several doses at 3–6 hr. intervals previous to operation, *intravenously*, 2–5 cc before or after operation; repeated if necessary.

Normal Horse Serum—as hemostatic; 30–100 cc repeated in 12–24 hr., orally; *subcutaneously* or *intramuscularly*, 10–20 cc daily until 100 cc are given.

Para-Thor-Mone—to increase blood coagulability; 38–40 units *subcutaneously*.

Theelin—as hemostatic in hemophilia; 1 or 2 ampules *subcutaneously* or *intramuscularly;* at night, 1 suppository on retiring.

Thromboplastin—as hemostatic; *subcutaneously* or *intramuscularly*, 10–20 cc, repeated if necessary.

BLOOD PRESSURE DISORDERS: *See* "Hypotensors," "Arteriosclerosis." *Chap. XI.*

BRONCHIAL AFFECTIONS: (*Bronchitis, Bronchiolitis, Bronchial pneumonia, Tracheitis, Emphysema*)

Anastil—antiseptic expectorant; *intramuscularly* 1 cc every 2–3 days; *intravenously* 1 cc in 3–5 cc saline, slowly injected every 2–3 days.

Bromoform Bronchial Anodyne Compound—as expectorant; 1 teaspoonful every 2 hr.

Bronchol—as expectorant; 1–2 capsules three to four times daily after meals.

Calcidin—as expectorant; 1–5 tablets four times daily.

Cheracol with Codein—1–3 teaspoonfuls every 3–4 hr.

Coci-Codeine—as expectorant; 2 teaspoonfuls every 3–4 hr.

Creo-terpin—as expectorant; half teaspoonful every 20–30 min.

Di-Efrin—as expectorant and sedative; 1–2 teaspoonfuls as often as indicated.

Dionin—as sedative and antispasmodic; ⅙–1 gr two to three times daily; *subcutaneously*, same dosage.

Ethyl Morphine and Ephedrine Compound—as antispasmodic expectorant; 1 teaspoonful four to eight times daily.

Euphillana—as expectorant, 1–2 teaspoonfuls every 4 hr.

Glypectus—as expectorant; 1–2 teaspoonfuls as required.

Guaiacose—as deodorizing expectorant; 1 teaspoonful three to four times daily.

Guaiaphedra Syrup—as deodorizing expectorant; 1–2 teaspoonfuls as required.

Guaiaphon—as deodorizing expectorant; 1–2 teaspoonfuls as often as required.

Hyotole—as expectorant; 1–2 dr. in water, every 3 hr.

Kresival—as expectorant; 2–4 teaspoonfuls three to four times daily.

Lumodrin—as antispasmodic; 1–2 tablets three times daily.

Orthoben—as disinfectant expectorant; 1–2 teaspoonfuls every 2–3 hr.

Phedros—as sedative expectorant; 1–2 teaspoonfuls, repeated in 2 hr. if necessary.

Pine and Somnos Cordial—as expectorant; 1 or 2 teaspoonfuls, repeated when necessary.

Sanguinaria Compound—as expectorant; 1–2 tablets dissolved on tongue every 2–3 hr.

Sedaco—as bronchial sedative; 1–2 teaspoonfuls as required.

Tolyphen—as expectorant; 2–4 teaspoonfuls as often as required.

Tritussis—as antispasmodic and expectorant; ½–1 teaspoonful; diluted, as often as required.

Yersanco—as expectorant; 1–4 teaspoonfuls as required.

BUBONIC PLAGUE: *See*—"Bubonic Plague Vaccinotherapy," *Chap. VI.*

BURNS: (*Sunburn, Scalds, Chemical burns*)

Amertan—applied liberally ½ in. thick, with or without dressing, until tanning occurs; oily and greasy substances are previously removed.

Butesin Picrate—applied locally, one or two times daily.

Dermalin—to promote granulation; applied freely and covered with gauze.

Iodomuth—as soothing and protecting dressing; applied as dusting powder or 40% ointment.

Parresin—as analgesic and protective; applied in thin layer by spray; covered with cotton, resprayed and bandaged.

Picratol—as germicide and styptic; applied once or twice daily.

Scarlet R Salve "Biebrich"—as desiccant and epitheliant; applied as liquid or ointment spread on gauze, dressed every 1–2 days, alternating with some bland ointment.

Vioform—as antiseptic; dusted or sprinkled locally, as often as required.

See also—"Ointments," "Liquid antiseptics," *Chap. X;* "Local analgesics," *Chap. XI.*

CALCIUM DEFICIENCY DISORDERS: (*Rickets, Tetany, Osteomalacia, Fragilitas ossium, Dental caries, Delayed fracture union, Pregnancy, Lactation, Scrofula, Blood calcium deficiencies, Spasmophilia, Chronic ulceration, Allergic disturbances*)

Afenil—as calcium therapy; *intravenously*, slowly, 10 cc of 10% aqueous solution; daily or several times weekly.
Calcilact—as calcium therapy; 1 teaspoonful in glass of cold water three times daily before meals, increased or decreased if necessary.
Calcionates—1 dr. three times daily between meals.
Calcium Gluconate—1 dr. three times daily after meals; *intravenously* or *intramuscularly*, 1 ampule every 1–2 days.
Calcium Granular—2 teaspoonfuls in glass of water, during meals.
Calglucon—1 or 2 tablets three times daily; *intramuscularly* or *intravenously* 10 cc or more every 1–3 days.
Chloro-Calcium—1–2 dr. as often as required.
Collosol Calcium—1 cc two to three times weekly, intravenously.
D.C.P. 340—½–¾ teaspoonful daily ½ hr. before or 2 hr. after meals; increased if necessary.
Fortossan—4 measurefuls four times daily.
Mineral Mixture Tablets 85—as mineralizer; 6 tablets daily.
Parathyroid with Calcium Lactate—1–2 tablets three times daily, or as necessary.
Syrup Hypophosphite of Calcium—1–2 teaspoonfuls after meals.
Tetanol-Collosol—as anticonvulsive; *intramuscularly* or *intravenously*, 1 ampule as often as necessary.
Thyrocalx—3 tablets daily, gradually reduced to 1 tablet.
Phytine—as calcium phosphorus therapy; 1–4 tablets daily, with meals.
See Also—"Cod liver oil preparations," "Vitamines," *Chap. XI*.

CANCER

Acidol and Acidol Pepsin—in gastric cancer, for anacidity; 1–2 tablets after each meal.
Acidulin—in gastric cancer, for anacidity; 1–2 pulvules after meals.
Aurocol—as palliative in malignancy; 1/40–1/10 gr, orally; *hypodermically*, ⅛–1 cc of solution.
Aurol—as palliative; 15 m three times daily; *intravenously* or *intramuscularly*, 1–5 cc three times weekly.
Collosol Cuprum—in epithelioma and carcinoma, as palliative; *intramuscularly*, 3 cc on first, fourth, seventh and twelfth days; then weekly until symptoms improve, thereafter once monthly; orally, 1 teaspoonful diluted.
Collosol Selenium—postoperatively and in inoperable cases; *intramuscularly*, 5 cc twice weekly for 2 weeks and once weekly for 10 additional weeks; *intravenously*, 5 cc first and third day, 10 cc fifth, eighth, tenth, twelfth days; after 1 mo. rest—10 cc twice weekly for 5 weeks till a total of 100 cc have been injected; orally, 1 dr. in water three times daily, between meals.
Lead Selenide—as palliative; *intravenously*, 5 cc, gradually increased to 15 cc, preceded and followed at each injection by 5% glucose solution; weekly for 8–12 weeks; after 3 mo. rest period—repeated if necessary.
Plumbicol—as palliative; orally ½–2½ gr; *hypodermically* ¼–2 cc; as often as required.
Radon—as therapy; by implantation and topical application by special technic.
Selenium "Oefele"—as prophylactic; 4 tablets daily.
Selencol—as palliative; *hypodermically*, 0.25–2 cc as often as required.

CARDIAC DISORDERS: *See* "Cardiology," "Diuretics," "Vasodilators" *Chap. XI*

CARIES: Dental—*See* "Calcium Deficiency Disorders" and "Dentistry," *Chap. XI*

CATARRHAL DISEASES: *See* "Catarrhal Respiratory Vaccinotherapy," *Chap. VI*; "Bronchial Affections"—"Infections, Acute," *Chap. XI*

CEREBRAL SPASM, VASCULAR: (*Vertigo, Cephalalgia, Tinnitus, Spasm arteriae retinae centralis, Insomnia*)

Acecoline—as vasodilator; *subcutaneously* or *intramuscularly*, 0.1–0.2 cc one or two times daily.

Anabolin—as hypotensive; 1 tablet three times daily.
Atomidine—as diuretic and alterative; 5–20 drops several times daily.
Cucurbocitrin—as hypotensor; 1–5 capsules daily before meals.
Dicitурin—as hypotensor; 60 gr daily.
Diuretin—as vasodilator; up to 80 gr daily.
Haimased—as antispasmodic; 1 teaspoonful two to three times daily for 1 week. then on alternate days.
Hepvisc—as hypotensor; 3–6 tablets daily, increased or decreased as required.
Metaphyllin—as hypotensor; 1–2 tablets two to three times daily in water.
See also—"Vasodilators," "Antispasmodics," "Sedatives" and "Hypnotics," *Chap. XI.*

CHLOROSIS: "*See* Anemia," *Chap. XI*

CHOLERA (Morbus and Infantum): See "Cholera Vaccines," *Chap. VI;* "Intestinal Astringents and Antiseptics," *Chap. XI*

CHOREA: *See* "Antispasmodics," "Sedatives," *Chap. XI*

CLIMACTERIC DISTURBANCES: *See* "Endocrines," *Chap. IV;* "Menstrual Disorders," "Sedatives," *Chap. XI*

COLDS, CORYZA: *See* "Infections, Acute," *Chap. XI*; "Vaccines," *Chap. VI*

COLIC: (*Biliary, Intestinal, Ureteral*)
Benzyl Benzoate—as intestinal antispasmodic, also biliary; 5–7 m increased to 20 or 30 m, repeated as necessary.
Calomel Camphor Compound—as intestinal antispasmodic; 1 tablet every hour for 4 days, then every 2–3 hr.
Esterol— as antispasmodic; initial dose 4 tablets, followed by 2 tablets every hour until relieved.
Papaverine—as narcotic for all colics, orally or hypodermically; ½–1½ gr per dose; daily dose up to 7½ gr.
Papaverine Hydrochloride—for all colics; ¾–1⅓ gr, up to 4 gr daily; *subcutaneously*, gr ¾–1½ as single injection; *intravenously* 1/12–⅙ gr up to ⅔ gr per day.
See also—"Antispasmodics," "Narcotics," "Sedatives," *Chap. XI*

COLITIS: *See* "Colon Vaccinotherapy," *Chap. VI*

CONJUNCTIVITIS: *See* "Ophthalmology," *Chap. XI*

CONSTIPATION: (*Spastic, Atonic, Functional*)
Agar—as mechanical stimulant; 1–4 dr. with water, between meals.
Agar-Agar—as mechanical stimulant; 1 teaspoonful to 1 tablespoonful as required.
Albagar—as mechanical lubricant; 1 tablespoonful at bedtime.
Albolene—as intestinal lubricant; 1–4 tablespoonfuls at bedtime.
Albomalt—as mechanical lubricant; 1 tablespoonful at bedtime.
Analax—as mechanical lubricant; ½–1 tablespoonful at bedtime.
Bile Salts Compound—as cholagogue and choleretic; 2 tablets night and morning in hot water.
Brandreth's Pills—as laxative; 1–3 pills at night.
Collosol Sulphur-paraffin Emulsion—as lubricating laxative; 1–2 tablespoonfuls twice daily.
Coreine "Daniel-Brunet"—1–2 dr. in water or milk after meals; in fermentative diarrhea, larger doses more often desirable.
Evacuant Medicone—as biliary laxative; 1–2 pills at bedtime.
Isacen—as purgative; 2 tablets or more at bedtime
Kasagra—as laxative; ½ dr. ½ hr. before meals; as cathartic, double dosage.
Kaylene—as lubricating laxative; 1 tablespoonful in water before meals.

Kondremul—as laxative; 1 tablespoonful at night and in morning.
Lapactic Pills—as laxative; 1 or 2 pills at bedtime.
Liquid Petrolatum with Agar—as intestinal lubricant; 1–2 tablespoonfuls mornings and evenings.
Mineral Oil Emulsion—as lubricating laxative; 1 tablespoonful one or two times daily.
Ovogal—as cholagogue laxative; 2 capsules three times daily after meals, with water.
Para-Psyllium—as mild laxative; 1–4 teaspoonfuls one or two times daily after meals.
Paroleine—as intestinal lubricant; 1–3 teaspoonfuls before meals.
Peristaltine—as intestinal stimulant; 1–2 tablets at bedtime; in persistent cases, several times daily; in prophylaxis of intestinal stasis, *subcutaneously* or *intramuscularly;* postoperatively—1 cc repeated in 12 hr. if necessary.
Petrobran—as mechanical laxative; 1–2 tablespoonfuls at bedtime.
Petrolagar—as mechanical lubricant; 1 tablespoonful night and morning; rectally 2–4 oz. in pint of warm water.
Phenobilin—as cholagogue laxative; 1 or 2 tablets after meals.
Pheno-sagra—laxative and carminative; 1 or 2 tablets as often as indicated.
Psyllium Seed—mechanical laxative; 1–4 dr. in fruit juice, hot water, one to three times daily after meals.
Pthalox—as cholagogue laxative; 1–2 tablets at night.
Saraka—as mechanical lubricating laxative; 1 teaspoonful half hour after meals.
See also—"Intestinal stimulants," "Digestives," Acidophilus preparations," *Chap. XI*

CONVULSIONS

Calcium Levulinate—*intravenously* 10–20 cc warmed, slowly injected, as indicated; *intramuscularly* 2 cc as indicated.
Chloretone—3–30 gr repeated as necessary; in convulsions of tetanus 40–60 gr in olive oil, as retention enema.
Collosol Palladium—*intramuscularly* ½–1 cc as indicated.
Ethyl Iodide—by inhalation; initial dose 1½ cc, average 3 cc, maximum 5 cc; slowly inhaled 10 min. for each cubic centimeter.
Pentobarbital-sodium—gr 3; repeated if necessary.
Phenobarbital-sodium—*hypodermically,* 5 gr repeated if necessary.
Sodium-amytal—2–4 pulvules till convulsions are controlled.
Tetanol-collosol—*intravenously* 1–2 ampules; *intramuscularly* 2 cc repeated if necessary.

CORONARY DISEASE: *See* "Cardiology," "Arterial Diseases," "Vasodilators," *Chap. XI*

CYSTITIS: *See* "Urology," "Urinary preparations," *Chap. XI*

DIABETES INSIPIDUS

Infundin—*intramuscularly* 5–10 International Units; rectally as saline retention enema.
Pitressin—*hypodermically* 3–5 m per dose; *intranasally* by spray or saturated pledget or as jelly.
Pituitary Extract—3–4 units, increasing dose daily until intestinal reaction is obtained.

DIABETES MELLITUS

Adrenalin—as stimulant in collapse; 5 drops 1:1,000 sol. *intravenously* in normal saline, or 10–15 drops *subcutaneously.*
Cellasin "Barr"—as oral therapy, 12–15 tablets daily in divided doses 1 or 2 hrs. after meals until urine is sugar free, then decreased; *maintenance dose* 4–6 tablets daily.

Dextrose—in insulinemia; *intravenously*, slowly injected in quantities indicated in each case.

Fer-Iodine—as inhibitor of diastatic fermentation in oral diabetic therapy; 1–2 tablets every 2 hr.

Insulin and Iletin—as specific therapy; *subcutaneously* in units calculated per 2 dr. of carbohydrates, blood, urine or food, given 15–30 min. before meals.

Panteric Tablets and Capsules—in oral diabetotherapy; 2–3 capsules or tablets three times daily after meals.

Protonuclein Special Tablets—2–4 tablets three to four times daily.

Saxin—as sugar substitute; as much as required.

See also—"Oral diabetic drugs," *Chap. XI;* "Foods," *Chap. VIII;* "Endocrines," *Chap. IV*

DIARRHEA: (*Simple enteritis, Enterocolitis, Dysentery, Intestinal tuberculosis, Children's diarrhea, Typhoid fever, Fermentation diarrhea*)

Bismogen—as astringent; 1–2 teaspoonfuls every 2–3 hr.

Bismuth Hydrate Compound—as astringent; 1–2 teaspoonfuls every half hour for 6–8 doses.

Bismutose—as astringent and antiseptic; 1 or more teaspoonfuls three times daily.

Calomel Camphor Compound—as astringent; 1 tablet every hour for 4 doses, then every 2–3 hr.

Eldoform—as astringent; 2–3 tablets three to four times daily, thoroughly chewed before swallowed.

Enteri-Drastis—as astringent; 2 tablets, three to four times daily, as indicated.

Iodomuth—as antiseptic astringent in ulcerative colitis and tubercular diarrheas; 10–30 gr every 2–3 hr.

Kaomin—as intestinal sedative; 1 level tablespoonful every morning in ½ glass of water.

Orphol—as antiseptic; astringent in tubercular diarrhea and dysentery; 1–2 teaspoonfuls daily.

Protan—as astringent; 10–30 gr every 2 hr. until effect is obtained.

Sulphodine—as intestinal astringent; 2 tablets first, then 1 every 2 hr.

Tannalbin—as astringent; ½–1 teaspoonful of powder, or 3–6 tablets several times daily.

Tannigen—as astringent; 8–15 gr reduced upon improvement.

Tannismut—as astringent; 1–2 tablets three to five times daily, chewed before swallowed.

See also—"Intestinal diseases," "astringents" and "antiseptics," *Chap. XI*

DIPHTHERIA: See "Antitoxins," "Toxins," "Toxoids" and "Schick Test," *Chap. VI*

Mercury Cyanide—as antiseptic gargle; in 0.01% solution as frequently as desired.

Trypsin—as membranous solvent; in 10% solution of 1:1,000 salicylic acid, applied topically by swab.

DROPSY: *See* Anasarca, *Chap. XI.*

DRUG ADDICTIONS: *See* Psychiatry, *Chap. XI.*

DRUG POISONINGS

Acetylcholine and Acetylcholine Bromide—in lead poisoning for relief of pain and spasm; *intramuscularly*, also *subcutaneously*, *never intravenously*, 0.05–0.2 Gm daily, as 5% solution in increasing dosage.

Alpha Lobelin—as respiratory stimulant in veronal, cocaine, scopolamine, morphine, carbon monoxide, chloral, cyanide and similar poisonings; ¼ gr *intramuscularly* or *subcutaneously; intravenously* 1/12–⅙ gr.

Carbon Dioxide-Oxygen Mixtures—for resuscitation in carbon monoxide and other gas poisoning; administered by special inhalation apparatus in proper percentage.

Collosol Iodine—in lead and mercury poisoning; 1–3 teaspoonfuls of the Iodine Aqueous three times daily after meals; *intramuscularly* 1 cc, 1% solution every fourth day; also given *intravenously*.

Coramin—as cardio-respiratory stimulant, in cresol, phenol, chloral, morphine, barbital, carbon monoxide and other asphyxias; *subcutaneously* or *intramuscularly*, in severe cases *intravenously*, 1 or 2 or more ampules, as required.
Dextrose—as detoxicant and nutrient; in 50% solution, 50 cc slowly administered.
Hepatrat—as hematopoietic in lead, bismuth, salvarsan and other metallic intoxication; *intramuscularly* 3–6 cc daily.
Homocamphin—as cardio-respiratory stimulant; *intramuscularly* 1 to 2 cc as necessary; *intravenously* 1 cc.
Luminal-Sodium and Phenobarbital Sodium—in cocaine and other intoxications, as antispasmodic and sedative; *hypodermically*, 1 ampule as often as required.
Methylene-Blue Medicinal (Methylthionine)—as antidote in the treatment of carbon monoxide poisoning; intravenously 5–10 cc well diluted, given slowly.
Ortal Sodium—as sedative and hypnotic; gr 3–6, repeated as required, to allay excitement and discomfort during withdrawal of habit-forming drugs.
Sodium Thiolsulphate—in metallic poisonings; 1 ampule *intravenously* three to four times daily.
Sulfactol—in mercury, bismuth and arsenic poisoning; *intravenously* gr 10–15 well diluted, daily.
Veronal-Sodium—in acute alcoholism; orally or rectally, gr 10, as necessary.
See also—"Stimulants," "Intoxicants," *Chap. XI*

DYSENTERY: *See* "Sera," "Vaccines," *Chap. VI;* "Intestinal Disorders," *Chap. XI*

DYSMENORRHEA: *See* "Menstrual Disorders," *Chap. XI*

EAR DISEASES: *See* "Otology," *Chap. XI*

EARACHE: *See* "Ear Drops," *Chap. XI*

ECLAMPSIA: *See* "Obstetrics," *Chap. XI*

ECZEMA: *See* "Dermatology," *Chap. XI*

ENDARTERITIS: *See* "Arterial Diseases," *Chap. XI*

ENDOCARDITIS: *See* "Cardiology," *Chap. XI*

ENDOCRINE DISORDERS: *See* "Endocrine Preparations," *Chap. IV*

EPIDIDYMITIS: *See* "Urology," *Chap. XI*

EPILEPSY: *See* "Spasmodic Diseases," *Chap. XI*

EYE DISORDERS: *See* "Ophthalmology," *Chap. XI*

FURUNCULOSIS: *See* "Biologicals," "Vaccines" and "Staphylocides," *Chap. VI*

GANGRENE: (*Senile, Diabetic*) *See* "Arterial Disease," *Chap. XI*

GAS-GANGRENE: *See* "Biologicals," "Anti-toxins and Sera," *Chap. VI*

GASTRIC DISORDERS

Hypacidity (*Subacidity, Achylia Gastrica, Pernicious anemia, Gastric cancer, Chronic dyspepsia, Gastrogenous diarrhea*)
Acidol and Acidol Pepsin—as acidifier; 1 or 2 tablets after each meal.
Acidone—as digestant; 2–4 tablets, after meals, increased where necessary.
Acidulin—as acidifier; 1 or 2 pulvules after meals.
Betaine Hydrochloride; as HCl substitute; gr 8 dissolved in water, after meals.
Dry Peptonoids—as nutrient; 2–4 teaspoonfuls in milk, broth or other fluids.
Enzymatase—to assist protein and starch digestion; 1–2 teaspoonfuls after meals.
Essence of Pepsin—as digestant; 1–2 teaspoonfuls after meals.

Gastron—as digestant; 2–4 teaspoonfuls after meals.
Holadin—as digestant; 1 or more capsules after meals.
Lactopeptin—as digestant; 1 tablespoonful after meals.
Liquid Peptonoids—as digestant and nutrient; 1 or 2 teaspoonfuls after meals.
Liquor Diastos—as digestant; 1–2 teaspoonfuls after meals.
Oxyntin—as HCl substitute; 5–15 gr, ½–1 hr. after meals.
Pan-Peptic Elixir—as digestant; 1 or 2 dessertspoonfuls after meals.
Panpeptic Elixir—as digestant; 1 tablespoonful after meals.
Papain—as proteolytic digestant; 1 or 2 tabloids, two to three times daily, half hour before meals.
Pepana—as digestant; 1–3 tablets, two to three times daily after meals.
Pepsencia—digestant; 1 teaspoonful or more after meals.
Peptenzyme—digestant; 1–2 teaspoonfuls after meals.

Hyperacidity: (*Peptic ulcer, Gastrosuccorrhea, Nervous dyspepsia, Pylorospasm, Acid Dyspepsia, Gastralgia, Gastrodynia*)
Activin—as non-specific agent in gastric ulcer; *intramuscularly*—0.5 cc gradually increased, twice weekly.
Alcaroid—as antacid; 1–2 teaspoonfuls, half hour after meals.
Alkarhein—as antacid; 1–4 teaspoonfuls in hot water every half to 2 hr.
Alvesen—as sedative and antacid; 1–2 tablets in water, as required.
Alucol—as adsorbent and sedative; 2 tablets or 15 gr of powder, 20 min. after meals, repeated if necessary.
Anesthesin—as analgesic and sedative; 5–8 gr, two to three times daily after meals.
Apothesin—as local anesthetic, analgesic and antinauseant; ½ gr as frequently as necessary.
Belladenal—as antispasmodic; 1–2 tablets half hour after meals.
Bellafoline—as antispasmodic and analgesic; 1–2 tablets or 10–20 drops of solution after meals; *subcutaneously* ½–2 cc daily.
Beta-Eucaine Lactate and Beta-Eucaine Hydrochloride—as anesthetic and analgesic; ⅛–½ gr as necessary.
Bismolate—as sedative and antacid; 1–2 tablets, two to three times daily, after meals.
Bismuth and Anesthesin Compound—as sedative and anesthetic; 1–2 tablets or capsules as required.
Bismutose—as antacid; ½–1 or 2 teaspoonfuls, three times daily, after meals.
Cal-Bis-Ma—as antacid, 1 teaspoonful several times daily.
Calcium Phosphate Tribasic—as antacid, 1 teaspoonful, half hour after meals.
Cerogen—as antacid; 1–2 tablets as often as required.
Coagulen—as hemostatic; 5–10 Gm dissolved in ¼–1 glass of water, sipped slowly; *subcutaneously* or *intramuscularly*, 1½–5 cc; *intravenously* 1–2 cc as necessary.
Collosol Lactalumina—as sedative and antacid; 1–4 teaspoonfuls half hour before or after meals.
Collosol Lactomagnesia—as sedative and antacid; 1–2 teaspoonfuls after meals.
Cremo-Carbonates—as antacid; 1–2 teaspoonfuls several times daily; increased if necessary.
Gastric Mucin—as sedative; 1–2 tablespoonfuls half hour before meals, repeated in 1 hr.; also 1 teaspoonful in small amount of water before meals.
Gastrosan—as sedative and antiseptic; daily dosage 3 Gm, single dose ½–1 Gm.
Hemosan—as antacid; 1 teaspoonful several times daily in water, after meals.
Iodomuth—as antiseptic, astringent; 10–30 gr every 2–3 hr.
Kaylene—as adsorbent and sedative; 1 tablespoonful in water before meals.
Macarbo—as antacid; 1 teaspoonful in water after meals.
Magnesium Peroxide—as antacid and antiseptic; 5–20 gr after meals.
Magnesium Phosphate Tribasic—as antacid; 15–75 gr several times daily after meals.
Menthol Y—as sedative in vomiting; ⅙–3 gr as indicated.
Milk of Magnesia—as antacid; 2–4 teaspoonfuls after each meal.

Neogestin—as antacid; 1 powder before or after meals, as required.
Neutralon—as sedative; 1 teaspoonful three times daily after meals.
Neutralon-Belladonna—as antispasmodic; 1 teaspoonful after meals.
Orthoform—as anesthetic and analgesic; 8–15 gr in emulsion.
Oxinol—as sedative; ½–2 teaspoonfuls every 2 hr.
Oxycaine—as antacid and sedative; 1 or 2 tablets after meals.
Pan-Bis-Cal—as digestant and antacid; 2–4 teaspoonfuls after meals.
Papaverine—as antispasmodic; orally or *hypodermically*, ½–1½ gr per dose; daily dosage up to 7½ gr.
Parathesin—as analgesic and anesthetic; 3–5 gr before meals.
Peroxoids—as antifermentative and analgesic; 2–3 tablets or ½–1 teaspoonful stirred in water before meals.
Silver Nitrate-Anesthesin Compound—as analgesic and sedative; 1–2 tablets three times daily after meals.
Sodinco—as antacid; 1 teaspoonful between meals.
Synodal—as non-specific therapy agent in ulcer; *intravenously* 1 ampule twice weekly; in severe cases more frequently, with intervals after sixth dose.

GLANDS: *See* "Adenitis," *Chap. XI*

GOITRE: *See* "Thyroid Disorders," *Chap. XI*

GOUT: (*Uric acid diathesis, Dermatoses*)
Befsal—as uricolytic; 2–3 dr. daily or 4–6 tablets, four times daily.
Chloroxyl—as uricolytic; 5–15 gr repeated as frequently as needed.
Cinchophen—as antiarthritic and uricolytic; 1–2 tablets every 4 hr.
Iodoxyl—as analgesic and antiarthritic; 2 capsules three times daily after meals with water.
Neo-Cinchophen—as uricolytic and analgesic; 1 or 2 tablets three or four times daily or oftener, with much water, after meals.
Organidin—as alterative; 5–20 drops, three times daily before meals.
Oxyl-Iodide—as alterative; 2 tablespoonfuls with water after meals.
Salit—as antiarthritic; in form of cream or oil, is rubbed in twice daily, after cleansing parts with alcohol.
Spirosal—as local analgesic; applied diluted in 2–3 parts alcohol or with olive oil 10%.
Synodal—as non-specific therapy agent; *intravenously*, 1 ampule, twice weekly, more frequently in severe cases; maximum course 10 injections, with intervals of 6–8 weeks between courses.
Panalgyn—as antiarthritic and analgesic; 1–4 teaspoonfuls every 3–4 hr. with plenty of water.
Piperazine—uricolytic; 15–20 gr daily with abundance of water.
See Also—"Uricolytics," "Intestinal detoxicants," "Analgesics" and "Topical analgesics," *Chap. XI.*

HAY FEVER: *See* "Allergens," *Chap. VI*

HEADACHE: *See* "Analgesics"; "Sedatives," *Chap. XI*

HEMOPHILIA: *See* "Blood Diseases," *Chap. XI*

HEMOPTYSIS: *See* "Pulmonary, Gastric, Intestinal, and Blood Diseases," "Hemostatics," *Chap. XI*

HEMORRHOIDS: *See* "Proctology," *Chap. XI;* "Rectal Suppositories" and "Ointments," *Chap. X*

HYPEREMESIS GRAVIDARUM: *See* "Obstetrics," *Chap. XI*

HYPERTENSION: *See* "Hypotensors," "Arteriosclerosis," *Chap. XI*

HYPERTHYROIDISM: *See* "Thyroidal disorders," *Chap. XI*

HYSTERIA: *See* "Neurology," *Chap. XI*

INFECTIONS, ACUTE: *(Colds, Grippe, Influenza, Tonsillitis, Early stages of all acute infectious diseases)*

Amertan—as antipyretic and analgesic; 1–3 tablets, three times daily.
Amosal—as antipyretic and diaphoretic; 1 tablet or capsule as frequently as necessary.
Ampydin—as antipyretic and analgesic; 5 gr repeated only as necessary.
Antifebrin—as antipyretic, analgesic; 1 tablet every 2–3 hr., with caution.
Barmiphen—as antipyretic; 1–2 capsules, three times daily, in water, given with bicarbonate.
Blandine-Compound—as respiratory emollient; for topical swabbing or spraying.
Camphor Compound—as analgesic and antipyretic; 1–2 tablets every half hour until relieved.
Caseosan—as non-specific therapy; *intravenously* or *intramuscularly*, 0.5–3 cc, 0.25–2 cc, at 1–3 day intervals.
Chlorine Gas "Roehling"—for inhalation as per directions.
Cibalgen—as analgesic and febrifuge; 1–3 tablets every 2–4 hr.
Cinchophen—as analgesic; 7½–15 gr three to four times daily.
Colchicum Compound—as antipyretic and analgesic; 1 tablet every half hour in water for 6 doses, less frequently thereafter.
Colsul—as non-specific agent; *hypodermically* ½ cc increased by ½ cc to *maximum* of 5 cc, at intervals in accordance with reaction.
Cryogenine—antipyretic and analgesic; 15–45 gr daily.
Empirin—as antipyretic and analgesic; 1–3 tabloids in water several times daily; as analgesic, 15 gr.
Euquinine—as antipyretic; 4–8 gr several times daily.
Guphen—as analgesic and antipyretic; 1–2 tablets three to four times daily.
Kola "Astier"—as stimulant and tonic; 2 teaspoonfuls daily, in water or other liquid.
Magnespirin—as antipyretic and analgesic; 1 tablet every 2–3 hr.
Methenos—as analgesic and antipyretic; 1 or 2 teaspoonfuls every 3–4 hr. in water.
Neocinchophen—as analgesic; 1–2 tablets every 3–4 hr., with abundance of water.
Nopirine—as analgesic and antipyretic; 1 tablet repeated in accordance with requirements.
Novaspirin—as analgesic and antipyretic; 10–15 gr several times daily, increased as necessary.
Phenacetin—as antipyretic and analgesic; 1 or 2 tablets as required.
Pyramidon—analgesic and antipyretic; 3–5 gr repeated in 3–4 hr.
Quinine Camphor Compound—as antipyretic; 1 tablet every hour, later every 2–3 hr. if required.
Quinisal—as antipyretic and analgesic; 1–2 tablets every 2 hr.
Saladin—as antipyretic; 1 tablet every 3 hr. or 2 at bedtime.
Sal-Ethyl Carbonate—as antipyretic and analgesic; 5–15 gr as required.
Salicin—as antipyretic and analgesic; 1–4 tablets on full stomach.
Salicionyl—as antipyretic; 1 dr. in 6 oz. of water every 1–2 hr. until relieved.
Salipyrin—as antipyretic and analgesic—7½–15 gr on empty stomach followed by water; several times daily.
Salophen—as analgesic, 15 gr three to four times daily.
Salysal—as analgesic—1–3 tablets three times daily in water.
Silosan—as analgesic and antipyretic, 1–3 tablets, repeated as indicated.
Tolysin—as analgesic and antipyretic, 1–2 tablets every 3 hr., as indicated.
Valital—as analgesic, 1 tablet every 3 hr.

INFLUENZA: *See* "Biologicals," *Chap. VI;* "Infections—Acute," *Chap. XI*

INSOMNIA: *See* "Hypnotics and Sedatives," *Chap. XI*

INTESTINAL DISORDERS: (*Intestinal indigestion, Flatulence, Catarrh, Ulceration; Enteritis, Intestinal complications of infectious diseases, Colic, Colitis, Toxemia, Ileus*)

Allisatin—as antispasmodic in colic, colitis; 2 tablets three times daily after meals.
Anayodin—as disinfectant in bacillary colitis; 1 pill three times daily for 30 days; after rest period of 7 days is repeated.
Bellafoline—as antispasmodic and analgesic in colic; 1–2 tablets or 10–20 drops, three times daily; *hypodermically* ½–2 cc daily.
Benzosol—as intestinal antiseptic; 3–10 gr three to four times daily.
Benzyl Benzoate—as antispasmodic in colic, 1 capsule as often as demanded.
Benzyl Fumarate—as antispasmodic in colic; 1 capsule every half hour until relieved.
Beta Lactose "National"—for acidophilus implantation, 3–9 oz. daily; as laxative, 2 tablespoonfuls in ½ glass of water, once or twice daily.
Betanaphthol Benzoate—as intestinal antiseptic; 3–8 gr, *maximum daily dose* 34 gr in divided doses.
Betanaphthol Compound—as antiseptic; 1–3 tablets as required.
Calcreose—as intestinal antiseptic; 1–2 teaspoonfuls or 4–8 tablets several times daily.
Cerevisine "Chapelle"—to change intestinal flora; 1 tablet every hour.
Collosol Ichthyol—as colloidal antiseptic; 5–10 gr in capsules, daily.
Collosol Kaolin—as colloidal adsorptive; 1 dessertspoonful to 1 oz. of water, morning and evenings; as colonic irrigation, 1–2 heaping tablespoonfuls to gallon of warm water.
Collosol Lactalumina—as antacid and laxative; 1–4 teaspoonfuls in water before or after meals.
Coryfin—as carminative; several drops on lump of sugar as often as desired.
Creosote Carbonate—as intestinal antiseptic; 5–20 m increased to 80 m several times daily; average dose 15 m.
Di-hydranol—intestinal germicide; 2–3 capsules or 1–2 dr., three to four times daily.
Dimol—as antiseptic; 2–4 pulverettes after meals, with water.
Duotal—as intestinal antiseptic, gr 5–15, three times daily.
Esterol—as antispasmodic in colic; initial dose 4 tablets, followed by 2 tablets every hour until relieved.
Isarol—intestinal antiseptic; 5–30 m in capsules, two to three times daily as required.
Panteric Tablets and Capsules—as digestant, in intestinal disorders of diabetic; 1 or 2 tablets or capsules several times daily after meals.
Peroxoids—as antacid and analgesic; 2–3 tablets or ½–1 teaspoonful as often as required.
Pitressin—as peristaltic stimulant; *hypodermically* 3–5 m as required.
Prostigmin—as intestinal peristaltic in atony and ileus; 1 ampule *subcutaneously* or *intramuscularly*, followed if necessary in 30 min. by enema of glycerin 150–200 cc; repeated where demanded after 4–5 hr.
Salophen—as antiputrefactive; 15 gr three to four times daily.
Soricin—as detoxifier; 40–60 gr daily with ice water, 20 min. before meals and on retiring; as colon irrigation in ¼–1 % solution.
Sulfactol—as detoxifier in metallic poisoning and as supplement to intravenous therapy; 1–2 tablets, three times daily before meals.
Taka-Diastase—as starch digestant; from 2½–5 gr as often as necessary.
Xeroform—as intestinal antiseptic; 15–45 gr daily.
See Also—"Acidophilus Therapy"—"Laxatives"—"Astringents," "Digestants," *Chap. XI*

KERATITIS: *See* "Ophthalmology" and "Antiluetics," *Chap. XI*

LEAD POISONING: *See* "Drug Poisoning," *Chap. XI*

LEPROSY

Chaulmestrol—1–5 cc, more if necessary, daily after meals, in warm drinks; *intramuscularly* and *intravenously*, 1 cc increased by 1 cc every second and third injection until 5 cc is administered.

Collosol Antimony—as parasiticide, 2 cc increased to 10 cc once or twice weekly.

Moogrol—1–5 cc daily, in increasing doses; *intramuscularly* once weekly, 1 cc increased by 1 cc to a maximum of 5 cc.

LEUKEMIA: See "Blood Diseases," *Chap. XI*

LIVER DISORDERS: See "Biliary Derangements," *Chap. XI*

LUMBAGO: See "Arthritis," *Chap. XI*

LUPUS ERYTHEMATOSUS: See "Dermatology," *Chap. XI*

MALARIA: (*Black Water Fever, Malarial Anemia, Cachexia, Hemoglobinuric fever*)

Chinoplasmin—as antimalarial; 2 tablets three to four times daily after meals.

Euquinine—as prophylactic; 4–8 gr, two to three times daily.

Ferro Sajodin—in anemia; 1–3 tablets, three times daily.

Optarson—as alterative; *subcutaneously* or *intramuscularly*, 1 ampule every second day.

Plasmochin—as antimalarial; 1 tablet three times daily; course directed as required. *See Chap. I.*

Quinarsin—as antimalarial; 1–2 teaspoonfuls, three to four times daily.

Solarson—*intramuscularly* or *subcutaneously*, 1 ampule every 2 days for 10–12 injections; repeated after rest period of 1 week.

See Also—"Hematinics," *Chap. XI* and "Ampule medication," *Chap. V.*

MALNUTRITION: *See* "Nutritional deficiencies," *Chap. XI*

MENINGITIS: *See* "Biologicals," *Chap. VI;* "Infections, Acute," *Chap. XI*

MENSTRUAL DISORDERS: (*Amenorrhea, Dysmenorrhea, Menorrhagia, Menopause, Sterility, Psychoses, Maldevelopment*)

Hormone preparations:

Agomensin—in ovarian hypofunction and manifestations; 1–3 tablets, three times daily, supplemented by *subcutaneous* or *intramuscular* injection of 1 ampule every second day.

Amniotin—in dysmenorrhea and menopausal psychoses; in recent menopause—1 cc *subcutaneously* two or three times weekly, or 10 drops orally twice daily, or 3 pessaries weekly; in protracted menopause, about double dosage. In dysmenorrhea—10 drops twice daily, or 1 pessary daily for 6–8 days, 15 days preliminary to menstrual onset; also *hypodermically* 1 cc every second day.

Anteri-cole—as menstrual flow regulator; *subcutaneously* 1 cc, one to two times daily for 8–10 days following menstruation; in menorrhagia is continued until bleeding is controlled; in frigidity, 1 injection every 1 or 2 days.

Antuitrin-S—as menstrual regulator in hypoovarianism; 50–200 rat units daily for about 2 weeks, later 100 units three times weekly, with rest periods.

Antophysin—as menstruation regulator in ovarian hypofunction; *intramuscularly*, 100 to 300 rat units daily, beginning on due menstruation date and continued for 2 weeks.

Follutein—in amenorrhea, 5–10 cc daily for 5 days, beginning 2 days after expected stoppage of flow; course repeated for several months; in sterility, 3–5 cc 1 injection on fifteenth day of cycle, repeated for several months; in menorrhagia 1–3 units; in premature menopause 5–10 units.

Ovacoids—in hypoovarism; 2–6 tablets three times daily; Ampacoids Ovary given *subcutaneously* or *intramuscularly*, 1 ampule three to six times weekly, more frequently where required.

Ovarialhormon Folliculin Menformon—*subcutaneously, intramuscularly, intravenously*, 1–2 ampules daily for 30 injections or 1–2 dragees orally.

Paroidin—in disturbances with parathyroidal symptoms; *intramuscularly* 30–60 units for 5–6 days.

Progynon—1 tablet three times daily for 10 days, or 1 ampule daily 10 days prior to menstrual period; in menopause 1 tablet three times daily.

Sistomensin—as ovarian therapy; 1–3 tablets three times daily, supplemented by *intramuscular* injections 1 or 2 ampules two to three times weekly.
Theelin—in ovarian deficiencies; subcutaneously or intramuscularly 1 or 2 ampules, suppositories—1 at night on retiring.
Theelol—1–3 kapseals daily in intervals between Theelin injections.
Thelestrin—1–2 ampules *subcutaneously* daily, as required.

Drugs

Antifebrin—as antispasmodic; gr 3 as often as required.
Belladenal—in dysmenorrhea; ½ tablet every hour until relieved.
Bellafoline—in dysmenorrhea, 1–2 tablets or 10–20 drops or ½–2 cc *hypodermically.*
Benzyl Aromatic—in dysmenorrhea; 2–3 capsules, two to three times daily.
Benzyl Benzoate—in dysmenorrhea; 5–8 m are required.
Calcilact—in menorrhagia; 1 teaspoonful three times daily 1 hr. before meals.
Collosol Ferro-Manganese—in anemia and dysmenorrhea; 1 teaspoonful three times daily or *intramuscularly* 1–2 cc twice weekly.
Dioviburnia—to relieve uterine colic; 2 teaspoonfuls in water, three times daily after meals.
Dysco—as antispasmodic; 2 tablets, then 1 tablet every 4–6 hr.
Dysmenatone—as uterine sedative; 1–2 tablets, three times daily.
Emmenagogue—in amenorrhea—3–4 pills after meals for 1 day only near period.
Esterol—as antispasmodic; 3–4 tablets in hot water, repeated in 1 hr. if necessary.
Genitone—as uterine sedative, in threatened abortion; 1–2 teaspoonfuls three times daily.
Gynergen—in excessive menstruation; 1–2 tablets or 15 drops three to four times daily.
Neo-Ergot—in menorrhagia and metrorrhagia; 10–30 m as frequently as required.
Ovaritone—as antispasmodic; 1 or 2 dr. four to five times daily if necessary; as tonic, 2 dr. three times daily.
Papaverine Hydrochloride—as anodyne; ¾–1½ gr daily, *subcutaneously; intravenously* 1/12–⅙ gr.
Peralga—as analgesic in dysmenorrhea; 1 tablet repeated as often as necessary.
Utros—as uterine sedative; 1–2 teaspoonfuls every 3–4 hr.
Valital—as antispasmodic; 1–2 tablets every 4 hr.; more frequently in severe cases.
Viburno—as uterine sedative; 1 teaspoonful, three to four times daily before meals.
Yohimbin—as uterine regulator and aphrodisiac; 1 tablet three times daily after meals; ampules, *hypodermatically.*

MENTAL DISORDERS: *See* "Psychiatry," *Chap. XI*

METALLIC POISONING: *See* "Drug Poisoning," *Chap. XI*

MIGRAINE

Acetidine—as analgesic; 1–2 tablets repeated in 2 hr. if not relieved.
Gynergen—in migraine of hepatic origin; 2 tablets at onset of attack, continued with 2 or 3 tablets daily for 3 days, where necessary.
Spiroform—as analgesic; 15–20 gr in tablet or powder form three or four times daily.
See Also—"Intestinal Detoxicants," "Sedatives," "Analgesics" and "Hypnotics," *Chap. XI*

MIXED INFECTIONS: *See*—"Vaccines" and "Bacteriophages," *Chap. VI;* "Systemic Antiseptics," *Chap. XI*

MYOCARDITIS: *See* "Cardiology," *Chap. XI*

NARCOTIC ADDICTION: *See* "Drug Poisoning," *Chap. XI*

NEPHRITIS: *See* "Renal Diseases," *Chap. XI*

NEURALGIA, NEURASTHENIA, NEURITIS: See "Neurology," *Chap. XI*

NEUROSYPHILIS: See "Neurology," *Chap XI*

NON-SPECIFIC THERAPY: (*Arthritis, Purulent Sinusitis, Iritis, Iridocystitis, Peptic ulcer, Epididymitis, Prostatitis, Adnexitis, Puerperal and other septic diseases, Respiratory affections, Certain dermatoses*)

Activin—*intramuscularly,* 0.5 cc gradually increased twice weekly; larger doses in acute, smaller in chronic conditions.

Aolan—*intramuscularly,* 10 cc at 5-6 day intervals; *intradermally,* 0.2–0.3 cc, sufficient for 2 wheals.

Caseosan—*intramuscularly* and *subcutaneously,* 0.5–2–3 cc at 1–3 day intervals; *intracutaneously* 0.25–2 cc; *intravenously* 0.3–1 cc—same intervals.

Collargol—*intravenously,* 10–20 cc of sterile 2 % suspension, every 3–4 days.

Lac-proteinate—*subcutaneously,* 0.5–2 cc, increased by 1–2 cc until 5–10 cc are injected; administered from 12–72 hr.

Lactigen—*intramuscularly,* from 1–10 cc in gradually increasing dosage every 3–5 days.

Man-Na-Gluconate—*subcutaneously* or *intramuscularly,* 0.5 cc increased to 2 cc every fourth day for 6–12 injections.

Omnadin—*intramuscularly,* 1 ampule daily, repeated in accordance with reaction.

Peptone Solution 5 % Sterile—*intravenously,* 1 cc, increased by 0.5 cc until 5 cc are given, every four to five days; also *intramuscularly.*

Stannoxyl—1–2 tablets every 3 hr.

Tinpronate—2 tablets every 3 hr. first day, every 4 hr. second day, 1 tablet every 3 hr. thereafter.

See Also—"Vaccines," *Chap. VI*

NUTRITIONAL DEFICIENCIES: (*Pregnant and nursing mothers, Convalescents, Invalids, the Aged, Malnutrition*)

Adex Tablets 10D—for vitamin, phosphorus and calcium deficiency; 1–3 tablets daily with fluids, at meals; increased to 6 tablets daily.

Albomalt—as mild laxative and nutrient; 1 level tablespoonful twice daily.

Aurol—as alterative and tonic; 15 m three times daily; *intravenously* and *intramuscularly* 1–5 cc three times weekly.

Beef Peptone—as nutrient; 1 tablespoonful three times daily.

B Vitamins—in vitamine B deficiencies; 1–3 tabloids after meals.

Chocolate Flavored Vitavose—as nutrient; 2 teaspoonfuls to glass of hot or cold milk.

Coco-Vitamin—as nutrient, stimulant; 1–2 tablespoonfuls three times daily.

Codamines Tablets—in vitamin A and D deficiencies; 2–4 tablets three to four times daily.

Cod Liver Oil—as nutrient in vitamin A and D deficiencies; 1 teaspoonful to 1 tablespoonful several times daily.

Cod Liver Oil Concentrates—in vitamin A and D deficiencies; 1 tablet three to four times daily.

Dry Peptonoids—as nutrient, especially for rectal alimentation; 2–4 tablespoonfuls in milk or other liquid foods.

Halibut Liver Oil, with or without Viosterol—in vitamine A and D deficiencies; up to 20 m per diem.

Insulin and Iletin—in undernutrition; 10–15 m 15 min. before meals, twice daily.

Malt Extracts, Plain and Combinations—as nutrient in vitamin deficiencies; 1–4 teaspoonfuls three times daily after meals.

Maltine, Plain and Combinations—as above.

Manola—as tonic; 1–2 teaspoonfuls four times daily.

Metatone—as tonic; 1–4 teaspoonfuls three to four times daily after meals.

Myeladol—as tonic in vitamin deficiencies; 1–4 teaspoonfuls after meals.

Neobovinine-20—as hematinic tonic; 1 tablespoonful four times daily.

Neurophosphates "Eskay"—as tonic in phosphorus deficiencies; 2 teaspoonfuls three to four times daily.

Neurotrophol "Byla"—as tonic and appetizer, 1 tablespoonful twice daily after meals.

Novatone—as tonic; 1–2 tablets three times daily after meals.

Panopepton—as nutrient and digestive; in tablespoonful doses, hot or cold.

Phos-hepatic Extract—as tonic and hematinic; 1 tablespoonful three times daily after meals.

Tonicine—as endocrine stimulant; 2 teaspoonfuls several times daily, before meals.

Vitafood—as stimulant; taken ad libitum.

Vitamins "A" and "D"—10 drops or more daily.

OBESITY (*Exogenous, Endogenous*)

Dextrettes "Eskay"—1 tablet every half hour between meals; about 10–12 daily.

Dinitrenal Capsules—1 or 2 capsules daily with meals, with water; increased cautiously to 3–4 capsules a day.

Iodobesin—2 opocrins daily for 10 days, then 3–4 daily for next 10 days, resumed after 10 day, rest period.

Phytolacca Compound—1 pulvoid 3 times daily, increased to 2 pulvoids after third week.

Remolysin—1–3 tablets after meals.

Riodine—2–6 capsules daily after meals.

See Also—"Endocrines," *Chap IV;* "Foods," *Chap. VIII;* "Mineral Waters," *Chap. IX*

OPHTHALMIA: *See* "Ophthalmology," *Chap. XI*

OSTEOMALACIA: *See* "Calcium Deficiencies," *Chap. XI*

OXYURIASIS: *See*—"Parasiticides," *Chap. XI*

PARASITIC INFESTATION

Antimony Sodium Thioglycollate—as trypanosomicide; ½–1 gr in 10–20 cc sterile water, *intramuscularly* or *intravenously*, twice weekly, for 15–25 injections.

Antimony Thioglycollamide—as trypanosomicide; 1–2 gr in 10–20 cc of sterile solution, *intramuscularly* or *intravenously*, twice weekly, for 15–25 injections.

Benzene (Benzol) Medicinal—in pin and tapeworm infestation, trichinosis, pediculosis; 2–10 m in emulsion or capsules every 3 hr.; *maximum single dose* 45 m, *maximum daily*—75 m; as enema, 3–8 gr in 500 cc of water.

Betanaphthol Benzoate—in ankylostomiasis; 3–8 gr, average dose 4 gr, *maximum single dose* 15 gr, *maximum daily dose* 34 gr; given in divided doses.

Butolan—in oxyuriasis; 1 tablet three times daily for 1 week, with enema of 1 tablespoonful of liquor aluminis acetatis to quart of water or limewater.

Calcidin—in actinomycosis; 5 gr four to six times daily.

Carbon Tetrachloride—in oxyuris, ascaris lumbricoides and trichocephalus dispar infestation; single dose only, 30–45 m, in water, milk or capsules, on empty stomach; followed in 3 hr. by epsom salts; not to be repeated within 3 weeks; not given to alcoholics.

Chinoplasmin—in malarial infestation; 2 tablets three to four times daily after meals.

Collosol Antimony—in Leishmaniasis, sleeping sickness, bilharziasis; *hypodermically*, 2–10 cc one to two times weekly.

Collosol Arsenic—in trypanosomiasis, blackwater fever; ½–1 dr. two to three times daily after meals; *intramuscularly*, 1 cc twice weekly for 10 doses.

Formin—for trypanosomiasis; 5–15 gr two to three times daily.

Larkspur Lotion—in pediculosis; as scalp massage each evening, 3–4 treatments.

Neostam—in kala-azar, filariasis, bilharziasis; *intravenously*, 0.1 Gm per 100 lb. of bodyweight, every 3 days.

Pelletierine Tannate—in tapeworm, hookworm, tenia solium infestation; 1–4 tabloids on empty stomach; after 2 hr.—1 oz. castor oil; repeated in 4 hr.

Phloridzin—in malaria, remittent and intermittent fever; 5–10 gr as often as necessary.
Plasmochin—in malaria, tertian, quartan, subtertian types in blackwater fever; 1 tablet three times daily.
Plasmochin Compound—2 tablets three times daily; after 1 week, rest period of 4 days.
Quassin—in oxyuriasis; introduced into rectum nightly, three to four times.
Quinarsin—in malaria, 1–2 dr. three to four times daily.
Quinidine—in malaria; 5 gr three times daily.
Sketofax—as insecticide, for local application.
Soamin—in trypanosomiasis; *hypodermically* 1–3 gr in sterile solution on alternate days; orally ¼–1 gr, maximum 3 gr, two or three times daily.
Solvochin—in malaria; 2 cc twice daily for 14 days, then continued at 1 cc for 14 additional days; in inoculation malaria—2 cc three times daily on first and third days.
Tryparsamide—for trypanosomiasis; 0.04–0.05 Gm per kilo body weight; *intravenously* and *intramuscularly*, once weekly for 8–16 doses.

PEPTIC ULCER: *See* "Gastric Hyperacidity," "Antacids," "Sedatives," "Non-specific Therapy," *Chap. XI*

PERNICIOUS ANEMIA
Cofron Liver Extract—3–5 capsules three times daily; elixir—half tablespoonful dosage.
Concentrated Liver Extract—1 tablespoonful three times daily, taken with beverages.
Erythgen Liver Extract—1–4 teaspoonfuls or 6 capsules three times daily; *intramuscularly* 2 ampules daily for 3–4 days; after rest period of 1 week, *maintenance dose* of 2 ampules weekly.
Extralin—3 vials daily in beverage; in some instances 6–8 vials; *intramuscularly* 2 cc daily.
Hepaticon—1 vial twice daily.
Hepati-cole—*intramuscularly*, 1–2 cc daily; *maintenance dose* 1 cc once or twice weekly.
Hepatrat—*intramuscularly* 3 cc, severe cases 6 cc, daily for 6–8 weeks; then oral therapy.
Liver Extract—in relapse, 300–400 Gm of liver equivalent, *maintenance dose* 200–300 Gm; in severe cases 300–500 Gm liver equivalent, for 10 days or longer until the desired blood changes are obtained; *intramuscularly* or *subcutaneously* where indicated.
Liver Extract E-29—1–2 tablespoonfuls three times daily, increased where necessary.
Liver Extract A-5—100 Gm liver equivalent three times daily, plain or in capsule form; mixed with beverages.
Liver Extract 100X, Concentrated—orally, 1 oz, three times daily; *maintenance dose* ½ oz. daily.
Liver Extract Subcutaneous—2.5 cc daily during remission period; *maintenance dose* 2.5 cc weekly.
Liver Extract 343—3–4 vials daily; *maintenance dose*—same dosage weekly.
Stomachon—1–2 vials per diem.
Ventriculin—1–4 vials daily in accordance with red cell count; in beverages.

PERTUSSIS: *See*—"Pertussis Vaccinotherapy," *Chap. VI;* "Antispasmodics," "Sedatives," *Chap. XI*

PLEURISY
Amatin—as analgesic and antipyretic; 1–3 tablets three times daily.
Analgine—as antipyretic and sedative; 1 or 2 tablets repeated in 2 hr. if necessary.
Aolan—for non-specific therapy; 0.2–0.3 cc *intradermally*, daily.
Guphen—antipyretic and analgesic; 1–2 tablets three to four times daily.
Iodalbin—as resorbent; 5 gr three times daily.
Iodotone—as resorbent; 1–2 teaspoonfuls three or four times daily before meals.

Katolox—as resorbent; 10–20 drops before meals; 2–3 doses; *intramuscularly,* 5 cc with 0.3 Gm sodium bicarbonate added.
Mervenol—as non-specific agent; 20 m every 3 hr. in water, between meals; in severe cases, *intramuscularly* and *intravenously* 2–3 cc daily.
Novaspirin—as analgesic and antipyretic; 5–10 gr three times daily.
Numotizine—as counterirritant; applied once or twice daily.
Optalidon—as analgesic; 1 tablet three to four times daily.
Quinisal—as antipyretic and sedative; 1–2 tablets every 2 hr.
Salophen—as analgesic and antipyretic; 15 gr three to four times daily.
Salysal—as analgesic and antipyretic; 1–3 tablets two times daily in water
See Also—"Anodynes," *Chap, XI;* "Intravenous therapy," *Chap. V.*

PNEUMONIA
Adenine Sulphate—to stimulate leucocytosis; 0.5 Gm in 20 cc normal saline, or 1 ampule *intravenously* twice daily.
Duotal—as deodorant antiseptic; 5–15 gr three times daily.
Formin—in septic conditions; *intravenously,* 4–30 gr in 25% solution, as often as required.
Optochin Base—as specific therapy; 4 gr with 5 fl. oz. of milk, five times daily day and night, continuously for 3 days; no other foods permitted.
Optochin Hydrochloride—as specific therapy in pneumococcic meningitis; spinal injection of 15 m of 1:1,000 solution in sterile saline, for each 2 kilos of body weight; given twice daily for 4–5 days; continued, 1 injection daily.
Pituitrin—as vasoconstrictor in circulatory collapse; *hypodermically,* 0.5–1 cc as demanded.
Quicamphol—as specific quinine therapy; 1–2 cc *intramuscularly,* daily for 7–14 days.
Solvochin—as specific quinine therapy; 2 cc *intramuscularly* for 3 successive days.
Syrup of Hydriodic Acid—as resolvent in resolution stage; ½–3 teaspoonfuls with plenty of water, several times daily.
See Also—"Antipneumococcus sera," *Chap VI;* "Expectorants," "Antipyretics," "Stimulants," "Nucleotides," *Chap. XI.*

POISON IVY and POISON OAK: *See*—"Plant Poisoning Serotherapy," *Chap. VI*

POLIOMYELITIS: *See*—"Poliomyelitis serotherapy," *Chap VI;* "Neurology," *Chap. XI*

POLLEN DISEASES: See "Allergens," *Chap. VII*

PROSTATIC DISORDERS: "*See* Urology," "Endocrinology," *Chap. XI*

PRURITUS (*General prurigo, Pruritus ani, Pruritus vulvae, Itching skin affections*)
Benacol Solution—as analgesic in pruritus ani; *subcutaneously* and *submucously,* 1 ampule injected slowly in fan shaped manner, repeated in 5 days.
Gynergen—in general pruritus of hepatic or renal origin; 1 tablet three or four times daily for 3 days; *intramuscularly,* 0.5 cc.
See Also—"Dermatology," "Antipruritics," *Chap. XI;* "Ointments," *Chap. X.*

PUERPERAL FEVER: See—"Puerperal Fever Serotherapy," *Chap. VI;* "Systemic Infections," "Systemic Antiseptics," "Obstetrics," *Chap. XI.*

PULMONARY DISEASES, *Severer Types* (*Abscess, Pulmonary gangrene, Bronchiectasis, Empyema, Emphysema pulmonum*)
Aolan—as non-specific agent; *intradermally,* 0.2–0.3 cc for 2 wheals; *intramuscularly,* 10 cc every 5–6 days.
Calcreose—as antiseptic expectorant; 1–2 teaspoonfuls or 4–8 tablets several times daily.
Cerose—as disinfectant expectorant; 1–2 teaspoonfuls three to four times daily.
Chlorazene—for Dakinization of empyema cavities, in 0.1% solutions, increased.

Creosotal—as disinfectant expectorant; ½–4 dr. daily, in divided doses.
Duotal—as stimulating expectorant; 5–15 gr three times daily.
Ethyl Iodide Vaporole with Chloroform—as antispasmodic; for inhalation of contents after crushing container.
Formin—as systemic antiseptic; *intravenously*, 4–30 gr only, in 25 % solution.
Lipoiodine—as alterative; 2 tablets daily.
Liquid Peptonoids with Creosote—as expectorant; 2–4 teaspoonfuls three to four times daily.
Mervenol—as non-specific therapy agent; 20 m every 3 hr., in water, between meals; *hypodermically*, in severe cases, 3 cc daily.
Proposote—as disinfectant expectorant; 5–10 m three times daily.
Riodine "Astier"—as resolvent; 2–6 capsules daily, after meals.
Soluble Iodine—as resolvent; 3–60 m three to four times daily, well diluted, in liquids; *intravenously*, same dosage, diluted in 20 parts distilled water.
Syrup Guaiacol Ammonium Compound—as expectorant; 1–2 teaspoonfuls every 2–4 hr.
Thiate—as sedative expectorant; 1 teaspoonful repeated as indicated.
Yatren-Casein—as non-specific therapy agent; *intravenously*, 1 cc weak solution, increased to 2 cc and repeated if necessary.
See Also—"Biologicals"—"Vaccinotherapy," *Chap. VI;* "Expectorants," "Systemic Antiseptics;" "Non-specific Therapy," *Chap. XI*

PYELITIS: *See* "Urology," *Chap. XI*

PYORRHEA ALVEOLARIS: See—"Pyorrhea Vaccinotherapy," *Chap VI;* "Dentistry," *Chap. XI*

RABIES: See "Rabies Vaccinotherapy," *Chap. VI;* "Antispasmodics," "Narcotics," "Stimulants," *Chap. XI*

RAYNAUD'S DISEASE: *See* "Arterial Diseases," *Chap. XI*

RENAL DISEASES: (*Nephritides, Nephroses, Albuminuria, Uremia, Cardionephritis, Albuminuria of pregnancy, Nephrolithiasis*)

Agurin—as diuretic in edemas; 8–15 gr in capsules, two to three times daily after meals.
Aminophyllin—as diuretic in anasarca; 1–2 tablets three to four times daily after meals; *intramuscularly* or *intravenously*, 1–3 ampules daily; rectally 2–4 suppositories.
Arbutin—as diuretic in effusions and edema; 1–2 tablets every 2 hr., in water.
Asparagus Compound—as diuretic; 1–2 teaspoonfuls in water as required.
Benzyl Benzoate—as antispasmodic in renal colic; 5–7 m in capsules, repeated as necessary.
Bromhosal—as salt substitute for flavoring food; ad libitum.
Calcilact—to promote osmosis in renal edema; 1 teaspoonful three times daily 1 hr. before meals.
Cymarin—as diuretic; 1–2 tablets daily; *intravenously* or *intramuscularly* 1 or 2 ampules.
Dialkalos—as uricolytic in prophylaxis of infections; 1 tablespoonful in water two to three times daily after meals.
Diuretin—as diuretic; 8–16 gr or 1–2 tablets three to four times daily after meals; *maximum daily dose* 80 gr.
Diurol—as diuretic; 2–4 dr. three to four times daily.
Erythrol Tetranitrate—as vasodilator in uremia; ¼–1 gr every 4–6 hr.
Euphydigtal—as diuretic, vasodilator; 1–2 tablets three to four times daily; rectally, 2–3 suppositories daily.
Glycine—as diuretic; 75 gr per diem, dissolved in 150 cc of fluid.
Hydragogin—as drastic diuretic; 3–15 drops every 3–4 hr.; in severe cases 15 drops every hour for 24–36 hr.

Kidnoids—as diuretic in edema and chronic pyelitis; 1–3 tablets three to four times daily.

Nephritin—as homostimulating hormone therapy; 4 tablets, from three to eight times daily; in uremia, 4 tablets every 2 hr. throughout attack.

Nitroscleran—as vasodilator; *subcutaneously*, 0.04 increased to 0.1 Gm for 8–15 injections; course repeated at intervals of 4–6 weeks.

Novasurol—as powerful diuretic; *intramuscularly, intravenously*, never subcutaneously; tolerance dosage 0.5 cc; treatment dose 1–2 cc once or twice weekly, with simultaneous administration of ammonium chloride or nitrate, 90–150 gr daily.

Phyllicin—as diuretic; 1 tablet two to four times daily after meals.

Piperazine—as uricolytic; 15–20 gr daily with abundance of alkaline water.

Salyrgan—as powerful diuretic; *intravenously* or *intramuscularly*, never subcutaneously; tolerance dose 0.5 cc; treatment dose 1 ampule every 3–4 days, in severe cases 2 ampules, with simultaneous administration of ammonium chloride or nitrate, 90–150 gr daily.

Scillaren—as cardiodiuretic; 2 tablets or 40 drops of oral solution three or four times daily.

Scillaren-B—as cardiodiuretic in urgent cases; *intravenously*, 1 cc daily, then decreased.

Theamin—as vasodilator and diuretic in uremia; 3–5 pulvules three to five times daily for several days.

Theocalcin—as diuretic; 1–3 tablets daily after meals; *maximum dosage* 60 gr daily.

Theocin—as diuretic; 1–2 tablets two to three times daily after meals, with abundance of fluid.

Thephyldine—as diuretic; 1–2 tablets three to four times daily after meals; *intramuscularly* and *intravenously*, 1–3 ampules; rectally 2–4 suppositories daily.

Thyractin—as hormone therapy in nephroses; 1–2 increased to 9 tablets daily.

Thyroxin—as hormone therapy in nephroses; 0.4 mg daily, *intravenously*, or orally 1 mg daily and increased.

Urea—as diuretic; 10–20 gr three times daily.

Verodigen—as stimulant; 1 tablet three times daily, reduced.

See Also—"Diuretics," "Cardiac stimulants," *Chap. XI*

RHEUMATISM: See "Vaccinotherapy," *Chap. VI;* "Arthritis," *Chap. XI*

RICKETS: *See* "Calcium deficiencies," "Vitamins," "Cod liver oil preparations," "Malt preparations," *Chap. XI*

SARCOMA: *See* "Coley's Toxins," *Chap. VI*

SCARLET FEVER: *See* "Scarlet Fever Serum and Vaccinotherapy," *Chap. VI.*

SCIATICA: *See* "Neurology," *Chap. XI*

SEA SICKNESS

Bellafoline—orally, 1–2 tablets or 10–20 drops three times daily; *hypodermically*, 0.5–2 cc daily; as antispasmodic

Bromipin 10%—as sedative; 1 teaspoonful three to four times daily.

Carbon Dioxide-Oxygen—as stimulant; administered by inhalation.

Chloretone—as sedative antispasmodic; 5–20 gr as necessary.

Neuronidia—as sedative; 1 teaspoonful two to three times daily.

Panopepton—as gastric sedative and nutrient; 1 tablespoonful in hot broth as required.

Papaverine Hydrochloride—as anodyne; ½ gr as required, orally; *subcutaneously*, ¾–1½ gr.

See Also—"Gastric sedatives," "Antispasmodics," "Hypnotics," *Chap. XI*

SHOCK: *See* "Cardiac Stimulants," "Vasoconstrictors," *Chap. XI*

SINGULTUS: *See* "Antispasmodics," "Sedatives," "Hypnotics," *Chap. XI*—"Carbon Dioxide-Oxygen"—as inhalation mixture.

SMALLPOX: *See* "Smallpox Vaccinotherapy," *Chap. VI*

SNAKE POISONING: *See* "Bothrops Antitoxin," "Crotalus Antitoxin," *Chap. VI*

SPASMODIC DISORDERS: (*Asthma, Whooping cough, Spasmophilia; Ureteral, Intestinal and Biliary colics; Pyloric, Vesical and Vascular spasm, Chorea*)

Adalin and Adalin-Luminal—as sedatives, 5–10 gr two to three times daily.

Alurate—½–1 teaspoonful three to four times daily in wineglassful of water.

Aubromid—as sedative in whooping cough; 1 or 2 tablets according to age.

Avertin—as rectal anesthetic; 0.1 cc per kilogram body weight; *maximum dose,* male 9–10 cc, female 6–8 cc.

Belladenal—as antispasmodic; half tablet every hour for 8 doses.

Bellafoline—as antispasmodic; 1–2 tablets or 10–20 drops of solution three times daily; *hypodermically,* 0.5–2 cc daily.

Benzyl Succinate—as antispasmodic; 5–15 gr as indicated.

Bromural—as sedative and hypnotic; 1 tablet several times daily, or 2–4 tablets at bedtime.

Bulbocapnine Hydrochloride—as antispasmodic; 1½ gr orally or *hypodermically; maximum dose* 3 gr daily.

Calcium Granular—as antispasmodic; 2 teaspoonfuls in glass of water during meals.

Calcium Levulinate—10–20 cc warmed, slowly *intravenously; intramuscularly,* 2 cc; repeated as indicated.

Chloretone—as sedative and antispasmodic; 3–30 gr, repeated as necessary.

Coryfin—as antispasmodic; 4–5 drops on lump of sugar.

Cypress Oil "Schimmel"—as antispasmodic in whooping cough; for inhalation, diluted in 1–4 parts of alcohol, sprayed on bedsheets, pillows and underwear.

Elixir Ma Huang—as antispasmodic; 1–4 teaspoonfuls as often as indicated.

Ephcaben—as antiasthmatic; in prophylaxis; 1–2 tablets daily or every other day, in nocturnal types, dosage repeated in half hour and continued with 1 tablet till relief is obtained.

Ephedrine—as antispasmodic; orally, ⅜–¾ gr every 4–8 hr.; *hypodermically,* 0.5% solution—5–15 m.

Ephedrine and Amytal—as sedative in asthma; 1 pulvule three times daily before meals; to abort attack, 1–2 pulvules before retiring.

Ephetal Tablets—as antispasmodic; 1–2 tablets every 2–4 hr. as required.

Erythrol Tetranitrate—in asthma and vascular spasm; gr ¾–1 every 4–6 hr.

Esterol—as antispasmodic in colics and asthma; 4 tablets followed by 2 tablets every hour until relieved.

Euphorbia Compound Syrup—as antispasmodic in asthma; 1–2 teaspoonfuls repeated in 2 hr. if indicated.

Glyco-Cypress—as antispasmodic in whooping cough and asthma; 1–2 teaspoonfuls every 4–6 hr.

Lumodrin—as antispasmodic in pertussis and asthma; 1 or 2 tablets three times daily.

Naiodine "Logeais"—as alterative; 20–40 cc *intramuscularly* two to three times daily; 5–10 cc daily as *maintenance dose.*

Neonal—as sedative and hypnotic; ¾–6 gr in divided doses; *maximum daily dosage* 6 gr.

Papaverine—as antispasmodic in pylorospasm and colics; orally or *hypodermically,* ½–1⅓ gr per dose; *maximum daily dose* 7½ gr.

Para-Thor-Mone—as hormone therapy in spasmophilia, tetany; 28–60 units daily, hypodermatically.

Parathyroid with Calcium Lactate—as hormone therapy in tetany, etc.; 1–2 tablets three times daily.

Paroidin—as hormone therapy; *subcutaneously* and *intramuscularly*, not intravenously; 30–60 units every 12 hr. for 5–6 days; after rest period of 1–2 weeks, repeated if necessary.

Phenobarbital-Sodium—as hypnotic; 1½–5 gr orally; rectally, in 20% solution.

Phytine—as calcium therapy in tetany, spasmophilia, asthma; 1–4 tablets daily with meals.

Sodium Amytal—as sedative and hypnotic; 1–2 pulvules every 6 hr.; in convulsive seizures, double dosage.

See Also—"Antispasmodics," "Hypnotics," "Vitamins," *Chap. XI*

STERILITY: *See* "Endocrines"—"Aphrodisiacs," *Chap. IV*

STOMATITIS: *See* "Otolaryngology"—"Dental Section," *Chap. XI*

SYPHILIS

Acetarsone—as arsenical antiluetic; 2–3 tablets daily for 7–10 days; *intravenously*, 0.5–1 Gm three times weekly for 7–8 weeks.

Arsphenamine—as arsenical antiluetic; *intravenously*, 0.3–0.6 Gm as indicated, at weekly intervals.

Bicreol—as bismuth therapy; *intramuscularly*, 1–1.5 cc for 8 weekly injections; course repeated as indicated.

Biliposol—as bismuth antiluetic; *intramuscularly*, 1 ampule every second day first week, then twice weekly for 12 treatments; after rest period course is repeated.

Bi-Na-Gluconate—as bismuth antiluetic; 1 hyposol *intragluteally* every 5 days, in usual courses.

Bisempco Cream—as bismuth antiluetic; *intramuscularly*, 10 m increased to 40 m, 2 weekly injections.

Bismarsen—as bismuth and arsenical combination, especially in tertiary stage; *intramuscularly*, 0.1 Gm one or two times weekly.

Bismo-Cymol—as bismuth antiluetic for congenital and neural syphilis; *intramuscularly*, 2 cc twice weekly for 6–8 weeks; resumed after 4 weeks' rest period.

Bismodide—as bismuth antiluetic in combination with iodine therapy; 1 capsule per kilo of body weight, average dosage, increased or decreased in accordance with rest periods.

Bismogenol—as bismuth antiluetic; *intramuscularly* 0.5–2 cc twice weekly for 30 injections.

Bismoid—as bismuth antiluetic in arsenic-fast cases; *intramuscularly*, 1 ampule every 5 days for 12–15 injections; after month's rest period is repeated.

Bismol—as bismuth antiluetic; *intramuscularly*, 1 cc every 5 days for 6–15 injections.

Bismosol—as bismuth antiluetic; *intramuscularly* 1 cc every 2–7 days for 20 injections.

Bismuth Salicylate—as bismuth antiluetic; *intramuscularly*, 1 ampule twice weekly in Wassermann-fast cases.

Bismuthoidol "Robin"—as bismuth antiluetic; *intramuscularly*, every 2–3 days for 5–6 weeks, repeated after rest period.

Bismuth Sodium Tartrate—as bismuth antiluetic; *intramuscularly*, 1 ampule twice weekly for 6–10 weeks, followed by Arsphenamine treatment after rest period.

Bisocol—as bismuth antiluetic; 2–20 gr; *hypodermically* 0.25–2 cc of solution twice weekly.

Calomelol—as mercurial antiluetic; in ointment for inunction, 1½ dr. daily for 30 days; as powder on syphilitic sores, and as prophylaxis.

Colloidal Mercury Sulphide—as mercurial antiluetic; *intramuscularly* 2–5 cc twice weekly.

Collosol Hydrargyrum—as mercurial antiluetic; 1 teaspoonful three times daily after meals; *intramuscularly*, 3 cc three times weekly; also for local use.

Collosol Iodine—as alterative; 1–3 teaspoonfuls, aqueous, three times daily after meals; *intravenously*, 0.2% solution, 20–100 cc as indicated; *intramuscularly*, 1% solution, 1 cc every 4 days.

Diarsenol—as arsenical therapy; *intramuscularly,* 0.1–0.6 Gm every 5–7 days.

Ferro-Sajodin—as iodine alterative; 1–3 tablets three times daily, thoroughly chewed.

Flumerin-H—as mercurial antiluetic; *intravenously,* 0.002–0.005 Gm per kilogram of body weight, in 2 % sterile distilled water, every 3–4 days.

Iodalbin—as iodine alterative; 1 capsule several times daily after meals.

Iodobismitol—as combined bismuth and iodine therapy for tertiary syphilis; 1 ampule every 3 days for 10 injections; course repeated after several weeks' rest period.

Iodo-Bismuth of Quinine—as combined bismuth and iodine therapy for tertiary syphilis; *intramuscularly,* 2 cc three times weekly for 20 injections.

Iodo Bismuthate of Quinine—"Fraisse"—as combined bismuth and iodine therapy for neurosyphilis; *intramuscularly,* 0.2 Gm twice weekly for 20 injections.

Merciol—as mercurial antiluetic; 1/6–1/2 gr, respectively in capsules of 1 and 2 gr, as frequently as indicated; locally as 5 % ointment for ulcerations.

Mercurettes—as mercurial antiluetic for inunction two to three times weekly.

Mercurial Cream, Blue—*intramuscularly,* 1½ gr as often as indicated.

Mercuric Oxycyanide—mercurial antiluetic; *intravenously;* one to two times weekly, with caution.

Mercurocol—as mercurial antiluetic; 1/8–1/2 gr orally; 0.25–6 cc *hypodermically.*

Mercurol—as mercurial antiluetic; 1 or 2 tablets as indicated.

Mercurosal—as mercurial antiluetic; *intramuscularly,* 0.05 Gm or more every 3–4 days; *intravenously,* 0.1 Gm every 1–2 days for 15–20 injections.

Mercury Benzoate—as mercurial antisyphilitic; 1 cc *intramuscularly* every second day.

Mercury Cyanide—as mercurial antiluetic; 1/16–1/8 gr orally; *hypodermically,* 25–35 m, 1 % solution; locally, on sores, 1:4,000 to 1:2,000 solution.

Mercury Salicylate—as mercurial antiluetic; *intramuscularly,* 1 ampule every 3–5 days.

Mercury Salicylate Cream and Hypoloids—*intramuscularly,* 1 cc weekly.

Mercury Succinimide—as mercurial antiluetic; *intramuscularly,* 1/6–1 gr every 1–2 days; *subcutaneously,* 8–15 m of 2.5 % aqueous solution.

Mergal—as mercurial antiluetic in parasyphilis; 1 capsule three times daily after meals, increased if necessary, cautiously.

Mesurol—as mercurial antiluetic; *intramuscularly,* one or two times weekly, 0.5–1 cc for 8–12 injections.

Metallic Bismuth—as bismuth antiluetic; *intramuscularly,* 1–2 gr once weekly.

Neoarsphenamine—as arsenical antiluetic; *intravenously,* once or twice weekly, from 0.1–0.6 Gm; course of 15–20 injections.

Neodiarsenol—as above, *intramuscularly.*

Neo-Riodine "Astier"—as iodine alterative; *intramuscularly* or *intravenously;* 1–5 cc three to four times weekly, course of 8–10 injections; repeated as indicated.

Neosalvarsan—as arsenical antiluetic; *intravenously,* also *intramuscularly* 0.1–0.9 Gm; 1–2 injections weekly.

Oleo-Bi—as bismuth antiluetic; *intramuscularly,* 2 cc two to three times weekly for 12–20 injections.

Potassium Bismuth Tartrate—as bismuth antiluetic; *intramuscularly,* 0.1–0.2 Gm every 7 days, until 2.4 Gm are given.

Potassium Mercuric Iodide—as mercurial antiluetic; *intramuscularly,* 1 ampule every 3–4 days.

Quiniobine—as iodine alterative in visceral lues; 1 cc increased by 0.1 cc, twice weekly for 12–14 injections; intervals of 6 weeks between courses; *intramuscular* injections.

Red Mercuric Iodide—as mercurial antiluetic; *intramuscularly,* 0.25–1 cc every 1–5 days.

Salvarsan—as arsenical antiluetic; 0.1–0.6 Gm *intravenously,* at weekly intervals.

Silver-Salvarsan—in neurosyphilis and Wassermann-fast cases; *intramuscularly,* 0.1–0.2 Gm every 4 days or longer.

Sodium Diarsenol—as arsenical antiluetic; 0.1–0.9 Gm, *intravenously*, every fifth day.

Sol-Bi "Fraisse"—as bismuth antiluetic; *intramuscularly*, two to three times weekly for 12 injections; after monthly rests, another 2 series.

Sulpharsphenamine—as arsenical antiluetic; *intramuscularly*, 0.15–0.6 Gm once or twice weekly.

Tartro-Quiniobine—as iodine antiluetic; *intramuscularly*, 1–2 cc, 2–3 injections weekly; after 2 weeks, course repeated; in visceral neurosyphilis, a 7 weeks course.

Thio-Bismol—as bismuth antiluetic; *intramuscularly*, 1–2 cc twice weekly; course of 3–4 weeks.

Tryparsamide—in neurosyphilis; *hypodermically* only, 0.04–0.05 Gm per kilogram of body weight, once weekly for 8–16 injections.

SYSTEMIC INFECTIONS: (*Septicemia, Pyemia, Septic endocarditis, Undulant fever, Puerperal sepsis, Postoperative sepsis, Septic pneumonia, Gas-gangrene*)

Acriflavine Neutral—as systemic antiseptic in bacteremia; *intravenously*, 10–50 cc in 0.5 % warm saline solution, freshly prepared and filtered.

Argocol—as systemic antiseptic; 0.25–5 cc daily, *intravenously;* orally, 1–3 gr.

Collosol Argentum—*intravenously* or *intramuscularly*, 1 ampule two or three times weekly.

Collosol Aurum—*intramuscularly*, 1 ampule every 2–4 days.

Formin—*intravenously*, 4–30 gr in a 25 % solution.

Gentian Violet Improved Medicinal—*intravenously*, 1–5 mg per kilogram of weight, in 0.5 % dilution, cautiously and slowly.

Mercurochrome—*intravenously*, in 0.4 % solution, freshly non-boiled distilled water, 1–5 mg per kilogram of body weight.

Metaphen Ampules—*intravenously* in 1:1,000 solution, 10 cc.

Siocol—*intravenously*, 0.25–2 cc of 10 % ampule.

Orargol—*intravenously*, 5–20 cc every 1–2 days.

Rivanol—*intravenously*, 1:1,000 solution, 1 part of Rivanol to 2 parts of dextrose.

See Also—"Puerperal Fever Serotherapy," "Streptococcus, Staphylococcus and Mixed Vaccines," "Undulant Fever Serotherapy," "Van Cott's Vaccines," *Chap. VI;* "Non-specific Therapy," *Chap. XI*

TABES DORSALIS: *See* "Neurosyphilis," *Chap. XI*

TETANUS AND TETANUS-GAS GANGRENE: *See* "Biologicals," *Chap. VI*

THYROID DISORDERS: (*Cretinism, Myxedema, Graves' disease, Hypothyroidism, Hyperthyroidism, etc.*)

Amytal—as sedative; ¾ gr two to three times daily.

Atomidine—as iodine therapy; 5–10 drops in water two to three times daily.

Calcidin—as iodine therapy; 1–5 gr four to five times daily with large amounts of water.

Collosol Iodine—as iodine therapy; orally, 1–3 teaspoonfuls, aqueous, three times daily after meals.

Dial—as sedative; 1½ gr or ½ dr. of elixir one to four times daily.

Ethidol—as iodine therapy; applied locally to thyroid by inunction.

Ferro Sajodin—as iodine therapy; 1–3 tablets three times daily.

Gynergen—as vasomotor sedative; 1 tablet three times daily.

Iodalbin—as iodine therapy; 5 gr after meals.

Iodicalcium—as iodine therapy; 1 tablet two to three times daily.

Iodicin—as iodine therapy; in prophylaxis of simple goitre—1 tablet weekly or 2–3 tablets weekly for 1 mo. only.

Iodostarin—as iodine therapy; prophylaxis, simple goitre—1 tablet weekly.

Iodotone—as iodine therapy; 1–2 teaspoonfuls three to four times daily before meals.

Lumalgin—as sedative; 1–3 tablets as required.

Luminal—as sedative; ½–1 gr two to three times daily.
Organidin—as iodine therapy; 5–20 drops three times daily.
Oridine—as iodine therapy; in prophylaxis of simple goitre; 1–3 tablets daily for 40 days.
Riodine "Astier"—as iodine therapy; 2–6 capsules daily after meals.
Sajodin—as iodine therapy; 5–15 gr three to four times daily 1 hr. after meals.
Sol. Iodine—as iodine therapy; 5–15 drops three times daily.
Stearodine—as prophylaxis in simple goitre; 1 tablet weekly or 2 tablets weekly for 2 mo. twice a year.
Thyracoids—as hormone therapy; ¼–½ gr one to two times daily.
Thyractin—as hormone therapy in hypothyroidism; 2–3 tablets three times daily.
Thyroxin—as hormone therapy in hypothyroidism; orally, 1 mg daily 1 hr. before meals; *intravenously*, 0.4 mg daily.
Thyroxine Synthetic—as hormone therapy in hypothyroidism; 2–4 tablets or 1–2 ampules daily.
See Also—"Endocrines," *Chap. IV*

TONSILLITIS: See "Rhinolaryngology," "Antipyretics," "Analgesics," *Chap. XI;* "Liquid Antiseptics," *Chap. X.*

TORTICOLLIS: See "Neuralgia," "Arthritis," *Chap. XI.*

TROPICAL DISEASES: (*Trypanosomiasis, Filiariasis, Kala-azar, Granuloma inguinale, Bilharziasis, Leishmaniasis, Ulcus molle serpigiosus, Blackwater fever*)
Anticol—as parasiticide in Leishmaniasis and Bilharziasis; orally, ½–5 gr two to three times daily; *hypodermically*, 0.25–3 cc every 1–2 days.
Antimony Sodium Thioglycollate—as trypanosomicide in trypanosomiasis, filiariasis, granuloma inguinale; ½–1 gr in 20 cc sterile water, *intramuscularly* or *intravenously* twice weekly for 15–25 injections.
Antimony Thioglycollamide—as trypanosomicide; 1–2 gr in 10–20 cc of sterile solution, *intravenously* or *intramuscularly*, twice weekly for 15–25 injections.
Arsphenamine—as trypanosomicide; *intravenously*, 0.3–0.4 Gm weekly, increased as indicated.
Collosol Antimony—as parasiticide in leishmaniasis; *hypodermically*, 2 cc increased to 10 cc once or twice weekly; orally, 0.5–1 cc two to three times daily.
Collosol Arsenic—as spirillicide in trypanosomiasis, blackwater fever; *intramuscularly*, 1 cc twice weekly, course of 10 doses; orally, ½–1 teaspoonful two to three times daily after meals.
Collosol Chrysarobin—as parasiticide in skin affections; orally, ½–1 teaspoonful in water two to three times daily; *intramuscularly* or *intravenously*, 1–3 cc weekly.
Formin—as trypanosomicide; *intravenously*, 4–30 gr in 25% solution; orally, 5–15 gr two to three times daily with large amounts of water.
Germanin—as trypanosomicide, *intravenously, subcutaneously* or intraperitoneally, 0.5–1.0 Gm in 5–10% solution.
Neostam—as parasiticide in filiariasis, bilharziasis; *intravenously*, 0.1 Gm per 100 lb. of body weight, in 4% solution, on alternate days, until 3 Gm per 100 lb. of body weight have been given.
Soamin—as trypanosomicide; *subcutaneously* or *intramuscularly*, 1–3 gr on alternate days; orally, ¼–1 gr two to three times daily after meals.
See Also—"Parasiticides," *Chap. XI*

TUBERCULOSIS: (*Pulmonary, Intestinal, Glandular*)
Acecoline—in tubercular hyperidrosis; 0.02 Gm daily.
Acetylcholine and Acetylcholine Bromide—as anhidrotic; *intramuscularly* or *subcutaneously*, never intravenously; 0.05–0.2 Gm daily in 5% solution.
Anesthesin Powder—as analgesic in tubercular laryngitis by insufflation.
Allochrysine—as phthisis therapy and tonic; *intramuscularly*, 2 cc mixed with 8 cc of artificial serum once or twice weekly, for 10–15 weeks.
Bellafoline—as anhidrotic; 1–2 tablets or 10–20 drops three times daily; *hypodermically*, 0.5–2 cc daily.

Benzosol—as pulmonary antiseptic; 3–10 gr as powder, pill or emulsion, three to four times daily.
Calcreose—as deodorant expectorant; 1–2 teaspoonfuls or 4–8 tablets several times daily.
Calglucon—as calcium therapy; *intramuscularly* and *intravenously*, 10 cc every 1–3 days.
Chaulmestrol—as phthisis therapy; *intramuscularly*, 0.5–6 cc every fifth day; *intravenously*, in smaller dosage.
Chocolate Flavored Vitavose—as vitamin B nutrient; 2 teaspoonfuls to glass of hot or cold milk as frequently as desired.
Coagulen—in pulmonary hemorrhage; *intravenously*, 2–3 cc, repeated if necessary.
Codamines Tablets—as vitamin A and D nutrient; 2–4 tablets three to four times daily.
Cod Liver Oil Concentrates—as vitamin A and D nutrient; several tablets daily.
Collosol Antimony—as phthisis therapy; *hypodermically*, 0.5–1 cc weekly. *See Chap. I.*
Collosol Calcium—in hemoptysis; *hypodermically*, 0.3–0.7 cc every 5–7 days.
Creosotal—in phthisis therapy; ½–4 dr. daily in divided doses.
Creosote Carbonate—in phthisis therapy; orally, 5–20 m increased to 80 m, several times daily.
Creosotide—in phthisis therapy; 1–2 tablets two to three times daily.
Dionin—as sedative and antispasmodic; orally and *subcutaneously*, ⅙–1 gr several times daily; evenings as hypnotic, ½–¾ gr.
Duotal—in phthisis therapy; 5–15 gr three times daily.
Firolyptol—as nutrient; 1–2 teaspoonfuls three to four times daily after meals.
Gold Sodium Thiosulphate—in lupus therapy; *intravenously* or *intramuscularly*, ⅙ gr, increased by gr ⅙ at weekly injections, with frequent rest periods; *maximum dosage* for *male* 100 mg, for *female* 75 mg.
Guaiacose—as disinfecting expectorant; 1–2 capsules two to three times daily before meals.
Haliver Oil Plain—as vitamin A nutrient; 10–20 m daily.
Homatropine Hydrochloride—as anhidrotic; 1/120–1/60 gr; *maximum daily dose* 1/20 gr.
Hydrastinin—as hemostatic in pulmonary hemorrhage; 1 tablet three to four times daily, or 20–40 drops several times daily.
Iodomuth—as intestinal astringent in tubercular diarrheas; 10–30 gr every 2–3 hr.
Kresival—as disinfecting expectorant; 2–4 teaspoonfuls three to four times daily.
Liquid Peptonoids with Creosote—as nutritive expectorant; ½–1 tablespoonful several times daily.
Malt Extracts, Plain, in Combinations, also with Creosote—as nutrient; 2–4 teaspoonfuls several times daily.
Neofosfan—as mineral metabolizer; *intramuscularly* or *subcutaneously*, 1 ampule every 1–3 days; 20–40 injections.
Papaverine Hydrochloride—in hemoptysis; *subcutaneously*, 0.75–1.5 cc; orally, ½ gr; twice daily.
Proposote—as expectorant; 5–10 m three times daily after meals.
Thiocol—as sedative expectorant; 1–2 teaspoonfuls every 2–3 hr., or 5–10 gr per dose.
See Also—"Tuberculins," *Chap. VI;* "Vitamins," "Cod liver oils," "Haliver oils," "Nutrients and Tonics," *Chap. XI.*

TYPHOID and PARATYPHOID FEVER: *See* "Biologicals," *Chap. VI.*

ULCERATIVE COLITIS: *See* "Biologicals," *Chap. VI;* "Intestinal Disorders," *Chap. XI*

UNDULANT FEVER: *See* "Biologicals," *Chap. VI;* "Systemic Infections," *Chap. XI*

URTICARIA: *See* "Allergy," *Chap. VII;* "Dermatology," *Chap. XI*

VARICOSE VEINS: *See* "Sclerosing Agents," *Chap. XI*

VASOMOTOR RHINITIS: *See* "Allergy," *Chap. VII.*

VENEREAL PROPHYLAXIS: *See* "Vaginal Antiseptics," "Urology," "Syphilis," "Gynecology," *Chap. XI*

VINCENT'S ANGINA: *See* "Angina," *Chap. XI*

VITAMIN DEFICIENCIES: (*Rickets, Sprue, Beri-beri, Polyneuritis, Xerophthalmia, Xerosis, Hemeralopia, Pellagra*)

Bemax—in vitamin B deficiency, beri-beri and polyneuritis; 1 heaping tablespoonful daily, cooked or uncooked.
Cod Liver Oil Concentrates—as for cod liver oil; several tablets daily.
Cod Liver Oil with Viosterol 10D—in vitamin A and D deficiencies; ½–1 teaspoonful three times daily.
Cod Liver Oils—1–4 teaspoonfuls several times daily after meals.
Emulsion of Cod Liver Oil—as for cod liver oil; 3 tablespoonfuls daily.
Irradol A—in vitamin D deficiencies and as nutrient; 1 tablespoonful several times daily after meals.
Malt Extract with Cod Liver Oil—in vitamin A, B and D deficiencies, and as nutrient; 1–3 capsules or 1–4 teaspoonfuls several times daily after meals.
Maradol—as tonic and vitamin therapy; 2–4 teaspoonfuls three times daily.
Marinol—as for cod liver oil; tablespoonful doses several times daily.
Myeladol—as tonic and vitamin therapy; 1–2 dessertspoonfuls after meals.
Natural Vitamin D—in vitamin D deficiencies; prophylactic, 10 drops daily; curative, 15–30 drops.
Oscodal—in vitamin therapy; 2–3 tablets several times daily before meals.
Super D Cod Liver Oil—in vitamin D deficiencies; 1–4 teaspoonfuls three times daily.
Undiluted Halibut Liver Oil—in vitamin A diseases; 1–2 teaspoonfuls daily.
Viosterol in Oil 250D—as prophylactic, 8–10 drops daily; curative, 20 drops daily.
Vitafood—in vitamin B deficiencies; 1–3 teaspoonfuls with food.
Yeast Bouillion Cubes—in vitamin B deficiency; 2 tablets three times daily, served as broth.
Yeastone—in vitamin B therapy; 1–3 pills three times daily.

WHOOPING COUGH: *See* "Pertussis Vaccinotherapy," *Chap. VI;* "Antispasmodics," "Sedatives," *Chap. XI*

CHAPTER XII

BIBLIOGRAPHY

This Bibliography is not complete; numerous additional references have in most instances been purposely omitted. It is designed to facilitate only, where desired, a somewhat broader study of a preparation or its allied topic, and is limited therefore to but few of the later contributions, principally in English, and presented in chronological sequence.

ABASIN

Gudden, H.: Med. Klin., 1924, No. 28.
Jehle, L.: Wien. med. Wochensch., 1924, No. 12.
Koritschan, A.: Wien. klin. Wochensch., 1924, No. 12.
Laband, L.: Therap. d. Gegenw., July, 1924.
Funfgeld, E.: Klin. Wochensch., 1925, No. 16.
Henius, K.: Klin. Wochensch., 1925, No. 30.
Bogner, F.: Therap. d. Gegenw., 1925, No. 2.
Weisbart, M.: Aerzt. Rundschau, 1926, No. 5.

ACECOLINE

Bailliart, M. P.: A case of Spasmodic Obliteration of the Central Artery; Bull. Soc. d'opht. de Paris, pp. 245–250, 1928.
Villaret, M. and Justin-Besancon, L.: The Therapeutic application of Acecoline; Lancet, 1929, 1:493.
Guns, P. and Coene, R.: New treatment for Atrophic Rhinitis; Ann. d. mal. de l'oreille, du larynx, 1929, 48:414.
Castellotti, F.: Clinical Study of Acrocyanosis: Acecoline Therapy; Biochim. e terap. sper., 1929, 16:385.
Heitz, J.: Critical review of the diagnostic and therapeutic uses of Acecoline; Arch. d. mal. du coeur, 1929, 22:383. As reported in the Brit. Med. Jour., Oct. 12, 1929, p. 56.
Douthwaite, A. H.: The Treatment of Hyperpiesia; Brit. Med. Jour., 1929, 2:844.
Abel, A. Lawrence: Acetylcholine in relation of Abdominal Surgery; Lancet, 1:459, March 1, 1930

ACETARSONE

Horster: Med. Klin; 1921, No. 14, p. 511.
Sezary and Barbe: Presse Medicale, January 2, 1929, p. 1.
Raiziss and Severac: J. of Chemoth., April, 1930.
Sezary: Ibid., September, 1931, No. 77, p. 1423.
Raiziss and Severac: Arch. of Dermat. and Syph., 1932.
Kolmer and Rule: Am. J. Syphilis, January, 1932, p. 53.

ACETYLCHOLINE

Hunt, R. and de Taveau, M.: The Toxicity of Choline Derivatives; J. Pharm. and Exper. Therap. 1910, 1:303.
Dale, H. H. and Ewins, A. J.: Cholinesters and Muscarine; J. of Phys., 1914, 48:24.
Dale, H. H. and Richards, A. N.: The vasodilator action of histamine and of some other substances; J. of Phys., 1918, 52:110.
Villaret, M., Schiff-Wertheimer and Besancon, L. J.: Compt. rend. Soc. Biol., 1928, 98:909.
Villaret, M. and Even, R.: Acetylcholin and tuberculous sweats; Pres. Medicale, 1928, 1561.
Kalt, M.: Restoration of macular vision; Pres. Medicale, 1928, 1065.
Guns, P. and Coene, R.: A new treatment of rhinitis atrophica; Journ. belge d'Oto-Rhino-Laryngologie, 1929, No. 2, 128–140.
Dainow, J.: Treatment of varicose ulcers with Acetylcholin; Ann. de Dermat. et de Syphiligraphie, 1930, No. 3, 270–282; Pres. Medicale, 1930, No. 42, 716.

ACETYLCHOLINE BROMIDE

Dale, H. H. and Richards, A. N.: J. of Phys., 1918, 52:110.
Learmonth, J. R. and Braasch, W. F.: Resection of Presacral Nerve in Treatment of Cord and Bladder: Surg., Gynec. and Obst., 1930, 51:494.
Perrin, M. and Kuntz, M.: Paris Med., 1931, 1:494.
Villaret, M. and Justin-Besancon: La Presse Med., 39:601, April 25, 1931; Med. Jour. and Record, 1930, 132:35.
Hunt, Reid: Bulletin No. 73, Treasury Dept. Hygienic Lab.

ACIDULIN

Criep, L. H. and McElroy, W. S.: Atopy; Arch. Int. Med., 1928, 42:865.
Beckman, H.: Allergy and the Acid-Base Balance; J. A. M. A., 1930, 95:1582.
Bray, G. W.: The Hypochlorhydria of Asthma in Childhood; Quart. J. Med., 1931, 94:181.
Davidson, L. S. P. and Gulland, G. L.: Pernicious Anemia; C. V. Mosby Co., St. Louis, Mo.

ACRIFLAVINE

Hull: Klin. Wochensch., 1918.
Neuschaeffer: Med. Klin., 1918, 14:839.
Templeton, Wm. and Carelaw, R. B.: Lancet, May 4, 1918, 1:634.
Feibusch, Carl: Use of Acriflavine in Dentistry; Deut. Zahnaertz. Wochensch., 1918, No. 28.
Werner, S.: Acriflavine Treatment of Coccogenic Pyodermias; Deut. med. Wochensch., 1918, 51: 1439.
Stowell, T. E. A.: Brit. Med. Jour., 1919, 1:244.
Heinrichsen: Klin. Wochensch., 1919, No. 36, 56:852.
Spencer, J. C.: Acriflavine, A New Gonococcicide; Calif. State Jour. Med., 1919, 17:404.
Quackenbos: Use of Acriflavine; J. A. M. A., Nov. 22, 1919, 73:1629.
Mendel, James H.: Acriflavine and Neutral-Acriflavine; Their History and Use in Aural Surgery; The Laryngoscope, June, 1924.
Martindale, W. H. and Wescott, W. W.: Extra Pharmacopoeia, 17th Ed., Vol. I, 293.

ACRIFLAVINE NEUTRAL

Strohm: J. A. M. A., Dec. 7, 1920, p. 1828.
Scal: J. A. M. A., Oct. 1, 1921, p. 1102.
Crohn and Rosenberg: J. A. M. A., Aug. 2, 1924, p. 326.
Davis: J. Urol., Jan., 1924, p. 29.
Herrold and Culver: J. A. M. A., Feb. 12, 1927, p. 459.
Patton: Canad. Med. A. J., Apr., 1927, p. 436.
Tinker and Sutton: J. A. M. A., May 14, 1927, p. 1560.
Verdier: New Orleans Med. and Surg. J., Aug., 1927, p. 109.
Jeck: J. A. M. A., July 27, 1929, p. 253.
Boyd: Urol. and Cut. Rev., May, 1930, p. 303.
Hoffman: J. A. M. A., Sept. 6, 1930, p. 747.

ACRIVIOLET

Churchman, John W.: Acriviolet in Otolaryngology; Jour. Urol., 1924, 11:12.
Abraham, Joseph H.: Treatment of Infections of Upper Respiratory Tract and Ear; Laryngoscope, August, 1924.
Herzig, Arthur J.: Treatment of Infections of Upper Respiratory Tract and Ear; Laryngoscope, June, 1926.
J. A. M. A., February 6, 1932, p. 480; Reports Council Pharm. and Chem., 1931, p. 7.

ACTIVIN

Boyd, W.: Some uses of non-specific protein therapy; J. Lab. Clin. Med., 1919, vol. 88.
Schmidt, R.: Protein therapy in disturbances of digestive apparatus and of metabolism; Med. Klin., 1924, 20:1678.
Holzbach, E.: Protein therapy in abdominal operations, with report on 181 cases; Zentralb, f. Gynaek., 1924, 48:2730–2732, ab. J. A. M. A., 1925, 84:326.
Mohler, R. W.: Foreign proteins as adjuvants in treatment of obstinate pelvic infections; Am. J. Obst. and Gynec., 1925, 9:365–368.
Lederer, E.: Question of protein therapy and shock treatment; Munch. med. Wochensch., 1925, 72:83–86.
Merklen and Wolf: Shock in therapeutics; protein anaphylactic shocks; Medicine, 1924, 6:196–201, ab. J. A. M. A., 1925, 84:631, 1925.
Ling, C. Y.: Mechanism of reaction of non-specific protein agents in treatment of disease; influence of various agents on mobilization of blood antibodies; Arch. Int. Med., 1925, 35:740–751.
Golay, F. and Starobinsky, A.: Protein therapy in dermatology; Ann. de dermat, et. syph., 1925, 6:248–259.
Ducourcy, C.: Ohio State Med. Jour., February, 1925.
Spangler, R. H.: Med. Jour. and Rec., Sept. 16, 1925 and Oct. 15, 1925.
J. A. M. A., May 11, 1929, p. 1783.
Pugh, W. S.: Non-specific Therapy, Med. Review of Reviews, May, 1930.

ADALIN

Merzbach, Joseph: Long Island Med. Jour., October, 1912.
Masarey: N. Y. Med. Jour., Aug. 22, 1914.
Eager, Richard: Jour. of Mental Science, July, 1914.
Dercum, F. X.: J. A. M. A., March 13, 1915.
Gudden, H.: Therap. d. Gegenw. October, 1918.
Gaines, Lewis M.: South. Med. Jour., May, 1921.

Melchior, E.: Berl. klin. Wochensch., No. 51, 1921.
Rosin, H.: Deut. med. Wochensch., No. 41, 1921.
Kauffmann: Deut. med. Wochensch., No. 13, 1924.
Grote, L. R.: Zentralb. f. inn Mediz. No. 1 & 2, 1924.

ADENINE SULPHATE

Reznikoff, Paul: Nucleotide Therapy in Agranulocytosis; J. Clinical Invest., Vol. 9, No. 3, December 20, 1930.

ADEX TABLETS—10D

Daniels, Hutton and Armstrong: J. A. M. A., 1923, 81:828.
Bloch, C. E.: Am. J. Dis. Child., 1924, 27:139.
Daniels: Proc. Soc. Exp. Biol. Med., 1926, 23:824.
J. A. M. A., March 19, 1932, p. 983; Reports Council Pharm. and Chem., 1932, p. 69.

ADRENALIN

Aldrich: J. Am. Chem. Soc., September, 1905.
Reports Council Pharm. and Chem., 1925, p. 19.
J. A. M. A., Jan. 17, 1925, p. 220.

ADSORGAN

Hofmann, Paul: Berl. Tieraerztl. Wschr., 1930, No. 1, p. 2.
Bechhold, H. and Schlesinger, M. Z.: Exp. Med., 1931, No. 1 and 2, page 96.
Bauer, K. H. and Rauscher, K.: Pharm. Zentralb., 1932, No. 9.

AGOMENSIN

Seitz, Wintz and Fingerhut: Munch. med. Wochensch., 1914, 61:1657; 1914, 61:1734–1738.
Wintz: Archiv. für Gynaekologie, 1920, 113:47.
Wintz: Deut. med. Wochensch., 1924, 50:67.
Faust, E. S.: Schweiz. med. Wochensch., 1925, 55:575.
Hartmann and Isler: Biochem. Zeitschr., 1926, 175:46.
Hartmann: Klin. Wochensch., 1926, 5:2152.
Mahnert and Siegmund: Wien. klin. Wochensch., 1927, 40:281.

AFENIL

Rose: Heufieberbehandlung mit Afenil; Ber. 21, 22, 24, des Heufieberbundes, 1919, 1920, 1922; Berl. klin. Wochensch., 1917, Nr. 43.
Pulay: Ekzematisation als eine vegetative (vagotonische) Manifestation; Med. Klin., 1921, No. 27.
Pulay: Eine modifizierte Salvarsantherapie der Lues der Inneren Organe (Herz-und Gefaessystem) und des Nervensystems; Deut. med. Schnschr., 1922, Nr. 7.
Rosenow: Offizielles Protokoll einer Sitzung des Vereins fuer wissenschaftliche Heilkunde; Deut. med. Wochensch., 1922, No. 16.
Stuempke: Ueber Afenil zur Verhuetung gewisser Salvarsanschaeden; Med. Klin., 1922, No. 30; Muench. med. Wochensch., 1924, No. 3.
Joseph: Die therapeutische Technich in der Dermatologie; Deut. med. Wochensch., 1924, No. 10.
Stuempke: Ueber Salvarsandermatitis; Med. Klin., 1926, No. 4.
Vollbracht: Heufieber; Med. Klin., 1929, No. 31.
Vollbracht: Pathogenese und Therapie des Bronchialasthmas; Wien. med. Wochensch., 1924, No. 2.
Monatschr. f. Ohrenhlk. u. Laryngo-Rhinolog., 1929, No. 5.

AGO-CHOLAN

Seiler: Erfahrungen mit einem neuen Gallensteinmittel; Med. Klin. No. 25. 1913.
Eberschweiler: Zur Therapie der Gallensteinerkrankungen; Schweiz. Rundsch. f. d. Medizine No. 49, 1921.
Henius: Zur Behandlung der Gallensteinerkrankungen; Klin. Wochensch. No. 4, 1921.
Schaefer: Zur Bekampfung von Gallensteinleiden und Erkrankungen der Gallenwege mit Agocholan; Deut. med. Wochensch. No. 40, 1923.
Runck and Werner: The Treatment of Cholelithiasis; Med. Progress, November, 1924.
J. A. M. A., Sept. 10, 1927, p. 901.

ALACTA

Kerley, C. G.: The Practice of Pediatrics, W. B. Saunders Co., Philadelphia, 1919, p. 214.
Muls, G.: Powdered milk as food for nursing children, Gaceta medica de Tampico, 1926, 2:327.
Reed, J. W.: The etiology and treatment of diarrhoeas of infancy; Virginia Med. Mo., 1927, 53:732.
Hess, J. H.: Feeding and the Nutritional Disorders in Infancy and Childhood; F. A. Davis Co., Philadelphia, 1928, p. 113.
Hunter, W. B.: Infantile diarrhea; West Virginia M. J., 1928, 24:382.

Kugelmass, I. N.: Feeding in Infancy and Childhood, J. B. Lippincott Co., Philadelphia, 1930, p. 76.
Marriott, W. M.: Infant Nutrition, C. V. Mosby Co., St. Louis, 1930, p. 231.
Nixon, S. H.: Diarrhea of infants, Virginia Med. Mo., 1931, 57:642.
Moore, H. L.: A clinical observation of nutritional injuries in infants; South. Med. Jour., 1931, 24:109.
Giblin, J. and von Pourtales, J. H.: Dried powdered milk preparations in the feeding of infants; Am. J. Dis. Child., 1931, 41:1100.
Parsons, L. G.: Coeliac disease; Lancet, 1931, 1:61.
Idem: Celiac disease; Am. J. Dis. Child., 1932, 43:1294, Pt. 2.

ALKARHEIN

Hommell, P. E.: Rhubarb and Soda Mixture, Merck's Report, February, 1914.
Solomon Solis-Cohen and Thomas Stotesbury Githens: Pharmacotherapeutics, Materia Medica and Drug Action.

ALLERGENS, HAY FEVER

Hitchens, A. P., Brown, C. P.: Hay Fever and Certain Other Local Anaphylactic Phenomenon Referable to the Respiratory Mucous Membrane; J. Lab. Clin. Med., Vol. 1, No. 7, 1916.
Walkler, I. C.: Frequent Causes and the Treatment of Seasonal Hay Fever; Arch. Int. Med., 1921, 28:71.
Bernton, Harry S.: J. A. M. A., 1923, 80:1301.
Armstrong, C. and Harrison, W. T.: A Study of Ragweed Pollen Extracts for Use in the Treatment of Ragweed Pollen Hypersensitiveness; Pub. Health Rep., 1924, 39:2422.
Brown, G. T.: Late Spring or Summer Hay Fever in the District of Columbia and Vicinity; Arch. Int Med., Vol. 1, No. 3, 1927.
Ramirez, M. A.: Statistical Report on the Treatment of Hay Fever; Am. J. M. Sc., Dec., 1928.
Spain and Hopkins: J. of Allergy, 1930, 1:209.
Duke, W. W.: J. A. M. A., 1930, 94:767.
Thommen: Asthma and Hay Fever in Theory and Practice, Chas. C. Thomas, 1931, p. 9.
Stull, Cooke and Barnard: J. of Allergy, 1932, 3:352.
Brown: J. of Allergy, 1932, 3:542.
Cooke and Stull: J. of Allergy, 1933, 4:87.

ALLISATIN

Roos, E.: Munch. med. Wochench. No. 39, 1925, p. 1637.
Wolf, J. E.: Schw. med. Wochench., 57, No. 21, 1927.
May, S.: Fortsch. d. Therapie, No. 21, Nov. 1927.

ALPHA LOBELIN

Wieland, Hermann: Pharmacological Studies of Reaction of the Respiratory Center; Arch. f. exper. Pathol. u. Pharmakol., 1915, 79:95.
Wieland, Hermann and Mayer: Pharmacological Studies of Reactions of the Respiratory Center; 11. Arch. f. exper. Pathol. u. Pharmakol., 1922, 92:195.
Eckstein, A., Rominger E. and Wieland, H.: Pharmacological and Clinical Observations of the Action of Crystalline Alpha-Lobelin on the Respiratory Center; Ztschr. f. Kinderh., 1921, 28:218.
Frommer, E. M.: The After Treatment in Abdominal Surgery; Med. Rev. of Reviews, October, 1925.
Reichle, Herbert S.: Alpha-Lobelin as a Specific Respiratory Stimulant with Special Reference to Its Use in Connection with Anesthesia; Anesthesia and Analgesia, August, 1925.
Oberbeck, August: Alpha-Lobelin in the Treatment of Asphyxia Neonatorum; Med. Jour. and Record, July 1, 1925.
Cox, Walter A.: The Use of Alpha-Lobelin in Asphyxia Neonatorum: A Case Report; Clin. Medicine, October, 1925.
Hofmeister, O., and Reichle, H. S.: Resuscitation with Alpha-Lobelin. New Specific Stimulant of the Respiratory Center; Med. Jour. and Record, October 21, 1925.
Manasse, H.: Drowning and Electric Shock treated with Alpha-Lobelin; The Amer. Physician, July, 1926.
Wilson, Robert A.: The Treatment of Asphyxia Neonatorum by the Injection of Alpha-Lobelin into the Umbilical Vein; Amer. J. Obst. and Gynec., September, 1928.
J. A. M. A., June 17, 1933, p. 1933.

ALUCOL

Revue Medical De La Suisse Romande, No. 4, April, 1924.
L'Echo Medical Du Nord, Oct. 10, 1925, No. 41.
Clinic. Medicine, April, 1925.
J. Lab. Clin. Med., Vol. 14, No. 7, April, 1926.
J. A. M. A., June 9, 1928, p. 1871; Reports Council Pharm. and Chem., 1928, p. 9.

ALYCIN

Lees, D. B.: The Effective Treatment of Acute and Subacute Rheumatism; Proc. Roy. Soc. Med. (Therap. Sect.), 1908-1909, 2:38-40.

Danielopolu: Treatment of Polyarticular Rheumatism; Presse Med., 1923, 31:1045, Abst. J. A. M. A., 1924, 82:424.
Hanzlik, P. J.: Action and Uses of the Salicylates and Cinchophen in Medicine; Medicine, 1926, 5:354.
Caussade, C. and Tardieu, A.: Method for Salicylate Therapy of Rheumatism; Presse Med., 1926, 34:1057; Abst. J. A. M. A., 1926, 87:1339.
Peters, J. R.: Large Doses of Sodium Salicylate in Treatment of Acute and Chronic Rheumatic Polyarthritis; Deut. med. Wochensch., 55:1086, 1929; Abst. J. A. M. A., 1929, 93:958.

ALYPIN

Bremerman, L. W.: Am. J. of Urology, June, 1909.
Bier, A.: Anesthesia in Urology; Munch. med. Wochensch., No. 27, 1914.
Stern, M.: Am. J. of Urology and Ven. and Sexual Dis., July, 1914.
Crosbie, Arthur: Boston Med. and Surg. Journal, Feb. 18, 1915.
Kofler, K.: Wien. med. Wochensch., No. 4, 1922.
Birkholz: Med. Klin., No. 45, 1922.
Finder: Deut. med. Wochensch., No. 51, 1922.
Neumann, H.: Zeitsch. f. Hals, Nasen, u. Ohrenheilk. Bd. 8, 1924.

AMBAZIN

Rudnick, Dorrin F.: Urinary Antisepsis—Introduction of a New Product for Oral Use; Illinois Med. Jour., August, 1932.
Brasch and Bumpus: Intravenous Chemotherapy in Urinary Infections; J. Urol., April, 1926, p. 341–349.
Boyd, Montague: Urinary Infections and Urinary Antiseptics; South. M. J., 1929, 22:719–722.

AMERTAN

Beck, C. S., and Powers, J. H.: Burns Treated by Tannic Acid; Ann. Surgery; 1926, 84:19.
Wilson, W. C.: Treatment of Burns and Scalds by Tannic Acid; Brit. Med. Jour., 1928, 2:91.
Montgomery, A. H.: The Tannic Acid Treatment of Burns in Children; Surg., Gynec. and Obst., 1929, 48:277.
Davidson, E. C.: The Use of Tannic Acid in Burns of Children; Minnesota Med., 1930, 13:775.
Bancroft, F. W.: The Treatment of Cutaneous Burns; New England J. Med., 1930, 202:811.
Robitshek, E. C.: The Tannic Acid Treatment of Cutaneous Burns; Lancet, 1930, 50:470.
Christopher, F.: The First-Aid Treatment of Burns with Tannic Acid; Lancet, 1930, 50:317.
Cutting, R. A.: The Immediate Treatment of Extensive Superficial Burns; Am. J. Surg., 1931, 14:705.
Reports Council Pharm. and Chem., 1932, p. 7.

AMFETIN

Warren, S.: Effects of Amniotic Fluid on Serous Surfaces; Arch. of Path., 1928, 6:860.
Johnson, Herbert L.: Amniotic Fluid Concentrate in the Prevention of Adhesions; New England J. Med., 1928, 199:661.
David, V. C. and Sparks, J. L.: The Peritoneum as related to Peritonitis; Ann. Surgery, 1928, 88:672.
Lacey, James T.: Prevention of Peritoneal Adhesions by Amniotic Fluid; Ann. Surgery, 1930, 92:281.
Johnson, Herbert L.: Asepsis: A Possible Interference with the Physiology of Repair; New England J. Med., 1931, 204:535.

AMINOPHYLLIN

Askanazy, S.: Klinisches uber Diuretin; Deut. Archiv. fur klin. Medizin, 1895, 56:209.
Breuer, R.: Munch. med. Wochensch., 1902, 49:1604.
Throhari, A.: Theophyllin in the treatment of Arterial Hypertension and Angina Conditions; Arch. des Maladies du coeur, 1923, 16:481.
Dock, W.: The use of Theobromine for pain of Arteriosclerotic Origin; Calif. and West. Medicine, 1926, 25:636.
Musser, J. H.: J. A. M. A., 1928, 91:1242.
Gilbert, N. C. and Kerr, J. A.: Clinical Results in the Treatment of Angina Pectoris with Purine Base Diuretics; J. A. M. A., 1929, 92:201.
Schmitt, P. W.: J. Amer. Pharm. Assoc., 1930, Vol. 19, No. 8.
Lambert, A.: Ann. of Int. Med., 1931, 5:256.
Wood, F. C., Wolferth, L. C. and Livesey, Mary M.: Arch. Int. Med., 1931, 5:256.

AMIODOXYL BENZOATE

Young and Youmans: J. A. M. A., 1926, 87, 746.
Smith: Boston Med. and Surg. J., 1927, 196:590.
Trauba: J. A. M. A., 1927, 89:1124.
Schauffler: J. A. M. A., Nov. 19, 1927, p. 1748.
Thomas: J. A. M. A., 1927, 89:2174.
Cottrell, J.: Am. J. M. Sc., Nov. 1927, p. 623.
Jeffery, R. L. and Burns, K. S.: Northwest Med., Dec., 1927, p. 623.
Bowers, J. M.: Clin. Va. Mason Hosp., Feb., 1928, p. 82.

Youmans: Ann. of Int. Med., Jan., 1928, p. 825.
Young, A. G.: J. Lab. Clin. Med., 1930, 15:1231.
J. A. M. A., March 19, 1932, p. 983; Reports Council Pharm. and Chem., 1932, p. 56.

AMI-SALOX

Ellis, Henry Augustus: Med. Jour. and Record, April 6, 1927.
Collins, Harold: Am. Med., Nov. 1927.

AMNIOTIN

Frank, R. and Goldberger, M. A.: J. A. M. A., 1926, 87:1719.
Hofbauer, J. I.: J. A. M. A., 1927, 89:24; Am. J. Obst. and Gynec., 1927, 14:137.
Macht, D. I.: J. of Pharmac. and Exp. Ther., 1928, 34:137.
Pratt, J. P., and Smeltzer, M.: Endrocrinology, 1929, 13:320.
Sevringhaus, E. L., and Evans, J. S.: Am. J. M. Sc., 1929, 178:638.
Powers. H. H., Varley, J. R. and Morrell, J. A.: Endocrinology, 1929, 13:395.
Morrell, J. A., Powers, H. H., Varley, J. R., and DeFrates, J.: Endocrinology, 1930, 14:174.
Allen, E., and Baker, D.: Am. J. Obst. and Gynec., 1930, 20:85.
Kennedy, W. P.: Brit. Med. Jour., 1932, 746.
Kurzrok, R.: Proc. Amer. Anat. Soc., March, 1932.
Kurzrok, R.: Endocrinology, 1932, 16:361, 366.
Mazer, C. and Goldstein, L.: Clinical Endocrinology of the Female. W. B. Saunders, Philadelphia, 1932.

AMPYDIN

Brown, L.: Osler's Modern Medicine, Phila., 1925, 1:469.
Feinblatt, H. M. and Eggerth, A. H.: Clin. Lab. Medicine; Wm. Wood and Co., N. Y., 1925, p. 140.
Githens, T. S.: The Mechanism of the Action of Antipyretic Drugs; J. Pharm. and Exper. Therap., 1925, 25:309.
Januschke, H. and Lasch, F.: Amidopyrine and the Intestine; Klin. Wochensch., 1926, 5:321.
Wilcox, R. W.: Materia Medica and Therapeutics including Pharmacy and Pharmacology; Phila., 1926, p. 542.

AMYLSOL

Johnson and Rettger: J. A. M. A., 1913.

AMYTAL

Drabkin, D. L., Page, I. H. and Edwards, D. J.: Blood Concentration in Insulin Hypoglycemia; Proc. Soc. Exp. Biol. Med., 1924, 21:309.
Collens, W. S.: The Blood Supply to the Pancreas; J. Biol. Chem., 1925, 64:461.
Nelson, H. B.: A Preliminary Report on the Use of Sodium Amytal and Scopolamine Anesthesia during Labor; Am. J. Obst. and Gynec., 1932, 23:752.
Littell, G. S.: The effect upon the New-born Child of Sodium Amytal when Used as an Obstetric Analgesic and Anesthetic; Am. J. Obst. and Gynec., 1932, 22:741.
Dodek, S. M.: A New Method for Graphically Recording the Contractions of the Parturient Human Uterus; Surg., Gynec. and Obst., 1932, 55:45.

ANASTIL

Unger, R.: Med. Klin., 1924, Nr. 39.
Hamburger, E. und H.: Med. Klin., 1926, Nr. 35.
Lindemann: Fortsch. d. Therapie, 1926, Nr. 4.
Basch: Munch. med. Wochensch., 1927, Nr. 3.
Engelen: Therap. d. Gegenw., 1928, Nr. 3.
Crohn: Med. Klin., 1929, Nr. 12.

ANAYODIN

Johns, F. M.: Amebiasis, with special reference to its treatment with Iodo-oxy-quinolin sulphonic acid; Med. Clin. of N. A., 1929, 12:1307–1314.
Jones, P. H. and Turner, R. H.: Iodoxyquinolin sulphonic acid in the treatment of Amebic Dysentery; J. A. M. A., 1929, 93:583–586.
J. A. M. A., Oct. 5, 1929, p. 1065; Reports Council Pharm. and Chem., 1929, p. 9.
O'Connor, F. W. and Hulse, C. R.: The Treatment of Amebiasis with Anayodin; Dept. of Medicine, Presbyt. Hosp., Columbia Univ., New York.
Thonnard-Neumann, Ernst and Valera, F.: United Fruit Company Hospital, Santa Maria, Colombia, South America.

ANGIER'S EMULSION

J. A. M. A., Sept. 12, 1914, p. 962; Reports Council Pharm. and Chem., 1914, p. 48; Reports Chem. Lab., 1914, p. 55; Propaganda, vol. 1, p. 169.

MacDowell, A.: Am. Rev. Tub., Feb., 1932.
Nalblant, J. P.: Am. Rev. Tub., May, 1932.
Carter, William Wesley: Med. Times and L. I. Med. J., May, 1932.
Lewis, H.: South African Med. J., June, 1932.
Brown, Samuel: J. Med., June, 1932.
Cowan, John, et al: Lancet, July 2, 1932.
Elterich, Theodore O.: Arch. Pediat., September, 1932.
Casey, Albert E. and Rosahu, Paul D.: J. Lab. Clin. Med., September, 1932.
Matthews, Warren B. and Dragstedt, Lester R.: Surg., Gynec. and Obst., September, 1932.
McDonagh, J. E. R.: Clin. Med. and Surg., September, 1932.
Kretschmer, Herman L.: Illinois Med. J., September, 1932.
Averett, Leonard, et al: Am. J. Obst. and Gynec., September, 1932.

ANTIFORMIN

Klebs: Ueber die therapeutische Verwendung des Antiformin; Berl. klin. Wochensch., 1909, Nr. 29.
Linke: Antiformin; Therapeutische Neuheiten, January, 1910.
Patterson, R. C.: Use of Antiformin for detection of Tubercle Bacilli in Sputum, etc.; J. Med. Res. Boston, Mass., April, 1910.
Tint, L. J. and Breskman, L. A.: Study of Acid-fast and Acid-semifast tubercle Bacilli (Human); J. A. M. A., May 14, 1910.
Koslow: Aether-acetonische Kombination der Antiformin Methode; Berl. klin. Wochensch., June 20, 1910.
Brown, Lawrason and Smith, Daniel: The Cultivation of Tubercle Bacilli Directly from Sputum by the use of Antiformin; J. Med. Research, Boston, Mass., June, 1910.
Philiph, R. W. and Porter, A. E.: Tubercle Bacilli in the Feces of Tuberculous patients; Brit. Med. Jour., July 23, 1910.
Arndt, G.: Ueber den Nachweis von Tuberkelbacillen bei Lupus miliaris disseminatus facili und Acnitis; Berl. klin. Wochensch., July 25, 1910.
Schmitt: Untersuchungen ueber die Desinfektionskraft des Antiformin; Zeitsch. f. Infectionskrankheiten, parasitaere Krankheit u. Hyg. d. Haustiere. Bd. 11, Heft 2 u. 3.

ANTI-MENINGOCOCCIC SERUM

Blackfan: J. A. M. A., 1921, January 1, p. 36.
Report Council Pharm. and Chem., 1917, p. 146; 1927, p. 42.

ANTIPHLOGISTINE

J. A. M. A., June 1, 1907, p. 1875; Feb. 23, 1918, p. 557; Propaganda, vol. 2, p. 409.
Veiel, Fritz: Die Behandlung von Rontgen Geschwuren mit warmen Breiumschlagen; Klin. Wochensch., July 9, 1925.
Broncho-Pneumonia; Lancet, January 19, 1929.
Singer, Gustav: Die Reizkorperbehandlung des Diabetes, Vienna, 1929.
Taylor: Practice of Medicine, 12th Edition, edited by E. B. Poulton.

ANTIPNEUMOCOCCIC THERAPY

Felton: A Method of Concentration of Pneumococcus Antibody; J. Inf. Dis., 1928, 43:543; The Concentration of Antipneumococcus Serum; J. A. M. A., 1930, 94:1893; The Units of Protective Antibody in Antipneumococcus Serum and Antibody Solution; J. Inf. Dis., 1928, 43:531.
Park, Bullowa and Rosenbluth: The Treatment of Lobar Pneumonia, with Refined Specific Antibacterial Serum, J. A. M. A., November 17, 1928, p. 1503.
Heffron, Roderick: New England J. Med., July 28, 1932.
Cecil and Sutliff: The treatment of Lobar Pneumonia with Concentrated Antipneumococcus Serum; J. A. M. A., December 29, 1928, p. 2035.
Sabin: The Stained Slide Microscopic Agglutination Test: Application to (1) Rapid Typing of Pneumococci: (2) Determination of Antibody: Proc. Soc. Exp. Biol. Med., 1929, 26:492.
Cecil and Plummer: A Study of 1161 Cases of Pneumococcus Type 1 Pneumonia with Especial Reference to Specific Therapy; J. A. M. A., 1930, 95:1547; J. A. M. A., March 5, 1932.
Cecil, Baldwin and Larsen: Lobar Pneumonia: A Clinical and Bacteriologic Study of 2,000 Typed Cases; Arch. Int. Med., September, 1927, p. 253.
Baldwin and Rhoades: The Protective Substance in Pneumococcus Pneumonia with special reference to Bacteremia and Specific Treatment; Hyg. Lab. Bull. No. 141, April, 1925, p. 43; The Specific Therapy of Pneumococcus Type 11 Pneumonia; Am. J. M. Sc., August, 1927, p. 191.

ANTUITRIN-S

Hamblem, E. C.: Endocrinology, 1931, 15:184.
Smith and Smith: J. A. M. A., 1931, 97:1857.
Novak and Hurd: Am. J. Obst. and Gynec., 1931, 22:501.
Snyder and Wislocki: Bull. Johns Hopkins Hosp., 1931, 49:103, 106.
Reynolds, S. R. M.: Am. J. Physiol., 1932, 100:545.
Friedman, M. H.: Am. J. Physiol., 1932, 99:332.
Saiki, S.: Am. J. Physiol., 8 March, 1932.

Anspach and Hoffman: Am. J. Obst. and Gynec., 1932, 24:3.
Pratt, J. P.: Endocrinology, 1932, 16:45.
Smith and Smith: Am. J. Physiol., 1932, 100:553.

AOLAN

Hampel, F.: Protein Therapy for Gastric Ulcer; J. A. M. A., 1923, 81:1059.
J. A. M. A., Nov. 8, 1924, p. 1526; Reports Council Pharm. and Chem., 1924, p. 8.
Graves, K. D.: Milk injections without local reactions; J. A. M. A., 1924, 83:1505.
Gellhorn, George: Milk injections in Gynecology and Obstetrics; Am. J. Obst. and Gynec., 1924, 8:535; New Orleans, M. and S. J., 1926, 78:557.
Eidelsberg, Joseph: Nonspecific Protein, M. J. and Record; 1925, 121:674.
Bryce, D. A.: Hypoleucocytosis Reversed by Nonspecific Protein Reaction; M. J. and Record, 1926, 123:584.
Cherry, Thomas H.: The treatment of Pelvic Infections; Surg., Gynec. and Obst., 1926, 42:600.
Hall, E. R.: Nonspecific Protein Therapy in Dermatology; South. M. J., 1926, 19:731.
Herrold, R. D.: Protein as an Adjunct in Treatment of Resistant Syphilis; J. A. M. A., 1926, 86:413.
Jarcho, J.: Nonspecific Protein Therapy in Pelvic Infections; M. J. and Record, 1926, 123:237.

ARGOLAVAL

Casper, L.: Zeitsch. f. Urol., 1926, Vol. 20; Zeitsch. f. Urol., Vol. 23, Nr. 3.
Schlueter, Hans: Dermatolog. Wochensch., 1927, Nr. 20.
Schirokauer, Hans: Therap. d. Gegenw., 1928, Nr. 2.
Heimann, Ernst: Deut. Med. Wochensch., 1928, Nr. 13.
Fuss, Ernst Martin: Med. Klin., 1929, Nr. 44.
Casper, L.: Deut. med. Wochensch., 1929, Nr. 18.
Picard, Edwin: Fortsch. d. Therapie, 1930, Nr. 10.
Blank, Adolf: Klin. Monatsblatter fur Augenheilkunde, August, 1930.
Pick: Therap. d. Gegenw., 1930, Nr. 10.
Hanke, Victor: Aerztl. Korrespondenz, 1930, Nr. 6.
Waegner, Alfred: Fortsch. d. Therapie, 1931, Nr. 16.

ARMERVENOL

Hille, Hermann.: Clin. Med. and Surg., January, 1927.
Ferguson, Burr: Clin. Med. and Surg., February, 1928.
Wakerlin, G. Earle: Am. J. Syphilis, Vol. 12, No. 3, July, 1928.
Wakerlin, G. Earle: Arch. of Dermat. and Syph., June, 1929.
Hille, Hermann: Medical Life, March, 1930.
Hille, Hermann: Clin. Med. and Surg., April, 1930.
Klein, H. P.: Clin. Med. and Surg., Vol. 38, No. 2, Feb., 1931.
Moritz, Gustave: The Eye, Ear, Nose and Throat, Monthly, Aug., 1931.
Colloidal Chemistry, Vol. 1, No. 1, 2 and 3.

ARSPHENAMINE

Moore, Joseph E. and collaborators: U. S. Public Health Service, Reprint No. 13; Venereal Disease Information, 1929, 10:12–18.

ARTHRITIS

Cecil, R. L., Nicholls, E. E. and Stainsby, W. J.: The Etiology of Rheumatoid Arthritis, Am. J. M. Sc., 1931, 181:12.
Cecil, R. L.: Ann. of Int. Med., July, 1931, p. 23.
Cecil, R. L.: N. Y. State J. Med., Nov. 1, 1932, p. 1245.

ASTHMOLYSIN

Weiss, O.: The Treatment of Bronchial Asthma; Zeitsch. fur med. Chemie IV, 1926, Nr. 5.
J. A. M. A., October 17, 1925, p. 1234; March 12, 1927, p. 858.

ATOQUINOL

Uhlmann: Schw. med. Wochensch., 1921, 51:416.
Hotz: Dissertation Zurich, 1922, Verlag Gebr. Leemann and Co., Zurich, 1922, p. 66.
Reynaud: Dissertation Paris, 1925, Verlag Jouve and Co., Paris, 1925, p. 96.
Kahn and Cohn: Am. J. M. Sc., 1926.
Merson, L.: LeConcours Medical, 49; 1927, 49:384.
Hirschfeld: Deut. med. Wochensch., 53, 1927, 53:969.

AURALGAN

Obermuller: On Conservative Treatment of Acute Otitis Media; Munch. med. Wochensch., 1908.
Obermuller: Therap. Monatshefte, 1911.

Kessel: Mediz. Correspondenzblatt, 1912, No. 26.
Schroeder: Moderne Medizin, 1922, No. 1.
Obermuller: Med. Klin., 1927, No. 3.

AUROL

Stoll, John E.: Clin. Med. and Surg., April, 1928.
Wakerlin, G. Earle: Am. J. Syphilis, July, 1928.
Wakerlin, G. Earle: Arch. Derma. and Syph., June, 1929.
Martin, T. A.: Clin. Med. and Surg., October, 1929.
Hille, Hermann: Med. Life, March, 1930.
Hille, Hermann: Clin. Med. and Surg., April, 1930.

AVERTIN

J. A. M. A., Sept. 8, 1928, p. 745.
Bailey, Fred. W.: Internat. J. Med. and Surg., 1931, 44:18.
Scott, W. J. Merle: New York State J. Med., 1931, 31:135
DeLee, Joseph B.: J. A. M. A., 1931, 96:1007.
Chipman, Clive N.: Anesth. and Anal., 1931, 10:206.
Dill, W. W.: Anesth. and Anal., 1931, 10:219.
Duff, James A.: Internat. J. Med. and Surg., 1931, 44:421.
Angle, Lewis W.: Avertin as a Rectal Anesthetic; J. Kansas M. Soc., 1931, 32: 399.
Hathaway, Starke and Rasmusen, Grant L.: Proc. Soc. Exp. Biol. Med., 1932, 29:412.
Stumpf, Elmer H.: N. Y. State J. Med., 1932, 32:126.
J. A. M. A., Feb. 4, 1933, p. 443; June 28, 1933, p. 2038.

BABY RALSTON

Macy, I. G., Outhouse, J., Graham A. and Long, M. Louisa: Human Milk Studies III, The Quantitative Estimation of Vitamin B; J. Biol. Chem., 1927, 73:189.
Plimmer, R. H., Rosedale, J. L., Raymond, W. N. and Lowndes, J.: Comparative Vitamin B value of Foodstuffs: Cereals I; Biochem. J., 1927, 21:1141.
Hunt, C. H. and Kraus, W. E.: The Relative Antineuritic and Antipellagric Potency of Cow's Milk; J. Biol. Chem., 1928, 79:733.
Hoobler, B. R.: Symptomatology of Vitamin B Deficiency in Infants; J. A. M. A., 1928, 91:307.
Dennett, Roger H.: Routine Use of the Vitamin B Factor in Infant Feeding; J. A. M. A., 1929, 92:10.
Rice, C. V.: The Treatment of Celiac Disease from the Standpoint of "Vitamin Deficiency"; Arch. Pediat., September, 1930, p. 572.
Metzger, Harry C.: Malnutrition in Children; J. Mich. Med. Soc., 1930, 29:896.
Morgan, A. F. and Barry, M. M.: Underweight Children: Increased Growth Secured Thru the Use of Wheat Germ; Am. J. Dis. Child., 1930, 39:5, 935–947.
McCollum, E. V., Simmons, N. and Pitz, W.: The Nature of the Dietary Deficiencies of the Wheat Embryo; J. Biol. Chem., 25:105.

BACILLUS ACIDOPHILUS

Cheplin, H. A. and Wiseman, John C.: Observations on the Effect of B. acidophilus Upon Cases of Chronic Constipation; Boston Med. and Surg. J., 1921, Vol. 185.
Rettger, L. F., and Cheplin, H. A.: A Treatise on the Transformation of the Intestinal Flora with Special Reference to the Implantation of Bacillus Acidophilus; Yale University Press, New Haven, Conn. 1921.
Rettger, L. F. and Cheplin, H. A.: Bacillus acidophilus and its Therapeutic Application; Arch. Int. Med., 1922, 29:357–367.
Bass, C. C.: Transformation of the Intestinal Flora; Annals Clin. Med., 1, 25–32. Transformation of the Intestinal Flora; South. Med. Journ. Jan., 1923.

BACILLUS ACIDOPHILUS CULTURE

J. A. M. A., Dec. 20, 1919, p. 1895; Report Council Pharm. and Chem., 1919, p. 51.
Rettger and Cheplin: Intestinal Flora; Yale University Press, 1921.
Kopeloff: Lactobacillus Acidophilus; Williams and Wilkins, 1926.
Portus and Albus: A Clinical and Laboratory Study of the Therapeutic Value of Lactobacillus Acidophilus; Am. J. Surg., Apr., 1931.
Kopeloff, Blackman and McGinn, L.: Acidophilus in Patients with Mental Diseases; Psych. Quart., Oct., 1931.

BACTERIOPHAGES

D'Herelle: The Bacteriophage and its Behavior, Williams and Wilkins, Baltimore, 1926.
Grenet, H. and Isaac-Georges, P.: Therapeutic Attempts with D'Herelle's Bacteriophage; Presse Med., 1928, 36:1089.
Smith, George H.: Bacteriophage and Phagocytosis; J. Immunol., 1928, 15:125.
Rice and Harvey: J. Lab. Clin. Med., 1928, 14:1.
Larkum: J. Inf. Dis., 1929, 45:34.

Albee, F. H.: The Principles of the Bacteriophage Applied to Osteomyelitis; Internat. J. Med. and Surg., 1929, 42:1.
Morison, J. and Vardon, A. C.: A Cholera and Dysentery Bacteriophage; Indiana J. Med. Research, 1929, 17:48.
Sauve: The Bacteriophage in Surgery; Medicine, 1930, 11:737.
Albee, F. H.: The Bacteriophage in Surgery; Internat. J. Med. and Surg., 1930, 43:461; Am. J. Surg., 1932, 15:228.
Cipollaro, A. C.: Bacteriophage. Its Application in Dermatological Practice; N. Y. State J. Med., 1931, 31:349.
Hauduroy, P.: Bacteriophage Treatment; Presse Med., 1931, 39:168.
Schultz, E. W.: Bacteriophage as Therapeutic Agent in Genito-Urinary Infections; Calif. and West. Med., 1932, Vol. 36, Nos. 1 and 2.

BANANA POWDER

Pease, M. C. and Rose, G. R.: Bananas as a Food for Children; Am. J. Dis. Child., 1917, 14:379.
Prescott, Samuel C.: The Banana: A Food of Exceptional Value; Scient. Monthly, Vol. 6, 1918.
Sugira, K. and Benedict, S. R.: Nutritive value of the Banana; J. Biol. Chem., Vol. 40, 1919.
Haas, Sidney V.: Value of the Banana in Treatment of Celiac Disease; Am. J. Dis. Child., 1924, 28:421.
Irish, H. E.: A Case of Celiac Disease with Banana Treatment; Arch. Pediat., 1926, 43:533.
Stross, Josephine: Coeliapie-Behandlung mit Bananen; Wien. med. Wochensch., 1928, 78:818.
Siperstein, David: New Trend in the Diet of Infants; Lancet, May 1, 1931, p. 257.
Haas, Sidney V.: Powdered Ripe Bananas in Infant Feeding; Arch. Pediat., 1931, 48:248.

BARB-ETH-OIL

Axelrod, M. L.: The Rectal Instillation of Certain Barbiturates in Ether and Oil with Quinine for Obstetrical Analgesia; Anesthesia and Analgesia, 1931, 10:64.

BEFSAL

Ott, Lambert: Cumulative Evidence of Curative Values of Befsal for Arthritis; Am. Physician, August, 1922.
Rentschler, Walter R.: The Etiology and Treatment of Arthritic and Rheumatic Conditions; Med. World, November, 1923.
J. A. M. A., February 21, 1925, p. 611; Reports Chem. Lab , 1924–5, p. 118.
Sherger, John A.: Metabolic Deficiency Caused by Rheumatic Poison; Med. Rev. of Reviews, February, 1926.
Carmichael, T. H.: Treatment of Arthritis; Med. Rev. of Reviews, October, 1926.
Beates, Henry M.: A Remedy for Rheumatism; Med. Life, April, 1927.
Collins, Harold: Rheumatoid Arthritis; Am. Med., November, 1927.

BELLADENAL

Viguier: Thesis, Paris, 1925.
Marchand and Viguier: Sciences Medicales, June 30, 1925.
Rue: Thesis, Paris, 1927.
Bohec: Presse Med., January 4, 1930.

BELLAFOLINE

Rothlin, E.: Schw. med. Wochensch, No. 48, 1924.
Loeffler, W.: Schw. med. Wochensch, No. 29, 1926.
Kalk and Siebert: Arch. f. Verdauungskr., 40, No. 56, 1926.
Ries, A.: Fortsch d. Therapie, No. 21, Nov. 1926.

BENZEDRINE INHALER

Berbolct, J. A.: Med. Jour. and Record, July 30, 1932.

BENZYL BENZOATE

Litzenberg, Jennings, C.: The use of Benzyl Benzoate in dysmenorrhea; J. A. M. A., Aug. 23, 1919, pp. 601–3.
Spach, A. B.: Angina Pectoris—A Survey of treatment with a new remedy, Benzyl Benzoate; Ill. Med. Jour., January, 1921, p. 28.
Ludwig, Fritz: Schweiz. Klin. Wochensch., Dec. 28, 1922, p. 1200.
Mundell, J. J.: Surg., Gynec., and Obst., November, 1922, p. 652.
Quack, D.: Med. Klin., 1923, 8:241.
Meeker, Samuel: Boston Med. and Surg. Jour., June 21, 1923, p. 100–105.
J. A. M. A., April 17, 1926, p. 1233; Reports Council Pharm, and Chem., 1926, p. 21.
J. A. M. A., March 19, 1927, p. 944; Reports Council Pharm. and Chem., 1927, p. 11. Reports Council Pharm. and Chem., 1931, p. 27.
J. A. M. A., March 4, 1933, p. 661.

BENZYL FUMARATE

Volwiler and Vliet J. A.: Chem. Soc., 1921, 43:1672.
J. A. M. A., March 4, 1933, p. 661.

BETA LACTOSE

Potter, Philip S.: Metabolism in Infancy; Arch. Pediat., 1928, 45:7–12.
Kopeloff, Nicholas: Man versus Microbes; Knopf, Inc. N. Y. 1930.
McCord, Mather, M.; Feeding Convalescent Cases of Colitis; Arch. Pediat., November, 1930.
Boros, Edwin: The Use of Lactose in the Treatment of Constipation; Med. Jour. and Record, August 5, 1931.
Frost, William D. and Butterworth, T. H.: Present Status of Acidophilus Milk; Amer. J. Publ. Health, Vol. 21, No. 8, August, 1931.
Stewart, C. E.: Practical Dietetics in the Light of Modern Scientific Research; J. Mich. Med. Soc., 28; No. 12, p. 835.

BICARBONATE OF SODA

Sippy, B. W.: Gastric and Duodenal Ulcer; J. A. M. A., 1915, 64:1625.
Abt, I. A.: Pediatrics, Yearbook 1926, pp. 367, 1927, pp. 392, 1929, pp. 411; 1930, pp. 122, 352.
Kitlowski, E. A.: The Pre-operative and Post-operative Care of Congenital Clefts of the Lip and Palate; Ann. Surgery, March, 1932.
Solis-Cohen and Githens: Pharmacotherapeutics, pp. 511, 519, 522, 524, 526, 1141, 1344.
Mariott, W. McKim: Infant Nutrition, p. 52.
Beckman: Treatment in General Practice, pp. 733, 423, 427, 21.

BICHLORACETIC ACID

Ill. Med. Jour., August, 1932.

BICREOL

Annales de L'Institut Pasteur, January, 1922.
Lancet, January 6, 1923, p. 39.
Anuil-Davies: Lancet, Jan. 15, 1927.

BILIVAL

Lusena: Biochem. Centr. J., 1904, 2:1526.
Slowtzoff: Contributions to Chemical Physiology and Pathology, 1906, 7:508.
Franchini: Biochem. J., 1907, 6:213.
Apel: The Action of Lecithin-Choleic Acid in Cholelithiasis, Deut. med. Wochensch. 9–1923.
M. R. Bonsmann: Results from Bilival; Therapie der Gegenwart, November, 1923.
Lepehne: Cholagogues and their application; Deut. med. Wochensch., 978–1923.
Bolt and Heeres: Pflinger's Archives of Physiology, 193, 449.
Legene, Cardozo: Clin. Jour., N. 10, 1924.

BISMARSEN

Stokes, J. H. and Chambers, S. O.: Bismuth Arsphenamine Sulphonate; J. A. M. A., 1927, 89:1500.
Tobias, Norman: Clinical Results from the Use of Bismarsen in Tabes Dorsalis; Am. J. Syphilis, 1928 12:536.
Templeton, H. J.: Bismarsen, An Addition in the Therapy of Syphilis; Cal. and West. Med., January, 1929, v. 30, No. 1.
Shivers, C. H. de T.: The Clinical Value of Bismarsen in the Treatment for Syphilis; Arch. of Derm. and Syph., 1930, 22:462–469.
Kolmer, J. A.: Bismuth Arsphenamine Sulphonate (Bismarsen) in the Treatment of Syphilis and of Other Spirochetic Infections; Arch. of Derm. and Syph., 1930, 21:394–412.
Sheppe, Wm. M.: The Treatment of Neurosyphilis; W. Va. Med. J., 1930, 26:662–669.
Stokes, J. H., Miller, T. H. and Beerman, H.: An Appraisal of the Newest Arsphenamine, Bismarsen, in the Treatment for Syphilis; Arch. of Derm. and Syph., 1931, 23:624–643.

BISMO-CYMOL

Kolmer: Am. J. Syphilis, April, 1931.

BISMOGENOL

Wittgenstein: Klin. Wochensch., No. 49, p. 2271, 1924.
Wodtke: Deut. Archiv. fur klin. Medizin, July, 1924.
Zieler: Munch. med. Wochensch., No. 47, p. 1670, 1924.
Saloncky: Pharmacotherapeutica Ertevito, 1925, No. 2.
Pinkus: Med. Klin., 1926, No. 6.
Oppenheim: Wien. klin. Wochensch., 1926, No. 22.

Oppenheim: Wien. Dermat. Gesellschaft, November, 7, 1927.
J. A. M. A., March 19, 1927, p. 944; Reports Council Pharm. and Chem., 1927, p. 16.
Ritter and Karrenberg: Lancet, November 9, 1929.

BISMUTH SALICYLATE

Rathery, F. and Richard, Jacques Charles: Paris Med., 1923, 13:101.

BISMUTH SODIUM TARTRATE

Hanzlik, et al.: Clinical Excretion of Bismuth Sodium Tartrate; Arch. of Derm. and Syph., 1920, 22:850.
Voegtlin, C. and Dyer, H. A. and Leonard, C. S.: Public Health Report 1923, 38:1882.
Kober, P. A.: J. Lab. Clin. Med., 1927, 12:962.
Habler, C. and Hummel, R.: Klin. Wochensch; 1928, 7:2151.
Engelhardt, W.: Arch. f. Dermat. u. Syph., 1928, 156:1.
Beinhauer, L. G., and Jacob, F. M.: Am. J. Syphilis, 1928, 12:61.
Yoe, J. H. and Mote, J. H.: J. Amer. Pharm. Assoc., 1929, 18:450.

BISMUTH VIOLET

Effect of Bismuth Violet on Certain Pathogenic Organisms; South. Med. Jour., 1928, 21:914.
The Use of Bismuth-Violet in the Prevention of Wound Infections; South. Med. and Surg., Sept., 1929.
The Value of Bismuth-Violet in Oto-Rhino-Laryngologic Practice; South. Med. Jour., 1930, 23: 140.
The Destruction of the Common Pathogenic Bacteria with Bismuth Violet; New York Med. J. and Rec., June 18, 1930.
Wounds and Their Treatment; South. Med. Jour., 1931, 24:837.
The Value of Bismuth-Violet in the Treatment of Vincent's Disease and Dry Socket; J. Amer. Dental Assoc., Dec., 1931.

BI-SO-DOL

Smithies, F.: Nature, Diagnosis and Clinical Management of Gastric Ulcer; Am. J. M. Sc., 1923, 166:781.
Bastedo, W. A.: Med. Treatment of Duodenal Ulcer; Med. Jour. and Record, 1924, 119:381.
Bolton, C.: Principles of Treatment of Gastric Ulcer in view of Recent Work; Brit. Med. Jour., 1924, 1:139.
Editorial: Alkalosis as a Clinical Condition; J. A. M. A., 1924, 83:615.
Sollmann, Torald: The Normal Diet; C. V. Mosby Co., 2nd Edition, pp. 44 and 45, 1928.
J. A. M. A., March 10, 1928, p. 793; Oct. 29, 1932, p. 1511; Reports Council Pharm. and Chem., 1932, p. 12.

BREWERS' YEAST

Bargen, J. A. and Victor, S. M.: Diet in Intestinal Disorders; J. A. M. A., 1931, 97:151.
Waring, J. I.: Vitamin B Feeding of Infants; J. South Carolina M. A., 1931, 27:322.
Hoerner M. T.: Use of Vitamin B in Diets of Infants, J. A. M. A., 1931, 96:675.
Henricke, S. G.: The Vitamin B Complex: Its Role in Infant Feeding in the Light of our Present Knowledge; Northwest Med., 1932, 31:165.
Kahn, B. L.: Dermatoses in Childhood; Arch. Pediat., 1932, 49:512.
Langhorst, H. F.: Vitamins: Their Role in the Prevention and Treatment of Disease; Med. Jour. and Record, 1932, 135:326.
Melcer, A. S.: Vitamin B Therapy of Diabetes Mellitus; Polska gaz. lek., 1932, 11:89.
Ross, J. R. and Robertson, E. C.: The Effect of Vitamin B Complex on the Resistance of Rats to Enteritidis Infection; Am. J. Dis. Child, 1932, 43:547.
Wheeler, G. A. and Sebrell, W. H.: The Control of Pellagra; J. A. M. A., 1932, 99:95.

BROMHOSAL

R. von den Velden: Clin. Med. and Surg., 1932, 39, 257.
J. A. M. A., July 22, 1933, p. 280.

BROMINOL

Rad: Wien klin. Wochensch., 1926, 39, 1011.
Belfield and Rolnick; J. A. M. A., 1926, 86, 1831.
Iglauer: J. A. M. A., 1926, 86, 1879.
Singer: J. A. M. A., 1926, 88, 1298.
Spielberg: Arch. Otolaryng., 1927, 5, 334.
Garnett and Greenbaum: J. A. M. A., 1927, 89, 1443.
Jackson: Surg., Gynec. and Obst., 1927, 46, 795.
Archibald and Brown: J. A. M. A., 1927, 88, 1310.
Proetz and Ernst: Ann. Otol. Rhin. and Laryngol, 1927, 36, 978.
Iglauer and Kuhn: J. A. M. A., 1928, 90, 1278.
Todd: Laryngoscope, 1928, 38, 688.
Tabern, Hansen, Volwiler and Crandall: Radiology, 1930, 14, 364.

BROMURAL

Krieger, u. v. d. Velden: Zur Beruhigungs-u. Einschlaferungs-Therapie; Deut. med. Wochensch., 1907, No. 6.
Renz: Ein neues Sedativum; Calif. State J. of Med., May, 1908.
Sollmann and Hatcher: A Comparative Study of the Dosage and Effects of Chloralhydrate, Isopral and Bromural on Cats; J. A. M. A., 1908. No. 6.
Boldt: Ueber bewahrte Arzneimittel in der Frauenpraxis; N. Y. Med. J., 1909, No. 8.
Moench: The Etiology, Pathology and Treatment of Dysmenorrhea; Med. Herald & Physiotherapist, April, 1924, p. 13.
Solis-Cohen and Githens: Pharmaco-Therapeutics; D. Appleton and Co., 1928.
Wolf, W.: The Scope of Sedative Medication; Memphis Med. J., May, 1930, p. 88.
Nervous Indigestion; Collected Papers of the Mayo Clinic, 1927, 19:73; publ. Paul B. Hoeber, Inc., New York, 1930.

BROSEDAN

Pfaff, Georg: Treatment with Brosedan; Med. Klin., 1930, No. 31.
Schierenberg, F.: Therapy by Means of Brosedan; Med. Klin., 1930, No. 35.
Bendiz, B.: Treatment of Nervous Disturbances and Convulsive Attacks in Children with Brosedan; Therap. d. Gegenw., 1931, No. 5.

BULBOCAPNINE

De Jong and Herman: The Action of Bulbocapnin in Three Cases of Paralysis Agitans and One Case of Tremor of Paralysis Agitans Type; Arch. Neurol. and Psychiat., 1926, 26:55.
De Jong und Schaltenbrand: Untersuchungen mit Bulbocapnin bei Erkrankungen des Nervensystems; Deut. Zeit. fur Nervenheil., 1927, Nr. 3.
Kuttner, H.: Bulbocapnin bei der Behandlung der Chorea Minor; Deut. med. Wochensch., April 12, 1929, Nr. 15, S. 616.
Hill, E. R.: Der Wert des Bulbocapnins bei Encephalitis und Dyspituitarismus; Lancet, December 14, 1929, p. 1262.
Neville, W. S. Thacker: Meniere's Disease; Brit. Med. Jour., July 11, 1931, p. 54.
Vogel, Claus: Bulbocapnin bei Menierescher Erkrankung; Zeit. fur Laryngol., Rhinol., Otol., 1932, Bd. 22, H. 2–3.
Lewy, F. H.: Experiences with the Action of Bulbocapnine in Tremor; The II. Mediz. Univ.—Klin. der Charite, Berlin.

BULBOCAPNINE PHOSPHATE

Lancet, May 11th, 1929, p. 968.

BUTESIN PICRATE

Taylor, F. R.: Southern Med. and Surg., Oct. 1926, p. 682.
Parsons, J. G.: Northwest Med., June, 1926, p. 322.

BUTOLAN

Francke: Med. Klin., No. 29, 1920.
Soslowsky, S.: Deut. med. Wochensch., No. 14, 1920.
Schule: Med. Klin., No. 36, 1920.
Disque, L. Jr.: Med. Klin., No. 30, 1921.
Selter: Deut. med. Wochensch., No. 29, 1921.
Bonniger, M.: Therap. Halbmonatsh., Feb. 1, 1921.
Brann, O.: Med. Klin., No. 8, 1922.
Satke, V.: Aerztl. Reform-Ztg., No. 9, 1923.

BUTYN

Gradle, H.: Illinois M. J., Nov. 1921.
Bulson, A.: Ann. Otol., Rhinol. & Laryngol, 1922, 31:131.
Oaks and Merill: Eye, Ear, Nose and Throat Monthly, January, 1925.
Carlton, Albert C.: Clin. Med. and Surg., 1926, 33:249.
Robinson: Bull. Ambulant Proctol., November, 1927.
Reaves, R. G.: Clin. Med. and Surg., January, 1928.
O'Brien, C. S.: J. A. M. A., 1928, 90:8.
Drueck, C. J.: Am. J. Surg., 1928, 4:491.
Chapman, T.: J. Tennessee St. M. A., 1929, 21:382.
Hughes, L. W.: J. Med. Soc. New Jersey, 1929, 26:842.
Chaignon: Paris Med., 1929, 19:377.
La Rochelle, F. D. and A. H.: Am. J. Surg., 1929, 7:270.
Canuyt and Joublot: L'Anesthesie locale en Oto-Laryngologie, Paris, 1930.
Byrd, H.: J. Michigan St. M. S., 1930, 29:294.
Tovell, R. M.: Anesth. and Anal. May-June, 1931.
McCannel, A. D.: Lancet, 1931, 51:559.

B VITAMINS

Bloxson, A. P.: Am. J. Dis. Child., 1929, 37:1161.
Sure, Barnett: J. Biol. Chem., 1929, 76:763.
Hoobler, B. R.: J. A. M. A., Vol. 91. p. 307.

BY-KEM

Morse, W.: Applied Bio-Chemistry, p. 145, 1927.
The Influence of Sodium Taurocholate and Copper Sulphate on Lipase; J. Biol. Chem., Vol. XCII. No. 1, June, 1931.
Influence of Lactic Acid on Hemolysis; J. Pharm. and Exper. Therap., Vol. 43, No. 2, October, 1931.
Pavloff and Zeleny: Soc. Biol., 1932.
Physiological Etiology of Anemia Produced by Pancreatic Juice; Am. J. Physiol., 93:636.
Mayerhof and Lohman: Biochem. Zeitschr., 171, 381.

CACTINA PILLETS

J. A. M. A., Sept. 21, 1907, p. 1021; March 21, 1908, p. 956; April 4, 1908, p. 1140; March 12, 1910, p. 888; Aug. 6, 1910, p. 455; Jan. 19, 1918, p. 185; July 9, 1927, p. 138; Reports Council Pharm. and Chem., 1910, p. 41; Propaganda, vol. 1, p. 37.
Solis-Cohen: Pharmacotherapeutics and Materia Medica, 1928.
Parsonnet and Hyman: J. Med. Soc. New Jersey, Nov., 1931.

CADECHOL

Boehm: Munch. med. Wochensch., 1920, no. 29, p. 833–835.
Nonnenbruch: Munch. med. Wochensch., 1920, No. 29, p. 835.
Engelen: Allgemeine med. Wochensch., 1922, 10:55.
Pototzky: Deut. med. Wochensch., 1922, No. 22.
Pribram: Deut. med. Wochensch.. 1922, No. 31.
Fahrenkamp: Med. Klin., 1923, p. 1635.

CALCILACT

McCollum, E. V., Simmonds, N. and Parsons, H. T.: J. Biol. Chem.; 1919, 38:113.
Singer, G.: Wien. med. Wochensch., 1921, 34:247.
Telfer, S. V., Quart. J. Med., 1924, 17:245.
Brown, G. T. and Hunter, O. B.: Ann. Clin. Med., 1925, 4:299.
Scott, H. H.: Ann. Trop. Dis., 1925, 19:23.
Reid, William D.: Boston Med. and Surg. J., 1925, 192:883.
Lowenstein, W.: Klin. Wochenschr., 1926, 5:354.
Roe, J. H. and Kahn, B. S.: J. A. M. A., 1926, 86:1761.
Irving, J.: J. Biol. Chem., 1926, 68:513.
Bergeim, O.: J. Biol. Chem., 1926, 70:29.

CALCIUM BENZIODOXYL

Gasser, H. S. and Loevenhart.: J. Biol. Chem., 1912–13, Vol. 14, p. 30.
Loevenhart, A. S.: Arch. f. Gesamte Physiologie, 1913, p. 379 to 389.
Loevenhart, A. S.: Arch. Int. Med., 1915, 15:1059.
Thompson, J. L.: Virginia M. Monthly, 1929, 5:32.
Harbinson, J. E.: California and West. Med., 1929, 31:24.
Bowers, J. M.: Northwest Med., 1929, 28:298.
Niehgbors, D.: Texas State J. of Med., 1930, 25:672.

CALCIUM GLUCONATE

Kottman, K.: Calcium Gluconate and Calcium Therapy; Schw. med. Wochensch., 1927, 57:409–411.
Klare, K.: Lime Therapy for Children; Munchen. med. Wochenschr., 1928, 75:2135–2136, 1928; Abstr. J. A. M. A., 1929, 92:762.
Steger, M.: The Use of Calcium Gluconate in Neurological Practice; Munch. med. Wochenschr., 1928, 75:1795–1796.
Karrenberg, C. L.: Therapeutic Use of Calcium Gluconate in Dermatology; Dermat. Wochensch., 1928, 86:540–545.
Alonza, F.: Calcium Gluconate Therapy; Arch. di pat e clin. med., 1928, 7:1–4.
Luttinger, P.: Calcium Metabolism and Therapy; Med. Rev. of Reviews, 1928, 34:579, 1929, 35:19, 1929, 35:189, 1929, 35:239.
Bardenheuer, F. H.: Prophylaxis of Postpartum Hemorrhage with Calcium; Zentralb. f. Gynaek., 1929, 53:1826; Abstracted J. A. M. A., 1929, 93:1186.
Herrold, R. D.: Complications of Gonococcus Infection treated by Calcium Gluconate; Venereal Disease Information, 1930, 11:55.
Hedge, W. M.: The Blood in Psoriasis; Arch. of Derm. and Syph., 1931, 24:201.

CALGLUCON

Wangensteen: Ann. Surgery, 1928, Vol. 88, p. 845.
Karrenberg: Dermat. Wochensch., Apr. 21, 1928; Clin. Med. and Surg., September, 1931.
Minot and Cutler: Proc. Soc. Exp. Biol. Med., April, 1929.
Zelewski: Praxis, 1929, December 10 and 24.
Stokes: J. A. M. A., April 15, 1930.
Ivy, A. C.: J. A. M. A., October, 11, 1930.
Bauer, Salter and Aub: J. A. M. A., April 11, 1931.
Downing and Blumenfeld: N. E. Med. Journ. February 5, 1931.
Diasio: Med. Jour. and Record, September 8, 1931.
O'Donnell and Levin: J. A. M. A., March 14, 1931, p. 837.
Kugelmass, I. N.: J. A. M. A., September 10, 1932.

CALMITOL

Jadassohn, J.: Fortsch. d. Therapie, No. 1., January, 1925.
Rabow: Arzneiverordnungen, Bd. 1, 1926, Bd. 11, 1927.
Franck: Moderne Therapie; Handbuch der medikamentosen, physikalischen und diathetischen Behandlungsweisen der letzten Jahre, 1926.
Winkler: Prurigo, Strophulus, Pruritus; Handbuch der Haut-und Geschlechtskkrankheiten, 1927, p. 353–355, 359.

CALSOMA

Steel, M. and Gies, W.: J. Physiol, 1908, 20:343.
Lothrop, A. P.: Am. J. Physiol, 1909, 24:297.
Hardt, L. L. and Rivers, A. B.: Arch. Int. Med., February 1922, p. 171.
J. A. M. A., 1923, 81:816.
Addis, T., Mackay, E. M. and Mackay, L. L.: J. Biol. Chem., December, 1926, p. 157.
Palmer, Walter Lincoln: Arch. Int. Med., January 15, 1927, p. 109.
Greenwald, I.: Proc. Soc. Exp. Biol. Med., Vol. 20, p. 436.

CAPROKOL

Leonard, Veader: J. A. M. A., 1924, 83:2005–2011; J. Urol., Vol. 12, No. 6, Dec. 1924, J. A. M. A., 1925, 85:1855–1861.
Henline, Roy B.: J. Urol., Vol. 14, No. 2, August, 1925.
Elliott, David C. and Barbour, Henry G.: Canad. Med. A. J., 1925, 15:787–788.
McCurry, W. E.: J. A. M. A., June 20, 1925, p. 1950.
Frobisher, Martin and Leonard, Veader: J. Urol., 1926, 15:1–10.
Scott, Wm. J. and Leonard, Veader: Am. J. Dis. Child., February, 1926, 31:241.
Brown, Damon A.: J. A. M. A., 1926, 86:668.
Wynne, H. M. N.: Minnesota Medicine, 1926, 9:156–160.
Feirer, Wm. A. Meader, Percy D. and Leonard, Veader: J. Urol., Vol. 16, No. 2 August, 1926.
Feirer, Wm. A. and Leonard, Veader.: J. Pharm. and Exper. Therap., Vol. 28, No. 3, September, 1926.

CARBARSONE

Brown, P. W.: The Nature, Incidence and Treatment of Endamebiasis; J. A. M. A., 1926, 86:457.
Chen, M. Y., Anderson, H. H. and Leake, C. D.: Rate of Urinary Arsenic Excretion after giving Acetarsone ("Stovarsol") and "Carbarsone" by Mouth; Proc. Soc. Exp. Biol. Med., 1930, 27:174.
Anderson, H. H. and Reed, A. C.: Amebiasis; Cases comparing various Amebacides; Cal. and West. Med., 1931, 35:439.
Craig, C. F.: The Pathology of Amebiasis in Carriers; Am. J. Trop. Med., 1932, 12:285.
Reed, A. C., Anderson, H. H., David, N. A. and Leake, C. D.: Carbarsone in the Treatment of Amebiasis; J. A. M. A., 1932, 98:189.
Leake, C. D.: Chemotherapy of Amebiasis; J. A. M. A., 1932, 98:195.

CARBON DIOXIDE—OXYGEN MIXTURES

Henderson, Yandell and Haggard, H. W.: J. A. M. A., 1922, 79:1137.
McCurdy, J. R.: Atlantic Med. Jour., April, 1923.
Brown, W. E., Henderson, V. E., Kennedy, A. S. and Lucas, G. H. W.: Cur. Res. in Anes. and Anal., 1930, 60:136.
Henderson, Yandell: J. A. M. A., 1931, 96:495.

CARITOL

Euler and Karber: Biochem. Z., 1929, 209:240–5.
Green and Mellanby: Brit. J. Exptl. Path., 1930, 11:81–9.
Goldblatt and Barnett: Proc. Soc. Exp. Biol. Med., 1932, 30:201–4.
Eusterman and Wilbur: J. A. M. A., 1932, 98:2054.

CASEC

Wilcox, H. B.: Clinical Pediatrics; D. Appleton and Co., New York, 1928, Vol. 12, p. 36.
Goldbloom, A.: Special Feeding Methods for Infants; Canad. Med. A. J., 1930, 23:807.
Kerley, C. G.: Treatment of Celiac Disease without the Use of Cow's Milk; Arch. Pediat., 1931, 48:326.
Parsons, L.: Celiac Disease; Lancet, 1931, 1:61.
West, J. H.: Low Fat High Starch Evaporated Milk Feeding for the Marasmic Baby; Arch. Pediat., 1931, 48:189.
Zahorsky, J.: The Treatment of Gastroenteric Intoxication in Infants; Ill. Med. Jour., 1931, 65:510.
Dalldorf, G. and Russell, H. K.: Anemia in the New Born; N. Y. State J. Med., 1932, 32:839.
Freedman, H. J.: Disturbances of Function of the Suprarenal Glands in Children; Am. J. Dis. Child., 1932, 44:1285.
Haas, S. V.: Celiac Disease, Its Specific Treatment and Cure without Nutritional Relapse; J. A. M. A., 1932, 99:448.
Parsons, L.: Celiac Disease; Am. J. Dis. Child., Part II, 1932, 43:1293.
Queries and Minor Notes: Diarrhea in Children; J. A. M. A., 1932, 99:849.
Sauer, L. W.: Simplified Feeding Technic for the Small Prematurely Born Infant; Am. J. Dis. Child., 1932, 44:106.

CASEOSAN

Lindig: Munch. med. Wochensch., 1919, Nr. 33, S. 921; Fortsch. d. Medizin, 1920, Nr. 2, S. 55; Munch. med. Wochensch, 1920, Nr. 34, S. 982; Deuts. med. Wochensch., 1921, Nr. 21, S. 585.
Von Jaschke, R.: Deut. med. Wochensch., 1920, Nr. 28, S. 785, Therap. Halbmonatschefte, 1921, Nr. 17, S. 539.
Hille, Max: Inaug. Diss. Halle, 1921; Deut. Zahnaertz. Wochen., 1922, Nr. 13.
Hecht, Nowawes: Med. Klin. 1923, Nr. 17, S. 578.
Singer, Gustav: Wien. klin. Wochensch., 1924, Nr. 7, S. 155; Klin. Wochensch., 1924, Nr. 51, S. 2361; Klin. Wochensch., 1925, Nr. 8, S. 380; Med. Klin., 1926, Nr. 16, S. 634.
Dollinger, Bela: Wien. klin. Wochensch., 1925, Nr. 47, S. 1260.

CATARRHAL RESPIRATORY VACCINES

J. A. M. A., June 22, 1918, p. 1967; Reports Council Pharm. and Chem., 1918, p. 11; Propaganda, vol. 2, p. 187.
Kolmer: Arch. Pediat., January, 1929.

CEANOTHYN

Clark, A. H.: Amer. Jour. Pharm., Vol. 98, No. 3, pp. 147–156; Vol. 100, No. 4, pp. 240–242.
Tharaldsen and Krawetz: Amer. J. Physiol., Vol. 79, No. 35, pp. 545–552.
Payne, R. J.: Ann. Otol. Rhin. and Laryngol., Vol. 35, No. 3, pp. 769–790.
Payne and O'Bannon: Clin. Med. and Surg., Vol. 35, No. 1, pp. 52–53.
Wirth, E. H.: Amer. Jour. Pharm., Vol. 98, No. 10, pp. 503–514.
Koppanyi, Theodore: J. Amer. Pharm. Assoc., Vol. 17, No. 6, pp. 528, 529.
Taylor, G. C.: Amer. Jour. Pharm., Vol. 99, No. 4, pp. 214–232.
Spotts, W. B.: Dental Survey, Vol. 5, No. 1, pp. 43–44.
J. A. M. A., March 20, 1926, p. 890, Feb. 8, 1930, p. 410; Reports Council Pharm. and Chem., 1926, p. 23, 1930, p. 16.

CEREALS

Tisdall, F. F., T. G. H. Drake and A. Brown: A New Cereal Mixture containing Vitamins and Mineral Elements; Am. J. Dis. Child., 1930, 40:791.
Crimm, P. D.: Dietary of Childhood Tuberculosis: Cereal as a Source of Added Mineral and Vitamin Elements; J. Ind. M. A., 1932, 25:205.
Henricke, S. G.: The Vitamin B Complex. Its Role in Infant Feeding in the Light of our Present Knowledge; Northwest Med., 1932, 31:165.
Langhorst, H. F.: Vitamins: Their Role in the Prevention and Treatment of Disease; Med. Jour. and Record, 1932, 135:326.
Morse, J. L.: Fads and Fancies in Present Day Pediatrics; Penna. M. J., 1932, 35:279.
Silverman, A. C.: Celiac disease; N. Y. State J. Med., 1932, 32:1055.
Sneed, W.: Ununited and Delayed Union of Fractures; Ky. M. J., 1932, 30:363.
Summerfeldt, P.: The Value of an Increased Supply of Vitamin B_1 and Iron in the Diet of Children: Am. J. Dis. Child., 1932, 43:284.
Summerfeldt, P., F. F. Tisdall and A. Brown: The Curative Effects of Cereals and Biscuits on Experimental Anaemias; Canad. Med. A. J., 1932, 26:666.
Troutt, L.: Quality Studies of Therapeutic Diets: I. The Ulcer Diet; J. Am. Dietet. A., 1932. 8:25.

CHAULMESTROL

Beasley, Thomas J.: N. Y. Med. Jour., September 21, 1921.
Hollmann, H. T.: Arch. of Derm. and Syph., January, 1922.
Aronstam, N. E.: Urol. and Cut. Rev., December, 1922.
Cown, Robert L.: Urol. and Cut. Rev., December, 1922.

Corlett, Wm. T.: J. A. M. A., August 5, 1922.
Brown, Philip King: Calif. State J. of Med., August, 1923.
Freudenthal, Wolff: The Laryngoscope, March, 1923.
Gavino, Catalino and Tietze, Samuel: Philippine Isl. Med. Assn. Jour., February, 1925.
Wilson, R. M.: South. Med. Jour., August, 1926.

CHINIOFON

Duhrasen, A.: Munch. med. Wochensch., 1922, 69:506.
Schneider, P.: Deut. med. Wochensch., 1926, 52:1047.
Bach, F. W. and Steinhauser, H.: Munch. med. Wochensch., 1926, 73:865.
Rehbein, M.: Arch. f. Schiffs u. Tropen Hyg., Vol. 30, July, 1926.
Williamson, C. S., Kaplan, B. and Geiger, J. C.: J. A. M. A., 1929, 92:528.
Dimetrakoff, K.: Arch. f. Schiffs u. Tropen Hyg., 1930, 34:54.

CHINOPLASMIN

See "Plasmochin" References.

CHOLE-CYSTO-COL

Fantus, Bernard: J. A. M. A., July 16, 1927.

CHOLEVAL

Koltonski, Hermann: Choleval als Prophylaktikum gegen die Blennorrhoe der Neugeborenen; Berl. klin. Wochensch., 1920, Nr. 40, S. 954.
Pranter, Viktor: Zur Behandlung von Hauterkrankungen mit Choleval; Wien. klin. Wochensch., 1920, Nr. 29.
Goldsmith: Choleval bei infektiosen Hauterkrankungen; Therap. d. Gegenw., September, 1921.
Friedberg, W.: Über Cholevalbehandlung in der Rhino-Oto-Laryngologie; Deut. med. Wochensch., 1922, Nr. 40.
Vogel, W.: Ueber Neuere Antigonorrhoika und Antisyphilitika; Deut. med. Wochensch., 1925, Nr. 27, S. 1119.
Pezold: Kritisches Sammelreferat über Gonorrhoebehandlung mit Silber-praparaten; Deut. med. Wochensch., 1925, Nr. 51, S. 541.
Anschel, Norbert: Beitrage zur internen Therapie der Erkrankungen der Leber und der Gallensystems; Archiv. Verdauungshr., 1927, Bd. 40, Heft 5/6.
Ullmann, K.: Über den Wert des kolloidal Silberpräparates Choleval fur die Behandlung der Gonorrhoe; Med. Klin., 1929, Nr. 40.
Ullmann, K.: Choleval in Gonorrhea; E. Merck's Report, 1930, Part I, p. 34–40.

CIBALGINE

Pick, E.: Med. Klin., 1925, 21:1141.
Wimmer and Schwarzbrod: Wien. klin. Wochensch., Vol. 38, No. 38, 1925, 38:1038.
Löwenthal: Deut. med. Wochensch., 1926, 52:963.
Gembicki: Zahnärztliche Rundschau, July 11, 1926, 35:491.
Friedrich: Deut. zahnarzt. Rundschau, 1926, 29:333.
Foster, G.: Med. Jour. and Record, 1930, 131:527–528.

CINCHOPHEN

Nicolaier and Dohrn: Deut. Archiv fur klin. Medizin, 1908, 93:331.
McLester: Arch. Int. Med., 1913, 12:739.
Fine and Chace: Proc. Soc. Exp. Biol. Med., 1914, 11:111, J. Pharm. and Exper. Therap., 1914, 6:219.
Denis: J. Pharm. and Exper. Therap., 1915, 7:612.
Smith and Hawk: Arch. Int. Med., 1915, 15:181.
Chace, Myers and Killian: J. A. M. A., 1921, 77:1230.
Barbour, H. G. and Lozinsky, E., J.: Lab. and Clin. Med., 1923, 8:217.
Barrow, Moses: J. A. M. A., 1924, 82:2010.
Med. Jour., p. 528, April 7, 1928.
Lowenthal, L. J., Macay, W. A. and Lowe, E. C.: Brit.

CITABS

Blatherwick, N. R. and Long, M. L.: J. Biol. Chem., 1922, 53:103.
Hess, A. F., and Matzner, M. J.: J. A. M. A., 1924, 82:1604.
Meyer, S.: Arch. f. Kinderh., 1927, 82:241.
Weissenberg, H.: Arch. f. Kinderh., 1926, 78:276, 1928, 84:200.
Behrens, R.: Arch. f. Kinderh., 1929, 86:90.
Marcus, J. H.: J. Med. Soc. New Jersey, 1930, 27:699.
Gonce, J. E. and Templeton, H. L.: Am. J. Dis. Child. 1930, 39:265.

CITRIN

Thorne, Leslie, and Starling, E. H.: Relation of the Cardiac Systole to Arterial Tension; Practitioner, 1912, 88:593.

Patterson, S. W.: Mechanical Factors which Determine the Output of the Ventricles; J. of Phys., 1914, 48:357.
Robinson, G. Cranby: The Relation of the Respiration and the Circulation; Ill. Med. Jour., 1924, vol. 416.
Hering, H. E.: Med. Wcheft, 1925, 72:339.
Bordley, James and Baker, Jr.: Johns Hopkins Hosp. Bull., 1926, 39:229.
Barksdale, I. S.: Studies on the Blood Pressure Lowering Principles in the Seed of the Watermelon; Am. J. M. Sc., 1926, 171:11.

COAGULEN

Fonio, A.: Zeitsch. f. Chirurgie, 1912, 117:176–194.
Kocher, Th.: Schweiz. Rundsch. für Mediz., 1913, 14:239.
Fonio: Mitteil. aus den Grenzgeb. der Mediz. und Chir., 1914, 27:642.
Rottenbiller: Oesterreichi. ungari. Vierteljahrsschr. f. Zahnheilkunde, 1915, 31:139.
Brem, Bolling & Casper: J. A. M. A., 1918, 71:2138.
Reports Council Pharm. and Chem., 1920, p. 53; Propaganda, vol. 2, p. 290.
Davis, R. H. and W. D.: Arch. of Derm. and Syph., Vol. 8, No. 5, November, 1923.

CODAMINES TABLETS

McCollum, E. V., and Davis, Marg.: J. Biol. Chem., 1913, 15:167.
Osborne, T. B., and Mendel, Lafayette: J. Biol. Chem., 1913, 15:311, 16:423.
Hess, A. F. and Weinstock: J. A. M. A., 1920, 80:687–690.
Werkman, C. H.: J. Inf. Dis., 1923, 32:255.
Steenbock, H. and Black, A.: J. Biol. Chem., 1924, 61:405.
Steenbock, H. and Nelson: J. Biol. Chem., 1924, Vol. 62:209–216.
Hess, A. F.: J. A. M. A., 1924, 83:1845.
Sherman, H. C., Macleod, F. L.: J. Am. Chem. Soc., 1925, 47:1658.
Hawk, P. B. Bergeim, Olaf: Practical Physiological Chemistry, 9th Ed., 1927, 820–838.
Grant, A. H., Suyenga, B. and Stegeman, D. E.: Am. Rev. Tub., 1928, 16:628.

COD LIVER OIL

Blunt, K. and Cowan, R.: Distribution of Vitamin D: Cod Liver Oil; J. A. M. A., 1929, 93:1219.
Caffey, J.: Changes in Human Rickets after Viosterol Therapy; J. Med. Soc. New Jersey, 1931, 28:21.
Boyd, J. O. and Drain, C. L.: The Arrest of Dental Caries; Am. J. Dis. Child., 1932, 44:691.
Brown, G. T.: Perennial Hay Fever; Arch. Otolaryn., 1932, 15:202.
Clein, N. W.: Cod-Liver Oil and Viosterol. Uses and Abuses; Northwest Med., 1932, 31:430.
Clouse, R. C.: Vitamin D; J. A. M. A., 1932, 99:215; 1932, 99:301.
Council on Pharmacy and Chemistry: Average Optimum Dosage of Cod Liver Oil; J. A. M. A., 1932, 98:316.
Luck, M. J.: Annual Review of Biochemistry; Stanford University Press, California, 1932.
McCollum, E. V.: International Clinics, Series 42, Vol. 2, June, 1932, p. 1.
Porter, L. and Carter, W. E.: Management of the Sick Infant, C. V. Mosby Co., St. Louis, 1932. pp. 136, 479.
Sincock, H. A.: Calcium Deficiencies in Pregnancies and Its Influences upon the Child; Wisconsin M. J., 1932, 31:838.
Ullmann, E. V.: Chronic Sinus Diseases; Northwest Med., 1932, 31:240.

COD LIVER OIL CONCENTRATE

Editorials, J. A. M. A., 1930, 94:414; 1930, 95:38, 1930, 95:798, 1931, 97:782.
J. A. M. A., January 2, 1932.

COD LIVER OIL WITH VIOSTEROL

Rosenheim, O. and Webster, T. A.: Lancet, 1927, i:306.
Vogt, E.: Munch. med. Wochensch., 1928, 75:721.
Green, H. M. and Mellanby, E.: Brit. Med. Jour., 1928, 11:691.
Hess, A. F. and Lewis, J. M.: J. A. M. A., 1928, 91:783.
Mellanby, M. and Pattison, C. L.: Brit. Med. Jour., Dec. 15, 1928.
Sobel, J. and Claman, I.: Arch. Pediat., 1929, 46:1.
Hess, A. F., Lewis, J. M. and Rivkin, Helen: J. A. M. A., 1930, 94:1885.
Hess, Julius H., Poncher, H. G., Dale, M. L. and Klein, R. L.: Viosterol; J. A. M. A., 1930, 95:316.

COFRON

Whipple, G. H. and Associates: Am. J. Physiol. 72, 1925.
Whipple, G. H. and Robscheit-Robbins: Am. J. Physiol., 1927, 79:260.
Hart, E. B., Steenbock, H. and Associates: J. Biol. Chem., 1928, 77:797.
McKay, Helen M. M.: Arch. Dis. Child., 1928, 3:117.
Middleton, W. S.: J. A. M. A., 1928, 91:857.
Meyers, V. C. and Beard, H. H.: J. A. M. A., 1929, 93:1210.
Mills, E. S.: Canad. Med. A. J., 1930, 22:175.

Dwyer, H. V.: J. Mich. State Med. Soc., 1930, 29:420.
Josephs, H. W.: South. Med. Jour., 1930, 23:1135.
Powers, J. H. and Murphy, W. P.: J. A. M. A., 1931, 96:504.
Vaughan, Janet M.: Lancet, 1932, 222:565.

COFRON ELIXIR

Hart, E. B., Steenbock, H. and Associates: J. Biol. Chem., 1928, 77:797.
Josephs, H. W.: South. Med. Jour., 1930, 23:1135.
Powers, J. H. and Murphy, W. P.: J. A. M. A., 1931, 96:504.

COLALIN

Jolin: Zeitsch. f. physiolog. Chemie, 1887, 11:417; 1888, 12:512; 1889, 12:223.
Howell, William H.: A Text Book on Physiology, 1915.
Reports Council Pharm. and Chem., 1918, p. 52; Propaganda, vol 2, p. 203.
Cushny, Arthur C.: A Text Book on Pharmacology and Therapeutics, 1924.

COLLODAURUM

Ochsner, Edw. H.: Colloidal Gold in Inoperable Cancer, Clin. Medicine, Oct. 1924.
J. A. M. A., Sept. 26, 1925, p. 997.
Ill. Med. Jour., July, 1926.
Wis. Med. Jour., March, 1926.
Internat. J. Med. and Surg., March, 1927.
Clin. Med. and Surg., Jan., 1929.

COLLOIDAL MERCURY SULPHIDE

Wakerlin, G. E. and Eisemann, C.: Am. J. Syphilis, 1928, 12:3.
Council on Pharm. and Chem., J. A. M. A., 1929, 92:1349.
Wakerlin, G. E.: Arch. of Derm. and Syph., 1929, 19:878–890.
Medical Life, March, 1930, pp. 111–164.
Freeman, M. J., Taylor, G. G. and White, C. J.: Am. J. Syphilis, 1931, 15:207.
Archiv. f. Dermat. und Syph., 1932, 165:209.
Am. J. Syphilis, 1932, 16:198.
Schw. med. Wochensch., April 16, 1932, pp. 378–380.

COLLOSOL ARGENTUM

Phillips, Sidney: Carbuncles; Lancet, January 8, 1921.
Kid, F.: Pyelography; Brit. Med. Jour., May 13, 1922.
Hedley, J. P.: Vaginitis; Dictionary of Practical Medicine, 1923.
Fine, J.: Septicemia following Abortion; Brit. Med. Jour., November 28, 1925.
Weir, R. S.: Cellulitis of the Scalp; Brit. Med. Jour., January 22, 1927.
Rorke, Margaret: Chronic Gonorrhoea in Women; Lancet, June 4, 1927.
MacDonald, Val.: Gonorrhea in the Male; Brit. Med. Jour., May 3, 1930.
Spence, H. D. Livingstone; Lancet, January 4, 1930.
Ford, R. Nelson: Midwifery; Brit. Med. Jour., November 11, 1930.
Simpson, G. A. Garey: Post-Influenzal Cough; Brit. Med. Jour., May 16, 1931.
Elliot, R. H.: Glaucoma; Brit. Med. Jour., December 26, 1931.

COLLOSOL BROMOFORM COMPOUND

Young, R. A.: Cough; Lancet, March 8, 1924.

COLLOSOL CALCIUM

Francis, L. A.: Urticaria; Brit. Med. Jour., Dec. 21, 1929.
Prest, E. E.: Therapeutic Action; Med. Press and Circular, April 3, 1929.
Fraser, Kenneth: Pulmonary Tuberculosis; Brit. Med. Jour., May 24, 1930.
Wheeler, Sir W. I. de C.: Perforative Diverticulitis of the Colon; Brit. Med. Jour., Jan. 4, 1930.
J. A. M. A., March 22, 1930, p. 920; Reports Council Pharm. and Chem., 1930, p. 20.
Drummond, J. C.: The Subcutaneous Administration of Vitamin D; Lancet, Oct. 24, 1931.
Graves, T. C.: Mental Disorder; Lancet, July 9 and 16, 1932.

COLLOSOL CHRYSAROBIN

Heaney, J. D.: Psoriasis; Brit. Med. Jour., December 17, 1927.
Sibley, W. Knowsley: Med. Press and Circular, February 13, 1929. Post-Grad. Med. J. April, 1932.

COLLOSOL CUPRUM

Rae, J.: Malignant Disease; Brit. Med. Jour, May 9, 1914.
Drage, L.: Malignant Disease; Lancet, June 6, 1914.

MacCarthy, T. M.: Malignant Disease; Brit. Med. Jour., July 28, 1917.
Thomson, Sir St. Clair: Dictionary of Practical Medicine, 1923.
Brierley, E. E.: Lancet, December, 1924.
Forsdike, Sidney: Brit. Med. Jour., November, 7, 1925.
Roper, F. A.: Brit. Med. Jour., April 17, 1926.
Mummery, J. Lockhart: Lancet, December 25, 1926.

COLLOSOL FERRO-ARSENICUM

Myers, Bernard: Practical Handbook Diseases of Children.

COLLOSOL FERRO-MANGANESE

Monypeny, H. J.: Practitioner, June, 1923.

COLLOSOL ICHTHYOL

Haler, D. H.: Medical Annual, 1932.

COLLOSOL IODINE

Journal A. M. A., September 8, 1917, p. 841; Reports Council Pharm. and Chem., 1917, p. 49; Propaganda, vol 2, pp. 144, 223.
Castellani, A.: Classification of Tonsillo-Mycosis; J. Trop. Med. and Hygiene, June 16, 1930.
Benson, W. T.: Erysipelas with Vaccines; Lancet, December 13, 1930.
Green-Armytage, V. B.: Habitual Abortion; Ind. Med. Gazette, February, 1931.
Mutch, N.: Chronic Arthritis; Brit. Med. Jour., March 7, 1931.
Hay, J.: Raised Blood Pressure; Brit. Med. Jour., July 11, 1931.
Mecredy, Gerald G.: Pulmonary Blastomycosis; I. J. Med. Sci., November, 1931.
Joynt, H. F.: Gumma of Mediastinum; Lancet, December 12, 1931.
Hassan, Bey Shaheen: Rheumatoid Arthritis; Brit. Med. Jour., January, 2, 1932.

COLLOSOL KAOLIN

Wynn, W. H.: Intestinal Toxaemia; Lancet, September 22, 1923.
Pirie, J.: Intestinal Toxaemia; Brit. Med. Jour., November 24, 1923.
Pope, Sir Wm. and Haines, R. T. M.: Lancet, May 23, 1925.
King, J. W.: Mucous Colitis; Brit. Med. Jour., October 23, 1926.
Russell, A. V.: Fistula; Brit. Med. Jour., August 11, 1928.
Kunstler, Monroe Bradford: Colitis; Med. Jour. and Record, May 4, 1932.
J. A. M. A., May 3, 1930, p. 1406; Reports Council Pharm. and Chem., 1930, p. 23.

COLLOSOL LEAD

Coke, W. F. H. and Cooke, J. B.: Malignant Disease; Brit. Med. Jour., March 6, 1926.
Talbot, E.: Cancer; Brit. Med. Jour., December 8, 1928.

COLLOSOL MANGANESE

Cutner, Morris: Urticaria; Brit. Med. Jour., June 27, 1921.
Barooa, D. M.: Carbuncle; Ind. Med. Jour., 1927.
Leeming, A. N.: Lymphatic Obstruction; Brit. Med. Jour., March 24, 1928.
McCormick, H. L.: Acute Pneumonia; Brit. Med. Jour., March 3, 1928.
Bhattacherjee, N. C.: Angioneurotic Oedema; Ind. Med. Jour., September, 1929.
Clayton, E. B. and Livingstone, J. L.: Fibrositis; Lancet, June 28, 1930.
Kraemer, W. H.: Am. J. Cancer, April 9, 1931.
Barooa, M.: Boils and Carbuncles; Antiseptic, May, 1933.

COLLOSOL PALLADIUM

King-Turner, A. C.: Brit. Med. Jour., Sept. 7, 1918.
Walker, J.: Board of Control, Eighth Ann. Rep., 1921.

COLLOSOL SELENIUM

Watson-Williams, E.: Brit. Med. Jour., October 11, 1919.
Watson-Williams, E.: Brit. J. Surg., 1920.
Waller, H. E.: Prescriber, June, 1920.
Pinch, A. E. Hayward: Brit. Med. Jour., June 18, 1921.
Cope, V. Z.: Med. Press, November 23, 1921.
Norbury, L. E. C.: Proc. Roy. Soc. Med., No. 8, June, 1923.
Thomson, Sir St. Clair: Dictionary of Practical Medicine, 1923.
Brierley, B. E.: Lancet, December 27, 1924.
Roper, F. A.: Brit. Med. Jour., April 17, 1926.

COLLOSOL SULPHUR

MacKenna, R. W.: Dermatology; Brit. Med. Jour., November 13, 1920.
Wynn, W. H.: Chronic Arthritis; Lancet, September 22, 1923.
Rorke, M.: Syphilitic Oedema; Lancet, December 6, 1924.
Pemberton, H. S.: Rheumatic Conditions; Lancet, December 25, 1926.
McEwen, P.: Toxic Goitre; Brit. Med. Jour., December 28, 1929.
Mutch, N.: Chronic Arthritis; Brit. Med. Jour., March 7, 1931.
Sibley, W. K.: Alopecia; Post-Grad. Med. J., April, 1932.
Graves, T. G.: Mental Disorder; Lancet, July 9 and 16, 1932.

COMPRAL

Jaeger, F.: Zentralb. f. Gynaek., No. 26, 1926.
Rosenthal: Med. Klin., No. 27, 1926.
Saenger, H.: Deut. med. Wochensch., No. 13, 1926.
Schmidt, F.: Fortsch. d. Therapie, No. 16, 1926.
Eicheler: Therap. d. Gegenw., No. 10, 1927.
Gaschke, R.: Wien. med. Wochensch., No. 17, 1927.
Maass, W.: Fortsch. d. Medizin, No. 12, 1927.
Noodt, K.: Med. Welt., No. 25, 1927.
Wilke, H.: Med. Klin., No. 14, 1927.
Hanke, V.: Klin. Wochensch., No. 10, 1928.
Hillebrand, H.: Deut. med. Wochensch., No. 14, 1928.

CORAMINE

Faust: Schw. med. Wochensch., 1924, 54:229.
Thannhauser and Fritzel: Schw. med. Wochensch., 1924, 54:232.
Hartmann: Schweiz. Apotheker-Zeitung, 1924, 62:337; 1924, 62:355.
Uhlmann: Zeitsch. f. die gesamte exp. Mediz., 1924, 43:556.
Asher: Schw. med. Wochensch., 1926, 56:569.
Fahrenkamp: Mediz. Korrespondenz-Blatt für Württemberg, No. 46, 1927.
Schubel and Gehlen: Arch. f. exper. Pathol. u. Pharmakol., 1928, 133:295.
Maloney-Tatum: J. Pharm. and Exper. Therap., No. 3, 1930, 40:291.
Maloney, Fitch and Tatum: J. Pharm. and Exper. Therap., 1931, 41:465.

CREOLIN-PEARSON

Antisepsis: With Particular Reference to the Uses of Creolin-Pearson; Merck's Archives, August, 1908.
Montgomery, D. W. and Culver, G. D.: Treatment of Scabies; Med. Jour. and Record, October 1, 1930.

CRYSTALLINE CAROTENE

Euler and Karrer: Biochem. Zeitschr., 1929, 209; 240–5.
Green and Mellanby: Brit. J. Exptl. Path., 1930, 11:81–89.
Goldblatt and Barnett: Proc. Soc. Exp. Biol. Med., 1932, 30:201–204.
Eusterman and Wilbur: J. A. M. A., 1932, 98:2054.

CUPRIFERRUM

Guerithault, B.: Bull. soc. hyg. aliment: 1927, 15:387.
Hart, E. B., et al.: J. Biol. Chem., 1928, 77:769, 777, 797.
Mackay, H.: Lancet, 1928, 2:1140.
Editorial review: J. Nutrition, 1929, 1:545.
Hart, E. B., et al.: J. Biol. Chem., 1929, 83:243.
Galloway, C. E.: J. A. M. A., 1929, 93:1695.
Flinn, F. B. and Inouie, J. M.: J. Biol. Chem., 1929, 86:101.
McCollum, E. V. and Simmonds, N.: Newer Knowledge of Nutrition; MacMillan, New York, ed. 4, 1929.
Lindlow, C. W., Elvehjem, C. A., and Peterson, W. H.: J. Biol. Chem., 1929, 82:469.
Mills, Edward S.: Canad. Med. A. J., 1930, 22:175.
Dwyer, H. V.: J. Mich. State Med. Soc., 1930, 29:420.
Lewis, Milton Smith: J. A. M. A., 1931, 96:1135.

CUPROGLOBIN

Whipple, S. H.: Hemoglobin Construction within the Body; Am. J. M. Sc., June, 1928.
Waddell, J., Elvehjem, C. A., Hart, E. B. and Steenbock, H.: Copper Essential Synergist to Iron in Treatment of Nutritional Anemias; Biol. Chem., July, 1929.
Silberschmidt, Paul: Jahrb. f. Kinderh., September, 1930.
Gelston, C. F. and Sappington, E. E.: Am. J. Dis. Child., April, 1930.
Parson, Leonard G.: Research in Pediatrics; Arch. Pediat., Vol. 48, No. 7, 1931.
Josephs, H. W.: Treatment of Anemias of Infancy With Copper and Iron; John Hopkins Univ. Pediat. Clinic.

DECHOLIN

Neufeld: Zeit. f. Hyg. u. Infektionskrankh. 1900, 34:454; Arb. a. d. k. Gsndhtsamte, 1907, 25:494.
Castellanos y Gonzales, A.: Rev. de. med. y ciruj. de la Habana, 1929, 34:133.
Gehling, J.: Zur Verbesserung der roentgenologischen Darstellung der Gallenblase; Deut. med. Wochensch., 54:2055, 1928, and 1929, 55:1220.
Leischner, A. W.: Med. Klin., 1930, 26:1582.
Taterka, H.: Ueber eine Verbesserung der Rontgendiagnostik der Gallenblase; Med. Welt., 1930, 4: 1722.
Ziegler, E. E.: The Specific Effect of Bile Salts on Pneumococci and on Pneumococcus Pneumonia; Arch. Int. Med., 1930, 46:644-656.
Sterner, R. F., Bartle, H. J. and Lyon, B. B. V.: Am. J. M. Sc., 1931, 182:822.
Jankelson and Altman: New England Jour. of Med., 1932, 206-796, 799.
Appel, B.: Sodium Dehydrocholate in Arsphenamine Poisoning, Preliminary Report; Arch. f. Dermat. und Syph., 1933, 27:401.

DEXIN

Ruickshank, R. C.: Dextrin in the Diet; Brit. J. Exptl. Path., 1928, 9:318.

DEXTRETTES "ESKAY"

Missler, C. W. and Gordon B.: Penna. M. J., December, 1929.
Missler, C. W., En Shui Tai and Gordon, B.: N. Y. State J. Med., July 15, 1931.

DEXTRI-MALTOSE NOS. 1, 2 AND 3

Barton, D. J.: Congenital pyloric stenosis; J. South Carolina M. A., 1930, 26:281.
Marriott, W. M.: Infant Nutrition, C. V. Mosby Co., St. Louis, 1930, p. 44.
Weinfeld, G. F. and Floore, F. B.: Infant feeding with Unlimited Amounts of a Concentrated and a Dilute Cow's Milk Formula; Am. J. Dis. Child., 1930, 40:1208.
Daniels, A. L. and Forman, M. B.: Relation of Various Substances Used in the Artificial Feeding Mixtures of Infants to Nutritional Anemia; Proc. Soc. Exp. Biol. Med., 1931, 28:431.
Curry, C. A.: Hypertrophic Pyloric Stenosis; Medical Arts, 1932, 35:14.
Lynch, H. D.: Powdered Citric Acid Milk in Infant Feeding; Arch. Pediat., 1932, 49:763.
Sauer, L. W.: Nursery Guide, C. V. Mosby Co., St. Louis, 1933, p. 63.
Grulee, C. G. and Bonar, B. E.: Clinical Pediatrics, D. Appleton and Co., New York, vol. 2, p. 158.

DEXTRI-MALTOSE WITH VITAMIN B

Hoobler, B. R.: Symptomatology of Vitamin B Deficiency in Infants; J. A. M. A., 1928, 91:307.
Bloxsom, A. P.: Vitamin B Requirements in Infancy; Am. J. Dis. Child., 1929, 37:1161.
West, J. H.: Supplying the Breast-Fed Baby with Vitamin B; Arch. Pediat., 1929, 46:646.
Young, J. G.: The Effect of Infections upon Peristalsis and Appetite With an Outline of Appetite Management; Texas State J. M., 1930, 26:374.
Hoobler, B. R.: Use of Vitamin B in Diets of Infants; J. A. M. A., 1931, 96:675, 1931.
Waring, J. I.: Vitamin B Feeding of Infants; J. South Carolina M. A., 1931, 27:322.
Cowgill, G. R.: Vitamin B in Relation to the Clinic; J. A. M. A., 1932, 98:2282.
Henricke, S. G.: The Vitamin B Complex: Its Role in Infant Feeding in the Light of our Present Knowledge; Northwest Med., 1932, 31:165.
Langhorst, H. F.: Vitamins: Their Role in the Prevention and Treatment of Disease; Med. Jour. and Record, 1932, 135:326.

DEXTROSE—RINGER'S CONCENTRATE

Horsley, J. Shelton: The Influence of Physiologic Research on Modern Surgery; Virginia Med. Monthly, 1929, 55:790.
Horsley, J. Shelton: The Intravenous Administration of Dextrose in Ringer's Solution; J. of Tenn. State Med. Asso., 1930, 23:169.
Horsley, J. Shelton and Horsley, Guy W.: Continuous Intravenous Injection of Dextrose in Ringer's Solution; Arch. of Surg., 1931, 22:86.

DEXTRO-VITAVOSE

Hoffman, C. J.: Ind. Eng. Chem., 1925, 17:498.
Cowgill, G. R. et al.: Am. J. Physiol., 1925, 73:106.
McKee, J. H.: Atlantic Med. J., 1926, 29:618.
Macy, I. G. et al.: J. Biol. Chem., 1927, 73:189, 203.
Sure, B.: J. Biol. Chem., 1927, 74:37.
Sherman, H. C.: Chemistry of Food and Nutrition, Ed. 3, New York, The MacMillan Company, 1927.
Sherman, H. C. and Axtmayer, J. H., J. Biol. Chem., 1927, 75:207.
Goldberger, J. and Wheeler, G. A.: Pub. Health Rep., 1927, 42:2383.
Hoobler, B. R.: J. A. M. A., 1928, 91:307.
Mackay, H.: Lancet, 1928, 2:1140.
McCollum, E. V. and Simmonds, N.: The Newer Knowledge of Nutrition, Ed. 4, 1929.
Dennett, R. H.: J. A. M. A., 1929, 92:769.

DIAL

Hirschfeld: Deut. med. Wochensch., 1914, 40:1221.
Stern: Berl. klin. Wochensch., 1914, 51:1262.
Christoffel: Zeit. f. d. ges. Neurol. Psychiat., 1918, 43:49.
Bürgi: Therap. d. Gegenw., April and June, 1925, pp. 145–150 and 302–508.
Craig: Brit. Med. Jour., May 28, 1927, p. 983.
Gillespie, Stuart-Low and Craig: Brit. Med. Jour., June 18, 1927, pp. 1125–1127.
Fulton, Liddell and Rioch: J. Pharm. and Exper. Therap., 1930, 40:423.
Fulton, Liddell and Rioch: J. Phys., 1930, 70:23.

DIBROMIN

Fallis, Wm. E.: The Efficiency of Dibromin; Med. Standard, March, 1922, page 15.
Hawkins, J. A.: Spontaneous Gangrene of the Scrotum; Milit. Surgeon, April, 1922, pp. 419–22.
Niddrie, R. J.: Canad. J. of Med. and Surg., May, 1922, p. 205.
Pirkey, M. E.: Treatment of Maxillary Sinus Infections with Dibromin., Med. Times, May, 1922, p. 736.
DeMartigny, F.: "Dibromin" Improved Surgical Disinfectant; Canad. Pract. and Rev., May, 1922, pp. 209–211.
Roberts, D. Y.: Am. Physician, May, 1922, p. 355.
Ellars, L. R.: Treatment of Infected Wounds; Internat. J. of Surg., Feb., 1922, p. 72.
St. Pierre, Chas.: Therap. Gaz., June, 1922, p. 338.
Murray, W. B.: Conclusions from treating 500 cases; West. Med. Times, Dec., 1922, pp. 179–181.
Paul, C. M.: Treatment of Surgical Infections; Internat. J. of Surg., Jan., 1923, p. 40.

DIGIFOLINE

Hartung: Arch. f. exper. Pathol. u. Pharmakol, 1912, 69:149.
Hartung: Münch. med. Wochensch., 1912, 59:1944.
Chevalier: Bull. gen. de Therap. med. chir., obst. et pharm., 1913, 165:914–929.
Hartung: Pharmazeutische Post, 1913, 46:421.
Holste: Arch. f. exper. Pathol. u. Pharmakol., 1913, 73:457.
Bürgi: Jahreskurse für aerztliche Fortbildung, Augustheft, 1915, p. 18.
Bürgi: Jahreskurse für ärztliche Fortbildung, 1920, 11:3.

DIGIFORTIS

Eggleston, Cary: Arch. Int. Med., 1915, 16:1–32; ibid., 1922, 30:133–157; J. A. M. A., March 13, 1920, p. 733.
Pardee: N. Y. State J. of Med., March, 1922 and February, 1924.
Willius, F. R.: Northwest Med., March, 1924.
Reports Council Pharm. and Chem., 1925, p. 75.

DIGISMITH AND DIGILUTEA PREPARATIONS

White, Marx: Lancet, March 15, 1917, pp. 176–181.
Morris: Minnesota Med., April, 1918.
Morris: Arch. Int. Med., 1918, 21:740.
Eggleston: Arch. Int. Med., 1922, 30:133.
Starling, E. H. and Visscher, M. B.: The Regulation of the Energy Output of the Heart; J. of Phys., 1927, 62:243.
Bodo, R.: The Effect of Heart Tonics and Other Drugs on the Heart Tone and Coronary Circulation; J. of Phys., 1928, 64:365.

DILAUDID

Gottlieb: Vergleichende Messungen ueber die Gewoehnung des Atemzentrums an Morphin, Dicodid und Dilaudid; Munch. med. Wochensch., 1926, Nr. 15, S. 595–597.
Krehl: Aerztliche Erfahrungen mit Dilaudid; Munch. med. Wochensch., 1926, Nr. 15.
Leyton: Dihydromorphinone Hydrochloricum (Dilaudid); Lancet, 1932, 1:835.
Alvarez: Dihydromorphinone Hydrochloride (Dilaudid) A Powerful Analgesic with Some Advantages over Morphine; Proc. of the Staff Meetings of the Mayo Clinic, August 17, 1932.
Menard: Dilaudid for Intractable Pain; Surgical Clinics of North America, 1933, 13:727.
J. A. M. A., April 1, 1933, p. 1031.

DIMAZON

Haass: Ophthalmology; J. for Therapeutics and Hygiene of the Eye, Dresden, 1913, No. 40.
Fischer, Franz: Dermatol. Journal, Leipzig, 17th year, No. 8.

DIMOL

Editorial; N. Y. Med. Jour. and Rec., April 18, 1923.
J. A. M. A., October 6, 1923, p. 1224.
Solis-Cohen and Githens: Pharmacotherapeutics, Materia Medica and Drug Action, 1928, p. 1205.

DIONIN

Dibailoff, S. S.: Beobachtungen uber Wirkung des Heroin und Dionin; Prakt. Wratsch, 1903, Nr. 34.
Deutsch, E.: Therapeutische Erfahrungen aus der Kinderpraxis. Einiges uber Pertussisbehandlung; Centralbl. f. Kinderh., 1904, Nr. 3.
Wiesner, A.: Neuere Arzneimittel gegen Keuchhusten; Heilmittel Revue, 1905, Nr. 9.
Lustwerk, E.: Zur kombinierten Verwendung von Veronal und Dionin; Allg. med. Centr.-Zeitg., 1907, Nr. 34.
Wilcox, D. D.: Dionin in Chronic Atrophic Rhinitis and Chronic Dry Pharyngitis; Virginia Med. Semi-Monthly, 1908, January 24.
Reif: Mitteilung uber die Anwendung von Dionin; Med. Klin. 1910, Nr. 9.
Apostolides: On the Treatment of Bronchial Asthma; April–July, 1911, Folia Therap.
Lindenmayr, J.: Zur Therapie des Schnupfens und seiner Komplikationen; Berl. klin. Wochensch., 1912, Nr. 17.
Rosenthal, H.: Zur Behandlung des Schnupfens; Deut. med. Wochensch., 1915, Nr. 13.

DIPHTHERIA ANTITOXIN

Reports Council Pharm. and Chem., 1917, p. 146; 1921, p. 23; 1922, p. 30.
Tuft, L.: Rate of Absorption of Horse Serum; J. A. M. A., 1929, 92:1667.
Cecil, R. L.: Textbook of Medicine; W. B. Saunders Co., Philadelphia, 1929, pp. 39, 472.
Park, William H.: Serum Therapy; Am. Med., 1931, 37:5 (supplement).

DIPHTHERIA TOXIN

Bunney, William E.: J. Immunol., 1931, 20:71.
White, Bunney and Malcolm: J. Immunol., 1932, 22:93.

DIPHTHERIA TOXOID

Dick: J. A. M. A., June 8, 1929, p. 1901.
Moloney, P. J.: Am. J. Pub. Health, 1926, 16:1208.
Ramon and Helie: J. A. M. A., 1928, 91:1028.
Thompson: J. Ind. M. A., 1929, 22:522.
Barnes, D. J.: J. Mich. Med. Soc., 1931, 12:949.
Hartzell, Ray H.: Am. J. M. Sc., 1931, 182:251.
Greengard, Joseph: J. A. M. A., 1931, 97:228.
Harrison, W. T.: Am. J. Pub. Health, 1932, 22:17.
Park and Schroder: Am. J. Pub. Health, 1932, 22:7.

DISKETS SODIUM BROMIDE COMPOUND

Nelson, E. S. and Keeton, R. W.: The Treatment of Nausea and Certain Related Circulatory Sensations; J. A. M. A., 1928, 90:683.

DIURETIN

Breuer: Treatment and Pathogenesis of Stenocardia and Allied Conditions; Munch. med. Wochensch., 1902, No. 39, 40 and 41.
Askanazy: Clinical Notes on Diuretin; Deut. Archiv. fur klin. Medizin, 1905, 56:209.
Journal A. M. A., April 4, 1914, p. 1108; Reports Chem. Lab., 1914, p. 7; Propaganda, Vol. 1, p. 251.
Heathcote: Action of Caffeine, Theobromine and Theophylline on the Mammalian and Batrachian Heart; J. Pharm. and Exper. Therap., 1920, 16:327.
Marriott, McK: Gebrauch von Theobromin-natr. sal (Diuretin) zur Behandlung von Hydrocephalus; Am. J. Dis. Child., 1924, Vol. 28, No. 4.
Gilbert and Fenn: The Effect of the Purine Base Diuretics on the Coronary Flow; Arch. Int. Med., 1929, 44:118.

DRYCO

Andresen, O.: Irradiated Milk in the Treatment of Rickets; Arch. f. Kinderh. 90:65, 1930; Abs. Am. J. Dis. Child., Jan., 1931, Vol. 41, No. 1.
Davies, W. L.: The Action of Strong Sunlight on Milk; Certified Milk, May, 1931.
Davies, A. G., Armstrong, G. L. and O'Brien, Brian: Combined Bactericidal and Antirachitic Effects Induced in Milk Through Carbon Arc Irradiation; Part 1, Certified Milk, Feb., 1931.
Editorial: Colorado Sunshine; J. A. M. A., March 28, 1931, Vol. 96, No. 13.
Hess, A. F. and Smith, Philip E.: Excessive Ultra-violet Irradiation; Am. J. Dis. Child., April, 1931, Vol. 41, No. 4.
Watson, Chalmers: Irradiated Milk—What It Is—What It Can Do; Certified Milk, April, 1931.
Sperti, George: Vitamin D (Antirachitic) Content of Milk Increased by Selective Rays; Certified Milk, Feb., 1931.

DYSCO

Lang, O.: Zentralbl. f. Gynaek., 1927, 51:1043.

EKZEBROL

Nobl: Wien. klin. Wochensch., 1925, No. 43.
Loewenfeld: Med. Klin., 1925, No. 40.
Lennartz: Munch. med. Wochensch., 1925, No. 17.
Minami, S.: Jap. J. of Dermat. and Urology, 1926, No. 4.
Hehner: Borgyogaszati Urologiai es Venerologiai Szemle, 1926, No. 12.
Kadisch and Ritter: Therap. d. Gegenw., January, 1927.
Nees: Munch. Med. Wochensch., 1927, No. 36.
Esser: Der Landarzt, 1927, No. 42.

ELDOFORM

Heidingsfeld, H.: Munch. med. Wochensch., No. 32, 1922.
Bassenge, E.: Therap. d. Gegenw., No. 9, 1923.
DeRudder, B.: Klin. Wochensch., No. 20, 1923.
Weber, H.: Med. Klin., No. 22, 1924.
Kern, H.: Therap. d. Gegenw., Feb. 1924.
Mader, E. J.: Munch. med. Wochensch., No. 18, 1925.

EMBO

Cooper, E. H.: The Protective and Curative Properties of Certain Foodstuffs Against Polyneuritis Induced in Birds by a Diet of Polished Rice; J. Hyg., 1912, 12:436.
Chick, H. and Hume, E. M.: Proc. Roy. Soc., London (Ser. B.), 1917, 90:44.
Bell, M. and Mendel, L. B.: Distribution of Vitamin B in Wheat Kernel; Am. J. Physiol., 1922, 62:146.
Waddell, J. and Steenbock, H.: The Destruction of Vitamin E in a Ration Composed of Natural and Varied Foodstuffs; J. Biol. Chem., 1928, 80:431.
Waring, J. I.: Beriberi in Infants; Am. J. Dis. Chil., 1929, 38:52.
Szarka, A.: Die Wirkung von "E" Vitamin auf die ovarialfunktion; Pfluger's Arch., 1929, 223:657.
Aykroyd, W. R. and Roscoe, M. H.: Distribution of Vitamin B in Certain Foods; Biochem. J., 1929, 23:483.
Tisdall, F. F., Drake, T. G. H. and Brown, A.: A New Cereal Mixture Containing Vitamins and Mineral Elements; Amer. J. Dis. Child., 1930, 40:1.
Aykroyd, W. R. and Roscoe, M. H.: The Effect of Parboiling and Milling on the Antineuritic Vitamin B and Phosphate Content of Rice; J. Hyg., 1932, 52:184.

ENDOMIN TABLETS

Beard, H. H., Baker, R. W. and Myers, V. C.: Studies in the Nutritional Anaemia of the Rat. V. The Action of Iron and Iron Supplemented with Other Elements Upon the Daily Reticulocyte, Erythrocyte, and Hemoglobin Response; J. Biol. Chem., 1931, 94:123.
Beard, H. H.: Studies in the Nutritional Anaemia of the Rat. VI. The Effect of Inorganic Elements Upon the Rate of Blood Regeneration and Growth; J. Biol. Chem., 1931, 94:135.
Josephs, H.: Treatment of Anaemia of Infancy with Iron and Copper; Johns Hopkins Hosp. Bull., 1931, 49:246.
Orten, J. M., Underhill, F. A., Mugrage, E. R. and Lewis, R. C.: Production of Experimental Polycythemia with Cobalt; Proc. Soc. Exp. Biol. Med., 1931, 29:174.
Editorial, Nutritional Anaemia; J. A. M. A., 1932, 98:320.
Elvehjem, C. A. and Hart, E. R.: The Necessity of Copper as a Supplement to Iron for Hemoglobin Formation in the Pig; J. Biol. Chem., 1932, 95:363.
Leichsenring, J. M. and Flor, I. H.: The Iron Requirement of the Pre-School Child; Jr. of Nutrition, 1932, 5:141.
Josephs, Hugh W.: Studies on Iron Metabolism and the Influence of Copper; J. Biol. Chem., 1932, 96:55.

EPHEDRINE

Chen, K. K. and Schmidt, C. F.: Action and Clinical Use of Ephedrine; J. A. M. A., Sept. 11, 1926, p. 836.
Chen, K. K.: A Study of Ephedrine; Brit. Med. Jour., Oct., 1927, p. 593.

EPHEDRINE AND SALTS

Miller, T. G.: A consideration of the clinical value of Ephedrine; Am. J. M. Sc., 1925, 170:157.
Thomas, W. S.: Clinical Uses of Ephedrine; N. Y. State J. Med., 1927, 27:831.
Rudolpe, R. D. and Graham, J. D.: Notes of Sulphate of Ephedrine; Am. J. M. Sc., 1927, 173:399.
Pitkin, G. P.: Controllable Spinal Anesthesia; J. Med. Soc. N. J., 1927, 24:425.
Dittman, G. C.: Newer Methods of Ocular Therapeusis; Am. J. Ophth., 1927, 10:362, Series 3.
Ramirez, M. A.: Statistical Report on the Treatment of Hay Fever; Am. J. M. Sc., 1928, 176:856.
Babcock, W. W.: Spinal Anesthesia; Am. J. Surg., 1928, 5:571.
Wallace, H. K.: Use of Ephedrine in Spinal Anesthesia; J. A. M. A., 1928, 90:144.
Schoenberg, M. J.: Experience with Ephedrine in Ophthalmic Practice; Arch. Ophth., 1928, 57:272.
Barlow, A.: Ephedrine and Glaucoma; Am. J. Ophth., 1930, 13:687, Series 3.
Editorial: Ephedrine and Habit Formation; J. A. M. A., 1930, 95:731.

Seevers, M. H.: Some observations on Ephedrine Addiction in Laboratory Animals; J. Pharm. and Exper. Therap., 1930, 39:251.

ERYSIPELAS STREPTOCOCCUS DISEASE

Tunnicliff, Ruth: J. A. M. A., 1920, 75:1339.
Birkhaug: Bull. Johns Hopkins Hosp., 1925, 36:248. Proc. Soc. Exp. Biol. Med., 1925, 23:201.
Rivers and Tillett: J. Exper. Med., 1925, 41:185.
Stevens and Dochez: J. Exper. Med., 1926, 44:439.
Musser: J. A. M. A., 1927, 88:1125.
Symmers and Lewis: J. A. M. A., 1927, 89:880.
Platou, Schultz and Collins: Am. J. Dis. Child., 1927, 34:1030.
Allan: Proc. Staff Meetings, Mayo Clinic, 1928, 3:23.
Symmers: J. A. M. A., 1928, 91: 535.
Tauber, E.: J. Med., December, 1928.
Gordon, J. E. and Young, D. C.: I. Mich. State Med. Soc., May, 1929.
J. A. M. A., October 11, 1924, p. 1184; Reports Council Pharm. and Chem., 1924, p. 57.
J. A. M. A., January 5, 1929, p. 55; Reports Council Pharm. and Chem., 1928, p. 43.

ERYTHROL TETRANITRATE

Wallace and Ringer: The Lowering of Blood Pressure by the Nitrite Group; J. A. M. A., 1909, 53:1629.
Matthew; Quart. J. Med., 2:261, 1909.

ESCHATIN

Swingle, W. W. and Pfiffner, J. J.: Science, 1930, 71:321–322, 489–490; 1930, 72:75–76; Amer. J. Physiol. 1931, 96:153–163, 164–179; Proc. Soc. Exp. Biol. Med., 1931, 28:510–512.
Pfiffner, J. J. and Swingle, W. W.: Amer. J. Physiol., 1931, 96:180–190; Endocrinology, 1931, 15:335–340.
Rowntree, L. G., Greene, C. H., Swingle, W. W. and Pfiffner, J. J.: J. A. M. A., 1931, 96:231; Science, 1930, 72:482.
Swingle, W. W., Pfiffner, J. J. and Webster, B.: Proc. Soc. Exp. Biol. Med., 1931, 28:728.
Harrop, G. A., Pfiffner, J. J., Weinstein, A. and Swingle, W. W.: Science, 1931, 73:683; Proc. Soc. Exp. Biol. Med., 1932, 29:449.
Webster, B., Pfiffner, J. J., Swingle, W. W. and Pfiffner, J. J.: Am. J. M. Sc., 1932, 183:1.

ESTIVIN

J. A. M. A., November 12, 1921, p. 1595; January 23, 1932, p. 340; vol. 2, p. 466.
Newton, F.: Internat. J. Med. and Surg., Vol. 39, No. 9.

ETHYL IODIDE

Lawrence, R. M.: Boston Med. and Surg. Jour., 1880, 102:428.
Henderson, Y. and Haggard, H. W.: Am. J. Physiol., 1925, 73:193.
Swartz, J. H., Blumgart, H. L. and Altschyle, M. D.: Arch. of Derm. and Syph., 1930, 21:182.

EUQUININE

Hartigan, W.: Euquinine in Blackwater Fever; W. J. J. Trop. Med., Jan. 15, 1906.
Grande, Emanuel: Quinine Salts and Euquinine in Malaria Infection during Pregnancy; Gazz. d. osp., 1909, No. 9.
Smith, L. E.: Treatment of Malaria; Ky. M. J., April, 1931, p. 170.
Manson-Bahr, Philip: Quinine Therapy in Malaria; Lancet, April 18, 1931, p. 844.

EURESOL

Powell: Treatment of Intractable Skin Diseases with Euresol; Merck's Arch., September, 1908.
White: Alopecia and Seborrhea; J. A. M. A., Sept. 24, 1910.
McCafferty: Alopecia and its Treatment; N. Y. Med. Jour. and Rec., Oct. 4, 1922.
Nobl: Zur Behandlung juckender Dermatosen; Sonderbeilage der Wien. Klin. Wochr. No. 43, 1925.
Goodman: Treatment of Common Skin Diseases; Medical Lay Press, New York, 1932.

EXICOL

Copher and Kodama: Arch. Int. Med., Vol. 38, No. 5, November, 1926.
Ivy, A. C.: Am. J. M. Sc., No. 4, April, 1927.
Levinson, B.: Med. Jour. and Record, No. 12, June, 1927.
Whitaker, L. R.: J. A. M. A., Vol. 88, No. 23, June, 1927.
Stewart and Ryan: Am. J. Roentg. and Rad. Ther. 19, No. 4, April, 1928.
Ivy, A. C., and Oldberg, E.: Am. J. Physiol., 1928, 86:599–613.
Ivy, A. C.: Am. J. Surg., Oct., 1929, pp. 455–459.
Stewart, Wm. H. and Ryan, E. J.: Am. J. Roentg. and Rad. Ther. 19, No. 4, April, 1928.
Crandall: Arch. Int. Med., 1931, 48:1217.
J. A. M. A., July 16, 1932, p. 224; Reports Council Pharm. and Chem., 1932, p. 45.

EXTRALIN

Minot, G. R. and Murphy, W. P.: Treatment of Pernicious Anemia by Special Diet; J. A. M. A., 1926, 87:470.

Cohn, E. J., Minot, G. R., Alles, G. A. and Salter, W. T.: Nature of Material in Liver Effective in Pernicious Anemia; J. Biol. Chem., May, 1928, p. 325.

Cohn, E. J., McMeekin, T. L. and Minot, G. R.: The Nature of the Material Effective in Pernicious Anemia; J. Biol. Chem., 1930, 87:49.

West, R. and Howe, M.: Material from Liver Active in Pernicious Anemia; J. A. M. A., 1931, 97:685.

Castle, W. B., Townsend, W. C. and Heath, C. W.: Observations on the Etiologic Relationship of Achylia Gastrica to Pernicious Anemia, III; Am. J. M. Sc., 1930, 180:305.

Walden, G. B. and Clowes, G. H. A.: On the Treatment of Pernicious Anemia; Proc. Soc. Exp. Biol. Med., 1932, 29:873.

Minot, G. R., Cohn, E. J., Murphy, W. P. and Lawson, H. A.: Treatment of Pernicious Anemia with Liver Extract; Am. J. M. Sc., 1928, 175:599.

Sturgis, C. C. and Isaacs, R.: Clinical and Experimental Observations on Treatment of Pernicious Anemia with Desiccated Stomach and with Liver Extract; Ann. Int. Med., 1931, 5:131.

Zerfas, L. G.: Liver Extract for Pernicious Anemia: Blood Changes During First Month; Report of 101 Cases; Arch. Int. Med., 1931, 47:135.

FARASTAN

Ross, Joseph G.: Med. Rev. of Reviews, Aug., 1929.

Fahlstrom, Stanley: Arthritis; Ill. Med. Jour., Sept., 1930.

J. A. M. A., February 15, 1930, p. 484; Reports Council Pharm. and Chem., 1930, p. 33.

Rudnick, D. E. and Burstein, H. J.: Ill. Med. Jour., June, 1931.

Fitch, Wm. E.: Neuritis; Clin. Med. and Surg., Apr., 1931.

Markson, D. E.: Am. Med., Feb., 1931.

Geckeler, Edwin O. and Vischer, Carl V.: The Hahnemannian Monthly, Jan., 1931.

White, E. P. Corson: J. Lab. and Clin. Med., Oct., 1931.

Bloomfield, M. D.: A Basic Treatment for the Relief of Persistent, Agonizing, Neural Pains; Am. Med., Sept., 1932.

FELAMINE

Larcher: Sciences Medicales, March 15, 1923.

Oppenheimer: Munch. med. Wochensch., 50, 1923.

Skutetsky: Wien. med. Wochensch., 7, 1923.

Pfaff: Deut. med. Wochensch., 52, 1923.

Vialard: Sciences Medicales, 31, 1924.

Kaiser: Prakt. Artz, 191, 1925.

Rivaz Hunt: Lancet, Oct. 23, 1926.

Calcaterra: Azione Sanitaria, 3, 1927.

Zahn: Klin. Wochensch., 32, Vol. 1.

FELSOL

Schw. med. Wochensch., No. 36, Sep. 4, 1924.

J. A. M. A., May 28, 1927, p. 1750.

Magyar Orvos, Budapest, July 15, 1932.

Fortsch. d. Medizin, Berlin Jahrgang 41, No. 5.

Fortsch. d. Medizin, Berlin, No. 17, October 24.

Mediz. Welt, Berlin, Jahrgang 4, No. 13.

FERMOGEN

Kelemen: Clinical Results with Fermogen; Magyar Urvos, March, 1932.

J. A. M. A., July 29, 1933, p. 389.

FERROPHYTINE

Rosner: Przeglad Dentystyczny, No. 7, pp. 188–192, 1929.

Szilagyi: Monatssch. Ungar. Mediziner, 1929, 3:41.

Meurisse: Le Progress Medical, No. 28, pp. 308–310, July 10, 1930.

FIBROLYSIN

Luedde, W. H.: Fibrolysin; Tr. Am. Ophth. Soc., 1919, XVII.

Greenbaum, Sigmund S.: Thiosinamin in the Treatment of Arsphenamin Dermatitis; J. A. M. A., 1924, 83:38–40.

Kretschmer, H. L. and Fester, G. M.: Plastic Induration of the Penis; J. Urol., 1926, 16:497–514.

Pugh, W. S.: Stricture of the Urethra; Internat. Clin., Vol. 4, Series 37, 1927.

Shalluck, H. P.: Postcicatricial Keloid; Clin. Med., Aug. 1928, pp. 603–604.

Kovacevic, Z.: 1,000 cases of Pulmonary Tuberculosis Treated with Fibrolysin; Aerztl. Rundschau. No. 26.

FERRO SAJODIN

See references for "Sajodin."

FIBROGEN ORAL AND SUBCUTANEOUS

Mills, C. A.: The Activity of Lung Extract as Compared to Extracts of Other Tissues in Inducing Coagulation of the Blood; J. Biol. Chem., 1919, 40:425.
Mills, C. A.: The Action of Tissue Extracts in the Coagulation of the Blood; J. Biol. Chem., 1921, 46:167.
Mills, C. A.: Chemical Nature of Tissue Coagulins; J. Biol. Chem., 1921, 46:135.
Mills, C. A., Dorst, S. E., Mychenberg, George and Nayakama, Joseph: Absorption from the Intestine and Excretion from the Kidney of an Unaltered Complex Protein Substance, Tissue Fibrinogen; Am. J. Physiol., 1923, 63:484.
Mills, C. A.: Hemorrhages: Their Significance and Methods of Treatment; Am. J. M. Sc., 1926, 172:71.

FOLLUTEIN

Zondek, B. and Aschheim, S.: Klin. Wochensch., 1928, 7:831.
Friedman, M. H.: Am. J. Physiol., 1929, 90:617.
VanDyke, H. B. and Wallen-Lawrence, Z.: J. Pharm. and Exper. Therap., 1930, 40:413.
Hill, M. and Parkes, A. S.: J. Physiol., 1930, 68:33.
Jares: Anat. Rec., 1930, 45:264.
Graves, W. P.: Am. J. Obst. and Gynec., 1930, 20:500.
Reichert, F. L., Pencharz, R. I., Simpson, M. E., Meyer, K. and Evans, H. M.: Proc. Soc. Exp. Biol. Med., 1931, 28:843.
Evans, H. M. and Simpson, M. E.: Am. J. Physiol., 1931, 95:511.
Burch, U. C., Williams, W. L., and Cunningham, R. S.: Surg., Gynec. and Obst., 1931, 53:338.
Novak, E. and Hurd, G. B.: Am. J. Obst. and Gynec., 1931, 22:501.
Evans, H. M., Meyer, K. and Simpson, M. E.: Am. J. Physiol., 1932, 100:141.
Mazer, C. and Goldstein, L.: Clinical Endocrinology of the Female, W. B. Saunders Co., Phila., 1932.

FOOD FERRIN

Mitchell: J. Biol. Chem., 1927, 75:123; 1929, 85:355.
Hughes: J. Biol. Chem., 1928, 80:565; 1929, 83, 463.
Hart, Steenbock, Waddell and Elvehizen: J. Biol. Chem., 1928, 77:797; 1929, 83:251.

FORTOSSAN

Streffer: Therapeutische Neuheiten, 1907, 2:169.
Loeb: Zentralbl. f. die gesamte Therapie, 1908, 26:602–604.
J. A. M. A., January 30, 1915, p. 456; Reports Council Pharm. and Chem., 1915, p. 131; Propag., vol. 1, p. 178.
Molinery: Le Concours Medical, 1917, 39:999.
Kovacz: Polska Gazeta Lekarska, 1927, 6:465.
Savigny: LaVie Medicale, 1930, 11:31.
Colas-Pelletier: Le Bulletin Medical, p. 659–660, 1931, 45:659.

GAS-GANGRENE ANTITOXIN

Flaum, A.: Compt. rend. Soc. de Biol., 1926, 95:1518.
Weintrob and Messeloff: Gas-Gangrene in Civil Practice; Am. J. M. Sc., 1927, 174:801–819.
Tenopyr, J.: Treatment of Aerogenes Capsulatus; N. Y. State J. Med., 1927, 27:16–18.
Bower and Clark: Bacillus Welchi; Am. J. M. Sc., 1928, 176:97–102.
Smith, G. A.: J. A. M. A., Dec. 14, 1929.
Boland, Frank J.: Ann. Surgery, Oct., 1929.

GASTRIC MUCIN

Klug, F.: Arch. Internat. de physiol., 1907, 5:297.
Ivy, A. C. and Oyama, Yutaka: Am. J. Physiol., 1921, 57:51.
Lim, R. K. S.: Am. J. Physiol., 1924, 69:318.
Hardy, T. L.: Lancet, 1929, I:711.
Palmer, W. L.: Arch. Int. Med., 1930, 46:165.
Kim, M. S. and Ivy, A. C.: J. A. M. A., 1931, 97:1511.
Fogelson, S. J.: J. A. M. A., 1931, 96:673.
Atkinson, A. J.: J. A. M. A., 1932, 98:153.
J. Am. Dietet. A., 1932, 7:359.
Whitlow, J. E.: The Protective Action of Mucus; Masters Thesis Loyola University (Unpublished).

GENTIAN VIOLET IMPROVED MEDICINAL

Abraham, Joseph H.: Laryngoscope, August, 1924.
Churchman: J. A. M. A., Vol. 70, p. 1047.

Churchman: J. A. M. A., Vol. 74, pp. 145–148.
Smith and Casparis: J. A. M. A., Vol. 81, p. 2184.
Waters: Amer. Rev. Tub., Vol. 4, p. 875.

GLUCO-CALCIUM

Cameron, A. T.: The Biochemistry of Calcium; Canad. Med. A. J., 1926, 16:753.
Cameron, A. T.: The Practical Application of Our Present Knowledge of Calcium Metabolism; Canad. Med. A. J., 1926, 16:759.
Kahn, B. S. and Roe, J. H.: Calcium Absorption from the Intestinal Tract in Human Subjects; J. A. M. A., 1926, 86:1761.
Collip, J. B.: The Therapeutic Value of the Parathyroid Hormone; J. A. M. A., 1926, 87:909.
Libermann, A. L.: Comparative Studies on Calcium Gluconate and Other Calcium Salts; J. A. M. A. 1931, 97:15.

GLYCINE

Milhorat, Techner and Thomas: Proc. Soc. Exp. Biol. Med., Feb., 1932.

GLYCOTAURO

Joslin: J. Exper. Med., 1900, 5:513.
Okada: J. of Phys., 1915, 50:457.
Hooper and Whipple: Am. J. Physiol., 1917, 42:264.
Lewis: South. Med. Jour., Dec, 1929, p. 868.
Palfrey: Boston Med. and Surg. Jour., 1922, 187:527.
Frazer: J. A. M. A., 1922, 79:1594.

GOLD SODIUM THIOSULPHATE

Mollgaard: The Chemotherapy of Tuberculosis, 1924.
Schamberg and Wright: Arch. of Derm. and Syph., 1927, 15:119.
Manley, W. F.: Virginia Med. Monthly, July, 1929, p. 255.
Markley, A. J. and Philpott, O. S.: Colorado Med., 1929, 26:177.
Saunders, H. C.: N. Y. State J. Med., 1929, 29:942.
Miller: Cal. and West. Med., October, 1929.
Towle, H. P. and Grund, J. L.: New England Jour. of Med., January 30, 1930.
Bernard, L.: Results of the Treatment of Pulmonary T. B. by Thiosulphate of Gold and Sodium; Ill. Med. Jour., 1931, 9:119.
Driver, J. R., Weller, J. N.: Untoward Results from the Use of Gold Compounds; Arch. of Derm. and Syph., 1931, 23:87.
Rutledge, W. U.: Lupus Erythematosus; Treatment with Gold Preparations; Arch. of Derm. and Syph., 1931, 23:874.

GONOCOCCUS VACCINOTHERAPY

Hyman, A.: Trans. Sect. on Gen.-Urin. Surg. of N. Y. Acad. of Med.; Internat. J. of Surg., October, 1921.
J. A. M. A., Jan. 17, 1925, p. 220; Reports Council Pharm. and Chem., 1924, p. 20.
J. A. M. A., Sept. 17, 1924, p. 984; Reports Council Pharm. and Chem., 1927, p. 37.
Reports Council Pharm. and Chem., 1928, p. 43.

GONOSAN

Boss, S.: Deuts. Med. Zeitung, 1902, p. 1153.
J. A. M. A., October 13, 1917, p. 1287; Reports Council Pharm. and Chem., 1917, p. 57; Propaganda vol. 2, p. 150.
Morton, H. H.: G. U. Diseases and Syphilis, 1918, p. 144–146.
Geiringer, D. and Campuzano, J.: Tice's Pract. of Med., 1920, p. 478.
Wolbarst, A. L.: Gonococcal Infection in Male, 1927, p. 64.
Neisser: Med. Klin. No. 14.

GYNERGEN

Stoll and Rothlin: Schw. med. Wochensch., November 5, 1927.
Hellman: Med. Jour. and Record, January 19, 1927.
Fohr: Zentralb. f. Gynaek., No. 3, 1927.
Nelson and Pattee: Am. J. Obst. and Gynec., July, 1928.
Rothlin: J. Pharm. and Exper. Therap., August, 1929.
Thompson: J. Amer. Pharm. Assoc., 1930.
Smith and Stohlman: J. Pharm. and Exper. Therap., 1930.
Lichtman: J. A. M. A., November 14, 1931.
Ignelzi: Med. Jour. and Record, May 4, 1932.
Report, Council Pharm. and Chem., New and Non-official Remedies, 1932, p. 190.

HALAZONE

Marshall: J. A. M. A., 1916, 67:1033.

HALIVER OIL PLAIN AND WITH VIOSTEROL 250D

Wolbach, S. B. and Howe, P. R.: J. Exper. Med., 1925, 42:753.
Mellanby, M. and Pattison, C. L.: Brit. Med. Jour., 1928, 2:1709.
Schmidt-Nielsen, S. and S.: Biochem. J., 1929, 23:1153.
Lassen, H. C. A.: J. Hyg., 1930, 30:300.
Tilden, E. B. and Miller, E. G.: J. Nutrition, 1930, 3:121.
Seifried, O.: J. Exper. Med., 1930, 52:519.
Sherman, H. C.: J. A. M. A., 1931, 97:1425.
Editorial: J. A. M. A., 1931, 97:782.
Hanke, Milton Theo.: J. Nutrition, 1931, 3:433.
Mellanby, E.: J. A. M. A., 1931, 96:325.
Wolfe, J. M. and Salter, H. P.: J. Nutrition, 1931, 4:185.
Sherman, H. C. and Smith: The Vitamins, 2nd edition.
Mendel, Lafayette B.: J. A. M. A., Jan. 4, 1932.

HELMITOL

Thompson, J. M.: Med. Record, Dec. 30, 1905.
Prentice, A. C.: Med. Rev. of Reviews, Dec., 1906.
Williams, J. A.: Brit. Med. Jour., May 18, 1907.
Garceau, Edgar: Am. J. Obst., Sept., 1907.
Lawson, Arnold: Med. Press, July 26, 1911.
Macklem, Glen Edrie: N. Y. Med. Jour., May 8, 1915.
Aronstam, N. E.: Med. Council, July, 1920.
J. A. M. A., January 22, 1921, p. 260; Reports Council Pharm. and Chem., 1920, p. 49; Propaganda vol. 2, p. 295.
Poulsen, Valdemar: Am. J. Dis. Child., July, 1923.
Beyea, Henry D.: Internat. Clinics, Vol. 2, Series 21.

HEPVISC

Chevalier: C. R. Acad. des Sciences, November, 1907.
Fabini and Antonini: C. R. Acad. de Medicine, Turin, May, 1911.
Mattei and Cavaroni: Pres. Medicale, August, 1926.
Major: J. A. M. A., July, 1926.
Langton and Macallum: Med. Jour. and Record, June, 1926.
O'Hart and Hoyt: Prog. Med., December, 1928.
Gley and Kisthinios: C. R. Soc. Biol. No. 12, 1929; Pres. Medicale, Oct., 1929.

HEXALET

Boxx, S.: Deut. med. Wochensch., No. 36, 1912.
Frank, S. Ernest R. W.: Munch med. Wochensch., No. 38, 1912.
Seegars, K.: Berl. klin. Wochensch., No. 38, 1912.
Kowanitz, Otto A.: Wien. klin. Wochensch., No. 1, 1913, p. 19.
Reports Council Pharm. and Chem., 1921, p. 27.

HEXYLRESORCINOL SOLUTION S.T. 37

Leonard, Veader and Feirer, Wm. A.: Bull. John Hopkins Hosp., 1927, 41:21; Surg., Gynec. and Obst., 1927, 45:603.
Feirer, W. A. and Leonard, Veader: Dent. Cosmos, June, 1927, p. 563.

HOLOCAIN

Wood, Casey A.: Am. Encyc. of Ophthal., 1913.
Fuchs, H. E.: Textbook of Ophthalmology, 1923, 7th ed.
May, Charles H.: Manual of Diseases of the Eye, 1924.
De Schweinitz, George E.: Diseases of the Eye, 1924.
Ball, James Moore: Modern Ophthalmology, 1926.

HOMOCAMFIN

Spengler, G.: Wien. med. Wochensch., No. 31, 1924.
Butzengeiger, O.: Munch. med. Wochensch., No. 37, 1924.
Kirch, Arnold: Wien. med. Wochensch., No. 14, 1924.
Lowinger, O.: Wien. klin. Wochensch., No. 15, 1924.
Kiefer, Robert: Arch. f. Kinderheilk., April 5, 1924.
Scheid, F.: Centralbl. f. Chirurg., No. 15, 1924.
Umber, F.: Munch. med. Wochensch., No. 2, 1924.

Grassman: Munch. med. Wochensch., July 17, 1925.
Fritz, W.: Wien. med. Wochensch., No. 25, 1925.
Hirschfelder, A. D.: Therap. Gaz., April, 1926.

HYCLORITE

Milroy, Thos. H.: Biochem. J., October, 1916, p. 453.
Taylor, H. D. and Austin, J. H.: The Solvent Action of Antiseptics on Necrotic Tissue; J. of Experim. Med., 1918, 27:155.
Cullen, G. E. and Taylor, H. D.: J. of Experim. Med., 1918, 28:681.
Hartwell and Butler: Surg., Gynec. and Obst., October, 1918, p. 82.

HYDROSAL

Sutton, Richard L.: Diseases of the Skin, 1928, pp. 126, 276, 407, 419, 1175.
Pusey, Wm. Allen and Rattner, Herbert: Arch. of Derm., Book 19, February 1, 1929.
Foote, E. Milton: Textbook of Minor Surgery.
Abt, Isaac A.: Diseases of the Skin, Vol. 8, pp. 52, 55, 149, 186, 374.
Politzer, Adam: Textbook of Diseases of the Ear, p. 210.
Ballinger, Wm.: Diseases of the Nose, Throat and Ear—Medical and Surgical, p. 101.
Smith, Harmon: Nursing in Diseases of the Eye, Ear, Nose and Throat, 4th Edition, pp. 203–204.

HYPOTAN

Sollman: Manual of Pharmacology, 3rd edition, 1926, p. 497.

ICHTHALBIN

Sack: Ueber weitere Erfahrungen mit Ichthalbin; Monatshefte f. prakt. Dermatologie, Bd. 25, 1897.
Wolf: Ichthalbin as a Substitute for Ichthyol; Merck's Archives, January, 1900.
Rolly: Ueber den Einfluss des Ichthalbin auf den Stoffwechsel und die Darmthätigkeit der Kinder; Munch. med. Wochnesch, No. 14, 1900.
Marcuse: Ueber Ichthalbin; Therap. d. Gegenw., March, 1903.
J. A. M. A., February 16, 1924, p. 565; Reports Council Pharm. and Chem., 1924, p. 30.

ICHTHYOL

Hirschman, L. J.: N. Y. Med. Jour., 253, July 29, 1905.
Macy, Frederick S.: N. Y. Med. J., April 28, 1906.
Hirschkron, J.: Deut. Aerzte Ztg., No. 1, 1907.
Zingler, K.: Wien. klin. Rundschau, No. 11, 1909.
Lautembacher: Rene, Rev. Internat. de Méd. et Chir., No. 2, 1912.
Daman, F. W. A.: The Use of Glycerin and Ichthyol in Septic Wounds; Brit. M. J., November 11, 1916.
Osborne, Olive J.: The Principles of Therapeutics, 1921.
Low, R. Cranston: The Association of Eye Lesions with Rosacea; Brit. J. Dermat., 1922, 34:275.
Pisko, Edward: Diagnosis and Treatment of More Common Diseases of the Skin; N. Y. Med. Jour., 116, Oct. 4, 1922.
Strandberg, J.: Erythrodermia Desquamativa; Urologic and Cutaneous Review, 1923, 27:529.
Montgomery, Douglass W. and Culver, George D.: Eczema of the Breast; Med. Jour. and Record 119:93, 1924.
J. A. M. A., February 16, 1924, p. 565; Reports Council Pharm. and Chem., 1924, p. 30.

IDOZAN

Lichtenstein: Haematolog, Stockholm, 1917; Jahrbuch f. Kinderheilk, 1918.
Alder, Arneth, Leube and Otten: Schw. med. Wochensch., 1920.
Meulengracht, E.: Acta Medica Scandinavica, Vol. 58, September 25, 1923.
J. A. M. A., April 17, 1926, p. 1233; Reports Council Pharm. and Chem., 1917, p. 18.

INSULIN

Benedict and Hendry: Basal Calories for Girls; Boston Med. and Surg. Jour., 1921, 184:329.
Benedict and Talbot: Basal Calories for Boys; Carnegie Inst. Wash. No. 302, 1921, p. 206.
Boothby and Sandiford: Basal Calorie Chart; J. A. M. A., 1922, 78:1878.
Joslin, E. P.: The Treatment of Diabetes Mellitus, Lea and Febiger.
Lusk, Graham: The Science of Nutrition, W. B. Saunders Co.

IODEIKON

Buxbaum, A.: Ueber die Photographie von Gallenstein in vivo; Wien. med. Presse, 1898, 39:534.
Graham, Evarts: Roentgenological Examination of the Gall Bladder; Canad. Med. A. J., 1927, 17:1019.
George, A. W., and Leonard, R. D.: Roentgen Diagnosis of Pathological Gall Bladders; Am. Jour. Roentgenol., 1917, 4:321.
Copher, G. H.: Cholecystography—Appearance and Disappearance of the Shadow; J. A. M. A., 1925, 84:1563.

Graham, Cole, Moore and Copher: Cholecystography; J. A. M. A., 1925, 85:953.
McLeary, C. C., and Graham, R. S.: Experiences with Cholecystography; J. A. M. A., 1926, 86:1899.
Kirklin, B. R.: Certain Practical Phases of Cholecystography by Oral Method; Wis. Med. Jour., 1927, 26:356.
Zink: The Value of Cholecystography in Gall Bladder Tract Disease; Am. J. Roentg. and Rad. Ther., 1928, 20:118.
McMillan, J. C., and Wheeler, Digby: Administration of Sodium Tetraiodophenolphthalein; Canad. Med. A. J., 1929, 20:390.
Case, James T.: Evaluation of Cholecystography; J. A. M. A., 1929, 92:219.

IODOBESIN

Wilcox, Reynold Webb: Materia Medica and Therapeutics, 12th ed., 1929.

IODOBISMITOL

Grund, J. L.: Bismuth Eruptions: Disorders of Skin following Intramuscular Administration of Bismuth Compounds in Treatment of Syphilis; Boston Med. and Surg. Jour., 1927, 196:998.
Lomholt, S.: Different Preparations of Bismuth in Syphilis Therapy: Rate of Absorption as Guide to Employment; Brit. Med. Jour., 1929, 2:887.
The Management of Syphilis in General Practice; Venereal Disease Information, Vol. 10, No. 2, February 20, 1929.
Stokes, J. H.: Critical Treatment Problems in Today's Syphilology; J. A. M. A., 1930, 94:1029.
Levaditi, C.: Bismuth in the Treatment of Syphilis; Am. J. Syphilis, 1930, 14:156.
Hanzlik, P. J. and Mehrtens, H. G.: J. A. M. A., February 13, 1932.

IODO-BISMUTH OF QUININE

Sazerac and Levaditi: Report to French Academy of Sciences, 1921.
Extrait Comptes rendus des seances de la Societe de Biologie., 29 April, 1922, Tome 86, p. 817, and seance du 6 Mai, 1922, Tome 86, p. 908.
DeGave: Communication faite a la Societe Belge de Dermatologie et Syphiligraphie, le 12 Nov., 1922; Bruxelles Medical, 1923.
Fournier, Guenot, Schwartz and Jovanovitch; Annales de l'Institut Pasteur, 1923, 38:240.
Hopkins, J. G.: J. A. M. A., 1924, 83:2087.

IODOCHLOROL

Wolf, George D.: N. Y. State J. Med., 1929, 29:193–198.
Zalewski, F.: Press. Medical, 1930, 38:779.
Faulkner, W. B. Jr.: J. A. M. A., 1930, 95:1324–1328.
Soresi, A. L.: Am. J. Surg., 1930, 8:272–274.
Yantzen, Ernst and Tiedke, Carl: J. Prakt. Chem., 1930, 127:277–291.
Jones, E. L.: Arch. Otolaryngol, 1930, 11:475, 484.
Wood, W. B.: Lancet, 1930, 1:1339, 1340.
Taylor, Fred: J. Biol. Chem., 1931, 91:541–550.
Crandall, L. A., Jr., Holinger, Paul H., and Walsh, Eugene L.: J. Pharm. and Exper. Therap., 1931, 41:347–354.
Deuss, H. O.: The Use of Iodized Oils in Bronchitis and Bronchiectasis; Ill. Med. Jour., July, 1932.
Greenbaum, F. R.: Jr. of Radiology, 1932, 18:1115.

IODOMUTH

Spencer: Am. J. of Otology, 1870.
Jones, H. McNaughton: Lancet, 1889, vol. 2.
Mudgett, John Herbert: An Unusual Case of Tertiary Syphilis; Med. Council, April, 1904.
J. A. M. A., Sept. 5, 1908, p. 818; May 8, 1909, p. 1511; Reports Council Pharm. and Chem., 1905–8, p. 166; 1909, p. 75.
Burnett: Treatment of the Ear, pp. 472, 473.
Rankin and Matthewson: Boston Med. and Surg. Jour., 92:21.

IODOSTARINE

Kimball: Am. J. Publ. Health, Feb., 1923.
Kimball, O. P.: J. Mich. State Med. Soc., 1923, 22:390, 393.
Jackson, Arnold S.: Wis. Med. Jour., Aug., 1924.
Kimball: J. A. M. A., November 28, 1925, p. 1710.

IODOTONE

J. A. M. A., Dec. 12, 1914, p. 2149; Reports Council Pharm. and Chem., 1914, p. 72; Propag., vol. 1, p. 113.
Canan, C. W.: Med. Rev. of Reviews, Sept., 1927.

IODOXYL

Marcovici: Am. Med., April, 1931.

IPRAL CALCIUM

Jackson, D. E.: The Pharmacological Action of Ethylisopropylbarturic Acid; J. Lab. Clin. Med., 1922, 8:23.
Lurie, Louis A.: A New Hypnotic Ethylisopropylbarbituric Acid; Cincinnati Jour. Med., March. 1923.
Jackson, D. E. and Lurie, L. A.: Experimental and Clinical Observations on the Action and Therapeutic Uses of Ethylisopropylbarbituric Acid; J. Lab. Clin. Med., 1925, 11:116.
Maxwell, Alice F.: Clinical Study of Post-Operative Value of Barbituric Acid Hypnotics; Am. J. Obst, and Gynec., 1931, 22:579.

IRRADOL-A

Mendel: J. A. M. A., June 4, 1932.
Eusterman and Wilbur: J. A. M. A., June 11, 1932.
Orton, Underhill and Lewis: J. Biol. Chem., April, 1932.

ISAROL

Hosslin: Dissertation Basel; Verlag Buchdruckerei J. Frehner, Basle, 1900, p. 68.
Goliner: Therap. Monatshefte, 1903, 17:151.
Blanchod: F. Consultations du medecin praticien. Guide de pratique medico-chirurgicale journaliere; J.-B. Bailliere and fils, Paris, 1925, p. 584.
Puckner, W. A.: J. A. M. A., 1929, 93:33.

ISO-IODEIKON

Graham, E. A.: Gall Bladder Diagnosis from the Standpoint of the Surgeon; Radiology, Apr., 1926.
Graham, Cole, Copher and Moore: J. A. M. A., Feb. 13, 1926, p. 467; June 19, 1926, p. 1899. April 7, 1928, p. 1111; Nov. 17, 1928, p. 1549.
Kirklin, B. Y.: Cholecystography; Arch. of Surg., June, 1929, p. 2246.

KALMERID GERMICIDAL TABLETS

Macfarlan, Douglas: Notes in the Study of Potassium-Mercuric-Iodid; J. A. M. A., 1914, 62:17.
Macfarlan, Douglas: A Rationale of a New Treatment for the Acute Frontal Sinusites; J. Ophth., Otol., and Laryng., 1915, 21:777.
Watson, Cassius H.: An Improved Substitute for Iodized Catgut Sutures; Surg., Gynec. and Obst., 1916, 22:114; 23:629.
Macfarlan, Douglas: A Remarkable Antiseptic; Charlotte Med. Jour., 1919, 80:233.
Macfarlan, Douglas: New Suggestions in the Treatment of Atrophic Rhinitis and Pyorrhea Alveolaris; Jour. Ophth., Otol., and Laryng., 1920, 24:70.
Macfarlan, Douglas: The Germicidal Value of Potassium Mercuric Iodide; Amer. J. M. Sc., 1920, 159:586.
McKenna, W. F. and Fisher, H. A.: The Use of Potassium-Mercuric-Iodide for Skin Disinfection; Surg., Gynec. and Obst., 1920, 30:370.

KAOMIN

Braafladt, L. H.: The Effects of Kaolin on the Intestinal Flora in Normal and Pathologic Conditions; J. Inf. Dis., 1923, 33:454.
Antoine, E. and Rolland, P.: Arch. des Maladies de l'Appareil de la Nutrition, Paris, 1928, 18:730.

KONDREMUL

Randolph, N.: Therap. Gaz., 1885, 9:732.
Schmidt, A.: Munch. med. Wochensch., 1905, 52:1970.
Wood, N.: West London Med. Jour., 1906, 11:99.
Kast, L.: Nelson's Loose Leaf Medicine, 1930, 5:352.
Hurst, A. F.: Constipation and Allied Intestinal Disorders; Oxford Medical Publication, 2nd edition.

KRESIVAL

Baron, C.: Med. Klin., No. 11, 1923.
Fein, A.: Wurt. Med. Korr-Bl., No. 17, 1923.
Wunnerlich, A.: Med. Klin., No. 17, 1923.
Cohn, Walter: Deut. med. Wochensch., No. 18, 1923.
Schirp, K. and Wachter, R.: Munch. med. Wochensch., No. 26, 1923.
Kohler, R. and Schmidt, H.: Deut. med. Wochensch., No. 41, 1923.
Schultz, W.: Klin. Wochensch., No. 47, 1923.
Jehle, L.: Wien. med. Wochensch., No. 51, 1923.

Hochsinger, K.: Wien. med. Wochensch., No. 51, 1923.
Beck, W.: Therap. d. Gegenw., No. 12, 1923.

LACTIC ACID MILK POWDERED

Marriott, W. M. and Davidson, L. T.: J. A. M. A., Dec. 15, 1923.
Levine, V. E.: Arch. Pediat., Oct., 1926.
Schwartz, A. B.: Am. J. Nursing, Dec., 1926.
Calhoun, D. A.: An Excellent Substitute for Breast Milk; Am. J. Obst. and Gynec., 1927, 13:96.
Krauss, F. I.: J. Med. Soc. New Jersey, Dec., 1928.
Gluich, M.: Med. Jour. and Record, August 17, 1929.
Lash, A. L.: Ill. Med. Jour., Jan., 1930.
Hess, J. H., Chamberlain, I. M. and Robins, L. S.: J. A. M. A., Apr. 9, 1932.
Craig, J. D. and Tobey, J. A.: Arch. Pediatr., August, 1932.
Hess, J. H. and Lundeen, E. C.: Premature Infants; Ohio State M. J., 1932, 28:253.
Lynch, H. D.: Powdered Citric Acid Milk in Infant Feeding; Arch. Pediat., 1932, 49:763.
Myers, B.: Practical Points on Modern Infant Feeding; Practitioner, 1932, 128:425.

LACTIGEN

Guszmann, Josef: Dermat. Wochensch., 1918, No. 48, p. 808.
Zalewski, Edward and Muller, E. F.: Munch. med. Wochensch., Feb. 14, 1919.
Muller, E. F.: Med. Klin., 1920, 26:579.
Culver, H.: J. A. M. A., 1921, 76:312.
Krosl, H.: Therap. d. Gegenw., September, 1921.
Miller, Jos. L.: J. A. M. A., 1921, 76:309.
Mohler, R. W.: Am. J. Obst. and Gynec., 1925, 60:365.
Rawls: N. Y. State J. Med., 1925, 25:1108.
Weirauk, H. V.: Ohio State M. J., 1925, 22:305.
Fox, L. Webster: Surg., Gynec. and Obst., 1926, 42:481.
Gellhorn, G.: J. Ind. State M. A., June 1926.

LACTOBACILLUS

Clark and Perry: N. Y. Med. Jour. and Rec., December 19, 1923.

LAROSAN

Abt, Isaac A.: Infant Feeding; The Practical Medicine Series, Vol. 1, 1915.
De Sanctis, Adolph G. and Paider, Lillian V.: Value of Calcium Caseinate Milk in Fermentative Diarrhea; Arch. Pediat., April, 1921.
Lowenburg, Harry: Treatment of Acute Alimentary Disturbances of Infancy; N. Y. Med. Jour., August, 192'.
Stoeltzner, W.: Treatment of Digestive Disturbances of Infancy; Pediatrics, Vol. 27, No. 4.
Meigs, Grace: Artificial Feeding of the Sick Infant; Am. J. Dis. Child., Vol. 10, No. 1.
Gelhorn, W.: Casein-Milk Feeding in Infancy and Childhood; J. A. M. A., Vol. 65, No. 10.
Webster, F. P.: Twelve Cases of Spasmophilia; Arch. Pediat., Vol. 33, No. 9.
Hill, Lewis Webb: Fermentative Diarrhea in Infants; Boston Med. and Surg. Jour., Vol. 174, No. 14.

LENIGALLOL

Kromayer: Prinzipien u. Fortschritte in der Behandlung der nichtparasitaeren Hautkrankheiten, Wien. klin.-therap. Wochensch., No. 47, 1904; Fortschritte in der Ekzembehandlung; Wien. med. Wochensch., No. 3, 1905; Ekzem und Ekzembehandlung; Neue Deut. Klin., No. 11, p. 63, 1929.
Galewsky: Die Behandlung des Saeuglingsekzems; Med. Klin. No. 47, 1910; Moderne Teer-Therapie"; Fortsch. d. Therapie. No. 13, 1927.
Galewsky: The Treatment of Psoriasis in Children; Kinderaerztl. Praxis, No. 3, p. 108. 1931.
Simpson, C. A.: Infantile Eczema, J. A. M. A., April 6, 1916.
Nobl: Zur Behandlung juckender Dermatosen; Wien. klin. Wochensch., No. 43, 1925; Treatment of Psoriasis; Wien. med. Wochensch., No. 27, 1926.
Winkler and Unna: Das seborrhoische Ekzem; Handbuch der Haut—und Geschlechtskrankheiten, No. 6, 1927.
Leidler: Treatment of Diseases of the Ear, Urban and Schwarzenberg, 1928.
Engelhardt and Welcker: Das Lenigallol in der dermatologischen Praxis; Dermat. Wochensch. No. 2, 1930.
Downing, J. G.: Industrial Medicine, Sept., 1932.

LENNOX ETHYLENE

Luckhardt, A. B. and Carter, J. B.: J. A. M. A., 1923, 80:765.

LIPOIODINE

Loeb and Velden, von den: Munch. med. Wochensch., 1911, 58:2616.
Loeb and Velden, von den: Therap. Monatshefte, 1911, 25:209.

Schwarz: Orvosi Hetilap, 1913, 57:302.
Hassel: Therap. Monatshefte, 1914, 28:753.
Comroe: Penna. M. J., 1922, 25:482.

LIPOIODINE DIAGNOSTIC

Pugh, W. S.: Med. Jour. and Record, p. 675–678, December 18, 1929.
Fox, E.: Am. Med., 1931, 26:235.

LIPOLYSIN

Holste: New Remedies (Composition of Lipolysin); Deut. med. Wochensch., 1923, No. 18.
Lewy: The Hormonal Treatment of Obesity; Fortsch. d. Medizin, 1923, No. 10.
Low: Lipolysin, a Pluriglandular Reducer; Great-Berl. Aerstb., 1923, No. 41.
Schlesinger, O.: Treatment of Obesity on the Basis of Present Endocrine Knowledge; Med. Klin., 1923, No. 42.
Alexander, A.: Pluriglandular Obesity and its Treatment; Deut. med. Wochensch., 1924, No. 10.
Heise, W.: About Endogenous Obesity; Fortsch. d. Medizin, 1924, No. 4–5.
Porges: Treatment of Pluriglandular Obesity; Deut. med. Wochensch., 1924, No. 25.
Karcher, M.: The Treatment of Endocrine Obesity with Lipolysin, Allg. Med. Centr.-Ztg., 1925, No. 4.
Umber, F.: Diseases of Metabolism; Munch. med. Wochensch., 1925, No. 10.
Frankel, M.: Rejuvenating the Woman; Publ. Bircher-Bern.

LITHIUM SALICYLATE

Maingot, R. H.: Med. Press and Circular, Dec. 23 and 30, 1931.

LIVER EXTRACT

Koessler, Maurer and Loughlin: J. A. M. A., 1926.
Minot and Murphy: J. A. M. A., 1926–1927.
Koessler and Maurer: J. A. M. A., 1927, 89:768, 774.
Maurer, Richter and Koessler: Am. J. Syphilis, July, 1928.
Maurer, Greengard and Kluver: J. A. M. A., 1932, 98:1069.
Sargent: Lancet, January 30, 1932, pp. 230–232.
Richter, Meyer and Ivy: J. A. M. A., May 7, 1932.
Meyer, Richter and Ivy: Arch. Int. Med., October, 1932.

LIVER EXTRACT 55

Whipple, G. H.: Robscheit-Robbins, F. S. and Hooper, C. W.: Am. J. Physiol., 1920, 53:236.
Robscheit-Robbins and Whipple: Am. J. Physiol., 1925, 72:408; 1927–28, 83:76.
Vaughan, Janet: Lancet, 1928, 1:1063.
Minot, G. R. and Murphy, W. P.: Am. J. M. Sc., 1928, 175:581.
Whipple, G. H., Robscheit-Robbins, F. S. and Walden, G. B.: Am. J. M. Sc., 1930, 179:628.
Cohn, E. J., Minor, G. R., Fulton, J. F., Ulrichs, H. F., Sargent, F. C., Weare, J. H., and Murphy, W. P: Biol. Chem., Vol. 69, p. 74.
Knap, W. H. and Rehfuss, M. E.: Weekly Roster and Med. Digest, 1928, 23:5.
Sturgis, C. C., Isaacs, R. and Smith, M.: Ann. Int. Med., 1928, 1:983.
Report Medical Research Council: Brit. Med. Jour., March 10, 1928.
Dyke, S. C.: Lancet, 1929, 1:1192.
Cabot, R. C.: New England Jour. of Med., 1929, 201:1003, Case 15462.
Keefer, C. S. and Yang, C. S.: J. A. M. A., 1929, 93:575.

LIVER EXTRACT 343

Cohn, E. J., McMeekin, T. L. and Minor, G. R.: The Nature of the Substance Effective in Pernicious Anemia; Tr. A. Am. Phys., 1930, 45:343.
Zerfas, L. G.: Liver Extract for Pernicious Anemia; Blood Changes During First Month: Report of 101 cases; Arch. Int. Med., 1931, 47:135.
Castle, W. B. and Taylor, F. H. L.: Intravenous Use of Extract of Liver; J. A. M. A., 1931, 96:1198.
Smith, C. T., and Kinlaw, W. B.: Clinical Consideration of Anemia of Pregnancy and Puerperium; Ann. Int. Med., 1931, 4:939.
Schilling, V.: Gansslen's injizierbares Leberextrakt; Klin. Wochensch., 1931, 10:301.
Freeman, S. L.: Rectal Administration of Liver Extract; J. Missouri M. A., 1931, 28:268.
Beebe, R. T. and Lewis, G. E.: The Maintenance Dose of Potent Material in Pernicious Anemia; Am. J. M. Sc., 1931, 181:796.
Minot, G. R. and Murphy, W. P.: Treatment of Pernicious Anemia by Special Diet; J. A. M. A., vol. 87, p. 470.
Guha, B. C.: Vitamin B_2 and Pellagra; Brit. Med. Jour., 1931, 2:53.

LIVER MEAL

Leupold, E.: Untersuchungen uber die Mikrochemie und Genese des Amyloids; Beitr. z. Path. Anat u. z. Allg. Pathol., 1918, 64:347.

Kuczynski, M. H.: Neue Beitrage zur Lehre vom Amyloid, Klin. Wochensch., 1923, 11:727.
Bennhold, H.: Uber die Beziehungen des Kongorotes zur amyloiden Substanz und uber den Mechanismus der beschleunigten. Farbstoffausscheidung bei tuberkularen Nierenkrankheiten; Klin. Wochensch., 1924, 111:1711.
Dunham, R. W.: The Effect of Spleen Extract and Bone Marrow on the Blood Picture in Pulmonary Tuberculosis; Am. J. M. Sc., 1925, 170:394.
Smetana, H.: The Relation of the Reticulo-Endothelial System to the Formation of Amyloid; J. Exper. Med., 1927, 45:619.
Newton, H. F.: Uber die Beeinflussung sekundarer Anamien bei Tuberkulosen durch Leberextrakte; Klin. Wochensch., 1928, 7:1062.
Grayzel, H. G., Jacobi, M., Maslow, H. and Warshall, H. B.: Experimental Studies of Amyloidosis; Proc. Soc. Exp. Biol. Med., 1930, 28:172.
Ropschitz: Uber eine bequeme Durchfuhrungstechnik der Rohmilztherapie bei destruktiver Gelenkstuberkulose; Med. Klin., 1930, 26:166.
Whitbeck, Brainerd H.: Treatment of Amyloidosis in Surgical Tuberculosis; Journal of Bone and Joint Surgery, 1932, 14:85.

LUIZYM

Lampe, Arno E. and Schmidt-Ott, Albrecht: Munch. med. Wochensch., 1931, No. 44.
Weltz, G. A.: Observations on the Use of Luizym in X-Ray Work; Munch. med. Wochensch., 1931, No. 44.
Grassmann, Wolfgang and Rubenbauer, Hans: On Cellulase and Hemicellulase, with Special Reference to their Therapeutic Application, Munch. med. Wochensch., 1931, No. 43.
Silberschmidt, Karl: Experiments on the Action of Cellulase and Hemicellulase on Vegetable Substances in Vitro, Munch. med. Wochensch., 1931, No. 43.
Mezger, Hans: On the Preparation of Patients for Pyelography, by means of the Enzyme Preparation "Luizym"; Munch. med. Wochensch., 1932, No. 9.

LUMALGIN

Mendenhall, W. L. and Camp, H. F.: Boston Med. and Surg. Jour., February 21, 1925.
Hanzlik: J. A. M. A., November 1, 1919.

LUMINAL

Impens: Deut. med. Wochensch., 1912, No. 20.
Dosio, Enrico: Annal. di Freniat. e Sci. aff. del R. Manicomio di Torino, 1913, Vol. 23, No. 1.
Dercum, F. X.: Therap. Gaz., Sept. 15, 1919.
Grinker, Julius.: J. A. M. A., Aug. 20, 1920; Sept. 2, 1922.
Rowley, A. R.: Boston Med. and Surg. Jour., May 12, 1921.
Wright, Harold W.: Calif. State J. of Med., Apr. 1923.
Schultz, F. D.: Lancet, Oct. 1, 1924.
Hosslin, R. v.: Munch. med. Wochensch., Nov. 7, 1924.
Gruber, Charles M. and Baskett, Roy F.: J. Lab. Clin. Med., May, 1925; J. Pharm. and Exper. Med., Apr. 2, 1925.
Tscherning, R.: Munch. med. Wochensch., 1925, No. 35.
Guttman, M. Reese: Arch. of Otolaryngology, Oct., 1926.
Grinker, Roy R.: J. A. M. A., Oct. 19, 1929.
Bartlett, Willard: Surg., Gynec. and Obst., April, 1930.

LUNOSOL

Cobb, Ralph B.: J. Urol., July, 1921.
Ballenger, E. G. and Elder, O. F.: Surg., Gynec. and Obst., July, 1922.
Wakerlin, G. E. and Eiseman, C.: Am. J. Syphilis, July, 1928.
Wakerlin, G. E.: Arch. of Derm. and Syph., June, 1929.

MAGNESPIRIN

Winter and Barbour: Proc. Soc. Exp. Biol. Med., 1928, 25:587.
Podolsky and Goldstein: Med. Jour. and Record, Aug. 5, 1931.

MALTED MILK

Hunziker, O. F.: Condensed Milk and Milk Powder, 1926.
Rose, E. S.: Malted Milk; Amer. Jour. Pharm, 1927, 99:163.
Tobey, J. A.: A Carrier for Barium in Roentgenology; Med. Jour. and Record, 1929, 130:332.
Ballard, C. W.: The Estimation of Fat in Malted Milk; J. Amer. Pharm. Assoc., 1929, 18:122.
Crumbine, S. J. and Tobey, J. A.: The Most Nearly Perfect Food, Baltimore, Williams and Williams, 1929.
Quinn, E. J. and Brabec, L. B.: The Vitamin A, B and G Content of Malted Milk, J. Home Econ., February, 1930.
Peterman, M. J. and Hug, I.: The Nutrition of Sick Children; Am. J. Dis. Child., 1930, 40:305.
Tobey, James A.: N. Amer. Diet. Assoc., Vol. 6, No. 4, March, 1931.

MALTINE AND PREPARATIONS

Fischer, Louis: Diseases of Infancy and Childhood, 9th ed., Vol. 1, F. A. Davis Co., Philadelphia, 1922.
Olitsky, P. K. and McCartney, J. E.: Studies on the Nasopharyngeal Secretions from Patients with Common Colds; J. Exper. Med., 1923, 38:427.
Smiley, D. F.: A Study of the Acute Infections of the Throat and Respiratory System; J. A. M. A., 1924, 82:540.
Cowell and Mellanby: The Effect of Iodine on Hyperthyroidism in Man; Quart. J. Med., 1924, 18:1.
Dubois, E. F.: Basal Metabolism in Health and Disease, Lea and Febiger, 1924.
Bass and Denzer: Iron Therapy in the Anemias of Infancy; J. A. M. A., 1926, 86:938.
Berkeley, W. N.: Principles and Practice of Endocrine Medicine, Lea and Febiger, 1926.
MacKenzie, G. M.: Anemia in Hypothyroidism; J. A. M. A., 1926, 86:462.
Reports Council Pharm. and Chem., 1931, p. 62.
Gant, Samuel G.: Diseases of the Rectum, Anus and Colon, Vol. 3, W. B. Saunders Company, Philadelphia.

MANCUHEMIN

Elvehjem, C. A.: The Relative Value of Inorganic and Organic Iron in Hemoglobin Formation; J. A. M. A., 1932, 98:1047.

MERCUROCHROME 220 SOLUBLE

Condit: Minn. Med., 1931, 14:319.
Lash: Ill. Med. Jour., 1931, 59:473.
Burch: Jour. Tenn. State Med. Assoc., 1931, 24:377.
Sprague: R. I. Med. Jour., 1931, 14:55.
Offutt: Bull. Chicago Med. Soc., 1931, 33:26.
Walke: New Orleans Med. and Surg. J., 1931, 83:553.
Bessesen: Va. Med. Monthly, 1931, 57:682.
Emrich: Ky. M. J., 1931, 29:304.
Gillespie: Col. Med., 1931, 28:112.
Greenhill: Ill. Med. Jour., 1931, 59:349.
Sellers and Sanders: New Orleans Med. and Surg., 1931, 83:757.
Sharp: J. Med. Assoc. Ga., 1931, 20:229.

MERCUROCHROME, COLLOSOL BRAND

Eyre, J., Notton, H. E. F., Pope, Sir W. J.: Brit. Med. Jour., August 11, 1928.
Moxey, P.: Brit. Med. Jour., March 23, 1929.

MERCUROPHEN

Schamberg, Kolmer and Raiziss: J. A. M. A., 1917, 68:1458; J. Inf. Dis., 1919, 24:527.
Shivers: The Military Surg., Aug. and Sept., 1919, p. 15; J. Urol., July, 1922.

MEROXYL

Young, White, Hill and Davis: A Further Discussion of Germicides and Presentation of a New Germicide—Meroxyl; Surg., Gynec. and Obst., 1923, 36:508.

MERTHIOLATE

Powell, H. M., and Jamieson, W. A.: Merthiolate as a Germicide; Am. J. of Hygiene, 1931, 13:296.
Marshall, M. S.: Merthiolate; A New Antiseptic; Cal. and West. Med., 1931, 35:43.
Jamieson, W. A., and Powell, H. M.: Merthiolate as a Preservative for Biological Products; Am. J. of Hygiene, 1931, 14:218.
Buchsbaum, R., and Bloom, W.: Relative Toxicity of Antiseptics on Bacteria and Tissues in Cultures; Proc. Soc. Exp. Biol. Med., 1931, 28:1060.

MERVENOL

Reports Council Pharm. and Chem., 1919, p. 82; Propaganda, vol. 2., p. 249.
Hille, Hermann: Clin. Med. and Surg., Jan., 1927.
Wakerlin, G. E.: Am. J. of Syphilis, July, 1928.
Wakerlin, G. E.: Am. Dermat. and Syph., June, 1929.
Hille, Hermann: Clin. Med. and Surg., April, 1930.
Hille, Hermann: Med. Life, March, 1930.
Colloidal Chemistry: Vol. 1, No. 1, 2, 3.

MESUROL

Scherber, G.: Wien. med. Wochensch., No. 40, 1924.
Hoffmann, E. and Schreus, H. T.: Deut. med. Wochensch., June 20, 1924.
Dietel, F.: Munch. med. Wochensch., July 4, 1924.
Poschacher, A.: Acta Dermato-Venerol., Jan., 1925.

Schmidt, F.: Deut. med. Wochensch., Feb. 20, 1925.
Conighi, R.: Prog. di Terap., No. 1, 1926.
Rosenberg, P.: Therap. Berichte, No. 1, 1927.
Tanimura, T. and Koso, K.: Hifuka Kiyo, July, 1928.
Genovese, Serafino and Vero, Frank.: Am. J. Syphilis, Jan., 1930.

METAPHEN

Raiziss, G. W., and Severac, M.: J. Lab. Clin. Med., 1923, 9:71.
Raiziss, G. W., Severac, M. and Moetsch, J. C.: J. Pharm. and Exper. Therap., Jan., 1926, Vol. 26, No. 6.
Raiziss, G. W. and Severac, M.: J. Inf. Dis., 1927, 40:447.
Spotts, S. D.: J. Chemoth., July, 1927, p. 48.
Fisher, R.: Clin. Med. and Surg., 1927, 34:857.
Dubois, Leo C.: Clin. Med. and Surg., 1928, 35:331.
Bledsoe, R. E. B.: J. Chemoth., April, 1928, Vol. 5, No. 1.
Bernstine, J. B.: Am. J. Obst. and Gynec., 1929, 18:220.
Wright, H. N. and Hirschfelder, A. D.: J. Pharm. and Exper. Therap., May, 1930, Vol. 39.
Birkhaug, K. E.: J. A. M. A., Sept. 27, 1930, p. 917.
Levinson, A. and Perstein, M. A.: Arch. Pathol., Nov., 1931, p. 729.
Keeler, H. R.: Med. Clinics of N. A., Vol. 15, No. 2, Sept., 1931, Phila. Number.

METAPHYLLIN

Gibson: Discussions on the Treatment of Muscular Heart-Affections; Brit. Med. Jour., 1912, 2699.
Ludwig: Euphyllin in Coronary Sclerosis; Fortschritte der Medicin, 1925, 8.
Oberndorfer: The Anatomical Fundaments of Angina Pectoris; Munch. med. Wochensch., 1925, 36.
Cohn: Angina Pectoris; Med. Klin., 1926, 2⅝8.
Peritz: Zeitschrift f. d. gesamte Neurologie und Psychiatrie, 1926, Vol. 102, part ¾.
Fisher, Guggenheimer and Muller: Deut. med. Wochensch., 1928, Nr. 38.
Musser: J. A. M. A., Oct., 1928.
Hecht: Die Arztliche Praxis, 1929, Part 3.
Romberg: Munch. med. Wochensch., 1929, No. 19.
Boden: Angina Pectoris and its Treatment; Mediz. Welt, 1930, No. 4.
Konig: Zeitschrift fur Kreislaufforschung, 1930, No. 14.

METRAZOL

Johnston: Cardiazol, A Clinical Report; Bull. Johns Hopkins Hosp., 1928, 44:32.
Barker and Levine: Cardiazol, Some Experimental Effects of this Drug on the Cardiorespiratory Mechanism; Arch. Int. Med., p. 14, July, 1928.
Meinhardt: Cardiovascular Support in Pneumonia and other Diseases; Clin. Med. and Surg., Nov., 1929, p. 829.
Bartle: Acute Cardiac Dilatation; Am. Med., New Series, 1930, 25:518.
Phillips: The Effect of Stimulants on Drug Poisoning; Med. Jour. and Record, Oct. 15, 1930.
Fulton: The Sign of Babinski; Publ. C. T. Thomas, Baltimore, 1932.
Strasser: Metrazol as a Stimulant During Surgical Anesthesia; Ohio State M. J., 1932, 28:123.
Schwartz: Congestive Heart Failure; Ohio State M. J., 1933, 29:308.

METYCAINE

Rose, C. L.: Studies in the Pharmacology of Local Anesthetics. V. A Discussion of the Present Methods for Evaluating Local Anesthetics; Anesth. and Anal., 1931, 10:159.
Coles, H. W. and Rose, H. T.: Studies in the Pharmacology of Local Anesthetics. IV. The Examination of the Urine and Blood of Dogs Injected Subcutaneously with Neothesin (Metycaine); Anesth. and Anal., 1931, 10:103.
Laszlo, Alexander F.: Reducing the Strength of Cocain Solutions in Nose and Throat Practice; Ann. Otol. Rhin. and Laryngol., 1931, 40:259.
Hirschfelder, A. D. and Bieter, R. N.: Local Anesthetics; Physiol. Rev., 1932, 12:190.
Bieter, R. N., Harvey, A. McG and Burgess, W. W.: Spinal Anesthesia in Summer Frogs; J. Pharm. and Exper. Therap., 1932, 45:291.
Meeker, W. R.: A Comparison of the Vasoconstrictive Action of Adrenalin and Ephedrine Added to the Local Anesthetic Solution; J. Lab. Clin. Med., 1932, 17:773.

MINERAL MIXTURE

Mills, E. S.: The Treatment of Idiopathic (hypochromic) Anaemia with Iron and Copper; Canad. Med. A. J., 1930, 22:175.
Banyai, A. L.: The Dietary Treatment of Tuberculosis; Am. Rev. Tuberc., 1931, 23:546.
Cantarow, A.: Calcium Metabolism and Calcium Therapy, Lea and Febiger, Philadelphia, 1931.
Orent, E. R. and McCollum, E. V.: Effects of Deprivation of Manganese in the Rat; J. Biol. Chem., 1931, 92: 657.
Sheldon, J. H.: Some Considerations on the Influence of Copper and Manganese on the Therapeutic Activity of Iron, Brit. Med. Jour., 1932, 2:869.
Bogen, E. and Rachmel, W. Pulmonary Tuberculosis—its Dietary Treatment; Cal.; and West. Med., 1932, 37:292.

Cocheu, L. F.: Anemia, J. Am. Inst. Homeop., 1932, 25:802.
Editorial: Trace Elements in the Body, J. A. M. A., 1932, 98:1746.
Kruse, H. D., Orent, E. R. and McCollum, E. V.: Studies on Magnesium Deficiency in Animals; J. Biol. Chem., 1932, 96:519.
Sherbon, F. B.: Diet in Pregnancy; Med. Women's J., 1932, 39:111.

MOOGROL

J. Chem. Soc., 1904, p. 838, 851, 854; 1907, p. 557.
J. Cutan. Dis., 1919, Vol. 37, No. 6, p. 367.
J. Inf. Dis., 1920, Vol. 26, No. 3, p. 238.
J. of Am. Med. Assoc., Nov. 27, 1920, p. 1484; Jan. 22, 1921, p. 248; Apr. 16, 1921, p. 1121; May 28, 1921, p. 1470.

MUCIN

Fogelson, S. J.: J. A. M. A., Feb. 28, 1931, p. 673.
Kein and Ivy: J. A. M. A., Nov. 21, 1931, p. 1511.
Atkinson, A.: J. A. M. A., Apr. 2, 1932, p. 1153.
Brown, et al.: J. A. M. A., July 9, 1932, p. 98.

MYORGAL

Hubert, G.: Myorgal in Angina Pectoris; Fortsch. d. Therapie, No. 14, 1931.

MYOSTON

Schwarzmann, J. S.: A New Method of Treatment for Angina Pectoris; Munch. med. Wochensch., 1929, Nr. 43.
Schwarzmann, J. S.: Skeletal Muscle Extract as a Tonic; Wien. klin. Wochensch., 1929, Nr. 48.
Haberlandt, L.: On a New Therapy for Angina Pectoris; Munch. mediz. Wochensch., 1929, Nr. 50.
Fahrenkamp, K. and Schneider, H.: Med. Klin., 1930, Nr. 2.
Schwarmann, J. S.: Paris Medical, 1930, Nr. 10, p. 226.
Bagdassarjanz and Turkeltaub: Munch. med. Wochensch., 1930, Nr. 31.

NATURAL VITAMIN D

Zucker, T. F., Pappenheimer, A. M. and Barnett, Marion: Observations on Cod Liver Oil and Rickets; Proc. Soc. Exp. Biol. Med., 1921, 19:167.
Pappenheimer, A. M.: J. of Exp. Med., 1922, 36:335.
Zucker, T. F.: Further Observations on the Chemistry of Cod Liver Oil; Proc. Soc. Exp. Biol. Med., 1922, 20:136.
Zucker, T. F. and Barnett, Marion: Observations on the Distribution of Antirachitic Substances; Proc. Soc. Exp. Biol. Med., 1922, 20:375.
Zucker, T. F. and Matzner, M. J.: Pharmacological Action of the Antirachitic Active Principle of Cod Liver Oil; Proc. Soc. Exp. Biol. Med., 1923, 21:186.
Chaplin, Hugh: Clinical Experience with the Active Principle of Cod Liver Oil; Proc. Soc. Exp. Biol. Med., 1924, 21:332.

NEOCAINE

Weinstein and McHugh: One Thousand Cases of Spinal Anesthesia Without a Death Attributable to the Anesthetic; Med. Jour. and Record, June 1, 1932.
Bower, Clark, Wagoner and Burns: Spinal Anesthesia; Surg., Gynec. and Obst., June, 1932.
Jones: One Thousand Spinal Anesthesias; Ann. Surgery, July, 1932.
J. A. M. A., Jan. 21, 1933, p. 210.

NEOCINCHOPHEN

Bendix: Therap. d. Gegenw., 1912, 53:301.
Klemperer: Therap. d. Gegenw., 1913, 54:257.
Jokl: Prague Med. Wochensch., 1913, 38:465.
Chace and Associates: J. A. M. A., 1921, 81:1230.
Hanzlik: J. Pharm. and Exper. Therap., 1921, 17:385.
Barbour and Lozinsky: J. Lab. Clin. Med., January, 1923.
Barbour, Lozinsky and Clements: Am. J. M. Sc., 1923, 165:708.
Boots and Miller: J. A. M. A., 1924, 82:1028.
Sollmann: Manual of Pharmacology, 1926.
Derick, Hitchcock and Swift: J. Clinical Invest., April, 1928.
J. A. M. A.: 1931, 97:409.

NEO-ERGOT

Thompson, M. R.: J. Amer. Pharm. Assoc., Vol. 19, Mar., 1930.
Editorial, Am. Med., Vol. 36, May, 1930.

NEOROBIN

Ormsby, O. S.: Diseases of the Skin, 3d ed., 1927, p. 277.
Pusey, W. A.: Principles and Practice of Dermatology, 4th ed., 1924, p. 431.
Greenbaum, S. S.: Penna. M. J., Feb., 1928, 324.
Masucchi and Slothower: J. Amer. Pharm. Assoc., 1923, 12:335.

NEO-IOPAX

Swick, M.: Klin. Wochensch., 1929, No. 45.
Swick, M.: Am. J. Surg., Feb., 1930.
Lubash, S.: Am. J. Surg., June, 1930.
Wolbarst, A. L. and Hirsch, I. S.: Med. Jour. and Record, July 2, 1930.
Jaches, L.: J. A. M. A., Nov. 8, 1930.
Braasch, Wm. F. and Bumpus, H. C.: J. A. M. A., Nov. 8, 1930.
Cooke, R. V.: Lancet, No. 13, Vol. 2, Sept. 27, 1930.
Heritage, K.: Lancet, July 19, 1930, p. 132.
Kidd, F.: Brit. J. Urology, 1930, 11:47.
Roth, E. J. H. and Wright, H. W. S.: Brit. Med. Jour., April 26, 1930, pp. 778–780.
Von Lichtenberg, A.: Radiology, Dec., 1930, Vol. 15, No. 6.

NEOMAGNEPHEN

Trippe, C. M.: Clinical Results with a New Magnesium Compound; J. Med. Soc. New Jersey, October 1930.
Fox and Kaplan: Effect of Magnesium on the Clinical Action of Phenylcinchoninic Derivatives; Med. World, March, 1931.
Podolsky: Magnesium Synergism in Chronic Arthritis; Med. Jour. and Record, March 18, 1931.
Trippe, C. M.: An Analysis of 300 Cases of Pain Treated by Magnesium Combinations; J. Med. Soc. New Jersey, January, 1932.

NEO SILVOL

Ravich: J. Urol. Nov., 1924.

NEPHRITIN

J. A. M. A., October 5, 1907, p. 1198; Reports Council Pharm. and Chem., 1905–8, p. 79; April 21, 1923, p. 1167.
Backman, E. L.: Effet sur la Pression Arterielle de la Nephrectomie et la Role Probable des Riens dans le Systeme Endocrine; Compt. rend. Soc. de biol., 1916, 79:406.
Stern, L. and Rothlin, E.: Action des Extraits de Tissus Animaux sur les Organes a Fibres Musculaires Lisses; J. de Physiol. et de Path. Gen., 1919, 18:441.
Roger, H.: Action des Extraits d'Organes sur la Pression Sanguine; Pres. Medicale, 1921, 29:901.
Lematte, L.: L'Oportherapie du Praticien, A. Maloine and Fils, 1923, p. 64–66.
Martinet, A.: Clinical Therapeutics, Vol. 2, F. A. Davis Co., Philadelphia, 1925, pp. 1295–1298.

NEUROPHOSPHATES "ESKAY"

J. A. M. A., September 29, 1917, p. 1102; Reports Council Pharm. and Chem., 1917, p. 52; Propaganda, vol. 2, p. 146.
Wilcox: Materia Medica and Therapeutics, 11th ed. 1926, p. 734.
Solis-Cohen and Githens: Pharmaco-Therapeutics, 1928, p. 1413.

NEUROSINE

J. A. M. A., January 9, 1915, p. 165; April 27, 1918, p. 1251; Reports Council Pharm. and Chem., 1914, p. 86; Propaganda, ed 9, p. 139; Propaganda, vol. 2, p. 404; J. A. M. A., October 10, 1925, p. 1155.
Gerty, F. J.: Clinical Effects of So-called Moonshine Liquors; Am. J. Publ. Health, 1924, 14:603.
Brams, W. A. and Vaughan, R. T.: False, Acute Surgical Abdomen on an Alcoholic Basis; Ill. Med. Jour., 1925, 67:125.
Mallory, F. B.: Hemochromatosis and Chronic Poisoning with Copper; Arch. Int. Med., 1926, 37:336.
Richardson, J. L. and Blankenhorn, M. A.: New Clinical Aspects of Alcoholism, Am. J. M. Sc., 1928, 176:168.
Hunt, R.: Toxicity of Illicit Liquor; New England, J. Med., 1928, 198–230.
Cowles, E. S.: A New Pathology and Treatment of Chronic Alcoholism; Med. Jour., and Record, 1931, 133:417.

NEUTRALON

Alexander, Alfred: Berl. klin. Wochensch., 1909, No. 49.
Rosenheim, and Ehrmann: Deut. med. Wochensch., 1910, No. 3.
Hirsch, Paul: Deut. med. Wochensch., 1910, No. 3.
Singer, G.: Med. Klin., 1910, No. 51.
Schlessinger, J.: Munch. med. Wochensch., 1911, No. 41.

Schlessinger, Emmo: Zeitsch. f. experim. Pathol. und Ther., 1920, No. 21.
Friedrich, v.: Munch. med. Wochensch., 1921, No. 50.
Hofrat, Cramer: Munch. med. Wochensch., 1922, No. 17.
Boas, J.: Diagnostik und Therapie der Magenkrankheiten, 7th edition, pp. 359–360.

NIAZO

Neuberg, H.: Med. Klin., 1930, No. 43, p. 1602.
Warner, H.: Mediz. Welt, 1930, No. 39.
Niessing, G.: Fortsch. d. Therapie, 1931, No. 15, p. 476.
Pugh, W. Scott: Am. Med., 1931, 16:489.
Sugar, H.: Med. Jour. and Record, July 15, 1931, p. 66.
Vara-Lopez, R. and Bolado, I. L. I.: Progressos de la Clinica, 1931, Vo. 39, No. 10.
Rusche, K.: Am. J. Surg., March, 1932.

NITROSCLERAN SALTS

Kroschinski: Fortsch. d. Medizin, 1926, No. 11.
Jaensch: Klin. Monatsbl. f. Augenheilk, 1926, Vol. 77.
Mueller-Deham: Wien. klin. Wochensch., 1926, No. 44.
Hoefler: Wuerzburger Abhandlungen, 1927, No. 9.
Weiss: Die Medizin, Welt, 1927, No. 22.
Schlesinger: Die Aerztliche Praxis, 1927, No. 4; Deut. med. Wochensch., 1927, No. 8; 1929, No. 27; Med. Klin., 1929, No. 1.
Zetsch: Fortsch. d. Medizin, 1928, No. 11.
Senator: Deut. med. Wochensch., 1928, No. 42.
Goldscheider: Zeitschrift f. aerztl. Fortbild, 1928, No. 2.

NORMOLACTOL

Behrens and Naujoks: Ztschr. f. exp. Med., 1925, 47.
Naujoks and Behrens: Zbl. fur Gyn., 1926, p. 161.
Pribram: Deut. med. Wochensch., 1926, p. 1950.
Lahm: Jahreskurse f. arztl. Fortb., 1927, 18:49.
Schmechel: Zbl. fur Gyn., 1927, p. 2566.
Schroder: Deut. med. Wochensch., 1927, p. 1415.
Jager: Med. Klin., 1928, p. 104.
Hahn: Dissertation, Hamburg, 1928.
v. Jaschke: Klin. Wochensch., 1928, No. 22.

NOSTAL

Ruehl, A.: Nostal as a Hypnotic in Childbed; Munch., med. Wochensch., 1926, No. 21.
Kirschbaum, W.: Clinical and Psychiatric Experiences with Nostal; Psychiatr. u. Neurol. Wochenschr., 1926, No. 28.
Halberkann, J. and Reiche, R.: The Elimination of Various Frequently Used Barbiturates; Munch. med. Wochenschr., 1927, No. 34:1450.
Wottschall, B. and Ruge, W.: Clinical Experiences with Nostal; Med. Klin., 1927, No. 18.
Wottschall, B. and Wheeler-Hill: The Elimination of Nostal; Deut. med. Wochensch., 1928, No. 4.
Boedecker, F. and Ludwig, H.: Nostal and Pernocton; Arch. f. exper. Pathol. u. Pharmakal., 1929, 139:353, 357, 361.
Breithaupt: The Hypnotic Nostal, An Unsaturated Barbiturate; Munch. med. Wochensch., 1929, No. 9:375.
Lardschneider, H.: Experiences with Nostal in Neuropsychiatry; Wien. med. Wochensch., 1929, No. 45.
Fitch, R. H. and Tatum, A. H.: The Duration of action of the Barbituric Acid Hypnotics as a Basis of Classification; J. Pharm. and Exper. Therap.; 1932, 44:325.

NOVASPIRIN

Hare, Hobart: Practical Therapeutics, 19th Edition, 1925.

NOVASUROL

Eppinger, H.: Therap. d. Gegenw., March, 1921.
Doll, H.: Zentralbl. f. Herz u. Gefasskrankh, 1922, No. 22.
Kulcke, E.: Klin. Wochensch., 1922, No. 13.
Hassencamp, E.: Zentralbl. f. inn. Med., 1922, No. 6.
Haggeney: Med. Klin., 1922, No. 2.
Burwinkel, O.: Munch. med. Wochensch., 1922, No. 6.
Neuhof, Selian: Therap. Gaz., Jan. 15, 1924.
Rowntree, Leonard G., Keith, Norman M., and Barrier, Charles W.: J. A. M. A., Oct. 17, 1925.
Crawford, J. Hamilton and J. F. McIntosh: J. Clinical Invest., Apr., 1925.
Gilchrist, A. R. and Edin, Ch. B.: Lancet, Nov. 14, 1925.
Stokes, Albert J.: Chicago Med. Recorder, June, 1925.
Barbosa, Jose: Sciencia Medica, 1925, No. 3.

NOVATONE

Karr: J. Biol. Chem., 1920, 54:277.
Cowgill: Am. J. Physiol., 1921, 57:420.
Osborne and Mendel: J. Biol. Chem., 1922, 54:739.
Nelson, Baldwin, Riggs and Cunningham: Am. J. Physiol., 1925, 72:69.
Cowgill, Deuel, Plummer and Messer: Am. J. Physiol., 1926, 77:389.
Hawk and Bergeim: Practical Phys. Chem., 9th Edition, 1927.

NOVATROPIN

Mullern, Ch.: Wien. med. Wochensch., 1922, No. 19, 20.
Dalmady, Z.: Med. Jour. of Budapest, 1922, No. 2.
Pachner, F.: Wien. med. Wochensch., 1922, No. 45.
Purjesz, B.: Med. Jour. of Transylvania, 1923.
De Heiner, L.: Deut. med. Wochensch. 1924, No. 42.
Ritter, Fritz: Arch. f. Kinderheilkunde, 1925, No. 2, Vol. 76.
Pal, J.: Am. Med., December, 1926.
Pal, J.: Therap. d. Gegenw., 1926, No. 9.
Biehl, K.: Wien. med. Wochensch., 1926, No. 1.

NOVIFORM

Lamers, A. J. M.: Med. Klin., 1912, No. 45, p. 1834.
Engelhard, W.: Versuche mit Noviform; Prager med. Wochensch., 1912, Nr. 33, S. 487.
Guttmann, C.: Deut. Zehnaerztl. Wochsch., 1913, No. 33.
Frischberg, A. L.: Noviform als neuer Jodoformersatz in der Chirurgie; Nowoe e Medizinie, 1913, Nr. 7, s. 391.
Leo, H.: Deut. med. Wochensch., 1923, Nr. 51.
Gins, Heinrich Al.: Biologie, Bakteriologie und Serologie; Fortsch. der Zahnheilkunde, 1925, I. Band, S. 73.
Kayser: Arztliche Rundschau, 1925, Nr. 3.

NOVOCAIN

Braun, Heinrich: Die ortliche Betaubung, ihre wissenschaftlichen Grundlagen und praktische Anwendung, 1919.
Hartel, Fritz: Die Lokalanasthesie., 2nd ed., Stuttgart, Ferdinand Enke, 1920.
Lockhart-Mummery, J. P.: Diseases of the Rectum and Colon, London, Baillere, Tindall and Cox, 1923.
Hirsh, Caesar: Lehrbuch der Lokalanasthesie des Ohres und der oberen Luft-und Speisewege, Stuttgart, Ferdinand Enke, 1925.
Cade, Standford: Lancet, April 25, 1925, Vol. 208, p. 856.
Mumey, Nolie and George K. Dunklee: Colorado Medicine, 1926, 23:247.
King, James J.: Local Anesthesia in Otolaryngology and Rhinology, New York, Paul B. Hoeber, 1926.
Hertzler, Arthur E.: The Technic of Local Anesthesia, St. Louis, C. V. Mosby Co., 1928.
Farr, Robert Emmett: Practical Local Anesthesia, 2nd ed., 1929, Lea and Febiger.
Rose, William and Carless, Albert: Manual of Surgery, 13th ed., edited by P. G. Wakeley and John B. Hunter, New York, Wm. Wood and Co., 1930.
DeTakats, Geza: Local Anesthesia, Phila., W. B. Saunders Co., 1931.
DaCosta, John Chalmers: Modern Surgery, General and Operative, Phila., W. B. Saunders Co., 1931.

NUMOTIZINE

McKee, E. S.: Med. Bull., Feb., 1907.
Culbreth: Materia Med. and Pharmacology, Lea and Febiger, 1927, p. 774.
Solis-Cohen and Githens: Pharmaco-Therapeutics, D. Appleton and Co., 1928, p. 996.
Wooton: Chronicles of Pharmacy, MacMillan and Co., Vol. 2, p. 298.

NUPERCAINE

Hirsch: Munch. med. Wochensch., 1929, 76:1715.
Fränkel: Die mediz. Welt, 1929, 3:612; Deut. med. Wochensch., 1929, 55:853.
Keyes and McLellan: Am. J. Surg., 1930, 9:1.
Bond and Bloom: J. Lab. Clin. Med., 1931, 16:447.
Keyes and McLellan: J. A. M. A., 1931, 96:2085.
Israels and Macdonald: Brit. Med. Jour., Nov. 28, 1931, No. 3699, pp. 986–988.
Holder: Am. J. Obst. and Gynec., June, 1932, p. 862.
Deyton, Wilson and Zaus: J. of Dental Research, August, 1932.
Arnheim and Mage: Surg., Gynec. and Obst., 1932, 54:826.

OCTOZONE

Parkes, Oscar and Buckley, C. H.: Treatment by Octozone; Lancet, October 17, 1931, p. 849.
Parkes, Oscar: Treatment of Rheumatism by Octozone; Brit. J. of Phys. Med., Jan. 1932.
McColl, A. G.: Observations on Octozone Therapy; Med. World, April 22, 1932.
Fawcitt, Richard: Brit. J. of Phys. Med., June, 1932.
Malleterre, F.: Octozone Therapy; Lien Medical, May, 1932.

OMNADIN

Much: Deut. med. Wochensch., 1920. Nos. 18 and 29; 1929, No. 26.
Roos: Fortsch. d. Medizin, 1921, No. 20.
Ridder: Med, Klin., 1922, No. 52.
Boehnke and Ignee: Fortschr. d. Medizin, 1923, No. 5.
Reichmann, W.: Deut. med. Wochensch., 1924, No. 36.
Rosenau, W.: Deut. med. Wochensch., 1925, No. 45.
Yamagishi: Die Therap. in der Praxis, 1926, No. 61.
Brunthaler: Deut. med. Wochensch., 1926, No. 50.
Miyakawa, H.: Rinsho Igaku, Monatschr. f. klin. Med., 1926, No. 6.
Berlin, Ch.: Therap. Berichte, 1927, No. 2.
Berlowitz: Therap. Berichte, 1927, No. 6.
J. A. M. A., April 15, 1933, p. 1172.
Denk: Sonder-Beilage d. Wien. Klin. Wochensch., Band 38, Heft 49.

OPTALIDON

Bandler: Zahnartzl. Rundschau, June 15, 1930, No. 34.
Fulep: Monatsch. Ungar. Mediz., 1930, 9–10.
Hellinger: Deut. Zahnaerz. Wochensch., Nov. 5, 1930, No. 21.
Herzog: Deut. med. Wochensch., 1930, No. 45.
Hopush: Zahnartztl. Rundschau, Oct. 19, 1930, No. 42.
Michaud: Schw. med. Wochensch., 1930, No. 13.
Nussbaum: Deut. med. Wochensch., 1930, No. 27,
Wachtel: Munch. med. Wochensch., 1930, No. 44.
Floor and Rohr: Schw. med. Wochensch., 1931, No. 6.
Jacoby: Munch. med. Wochensch., 1931, No. 18.

OPTARSON

Klemperer, G.: Therap. d. Gegenw., 1921, No. 3.
Lange, J.: Deut. med. Wochensch., 1921, No. 17.
Eisner, G.: Therap. d. Gegenw., 1921, No. 6.
Schultes: Therap. d. Gegenw., 1921, No. 8.
Geronne: Therap. d. Gegenw., January, 1922.
Walther: Med. Klin., 1922, No. 29.
Hosch: Therap. d. Gegenw., 1923, No. 1.
Helwig: Therap. d. Gegenw., 1924, No. 5.
Cushny, Arthur R.: A Text-book of Pharmacology and Therapeutics, 1924.
Krekeler: Therap. d. Gegenw., 1925, No. 2.

OPTOCHIN BASE

Levy, R.: Berl. klin. Wochensch., 1912, 49, 2486.
Mendel, F.: Munch. med. Wochensch., 1915, 62:740.
Rosenow, G.: Deut. med. Wochensch., 1915, 51:791.
Mendel, F.: Therap. d. Gegenw., Aug., 1917.
Kolmer, J. A., Solis-Cohen, S. and Heist, G. D.: J. Inf. Dis., 1917, 20:293, 333.
Rosin, H.: Therap. d. Gegenw., June, 1917 (new issue 19), 580.
Jakbo: Munch. med. Wochensch., 1917, 64: No. 35.
Schneider: Munch. med. Wochensch., 1920, 67:1006.
Cahn-Bronner- Ergebn. der inn. Medizin, 1922.
Cross, F. B.: L. I. Med. J., 1927, 20:132.

ORGANIDIN

Kimball: J. A. M. A., 1928, 91:454.

ORTAL SODIUM

Dox, Arthur W. and Hjort, A. M.: The Relative Physiological Properties of Certain Trialkyl and Dialkyl Barbituric Acids; J. Pharm. and Exper. Therap., 1927, 31:455.
Dox, Arthur W. and Jones, Edward G.: New Derivatives of Barbituric Acid; J. Am. Chem. Soc., 1928, 50:2033.
Hjort, A. M. and Dox, Arthur W.: Some Relative Physiological Properties of Certain New 5,5-Dialkyl and 1-Aryl-5,5-Dialkyl Barbituric Acids; J. Pharm. and Exper. Therap., 1929, 35:155.
Dox, Arthur W. and Jones, Edward G.: Direct Substitution of the Nitrogen of 5,5-Dialkylbarbituric Acids; J. Am. Chem. Soc., 1929, 51:316.
Dox, Arthur W.: The Reaction Between Barbital (Diethyl-barbituric Acid) and Phosphorus Pentachloride; J. Am. Chem. Soc., 1931, 53:1559.
Dox, Arthur W.: Oxygen Ethers of Barbital; J. Am. Chem. Soc., 1931, 53:2741.

OSCODAL

Dubin and Funk: J. Met. Res., 1923, 4:467.
Heft, H. L.: J. Amer. Pharm. Assoc., 1927, 16:41.

Fischer, Louis: J. Met. Res., 1925, 4:481.
Cohen: Med. Jour. and Record, Sept., 1927.
Daniels and Brooks: Proc. Soc. Exp. Biol. Med., 1927, 24:972.
Kramer, Shelling and Shear: J. Biol. Chem., 1928, 79:147.

OXINOL

Aaron: Diseases of the Digestive Organs, 4th ed.; 1927, p. 279.
Solis-Cohen and Githens: Pharmaco-therapeutics; Materia Medica and Drug Action; 1928, pp. 488–489.

OXO-ATE AND OXO-ATE "B"

Jeffery, R. L.: Northwest Medicine, June, 1928.
Rhodenburg, G. L. and Reich, C.: Am. J. Surg., Oct., 1928.
Stern, L. G.: J. A. M. A., Oct. 27, 1928.
Shands, A. R.: Internat. J. Med. and Surg., Nov., 1928.
Young, A. G.: New England Jour. of Med., Dec. 13, 1928.
Pemberton, R.: Arthritis and Rheumatoid Conditions; Lea and Febiger, Phila., 1929, pp. 282–284.

PANCREPATINE

Bernstein, J.: Raw Pancreas by Mouth Compared with Insulin; Brit. Med. Jour., 1925, 2:844.
Dunn, W.: Treatment of Diabetes by Raw Fresh Gland (Pancreas); Brit. Med. Jour., 1925, 1:680.
Kelly, H. P.: Treatment of Diabetes by Raw Fresh Gland (Pancreas); Brit. Med. Jour., 1925, 1:921.
Young, R. R.: Treatment of Diabetes by Raw Fresh Gland (Pancreas); Brit. Med. Jour., 1925, 1:632.
Hollins, T. J.: Treatment of Diabetes by Raw Fresh Gland (Pancreas); Brit. Med. Jour., 1925, 1:503.
Blum, L. and Carlier, P.: Le traitement du diabete par la synthaline; Bull. et mem. Soc. med. d. hop. de Paris, 1927, 51:5.
Editorial; J. A. M. A., 1927, 88:34.
J. A. M. A., March 3, 1928, p. 714.

PANCRESAL

Williams, Leonard: Brit. Med. Jour., 16. V., 23.
J. A. M. A., May 27, 1933, p. 1686.

PANKREON

Thompson, Howard: The Regular Medical Visitor, 1903, No. 12.
Schmidt, A.: Deut. Archiv. fur klin. Medizin, 1906, Vol. 87.
v. Noorden: Klin. Therap. W., 1908, No. 36.
Herz, M.: Klin. Therap. W., 1909, No. 47; Wien. med. Wochensch., 1911, Nos. 12 and 13.
Nigoul: Concours Medical, 1910, No. 2.
Klemperer, G.: Therap. d. Gegenw., 1913, No. 8.
Minkowski: Med. Klin., 1913, No. 17.
Buttersack: Berl. klin. Wochensch., 1921, No. 29.
Jankowsky: Munch. med. Wochensch., 1925, No. 22.
Boas, J.: Diagnostics and Therapeutics for Stomach Diseases; Part 1, 5th Ed.

PANTHESINE

Spiess: Munch. med. Wochensch., 1905, 53.
Gaza and Brandi: Mitt. klin. Wochensch., 1927, 6.
Rothlin: Arch. f. exper. Pathol. u. Pharmakol., 1929, 144, Nos. 3 and 4.
Wild: Schw. med. Zahnh., 1929, 39, 3.
Gigon: Schw. med. Wochensch., 1931, 61.
Lutz and Kelterborn: Schw. med. Wochensch., 1931, 61.
Pflimlin: Klin. Mtsbl. f. Augenheilk, Feb., 1931.
Rothlin: Arch. Exp. Path. and Pharm. Vol. 144, No. 3, 4.
Benedict, Clark and Feedman: J. A. D. A., Dec. 1932.
Bieser, Harvey and Burgers: J. Pharm. and Exp. Therap. Vol. 45, No. 3, 1932.

PARAFFIN COMPOUND

deSandford, Barthe: Progress Medicale, Feb. 24, 1917.
Sollmann: J. A. M. A., 1917, p. 1800.
Brit. Med. Jour., Jan. 13, 1917, p. 37.
New Orleans Med. and Surg., J., April, 1917, p. 681.
J. A. M. A., Apr. 7, 1917, pp. 1037; May 19, 1917, pp. 1497.

PARA-THOR-MONE

McCann, W. S.: Parathyroid Therapy; J. A. M. A., 1924, 83:1847.
Powers, G. F.: Tetany as a Cause of Convulsions in Whooping Cough; Am. J. Dis. Child., 1925, 30:632.
Snell, A. M.: Parathyroid Extract in Treatment of a Case of Tetany; J. A. M. A., 1925, 85:1632.

Cameron, A. T.: The Biochemistry of Calcium; Canad. Med. A. J., 1926, 16:753.
Collip, J. B.: The Therapeutic Value of the Parathyroid Hormone; J. A. M. A., 1926, 87:908.
Hoag, L. A. and Rivkin, K.: Treatment of Infantile Tetany, with a Parathyroid Ext.; J. A. M. A., 1926, 86:1343.
Keith, N.: In Discussion on Collip's Paper; J. A. M. A., 1926, 87:909.
Mason, E. H.: A Case of Chronic Nephritis treated with Collip's Parathyroid Extract; Canad. Med. A. J., 1926, 16:538.
Gordon, B. and Cantarow, A.: The use of Parathyroid Extract in Hemorrhage; J. A. M. A., 1927, 88:1301.
Backus, H. L., Bank, J. and Wilkinson, S. A.: Neurogenic Mucous Colitis; Am. J. M. Sc., 1928, 176:813.
Flinn, F. B. and Seidlin, S. M.: Para-thor-mone in Treatment of Radium Poisoning; Bull. Johns Hopkins Hosp., 1929, 45:269.
Haskell, B. and Cantarow, A.: Calcium and Parathyroid Therapy in Chronic Ulcerative Colitis; Am. J. M. Sc., 1931, 181:180.

PARATHYROID WITH CALCIUM LACTATE

Grove, W. R. and Vines, H. W. C.: Brit. Med. Jour., May 20, 1922 (abstr.) Ill. Med. Jour., July, 1923.
Editorial; J. A. M. A., Aug. 25, 1923.

PAROIDIN

Hanson, Adolph M.: J. A. M. A., March 10, 1928.

PENTNUCLEOTIDE

Jackson, Parker, Rinehart and Taylor: J. A. M. A., 1931, 97:1436.
Doan: J. A. M. A., 1932, 99:194.
Jackson, Parker and Taylor: Am. J. M. Sc., Sept., 1932.

PENTOBARBITAL SODIUM

Magill, I. W.: Lancet, 1930, 220:74 (Jan. 10, 1930).
Volwiler, E. H. and Tabern, D. L.: J. Am. Chem. Soc., 1930, 52:1676.
Fitch, R. H., Waters, R. M. and Tatum, A. L.: Am. J. Surg., 1930, 9:110.
Lundy, John S.: Anesthesia and Analgesia, 1930, 9:210.
Tabern, D. L.: Clin. Med. and Surg., 1930, 37:809.
Lundy, J. S., McCuskey, C. F. and Tovell, R. M.: Proc. Staff Meetings Mayo Clinic, 1931, 6:2.
Shipway, F.: Lancet, 1931, 220:353.
Magill, I. W.: Lancet, 1931, 220:353.
Rowbotham, S.: Lancet, 1931, 220:439.
Riddell, J.: Lancet, 1931, 220:498.
Barlow, O. W., Duncan, J. T. and Gledhill, J. D.: J. Pharm. and Exper. Therap., 1931, 41:366.
Graham, J. D.: Lancet, 1931, 51:470.
Rowbotham, S.: Lancet, 1931, 221:743.

PEPTENZYME

Fantus, Bernard: J. A. M. A., March 6, 1926, Vol. 86, No. 10.
J. A. M. A., Feb. 9, 1907, p. 533; Oct. 5, 1907, p. 1198; Reports Council Pharm. and Chem., 1905, 8, p. 79.

PEPTONE SOLUTION

Auld, A. G.: Brit. Med. Jour., May 5, 1917.
Brit. Med. Jour., July 20, 1918.
Fatou, E.: Bull. Med., Sept. 30, 1922.
Vallery-Radot, P.: Bull. Med., Sept. 30, 1922.
Lancet, April 21, 1923.
N. Y. Med. Jour. and Record, June 20, 1923.
Schiff, N. S.: Am. J. M. Sc., Nov., 1923.
Wynn, W. H.: Lancet, Sept. 22, 1923.
Miller, J. L. and Raulston, B. O.: J. A. M. A., June 30, 1923.
J. A. M. A., Nov. 29, 1924, p. 1786; Reports Council Pharm. and Chem., 1924, p. 50.

PERISTALTINE

Pietsch: Dissertation Bern, p. 20; Therapeut. Monatshefte, Vol. 24, No. 1, Jan., 1910.
Tschirch and Monikowski: Archiv. der Pharmazie, 1912, 250:92.
Duhem: Journal de Medecine de Paris, 1913, 33:936.
Kastriner: Gyogyaszat, No. 51, pp. 891–892, Dec. 21, 1913 and Therap. d. Gegenw., Vol. 56, No. 7, July, 1915.
Flatau: Monatssch. f. Geburtsh. und Gynaek., 1914, 39:646.
Platau: Monatssch. f. Geburtsh. und Gynaek., 1916, 43:265.

PERNOSTON (Pernocton)

McKesson, E. I. and McCarthy, K C.: A Comparison of Sodium Amytal and Pernoston as Pre-Anesthetic Hypnotics; Brit. Med. Jour., November 29, 1930.
McCarthy, K. C.: Pre-anesthetic Hypnosis by Means of Pernoston; Anesthesia and Analgesia, 1930, 9:231.
Fitch, R. H., Waters, R. M. and Tatum, A. L.: The Intravenous use of the Barbituric Acid Hypnotics in Surgery; Am. J. Surg., 1930, 9:110.
Brown, R., Moloy, H. and Laird, M.: Pernoston as an Analgesic in Obstetrics and Gynecology; Amer. J. Obst. and Gynec., 1931, 22:225.
Friedlaender, B.: Pernoston Sleep; Am. J. Surg., 1931, 11:485.
Kautz, F. A. S.: Pernoston, A Hypnotic and Amnesic Agent; J. Med., 1931, 12:16.
Matters, R. F.: Pernoston in Obstetrics; Med. Jour. of Australia, Nov. 21, 1931.
J. A. M. A., October 3, 1931, p. 1001; Reports Council Pharm. and Chem., 1931, p. 77.
Poe, James G.: Modern General Anesthesia; F. A. Davis Co.; Philadelphia, 1932, pp. 200–203.
Saklad, Meyer: Anesthetic Agents; Am. J. Surg., 1932, 16:451.
Stedge, R. L.: The Use of Pernoston in Obstetrics; Guthrie Clinic Bulletin, 1932, 1:77–79.
Fitch, R. H. and Tatum, A. L.: The Duration of Action of the Barbituric Acid Hypnotics as a Basis of Classification; J. Pharm. and Exper. Therap., 1932, 44:325.
Green-Armytage, V. B.: Gynecology in the Tropics; Indian Medical Gazette, 1932, 1:26.
Costallo, M. A.: Pernoston Hypnosis in Obstetrics; New Engl. J. of Med. 1933, 209: 744.

PERTUSSIN

Camphausen: Fortsch. d. Medizin, Aug. 21, 1913.
J. A. M. A., March 8, 1913, p. 766; March 27, 1920, p. 905; Propaganda, vol. 1, p. 334; vol. 2, p. 467;
J. A. M. A., Feb. 20, 1926, p. 573.
Sommerfeld, Th.: Med. Klin., March 8, 1914.
Sollmann: A Manual of Pharmacology, 1927, p. 860.
Paulsen, Ernst: Die Tuberkulose, Feb. 10, 1928.
Poras, Josef: On Cough Specialties; Arztliche Rundschau, vol. 15, 1928.
Jungmann, M.: Allgem. mediz. Zentral-Zeitung, 1928, Jan. 28.
Kochmann, M.: Arch. f. exper. Pathol. u. Pharmakol., 1930, 150:23.
Gordonoff, T.: Med. Klin., 1931, 27:1794.
Schif, Erich: Arch. f. exper. Pathol. u. Pharmakol., 1932, 166:22.
Vollmer, Hubert: Klin. Wochensch., 1932, 11:590.

PERTUSSIS VACCINOTHERAPY

Luttinger: J. A. M. A., May 19, 1917.
Luttinger: N. Y. Med. Jour., Feb. 22, 1919.
Davies: Am. J. Dis. Child., May, 22, p. 423.
J. A. M. A., Oct. 11, 1924, p. 1184; Reports Council Pharm. and Chem., 1924, p. 58.
Aldrich: Am. J. Dis. Child., April, 1925, p. 486.

PETROLAGAR

Moore, I. H.: Northwest Medicine Vol. 25, No. 11, Nov., 1926.
Fantus, Bernard: Useful Cathartics; J. A. M. A., 1927.
Aaron, Chas. L.: Diseases of the Digestive Organs, Lea and Febiger, Phila., 1927.
De Lee, Joseph B.: The Principles and Practice of Obstetrics, W. B. Saunders, Phila.
Drueck, Chas. J.: Influence of Rectal Disease upon the Central Nervous System; Chicago Med. Recorder, April, 1927.
Montague, Joseph Franklin: The Modern Treatment of Hemorrhoids. J. B. Lippincott Company.
Bastedo, Walter A.: Rambles in the Field of Gastrointestinal Therapeutics; N. Y. State J. Med., Vol. 27, No. 21, Nov. 1, 1927.
Montague, J. F.: Suggested Modification in the Technic of X-Ray Examinations of the Gastrointestinal Tract; Med. Jour. and Record, N. Y., May 4, 1927, p. 602.

PHANODORN

Krieger, K. Isaac and Noah, G.: Med Klin., No. 18, 1925.
Pfannmuller: Munch. med. Wochensch. No. 46, 1925.
Meyer, Walter B.: Klin. Wochensch. No. 23, 1925.
Muller, P.: Munch. med. Wochensch. No. 35, 1925.
Weisz, E.: Therap. d. Gegenw., Dec., 1927.
Silzer, O.: Munch. med. Wochenschr. No. 49, 1928.
Mondre, O.: Wien. klin. Wochensch. No. 4, 1928.
Hamburger, H.: Med. Klin., No. 19, 1929.
Lackerbauer, J.: Zeitsch. f. d. ges. Neurol., u. Psychiat. Bd. 90, Hft. 1 and 2.

PHEDROCAINE

Lilienthal, Howard: Thoracic Surgery as a Specialty; Ann. Surgery, January, 1925.
Jackson, Chevalier: Bronchoscopy and Esophagoscopy; September, 1927, Sec. Ed.

McCullagh: Med. Jour. and Record, Sept., 1930.
Diasio, Joseph S.: Med. Jour. and Record, May 6, 1931.
Straatsman, C. R.: Med. Jour. and Record, April 20, 1932.
Haiman, J. A.: Med. Jour. and Record, May 18, 1932.

PHENOLSULPHONEPHTHALEIN

Rowntree and Geraghty: J. A. M. A., 1911, 57:811.
Roth, Max: Berl. klin. Wochensch., September, 1913, p. 1609.
Sohon, Michael Druck: Am. Chem. J., Vol. 20, No. 4, p. 263.
J. A. M. A., Vol. 62, No. 4, p. 298.
Abel and Rowntree: J. Pharm. and Exper. Therap., Vol. 1, No. 6, p. 595.

PHYLLICIN

Bliss and Morrison: A Comparative Study of Certain Xanthine Diuretics; J. of the Tennessee State Med. Assoc. 1932, 25:387-400.
Hyman and Parsonnet: The Failing Heart of Middle Life; F. A. Davis Co., Philadelphia, 1932.
Sutton and Lueth: Diseases of the Coronary Arteries; C. V. Mosby Co., St. Louis, 1932.
J. A. M. A., March 25, 1933, p. 886.

PHYTINE

Gilbert and Lippmann: Pres. Medicale, 1904, 69 and 73, pp. 545 and 577.
Winterberg: Aerztl. Central-Zeitung, 1905, 17:406; 1905, 17:420.
Renon: Journal des Practiens, No. 5, 1905, p. 65-68.
Cimbal: Med. Klin., 1926, 22:1727.
Negro: Journal des Praticiens, 1928, 42:1292.
Basch: Med. Klin., 1929, 25:151.
J. A. M. A., January 30, 1915, p. 456; Reports Council Pharm. and Chem., 1915, p. 131; Propaganda, vol. 1, p. 178.

PITOCIN

Ward, Lyons and Bemis: Proc. Soc. Exp. Biol. Med., December, 1928.
Bourne, A. W. and Burn, J. H.: Lancet, Oct. 6, 1928.
Clark: J. of Phys., Nov. 9, 1928.

PITUITRIN

Kamm, Aldrich, Grote, Rowe and Bugbee: J. A. M. A., Feb. 25, 1928.
J. A. M. A., August 17, 1929, p. 524; Reports Council Pharm. and Chem., 1929, p. 39.

PIXALBOL

Kromayer: Progress in the Treatment of Eczema; Canad. J. Med. and Surg., 1904; Wien. med. Wochensch. No. 3, 1905.
Simpson: Infantile Eczema; J. A. M. A., April 6, 1912.
Pusey: Principles and Practice of Dermatology, D. Appleton Co., 1924.
J. A. M. A., November 22, 1924, p. 1704; Reports Council Pharm. and Chem., 1924, p. 51.
Galewsky: Zehn Jahre Cignolin und seine therapeutische Verwendung in der Dermatologie; Dermat. Wochensch. No. 26, 1926.
Jadassohn: Treatment of Psoriasis; Allgem. Med. Zentralztg. No. 7, 1927.
Hoffman: Die Behandlung der Haut und Geschlechtskrankheiten. Textbook.

PLANT POISONING

Strickler, Albert: The Treatment of Dermatitis Venenata by Vegetable Toxins; J. Cutan, Dis. 1918, 36:327.
Strickler, Albert: The Toxin Treatment of Dermatitis Venenata; J. A. M. A., 1921, 77:910.
Strickler, Albert: The Value of the Toxin (Antigen) of Rhus venenata in the Treatment and Desensitization of Patients with Dermatitis Venenata; J. A. M. A., 1923, 80:1588.
Bivings, F. Lee: Successful Desensitization and Treatment of Poison Ivy and Poison Oak Poisoning; Arch. of Derm. and Syph., 1924, 9:602.
Alderson, Harry E.: Treatment of Poison Oak Dermatitis; Cal. and West. Med. 1925, 23:982.
Spain, W. C. and Cooke, R. A.: Studies in Specific Hypersensitiveness; XXVII. Dermatitis Venenata: Observations Upon the Use of a Modified Extract from Toxicodendron Radicans (L); J. Immunol., 1927, 13:93.

PLASMOCHIN

Clark, H. C.: Am. J. Trop. Med., 1927, 7:15.
Djokic, A. and Stambuk, Dinko: Beihefte z. Arch. f. Schiffs-u. Tropen-Hyg., 1927, 31:117.
Hegner, R. and Manwell, R. D.: Am. J. Trop. Med., 1927, 7:279.
Roehl, W.: Beihefte z. Arch. f. Schiffs-u. Tropen-Hyg., 1926, 30:311; 1927, 31:48.

Vad, B. G. and Mohile, G. B.: Ind. Med. Gazette, 1927, 62:430.
Bhattacharyya, P. and Chowdhury, S. P. Roy: Ind. Med. Gazette, 1928, 63:630.
Krauss, William: South. Med. Jour., 1928, 21:729; 1929, 22:359.
Connor, R. C.: Texas J. Med., 1929, 25:219.
Ejercito, A.: J. Philippine Med. Assoc., 1929, 9:229.
Smith, S.: J. Roy. Army Med. Corps, 1929, 53:81.
Miller, R. L.: J. Med. Assoc. Georgia, 1930, 19:363.
Sinton, J. A.: Ind. Med. Gazette, 1930, 65:603.

POLYGALYSATE

Handovsky, H.: Deut. Med. Wochensch. 1925, No. 32.
Oppenheim, H.: Med. Klin., 18th year, No. 12.
Levisohn, Hugo: Med. Wochensch., 73d year, No. 43.

POTASSIUM IODO-THEOCALCIN

Askanazy: Ueber Iod. Calcium-Diuretin; Med. Klin., 7, 1925.

PROCAINE BORATE AND EPINEPHRIN

Dailey, H. T. and Benedict, H. C.: Studies in Local Anesthetics; Dental Cosmos, 1929.

PROGENE

Weil, Arthur: The Chemical Causes of the Motility of Spermatozoa; Archiv. f. Frauenheilkunde und Eugenetik, Nr. 3, Bd. VII, 1921.
Bandler, S. W.: The Endocrines, Saunders, 1921.
Huhner, Max: Diagnosis and Prognosis of Sterility in both Sexes; Am. Med., February, 1925.
Muschat, Maurice: The Effect of Variations of Hydrogen Ion Concentration on the Motility of Human Spermatozoa; Surg., Gynec. and Obst., June, 1926.
Meaker, S. R. and Glaser, W.: The Hydrogen Ion Concentration of the Endocervical Secretions, with Special Reference to Chemical Factors in the Causation of Sterility; Surg., Gynec. and Obst., 1929, 48:73.
Meaker, Samuel R.: The Need for Complete investigation in Cases of Sterility; J. Med., September, 1930.
Meaker, Samuel R.: A Survey of Causative Factors in Sterility; Am. J. Obst. and Gynec., 1930; 20:758.

PROGYNON

Streck, A. and Wurzburg: Klin. Wochensch., 1929, No. 25, p. 1172.
Sajitz, R.: Hormone Therapy in Ovarian Hypofunction; Mediz. Welt., Berlin, 1930, No. 44, p. 1585.
Schoeller, W., Dohrn, M. and Hohlweg, W.: The Peroral Effect of Follicular Hormones; Med. Jour. and Record, Nov. 19, 1930.
Hacker, Raymond C.: Report of a severe case of Dysmenorrhea relieved with Progynon, an Allen-Doisy Female Sex Hormone; Med. Jour. and Record, Sept. 2, 1931.
Dodds, E. C.: The Clinical Importance of the Sex Hormones; Am. J. Obst. and Gynec., 1931, 22:520.
Mazer, Chas. and Ziserman, A. J.: Present Status of Female Sex Hormone Therapy; Med. Jour. and Record, Jan. 6, 1932.
Hall, George, Joyce: Endocrine Therapy in Menstrual Disorders; Am. Med., new series, Vol. 27, No. 8, June 1932.
Smith, Geo. Van S. and Smith, O. Watkins: The Excretion of Oestrin by Women; Am. J. Physiol., Vol. 100, No. 3, May, 1932.
Stein, Irving F., and Leventhal, Michael L.: Infertility and Sterility; J. A. M. A., Feb. 20, 1932.
Saxon, Leon: Endocrine Aspects of Chronic Arthritis; Med. Jour. and Record, Jan. 4, 1933.

PROKLIMAN

Keip: Deut. med. Wochenschr., No. 34, 1927.
Kerstan: Med. Klin., No. 22, 1927.
Weiss: Fortsch. d. Medizin., No. 16, 1927.
Braun: Zentralb. f. Gynaek., No. 37, 1927.
Hertel: Zentralb. f. Gynaek., No. 12, 1928.

PROTARGOL

Chetwood, Charles H.: Practice of Urology, 1913.
Coryell, John R.: Lancet, May 15, 1915.
Strouse, A. N.: Bull. Dept. Public Charities, October, 1916.
Jones, W. Ray: Med. Record, June 2, 1917.
Copridge, W. M.: Charlotte Med. Jour., September, 1919.
Peacock, Alexander H.: Northwest Medicine, March, 1920.
Michelson, H. E.: Lancet, Jan. 15, 1920.
Schapira, S. William and Joseph Wittenberg: Am. Med.. June. 1921.
Bourne, A. W.: Lancet, Feb. 24, 1923.

Roblee, Lawrence H.: Urol. and Cut. Rev., Sept., 1924.
Bierhoff, Frederick: Therap. Gaz., 3, 15, 1924.
Kurzweil, P. M. and Saxl, N. T.: Arch. Pediat., March, 1925.

PROTEIN MILK, POWDERED

Haas, S. V., Bargenberg, L. H. and Bloomberg, M. W.: Protein Milk as an Infant Food; Arch. Pediat., 1924, 41:741.
Hucker, G. J. and Hucker, A. M.; Organisms Associated with Commercially Prepared Infant Foods; Am. J. Dis. Child., 1929, 38:310.
Abt, A. F. and Feingold, B. F.: The Use of Powdered Milk and Milk Derivatives in the Concentration of Infant Foods; Arch. Pediat., 1930, 47:603.
Goldbloom, A.: Special Feeding Methods for Infants; Canad. Med. A. J., 1930, 23:807.
Hill, N. and Mellor, A. W. C.: Protein Milk in Infant Feeding; Lancet, 1930, 2:398.
Hodges, G. C.: Celiac Disease; West Virginia M. J., 1930, 26:471.
Parsons, L. G.: Celiac Disease; Lancet, 1931, 1:61.
Haas, S. V.: Celiac Disease: Its Specific Treatment and Cure Without Nutritional Relapse; J. A. M. A., 1932, 99:448.
Moore, H. L.: The Medical Treatment of Congenital Pyloric Stenosis; Texas State M. J., 1932, 28:459.
Porter, L. and Carter, W. E.: Management of the Sick Infant, G. V. Mosby Co., 1932, p. 59.
Silverman, A. C.: Celiac Disease; N. Y. State J. Med., 1932, 32:1055.

PROTOLAC

Dennett, R. H.: Simplified Infant Feeding.
Marriotte. Wm.: Infant Nutrition, etc.

P-THIOCRESOL

J. A. M. A., May, 1930.
Ann. Surg., February, 1931.

PYRAMIDON

Januschke, H.: Wien. klin. Wochensch., No. 13, 1927.
Bodenstab: Deut. Archiv. fur klin. Medizin, 1928, 159:171.
Korobkoff: Vratchebnaya Gazeta, 1930, 34:1745.
Schultz: Arch. of Int. Med., 1931, 48:1138–1145.

PYRIDIUM

Jones, H. F. H.: Renal Infections Complicating Pregnancy; Jour. Arkansas Med. Soc., November, 1928.
Pugh, W. S.: The Prostate Gland; Am. Med., 1928, 23:504–508.
Wolbarst, A. L.: The Present Day Treatment of Acute Gonorrhea in the Male; Am. J. Surg., 1928, 4:280–287.
Wagner, O.: Oral Treatment of Gonorrheal Diseases; Wien. med. Wochensch., No. 50, 1929.
Russo: T. Pyridium; Zahnarztl. Rundschau 38: Dec. 29, 1929.
Neuburger, J.: Pyridium, a New Urinary Antiseptic; Munch. med. Wochensch., 1930, 77:1016–1017.
Louda, V.: Pyridium; Fortsch. d. Medizin, 48: Sept., 1930.
Wyman, H. E.: Backache in the Male; J. South Carolina M. A., 1931, 27:113, April, 1931.
Ludden, R. H.: Cervicitis; Wis. Med. Jour., 1931, 30:903–908.
Helmholz, H. F.: Diagnosis and Treatment of Infection of Urinary Tract in Childhood; Lancet, 1932, 52:295–297.
Stokes, P. B.: Cystitis; Texas State J. Med. 1932, 27:728–730.
Young, H. M.: The Management of Chronic Prostate; J. Missouri State Med. Assoc., 1932, 29:300–305.

QUICAMPHOL

K. Radicke: Therap. d. Gegenw., December, 1926, 67:537.
Rossius: Fortsch. der Therapie, July, 1926, No. 13.
Wolfer: Schw. med. Wochensch., 1926, No. 25.
A. Müller-Deham: Wien. klin. Wochensch., Suppl. No. 33, 1926, 39:1; 1927, No. 3.
Hummelet: Tierarztliche Rundschau, 1926, No. 50.
Cahn-Bronner: Therap. d. Gegenw., 1927, 68:97.
Newton and Heine: Am. Rev. of Tub., November, 1928.
Lolita M. Flewelling: Med. Jour. and Record, 1929, 129:446.
J. A. M. A., November 9, 1929, p. 1471; Reports Council Pharm. and Chem., 1929, p. 40.

QUINIDINE

Brit. Med. Jour., Jan., 1921, p. 521.
Lancet, Jan., 1921, p. 374.
Brit. Med. Jour., Nov., 1921, p. 576.
Lancet, Nov., 1921, p. 894.
J. A. M. A., Nov. 25, p. 1091.
J. A. M. A., Nov. 25, p. 1159.

QUININE HYDROCHLORIDE AND URETHANE

Aaron, Chas. D.: N. Y. Med. Jour. and Med. Rec., Dec. 20, 1922.
Howard, C. The Lancet, Jan. 5, 1929.

QUINIOBINE

Müller, Hugo and Kohlenberger: Munch. med. Wochensch., 1927, 74:1491.
Curth, W. and Curth-Ollendorf, H.: Dermat. Wochensch., 1928, 87:1395.
Dörffel, J. and Pachur, R.: Dermat. Zeitschrift, 1929, 55:131.
Mignot, René: Pres. Medicale, 1929, 37:332.
Curth, W.: Therap. d. Gegenw., 1930, 71:28.

QUINISAL

Cushny: Pharmacology and Therapeutics, 7th edition, 1918.
Sollman: Manual of Pharmacology, 1922.

QUINOXYL

Jones and Turner: J. A. M. A., Aug. 24, 1929, p. 583.

RABIES VACCINE

Semple, Sir David: The Nature of Rabies and Anti-Rabic Treatment; Brit. Med. Jour., Vol. 7, Sept. 20, 1919.
Harvey, W. I. and Acton, H. W.: An Examination Into the Degree of Efficiency of Anti-Rabic Treatment; Indian J. M. Res. Calcutta, 10.020, April, 1923.

RADIUM SALTS

Farrar: Am. J. Obst. and Gynec., 1925, 10:205.
Murphy, Ignatius J.: Radiotherapy for Skin Lesions; Radiol. Rev. and Chicago Med. Rec., March, 1928.
Pfahler, George E.: The X-Rays and Radium in the Control of Cancer; Radiol. Rev. and Chicago Med. Rec., March, 1928.
MacKee, George M.: Cutaneous Roentgen-Ray and Radium Therapy; J. A. M. A., 1928, 90:28.
Ward: Am. J. Obst. and Gynec., 1929, 17:8.
Ward, George Gray and Farrar, Lillian K. P.: Eleven Years' Experience with the Radium Treatment of Carcinoma of the Cervix at the Woman's Hospital; Surg., Gynec. and Obst., February, 1931, p. 556.

RADON

Eller, Joseph Jordan and Fox, Everett C.: Treatment of Skin Cancer; N. Y. State J. of Med., Nov. 15, 1930.
Bowing: Am. J. Roentg. and Rad. Ther., May, 1931.
Dean, Archie L., and Quimby, Edith H.: Radiation Therapy of Carcinoma of the Bladder; Surg., Gynec. and Obst., 1931, 53:89–96.
Ferguson, Russell S.: Cancer of the Prostate; Am. J. Cancer, Vol. 16, No. 4, July, 1932.
Burton, J. Lee, Pack, George T, Quimby, Edith H., and Stewart, Fred W.: Irradiation of Mammary Cancer, with Special Reference to Measured Tissue Dosage; Arch. of Surg., 1932, 24:339–410.

RECOLAC

Courtney, A. M. and Brown, A.: A Comparison of the Buffer Capacity of Various Milk Mixtures Used in Infant Feeding; Canad. Med. A. J., 1928, 19:51.
Gladstone, H. B.: Clinical Observations on Infant Feeding and Nutrition, William Heinemann, Ltd., London, 1928.
Hucker, G. J. and Hucker, A. M.: Organisms Associated with Commercially Prepared Infant Foods; Am. J. Dis. Child., 1929, 38:310.
McClanahan, H. M.: Pediatrics for the General Practitioner, J. B. Lippincott Co., Philadelphia, 1929, p. 114.
Shapero, A. A.: Infant Diet and Hygiene During the First Year; Ky. M. J., 1929, 27:192.
Braithwaite, J. V. C.: Infant Feeding in General Practice, William Wood and Co., New York, 1930, p. 64.
Sellew, G.: Pediatric Nursing, W. B. Saunders Co., Philadelphia, 1931, p. 54.
Sauer, L. W.: Nursery Guide, C. V. Mosby Co., St. Louis, 1933, p. 63.

RECVALYSATE

Liepelt, K.: Deut. med. Wochensch., 1916, No. 2.
Maass, R.: Fortsch. d. Medizin, 1925, No. 16.
Steiner: Fortsch. d. Medizin, 1925, No. 24.
Lorenz: Landarzt, 1925, No. 25.
Spiethoff, B.: Fortsch. d. Therapie, 1925, No. 3.
Lenhardt, K.: Therap. d. Gegenw., 1926, No. 8.

Braun, G.: Klin. Wochensch., 1927, No. 50.
Graf, F.: Fortsch. d. Medizin, 1927, No. 11.
Arlt, F.: Medizin. Welt, 1928, No. 3.

REGULIN

Strasburger: Zeitsch. fur klin. Medizin, 1902, 46:413.
Lohrisch: Deut. Archiv. fur klin. Medizin, 1904, 79:383.
Simon-Lohrisch: Zeitsch. f. physikal. Chemie, 1904, 42:55.
Schmidt, Ad.: Munch. med. Wochensch., No. 41, 1905.

REMOGLAND

Hoskins and Hoskins: Arch. of Int. Med., 1918, 17:584.
Kingsburg, B. F.: Endocrinology, Jan., 1924.
Zondek: Deuts. Med. Wochensch., 339, March, 1923.
Jacoby: Med. Jour. and Record, June, 1924.
Weil: Med. Life, March, 1925.
Hulton: Ill., Med. Jour., Dec., 1926.
Molony: Jour. of Mental Science, Jan., 1927.
Lyons, Hunt: Med. Times, March, 1927.
Levy: Am. Med., Jan., 1928.
Vincent and Thompson: Endrokrinologie, 1929, 5:335.
Novak: J. A. M. A., 1930, 95:17.
Schapiro: Deuts. Med. Wochensch., 1930, 56:1599.

RIVANOL

Hill, Thomas Clement: Am. J. Surg., Jan., 1929.

ROOT-CANAL FILLING

Eisenberg, M. J. and Frost, W. S.: Dental Items of Interest, 1932, 54:833; Modern Dentistry, Jan. 1933.

SAJODIN

Barbier, P.: Revue de Pathol. Comparee, No. 40, 1907.
Barker, L. F.: Virginia Med. Semi-Month, Jan. 27 and Feb. 10, 1911.
Williamson, O. K.: The Lancet, Apr. 11, 1914.

SALIHEXIN

Corson-White, E. P.: Med. Jour. and Record, Dec. 5 and 19, 1928.

SALIPYRIN

Smith, Alfred John: Univ. Dublin; The Hospital, 1898, p. 290.
Hare: National Stand. Disp., 1908, p. 200.
Bellamy, Henry F.: West London Hosp. Folio Therapeutics, 119.
Potter, F. P.: Practical Therapeutics.

SALIT

Muller, Paul; Schmidt and Buch: Deut. med. Wochensch., 1904, No. 15.
J. A. M. A., June 5, 1909, p. 1852; Reports Council Pharm. and Chem., 1909, p. 106.
Salgo: Die Heilkunde, 1913, No. 5.
Brandes: Gross Berliner Aerzte Blatt, 1930, No. 35.
Schoenke: Dtsch. Aerzte Ztg., 1931, No. 272.
Kionka, H.: Klin. Wochensch., 1931, No. 34, p. 1570.

SALVYSATE

Koeniger, K.: Therap. d. Gegenw., 1923, No. 9, 10.
Katz, George: Therap. d. Gegenw., 1923, No. 2.
Loyko, E.: Orvosi Hetilap, 1925, No. 27.
Danzer, Leo: Munch., med. Wochensch., 1925, No. 37.
Zwerg: Deut. med. Wochensch., 1925, No. 42.
Unvericht: Klin. Wochensch., 1926, No. 31.
Weiss, F.: Fortsch. d. Therapie, 1926, No. 14.
Sternberg, T.: Wien. Kl. W., 1926, No. 43.
Mattausch, F.: Wien. Kl. W., 1927, No. 34.

SALYRGAN

Bernheim, F.: Therap. d. Gegenw., Nov. 12, 1924.
Rosenberg, M.: Klin. Wochensch., March 19, 1925.

Allen, F. M.: Maine Med. Jour., Sept., 1927.
Harvey G. Agnew: Canad. Med. A. J., Jan., 1928.
Bannick, Edwin G. and Keith, Norman M.: J. A. M. A., Dec. 22, 1928.
Barker, M. Herbert and O'Hare, James P.: J. A. M. A., Dec. 29, 1928.
Bannick, Edwin G. and Keith, Norman M.: Med. Clin. of North America, June, 1929.
Dwyer, Hugh L.: Jour. Kansas Med. Soc., May, 1929.
Funkhouser, W. L.: Arch. Pediat., March, 1929.

SANDOPTAL

Nielson, Higgins and Spruth: J. Pharm. and Exper. Therap. 5, 1925.
Mosbacher: Munch. med. Wochensch., 37, 1927.
Bamberger: Deut. med. Wochensch., 3, 1928.
Groszhaus: Monatsschr. Ungar. Med., 10, 1928.
Walker: Munch. med. Wochensch., 35, 1929.
Reinhardt: Zentralb. f. Gynaek., 44, 1930.

SANTYL

Powell: The Causes of Urethritis: Treatment with the New Balsam, Santyl; Merck's Archives, 1, p. 7, 1907.
Wolbarst: Genito-urinary Diseases, Acute Gonorrhea and Acute Posterior Urethritis; Internat. J. of Surg., April and May, 1908.
Jacoby: The Treatment of Vesical Tenesmus in various Gynecological Affections by Santyl; Med. Klin., 11, 1908.
Read: Acute Gonorrhea in the Male—Its Duration and Treatment; Long Island Med. Jour., February, 1910.
Mehlhorn: Ueber Santyl-Knoll; Zentralb. f. d. gesamte Therapie, Heft 8, 1911.

SARAKA

Lindner, Kurt: Deut. med. Wochensch., No. 6, 1924.
Maul, Nelly: Klin. Wochensch., 2nd year, 26.
Wachenheimer, H.: Med. Welt, No. 4, 1931.
Burrows, E. C. and Burrows, Walter C.: Am. Med., March, 1931.

SAVITA

Mason: Med. Times, 1921, p. 130.
Newton, C. Faust: Med. Jour. and Record, May 19, 1926.

SCARLET FEVER ANTITOXIN

Dick, G. F. and Dick, Gladys H.: A Skin Test for Susceptibility to Scarlet Fever; J. A. M. A., 1924, 82:265, 266.
Dick, G. F. and Dick, Gladys H.: The Control of Scarlet Fever; Northwest Med., 1926, 25:200–204.
Kolmer, J. A.: The Practical Value of Biologic Therapy in the Prophylaxis and Treatment of Scarlet Fever; Am. J. Dis. Child, 1926, 32:556–563.
Lewis, M. S.: Scarlet Fever, Prevention and Treatment; J. Tenn. Med. Assoc., 1926, 19:5–7.
Young, C. C. and Orr, P. F.: Dosage of Toxin for Active Immunization against Scarlet Fever; J. A. M. A., 1926, 86:1340–1343.
Gordon, J. E.: Treatment of Scarlet Fever with Streptococcus Antitoxin; J. A. M. A., 1927, 88:382.
Dick, G. F.: Methods for the Control of Scarlet Fever; W. Virginia Med. J., 1928, 24:441–447.

SCILLAREN

Okushina: Arch. f. Exper. Pathol. and Pharm., Vol. 95, 1922, p. 258.
Stoll: Arch. de Cardiol. y Hematol. 12, 1922, p. 478.
Fahrenkamp: Deut. Archiv. fur. klin. Medizin, Vol. 144, Nos. 1–2, 1924.
Burn: Pharm. Jour. and Pharmacist, March 26, 1927, p. 328.
Premankur de: J. Pharm. and Exper. Therap., Vol. 31, No. 1, May, 1927.
Rothlin: Schw. med. Wochensch., 1927, 57:1171.
Stoll, Suter and Kreis: Verhand. d. Schw. Naturforsch. Gessls., Basel, 1927, II. Teil, pp. 132–134; 1932 pp. 331–334.
Winton: J. Pharm. and Exper. Therap., Vol. 31, No. 2, June, 1927.
Eismayer: Munch. med. Wochensch., No. 27, 1928.
Rothlin: Arch. f. Exper. Pathol. and Pharm., Vol. 131, Nos. 3 and 4, 1928.
Stehle, Ross and Dreyer; J. Pharm. and Exp. Ther. May, 1931.
Chen and Chen: J. Pharm. and Exp. Therap., March, 1933.

SILARGEL

Suchanek, E.: Wien. med. Wochensch. No. 50, 1931.
Raabe, R.: Mediz. Welt. 1931, No. 30.
Heindl, A.: Wien. med. Wochensch. No. 6, 1932.
Jehle, L.: Wien. med. Wochensch. No. 1, 1932.

SILVOGON

VonZumbusch: Cyansilbercholat zur Gonorrhoebehandlung; Wien. med. Wochensch., 1925, No. 6.
Samuels, Saul S. and Scher, Isador: The Treatment of Acute Gonorrhea with Potassium Silver Cyanide; The Urologic and Cutaneous Review, Vol. 34, No. 9.

SISTOMENSIN

Faust, E. S.: Schw. med. Wochensch., 1927, 57:368.
Uhlmann: La Gynecologie, 1927, 26:65.
Faust, E. S.: Verhandl. des I. Internat. Kongresses f. Sexual-forschung, Berlin, 1926; I. Bd.
Kennedy and Thompson: Quart. J. of Exper. Physiol., 1929, 19:377.
Kennedy, W.: Quart. J. of Exper. Physiol., 1930, 20:71.
Kurzrok, R.: Endocrinology, 1932, 16:361 and 366.

SKIMMED MILK POWDERED

Persoff, L. E.: Arch. Pediat., November, 1928.
Ashton, L. O. Stringfield, O. L., and Martin, C. W.: Arch. Pediat., February, 1929.
Toby, J. A.: New England Jour. of Med., January 31, 1929.
Abt, A. F. and Feingold, B. F.: Arch. Pediat., October, 1930.
Giblin, J. and Von Pourtales, J. H.: Am. J. Dis. Child., May, 1931.
Amick, A. F.: W. Va. Med. J., May, 1932.
Martin, C. W.: N. Y. State J. Med., September, 1932.

SKIODAN

Pearse, H. E., Jr. and Warren, S. L.: The Roentgenographic Visualization of the Arteries of the Extremities in Peripheral Vascular Disease; Ann. Surgery, Dec., 1931.

SMALLPOX VACCINOTHERAPY

New England Jour. of Med., 1928, 198:464.
New England Jour. of Med., 1930, 202:937.
Public Health Reports, 1930, 45:2793.

SOAMIN

Reports Council Pharm. and Chem., 1919, p. 89; Propaganda, vol. 2, p. 253.
Lancet, July 3, 1926, p. 43.

SOBEE

Hill, L. W. and Stuart, H. C.: A Soy Bean Food Preparation for Feeding Infants with Milk Idiosyncrasy; J. A. M. A., 1929, 93:985.
Hill, L. W.: Infantile Eczema with Especial Reference to the Use of a Milk-Free Diet; J. A. M. A., 1931, 96:1277.
Krauss, F. I.: Diet in eczema of infants; J. Med. Soc. New Jersey, 1931, 28:217.
Baumhauer, J. H.: Allergy in Children with Particular Reference to Food Idiosyncrasy; J. M. A., Alabama, 1932, 2:195.
Bivings, L.: Eczema in Infancy and Childhood: Its Relation to Allergy; South. Med. Jour., 1932, 25:223.
The Infantile Eczema Problem; New England Jour. of Med., 1932, 207:655.
Kahn, B. L.: Dermatoses in Childhood; Arch. Pediat., 1932, 49:512.
Levy, J. and Finkelstein, A. S.: Treatment of Eczema in Infants by a Milk-Free Diet; J. Med. Soc. New Jersey, 1932, 29:189.
MacDonald, W. J.: Etiology of Eczema; New England Jour. of Med., 1932, 207:940.

SODIUM AMYTAL

Eddy, N. B.: Studies on Hypnotics of Barbituric Acid Series; J. Pharm. and Exper. Therap., 1928, 33: 43.
Mulinos, Michael G.: Amytal as a Laboratory Anesthetic for Cats; J. Pharm. and Exper. Therap., 1928, 34:425.
Robbins, A. R., McCallum, J. T. C., Mendenhall, A. M., and Zerfas, L. G.: The Use of Sodium Amytal in Obstetrics; Am. J. Obst. and Gynec., 1929, 18:406.
Cullen, Paul K.: Sodium Amytal in Internal Medicine; Indianapolis M. J., 1930, 33:356.
Sloan, Harry G.: Amytal as Anesthetic in Operations for Goitre; Ann. Surgery, 1930, 91:901.
Sise, L. F. and Woodbridge, P. D.: Choice of Anesthesia; Med. Jour. and Record, 1930, 131:575.
Mason, J. Tate, and Baker, Joel W.: Experience with Sodium Amytal as an Intravenous Anesthetic; Surg., Gynec. and Obst., 1930, 50:828.
Brown, Rexwald: Experiences with Sodium Amytal as a General Anesthetic; Ann. Surgery, 1930, 91:492.
Moore, John H.: Sodium Amytal in Treatment of the late toxemias of Pregnancy; Am. J. Obst. and Gynec., 1930, 19:544.

SODIUM GLYCOCHOLATE COMPOUND

Hoppe-Seyler: Physiologische Chemie, 2nd Part; p. 301; Berlin, 1878.
Frerichs: Hammarstens' Physiological Chemistry; J. A. Mandel translation, 3rd Ed. p. 239, Wiley and Sons, 1901.
Hope: Ch. F. in U. S. Dispensatory, 21st Ed., p. 1481, J. Lippincott, Phila., Pa., 1926.
Solis-Cohen and Githens: Pharmacotherapeutics, p. 1186, D. Appleton and Co., New York, 1928.

SODIUM MORRHUATE

J. A. M. A., March 8, 1924, p. 813; Sept. 27, 1924, p. 1022.
McEvedy, Peter: Lancet, 1930, 2:902.
Levy, David: Lancet, July 5, 1930, p. 16.
Delville, P. M.: Brit. Med. Jour., Dec. 13, 1930.
Patey, David H. and Loud, M. S.: Lancet, Aug. 8, 1931, p. 289.
Higgins, T. Troistington and Kirtel, P. B.: Lancet, Jan. 11, 1931, p. 68.
Porrett, A. E.: Proc. Roy. Soc. Med., Vol. 24, No. 7, May, 1931.
Kilbourne, Norman J. Dodson, Wm. and Zeiler, A. H.: Surg., Gynec. and Obst., 1932, 54:640.
Shands, H. R.: The Southern Surgeon, 1932, 1:51.
Tunick, Isidor S. and Nach, Robert: Ann. Surgery, May, 1932.

SOLARSON

Bogner, F.: Therap. d. Gegenw., January, 1917.
Sussman, M.: Therap. d. Gegenw., Nov. 1918.
Gang, M.: Wien. med. Wochensch., No. 16, 1920.
Strauss, W.: Therap. d. Gegenw., No. 4, 1923.

SOLUBLE IODINE

Morse, F. H.: Galvanism and Sine Current Technique; 1930 ed. p. 18.
Jorgenson, G. E.: Clin. Med. and Surg., March 1930.
Redewill, F. H.: Urol. and Cut. Rev., p. 620, Oct. 1931.
Eisenberg, M. J. and Frost, W. S.: Dent. Items of Int., p. 833, 1932; Modern Dentistry, Jan. 1933.
J. A. M. A., July 1, 1933, p. 33.

SOLVOCHIN

Cahn-Bronner: Zeitsch. fur klin. Medizin, 1919, 87:292.
Cahn-Bronner: Therap. d. Gegenw., 1927, 68:97.
Vonkennel: Die Malariabehandlung der Fruhsyphilis; Karger, 1927.
Deckert: Therap. d. Gegenw., 1927, 68:533.
Lust: Diagnost. Therap. der Kinderkrankh., 1927.
von Ammon: Deut. med. Wochensch., 1928, 54:1465.
J. A. M. A., May 2, 1931, p. 1577; Reports Council Pharm. and Chem., 1931, p. 88.

SORICIN

Morris, Roger S. and Dorst, Stanley E.: Sodium Ricinoleate in Allergic Disease of the Intestinal Tract; Am. J. M. Sc., 1929, 178:631–632.
Morris, Roger S. and Dorst, Stanley E.: The Use of Sodium Ricinoleate in Bacterial Hypersensitiveness of the Intestinal Tract; Ann. Int. Med., 1930, 4:396–397.
Dorst, Stanley E. and Morris, Roger S.: Bacterial Hypersensitivity of the Intestinal Tract. Its Treatment with Autogenous Vaccine and Sodium Ricinoleate; Am. J. M. Sci., 1930, 180:650–656.

SPASMOLYSIN

Bircher, E.: Die Organotherapie der postoperativen parathyreopriven Tetanie. M. K. I. 1910 Nr. 44.
Biedl: Innere Sekretion, Urban and Schwarzenberg, 1912.
Rudolph Klotz: Zur Aetiologie der Rachitis auf Grund ihrer therapeutischen Beeinflussung durch Hypophysenmedikation; M. v. W. 1912, 59.
Kurt Weiss: Zur Frage der Hypophysentherapie bei Rachitis; Therap. Monatshefte., 1913, 27.
Oswald Meyer: Zur Parathyreoidbehandlung der Spasmophilie; Therap. d. Gegenw., 1913, 8.
Aschenheim: Jb. f. Kindhlk., 1914, 79, 4.
Weiss: Spasmolysin for Epilepsy; Munch. med. Wochensch., 1922, Nr. 43, p. 1525.

SPLEEN LIQUID

Paul, T. M.: Urol. and Cut. Rev., Nov., 1929 and June, 1930.

STANNOXYL

Bruhl, I.: Bull. et mem. Soc. med. d. hop. de Paris, 1917, 41:892.
J. A. M. A., March 6, 1920, p. 692; Propaganda, vol. 2, p. 469.
Hoffmann, W.: Arch. f. klin. Chir., 1923, 123:51.

Canon: Deut. med. Wochensch., 1925, 51:951.
Fabry, J.: Munch. med. Wochensch., 1925, 72:2016.
Zechlin, Th.: Munch. med. Wochensch., 1926, 73:1742.

STREPTO-STAPHYLO COMBINED VACCINE

J. A. M. A., October 23, 1926.
Young's Practice of Urology, Vol. 1, pp. 222, 223.

STYPTYSATE

Petermayr, Joseph: Observations Concerning the Effects of Styptysate; Fortsc. d. Medizin, Jan. 13, 1928, Vol. 46, No. 2.
McAuliffe, George B.: Prevention of Tonsillar Bleeding; Med. Record, March 19, 1930, Vol. 131, No. 6.

SUFROGEL

Spiethoff, B.: Der Schwefel in der Gewebs-und Reiztherapie; Dermat. Wochensch., 1925, Nr. 29, S. 1077.
Klewitz, F.: Klinik der Proteinkorpertherapie. Innere Medizin; Deut. med. Wochensch., 1927, Nr. 41, S. 1719, spez. S. 1720.
Schlesinger, Hermann: Gonorrhoe und Lues als Ursache von Gelenkserkrankungen; Wien. klin. Wochensch., 1928, Nr. 18, S. 638, spec. S. 640.
Alwens, W.: Die praktische Therapie der Endocarditis lenta, der Infektarthritis und deren Folgezustande; Med. Klin., 1928, Nr. 27, S. 1035, spez. S. 1036.
Pincussen, Ludw. und Gornitzkaja, Edda: Zeitsch. fur klin. Medizin, 1928, Bd. 108, H. 1/3, S. 369.
Haebler, C. and Weitzenfeld, N.: Deut. med. Wochensch., 14, 1928.
Pfalz: Med. Klin., 1930, No. 52, p. 1933; also Klin. Wochensch., No. 7, p. 306; Arch. Gynaek., 1930, 143:376.

SULFIDAL

Joseph, M.: Derm. Zentralblatt, 1907, No. 12.
J. Nevinnys: Berl. klin. Wochensch., 1908, Nr. 42 and 43.
Carl Bruck: vergl. Zeitschrift f. exper. Path. u. Ther., 1909, Nr. 6, S. 700; Munch. med. Wochensch., 1911, Nr. 39; E. Neisser, Fortsch. d. Medizin, 1910, Nr. 22, S. 688.
A. Robin und L. C. Maillard: Le Bulletin Medical, 1913, No. 93, p. 1032.
Jastrowitz, H.: Deut. med. Wochensch., 1931, No. 23.

SULOPHEN

Trapesnikow, Th.: Therapeut. Blatter, 1893, Nr. 2.
Stetter, Georg: Monatssch. fur Ohrenheilkunde usw., Berlin, 1896.
Besold, Gustav: Munch. med. Wochensch., 1898, Nr. 26.
Baginsky, Adolf: Therap. d. Gegenw., June, 1900.
Bresgen, Maximilian: Die arztliche Praxis, 1900, Nr. 3 u. 4.
Schwarzenbach, Tramelau: Schweizer Arzte, 1905, Nr. 5, 6, 7.
Bethge, Hans: Deut. med. Wochensch., 1910, Nr. 2.

SUPSALVS

Sabouraud: La Clinique, 1913, 13, 4.

SYNEPHRIN TARTRATE

Doty, E. J.: Pharm. and Exp. Ther., 36, 519–1929.
Gordon, Samuel: J. Amer. Pharm. Assoc., Vol. 20, No. 5, May, 1930.
Tainter, M. L. and Seidenfeld, M. A.: J. Pharm. and Exper. Therap., Vol. 40, No. 1, Sept. 1930.
Trendelenburg, Paul: Deut. med. Wochensch., 1930, 1987.
Kuschinsky, G.: Arch. f. exper. Pathol., 1930, 156, 290.
Bulbring: Arch. f. exper. Pathol., 152, 257, 1930.
Tainter: J. Pharm., 40, 43, 1930.
Kottlors u. Faust: Med. Klin., 1931, 13.
Schunterman, C. E.: Klin. Wochensch., No. 38, 1931, p. 1764–1766.
Tainter: Anesth. and Anal., 1931, 10:224.
Fischer: Mntschr. Ohrenheilk. u. Laryngo-Rhinologie, 1931, 65, 2.
Simmel: Hans, Fortschritte der Ther., 1931, Vol. 19.

SYNODAL

Pitkin, George P.: A New Treatment of Peptic Ulcer; Am. J. Surg., June, 1931.
Hiatt, H. B.: Something New in Treatment of Peptic Ulcer; South. Med. and Surg., Sept., 1931

TANNIGEN

Morse, John Lovett: Boston Med. and Surg. Jour., Aug. 3, 1899.
Hemmeter, J. C.: Va. Med. Semi-Mo., March 8, 1901.

Tomovice: Jour. de Med. de Paris, Nov. 11, 1911.
Niles, George M.: J. South Carolina M. A., June, 1914.
Johnson, J. Clarence: Southern Med. Jour., April, 1915.
Roberts, Dudley: Am. J. M. Sc., Feb., 1916.
Lamb, F. H.: Ohio State M. J., May, 1916.
Tobeitz, A.: Wien. med. Wochensch., No. 1, 1927.
Koplik, Henry: Diseases of Infancy and Children, 3d ed.

TANNISMUT

Wertheimer, R.: Deut. Med. Wochensch. 1925, No. 45.
Lehndorff, Heinrich: Wien. klin. Wochensch., 1930, No. 3.
Kuettner and Scherk, C.: Fortsch. Therapie., 1930, No. 1.
Steindl, Hans: Wien. med. Wochensch. 1931, No. 40.

TARGESIN

Wreszynski, E.: Klin. Wochensch., 1926, No. 13.
Scheuer: Munch. med., Wochensch., 1926, No. 12.
Wolfes, Ernst: Med. Klin., 1926, No. 28.
Kloeppel, F. W.: Fortsch. d. Therapie, 1926, No. 13.
Ullmann, Karl: Wien. klin. Wochensch., 1926, No. 29.
Portmann, F. W.: Dermat. Wochensch., 1926, No. 39.
Abelsohn, Hans: Therapie d. Gegenw., 1926, No. 8.
Polland, Rudolf: Dermat. Wochensch., 1926, No. 33.
Mayr, J. K.: Munch. med. Wochensch., 1926, No. 40.
Dietel, Friedrich: Deut. med. Wochensch., 1926, No. 40.
Krechel, J.: Munch. med. Wochensch., 1926, No. 46.
Siebert, C. and Cohn, Henry: Zeitsch. f. Urol., 1926, Vol. 20, No. 8.

TAROXIDE

Brocq: Ann. de dermat. et syph., vol. 40, 1, 1909.
White, C. J.: Boston Med. and Surg., vol. 175, 5, 1918.
Abt: "Pediatrics," vol. 8, 183, 1926.
Nelson, M. O. and Osterberg, A. E.: Arch. of Derm. and Syph., vol. 15, 669, 1927.

TARTRO-QUINIOBINE

Fraenkel, E.: Med. Klin., 1923, 19:1524.
Reicher, K.: Therap. d. Gegenw., 1923, 64:450.
Baer, Th.: Fortsch. d. Medizin., 1924, 42:7.
Nathan, E.: Munch. med. Wochensch., 1924, 71:647.
Feldhaus, E.: Die Behandlung der Spätsyphilis mit Spirobismol; Treatise, Berlin, July, 1924.
Cardoso: Klin. Wochensch., 1924, 3:1674.
Bogdanow, S.: Dermat. Wochensch., 1925, 80:25.
Levy and Selter: Archiv für Kinderheilkunde, 1925, 75:241, 281.
Robitschek: Med. Klin., 1926, 22:1034.
Lucke: Deut. med. Wochensch., 1927, 53:929.
Delbanco, E.: Med. World, Nov. 7, 1930.

TAUROCOL

J. A. M. A., April 24, 1915, p. 1441; Reports Council Pharm. and Chem., 1915, p. 143; Propaganda, ed. 9, p. 198.
Sollmann: Manual of Pharmacology, 1927, p. 230.

TENAMIN

Marino, Alessandro: La Ginecologia, No. 11, 1914.
Jaeger, F.: Zentralb. f. Gynaek., No. 29, 1919.
Katz, G.: Therap. d. Gegenw., May, 1921.

TEROGON "SCHUFTAN"

Schuftan, Adolf: Dermat. Zeitschrift, Volume 29, No. 5.

TERPICHIN

Sfakianakis, J.: On Experiences with Terpichin in Dermatology; Deut. med. Wochensch., 1920, No. 49.
Lenzmann: On Terpichin; Der Praktische Arzt, 1920, No. 7.
Karo, W.: Terpichin in Inflammatory Affections of the Urinary Passages; Therap. d. Gegenw., 1920, No. 3.
Umberto, M: Terpichin in Treatment of Affections of the Adnexae; Atti della Societa Italiana, 1921.

Arnold: On the Treatment of Gonorrheal Prostatitis with Arthigen and Terpichin; Munch. med. Wochensch. 1922, No. 17.
Klingmuller, V.: A Further Contribution to Turpentine Treatment; Munch. med. Wochensch. 1923, No. 21.

TETROPHINE

Foerster, O.: The Therapeutic Usefulness of Tetrophine; Klin. Wochnschr, 1925, No. 2.
Friedlaender, K.: Experiences with Tetrophine in a Number of Diseases of the Nerves; Muench. med. Wochnschr., 1927, No. 10:411.
Kardos, G.: Tetrophine in Pediatrics; Fortschr. d. Medizin., 1933, 51:402.
Langstein, L.: Therapy of Poliomyelitis; Kinderaerztl. Praxis, 1932, 3:537.
Ochsenius, K.: The Early Treatment of Poliomyelitis; Muench. med. Wochnschr., 1933, 80:891.
Ostman: Clinical Studies Regarding the Action of Tetrophine; Deutsche med. Wochnschr. 1925, No. 49.
Schneideberger, H.: Experiences with Tetrophine; Therapie der Gegenwart. 1932, No. 6:287.
Stark, K.: The Treatment of Encephalitis Epidemica Chronica; Psych.-Neurolog. Wochnschr. 1932, No. 5:58.

THEELIN

Allen, E., Doisy, E. A., et al.: Am. J. Anat., 1924, 34:133.
Allen, E.: Anat. Record, 1926, 32:226.
Doisy, E. A., Thayer, S. A., and Veler, C. D.: J. Biol. Chem., 1930, 86:499.
Robertson, D. C., Maddux, W. P. and Allen, E.: Endocrinology, 77, 1930, 14:77.
Veler, C. D., Thayer, S. A., and Doisy, E. A.: J. Biol. Chem. 1930, 87:357.

THEELOL

Allen, E., Doisy, E. A., et al.: Am. J. Anat., 1924, 34:133.
Allen, E.: Anat. Record, 1926, 32:226.
Doisy, E. A., Thayer, S. A., and Veler, C. D.: J. Biol. Chem., 1930, 86:499.
Doisy, E. A., Curtis, J. M., Levin, L., Katzman, P. A., and Thayer, S. A.: Proc. Soc. Exp. Biol. Med., 1930, 28:216.
Robertson, C. D., Maddux, W. P., and Allen, E.: Endocrinology, 1930, 14:77.
Veler, C. D., Thayer, S. A., and Doisy, E. A.: J. Biol. Chem., 1930, 87:357.
Thayer, S. A., Levin, L., and Doisy, E. A.: Biol. Chem., 1931, 91:665.
Slawson, C. B.: J. Biol. Chem., 1931, 91:665.
Melchionna, R.: J. Biol. Chem., 1931, 91:653.
Doisy, E. A., and Thayer, S. J.: Biol. Chem., 1931, 91:647.
Curtis, J. M. and Doisy, E. A.: J. Biol. Chem., 1931, 91:647.

THEOCALCIN

Askanazy: Uber Iod. Calcium-Diuretin; Med. Klin., 7, 1925.
Love: A Clinical Survey of the Action of Theocalcin; Bulletin of the School of Med., Univ. of Md., January, 1930.
Preble: Recent Advances in the Therapy of Heart Failure; Internat. J. Med. and Surg., August, 1930, pp. 418–421.
Stewart: The Use of Theocalcin in the Treatment of Heart Failure of the Congestive Type; Am. J. Clin. Inv., 1930, 8:389.
Paul D. White: The Treatment of Congestive Heart Failure; Maine Med. J., 1931, 22:182.
Viko: Arteriosclerotic Heart Disease; Cal. and West. Med., December, 1931, pp. 433–438.
Nathanson: Diagnosis and Management of Coronary Arterial Disease; Minn. Med., March, 1932, pp. 150–162.
Bliss and Morrison: A Comparative Study of Certain Xanthine Diuretics; Jour. Tenn. State Med. Assoc., 1932, 25:387.

THEOCIN

Miller, Joseph L.: J. A. M. A., June 22, 1912.
Bond, George S.: Jour. Iowa State Med. Soc., Feb., 1926.
Christian, H. A.: Boston Med. and Surg. Jour., Oct. 13, 1927.

THEOMINAL

Strauss, H.: Therap. Monatshefte., August, 1917.
Roemheld, L.: Therap. d. Gegenw., November, 1923.
Gruber, Shackelford and Ecklund: Arch. Int. Med., Sept. 15, 1925.
Wiechmann, E.: Munch. med. Wochensch. No. 16, 1925.
Muller, H.: Munch, med. Wochensch., June 18, 1926.
Schmilinsky, K.: Klin. Wochensch., No. 46, 1926.
Schlayer, C. R.: Munch. med. Wochensch., May 21, 1926.
Heinmann, W., Hatry: Med. Klin., No. 39, 1926.

THEPHYLDINE

Smith, F. M., Miller, G. H. and Graber, B. C.: J. Clinical Invest., Dec., 1925, pp. 157–166.
Smith, F. M., Graber B. C. and Miller, G. H.: Sect. Pharmacol. and Therap. A. M. A., 1926, p. 171.
Musser, J. H.: J. A. M. A., 1928, 91:1242.
Bannick, E. G. and Keith, N. M.: J. A. M. A., 1928, 91:1944.
Gilbert, N. C. and Kerr, John Austin: J. A. M. A., 1929, 92:201.
Curtis, George M.: J. A. M. A., 1929, 93:2016.
Levine: J. A. M. A., 1932, 99:1737.
Herrmann: J. A. M. A., 1932, 99:1647.

THIOCYAN-ELIX

Gager, Leslie T.: J. A. M. A., Jan. 14, 1928.

THOROTRAST

Allen, E. V. and Camp, J. D.: Proc. of Staff Meetings of Mayo Clinic, Nov. 16, 1932.
Dickson, W. H.: Canad. Med. A. J., August, 1932.
Einhorn, Max, Stewart, William H. and Illick, Earl H.: Med. Jour. and Record, July 15, 1932.
Gottlieb, R.: Canad. Med. A. J., Oct., 1932.
Dudley, A. Irwin: Canad. Med. A. J., August and October, 1932.
Silvije Kadrnka: Radiology, February, 1932.
Lewisohn, Richard: Surg., Gynec. and Obst., July, 1932.
MacDonald, Ian G.: Canad. Med. A. J., Aug., 1932.
Menville, Leon J. and Ane, J. N.: J. A. M. A., May 21, 1932.
Wiltrakis, George A.: Bull of Ill. State Psych. Inst., July, 1932.
Warfield, C. H.: Radiology, November, 1932.

THROMBOPLASTIN

Hess, Alfred F.: J. A. M. A., April 24, 1915.
Cronin, John J.: J. A. M. A., Feb. 19, 1916.
Hanzlik, P. J. and Weidenthal, C. M.: J. Pharm. and Exper. Therap., Oct. 1919, p. 173.
J. A. M. A., Jan. 9, 1932, p. 143; Reports Council Pharm. and Chem., 1932, p. 89.

THYRACTIN

Dehner, Walter: Deut. med. Wochensch., 1931, 57:278.
Guttman, David: Therap. d. Gegenw. No. 1, 1931.
Noorden, V. Wien. med. Wochensch., No. 1, 1931.

THYROCALX

Novak and Hollender: J. A. M. A., Dec. 15, 1923, p. 2003.
Vines: American Medicine, Vol. 18, 1923.
Scott: China Med. Jour., July, 1923, and Brit. Med. Jour., Dec. 15, 1923 and Aug., 1924.
Brown and Hunter: Ann. Clin. Med., 1925, 4:299.

THYROXIN

Warfield, L. M.: J. A. M. A., 1930, 95:1076.
Hoge, Albert H.: W. Va. Med. J., 1931, 27:461.
Bram, Israel: Med. Times and L. I. Med. J., 1931, 59:241.
Nissler, Tai and Gordon: N. Y. State J. Med., 1931, 31:887.
Evans and Strang: J. A. M. A., 1931, 97:1063.
Beach, George C.: Military Surg., 1931, 69:483.
Schittenhelm, A. and B. Eisler: Klin. Wochensch., 1931, 10:680.
Helfors, Alfred: Munch. med. Wochensch., No. 20, 1931, p. 826.

TISSUE EXTRACT 568

Frey, E. K. and Kraut, H.: Ein neues Kreislaufhormon und seine Wirkung; Arch. f. exper. Path. u. Pharmakol., 1928, 133:1–56.
Gley, P. and Kisthinios, N.: Recherches sur la Substance Hypotensive du Pancreas; Pres. Medicale. 1929, 37:1279–82.
Elliot, A. H. and Nuzum, F. R.: J. Pharm. and Exper. Therap., 1931, 43:3.
Wolffe, J. B., Findlay, D. and Dessen, E.: Ann. of Int. Med., November, 1931, p. 625–42.
Wolfee, J. B.: Trans. Am. Therap. Soc., 1931.

TOLYSIN

Hanzlik, Scott, Weidenthal and Fetterman: J. A. M. A., 1921, 76:1728.
Chace, Myers and Killian: J. A. M. A., 1921, 77:1230.
Barbour and Lozinsky: J. Lab. Clin. Med., 1923, 8:217.

Barbour, Lozinsky and Clements: Am. J. M. Sc., 1923, 165:708.
Reports Council Pharm. and Chem., 1924, p. 73.
Miller and Boots: J. A. M. A., 1924, 82:1028.
Grahm: Lancet, 1926, 211:856.
Spurling and Hartman: J. Pharm. and Exper. Therap., 1926, 30: 185.
Solis-Cohen: Text Book of Pharmaco-Therapeutics; D. Appleton and Co., 1928, p. 1433.
Spurling and Hartman: J. Lab. Clin. Med., June, 1928.
Lukens, Jr.: Clin. Invest., 1928, 6:319.
J. A. M. A., April 26, 1924, p. 1381; Apr. 9, 1932, p. 1322.

TRICHLORETHYLENE

Lehmann: Arch. f. Hyg., 1911, 74:1.
Plessner: Klin. Wochensch., 1916, 53:25.
Saphier: Munch. med. Wochensch., 1920, 67:133.
Bab: Klin. Wochensch., 1923, 2:474.
Joachimoglu: Klin. Wochensch., 1921, 58:147.
Blumenthal: Deut. med. Wochensch., 1924, 5:140.
Oljenick: J. A. M. A., October 13, 1928, p. 1088.
Glaser: J. A. M. A., 1931, 96:916.
Duffield-Fahy: Dental Cosmos, September, 1931.

TRIPHAL

Throne, Binford, Clark, A. Schuyler, Van Dyck, Laird S. and Myer, C. N.: N. Y. State J. Med., Oct. 1, 1927.
Katz, E. Wagner: Deut. med. Wochensch., No. 24, 1927.
Olah, O.: Wien, klin. Wochensch., No. 23, 1927.
Mohrmann, B. H. U.: Munch. med. Wochensch., No. 35, 1927.
Kall, Kurt: Deut. med. Wochensch., No. 49, 1928.

TRYPARSAMIDE

Hanschell, H. M.: Tryparsamide; Brit. Med. Jour., 1923, 2:87.
Brown, W. H. and Pearce, L.: Tryparsamide. Its Action and Use; J. A. M. A., 1924, 82:5–9.
Lorenz, W. F., Loevenhart, A. S., Reitz, T. F. and Eck, C. P.: The Use of Tryparsamide in Neurosyphilis; Am. J. M. Sc., 1924, 168:157–165.
Viner, Norman: Tryparsamide in Late Neurosyphilis; Canad. Med. A. J., 1924, 14:978.
Hecht, S.: Treatment of Neurosyphilis; Med. Jour. and Record, 1927, 125:403.
Fong, T. C. C.: Tryparsamide Therapy in Treatment of Neurosyphilis; Med. Jour. and Record, 1928, 128:85–88.
O'Leary, P. A. and Brunsting, L. G.: Nonspecific Treatment of Neurosyphilis; J. A. M. A., 1930, 94:452–4.
Lorenz, W. F.: Neurosyphilis; Wis. Med. Jour., 1930, 29:372–378.
Weigner, W. C.: Remarks on Treatment of Neurosyphilis; Rhode Island M. J. 1930, 13:130–134.
Sheppe, Wm. M.: Treatment of Neurosyphilis; West Virginia M. J., 1930, 26:662–669.
Solomon, H. C. and Epstein, S. H.: Tryparsamide in Treatment of Neurosyphilis; N. Y. State Med. J., 1931, 31:1012–1016.
Lichtenstein, Julia V.: Tryparsamide Therapy; Arch. of Derm. and Syph., 1931, 24:182–195.

TUTOCAINE

Heuss, H.: Med. Klin., Nov. 22, 1924.
Chetwood, Chas. H. and Cooney, John D.: Am. J. Surg., May, 1925.
Fauvet, Egen: Zentralb. f. Chir., No. 7, 1928.

UMBRATHOR

Kalkbrenner: Fortschr. a. d. Gebieten d. Roentgenstr., 1928, Bd. 38, H. 2, S. 325.
Regelsberger: Roentgenpr., 1930, No. 19, p. 876.
Regelsberger: Munch. med. Wochensch., 1930, No. 38, p. 1649.
Weiser: Wien. med. Wochensch., 1930, No. 44, p. 1427.
Ritter and Rattner: Am. J. Roentg., Nov., 1932, p. 629.

UNDILUTED HALIBUT LIVER OIL

Schmidt-Nielsen, Signe and Sigval Schmidt-Nielsen: Some Liver Oils Yielding a Strong Colour Reaction with Antimony Trichloride; Biochem. J., 1929, 23:1153.
Wilbur, D. L.: Significance of Diet in the Practice of Medicine; Lancet, 1932, 52:564.
Schlutz, F. W.: The Clinical Significance of Vitamin D in Infancy and Childhood; J. A. M. A., 1932, 99:384.
Heilbron, I. M., Heslop, R. N., Morton, R. A., Webster, E. T., Rea, J. L. and Drummond, J. C.: Characteristics of Highly Active Vitamin A Preparations; Biochem. J., 1932, 26:1178.
Eusterman, G. B. and Wilbur, D. L.: Clinical Features of Vitamin A Deficiency; J. A. M. A., 1932, 98:2054.
Edisbury, J. R., Gillam, A. E., Heilbron, I. M., and Morton, R. A.: Absorption Spectra of Substances Derived from Vitamin A; Biochem. J., 1932, 26:1164.

Ender, F.: The Reaction of Fish-Liver Oils with Antimony Trichloride; Biochem. J., 1932, 26:1119.
Clein, N. W.: Cod-liver Oil and Viosterol. Uses and Abuses; Northwest Med., 1932, 31:430.

UNDULANT FEVER VACCINE

J. A. M. A., April 26, 1930, p. 1304.

UROCEDROL

Lautier: Bull. Soc. de Ther., Oct. 12, 1921.
Brit. Med. Jour., January 14, 1922, No. 3185, p. 84.

UVALYSATE

Knust: Fortsch. d. Therapie., 1925, No. 23.
Lenhardt, K.: Der Landarzt, 1926, No. 24.
Isaak: Fortsch. de Medizin, 1926, No. 10.
Beckmann, K.: Therap. d. Gegenw., 1926, No. 7.
Schubert: Dermat. Wochensch., 1927, Vol. 85, No. 37.
Mayr, J.: Munch. med. Wochensch., 1926, No. 8; Med. Klin., 1928, No. 9, p. 341.

VARI-CHLOR-OSE

Nobl, Gabor: Die Calorose als Verordnungsmittel varikos entarteter Venen, d. Wien. klin. Wochensch., 1926, No. 4.
Nobl, G.: Varices der Venen der unteren extremitaten mit Injektionen von Calorose Losungen zwecks kunstilicher Trombose behandelt.; Wien. med. Wochensch., 1926, 76:1880.

VENTRICULIN

Levine and Ladd: Johns Hopkins Bull., 1921, 32:254.
Warthin: J. A. M. A., June 30, 1928.
Minot: Am. J. M. Sc., May, 1928.
Sturgis and Isaacs: J. A. M. A., Sept. 7, 1929.

VERONAL

Saundby, R.: Brit. Med. Jour., Oct. 20th, 1906.
Rowland, F. M.: Brit. Med. Jour., Nov. 24, 1906.
Hutchison, Robert: The Clin. Jour., Aug. 9, 1911.
Ranson, S. Walter and Scott, D. G.: Am. J. M. Sc., May, 1911.
Meyers, Sidney J.: Louisv. Mo. Jour. of Med. and Surg., May, 1912.
House, William: Therap. Gaz., May, 1913.
Barker, Lewellys F.: Am. J. M. Sc., January, 1913.
Howell, C. H.: J. A. M. A., Oct. 17, 1914.
Gelhorn, George: J. A. M. A., Oct. 11, 1914.
Bram, I.: N. Y. Med. Jour., Nov. 27, 1915.
Lahey, Frank H.: Boston Med. and Surg. Jour., Oct. 19, 1916.
Lind, John E.: N. Y. Med. Jour., Feb. 3, 1917.

VIOFORM

Tavel: Deut. Zeits. f. Chirurgie, 1900, 55:558.
Thomann: Schw. Wochensch. für Chemie und Pharmacie, No. 27, 1905, pp. 361–366.
Tavel: Correspondenz-Blatt für Schweizer Aerzte, No. 28, 1910, pp. 881–892.
Takahara: Ciba-Jiho, Sept. 1929, p. 25.
Anderson and Koch: Proc. Soc. Exp. Biol. Med., 1931, 28:838.
Anderson, David and Koch: Proc. Soc. Exp. Biol. Med., 1931, 28:484.
Leake, C. D.: J. A. M. A., 1932, 98:195.

VIOSTEROL

Hartley, E. C.: Am. J. Obst. and Gynec., 1930, 19:54.
Dorsett, E. Lee: Am. J. Obst. and Gynec., 1930, 19:709.
Mellanby, E.: J. A. M. A., 1931, 96:325.
Richardson, Garwood C.: The Role of Viosterol in Pregnancy; Ill. Med. Jour., June, 1931.
Sincock, Henry A.: Calcium Deficiencies in Pregnancies and Influences Upon the Child; Wis. Med. Jour., December, 1932.
Agnew, Mary Caldwell, Agnew, R. Gordon and Tisdall, Frederick F.: The Production and Prevention of Dental Caries; J. Amer. Dent. Assoc., 1933, 20: 193; J. of Pediat., February, 1933.

VIOSTEROL IN OIL 250D

Mcbane, D. C.: The Prevention and Treatment of Infantile Eczema; Ohio State M. J.; 1930, 26:834.
Caffey, J.: Changes in Human Rickets After Viosterol Therapy; J. Med. Soc. New Jersey, 1931, 28:21.

Crimm, P. D.: Vitamine Therapy in Pulmonary Tuberculosis. I. The Effect of Activated Ergosterol on the Calcium and Inorganic Phosphorus in the Blood Serum; Am. Rev. Tub., 1931, 23:576.
Flinn, F. B.: Elimination of Radium Salts from the Human Body; J. A. M. A., 1931, 96:1763.
Blatt, M. L. and Saffro, L. B.: Rachitic Osteomalacia. Report of Case Treated by Massive Doses of Viosterol; Arch. Pediat., 1932, 49:109.
Sincock, H. A.: Calcium Deficiencies in Pregnancy and its Influences Upon the Child; Wis. Med. Jour., 1932, 31:838.
Brown, G. T.: Perennial Hay Fever; Arch. Otolaryn., 1932, 15:202.
Clouse, R. C.: Vitamin D; J. A. M. A., 1932, 99:215; 1932, 99:301.
Clein, N. W.: Cod-liver Oil and Viosterol. Uses and Abuses; Northwest Med., 1932, 31:430.
Hess, J. H. and Lundeen, E. C.: Premature Infants; Ohio State M. J., 1932, 28:253.
Jampolis, M. and Londe, S.: The Need of Larger Doses of Viosterol in Severe Rickets (Osteomalacia Type); Comparative Study of Efficacy of Viosterol and Cod Liver Oil; J. A. M. A., 1932, 98:1637.
Jones, H. W. and Tocantins, L.: The Treatment of Purpura Hemorrhagica; J. A. M. A. (Soc. Proc.), 1932, 99:164.

VISCYSATE

Lenhardt, Kassel: Viscysate in the Treatment of High Blood Pressure; Med. Klin., No. 31, 1926.
Preuss, Leo: Experience with Viscysate in Hypertonia; Med. Klin., No. 8, 1927.
Bachem, C.: Zentralb. f. innere Medizin, No. 11, 1927.
Esser, Heinz: The Treatment of Hypertonia with Viscysate; Fortsch. d. Medizin, No. 13, 1928.
Grossmann, W.: The Treatment of Hyperpiesia with Viscysate; Med. Klin., No. 12, 1928.
Schlenck, Alfred, Munich: Viscysate as a Depressant of Blood Pressure; Munich med. Wochensch., No 3, 1928.
Orlowski, P.: The Use of the Mistletoe for Reducing the Blood Pressure; Wien. med. Wochensch., No 33, 1932.

WHOLE MILK POWDERED

Muls, G.: Powdered Milk as Food for Nursing Children; Gac. med. d. Tampico, 2:327, March, 1926; abstr. Int. M. Dig., September, 1926, p. 174.
Hess, J. H.: Feeding and the Nutritional Disorders in Infancy and Childhood, F. A. Davis Co., Philadelphia, 1928.
Hucker, G. J. and Hucker, A. M.: Organisms Associated with Commercially Prepared Infant Foods; Am. J. Dis. Child., 1929, 38:310.
Abt, A. F. and Feingold, B. F.: The Use of Powdered Milk and Milk Derivatives in the Concentration of Infant Foods; Arch. Pediat., 1930, 47:603.
Marfan, A. B.: The Use of Evaporated and Powdered Milk in Infant Feeding; Nourrisson, 18:1, Jan., 1930; abstr. Am. J. Dis. Child., 1930, 40:160.
Giblin, J. and von Pourtales, J. H.: Dried Powdered Milk Preparations Used in the Feeding of Infants; Am. J. Dis. Child., 1931, 41:1100.
Dennett, R. H. and Craig, J. D.: A Comparative Study of Infant Foods; Med. Jour. and Record, 1932, 136:133.
Kerley, C. G.: Substitute Breast Feeding; Med. Jour. and Record, 1932, 136:371.
Lynch, H. D.: Powdered Citric Acid Milk in Infant Feeding; Arch. Pediat., 1932, 49:763.
Mackay: Nutritional Anemia in Infancy; Med. Res. Counc. Spec. Rep. Ser. No. 157, H. M. S. O., London, 1931; abstr. New England J. M., 1932, 207:1050.
Martin, C. W.: Some Dried Foods Used in Infant Feeding; N. Y. State J. Med., 1932, 32:1012.
Nichamin, S.: Infants' and Children's Diet; Soc. Trans., Am. J. Dis. Child., 1932, 44:251.

YATREN-CASEIN

Bahr, Philip Manson and Sayers, E. G.: Brit. Med. Jour., September 17, 1927.
Craig, C. F.: J. A. M. A., April 28, 1928.
Jones, P. H. and Turner, R. H.: J. A. M. A., August 24, 1929.
Dougherty, Mark S.: South. Med. Jour., March, 1930.
Willoughby, Hugh: J. Roy. Naval Med. Serv., January, 1931.
Andrews, Justin and Paulson, Moses: Am. J. M. Sc., January, 1931.

CHAPTER XIII

DISTRIBUTORS' AND MANUFACTURERS' INDEX

This Index is intended to assist the physician in the choice of a remedy from a *favorite* concern. It presents in alphabetical order the names and addresses of the 342 Manufacturers and Distributors of the pharmaceutical preparations accorded description in this work, with listings of their products and abbreviations of names for the convenience of prescriber.

ABBOTT LABORATORIES (Abbott)

North Chicago, Ill.

A.B.D. Malt Extract
Acetarsone Ampules
Acetarsone Tablets
Acetylcholine Bromide Ampules
Acne Bacterin
Acriflavine Neutral Ampules
Acriflavine Neutral Jelly
Acriflavine Neutral Ointment
Acriflavine Neutral Powder
Acriflavine Neutral Suppositories (1:2000)
Acriflavine Neutral Tablets, Plain, Enteric coated
Acriflavine Neutral Tablets
Acriflavine Neutral Suppositories
Allergens—Foods
Allergens—Miscellaneous, Epidermals
Allergens—Pollens, Group
Allergens—Pollens, Individual
Allergens—Protein Extracts
Amiodoxyl Benzoate
Aneskreme
Anespray
Anesthesin Powder
Anesthesin-Calcidin Troches
Anesthesin and Cerium Oxalate Compound Tablets
Arbutin Powder
Arbutin Tablets
Argyn Powder
Argyn Tablets
Arsphenamine Ampules
Bacteriophage-Staphylococcus
Bacteriophage-Staphylococcus-Coli
Barb-eth-Oil Surgical
Barb-eth-Oil Obstetrical
Benzyl Benzoate Elixir 20%
Benzyl Benzoate Tablets
Benzyl Fumarate Tablets
Bilein Tablets
Bismarsen Ampules
Bismo-Cymol Ampules
Bromhosal
Brominol Heavy
Brominol Light
Butesin Powder
Butesin Compound Suppositories
Butesin Picrate Powder
Butesin Picrate Ointment
Butyn Tablets
Butyn Tablets Hypodermic
Butyn Powder
Butyn Ephedrine Solution
Butyn and Epinephrine Chloride Solution Ampules 2%
Butyn Solution
Calcidin Powder
Calcidin Tablets
Calcidin Troches
  Salicylic Acid and Calcidin Compound
  Camphor and Calcidin Compound
Calcilact
Calcium Gluconate Ampules
Calsoma Plain
Calsoma Mint Tablets
Campiodol Emulsion
Campiodol Solution
Chlorazene Tablets
Chlorazene Powder, Aromatic
Chlorazene Surgical Powder
Chlorazene Surgical Cream
Chlorazene Surgical Gauze
Chole-Cysto-Col
Cinchophen Tablets
Citro-Soda
Cod Liver Oil with Viosterol 10D
Cofron Capsules
Cofron Elixir
Corpus Luteum Ampules
Corpus Luteum Capsules
Dextrose Ampules
Dextrose-Ringer's Concentrate Ampules

Digipoten Tablets
Dysco Tablets
Ephedrine Butesin Jelly
Ephedrine Butesin Spray
Ephedrine Hydrochloride Ampules
Ephedrine Hydrochloride Capsules
Ephedrine Hydrochloride Elixir
Ephedrine Hydrochloride Inhalant 1%
Ephedrine Hydrochloride Nasal Ointment
Ephedrine Hydrochloride Solution 3%
Ephedrine Hydrochloride Syrup; Plain and Double Strength
Ephedrine Hydrochloride Tablets
Ephedrine Inhalant 66
Ephetal Tablets
Epinephrine Hydrochloride Ampules
Erysipelas Bacterin
Ethyl Morphine and Ephedrine Compound
Furunculosis Bacterin
Gold Sodium Thiosulphate Ampules
Gonococcus Vaccine
Gonorrhea Bacterin
Halazone
Haliver Oil Plain Capsules
Haliver Oil Plain Liquid
Haliver Oil with Viosterol 250 D Capsules
Haliver Oil with Viosterol 250 D Liquid
Hepasol Ampules
Hosal
Influenza Bacterin
Iodeikon Capsules
Iodeikon Emulsion
Iodeikon Powder
Islands of Langerhans Capsules
Lactigen Ampules
Mercuric Potassium Iodide Ampules
Mercury Biniodide Ampules
Mercuric Oxycyanide Ampules
Mercuric Salicylate Ampules
Mercury Benzoate Ampules
Mercury Succinimide Ampules
Metaphedrin Inhalant
Metaphedrin Inhalant #99
Metaphen Ampules
Metaphen Aqueous Ointment 1:5,000
Metaphen 2,500
Metaphen in Oil C
Metaphen Eye Ointment 1:3,000
Metaphen Antiseptic Bar Soap 1:500
Metaphen Inhalant 99
Metaphen Liquid Soap 1:1,000
Metaphen in Oil-A 1:5,000
Metaphen in Oil-B 1:1,000
Metaphen Tincture
Metaphen Suppositories
Metoso
Mineral Oil Emulsion
Mixed Furunculosis Bacterin
Neisser Bacterin
Neoarsphenamine Ampules
Neocinchophen Powder
Neocinchophen Tablets
Neo-Ergot
Neonal Powder
Neonal Tablets
Neorobin
Ophthalmic Ointments:
  Ammoniated Mercury
  Argental
  Atropine Sulphate 1%, 2%
  Boric Acid 10%
  Boric Acid Compound
  Butesin Picrate 1%
  Butyn 2%
  Eserine ¼%
  Holocaine and Epinephrine
  Hyzin
  Mercuric Oxide Yellow ½%, 1%, 2%
  Mercuric Oxide Yellow Compound
  Mercury Bichloride 1:3000, 1:5000
  Metaphen 1:3000
  White's Ointment
  Zinc Sulphate
Orchic Substance Ampules
Orchic Pituitary Compound Capsules
Ovarian Substance Ampules
Ovarian Substance Capsules
Ovarian Substance Tablets
Ovarian Compound Capsules
Ovarian Thyroid Compound Capsules
Ovarian Pituitary Compound Capsules
Pancreas Substance Powder
Pancreas Substance Tablets
Para-Psyllium
Para-Psyllium with Phenolphthalein
Parathyrin Ampules
Parresine
Pentobarbital-Sodium Capsules
Pentobarbital-Sodium Powder
Pertussis Bacterin
Pituitary (Anterior) Capsules
Pituitary Solution U.S.P. Obstetrical Ampules
Pituitary Solution Double Strength Surgical Ampules
Pituitary (Whole) Capsules
Pneumonia Bacterin
Potassium Bismuth Tartrate with Butyn Ampules
Potassium Mercuric Iodide Ampules
Procaine Tablets
Procaine Tablets A-P 1
Procaine Tablets A-P 2
Proflavine
Respiratory Bacterin

Rheumatic Bacterin
Salihexin Ampules
Salihexin Capsules
Saline Laxative
Salithia
Sepsis Bacterin (Van Cott's)
Staphylococcus Mixed Bacterin
Strepto-Pneumo-Staph Bacterin
Sulpharsphenamine Ampules
Sunex
Taroxide
Typhoid Paratyphoid Bacterin
Typhoid Prophylactic
Undulant Fever Bacterin
Urethritis Bacterin
Viosterol in Oil 250 D
Whooping Cough Bacterin
Yohimbin and Orchic Compound Capsules
Also Ampules: Intravenous, 41 in 73 forms; Subcutaneous and Intramuscular, 29 in 36 forms; *See Chap. V*

ACES LABORATORY, INC. **(Aces)**
Peekskill, N. Y.

Mercurochrome Suppository

ADGENE, INCORPORATED **(Adgene)**
Patterson, N. J.

Adgene

AKATOS, INC. **(Akatos)**
55 Van Dam Street, New York City

Neo-Reargon
Reargon

THE ALKALOL CO. **(Alkalol)**
Taunton, Mass.

Alkalol
Irrigol

THE ALLCOCK MANUFACTURING CO. **(Allcock)**
Ossining, N. Y.

Brandreth's Pills

ALPHADEN CO. **(Alphaden)**
154 E. Erie Street, Chicago, Ill.

Betaphos Powder

AMERICAN AGENCY OF FRENCH VICHY, INC. **(American Agency)**
503 Fifth Avenue, New York City

Purgos
Vichy

AMERICAN ANTIFORMIN CO. **(American Antiformin)**
164—8th Street, Brooklyn, N. Y.

Antiformin

AMERICAN BIO-CHEMICAL LABORATORIES, INC.

(American Bio-Chem.)

235 Fourth Avenue, New York City

Euphagin

Homiodin Ampules

AMERICAN FELSOL CO. (American Felsol)

Lorain, Ohio

Felsol Powders

AMERICAN FERMENT CO. (American Ferment)

163 Adams Street, Buffalo, N. Y.

Alcaroid
Caroid Essence
Caroid Powder
Caroid Tablets, Plain
Caroid and Bile Salts Tablets
Caroid Laxative Tablets
Caroid and Bana Diastase Tablets
Caroid and Nux Vomica Tablets
Caroid and Soda Tablets
Caroid and Charcoal Tablets

AMERICAN ORGANOTHERAPY CO.

(American Organotherapy)

31 North State Street, Chicago, Ill.

Arsenoid
Corpus Luteum Comp. "Lowenthal" Capsules
Iodo-Alboid Tablets
Glandoid Compound "Lowenthal"
Lymph Comp. "Lowenthal" Ampules
Lymphoid Comp. "Lowenthal" 1 Capsules
Lymphoid Comp. "Lowenthal" 2 Capsules
Ova Mammoid Comp. "Lowenthal" Capsules
Phenobarboid Tablets
Pituitoid Comp. "Lowenthal" Capsules
Placentoid Comp. "Lowenthal" Capsules
Prostoid Comp. "Lowenthal" Capsules
Splenoid Comp. "Lowenthal" Capsules
Thyroid Gland "Lowenthal" Capsules
Tyloid Tablets
Yohimboid Tablets

AMTORG TRADING CORPORATION (Amtorg)

261 Fifth Avenue, New York City

Borjom

Narzan

THE ANACIN COMPANY (Anacin)

8134 McCormick Boulevard, Chicago, Ill.

Anacin Tablets

Sy-Lac

ANGIER CHEMICAL CO. (Angier)

Allston District, Boston, Mass.

Angier's Emulsion

Angier's Throat Tablets

ANGLO-FRENCH DRUG COMPANY (Anglo-French)
1270 Broadway, New York City

Acecolex
Acecoline Ampules
Allochrysine Ampules
Anti-Asthmatic "Hoeckel" Ampules
Bacteriophage:
  Bacte-Dysenteri-Phage Ampules
  Bacte-Intesti-Phage Ampules
  Bacte-Coli-Phage Ampules
  Bacte-Pyo-Phage Polyvalent Ampules
  Bacte-Staphy-Phage Ampules
  Bacte-Rhino-Phage Ampules
Cryogenine Tablets
Dimol Pulverettes
Dimol Syrup
Elixir Bromo Valerianate
Hepvisc
Hypotan Tablets
Iodobesin Dragees
Lead Selenide Ampules
Mersalv
Neocaine (Spinal) Ampules
Neocaine (Local and Regional)
Neocaine
Neocaine Surrenine Ampules
Neocaine Pure (without Surrenine) Ampules
Neocaine Pure (without Surrenine) Crystals
Orargol Noninjectable
Orargol Injectable Ampules
Orargol O.R.L.
Pancrepatine Globules
Sarcoptal
Stannoxyl Ampules
Stannoxyl Gauze
Stannoxyl Glycerine
Stannoxyl Liquid
Stannoxyl Ointment
Stannoxyl Tablets
Sulfarsenol Ampules
Suppositories "Erge"
Supsalve Suppositories
Urocedrol Capsules
Viosterol in Oil 250D
Also Ampules: Intravenous, 2 in 5 forms; Subcutaneous and Intramuscular, 11 in 16 forms; *See Chap. V*

AN-GLY LABOSATORIES (An-Gly Lab.)
624 Brighton Beach Avenue, Brooklyn, N. Y.

An-Gly-Flav

APOLLINARIS AGENCY COMPANY (Apollinaris)
503 Fifth Avenue, New York City

Apenta
Apollinaris

ARGY LABORATORY (Argy)
939 Main Street, Patterson, N. J.

Iodoxyl Capsules

ARLINGTON CHEMICAL COMPANY (Arlington)
Yonkers, N. Y.

Allergens—Foods
Allergens—Individual (Bacterials, Pollens, Foods, Furs, Miscellaneous)
Allergens—Groups, Pollen
Bacid Culture
Borolyptol
Cascara Peptonoids
Dry Peptonoids
Hemaboloids Liquid
Hemaboloids Tablets
Hemaboloids Arseniated with Strychnia
Iodo-Peptonoids
Lactopeptine Elixir
Lactopeptine Powder
Lactopeptine Tablets
Liquid Peptonoids
Liquid Peptonoids with Creosote
Neocultol

ARMOUR AND COMPANY (Armour)

Union Stock Yards, Chicago, Ill.

Adrenal Cortex Liquid—Ampules
Beef Peptone Powder
Bone Marrow Substance
Brain Substance
Chymogen Powder
Concentrated Liver Extract
Concentrated Liver Extract with Iron
Corpus Luteum Capsules
Corpus Luteum Powder
Corpus Luteum Tablets
Corpus Luteum Liquid—Ampules
Diastase Powder
Duodenin Powder
Duodenin Tablets
Elixir of Enzymes
Epinephrin Hydrochloride Ampules
Elixir of Lactated Pepsin
Essence of Pepsin
Extract of Red Bone Marrow
Kephalin
Kidney Substance
Lecithol
Liver Liquid Ampules
Liver Substance Powder
Liver Substance Tablets
Mammary Substance Powder
Mammary Substance Tablets
Orchic Substance Powder
Orchic Substance Tablets
Ovarian Residue Capsules
Ovarian Residue Powder
Ovarian Residue Tablets
Ovarian Substance Ampules
Ovarian Substance Capsules
Ovarian Substance Powder
Ovarian Substance Tablets
Parathyroid Substance Powder
Parathyroid Substance Tablets
Parathyroid with Calcium Lactate Powder and Tablets
Parotid Tablets
Peptonal
Peptone Solution Ampules 5%
Pineal Substance Powder
Pineal Substance Tablets
Pituitary Liquid, Obstetrical and Surgical—Ampules
Pituitary Liquid, Obstetrical—Ampules
Pituitary Liquid, Surgical—Ampules
Pituitary Substance Anterior—Ampules
Pituitary Substance Anterior—Powder
Pituitary Substance Anterior—Tablets
Pituitary Substance Posterior—Powder
Pituitary Substance Posterior—Tablets
Pituitary Substance Whole—Powder
Pituitary Substance Whole—Tablets
Placental Substance Powder
Placental Substance Tablets
Prostate Substance Powder
Prostate Substance Tablets
Red Bone Marrow
Rennet
Spinal Cord Substance
Spleen Liquid Ampules
Spleen Liquid Solution 40%, 150%
Spleen Substance Capsules
Spleen Substance Powder
Spleen Substance Tablets
Suprarenal Cortex Liquid Ampules
Suprarenal Cortex Substance Powder
Suprarenal Cortex Substance Tablets
Suprarenal Medulla Powder
Suprarenal Medulla Tablets
Suprarenal Substance Whole Gland Powder
Suprarenal Substance Tablets
Suprarenalin Crystals
Suprarenalin Ampules
Suprarenalin Solution
Suprarenalin Ointment
Thromboplastin
Thymus Substance Capsules
Thymus Substance Powder
Thyroid (U.S.P.) Powder
Thyroid (U.S.P.) Tablets
Trypsin Powder
Also Ampules: Intramuscular, 8 in 10 forms; *See Chap. V*

ARROWHEAD HOT SPRINGS CO. (Arrowhead)

Arrowhead Springs, Cal.

Arrowhead Hot Springs

BALMOGEN CHEMICAL CORPORATION (Balmogen)

898 Westchester Avenue, New York City

Balmogen
Glycerophan

BANFI PRODUCTS CORPORATION, INC. **(Banfi)**
140 Sixth Ave., New York City

Montecatini Salts

A. C. BARNES, INC. **(Barnes)**
New Brunswick, N. J.

Argyrol Crystals
Argyrol Tablets

BATES PRODUCTS, INC. **(Bates)**
941 Washington Avenue, Brooklyn, N. Y.

Cuproglobin

BATTLE AND COMPANY **(Battle)**
4026 Olive Street, St. Louis, Mo.

Bromidia
Echthol
Iodia
Papine

THE BATTLE CREEK FOOD CO. **(Battle Creek)**
Battle Creek, Mich.

Acidone Tablets
Food Ferrin, Sweetened
Food Ferrin, Unsweetened
Gluten Flour
Laxa Biscuit
Malted Nuts
Paralax
Paralax with Agar
Psylla White
Psylla White Wafers
Savita Bouillon Cubes
Savita Yeast Tablets
Spinach Concentrate

B. B. CULTURE LABORATORY, INC. **(B. B. Culture)**
Yonkers, N. Y.

Bacillus Acidophilus Culture
Bac. Bulgaricus Culture

GREAT BEAR SPRING CO. **(Great Bear)**
271 Church Street, New York City

Bear Lithia Springs

H. H. BEISNER **(Beisner)**
120 Wall Street, New York City

Asthmolysin Ampules
Brosedan
Posterisan "Kade" Ointment
Posterisan "Kade" Suppositories
Spasmolysin Ampules
Terpichin Ampules
Also Ampules: Subcutaneous and Intramuscular, 3 in 3 forms; *See Chap. V*

BELMONT LABORATORIES, INC. (Belmont)

4430 Chestnut Street, Philadelphia, Pa.

Mazon Soap
Mazon Ointment

BENZOINOL MANUFACTURING CO. (Benzoinol)

90 West Street, N. Y.

Benzoinol
Benzoinol and Resorcin Comp.
Benzoinol with Camphor
Benzoinol with Menthol
Benzoinol Camphor-Menthol
Benzoinol with Eucalyptol
Benzoinol with Carbolic Acid
Benzoinol with Iodine
Benzoinol with Iodine and Carbolic Acid
Dr. Douglas' Formula

BENZOL PRODUCTS COMPANY (Benzol)

237 South Street, Newark, N. J.

Neocinchophen
Oxyquinolin Sulphate
Phenobarbital-Sodium

ROBERT A. BERNHARD (Bernhard)

153 Anderson Avenue, Rochester, N. Y.

Saf-Fast
Saf-T-Top

BERWYN PHARMACEUTICAL CORPORATION (Berwyn)

Erie and Division Streets, North Tonawanda, N. Y.

Corpus Luteum Extract Ampules
Epinephrine Hydrochloride 1:1,000 Ampules
Epinephrine Hydrochloride 1:10,000 Ampules
Ovarian Extract Ampules
Ovarian Residue Extract Ampules
Pituitary Anterior Lobe—Ampules
Pituitary Extract U.S.P. Obstetrical Ampules
Pituitary Extract Double U.S.P. Surgical Ampules
Also Ampules: Intravenous, 25 in 39 forms; Subcutaneous and Intramuscular, 47 in 63 forms; *See Chap. V*

BETHLEHEM LABORATORIES, INC. (Bethlehem)

300 Century Building, Pittsburgh, Pa.

Hyclorite

BILHUBER-KNOLL CORPORATION (Bilhuber-Knoll)

154 Ogden Avenue, Jersey City, N. J.

Afenil Ampules
Ago-Cholan Tablets
Bromural Powder
Bromural Tablets
Calciphos Powder
Calciphos Tablets
Dilaudid Ampules
Dilaudid Powder
Dilaudid Suppositories
Dilaudid Tablets
Diuretin Powder
Diuretin Tablets
Euresol
Euresol Pro Capillis
Histosan Powder
Ichthalbin Powder
Ichthalbin Tablets
Lenigallol Powder

Lenigallol-Zinc Ointment 6%
Metrazol Ampules
Metrazol Powder
Metrazol Solution
Metrazol Tablets
Phyllicin Powder
Phyllicin Tablets
Pixalbol
Potassium Iodide-Theocalcin
Santyl Capsules
Santyl Liquid
Tannalbin Powder
Tannalbin Tablets
Theocalcin Powder
Theocalcin Tablets
Also Ampules: Intravenous, 1; Subcutaneous and Intramuscular, 2; *See Chap. V*

BIO MEDICO, INC. (Bio Medico)
62 West 14th Street, New York City

By-Kem Tablets

ERNST BISCHOFF CO., INC. (Bischoff)
135 Hudson Street, New York City

Activin Ampules
Activin Liquid
Alpha Lobelin Ampules
Anayodin Pills
Anayodin Powder
Bilival Pills
Cadechol Powder
Cadechol Tablets
Camphogen Ampules 1
Cardysate
Diatussin
Diatussin Syrup
Hydragogin
Normolactol Tablets
Polygalysate
Pronusin Ointment
Pronusin Suppositories
Recvalysate
Salvysate
Silvogon Powder
Silvogon Tablets
Spiroform Powder
Spiroform Tablets
Styptysate Liquid
Styptysate Tablets
Syrup Histosan
Uvalysate
Viscysate Liquid
Viscysate Tablets
Also Ampules: Intravenous 1; Subcutaneous and Intramuscular, 3 in 4 forms; *See Chap. V*

THE BISODOL COMPANY (Bisodol)
New Haven, Conn.

Bisodol

BISURATED, INC. (Bisurated)
Binghamton, N. Y.

Bisurated Magnesia

BLEACHO CO. (Bleacho)
174 Frank Street, Rochester, N. Y.

Berry Hill Mineral Springs

BLOOMFIELD LABORATORIES (Bloomfield)
Bloomfield, N. J.

Culture Lacto Bacillus
Hygem

BOERICKE AND RUNYON, INC.

(Boericke and Runyon)

518 Sixth Avenue, New York City

Asparagus Compound
Bile Salts Compound Tablets
Boerenzyme
Boro-Cap-Tol
Calcium Bismuth Compound
C. C. C. Tonic
Guaiacol Compound
Hema-Glycon Tablets
Painol
Yerba Santa-Creo Compound

BOERICKE AND TAFEL

(Boericke and Tafel)

1011 Arch Street, Philadelphia, Pa.

Corpus Luteum Capsules
Islands of Langerhans Capsules
Mammary Substance Capsules
Ovarian Substance Capsules
Pancreatin Capsules
Parathyroid Capsules
Parotid Gland Capsules
Pineal Gland Capsules
Pituitary Whole Capsules
Placenta Capsules
Prostate Gland Capsules
Spleen Capsules
Sulfax Powder
Sulfax Tablets
Sulfax Vaginals
Suprarenal Whole Capsules
Surgical Powder
Testicles Capsules
Thymus Capsules
Thyroid Capsules

BORCHERDT MALT EXTRACT CO.

(Borcherdt)

217 North Lincoln Street, Chicago, Ill.

Malt Extract Plain
Malt with Iron Iodide
Malt Extract with Cascara Sagrada
Malt Extract with Yerba Santa Compound
Malt Extract with Cod Liver Oil
Malt Extract, Cod Liver Oil with Iron Iodide
Malt Cod Liver Oil with Spleenmarrow
Malt Extract with Creosote
Malt Soup Extract
Malt Sugar

THE BORDEN COMPANY

(Borden)

350 Madison Avenue, New York City

(Merrell-Soule)

Malted Milk
Klim Powdered Whole Milk
Powdered Protein Milk
Powdered Skimmed Lactic Acid Milk
Powdered Skim Milk
Powdered Whole Lactic Acid Milk
Thompson's Double Malted Milk

BOVININE COMPANY

(Bovinine)

536 Lake Shore Drive, Chicago, Ill.

Neobovinine 20
Neobovinine with Malt and Iron

M. J. BREITENBACH COMPANY

(Breitenbach)

160 Varick Street, New York City

Pepto-Mangan "Gude" Liquid
Pepto-Mangan "Gude" Tablets

GEORGE A. BREON AND COMPANY (Breon)

319 West 50th Street, New York City or Kansas City, Mo.

Corpus Luteum Solution Ampules
Epinephrin Solution Ampules
Orchic Extract Solution Ampules
Ovarian Extract Solution Ampules
Pituitary Solution Anterior Ampules
Pituitary Extract Obstetrical Ampules
Pituitary Extract Surgical, Double strength, Ampules
Also Ampules: Intravenous, 34 in 57 forms; Subcutaneous and Intramuscular, 31 in 39 forms; *See Chap. V*

BREWER AND CO., INC. (Brewer)

Worcester, Mass.

Copral

BRISTOL-MYERS COMPANY (Bristol-Myers)

75 West Street, New York City

Analka
Gastrogen Tablets
Ipana Tooth Paste

BROOKLYN SCIENTIFIC PRODUCTS CO., INC. (Brooklyn Scientific)

313 Bedford Avenue, Brooklyn, N. Y.

Exicol Capsules
Exicol Capsules with Phenolphthalein
Novatone Tablets

BUCKHEAD SPRINGS CO. (Buckhead)

Buckhead Springs, Va.

Buckhead Spring Natural Waters

BUFFINGTON'S, INC. (Buffington)

300–306 Main Street, Worcester, Mass.

Chiquenia
Cupramin
Di-Efrin
Nasedra Aplikol
Vaginettes

C. D. BURCHARD, INC. (Burchard)

121 Varick Street, New York City

Duofoam Tubes

BURNHAM SOLUBLE IODINE COMPANY, INC. (Burnham)

Auburndale, Mass.

Alterative Compound
Amiodoxyl Benzoate
Ethyl Iodide
Iodine Ointment
Iodine Suppositories
Root Canal Filling
Soluble Iodine

BURROUGHS WELLCOME AND COMPANY

(Burroughs Wellcome)

9–11 East 41st Street, New York City

Alaxa
Alvesen Tabloids
Antifebrin
Antifebrin Compound Tabloids
Ascaridole
B Vitamins Tabloids
Bicreol
Bone Medulla Tabloids
Borofax
Bulbocapnine Phosphate Tabloids, Hypodermic
Butyl Chloral Hydrate et Gelsemium Tabloids
Calomel Cream
Cannabine Tannate
Cerebrine Tabloids
Cod Liver Oil "Kepler"
Dexin
Didymin
Diginutin
Digitalin (Amorphous) Tabloids Hypodermic
Digitalin (Amorphous) Tabloids Oral
Digitalin (Crystalline) Hypoloids
Digitalin (Crystalline) Tabloids
Empirin Tabloids
Empirin Compound Elixoid
Ephedrine Tabloid Comp.
Ephedrine Hydrochloride Solution
Ephedrine Hydrochloride Hypoloid
Ephedrine Hydrochloride Tabloid
Epinephrine Solution 1:1,000
Epinephrine Solution 1:1,000 Hypoloids
Epinine Solution 1:100
Epinine Tabloids Ophthalmic
Epinine Tabloid Compound
Epinine Nasal Jelly
Epinine Hydrochloride Hypoloids
Epinine Hydrochloride Enule 1:100
Ergamine Tabloids Hypodermic
Ergotoxine Tabloids Hypodermic
Ergotoxine Tabloids Hypodermic and Strychnine Sulphate
Ernutin Oral
Ernutin Hypoloids
Ethidol
Euphthalmin Hydrochloride Tabloids Ophthalmic
Fluorescein Tabloids Ophthalmic
Gingament Tabloids
Haemoglobin Tabloids
Haemoglobin Scales
Hazeline Cream
Hazeline Liquid
Hazeline Snow
Hazeline Soap
Hazeline Suppositories
Hydrargyri Succinimidi Hypodermic Tabloid
Ichthamol Tabloids
Infundin Hypoloids (5 I.U.)
Infundin Hypoloids (10 I.U.)
Iodicin Capsules
Iodicin Tabloids
Kepler Malt Extract with Hemoglobin
Kepler Cod Liver Oil with Malt Extract
Kepler Cod Liver Oil with Malt Extract and Creosote
Kepler Cod Liver Oil with Malt Extract and Hypophosphites
Kepler Cod Liver Oil with Malt Extract and Iron Iodide
Kepler Cod Liver Oil with Malt Extract and Phosphorus
Kepler Cod Liver Oil with Malt Extract and Haemoglobin
Kidney Substance Tabloids
Laxamel
Lymphatic Gland Tabloids
Lubafax
Malt Extract "Kepler"
Malt Extract with Cascara Sagrada
Malt Extract with Glycerophosphates
Malt Extract with Hypophos. of Calcium
Malt Extract with Iron Iodide
Malt Extract with Iron Pyrophos.
Malt Extract with Iron, Quinine and Strychnine Phosphate
Malt Extract with Phosphorus and Hemoglobin
Mammary Gland Tabloids "Mamos"
Mercurials
Mercurial Cream Blue
Mercury Salicylate Hypoloid
Mercury Salicylate Cream
Moogrol
Mucin
Neostam
Nizin Powder
Nizin Soloid
Nuclein Hypoloids
Nucleo-Lecithin Comp. Tabloids
Papain Tabloids
Parathyroid Tabloids
Paroleine
Paroleine Spray Compound
Pelletierine Tannate Tabloids
Pepana
Phenofax

Pituitary Gland Anterior—Tabloids
Pituitary Gland Posterior—Tabloids
Pituitary Whole—Hypoloids
Pituitary Whole—Tabloids
Prostate Gland Substance Tabloids
Quassin Suppositories
Quinine Compound Tabloid
Quinine and Urea Hydrochloride Tabloids
Quinine and Urethane Hypoloids
Quinoxyl Soloids
Quinoxyl Tabloids
Red Gum
Saxin Tabloids
Sketofax
Spleen Substance Tabloids
Suprarenal Whole Tabloids
Soamin Tabloids
Soamin Powder
Tabloid Hydrastine Comp. (Cannabine Tannate)
Tabloid Glandular Mixture 1 Male
Tabloid Glandular Mixture 2 Female
Tabloid Thyrovarium
Tabloid Varium
Thymus Tabloids
Thyroid Tabloids
Tyramine Tabloids Hypodermic
Tolamine Soloids
Vaporole Chloroform with Ethyl Iodide Compound.
Also Ampules: Intravenous, 22 in 27 forms; *See Chap. V*

CALCO CHEMICAL COMPANY (Calco
Bound Brook, N. J.

Cinchophen Powder
Cinchophen Tablets
Magnespirin Powder
Magnespirin Tabloids
Neomagnephen Tablets
Tolysin Powder
Tolysin Tablets
Trichlorethylene Tubes

CARLSBAD PRODUCTS COMPANY, INC.
154 West 14 St., New York City

Karlsbad Bath Salts
Karlsbad Sprudel Salt
Karlsbad Sprudel Spring Water
Karlsbad Muehlbrunn Water

CAMPBELL CEREAL COMPANY (Campbell)
Northfield, Minn.

Malto Meal

CAREL LABORATORIES (Carel)
Redondo Beach, Calif.

Alpha-Naphco Camphor Ointment
Alpha-Naphco Cones
Alpha-Naphco Jelly Capsules
Alpha-Naphco Liquid
Alpha-Naphco Menthol Suppositories
Alpha-Naphco Nasal Ointment
Alpha-Naphco Ointment
Alpha-Naphco Powder
Alpha-Naphco Suppositories Rectal
Alpha-Naphco Suppositories Vaginal
Alpha-Naphco Zinc Stearate
Alpha-Naphco Zinc Stearate Powder

G. W. CARNRICK COMPANY (G. W. Carnrick)

20 Mt. Pleasant Avenue, Newark, N. J.

Bilina Tablets
Corpus Luteum Ampules
Corpus Luteum Capsules
Corpus Luteum Powder
Corpus Luteum Tablets
Corpus Luteum Compound Capsules
Corpus Luteum Compound Tablets
Duodenal Substance
Epinephrine Powder
Epinephrine Chloride Solution 1:1,000—Ampules
Epinephrine Chloride Solution 1:10,000—Ampules
Erythgen Liver Extract Ampules
Erythgen Liver Extract Capsules
Erythgen Liver Extract Liquid
Glandular Compound Male Capsules
Glandular Compound Male Tablets
Glandular Compound Female Capsules
Glandular Compound Female Tablets
Hormotone Tablets
Incretone Solution
Kidney Substance
Kinazyme Capsules
Kinazyme Tablets
Liver Extract (Erythgen) Ampules
Liver Extract (Erythgen) Capsules
Liver Extract (Erythgen) Glycerin solution
Liver Substance Capsules
Liver Substance Powder
Liver Substance Tablets
Lymphatic Substance
Mammagen Capsules
Mammagen Tablets
Mammary Compound Capsules
Mammary Compound Tablets
Mammary Substance Capsules
Mammary Substance Powder
Mammary Substance Tablets
Orchic Substance Capsules
Orchic Substance Powder
Orchic Substance Tablets
Orchic-Prostate Compound Capsules
Orchic-Prostate Compound Tablets
Ovarian Substance Capsules
Ovarian Substance Powder
Ovarian Substance Tablets
Ovarian Compound Capsules
Ovarian Compound Tablets
Pancreas Substance Capsules
Pancreas Substance Powder
Pancreas Substance Tablets
Pancreatin U.S.P. Powder
Pancreatin and Soda Tablets
Parathyroid Substance Powder
Parathyroid Substance Tablets
Parathyroid Compound Capsules
Parathyroid Compound Tablets
Pineal Substance Powder
Pineal Substance Tablets
Pineal Compound Male Capsules
Pineal Compound Male Tablets
Pineal Compound Female Capsules
Pineal Compound Female Tablets
Pituitary Anterior, Powder
Pituitary Anterior, Tablets
Pituitary Posterior, Powder
Pituitary Posterior Tablets
Pituitary Posterior Obstetrical Ampules
Pituitary Posterior Surgical Ampules
Pituitary Whole Powder
Pituitary Whole Tablets
Placenta Substance Capsules
Placenta Substance Powder
Placenta Substance Tablets
Prostate Substance Capsules
Prostate Substance Powder
Prostate Substance Tablets
Renal-Pancreas Compound Capsules
Renal-Pancreas Compound Tablets
Rythmin
Secretogen Elixir
Secretogen Tablets
Spinal Cord Substance
Spleen Substance Capsules
Spleen Substance Powder
Spleen Substance Tablets
Spleen-Red Bone Marrow Compound Tablets
Suprarenal Cortex Capsules
Suprarenal Cortex Powder
Suprarenal Cortex Tablets
Suprarenal Medulla Tablets
Suprarenal Whole Powder
Suprarenal Whole Tablets
Suprarenal-Pituitary Compound Capsules
Suprarenal-Pituitary Compound Tablets
Thelestrin Ampules
Thymus Substance Capsules
Thymus Substance Powder
Thymus Substance Tablets
Thymus Compound Capsules
Thymus Compound Tablets
Thyroid U.S.P. Capsules
Thyroid U.S.P. Powder
Thyroid U.S.P. Tablets
Trypsogen Capsules
Trypsogen Tablets
Viriligen Ampules
Viriligen Capsules

Viriligen Tablets

Also Ampules: Subcutaneous and Intramuscular, 7 in 7 forms; *See Chap. V*

CAVENDISH CHEMICAL CORPORATION **(Cavendish)**
25 West Broadway, New York City

Anastil Ampules, Plain and Reinforced
Bismolan Ointment
Bismolan Suppositories
Cavosept Tablets
Elixir Neurogenic
Lipolysin Ampules
Lipolysin Tablets
Myoston Ampules
Myoston Liquid
Terogon "Schuftan" Tablets
Testogan Ampules
Testogan Tablets
Thelygan Ampules
Thelygan Tablets
Yohimbin Ampules
Yohimbin Elixir
Yohimbin Tablets
Also Ampules: Intravenous, 2; Subcutaneous and Intramuscular, 7; *See Chap. V*

CELLASIN COMPANY **(Cellasin)**
Buffalo, N. Y.

Cellasin "Barr" Tablets 1, 2

THE CENTRAL PHARMACAL COMPANY
(Central Pharmacal)
Seymour, Indiana

Bismodide Capsules

CERTIFOODS, INC. **(Certifoods)**
436 Eighteenth Street, Brooklyn, N. Y.

Sieved Vegetalbes

CHAPPEL BROTHERS, INC. **(Chappel)**
Rockford, Ill.

Hemo-S
Liver Extract—Oral
Liver Extract—Subcutaneous, Ampules
Also Ampules: Subcutaneous and Intramuscular, 1 in 1 form; *See Chap. V*

CHEMICO-BIOLOGIC LABORATORIES
(Chemico-Biologic)
101 Maiden Lane, New York City

Di-citurin Tablets

CHEPLIN BIOLOGICAL LABORATORY **(Cheplin)**
Taylor and King Streets, Syracuse, N. Y.

Bacillus Acidophilus Liquid
Bacillus Acidophilus Milk
Ovarian Substance Ampules
Also Ampules: Intravenous, 28 in 29 forms;
Subcutaneous and Intramuscular, 12 in 12 forms; *See Chap. V*

CHESEBROUGH MANUFACTURING COMPANY

(Chesebrough)

17 State Street, New York City

Vaseline Preparations:
"Vaseline"
"Vaseline" Borated Jelly
"Vaseline" Carbolated Jelly
"Vaseline" Camphor Ice
"Vaseline" Eucalyptol Jelly
"Vaseline" Mentholated Jelly

CHICAGO DIETETIC SUPPLY (Chicago Dietetic)

1750 W. Van Buren Street, Chicago, Ill.

Agar-Agar
Agar Dessert
Bouillon Cubes
Bran Breakfast Food
Bran Special Wafers
Bran Wafers
Canned Fruits
Canned Vegetables
Cellu Agar Jelly
Cellu Chili Sauce
Cellu Flour
Cellu Soy Beans in Tomato Sauce
Cellu Soy Crisp
D-Zerta
Gelatin Desserts
Mayonnaise
Mineral Oil Dressing
Noodles
One-Two-Three Flour
Psyllium Seed
Pulverized Washed Bran
Soy Bean Flour
Sugarless Sweetener
Washed Bran

CHURCH AND DWIGHT COMPANY, INC.

(Church and Dwight)

70 Pine Street, New York City

Bicarbonate of Soda (Arm and Hammer)

CIBA COMPANY, INC. (Ciba)

Greenwich and Morton Streets, New York City

Agomensin Ampules
Agomensin Tablets
Atoquinol Tablets
Cibalgine Ampules
Cibalgine Elixir
Cibalgine Tablets
Coagulen Ampules 3%
Coagulen Powder
Coramine Ampules
Coramine Oral
Dial Ampules
Dial Elixir
Dial Powder
Dial Tablets
Digifoline Ampules
Digifoline Liquid
Digifoline Tablets
Ferrophytine Pills
Fortossan Powder
Isarol
Lipoiodine Tablets, Plain and Sugar coated
Lipoiodine Diagnostic Ampules and Solution
Nupercaine Ampules
Nupercaine Ointment
Nupercaine Powder
Nupercaine Solution
Nupercaine Tablets
Nupercaine with Epinephrine Ampules
Peristaltine Ampules
Peristaltine Tablets
Phytine Tablets
Prokliman Tablets
Silosan Powder
Silosan Tablets
Silosan Compound Tablets
Sistomensin Ampules
Sistomensin Tablets
Vioform Powder
Also Ampules: Subcutaneous and Intramuscular, 9 in 16 forms; *See Chap. V*

HAROLD H. CLAPP, INC. **(H. H. Clapp)**
1328 Rochester Ave., Rochester, N. Y.

Baby Soups—Strained and Unstrained
Beef Broth
Liver Soup
Strained Fruit Pulps
Strained Vegetables
Vegetable Soup
Wheatheart Soup

OTIS CLAPP AND SON, INC. **(Otis Clapp)**
439 Boylston Street, Boston, Mass.

Obtundia
Obtundia Cream
Obtundia Ephedrine Inhalant
Obtundia Inhalant
Obtundia Nasal Cream
Obtundia Vagiobulbs
Obtundobulbs
Obtundorrhoids

CLINADOL COMPANY, INC. **(Clinadol)**
64 West 14th Street, New York City

Cod Liver Oil Concentrate

CLOVERDALE BEVERAGE COMPANY **(Cloverdale)**
50 East 9th Street, New York City

Cloverdale Lithia Springs

COLE CHEMICAL COMPANY **(Cole)**
3727 Laclede Avenue, St. Louis, Mo.

Anteri-Cole Ampules
Endocrine Compound 26, Capsules
Glycocholate-Pancreas Comp., Capsules
Gonad-Prostate Comp., Capsules
Hemoglobin Comp., Capsules
Hepati-Cole Ampules
Hepatic-Ovary Pancreas Comp., Capsules
Mammary-Ergotin Comp., Capsules
Mammary-Placenta Comp., Capsules
Neutralizing Sodium Potassium Comp., Capsules
Nucleinized Thyro-Iodide Comp., Capsules
Ovarian Comp. 24, Capsules
Ovarian Comp. 4, Capsules
Ovary-Mammary Comp., Capsules
Pancreas-Adrenal Comp., Capsules
Parathyroid-Spermin Comp., Capsules
Pituitary-Phosphate Comp., Capsules
Pituitary-Thymus Comp., Capsules
Placenta-Thyroid Comp., Capsules
Prostate-Spermin Comp., Capsules
Pulmo-Hemoglobin Comp., Capsules
Renal-Pancreas Comp., Capsules
Secretin-Pancreas-Myrtillin Comp., Capsules
Spermin-Pancreas Comp., Capsules
Suprarenal-Spermin Comp., Capsules
Thyro-Pituitary Comp., Capsules
Also Ampules: Subcutaneous and Intramuscular, 2; *See Chap. V*

THE COLEMAN AND BELL COMPANY, INC. **(Coleman and Bell)**
Norwood, Ohio

Gentian Violet Improved Medicinal Powder

COLLENE LABORATORIES, INC. **(Collene)**
77 White Street, New York City

Collene

COLUMBUS PHARMACAL COMPANY

(Columbus Pharmacal)

326–336 Oak Street East, Columbus, Ohio

An-nu-tol
Barbromid Tablets
Benzalba
Carbovescent
Chlomin
Golden Powder
Kaosyl
Loingia
Neutralizing Cordial
Oxachol
White Liniment

COLWELL PHARMACAL CORP. (Colwell)

106 East 19th Street, New York City

Adrenal Cortex Solution
Corpus Luteum Ampules
Corpus Luteum Crinogen
Epinephrin 1:1,000 Ampules
Epinephrin Chloride Solution 1:1,000
Folliculin (Ovarian Hormone) Ampules
Folliculin (Ovarian Hormone) Crinogen
Hormones Solution
Mammary Crinogen
Multicrinogen Ampules
Orchic Ampules
Orchic Crinogen
Orchic (Special Concentration) Ampules
Orchic (Special Concentration) Solution
Ovarialhormon Folliculin Menformon
Ovarian Residue Ampules
Ovarian Residue Crinogen
Ovarian Whole Ampules
Ovarian Whole Crinogen
Parathyroid Crinogen
Parathyroid Solution Ampules
Phedrocaine Oil 10%
Phedrocaine Tablets
Phedrocaine Suppositories
Pituitary Anterior Ampules
Pituitary Anterior Solution
Pituitary Solution Obstetrical Ampules
Pituitary Solution Surgical Ampules
Pituitary Whole Ampules
Pituitary Whole Crinogen
Placenta Crinogen
Placenta Substance Powder
Placenta Substance Tablets
Prostate Crinogen
Suprarenal Whole Solution
Thymus Crinogen
Thy-Ovarian Comp.
Thyroid Crinogen
Thyroid Solution Ampules

COOK LABORATORIES, INC. (Cook)

170 Varick Street, New York City

Ampules (Cartridges): Subcutaneous and Intramuscular, 13 in 19 forms

---

CRAZY WELL WATER CO. (Crazy Well)

Mineral Well, Texas

Crazy Mineral Wells
Crazy Water Crystals

CROOKES LABORATORIES, INC. (Crookes)

145 East 57th Street, New York City

Collosol Antimony Hypodermic
Calcium Levulinate Ampules
Cod Liver Oil Emulsion with Calcium
Cod Liver Oil Emulsion with Collosol Calcium
Cod Liver Oil Emulsion with Collosol Iodine
Cod Liver Oil Emulsion with Yeast
Colloplasma
Collosol Antimony Ampules
Collosol Antimony Oral
Collosal Antimony Hypodermic
Collosol Argentum Ampules
Collosol Argentum Liquidum

Collosol Argentum Beta 0.25%
Collosol Argentum Bougies
Collosol Argentum Dentifrice
Collosol Argentum Ophthalmic
Collosol Argentum Pasta 0.25%
Collosol Argentum Pessaries 0.25%
Collosol Argentum Soap
Collosol Argentum Suppositories 0.25%
Collosol Argentum Oil
Collosol Argentum Tampons
Collosol Argentum Unguentum 1%
Collosol Arsenic
Collosol Aurum 1:2,000 (Oral)
Collosol Aurum 1:8,000 Ampules
Collosol Aurum for Lange Colloidal Gold Test
Collosol Bromide Oral
Collosol Bromoform Compound
Collosol Calamine Lotion
Collosol Calcium Ampules
Collcsol Calcium Oral
Collosol Calcium with Lecithin Ampules
Collosol Calcium with Lecithin Oral
Collosol Calcium with Vitamin D Oral
Collosol Chlor-Carvacrol
Collosol Chrysarobin External 0.2%
Collosol Chrysarobin Oral 0.2%
Collosol Chrysarobin Intravenous—Ampules 1:1,000
Collosol Chrysarobin Intravenous—Bottles
Collosol Cuprum Ampules
Collosol Cuprum Hypodermic
Collosol Cuprum Oral
Collosol Cuprum Ophthalmic
Collosol Cuprum Paste
Collosol Cuprum Suppositories
Collosol Cuprum et Ferrum Ampules
Collosol Cuprum et Ferrum Oral
Collosol Cuprum et Ferro-Arsenicum Ampules
Collosol Cuprum et Ferro-Arsenicum Oral
Collosol Cuprum et Ferro-Manganese Ampules
Collosol Cuprum et Ferro-Manganese Oral
Collosol Ferro-Arsenicum Ampules
Collosol Ferro-Arsenicum Oral and Injection
Collosol Ferro-Arsenicum and Strychnine 0.1% Ampules
Collosol Ferro-Arsenicum and Strychnine Oral, Injection, Ampule
Collosol Ferromalt
Collosol Ferromalt and Hypophosphites
Collosol Ferromalt and Glycerophosphates
Collosol Ferromalt and Cascara
Collosol Ferromalt and Hemoglobin
Collosol Ferromalt and Manganese
Collosol Ferrum Ampules
Collosol Ferrum Oral and Injection
Collosol Ferro-Manganese Ampules
Collosol Ferro-Manganese Oral and Injection
Collosol Ferro-Manganese-Arsenic Ampules
Collosol Ferro-Manganese-Arsenic Oral and Injection
Collosol "F.C.V.D."
Collosol Hydrargyrum Ampules 1% and Injection
Collosol Hydrargyrum Oral 0.05%
Collosol Hydrargyrum Cream 5%
Collosol Hydrargyrum Vaginal Suppositories
Collosol Ichthyol Capsules
Collosol Ichthyol Glycerine 50%
Collosol Ichthyol Ointment 10%
Collosol Ichthyol Ointment with Resorcin
Collosol Ichthyol Ointment with Resorcin and Chrysarobin
Collosol Ichthyol Pessaries
Collosol Ichthyol Soap
Collosol Ichthyol Sodium (Granular)
Colossol Ichthyol Suppositories
Collosol Ichthyol Tampons
Collosol Iodine Ampules 1%
Collosol Iodine Ampules 0.2%
Collosol Iodine Ampules 0.4% (C.I.N.S.)
Collosol Iodine Ampules 0.8%
Collosol Iodine Oil
Collosol Iodine Oil with Methyl Salicylate
Collosol Iodine 0.2% Oral
Collosol Iodine Paste
Collosol Iodine Pessaries
Collosol Iodine Pigmentum
Collosol Iodine Pastilles
Collosol Iodine Pastilles with Black Currant
Collosol Iodine Suppositories
Collosol Kaolin
Collosol Kaolin with Phenolphthalein
Collosol Lactalumina
Collosol Lactalumina Laxative
Collosol Lactalumina with Bismuth
Collosol Lacto-Calamine
Collosol Lactomagnesia
Collosol Lead M.A. Ampules
Collosol Lead M.A. Liquid
Collosol Plumbum Ampules
Collosol Manganese Oral
Collosol Manganese "Single Sol" and "Double Sol" Ampules
Collosol Palladium Ampules
Collosol Palladium Oral and Injection

Collosol Scalp Lotion Oily
Collosol Scalp Lotion Non-Oily
Collosol Selenium Ampules
Collosol Selenium Oral and Injection
Collosol Silica with Drosera Rutondifolia
Collosol Soap
Collosol Stannum Ampules
Collosol Sulphur Ampules
Collosol Sulphur External
Collosol Sulphur Cream
Collosol Sulphur Oil
Collosol Sulphur Oral
Collosol Sulphur Pessaries
Collosol Sulphur Pigmentum
Collosol Sulphur Paraffin Emulsion
Collosol Transfusion Supplies:
  Glucose 5%, 10%, 20%, 50%
  Glucose 5% in normal saline
  Gum Saline
  Hypertonic Saline
  Normal Saline
Collosol Trimine Ampules
Collosol Trimine Oral
Collosol Zinc
Collosol Zinc Pipette Bottle
Collosol Zinc Cream
Colsul Aqueous Ampules
Colsul Oily Ampules
Episol Ampules
Halibut Liver Oil (Collosol Brand) Capsules
Halibut Liver Oil (Collosol Brand) Liquid
Ichthyol Ointment
Ichthyol Pessaries
Ichthyol Suppositories
Lithium Salicylate 30% with Tutocaine 1% Ampules
Manganese Butyrate Ampules and Injection
Mercurochrome (Collosol Brand) Pessaries
Mercurochrome (Collosol Brand) Pigmentum
Mercurochrome (Collosol Brand) Scales
Mercurochrome (Collosol Brand) Solution 2% Aqueous
Mercurochrome (Collosol Brand) Solution 5% Alcoholic
Mercurochrome (Collosol Brand) Solution 2% Isotonic
Mercurochrome (Collosol Brand) Solution 0.4% Intravenous Set
Mercurochrome (Collosol Brand) Tampons
Metallic Bismuth (Collosol Brand) 5%
Metallic Bismuth (Collosol Brand) 10%
Metallic Bismuth (Collosol Brand) 20%
Pastilles
Sodium Morrhuate (Collosol Brand) 5%—Ampules
Sodium Morrhuate (Collosol Brand) 10%—Ampules
Tannic Acid Spray Ampules
Tannic Acid Spray Adaptor
Tetanol-Collosol Ampules
Also Ampules: Intravenous, 9 in 19 forms; Subcutaneous and Intramuscular, 25 in 64 forms; *See Chap. V*

CURDOLAC FOODS COMPANY (Curdolac)

Waukesha, Wis.

Bouillon Cubes
Breakfast Cereal
Breakfast Food
Butter, Peanutless
Cakes, Cookies, Wafers, etc., 24 products
Casein Compound
Citric Acid
Delecto Dessert Powder
Improved Flour
Johnny Cake Flour
Mayonnaise
Noodles
Oil Dressing
Soya Flour
Soya Bran Flour
Wheat Soya Flour

THE CUTTER LABORATORY (Cutter)

Fourth and Parker Streets, Berkeley, Calif.

Acne Bacillus Vaccine
Allergens—Pollens, Individual
Allergens—Pollens, Stock mixtures
Antistreptococcus Serum Concentrated
Antistreptococcus Serum Unconcentrated
Bacillus Acidophilus
Colon Bacillus Vaccine
Diphtheria Antitoxin
Diphtheria Toxoid
Diphtheria Toxoid for Reaction Test
Diphtheria Toxin-Antitoxin Mixture
Diphtheria Toxin-Antitoxin Mixture (Goat)
Gonococcus Vaccine

Mixed Vaccine—Gonorrhea
Mixed Vaccine—Influenza
Mixed Vaccine—Respiratory
Mixed Vaccine—Respiratory, 4 count
Mixed Vaccine—Respiratory Prophylactic
Normal Horse Serum
Pertussis Vaccine
Pertussis Vaccine Special High Count
Pertussis Vaccine High Count, Fresh
Pertussis Prophylactic Vaccine
Pertussis Mixed Vaccine
Poisonivi
Poisonok
Polyanaerobic Antitoxin
Rabies Vaccine
Respiratory Infection Prophylactic Vaccine
Schick Test
Schick Test Dilution
Schick Test Control
Silver Nitrate Solution Ampules
Smallpox Vaccine
Staph-Acne Vaccine (Acne Combined Vaccine)
Staph-Acne Vaccine (Acne Combined Vaccine 4)
Staphylococcus Vaccine
Staph-Strep Vaccine
Streptococcus Vaccine
Tetanus Antitoxin Human
Thromboplastin Local
Toxivi
Toxok
Tuberculin Diagnostic
Tuberculin Dilutions O.T.
Tuberculin Concentrated (B.F.)
Tuberculin Bouillon Filtrate
Tuberculins Concentrated T.O.
Typhoid Vaccine
Typhoid Prophylactic
Typhoid-Paratyphoid Prophylactic
Ulcerative Colitis Vaccines
Van Cott's Combination
Also Ampules: Intravenous, 10 in 18 forms; Subcutaneous and Intramuscular, 6 in 11 forms; *See Chap. V*

DAVIES, ROSE AND CO., LTD. (Davies, Rose)
22 Thayer Street, Boston, Mass.

Shadocol

DAVIS AND GECK, INC. (Davis and Geck)
211–221 Duffield Street, Brooklyn, N. Y.

Kalmerid Germicidal Tablets

THE DAWSON SPRINGS WATER CO., INC.
Dawson Springs, Ky. (Dawson Springs)

Hamby's Genuine Dawson Springs

THE DENTINOL AND PYROZIDE COMPANY (Dentinol)
1480 Broadway, New York City

Dentinol
Pyrozide

THE DENVER CHEMICAL MFG. COMPANY
163 Varick Steet, New York City (Denver Chemical)

Antiphlogistine

DIARSENOL COMPANY, INC. (Diarsenol)
771 Ellicott Square, Buffalo, N. Y.

Diarsenol Ampules
Neodiarsenol Ampules
Sodium Diarsenol Ampules
Also Ampules: Intravenous, 3 in 21 forms; *See Chap. V*

DIETETIC FOOD COMPANY (Dietetic Food)

6205 Eighteenth Avenue, Brooklyn, N. Y.

Beverage Compound
Bran Cookies
Breakfast Food
Casein Lady Fingers
Casein Sponge Cookies
Dietetic Candy
Dietetic Casein Flour
Dietetic Cocoa Bars
Dietetic Pudding
Gluten Bread
Gluten Cookies
Gluten Noodles
Gluten Plus Bread
Gluto-Lax Breakfast Food
Golden Gluten Breadsticks
India Gum
Low Calory Cookies
Low Calory Flour
Neutralized Flour
Pure Gluten Flour
Snaps
Starch-free Bran

THE DICK X-RAY COMPANY (Dick X-Ray)

3974 Olive Street, St. Louis, Mo.

I-X Barium Meal
I-X Barium Meal Unflavored

DIOS CHEMICAL COMPANY (Dios Chemical)

3954 West Pine Blvd., St. Louis, Mo.

Dioviburnia
Neurosine
Palpebrine

DOHO CHEMICAL CORPORATION (Doho)

105 Fulton Street, New York City

Argolaval Eye Ointment
Argolaval Liquid
Argolaval Ointment
Auralgan

DREW PHARMACAL CO. (Drew Pharmacal)

Buffalo, N. Y.

Zilatone Tablets

DRUG PRODUCTS COMPANY, INC. (Drug Products)

26–01 Skillman Avenue, Long Island City, N. Y.

Bi-Na-Gluconate Ampules
Brain Substance Capsules
Calcium Gluconate Tablets
Calcium Gluconate Wafoids
Calcium Gluconate Hyposols
Calmoxide
Corpus Luteum Capsules
Corpus-Ova 1 Capsules
Dinitrenal Capsules
Ferro-Cu-Mang Hyposols
Ferro-Cu-Mang Pulvoids
Ferro-Cu-Mang Solution
Hemoglobin Compound 1 Capsules
Kidney Substance Capsules
Lecithin Compound 1 Capsules
Lymphatic Compound 1 Capsules
Lymphatic Substance Capsules
Mammary Capsules
Mammary Compound 1 Capsules
Man-Na-Gluconate Hyposols
Orchic Solution Ampules
Orchic Compound Capsules
Ovarian Capsules
Ovarian Solution Ampules
Ovarian Compound 1 Capsules
Ovarian Compound 2 Capsules

Pamol Plain
Pamol Compound
Parathyroid Capsules
Phytolacca Compound Pulvoids
Pitovaco Pulvoids
Pit-Ren Capsules
Pit-Ren Hyposols
Pituitary Solution Surgical and Obstetrical Ampules
Pituitary Solution Surgical Ampules
Pituitary Compound 1 Capsules
Pulvoids Digitalis Folium
Pulvoids Natrico
Secretin Compound Capsules
Taurophen Pulvoids
Thymus Capsules
Thyovaco Pulvoids
Thyroid Capsules
Thyroid-Ioform Compound Capsules
Also Ampules: Intravenous, 21 in 25 forms; Subcutaneous and Intramuscular, 18 in 20 forms; *See Chap. V*

THE DRY MILK COMPANY, INC. **(Dry Milk)**
205 East 42d Street, New York City

Dryco
Protolac

DUKE LABORATORIES, INC. **(Duke)**
200 Hudson Street, New York City

Aolan Ampules
Aquaphor
Liantral
Liantral Casein Ointment 5%
Also Ampules: Subcutaneous and Intramuscular, 2 in 3 forms; *See Chap. V*

EASTERN PHARMACAL CO., INC. **(Eastern Pharmacal)**
308 West 141st Street, New York City

Elixir Aspiral

EASTMAN KODAK COMPANY **(Eastman)**
Medical Department, Rochester, N. Y.

Acetyl Choline Bromide Ampules
Adenine Sulphate Ampules
Glycine
P-Thiocresol
Resorcinol Monoacetate
Tetrabromphenolphthalein Sodium Salt
Tetraiodophenolphthalein Sodium
Trichlorethylene
Also Ampules: Intravenous, 1; Subcutaneous and Intramuscular, 1; *See Chap. V*

EIMER AND AMEND, INC. **(Eimer and Amend)**
205–211 Third Avenue, New York City

Iodotone
Katolox
Myodine
Phosphorcin

ENDO PRODUCTS, INC. **(Endo)**
251 4th Avenue, New York City

Endo-Mangalac Ampules

ENERGEN FOODS COMPANY, INC. (Energen)

93 Chambers Street, New York City

Agar Bran Biscuit
Bismeal
Digestive Biscuit, 4 products
Endo Bran Biscuit
Energen Breads, 5 products
Nutrient Flour
Tapioca

EXCELSIOR SPRINGS MINERAL WATER AND BOTTLING CO. (Excelsior)

Excelsior Springs, Mo.

Siloam Springs

FAIRCHILD BROTHERS AND FOSTER (Fairchild)

Washington and Laight Streets, New York City

Bile Salts Capsules
Bile Salts Powder
Bile Salts with Phenolphthalein and Holadin Capsules
Bile Salts with Succinate of Soda and Holadin Capsules
Bile Salts with Succinate of Soda and Phenolphthalein Capsules
Bile Salts with Salicylate of Soda and Holadin Capsules
Carminzym
Diazyme Glycerole
Enemose
Enzymol
Extractum Pancreatis
Gastron
Gastron with Iron
Holadin Capsules
Holadin and Bile Salts Capsules Enteric coated
Lecibrin Capsules
Lecithin Glycerole
Liver Extract
Marinol
Oxyntin Capsules
Oxyntin Powder
Oxyntin with Pepsin Capsules
Oxyntin with Nux Vomica Capsules
Panopepton Plain
Panopepton Ferruginous
Pepsencia
Peptogenic Powder
Peptonizing Tubes
Trypsin

THE FARASTAN COMPANY (Farastan)

135 South 11th Street, Philadelphia, Pa.

Ambazin Capsules
Farastan Capsules

WM. A. FITCH, INC. (Fitch)

100 West 21st Street, New York City

Ampules: Intravenous, 48 in 72 forms

C. B. FLEET COMPANY (Fleet)

Lynchburg, Va.

Phospho-Soda

FLINT, EATON COMPANY (Flint, Eaton)

Decatur, Ill.

Ceanothyn

FOMOS LABORATORIES, INC. (Fomos)
207 Fourth Avenue, New York City

Fomos Tablets

THE FOSTER LABORATORIES (Foster)
Bloomfield, N. J.

Pheno-Bromate Powder
Pheno-Bromate Tablets

E. FOUGERA AND COMPANY (Fougera)
75 Varick Street, New York City

Aerophagyl "Beytout" Tablets
Alepsal Tablets
Ampoules "Reipar"
Bismuthoidol "Robin" Ampules
Camphro-Salyl "Fraisse" Ampules
Cerevisine "Chapelle" Granulated
Cerevisine "Chapelle" Tablets
Cerevisine "Chapelle" Tablets
Citrosodine "Longuet" Tablets
Coreine "Daniel-Brunet" Flakes
Coreine "Daniel-Brunet" Granules, Solution
Delbiase Ampules (Gelodelbiase)—Intramuscular
Delbiase Ampules Isotonic Solution—Subcutaneous
Delbiase Tablets
Digitaline "Nativelle" Ampules Intramuscular
Digitaline "Nativelle" Ampules Intravenous
Digitaline "Nativelle" Granules
Digitaline "Nativelle" Solution
Elixir I.A.S.
Ferruginous Compound "Fraisse" Ampules
Ferruginous Compound "Fraisse" Solution
Hypotens "Fraisse" Ampules
Hypotens "Fraisse" Oral
Inoton "Debat" Ointment
Inoton "Debat" Powder
Iodo Bismuthate of Quinine "Fraisse" Ampules
Iodo Bismuthate of Quinine "Fraisse" Liquid
Kaylene
Kaylene-Ol
Kaylene-Ol with Phenolphthalein
Lipiodol "Lafay" Ampules
Lipiodol "Guerbert" Ascendant Capsules
Lipiodol "Guerbert" Ascendant Flasks
Lipiodol "Guerbert" Ascendant Tablets
Lipiodol "Guerbert" Descendant Capsules
Lipiodol "Guerbert" Descendant Flasks
Lipiodol "Guerbert" Descendant Tablets
Morrhuol "Chapoteaut" Capsules
Morrhuol Creosote Capsules
Naiodine "Logeais" Ampules
Natibaine "Nativelle"
Neurinase Liquid
Neurinase Tablets
Neurotrophol "Byla"
Neusthenic "Fraisse" Ampules
Neusthenic "Fraisse" Liquid
Nopirine "Vicario"
Ouabaine "Arnaud" Ampules
Ouabaine "Arnaud" Tablets
Ouabaine "Arnaud" Solution
Quinicardine "Nativelle" Tablets
Sol-Bi "Fraisse" Ampules
Terpoflor
Tiodine "Cognet" Ampules
Tiodine "Cognet" Pills
Uraseptine "Rogier"
Also Ampules: Intravenous, 2;
Subcutaneous and Intramuscular, 14 in 21 forms; *See Chap. V*

HENRY FRANCK AND SONS, INC. (Franck)
131–33 Avery Avenue, Flushing, N. Y.

Tablets Chicory

FRASER TABLET COMPANY (Fraser)
251 Fourth Avenue, New York City

Antiseptic Gargle
Aphrodin Tablets
Barmidon Tablets
Barmiphen Capsules
Chamomilla Compound
Copfertabs
Dermalin
Digitabs
Eczemol
Elixir Barmival
Elixir Caricans
Ephedrine Inhalant Plain
Ephedrine Inhalant Compound
Ephedrine Sulphate Solution
Providin Tablets

FRITZSCHE BROTHERS, INC. (Fritzsche)
78 Beekman Street, New York City

Benzyl Benzoate
Cypress Oil "Schimmel"

GEO. C. FRYE COMPANY (Frye)
116 Free Street, Portland, Me.

Pancreo-Bismuth and Pepsin

GALLIA LABORATORIES, INC. (Gallia)
450 Seventh Avenue, New York City

Arheol "Astier" Pearls
Kola "Astier"
Neo Riodine "Astier" Ampules
Riodine "Astier" Capsules
Also Ampules: Intravenous, 1; Subcutaneous and Intramuscular, 1; *See Chap. V*

GANE AND INGRAM, INC. (Gane-Ingram)
43 West 16th Street, New York City

Alphebin Tablets
Calmitol
Eau de Botot
Ephedrine Hydrochloride
Ephedrine Sulphate
Guphen Tablets
Phenobarbital Sodium Tablets
Phenobarbital Sodium Powder

R. W. GARDNER (Gardner)
Orange, N. J.

Syrup Ammonium Hypophosphites
Syrup Hydriodic Acid
Syrup Hypophosphite of Calcium
Syrup Hypophosphite of Iron
Syrup Hypophosphites of Iron and Quinine
Syrup Hypophosphites of Lime and Soda
Syrup Hypophosphite of Manganese
Syrup Hypophosphite of Sodium

GENERAL MILLS, INC. (General Mills)
Chamber of Commerce Bldg , Minneapolis, Minn.

Embo

GERBER PRODUCTS DIVISION (Gerber)

Fremont Canning Company, Fremont, Mich.

Strained Cereal
Strained Vegetables

THE GILLILAND LABORATORIES, INC. (Gilliland)

Marietta, Pa.

Antimeningococcic Serum
Antipneumococcic Serum (I and II)
Antistreptococcic Serum
Catarrhalis Vaccine Mixed
Dilute Tuberculin (Mantoux Test)
Diphtheria Antitoxin
Diphtheria Schick Test Toxin
Diphtheria Toxoid
Diphtheria Toxin-Antitoxin Mixture
Gonococcic Vaccine
Gonococcic Vaccine Mixture
Influenza Vaccine Mixed
Normal Horse Serum
Pasteur Antirabic Vaccine
Pertussis Vaccine
Pertussis Vaccine Mixed
Pneumococcic Vaccine (I, II, III)
Rabies Vaccine
Scarlet Fever Streptococcus Antitoxin
Scarlet Fever Streptococcus Toxin
Schick Test
Schick Test Control
Staphylococcic Vaccine
Streptococcic Vaccine
Tetanus Antitoxin
Tuberculin Solution O.T. for Von Pirquet Test
Tuberculin Ointment for Moro Test
Tuberculin Original
Tuberculin Bacillen Emulsion
Tuberculin Bacillen Filtrate
Typhoid Vaccine
Typhoid-Paratyphoid Vaccine
Vaccine Virus (Smallpox Vaccine)

GLANDULAR LABORATORIES OF AMERICA (Glandular Lab.)

72 Cortland Street, New York City

Adrosil Tablets
Adrenal Cortex Capsules
Corpus Luteum Capsules
Duodenal Substance
Mammary Substance Capsules
Orchic Substance Capsules
Ovarian Substance Capsules
Pancreas Substance Capsules
Parathyroid Substance Capsules
Pineal Substance Capsules
Pituitary Anterior Capsules
Pituitary Whole Capsules
Prostate Substance Capsules
Suprarenal Substance Capsules
Thyroid Substance Capsules

GOVETT LIMITED (Govett)

141 East Avenue, Long Island City, N. Y.

Aquadine Solution 0.2%
Aquadine Tablets
Aquadine Ointment
Ferrodine
Manganese Dioxide

HAHN AND WESSEL (Hahn and Wessel)

316 East 21st Street, New York City

Abilena Wells
Alqua Water
Bassin de Vichy
Bedford Springs
Bethesda Mineral Springs
Biliner Sauerbrunn
Birmo
Braun Mineral Springs
Buckhorn Lithia Springs
Buffalo Lithia Springs
Capon Springs
Carabana

Contrexeville
Evian-Cachat
Fachingen
Franzensbad
French Lick Springs
Kissingen
Levico
Man-A-Cea
Manitou Springs
Marienbad
Mattoni "Giesshubler"
Mergentheim
Mountain Valley Springs
Neuenahr
Piyerazine
Poland Springs
Purgos
Rhens
Rubinat-Llorach
Saint-Galmier Badoit
Salvator
San Pellegrino
Saratoga Vichy
Veronica Springs
Villacabras
Vittel
White Rock Springs
White Sulphur Springs
Wildungen

THE HALEY M-O COMPANY **(Haley)**
Geneva, N. Y.

Haley's M-O

A. K. HAMILTON **(Hamilton)**
95 Wall Street, New York City

Antidolorin Glass Automatic Syphon Tubes
Antidolorin Glass Automatic Tubes
Antidolorin Metal Automatic Tubes
Antidolorin Metal Tubes 100 cc

HANCE BROTHERS AND WHITE, INC. **(Hance)**
Philadelphia, Pa.

Cerogen Tablets
Cod Liver Oil and Capsules
Cod Liver Oil and Creosote Capsules
Thyovaroid Tablets
Vagitories

JOHN F. HANCOCK AND SON **(Hancock)**
521 W. Lombard Street, Baltimore, Md.

Cocoanilid Lozenges
Guai-Ammon Lozenges
Guaiatan Lozenges

CHR. HANSEN'S LABORATORY, INC. **(Hansen)**
Little Falls, N. Y.

Junket Powder
Junket Tablets

THE HARRIS LABORATORIES **(Harris)**
Tuckahoe, N. Y.

Yeast Bouillon Cubes
Yeast Vitamin Powder
Yeast Vitamin Tablets

THE HARROWER LABORATORY, INC. (Harrower)

920 East Broadway, Glendale, Calif.

Accretin Capsules
Adreno-Cortin Solution Ampules
Adreno-Cortin Capsules
Adreno-Hypophysis Compound Sanitablets
Adreno-Ovarian Compound Sanitablets
Adreno-Spermin Capsules
Adreno-Spermin Sanitablets
Adreno-Spermin Compound 1A Ampules
Anabolin Tablets
Anabolin Solution Ampules
Anabolin Solution Fortior
Antero-Pituitary Compound Sanitablets
Apestrin Solution Ampules
Bile Salts Sanitablets
Chalomen Capsules
Chalomen Sanitablets
Endothyrin Tablets
Endothyrin Solution Ampules
Endovarin Ampules
Endovarin Tablets
Gonad Compound Sanitablets
Gonad Compound Solution Ampules
Gonad-Ovarian Compound Sanitablets
Heparhemin Ampules
Heparhemin Solution Liver Extract Ampules
Heparnucleate Liver Extract Tubes
Hepato-Splenic Compound Sanitablets
Iodized Thyroid Compound Sanitablets
Liquor Pituitarii Ampules
Lydin Ampules
Lydin Capsules
Mamma-Ovary Compound Sanitablets
Menocrin
Menocrin Solution Ampules
Pancreas Compound Sanitablets
Pansecretin Sanitablets
Paracalcin Tablets
Paracalcin Solution Ampules
Para-Spleen Compound Sanitablets
Para-Spleen Compound Solution 24A Ampules
Pituitary Compound
Pituitary Compound Solution Ampules
Pituthymin Solution Ampules
Placenta Compound Sanitablets
Placenta-Luteum Compound Ampules
Placento-Mammary Compound Sanitablets
Plestrin Capsules
Plestrin Solution Ampules
Prostate Compound Sanitablets
Renal Compound Sanitablets
Spermin Hemoglobin Sanitablets
Splenocrin Solution Ampules
Thymocrin Solution Ampules
Thyro-Pancreas Compound with Ovary Sanitablets
Thyro-Pancreas Compound with Spermin
Thyroid Compound Sanitablets
Thymus Spermin Sanitablets

E. J. HART AND CO., LTD. (Hart)

508–510 Charles Street, New Orleans, La.

Lac Bismo

HARVEY-PITTENGER COMPANY (Harvey-Pittenger)

5250 Market Street, Philadelphia, Pa.

Adrenapit Solution, Hypodermic
Adrenapit Solution, Local
Adrenapit Solution, Oral
Corpus Luteum Extract Capsules
Corpus Luteum Extract Powder
Corpus Luteum Extract Solution
Diabetan Capsules
Digipit
Ephedan Capsules
Galacan Capsules
Glandular Compound 1 Capsules
Glandular Compound 2 Capsules
Hemovaran Capsules
Mameran Capsules
Mammary Substance Capsules
Mammary Substance Powder
Orchan Capsules
Orchic Substance Capsules
Orchic Substance Powder
Ovarian Capsules
Ovarian Residue Capsules
Ovarian Residue Powder
Ovarian Residue Extract Solution
Ovarian Extract Solution
Ovarian Substance Capsules
Ovarian Substance Powder
Paracal Capsules
Pituitary Anterior Capsules

Pituitary Anterior Powder
Pituitary Extract (Posterior) Solution
Pituitary Substance (Whole) Capsules
Pituitary Substance (Whole) Powder
Suprarenal Whole Capsules
Suprarenal Whole Powder
Thyorcan Capsules
Thyovaran Capsules
Thyroid Capsules
Thyroid Powder
Also Ampules: Intravenous, 20 in 20 forms; Subcutaneous and Intramuscular, 27 in 33 forms; *See Chap V*

HEALTH PRODUCTS CORPORATION **(Health Products)**
113 North 13th Street, Newark, N. J.

Cod Liver Oil "White's" Tablets

HEILKRAFT MEDICAL COMPANY **(Heilkraft)**
321 Talbot Avenue, Boston, Mass.

Dimazon
Dimazon Oil
Dimazon Powder
Scarlet R Salve "Biebrich"
Siliform Ampules
Also Ampules: Subcutaneous and Intramuscular, 1; *See Chap V*

HEYDEN CHEMICAL CORPORATION **(Heyden)**
50 Union Square, New York City

Adsorgan Powder
Calomelol Powder
Calomelol Ointment
Caseosan Ampules
Collargol Crystals
Ichthynat
Noviform Powder
Salit Cream
Salit Oil
Salit Purum
Silargel Powder
Sillargetten Gum Pastilles
Sufrogel Ampules
Sulfidal Powder
Tannismut Powder
Tannismut Tablets
Thorotrast
Thorotrast Ampules
Umbrathor
Unguentum Credé
Also Ampules: Intravenous, 3 in 5 forms; Subcutaneous and Intramuscular, 3 in 4 forms; *See Chap V*

HILLE LABORATORIES **(Hille)**
1791 Howard Street, Chicago, Ill.

Armervenol Oral
Armervenol Injection
Aurol Oral
Aurol Intravenous
Colloidal Mercury Sulphide Oral 1%
Colloidal Mercury Sulphide 2% Hypodermic
Lunosol
Mervenol Oral
Mervenol Injection

THE CHAS. E. HIRES COMPANY **(Hires)**
206 South 24th Street, Philadelphia, Pa.

Root Beer Extracts

HIXSON LABORATORIES, INC. **(Hixson)**
22 West Gay Street, Columbus, Ohio

Diphtheria Antitoxin
Diphtheria Toxin-Antitoxin
Diphtheria Toxoid
Rabies Vaccine
Schick Test Diluted
Tetanus Antitoxin

HOFFMAN-LA ROCHE, INC. **(Roche)**
See page 1153

HOLLAND-RANTOS COMPANY, INC. **(Holland-Rantos)**
37–41 East 18th Street, New York City

H-R Vaginal Diaphragm
Hyva Sani-Tablets
Koromex
Progene

HOLLISTER-STIER LABORATORIES **(Hollister-Stier)**
476–481 Paulsen Medical and Dental Bldg., Spokane, Wash.

Acne Bacillus Vaccine
Allergens—Epidermals, Furs
Allergens—Foods
Allergens—Miscellaneous
Allergens—Pollens, Individual
Allergens—Protein Extracts
Bacillus Acidophilus Culture
Bacillus Acidophilus Culture (Dextrose Mixture)
Bacterial Vaccine (Bargen)
Colon Bacilli Vaccine
Gonococcic Vaccine
Mixed Vaccine—Gonorrhea
Mixed Vaccine—Influenza
Mixed Vaccine Respiratory Low Count
Mixed Vaccine Respiratory High Count
Pertussis Vaccine
Pertussis Mixed Vaccine
Poison Oak-Ivy Treatments
Staph-Acne Vaccine
Staph-Strept-Coli-Pneumo Vaccine (Van Cott's)
Staphylococcus-Streptococcus Vaccine
Staphylococcic Vaccine

HORLICK'S MALTED MILK CORP. **(Horlick)**
Racine, Wis.

Malted Milk

FRANK W. HORNER, INC. **(Horner)**
11 Liberty Square, Lynn, Mass.

Urasal

ADOLPHE HURST AND COMPANY, INC. **(Hurst)**
330 West 42 Street, New York City

Euphydigtal Tablets
Euphydigtal Suppositories
Lactin Preparations:
- Bololactin Powder
- Globulactin Compound
- Globulactin Pellets
- Globulactin c/Arg. prot.
- Stylolactin c/Arg. prot.
- Stylolactin Rods
- Tampolactin Compound
- Tampolactin c/Arg. Prot.
- Tampolactin Liquid

Metaphyllin Ampules
Metaphyllin Powder
Metaphyllin Tablets
Metaphyllin Suppositories
Metaphyllin with Calcium Tablets
Metaphyllin with Calcium Ampules
Metaphyllin with Calcium Suppositories
Metaphyllin with Calcium and Iodine Ampules
Metaphyllin with Calcium and Iodine Suppositories
Metaphyllin with Calcium and Iodine Tablets
Also Ampules: Intravenous, 3 in 3 forms; Subcutaneous and Intramuscular, 1; *See Chap V*

THE HUXLEY LABORATORIES, INC. (Huxley)

175 Varick Street, New York City

Betulol
Colchi-Sal
Iodo-Bismuth of Quinine Ampules
Iodo-Bismuth of Quinine Liquid
Quinbolin
Also Ampules: Subcutaneous and Intramuscular, 1; *See Chap V*

THE HYDROSAL COMPANY (Hydrosal)

Cincinnati, Ohio

Hydrosal Liquid
Hydrosal Ointment
Hydrosal Compound Ointment

HYNSON, WESTCOTT AND DUNNING, INC. (Hynson, Westcott and Dunning)

Baltimore, Md.

Antimony Sodium Thioglycollate Ampules
Antimony Thioglycollamide Ampules
Benzyl Benzoate Ampules
Benzyl Benzoate Globules
Benzyl Benzoate Liquid 20%
Benzyl Benzoate and Benzaldehyde 20%
Benzyl Succinate Tablets
Bromsalizol Tablets
Bromsulphalein Ampules
Flumerin-H Ampules
Flumerin-H Powder
Glycotauro Capsules
Glycotauro Tablets
Glycotauro with Cascara and Phenolphthalein
Lutein Solution Ampules
Lutein Tablets
Mercurochrome Powder
Mercurochrome Tablets
Mercurochrome Tubes
Mercury Salicylate Ampules
Meroxyl Tablets
Ouabain Ampules
Ovarian Residue Ampules
Ovarian Residue Powder
Ovarian Residue Tablets
Ovary (Whole) Ampules
Ovary (Whole) Powder
Ovary (Whole) Tablets
Phenolsulphonphthalein Ampules
Phenoltetrachlorphthalein Ampules
Red Mercuric Iodide Ampules
Thantis Lozenges
Thyroid Powder
Thyroid Tablets
Also Ampules: Subcutaneous and Intramuscular, 17 in 23 forms; *See Chap V*

CONRAD INGOLD COMPANY (Ingold)

168 Water Street, New York City

Rubinat-Llorach

INTRAVENOUS PRODUCTS CO. OF AMERICA, INC. (Intravenous Products)

251 Fourth Avenue, New York City

Endo Corpus Luteum Ampules
Endo Liver Extract Ampules
Endo Orchic Liquid Ampules
Endo Ovarian Liquid Ampules
Endo Paradin Ampules
Endo Pituitary Liquid Anterior Ampules
Endo Pituitary Liquid Obstetrical Ampules
Endo Pituitary Liquid Surgical Ampules
Endo Suprarenalin Solution 1:1,000 Ampules
Also Ampules: Intravenous, 53 in 77 forms; Subcutaneous and Intramuscular, 39 in 49 forms; *See Chap V*

IODENT CHEMICAL COMPANY (Iodent)
1535 Sixth Street, Detroit, Mich.

Iodent Tooth Paste

IRWIN, NEISLER AND COMPANY (Irwin, Neisler)
Morgan, North and Short Streets, Decatur, Ill.

Anuform Suppositories
Arsclero
Barbromide
Bismolate Tablets
Borolyptol
Camphaseptic
Camphaseptic Balm
Camphaseptic Nasal Oil
Camphaseptic Ointment
Camphaseptic Powder
Douchal Suppositories
Duo-Ban Suppositories
Ephedol
Glyco-Cypress
Hemol
Molan
Otalgyne
Petro-mul
Sodinco
Tinapo

WALTER JANVIER, INC. (Janvier)
121 Varick Street, New York City

Tasteless Castor Oil "Kellogg's"

JENSEN-SALSBERY LABORATORIES, INC.
(Jensen-Salsbery)
21st and Penn Streets, Kansas City, Mo.

Rabies Vaccine
Undulant Fever Bacterial Vaccine

JOHNSON AND JOHNSON (Johnson and Johnson)
New Brunswick, N. J.

Camphenol
Chlorine-Soda Ampules
J and J Analgesic Balm
Joncolia Burn Emollient
K Y Lubricating Jelly
Ortho-Gynol

THE KAHLENBERG LABORATORIES, INC. (Kahlenberg)
1316 River Street, Two Rivers, Wis.

Bichloracetic Acid
Collodaurum Ampules
Collodaurum Liquid
Vivargin
Also Ampules: Intravenous, 1 in 2 forms;
See Chap V

KALAK WATER COMPANY
6 Church Street, New York City

Kalak Water (Kalak)

KATHARMON CHEMICAL COMPANY (Katharmon)
101 N. Main Street, St. Louis, Mo.

Hagee's Original Cordial Compound

CHAS. B. KNOX GELATINE COMPANY, INC. (Knox)

Johnstown, N. Y.

Knox Jel

Sparkling Gelatin

A. W. KRETSCHMAR, INC. (Kretschmar)

396 Broadway, New York City

Amarbital
Ephcaben
Hepatrat Ampules
Kathesina "Heisler" Ampules
Kathesina "Heisler" Pills
Luizym Tablets
Novatropin Ampules
Novatropin Powder
Novatropin Solution
Novatropin Tablets
Ovarialhormon Folliculin Menformon Ampules
Ovarialhormon Folliculin Menformon Dragees
Pankreon "Rhenania" Powder
Pankreon "Rhenania" Tablets
Pansuline "Fornet" Pills (Concentrations 1, 2, 3)
Targesin
Thephyldine Ampules
Thephyldine Powder
Thephyldine Suppositories
Thephyldine Tablets
Thephyldine with Benzyl Succinate Tablets
Thephyldine with Calcium Lactate Suppositories
Thephyldine with Calcium Lactate Tablets
Thephyldine with Calcium Lactate and Potassium Iodide Tablets
Thephyldine with Calcium Lactate and Potassium Iodide Suppositories
Thephyldine with Calcium Salicylate and Potassium Iodide Ampules 10 cc
Thephyldine with Phenobarbital Tablets

LAFAYETTE PHARMACAL CO. (Lafayette)

Pharmaceutical Building, Lafayette, Ind.

Asexualism, Female Capsules
Asexualism, Male Capsules
Brain Capsules
Calcium Gluconate Powder
Calcium Gluconate Tablets
Cholepulvis Powder
Cholemulsion Vials
Corluroid Capsules
Corpus Luteum Capsules
Duobilad Capsules
Duodenal Capsules
Femex Capsules
Gonadrenal Capsules
Hemosplenic Capsules
Heart Muscle Capsules
Hepato-Bilad Capsules
Iodeikon Capsules
Kidney Capsules
Leci-Nuclein Capsules
Liver Capsules
Liver Concentrate Capsules
Lymphatic Capsules
Málex Capsules
Mammary Capsules
Mammary Mixture Capsules
Morrol with Suprarenal Capsules
Normalizer Capsules (1, 2)
Oralsulin Capsules A, B, C and D
Orálsulin with Duodenal Extract Capsules
Oralsulin Mixture Capsules
Orchic Capsules
Orchiroid Capsules (1, 2, 3)
Ovarian Capsules
Ovaroid Capsules (1, 2, 3)
Pancreas Capsules
Pancreatin Capsules
Parathyroid Capsules
Pineal Capsules
Pituitary Anterior Capsules
Pituitary Posterior Capsules
Pituitary (Whole) Capsules
Placental Capsules
Placental Mixture Capsules
Prostate Capsules
Pulvis Alkantis
Spleen Capsules
Suprarenal Cortex Capsules
Suprarenal Mixture Capsules
Suprarenal Whole Capsules
Thymus Capsules

Thyorchic Mixture Capsules
Thyovary Capsules
Thyroid Tablets
Yohimbin and Orchic Mixture Capsules
Yohimbin and Ovarian Mixture Capsules

THE LAKESIDE LABORATORIES, INC. **(Lakeside)**
1823 East Windsor Place, Milwaukee, Wis.

Chlorine Gas "Roehling" Ampules
Dextrose Ampules
Also Ampules: Subcutaneous and Intramuscular, 1; *See Chap. V*

L. H. LANG **(Lang)**
41 East 42nd Street, New York City

Brain Substance Extract
Corpus Luteum Extract
Corpus Striatum Extract
Duodenal Substance Extract
Kidney Extract
Lamb Liver Extract
Mammary Extract
Orchic Extract
Ovarian Residue
Ovarian Extract
Pancreas Extract
Parathyroid Extract
Pineal Extract
Pituitary Extract Anterior
Pituitary Extract Posterior
Pituitary Extract Whole
Placenta Extract
Prostate Extract
Spleen Extract
Suprarenal Cortex Extract
Suprarenal Extract Whole
Suprarenal Medulla Extract
Thymus Extract
Thyroid Extract

LAVORIS CHEMICAL COMPANY **(Lavoris)**
918—3 Street, North, Minneapolis, Minn.

Lavoris

LEDERLE LABORATORIES, INC. **(Lederle)**
511 Fifth Avenue, New York City

Abortion Test Antigen
Acne Vaccine
Acne Combined Vaccine
Allergens—Bacterials
Allergens—Combinations
Allergens—Epidermals
Allergens—Foods—Individual and Groups
Allergens—Inhalants, Individual and groups
Allergens—Miscellaneous
Allergens—Pollen Antigens, Spring Type
Allergens—Pollen Antigens, Ragweed Combined
Antianthrax Serum
Antidysenteric Serum
Antimeningococcic Serum
Antipneumococcus Serum (I, II, I and II, VII)
Antistreptococcus Serum
Bacillus Acidophilus Milk
Bacillus Bulgaricus Culture
Bile Salts Combined Tablets
Bile Salts Plain Tablets
Brucella Melitensis Vaccine
Bubonic Plague Vaccine
Catarrhal Combined Vaccine
Catarrhalis Influenza Glycerol Vaccine
Catarrhalis Influenza Vaccine
Cholera Vaccine
Combined Bacterial Vaccine (Van Cott)
Corpus Luteum Ampules
Corpus Luteum Tablets
Conjunctival Test
Digitalis Tablets
Diphtheria Antitoxin
Diphtheria Toxin for Schick Test
Diphtheria Toxoid
Diphtheria Toxin-Antitoxin Mixture (Horse)
Diphtheria Toxin-Antitoxin Mixture (Goat)
Ephedrin Inhalant

Ephedrine Hydrochloride Solution
Ephedrine Hydrochloride Tablets
Ephedrine Solution 3% Compound
Ephedrine Hydrochloride Ampules
Ephedrine Hydrochloride Vials
Epinephrine Hydrochloride Ampules
Erysipelas Streptococcus Antitoxin
Ferric Ammonium Citrate Capsules
Gas Gangrene Antitoxin
Gonococcus Vaccine
Gonococcus Glycerol Vaccine
Gonococcus Combined Vaccine
Influenza Combined Vaccine
Liver Extract Oral
Liver Extract Parenteral
Normal Horse Serum
Ovarian Residue Tablets
Ovarian Whole Tablets
Pertussis Glycerol Vaccine
Pertussis Vaccine
Pertussis Combined Vaccine
Pituitary Anterior Tablets
Pituitary Extract Posterior Tablets
Pituitary Extract Ampules
Pituitary Entire Tablets
Pneumococcus Vaccine
Pneumococcus Combined Vaccine
Poison Ivy Extract
Poison Oak Extract
Rabies Vaccine
Rheumatoid Arthritis Vaccine (Intramuscular & Intravenous)
Schick Test
Schick Test Control
Silver Nitrate Solution Ampules
Staphylococcus Combined Vaccine
Staphylococcus-Streptococcus Vaccine
Staphylococcus Vaccine
Staphylococcus Albus Vaccine
Staphylococcus Aureus Vaccine
Surgical Maggots
Streptococcus Vaccine
Tetanus Antitoxin
Terpal
Tetanus Gas-Gangrene Antitoxin
Thromboplastin
Thyroid Tablets
Triple Typhoid Vaccine
Tuberculin O.T.
Tuberculin Test Intracutaneous (Mantoux)
Tuberculin B.E.
Tuberculin B.F.
Von Pirquet Test
Typhoid Combined Vaccine
Typhoid Vaccine
Urethritis Treatment Vaccine
Vaccine Virus
Vaccine Virus Green
Also Ampules: Subcutaneous and Intramuscular, 2 in 4 forms; *See Chap V*

THOMAS E. LEEMING AND COMPANY, INC. (Leeming)
101 West 31st Street, New York City

Baume Bengue
Calmitol Liquid
Calmitol Ointment
Calmitol Suppositories
Valital Tablets

LEHN AND FINK, INC. (Lehn and Fink)
683 Fifth Avenue, New York City or Bloomfield, N. J.

Formula L-F
Lygel
Lysol
Yohimbin Tablets

ELI LILLY AND COMPANY (Lilly)
Indianapolis, Ind.

Acidulin Pulvules
Acne Mixed Vaccine
Alpha-Betamin Pulvules
Amertan Ointment
Amfetin Ampules
Amfetin Liquid
Ampule Glucose
Amytal Tablets
Amytal Crystals
Antimeningococcic Serum
Antistreptococcic Serum
Antistreptococcic Serum (Purified)
Antistreptococcic Serum (Erysipelas Concentrated)
Antistreptococcic Serum (Poliomyelitis)

Antistreptococcic Serum (Puerperal Fever)
Bismoid Ampules
Carbarsone Pulvules
Carbarsone Powder
Catarrhal Vaccine Combined
Chloroxyl Powder
Chloroxyl Tablets
Cholera Vaccine Prophylactic
Coco-Quinine
Coco-Vitamin
Coli Combined Vaccine
Colo-Jel Combined
Corpus Luteum Ampules
Corpus Luteum Pulvules
Corpus Luteum Powder
Corpus Luteum Tablets, Enteric coated
Corpus Luteum Tablets, Plain
Digiglusin Ampules
Digiglusin Liquid
Digiglusin Tablets
Diphtheria Toxoid
Diphtheria Toxin-Antitoxin
Diphtheria Antitoxin
Diskets Alkaline
Diskets Bromides
Diskets Sodium Bromide Compound
Diskets Sodium Salicylate Compound
Ento-Jel
Ento-Lysate
Ephedrine and Amytal Pulvules
Ephedrine Hydrochloride Crystalline
Ephedrine Compound Plain 1%
Ephedrine Sulphate Elixir
Ephedrine-Merthiolate
Ephedrine Sulphate Crystalline
Ephedrine Hydrochloride Pulvules, Syrup
Ephedrine Hydrochloride Tablets Hypodermic
Ephedrine Hydrochloride 3% Solution
Ephedrine Inhalant Compound 30
Ephedrine Inhalant Plain
Ephedrine Compound Ointment
Ephedrine Sulphate 3% Solution
Ephedrine Sulphate Jelly
Ephedrine Sulphate Pulvules
Ephedrine Sulphate Tablets Hypodermic
Erysipelas Antistreptococcus Serum
Extralin Powder
Extralin Pulvules
Extralin Ampules
Gas-Gangrene Antitoxin
Glucose
Gluco-Calcium
Gonococcus Vaccine
Gonococcus Mixed Vaccine
Hemagulen
Iletin (U 10, U 20, 40, and 80)
Influenza Mixed Vaccine
Influenza Pneumonia Vaccine
Iodeikon Pulvules
Kaomin
Liver Extract 343 Ampules
Liver Extract 343 Powder
Liver Extract with Iron 55 Powder
Mammary Substance Powder
Mammary Substance Pulvules
Mammary Substance Tablets Plain and Enteric coated
Merthiolate Solution 1:1,000
Merthiolate Tincture 1:1,000
Merthiolate Jelly 1:1,000
Merthiolate Ointment 1:2,000
Merthiolate Ophthalmic Ointment 1:5,000
Metycaine Tablets
Metycaine Solution 2%
Metycaine Powder
Metycaine Ampules
Metycaine and Adrenalin Ampules
Normal Horse Serum
Ophthalmic Ointments:
- Ammoniated Mercury
- Atropine Sulphate
- Boric Acid
- Copper Citrate
- Holocaine Hydrochloride
- Iodoform
- Mercuric Oxide and Atropine
- Mercuric Oxide and Ephedrine
- Mercuric Oxide Yellow ½%, 1%, 2%
- Mercury Bichloride
- Merthiolate
- Petrolatum, Sterile
- White's Ointment
- Zinc Sulphate

Orchic Substance Powder
Orchic Substance Pulvules
Orchic Substance Tablets, Plain, Enteric coated
Oridine Tablets
Ouabain Ampules
Ovarian Residue Powder
Ovarian Residue Pulvules
Ovarian Residue Tablets, Plain, Enteric coated
Ovarian Residue Extract Ampules
Ovarian Extract Ampules
Ovarian Substance Powder
Ovarian Substance Pulvules
Ovarian Substance Tablets, Plain, Enteric coated
Oxyl Iodide Tablets
Oxyl Iodide Compound
Para-Thor-Mone Ampules, Vials
Parathyroid Powder
Parathyroid Tablets, Plain and Enteric coated

Pertussis Vaccine
Pertussis Mixed Vaccine
Pineal Tablets Plain
Pineal Tablets Enteric coated
Pituitary Anterior Powder
Pituitary Anterior Tablets, Plain and Enteric coated
Pituitary Posterior Powder
Pituitary Posterior Tablets, Plain and Enteric coated
Pituitary Extract Obstetrical Ampules
Pituitary Extract Surgical Ampules
Pituitary Entire Powder
Pituitary Entire Tablets, Plain and Enteric coated
Placenta Powder
Placenta Pulvules
Placenta Tablets, Plain and Enteric coated
Plague Vaccine Prophylactic, Double
Plague Vaccine Prophylactic, Single
Pneumococcus Antigen
Pneumococcus Vaccine, Prophylactic
Pneumococcus Mixed Vaccine
Psyllium Seed
Pulvules Lextron 55
Rabies Vaccine (Harris)
Rectal Analgesia Gwathmey 1
Rectal Analgesia Gwathmey 2
Rectal Analgesia Gwathmey with Apparatus
Schick Test
Schick Test Control
Smallpox Vaccine Virus
Sodium Amytal Pulvules
Solution Invert Sugar
Staphylococcus Vaccine
Staphylococcus Aureus Vaccine
Staphylo-Jel
Staphylo-Lysate
Strepto-Jel
Strepto-Lysate
Streptococcus Vaccine
Streptococcus-Staphylococcus Vaccine
Suprarenal Whole Powder
Suprarenal Whole Pulvules
Suprarenal Whole Tablets, Plain and Enteric coated
Tetanus Antitoxin
Tetanus Gas-Gangrene Antitoxin
Theamin Pulvules
Thymus Powder
Thymus Tablets Chocolate and Enteric coated
Thyroid Powder
Thyroid Pulvules
Thyroid Tablets
Thyroid Tablets Enteric coated
Thyroid Tablets Chocolate coated
Tuberculin Old
Tuberculin Old Concentrated
Tuberculin Ointment (Moro)
Tuberculin Test (Von Pirquet)
Tuberculin Therapeutic
Typhoid Vaccine
Typhoid Mixed Vaccine
Also Ampules: Intravenous, 24 in 38 forms; Subcutaneous and Intramuscular, 60 in 84 forms; *See Chap. V*

LISTER BROS., INC. **(Lister)**
41 East 42nd Street, New York City

Dietetic Flour
Equalized Flour
Golden Spread
India Gum
Lister's Brittle
Starch Free Bran
Starchless Breakfast Food
Starchless Porridge Powder
Sugarless Sweetener

LIVERMEAL CORPORATION **(Livermeal)**
1006 Clinton Street, Hoboken, N. J.

Liver Meal
Phos-hepatic Extract

LLOYD BROS., PHARMACISTS, INC. **(Lloyd Bros.)**
300 West Court Street, Cincinnati, Ohio

Glyconda
Libradol
Libradol Mild

THE LOEB DIETETIC FOOD COMPANY (Loeb)
4378 Broadway, New York City

Aerated Gluten Bread
Aerated Gluten Rolls
Assortment Package
Baking Powder, Starch Free
Bran and Gluten Cereal
Chewing Gum
Dietetic Agar-Agar
Dietetic Almond Macaroons
Dietetic Canned Fruit
Dietetic Chocolate Bar
Dietetic Cocoa
Dietetic Cocoa Shells
Dietetic Grape Jelly
Dietetic India Gum
Dietetic Lady Fingers
Dietetic Gluten Breadsticks
Dietetic Gluten Crackers
Dietetic Gluten Zwieback
Dietetic Mayonnaise
Genuine Gluten Bread
Genuine Gluten Croutons
Genuine Gluten Flour
Gluten Breakfast Cereal
Gluten Butter Cookies
Gluten Cheese Tidbits
Gluten Cracker Meal
Gluten Noodles
Imitation Maple Syrup
Karlsbadder Biscotten
Prepared Soy Bean Flour
Self-Rising Gluten Flour
Starch Free Bran
Starch Free Bran Wafers
Supposidines
Unsweetened Chocolate

LOESER LABORATORY (Loeser)
22 West 26th Street, New York City

Ampules: Intravenous, 36 in 50 forms; Subcutaneous and Intramuscular 16

LORATE COMPANY, INC. (Lorate)
308 West 141st Street, New York City

Lorate

MACDOWELL BROTHERS (MacDowell)
Ogdensburg, N. Y.

D-Zerta
Dietetic Flour
Dietetic Wafers
Gluten Flour
India Gum Karaya
Merrillized Yeast
Psyllium (Plantago Seed)
Soy Bean Flour
Starch Free Bran
Sugar Free Beverages

MALLINCKRODT CHEMICAL WORKS (Mallinckrodt)
Second and Mallinckrodt Streets, St. Louis, Mo.

Arsphenamine Ampules
Benzyl Benzoate
Calcium Gluconate Ampules
Ichthymall
Iodeikon Ampules
Iodeikon Powder
Iso Iodeikon Ampules
Iso Iodeikon Powder
Mallophene Disks
Mallophene Powder
Mallophene Tablets
Neoarsphenamine Ampules
Sulpharsphenamine Ampules
Also Ampules: Intravenous, 4 in 16 forms; Subcutaneous and Intramuscular, 3 in 9 forms; *See Chap. V*

THE MALTBIE CHEMICAL COMPANY (Maltbie)

246 High Street, Newark, N. J.

Alka-Sal
Analgesic Balm
Anazyme Dusting Powder
Anazyme Ointment
Benzocomp Ointment
Calcreose Powder
Calcreose Solution
Calcreose Tablets Plain
Calcreose Tablets Enteric coated
Calcreose Compound 2
Calcreose Compound 3
Calcreose Euphorbia Compound
Calcreose with Iodine
Compound Syrup of Calcreose
Creomint Lozenge
Creodide Tablets
Ephedrine Nasal Jelly
Glandular Compound Female Capsules
Glandular Compound Female Tablets
Glandular Compound Male Capsules
Glandular Compound Male Tablets
Hemodal Ointment
Hemodal Suppositories
Iodahl Ointment
Islands of Langerhans Capsules
Islands of Langerhans Tablets
Liver Extract Capsules
Nasal Cream
Nuchol Tablets
Nuchol "B" Tablets
Ophthalmic Ointments:
  Atropine Sulphate
  Benzocaine
  Boric Acid
  Copper Citrate
  Mercury Yellow Oxide Compound
  Ophthalmic Cream
Pituitary Extract Obstetrical Ampules
Reso-Lanae Ointment
Thyroid Gland Tablets
Tricocide Ointment

THE MALTINE COMPANY (Maltine)

Eighth Avenue and 18th Street, Brooklyn, N. Y.

Maltine Plain
Maltine with Cascara Sagrada
Maltine with Cod Liver Oil
Maltine with Cod Liver Oil Concentrate
Maltine with Cod Liver Oil and Cascara Sagrada
Maltine with Cod Liver Oil and Iron Iodide
Maltine with Iron Iodide
Maltine with Creosote
Maltine Ferrated
Maltine with Hypophosphites
Maltine with Iron, Quinia and Strychnia
Maltine with Mineral Oil and Cascara Sagrada
Maltine with Spleen Marrow and Iron
Malto-Yerbine
Neoferrum

MANHATTAN EYE SALVE COMPANY (Manhattan)

Louisville, Ky.

Nasal Ointments:
  Carbolic Acid and Benzoinol
  Compound Camphor and Menthol
  Compound Eucalyptol and Gaultheria
  Compound Iodine and Glycerine
  Eucalyptol and Benzoinol
  Resorcinol
Ophthalmic Ointments:
  Argyrol
  Atropine Alkaloid 1 %
  Atropine (Alkaloid ½ %)
  Atropine (Sulphate 2 %)
  Atropine and Bichloride
  Bichloride
  Bichloride (White)
Ophthalmic Ointments:
  Butyn 1 %
  Butyn and Bichloride ½ %, 1 %
  Calomel 5 %
  Copper Citrate 5 %, 10 %
  Comp. Silver Iodide
  Comp. Yellow Oxide Mercury and Adrenalin
  Copper Sulphate ½ %
  Eserine
  Holocain
  Holocain and Bichloride 1 %, 2 %
  Iodoform Sterile
  Mercurochrome 1 %, 2 %
  Ointment 38

Ophthalmic Ointments:—(*Continued*)
- Ointment 39
- Petrolatum (White) Sterile
- Petrolatum (White) Sterile (Carbolate 1 %)
- Scarlet Red

Ophthalmic Ointments:
- Silver Nitrate 1 %
- Thiosinamine
- Yellow Oxide Mercury and Atropine
- Zinc Oxide 10 %
- Zinc Sulphate

THE MANOLA COMPANY (Manola)
4200 Laclede Avenue, St. Louis, Mo.

Manola
Mineralization Tablets

THE MARVELL PHARMACAL COMPANY (Marvell)
55 West 16th Street, New York City

Adrempco Capsules
Adrempco 100 Ampules
Adrenal Cortex Capsules
Adrenal Cortex Powder
Anterior Pituitary Sex Hormone Solution
Atoco Capsules
Benacol Solution Ampules
Bisempco Ampules
Bisempco Cream Capsules
Bisempco Cream Solution
Cardiac Substance Powder
Corpus Luteum Substance Powdered Extract
Corpus Luteum Substance Tablets
Corpus Luteum Substance Solution—Ampules
Duodenal Substance
Hemo-Nucleo-Spleen Compound Capsules
Interrenin Ampules
Islands of Langerhans Powder
Lar-Io-Ben
Mammary Compound Capsules
Mammary Substance Powder
Mammary Substance Tablets
Neurempco 3, 4, 8
Orchiben Compound Capsules
Orchiben Concentrated Ampules
Orchiben Solution Ampules
Orchic-Epinephrine Compound Ampules
Orchic Substance Powder
Orchic Substance Tablets
Ovamone Ampules
Ovamone Capsules
Ovarialhormon Folliculin Menformon Solution Ampules
Ovarialhormon Folliculin Menformon Dragees
Ovarian Solution Ampules
Ovarian Substance Powder
Ovarian Substance Tablets
Ovempco Capsules
Ovowop Tablets
Pancreas Substance Powder
Pan-Orch-Oid Capsules
Parathyroid Solution Ampules
Parathyroid Substance Powder
Parathyroid Substance Tablets
Pituitary Substance Anterior Powder
Pituitary Substance Anterior Tablets
Pituitary Solution Anterior Ampules
Pituitary Solution Whole Ampules
Pituitary Substance Whole Powder
Pituitary Substance Whole Tablets
Placenta Powder
Polempco Capsules
Polempco Ampules 96, 101, 102
Prostate Substance Powder
Prostate Substance Tablets
Seminal Vesicles Powder
Semvesco Capsules
Semvesco Solution 128 Ampules
Splenium "Oefele" Tablets
Suprarenal Substance Tablets
Testempco Tablets
Testempco Solution Ampules
Thyroid Substance Tablets
Vesix Capsules
Also Ampules: Subcutaneous and Intramuscular, 32 in 34 forms; *See Chap V*

MARCY COMPANY (Marcy)
Boston, Mass.

Veracolate Tablets
Veracolate with Pancreatin and Pepsin Tablets
Veracolate with Iron, Quinine and Strychnine Tablets

McKESSON AND ROBBINS, INC.

(McKesson and Robbins)

Bridgeport, Conn.

Albagar Compound
Albagar Plain
Albatum
Albolene
Albolene Solid
Albomalt
Albomist
Analax Tablets
Analgesic Balm
Antiseptic Solution 59
Aspiro-Lithine Tablets
Burntone
Camphor Ice
Copper-Iron Compound Liquid
Copper-Iron Compound Tablets
Darol Tablets
Emoleo Iodized
Emoleo Plain
Emoleo with Camphor and Menthol
Emulsion Cod Liver Oil
Glycerine Suppositories
I-Bath
Kigo
Lagarg
Larkspur Lotion
Mosquitone
Mustarx
Nasal Jelly
Norwegian Cod Liver Oil
Phospho-Vitamin B
Pinotol
Poison Ivy Lotion
Pyrozone
Rectal Ointment "Keno"
Soda Mint Tablets
Soda Mint Tablets with Pepsin
Sunburn Lotion
Tartarlithine Tablets
Toothache Drops
Vitamin Concentrate of Cod Liver Oil
Vitamin Concentrate Tablets of Cod Liver Oil

ROBERT McNEIL

(McNeil)

2900 North 17th Street, Philadelphia, Pa.

Alquinco Suppositories
Alquinco Tablets
Amifeine
Amifeine Compound 1
Amifeine Compound 2
Amifeine Elixir
Amifeine Tablets (Children)
Amosal Capsules
Amosal Tablets, Plain and Enteric coated
Amylgestin Tablets
Amylgestin Compound
Antiseptinol Ointment
Aspirofeine 1, 2, 3 Capsules
Aspirofeine 1, 2, 3 Tablets
Aspirofeine Tablets (Children)
Aubromid Tablets
Baramid 1, 2 Capsules
Baramid 1, 2 Tablets
Baramid Compound
Barlupulin Capsules
Bilox Tablets
Bisalco Tablets
Bromidonna Elixir
Bromiphen Elixir
Burn Ointment 2, 3
Cagestol
Chloro-Camphene
Chlorung Ointment
Cociphen Syrup
Corpus Luteum Ampules
Corpus Luteum Capsules
Corpus Luteum Tablets
Coteremul Capsules
Digestone Elixir
Digitalis "Duo-Test" Capsules
Digitalis "Duo-Test" Liquid
Elixir Ma Huang
Epinephrine Hydrochloride Solution 1:1,000
Ferri-Quin Capsules
Glandular Compound 2 (Male); 3 (Female); Capsules and Tablets
Glandular Compounds 4, 5, 7, 8, 9, 10 Capsules and Tablets
Glucal Emulsion
Glucal Lozenges
Guaiaphedra Syrup
Guaiaphon
- Syrup Guaiaphon
- Syrup Guaiaphon with Codeine Sulphate
- Syrup Guaiaphon Compound
- Syrup Guaiaphon Compound 1, 2, 3

Hemarestors
I-Lan-Glans Capsules
Iocol Compounds 1, 2, 3, 4
Iocol Syrup
Kacyan Capsules
Kacyan Elixir
Kacyan Tablets
Liver Extract Capsules
Liver Extract Powder
Liver Extract Concentrate Ampules
Liver Extract Solution Ampules
Liver Substance Capsules
Lotion Carmatal
Lubricant
Macarbo Powders
- Powder Macarbo with Bismuth Subcarbonate
- Powder Macarbo with Orthesin
- Lozenge Macarbo with Bismuth
- Tablets Macarbo
- Tablets Macarbo with Bismuth Subcarbonate
- Tablets Macarbo with Calcium and Magnesium Carbonate
- Tablets Macarbo with Orthesin
- Tablets Macarbo with Papain
- Tablets Macarbo with Phenolphthalein

Mammary Gland Capsules
Mammary Gland Tablets
Mebluco Tablets
Mentholyp
Mentholyp with Aromatics and Oil of Cassia Capsules
Mentholyp Solution
Mentholyp (Moulded) Tablets
Metabol
Nacitra Tablets
Nitrobar Tablets
Nitrocon Capsules
Nitrocon Tablets
Nitrophen Tablets
Ophthalmic Ointments:
- Acid Boric
- Adrenals Comp.
- Atropine
- Copper Citrate
- Mercuric Chloride, Corrosive
- Mercuric Chloride with Procaine
- Mercuric Oxide, Yellow
- Mercuric Oxide, Yellow with Ephedrine
- Procaine with Epinephrine
- Quinosol
- Silver Albuminate

Orchic Substance Capsules
Orchic Substance Solution
Orchic Substance Tablets
Orcon Ampules
Orcon Capsules
Orcon Compound 1, 2 Capsules
Orthosine-Epinephrine Compound
Orthosine-Iodine Troches
Orthosine-Quinosal Lozenges
Ovaracon Ampules
Ovarian Residue Ampules
Ovarian Residue Capsules
Ovarian Substance Whole Ampules
Ovarian Substance Whole Capsules
Ovarian Substance Whole Tablets
Ovarian Substance Capsules
Ovarian Substance Tablets
Paraco Gauze
Parathyroid Gland Capsules
Parathyroid Gland Tablets
Passiphen Tablets
Pheno-Sagra 1, 2
Pheno-Sagra Tablets
Phostone Elixir
Physilin
Pituitary Anterior Capsules
Pituitary Anterior Tablets
Pituitary Whole Capsules
Pituitary Whole Tablets
Pituitary Sex Hormone Solution Ampules
Pituitary Posterior Ampules and Vials
Pituitary-Thymus Ampules
Quinothesin Lozenges
Quinothesin Ointment 1, 2, 3
Quinothesin Powder
Quinothesin Tablets
Rectal Suppositories Hemastin
Rectal Suppositories Quinosal Orthesine
Sanpaiba Capsules
Solurea Tablets
Solurea Compound Capsules
Solurea Compound Tablets 2, 3, 4, 5, 6
Stanprotein Tablets
Sulophen
Sulophen Ointment 1, 2
Suprarenal Gland Capsules
Suprarenal Gland Tablets
Syrup Yersanco with Codeine Sulphate
Syrup Yersanco with Phenobarbital-Sodium
Syrup Yersanco with Codein and Phenobarbital
Thymephen Syrup
Thyroid Gland Capsules
Thyroid Gland Tablets
Toluphen
Triglucon
Yersanco
Also Ampules: Intravenous, 5 in 5 forms; Subcutaneous and Intramuscular, 23 in 34 forms; *See Chap. V*

MEAD JOHNSON AND COMPANY (Mead Johnson)
Evansville, Indiana

Alacta
Brewers' Yeast Powder
Brewers' Yeast Tablets
Casec
Cod Liver Oil "Newfoundland"
Cod Liver Oil with Viosterol 10D
Dextri-Maltose with Vitamin B
Dextri-Maltose 1, 2, 3
Mead's Cereal
Mineral Mixture Tablets 85
Powdered Lactic Acid Milk
Powdered Lactic Acid Milk with Dextri-Maltose
Powdered Protein Milk
Powdered Whole Milk
Recolac
Sobee
(Undiluted) Halibut Liver Oil
Viosterol in Halibut Liver Oil 250 D
Viosterol in Oil 250D

MEDICAL ARTS LABORATORY (Medical Arts)
Medical Arts Building, Oklahoma City, Oklahoma

Antirabic Vaccine

Also Ampules: 1 Subcutaneous and Intramuscular; *See Chap. V*

THE MEDICINAL PRODUCTS CORPORATION (Medicinal Products)
Forty-seventh Avenue and 11th Street, Long Island City, N. Y.

Citrosalven Ampules

Also Ampules: Intravenous, 1 in 2 forms; *See Chap. V*

MEDICONE COMPANY, INC. (Medicone)
12 John Street, New York City

Derma-Medicone Ointment
Emmenagogue Pills
Evacuant Pills
Rectal Medicone
Suppository—Vaginal

MELLIER DRUG COMPANY (Mellier Drug)
2112 Locust Street, St. Louis, Mo.

Tongaline Liquid
Tongaline Tablets
Tongaline with Lithia Tablets
Tongaline with Quinine Tablets

MENLEY AND JAMES, LTD. (Menley and James)
70 West 40th Street, New York City

Iodex Ointment
Iodex Liquid
Iodex Soap
Iodex with Methyl Salicylate

THE MENNEN COMPANY (Mennen)
345 Central Avenue, Newark, N. J.

Antiseptic Baby Oil
Borated Talcum

MERCK AND COMPANY (Merck)
Rahway, N. J.

Agar Powder
Agar Shreds
Arsenoferratose Liquid
Arsphenamine Ampules
Banana Powder
Benzene (Benzol) Medicinal Liquid
Benzyl Benzoate
Benzyl Succinate
Betanaphthol Benzoate
Bismosol Ampules
Bromipin 10%
Bromipin 33%
Bulbocapnine Hydrochloride Ampules
Bulbocapnine Hydrochloride Tablets
Butyl-Chloral Hydrate
Calcium Phosphate Tribasic
Chlorbutanol (Hydrous)
Chlorbutanol (Anhydrus)
Choleval Powder
Choleval Tablets
Clymocol
Creolin-Pearson
Digitan Ampules
Digitan Liquid
Digitan Powder
Digitan Tablets
Digitoxin
Dionin Powder
Dionin Tablets
Erythrol Tetranitrate Tablets
Ethyl Salicylate
Euquinine
Fibrolysin Ampules
Fluorescein
Formin Powder
Formin Tablets
Homatropine Hydrochloride
Ichthyol Liquid
Ichthalbin Powder
Ichthalbin Tablets
Ichthargan Powder
Iodipin 40% Ampules
Iodipin Tablets
Iodipin 40%
Iron Lactate
Kelene
Magnesium Phosphate Tribasic
Mercury Cyanide
Mercury Succinimide
Neoarsphenamine Ampules
Neocinchophen
Optochin Base Powder
Optochin Base Tablets
Optochin Hydrochloride
Ouabain
Papaverine Hydrochloride
Peroxoids Tablets
Phenobarbital Sodium
Phloridzin
Pyridium Ointment 10%
Pyridium Powder
Pyridium Solution 1%
Pyridium Tablets
Quinidine
Quinisal Powder
Quinisal Tablets
Salysal Powder
Salysal Tablets
Scarlet Red Medicinal "Biebrich"
Silver Lactate
Skiabaryt Oral
Skiabaryt Rectal
Sodium Peroxide
Stovarsol Tablets
Stypticin Powder
Stypticin Tablets
Stypticin Tablets Hypodermic
Sulpharsphenamine Ampules
Theobromine
Theobromine and Sodium Acetate
Tryparsamide Ampules
Urea
Verodigen Tablets
Veronal Powder
Veronal Tablets
Veronal-Sodium Powder
Veronal-Sodium Tablets
Yeastone Pills
Zinc Permanganate
Also Ampules: Intravenous, 3 in 15 forms; Subcutaneous and Intramuscular, 4 in 16 forms

MERCKENS CHOCOLATE COMPANY, INC. (Merckens)
Buffalo, N. Y.

Maltcao

THE WM. S. MERRELL COMPANY (Merrell)
Cincinnati, Ohio

Alkarhein
Alycin
Blenol
Cod Liver Oil Concentrate Tablets
Detoxol Paste
Fibrogen Oral
Fibrogen Subcutaneous Ampules
Fibrogen Local
Genitone
Natural Salicylates:
 Acid Salicylic Crystals
 Sodium Salicylate Ampules
 Sodium Salicylate Powder
Natural Salicylates:—(*Continued*)
 Sodium Salicylate Tablets
 Sodium Salicylate with Sodium Iodide Ampules
Nephroson
Pascarnata
Pentabromides
Soricin Capsules
Soricin Surgical 40%
Thiate
Thiate with Codein
Also Ampules: Subcutaneous and Intramuscular, 2 in 3 forms; *See Chap. V*

H. A. METZ LABORATORY (Metz)
170 Varick Street, New York City

Acidol Tablets
Acidol Pepsin 1 Tablets
Acidol Pepsin 2 Tablets
Alumnol Powder
Anesthesin Powder
Benzosol Liquid
Duotal
Gravocain Ampules
Holocain Powder
Holocain Solution 1%
Melubrin Powder
Melubrin Tablets
Neosalvarsan Ampules, Single Dosage
Neosalvarsan Ampules, Multiple Dosage
Novocain Crystals—Ampules, Vials
Novocain Solution 1%—Ampules
Novocain Solution 20%—Ampules
Novocain Tablets—Plain, F and D
Novocain-Suprarenin Solution 1%—Ampules "K"
Novocain-Suprarenin Solution 2%—Ampules "E"
Novocain-Suprarenin Solution 2%—Ampules "T"
Novocain-Suprarenin Solution Concentrated 20% Ampules
Novocain-Suprarenin Pluglets
Novocain-Suprarenin Tablets "A," "B," "C," "E," "H," "K," "T"
Omnadin Ampules
Ortho-Troches
Orthoform Powder
Orthoform Troches
Oscodal Tablets
Parathesin Powder
Parathesin Troches
Paroxyl (Spirocid) Tablets
Pyramidon Tablets
Pyramidon Salicylate Tablets
 Elixir of Pyramidon
Pyraminal Tablets
 Elixir Pyraminal
Rivanol Lactate Powder
Rivanol Powder
Rivanol Tablets
Rivanol with Dextrose Capsules
Salvarsan Ampules Single Dosage
Salvarsan Ampule Multiple Dosage
Salvarsan Glucose Solution Ampules
Salyrgan Ampules
Silver-Salvarsan Ampules
Spinocain Ampules
 Ephedrine Novocaine Solution Ampules
Sulfactol Ampules
Sulfactol Tablets
Sulpharsphenamine Ampules
Suprarenin Ampules
Suprarenin Solution
Suprarenin Tablets
Synodal Ampules
Trichophytin Extract
Triphal Ampules
Also Ampules: Intravenous, 7 in 29 forms; Subcutaneous and Intramuscular, 7 in 36 forms; *See Chap. V*

MICAJAH AND COMPANY (Micajah)
Warren, Pa.

Medicated Suppositories
Medicated Wafers

E. S. MILLER LABORATORIES, INC. (Miller)
743 Maple Avenue, Los Angeles, Calif.

Corpus Luteum Extract Ampules
Corpus Luteum Extract Capsules
Corpus Luteum Extract Powder
Corpus Luteum Extract Tablets Chocolate coated, Enteric coated
Dextrose Ampules
Digestive Enzymes Tablets
Duodenal Substance Powder
Kidney Extract Ampules
Kidney Substance Capsules
Kidney Substance Powder
Kidney Substance Tablets
Liver Extract Hematopoietic Capsules
Liver Extract Hypotensive Ampules
Mammary Substance Capsules
Mammary Substance Powder
Mammary Substance Tablets, Chocolate coated, Enteric coated
Mammary Compound 1 Capsules
Mammary Compound 2 Capsules
Orchic Capsules
Orchic Powder
Orchic Tablets
Orchic Extract Ampules
Orchic Extract Special ampules
Orchic Compound 1 Capsules
Orchic Compound 2 Capsules
Orchic Compound 3 Capsules
Ovarian Compound 1 Capsules
Ovarian Compound 2 Capsules
Ovarian Compound 3 Capsules
Ovarian Residue Compound Capsules
Ovarian Residue Extract Ampules
Ovarian Residue Capsules
Ovarian Residue Powder
Ovarian Residue Tablets
Ovarian Whole Capsules
Ovarian Whole Powder
Ovarian Whole Tablets, Chocolate coated, Enteric coated
Ovarian Extract Whole Ampules
Pancreas Substance Powder
Pancreatic Extract Ampules
Pancreatin Powder
Pancreatin Tablets
Parathyroid Compound Capsules
Parathyroid Powder
Parathyroid Tablets
Pituitary Compound Capsules
Pituitary Extract Anterior Ampules
Pituitary Anterior Capsules
Pituitary Anterior Powder
Pituitary Anterior Tablets Plain and Chocolate coated
Pituitary Anterior Tablets, Enteric coated
Pituitary Extract Obstetrical Ampules
Pituitary Extract Surgical Ampules
Pituitary Posterior Powder
Pituitary Whole Capsules
Pituitary Whole Powder
Pituitary Whole Tablets
Placenta Capsules
Placenta Powder
Placenta Tablets Chocolate coated, Enteric coated
Placenta Extract Ampules
Pluriglandular Compound 1 Ampules
Pluriglandular Compound 2 Ampules
Prostate Capsules
Prostate Powder
Prostate Tablets, Chocolate coated, Enteric coated
Prostatic Compound Capsules
Prostatic Extract Ampules
Spleen Substance Capsules
Spleen Substance Powder
Spleen Substance Tablets, Chocolate coated, Enteric coated
Spleen Extract Ampules
Suprarenal Cortex Capsules
Suprarenal Cortex Powder
Suprarenal Cortex Extract Ampules
Suprarenal Whole Capsules
Suprarenal Whole Powder
Suprarenal Whole Tablets
Suprarenal Whole Extract Ampules
Suprarenal Medulla Solution (Epinephrine) 1:1,000 Ampules
Suprarenal Medulla Solution (Epinephrine) 1:1,000 Solution
Suprarenal Medulla Capsules
Suprarenal Medulla Powder
Thymus Extract Ampules
Thymus Substance Capsules
Thymus Substance Powder
Thymus Substance Tablets
Thymus and Suprarenal Extract Ampules
Thyroid Extract Ampules
Thyroid Substance Tablets
Also Ampules: Intravenous, 37 in 64 forms; Intramuscular and Subcutaneous, 55 in 112 forms; *See Chap.*

MONSANTO CHEMICAL WORKS (Monsanto)
St. Louis, Mo.

Halazone Tablets

MORGENSTERN CHEMICAL COMPANY (Morgenstern)

12 John Street, New York City

Combinal Tablets
Neogestin Powders
Nervinal Tablets

THE MOROTOL COMPANY, INC. (Morotol)

68 Pennsylvania Avenue, Brooklyn, N. Y.

Morotol

MORRIS AND SCHRADER (Morris and Schrader)

8 Barclay Street, New York City

Bassin de Vichy
Biliner Sauerbrunn
Birmo
Bognanco
Contrexeville
Evian-Cachat
Fachingen
Kissingen
Levico
White Sulphur Springs
Wildungen

MOUNT CLEMENS MINERAL WATER PROD. CO. (Mount Clemens)

Mount Clemens, Mich.

Mount Clemens Mineral Springs

MT. VERNON LABORATORIES, INC. (Mt. Vernon Lab.)

209 Washington Street, Mt. Vernon, N. Y.

Virilus

Also Ampules: 1 Subcutaneous and Intramuscular; *See Chap. V*

M AND R DIETETIC LABORATORIES, INC. (M and R Dietetic)

Columbus, Ohio

Similac

MULFORD BIOLOGICAL LABORATORIES (Mulford)

Philadelphia, Pa.

Acidophilus Blocks
Acne Bacterin
Acne Bacterin Mixture
Acne Serobacterin
Acne Serobacterin Mixture
Allergens—Bacterials
Allergens—Combinations
Allergens—Epidermals
Allergens—Foods
Allergens—Miscellaneous
Allergens—Pollens, Individual
Allergens—Pollens, Groups
Antianthrax Serum
Antidysenteric Serum
Antigonococcus Serum
Antimelitensis Serum
Antimeningococcic Serum
Antipneumococcic Serum (Type I)
Antipneumococcic Serum (Type I and II)
Antipneumococcic Serum (Polyvalent)
Antistreptococcic Serum (Polyomyelitis)
Antistreptococcic Serum Concentrated
Antistreptococcic Serum Hemolytic
Antistreptococcic Serum Polyvalent

Antistreptococcic Serum Viridans
Bacillus Acidophilus Liquid
Bothrops Antitoxin
Catarrh "Cold" Bacterin Mixed
Catarrh "Cold" Serobacterin Mixed
Cholera Bacterin (Cholera Vaccine)
Cholera Vaccine Prophylactic
Cholera Serobacterin
Coli Bacterin
Coli Serobacterin
Crotalus Antitoxin
Diphtheria Toxin for Schick Test
Diphtheria Toxin for Schick Test Control
Diphtheria Antitoxin Superconcentrated
Diphtheria Antitoxin Bovine
Diphtheria Toxin-Antitoxin Mixture
Diphtheria Toxin-Antitoxin Mixed (Goat)
Diphtheria Toxoid
Erysipelas Streptococcic Antitoxin, Concentrated
Influenza "Cold" Bacterin Mixed
Influenza "Cold" Serobacterin Mixed
Ivyol—Poison Ivy Extract
Ivyol Poison Oak Extract
Meningo-Bacterin
Neisser Bacterin
Neisser Serobacterin
Neisser Bacterin Mixed
Neisser Serobacterin Mixed
Normal Horse Serum
Perfringens Antitoxin (Unconcentrated)
Perfringens Antitoxin (Concentrated)
Pertussis Bacterin
Pertussis Serobacterin
Pertussis Bacterin Mixed
Pertussis Serobacterin Mixed
Plague Bacterin
Pneumo-Strept-Serobacterin
Pneumococcus Antibody Globulin
Pneumococcus Antibody Solution (Type I and II Combined)
Pneumo-Strept-Bacterin
Pneumo-Bacterin Mixed
Pneumo-Serobacterin Mixed
Pyorrhea Serobacterin Mixed
Rabies Vaccine
S-C-A Soluble Antigen
Scarlet Fever Streptococcus Toxin
Scarlet Fever Streptococcus Toxin (Dick Test)
Scarlet Fever Streptococcus Antitoxin (Concentrated)
Smallpox Vaccine
Staphylo-Bacterin Mixed
Staphylo-Streptobacterin Mixed
Staphylo-Streptoserobacterin Mixed
Staphylo-Serobacterin Mixed
Streptococcus Antibody Globulin (Bargen Serum)
Strepto-Sero Bacterin
Tetanus Antitoxin (Bovine)
Tetanus Antitoxin (Superconcentrated)
Tetanus Gas-Gangrene Antitoxin
Tuberculin Intracutaneous (O.T. Human)
Tuberculin Intracutaneous (O. T. Bovine)
Tuberculin Concentrated Undiluted
Tuberculin Dilutions (O.T. Human)
Tuberculin Concentrates (B.E. Human) Undiluted
Tuberculin Dilutions (B.E. Human)
Tuberculin Dilutions (T.R. Human)
Typho-Bacterin
Typho-Serobacterin
Typho-Bacterin Mixed
Typho-Serobacterin Mixed
Von Pirquet Test (T.O. Human)

MULFORD COLLOID LABORATORIES (Mulford Colloid)

5109 Germantown Avenue, Philadelphia, Pa.

Anticol
Anticol Sol 10%
Argocol
Argocol Sol 10%
Argocol Ointment 10%
Armicol
Armicol Capsules
Arsenocol
Arsenocol Sol 10%
Aurocol
Aurocol Sol 10%
Bisocol
Bisocol Sol
Bromocol
Calcol
Calcol Capsules
Calcol Sol 10%
Cupricol Scales
Cupricol Sol 10%
Ferrocol
Ferrocol Sol 10%
Iodocol
Iodocol Sol 10%
Iodocol Soluble Capsules
Mangacol
Mangacol Sol 10%
Merciol
Merciol Capsules Soluble
Merciol Ointment 5%
Mercurocol

Mercurocol Sol 1%
Mercurocol Ointment 10%
Plumbicol
Plumbicol Sol 10%
Selencol Sol 10%—25 cc
Siocol
Siocol Sol 10%—25 cc
Siocol Ointment 10%
Sulphocol
Sulphocol Capsules Soluble
Sulphocol Ointment 10%
Sulphocol Sol 10%—25 cc
Vitacol (Liquor Ferrocol Comp.)
Zincol
Zincol Ointment 10%

WM. H. MULLER AND COMPANY, INC. (W. H. Muller)
122 East 42nd Street, New York City

Mattoni "Giesshubler"

NATIONAL ANILINE AND CHEMICAL COMPANY (National Aniline)
40 Rector Street, New York City

Acriflavine "National" Tablets
Acriflavine "National" Throat Troches
Acriviolet "National" Solution 1%
Acriviolet "National" Powder
Acriviolet "National" Tablets
Ampydin Crystals
Ampydin Tablets
Gentian Violet Medicinal "Churchman" Tablets
Malic Acid F.P.
Neutral Acriflavine "National" Ampules
Neutral Acriflavine "National" Ointment 1%
Neutral Acriflavine "National" Powder
Neutral Acriflavine "National" Tablets
Neutral Acriflavine "National" Troches
Proflavine
Scarlet Red Medicinal "Biebrich"
Tetradol Emulsion
Tetradol Powder

THE NATIONAL DRUG COMPANY (National Drug)
5109 Germantown Avenue, Philadelphia, Pa.

Acados
Acne Combined Vaccine
Allergens—Epidermals, Furs
Allergens—Foods
Allergens—Miscellaneous
Allergens—Pollens, Individual
Allergens—Pollens, Groups
Antimeningococcic Serum (Polyvalent)
Antipneumococcus Serum (Refined and Extra Concentrated)
Antistreptococcic Serum (Polyvalent)
Antistreptococcus Erysipelas Serum
Bismol
Calcium Gluconate Compound
Catarrhal Vaccine
Cholera Combined Vaccine
Coli Combined Vaccine
Colloidal Sulphur Compound
Combined Vaccine (Van Cott)
Corpus Luteum Ampules
Corpus Luteum Tablets
Corpus Luteum Compound Capsules
Dermalgen
Diphtheria Toxoid
Diphtheria Antitoxin
Drosine
Epinephrin 1:1,000 Solution
Epinephrin 1:1,000 Ampules, Ampulevials.
Erysipelas Vaccine
Influenza Combined Vaccine
Lac-Proteinate Ampules
Liver Extract Capsules
Mammary Capsules
Mammary Tablets
Meningococcic Vaccine
Neisser Vaccine (Neisser Bacterin)
Neisser Combined Vaccine
Neodyne
Normal Horse Serum
Orchic Compound Capsules
Orchic Compound Tablets
Orchic Compound Special Tablets
Orchic Substance Tablets
Orchic Extract Ampules
Ovarian Extract Ampules
Ovarian Compound Capsules
Ovarian Compound Tablets

Parathyroid Tablets
Parathyroidin Solution Ampules
Parotid Tablets
Peptone Solution Ampules
Pertussis Vaccine
Pertussis Combined Vaccine
Pineal Tablets
Pituitary Anterior Tablets
Pituitary Extract Anterior Ampules
Pituitary Extract Posterior, U.S.P. Ampules
Pituitary Liquor Obstetrical Ampules
Pituitary Posterior Tablets
Pituitary Whole Tablets
Pneumococcus Vaccine (Pneumo-Bacterin)
Pneumococcus Combined Vaccine
Prostate Tablets
Rabies Vaccine (Human, Semple Method)
Rhus Venenata Antigen
Rhus Toxicodendron Antigen
Scarlet Fever Streptococcus Antitoxin
Scarlet Fever Streptococcus Toxin (Dick Test)
Scarlet Fever Streptococcus Antitoxin (Refined and Concentrated)
Schick Test
Schick Test Control
Staphylococcus Vaccine
Sterile Peptone Solution 5% Ampules
Streptococcus Vaccine (Strepto-Bacterin)
Strept-Staphylo Combined (Strept-Staphylo Mixed Bacterin)
Suprarenal Tablets
Tetanus Antitoxin (Extra Refined and Concentrated)
Tetanus-Perfringens Antitoxin
Tetra-Citrates
Thymus Tablets
Thyroid Capsules
Thyroid Tablets
Toxin Antitoxin (Diphtheria Toxin-Antitoxin Mixed)
Tuberculin O.T. (Von Pirquet Test)
Tuberculin Intracutaneous (O.T.)
Tuberculin Old (O.T.) Human
Tuberculin O.T. Serial Dilutions
Tuberculin Old O.T.
Typhoid Vaccine
Typhoid-Paratyphoid-A Vaccine
Typhoid-Paratyphoid Mixed Vaccine
Undulant Fever Vaccine
Vaccine Virus
Vito-Lecithin
Also Ampules: Intravenous, 24 in 38 forms; Subcutaneous and Intramuscular, 39 in 74 forms; *See Chap. V*

THE NATIONAL BISCUIT COMPANY (National Biscuit)
449 West 14th, St. New York City

Breadstuffs, Crackers, Wafers.

NATIONAL MILK SUGAR COMPANY (National Milk)
205 East 42nd Street, New York City

Beta Lactose

NELSON, BAKER AND COMPANY (Nelson, Baker)
Detroit, Mich.

Argentiform Vaginal Cones
Argentiform Urethral Ointment 0.2%, 1%
Argentiform Ophthalmic Ointment 0.2%, 1%
Argentiform Urethral Pencils
Bromoform Bronchial Anodyne Compound
Chionacea
Creosotide Tablets
Creosotide and Bismuth Compound Tablets
Creosotide Bronchial Sedative
Creosotide, Iron and Arsenic Tablets
Creosotide and Pepsin Compound Tablets
Creosotide and Strychnine Tablets
Elixir Digitalin Compound
Eupeptic Hypophosphites
Gallo-Bismuth Compound
Iodosyl Capsules
Iodosyl Duster
Iodosyl Nasal-Points
Iodosyl Ointment, 6% Aseptic
Iodosyl Ointment—Ophthalmic

Iodosyl Ointment—Urethral
Iodosyl Ointment Compound—Hemorrhoidal
Iodosyl Ointment Compound—Urethral
Iodosyl Pencils
Iodosyl Pencils, Milder
Iodosyl Powder Blower
Ophthalmic Ointments:
  Argentiform
  Atropine and Iodosyl, 1 (Regular)
  Atropine and Iodosyl, 3 (Special)
  Iodosyl
  Mercuriform
  Mercuric Oxide, Yellow
Suppositories Compound Iodosyl

NESTLE'S MILK PRODUCTS, INC. **(Nestle)**
2 Lafayette Street, New York City

Hylac
Lactogen
Nestle's Food

N. Y. PHARMACEUTICAL COMPANY **(N. Y. Pharmaceutical)**
Bedford Springs, Bedford, Mass.

Hayden's Viburnum Compound

THE N. Y. QUININE AND CHEMICAL WORKS, INC. **(N. Y. Quinine)**
99 North 11th Street, Brooklyn, N. Y.

Menthol Y
Quinidine

THE NORWICH PHARMACAL COMPANY **(Norwich)**
Norwich, N. Y.

Dysmenatone Tablets
Euphillana
Euphillana with Dionin
Mobé
Norwich Douche Powder
Orchaton Tablets
Phenobilin Tablets
Scabiola
Unguentine
Unguentine Crayons with Protargol
Unguentine Rectal Cones
Unguentine Skin Cream
Unguentine Soap
Yeastamine Tablets

THE P. J. NOYES COMPANY **(Noyes)**
51 Main Street, Lancaster, N. H.

Boro-Glyceride with Neo-Silvol Suppositories
Enzymes Solution
Gaduol Cordial
Gaduol with Hypophosphites Compound
Hyos-Zea
Kidnoids Tablets
Nasal Cream
Nasal Cream with Procaine 1%
Nasal Cream with Ephedrine 1%
Ointment-Compound Ichthyol
Pan-Bis-Cal
Restophen
Suppositories Oxyquinoline
Syndrome Tablets
Tritussis

NUMOTIZINE, INC. **(Numotizine)**
900 N. Franklin Street, Chicago, Ill.

Numotizine

THE NUTRADIET COMPANY **(Nutradiet)**
155 Berry Street, San Francisco, Calif.

Berries
Fruit Juices
Fruits
Honey
Sun Dried Fruits
Vegetables

NUTRIVOID PRODUCTS SALES COMPANY **(Nutrivoid)**
76 Montgomery Street, Jersey City, N. J.

Flour

THE OAKLAND CHEMICAL CO. **(Oakland)**
59 Fourth Avenue, New York City

Dioxogen

OCCY-CRYSTINE LABORATORIES **(Occy-Crystine)**
Box 118, Grand Central Station, New York City

Occy-Crystine

OCTOZONE COMPANY OF AMERICA **(Octozone)**
270 Broadway, New York City

Octozone

OD PEACOCK SULTAN COMPANY **(Od Peacock)**
4500 Parkview, St. Louis, Mo.

Cactina Pillets
Neurilla
Peacock's Bromides
Sanmetto
Seng

THE OHIO CHEMICAL AND MANUFACTURING CO. **(Ohio Chemical)**
1177 Marquette Street, N.E., Cleveland, Ohio

Carbon Dioxide-Oxygen Mixtures
Dermalene
Lennox Ethylene

OLEOTHESIN CO. **(Oleothesin)**
68–70 E. Utica Street, Buffalo, N. Y.

Oleothesin Solution
Oleothesin Packing
Oleothesin Spray
Oleothesin Socket Paste
Oanda Ointment

OXINOL LABORATORIES, INC. **(Oxinol)**
308 West 141st Street, New York City

Oxinol

PANCRESAL SALES COMPANY, INC. (Pancresal Sales)
11 West 42nd Street, New York City

Pancresal Tablets

PARKE, DAVIS AND COMPANY (Parke, Davis)
Detroit, Mich.

Acne Vaccine Combined
Adrenalin Chloride Solution Ampules
Adrenalin Chloride Solution Dilute Ampules
Adrenalin Crystals
Adrenalin and Cocaine Tablets
Adrenalin Compound Suppositories
Adrenalin Compound Suppositories 1:6,000
Adrenalin Inhalant
Adrenalin Ointment
Adrenalin Ointment 1:1,000
Adrenalin Suppositories
Adrenalin Suppositories 1:1,000
Adrenalin Suppositories with Chloretone
Adrenalin Tablets
Adrephine Ampules
Adrephine Liquid
Adrephine Inhalant
Adrephine Ointment
Adrephine Suppositories
Adrocaine Ampules "A"
Adrocaine Tablets "A" and "B"
Adrocaine Solution
Allergens—Individual (Bacterials, Epidermals, Foods, Pollens, Miscellaneous).
Allergens—Groups (Pollens)
Anesthone Cream
Antianthrax Serum
Antidysenteric Serum
Antimeningococcic Serum
Antipneumococcic Serum (Felton)
Antipneumococcic Serum (Felton, High Concentration)
Antistreptococcic Serum (Polyvalent)
Antistreptococcic Serum (Polyvalent, Refined and Concentrated)
Antuitrin-S Ampules
Apothesine Solution 1.5%
Apothesine and Adrenalin Tablets (Dental)
Apothesine Tablets
Apothesine Tablets "B" Hypodermic
Apothesine and Adrenalin Tablets Hypodermic
Bismuth Salicylate Ampules
Brometone Capsules
Chloretone Capsules
Chloretone Emollient
Chloretone Inhalant
Carbon Tetrachloride Capsules
Catarrhal Vaccine
Catarrhalis Immunogen Combined
Cod Liver Oil with Viosterol 10D
Codrenin
Coley Toxins
Combined Bacterial Vaccine (Van Cott)
Combined Immunogen (Van Cott)
Corpora Lutea Ampules
Corpora Lutea Capsules
Corpora Lutea Emplets
Corpora Lutea Powder
Corpora Lutea Tablets
D.C.P. 340
Dextrose Ampules
Dibromin Capsules
Digifortis Kapseals.
Digifortis Liquid
Digifortis Tablets
Diphtheria Antitoxin
Diphtheria Toxoid
Diphtheria Toxin Antitoxin Mixture
Diphtheria Toxin for Schick Test
Diphtheria Toxin Control
Emulsion Metagen and Cod Liver Oil
Ephedrine Alkaloid
Ephedrine Hydrochloride Capsules
Ephedrine Inhalant Plain 1%
Ephedrine Inhalant Compound
Ephedrine Sulphate Capsules
Ephedrine Sulphate Solution 3%
Ephedrine Sulphate Ampules
Ergot Aseptic Ampules
Erysipelas Streptococcus Immunogen
Erysipelas Phylacogen
Erysipelas Streptococcus Antitoxin
Eschatin
Estrogen Ampules
Furunculosis Vaccine
Gas-Gangrene Antitoxin
Germicidal Discs Large, Small.
Glucose Ampules
Gonococcus Immunogen
Gonococcus Immunogen Combined
Gonorrheal Phylacogen
Gonococcus Vaccine Combined
Haliver Oil Plain Capsules, Vials.
Haliver Oil with Viosterol 250 D Capsules, Vials
Hemoprotein "Brooks"

Hemostatic Serum
Influenza Vaccine Combined
Influenza Pneumonia Vaccine
Insulin
Iodalbin Capsules
Iodalbin Powder
Iodalbin and Mercurol Tablets
Iron Citrate Green Ampules
Irradol A
Lipo-Lutin Ampules
Liver Extract Ampules, Vials
Locosthetic
Malt Extract with Cod Liver Oil Capsules
Mammary Substance Emplets
Mammary Substance Powder
Mammary Substance Tablets
Mercurettes
Mercuric Salicylate Ampules
Mercurol Tablets
Mercurosal Ampules
Mercury Succinimide Ampules
Metatone
Mixed Infection Phylacogen
Mycozol Ointment
Neo-Silvol Capsules
Neo-Silvol Ointment 5%
Neo-Silvol Powder
Neo-Silvol Suppositories 5%
Normal Horse Serum
Orchic Substance Emplets
Orchic Substance Powder
Orchic Substance Tablets
Ortal Sodium Capsules
Ovarian Residue Ampules
Ovarian Residue Capsules
Ovarian Residue Emplets
Ovarian Residue Powder
Ovarian Residue Tablets
Ovarian Substance Ampules
Ovarian Substance Capsules
Ovarian Substance Emplets
Ovarian Substance Powder
Ovarian Substance Tablets
Panteric Capsules
Panteric Tablets
Panteric Compound Tablets
Parathyroid Emplets, Tablets
Paroidin
Pineal Gland Emplets, Tablets
Pitocin Ampules
Pitressin Ampules
Pitressin Nasal Jelly
Pituitary Anterior Emplets
Pituitary Anterior Powder
Pituitary Anterior Tablets
Pituitary Posterior Emplets
Pituitary Posterior Tablets
Pituitary Whole Powder
Pituitary Whole Tablets
Pituitrin Ampules, Obstetrical
Pituitary Ampules, Surgical
Placenta Capsules
Placenta Emplets
Placenta Powder
Pertussis Immunogen
Pertussis Immunogen Combined
Pertussis Vaccine
Pertussis Vaccine Combined
Pneumococcus Immunogen Combined
Pneumonia Vaccine
Pneumonia Phylacogen
Proposote Capsules
Puerperal Septicemia Antistreptococcic Serum
Quinine and Urea Hydrochloride Ampules
Quinine Hydrochloride and Urethane Ampules
Rabies Vaccine
Rheumatism Phylacogen
Sal-Ethyl
Sal-Ethyl Carbonate Tablets
Sal-Ethyl Carbonate Tablets with Amidopyrine
Scarlet Fever Streptococcus Toxin
Scarlet Fever Streptococcus Toxin for Immunization
Scarlet Fever Streptococcus Antitoxin
Scarlet Red Sulph. Emulsion
Scarlet Red Sulph. Ointment A, B
Scarlet Red Ointment
Silver Nitrate Solution
Silvol Bougies
Silvol Capsules
Silvol Ointment
Silvol Powder
Silvol Suppositories
Skiagenol
Smallpox Vaccine
Staphylococcus Immunogen
Staphylococcus Vaccine
Stearodine Tablets
Streptococcus Immunogen
Streptococcus Immunogen Combined
Streptococcus and Staphylococcus Vaccine
Streptococcus Vaccine
Surgical Lubricant
Taka-Diastase Capsules
Taka-Diastase Liquid
Taka-Diastase Powder
Taka-Diastase Tablets
Taka-Diastase and Pancreatin Tablets
Taka-Diastase, Pancreatin, Nux Vomica Tablets
Taka-Diastase, Pepsin and Pancreatin Capsules

Taka-Diastase, Pepsin and Pancreatin Tablets
Taka-Diastase, Pepsin and Strychnine Tablets
Takazyme Tablets
Tetanus Antitoxin
Tetanus Gas-Gangrene Antitoxin, Combined
Theelin Ampules
Theelin Suppositories
Theelol Capseals
Thio-Bismol Ampules
Thyroid Capsules
Thyroid Emplets
Thyroid Powder
Thyroid Tablets
Thyroid Tablets, Enteric coated
Thymus Gland Emplets
Thymus Gland Tablets
Thymus Gland Powder
Thyroidectomized Horse Serum
Thyro-Protein Ampules
Thyro-Protein Tablets
Tuberculin Old (O.T.)
Tuberculin Old (Von Pirquet)
Tuberculin Old (Mantoux)
Tuberculin Old (Ophthalmic)
Tuberculin B.E.
Tuberculin B.E. Tablets
Tuberculin Residue (T.R.)
Tuberculin Residue Tablets
Typhoid Vaccine
Typhoid-Paratyphoid Vaccine
Typhoid Phylacogen
Ulcerative Colitis Antistreptoccic Serum
Ventriculin
Yellow Oxide of Mercury Ointment
Also Ampules: Intravenous, 17 in 25 forms; Subcutaneous and Intramuscular, 44 in 62 forms; *See Chap. V*

THE E. L. PATCH COMPANY **(Patch)**
Stoneham P. O., Boston, Mass.

Cod Liver Oil, Flavored
Kondremul
Kondremul with Phenolphthalein

PASTEUR INSTITUTE OF ST. LOUIS **(Pasteur)**
3514 Lucas Street, St. Louis, Mo.

Antirabic Virus

THE PEPSODENT COMPANY **(Pepsodent)**
919 North Michigan Avenue, Chicago, Ill.

Pepsodent Antiseptic
Pepsodent Tooth Paste

PET MILK COMPANY **(Pet Milk)**
St. Louis, Mo.

Pet Milk

PETROLAGAR LABORATORIES, INC. **(Petrolagar)**
8134 McCormick Blvd., Chicago, Ill.

Petrolagar Plain
Petrolagar Unsweetened
Petrolagar with Phenolphthalein
Petrolagar with Milk of Magnesia

PHARMEDIC CORPORATION **(Pharmedic)**
227 Thirty-fourth Street, Brooklyn, N. Y.

Aminophyllin Ampules
Aminophyllin Suppositories
Aminophyllin Tablets
Methatropin

THE CHAS. H. PHILLIPS CHEMICAL COMPANY **(Phillips)**
170 Varick Street, New York City

Dental Magnesia
Milk of Magnesia "Phillips," Liquid
Milk of Magnesia "Phillips," Tablets

PICKER X-RAY CORPORATION **(Picker X-Ray)**
300 Fourth Avenue, New York City

Keraphen A and B

GEO. P. PILLING AND SON **(Pilling)**
Arch and 23rd Street, Philadelphia, Pa.

Iodine-Boric Acid Dusting Powder "Sulzberger"

THE PINOLEUM COMPANY **(Pinoleum)**
52 West 15th Street, New York City

Pinoleum Liquid

PITMAN-MOORE CO. **(Pitman-Moore)**
Indianapolis, Ind.

Oxiphen Tablets

THE PAUL PLESSNER COMPANY **(Plessner)**
3538 Brooklyn Avenue, Detroit, Mich.

Taurocol
Taurocol Compound Tablets
Vera Perles

PROTEIN MINERAL CO., INC. **(Protein Mineral)**
18 E. 41st Street, New York City

PMC.

THE PURDUE FREDERICK COMPANY **(Purdue Frederick)**
135 Christopher Street, New York City

Gray's Glycerine Tonic
Hyperol Capsules

THE PURE GLUTEN FOOD COMPANY **(Pure Gluten)**
175 Fifth Avenue, New York City

Gluten Bran Flakes "Hoyt"
Gluten Special Flour "Hoyt"

PYCOPÉ, INC. **(Pycopé)**
531 Kentucky Avenue, Joplin, Mo.

Pycopé Tooth Powder

RADIUM CHEMICAL COMPANY (Radium Chemical)

1 East 42nd Street, New York City

Radium Salts as Radium Needles, Radium Tubes, Radium Plaques:
Radium Bromide
Radium Carbonate
Radium Sulphate
Radium Chloride

THE RADIUM EMANATION CORPORATION (Radium Emanation)

Graybar Building, Grand Central Terminal, New York City

Radon

RADON COMPANY, INC. (Radon Co.)

1 East 42nd Street, New York City

Radon

RALSTON PURINA COMPANY (Ralston)

Checkerboard Square, St. Louis, Mo.

Baby Ralston
Ralston Wheat Cereal
Rye Krisp

REED AND CARNRICK (Reed and Carnrick)

155 Van Wagenen Avenue, Jersey City, N. J.

Ampacoids Ovary
Ampacoids Prostate
Ampacoids Testicle
Analeptine
Corpus Luteum Powder
Corpus Luteum Tablets, Plain and Enteric coated
Endomin Tablets
Entacarb Tablets
Mammary Gland Powder
Mammary Gland Tablets, Plain and Enteric coated
Nephritin Tablets
Ovacoids Tablets
Ovarian Residue Powder
Ovarian Residue Tablets, Plain and Enteric coated
Panacoids Tablets
Pancreas Powder
Pancreas Tablets
Pancrobilin Pills Plain
Pancrobilin Pills Compound
Pancrobilin Liquid
Pancrobilin Pills with Cascara
Pancrobilin Pills with Phenophthalein
Pancrobilin Pills with Podophyllin
Parathyroid Powder
Parathyroid Tablets, Plain and Enteric coated
Parathyroid with Calcium Lactate
Peptenzyme Effervescent Granules
Peptenzyme Elixir
Peptenzyme Powder
Peptenzyme Tablets
Pineal Powder
Pineal Tablets, Plain and Enteric coated
Pituitary Anterior Powder
Pituitary Anterior Tablets, Plain and Enteric coated
Pituitary Posterior Powder
Pituitary Posterior Tablets, Plain and Enteric coated
Pituitary Whole Powder
Pituitary Whole Tablets, Plain and Enteric coated
Protonuclein Beta Cubes
Protonuclein Special Dusting Powder
Protonuclein Powder
Protonuclein Ointment
Protonuclein Tablets
Protonuclein Special Tablets
Roboline
Suprarenal Cortex Powder
Suprarenal Cortex Tablets, Plain and Enteric coated
Suprarenal Medulla Powder
Suprarenal Medulla Tablets, Plain and Enteric coated

Suprarenal Whole Gland Powder
Suprarenal Whole Gland Tablets, Plain and Enteric coated
Testacoids
Thymus Powder
Thymus Tablets
Thyracoids Tablets, Plain and Enteric coated
Thyroid Powder
Tonicine Male
Tonicine Female
Trophonine
Whole Ovary Powder
Whole Ovary Tablets, Plain and Enteric coated
Zymocide
Also Ampules: Subcutaneous and Intramuscular, 3 in 3 forms; *See Chap. V*

THE REINSCHILD CHEMICAL COMPANY (Reinschild)
18 Grand Street, New Rochelle, N. Y.

Bromo-Mangan
Ferro-Mangan Peptonized
Iodo-Mangan
Regulin

REMOGLAND CHEMICAL COMPANY (Remogland)
25 West Broadway, New York City

Forto-Testin Tablets
Remogland Ampules
Remogland Tablets
Remolysin
Also Ampules: Subcutaneous and Intramuscular, 1; *See Chap. V*

RIEDEL AND COMPANY (Riedel)
Barry and South 5th Streets, Brooklyn, N. Y.

Gonosan Capsules
Hexalet Powder
Hexalet Tablets
Mergal Capsules
Neo Bornyval Pearls
Ovogal Capsules
Salipyrin Powder
Salipyrin Tablets
Thiol Liquid
Thiol Powder

RIEDEL-DE-HAEN, INC. (Riedel-de-Haen)
105 Hudson Street, New York City

Decholin Tablets
Decholin-Sodium Ampules
Nostal Tablets
Pernoston Ampules
Tetrophine
Also Ampules: Intravenous, 2 in 4 forms; *See Chap. V*

HOFFMANN-LA ROCHE, INC. (Roche)
Nutley, N. J.

Acetylcholine Ampules
Allonal Tablets
Alurate Tablets
Alurate Ampules
Alurate Elixir
Betaine Hydrochloride
Digalen "Cloetta" Ampules
Digalen "Cloetta" Solution
Digalen "Cloetta" Tablets
Elixir Arsylen Compositum
Histamine
Histamine Ampules
Homatropine Hydrochloride
Iodostarine Tablets
Isacen Tablets
Larocaine
Larosan
Oleo-Bi Ampules
Pantopon Ampules
Pantopon Powder
Pantopon Tablets
Papaverine Sulphate Ampules
Papaverine Hydrochloride Powder
Prostigmin Ampules

Scopolamine Stable Ampules
Sedobrol
Sedormid Tablets
Thigenol
Theobromine
Theobromine Sodium Acetate
Thiocol Powder
Thiocol Syrup
Thiocol Tablets
Thyroxine Synthetic Ampules
Thyroxine Synthetic Crystals
Thyroxine Synthetic Liquid
Thyroxine Synthetic Tablets
Tyramine
Also Ampules: Subcutaneous and Intramuscular, 9 in 9 forms; *See Chap. V*

ROCKBRIDGE ALUM SPRINGS, INC. **(Rockbridge)**
P. O. Rockbridge, Alum Springs, Va.

Rockbridge Alum Springs

THE ROESSLER AND HASSLACHER CHEMICAL COMPANY, INC.
(Roessler and Hasslacher)
c/o E. T. Dupont, Wilmington, Del.

Calcium Peroxide
Magnesium Peroxide
Sodium Dioxide Dental
Sodium Perborate
Sodium Peroxide
Strontium Peroxide
Zinc Perborate
Zinc Peroxide

WM. H. RORER, INC. **(Rorer)**
267 South 4th Street, Philadelphia, Pa.

Adrenal Substance Powder
Asthmaglands Capsules
Calcium Lactate with Parathyroid Capsules
Cerebrolecithin with Nuclein Capsules
Cerebro-Orchic Compound Capsules
Combined Carbonates Compound
Corpora Lutea Ampules
Corpora Lutea Capsules
Corpora Lutea Powder
Corpora Lutea Tablets
Cretinglands Capsules
Diasystol
Digicardium
Glanditone Tablets
Glycosuretics Capsules, Plain and Enteric coated
Homoglands Capsules
Lacto-Protein Ampules
Liver Substance (1:20) Capsules
Mammary Substance Capsules
Mammary Substance Powder
Mammary Substance Tablets
Miscidine
Methylene Blue Ampules
Nurobromyds
Orchic Substance Capsules
Orchic Substance Powder
Orchic Substance Tablets
Ovarian Substance Capsules
Ovarian Substance Powder
Ovarian Substance Tablets
Ovaradysfunction Capsules
Parathyroid Capsules
Parathyroid Powder
Parathyroid Tablets
Pituitary Extract Obstetrical Ampules
Pituitary Substance Anterior Capsules
Pituitary Substance Anterior Powder
Pituitary Substance Anterior Tablets
Pituitary Substance Posterior Powder
Pituitary Substance Whole Capsules
Pituitary Substance Whole Powder
Prostate Substance Capsules
Prostate Substance Powder
Prostate Substance Tablets
Spleen Substance Capsules
Spleen Substance Powder
Spleen Substance Tablets Chocolate coated and Enteric coated
Thyroid Substance Capsules
Thyroid Substance Powder
Thyroid Substance Tablets
Vitaglands Capsules
Vulnerine
Also Ampules: Intraveous, 3 in 7 forms; Subcutaneous and Intramuscular, 17 in 19 forms; *See Chap. V*

RUBROL CO. **(Rubrol)**
460 W. 34th Street, New York City

Rubrol with Ephedrine

SANDOZ CHEMICAL WORKS, INC. **(Sandoz)**
61 Van Dam Street, New York City

Allisatin Tablets
Belladenal Tablets
Bellafoline Tablets
Bellafoline Ampules
Bellafoline Solution 1:2,000
Calglucon Ampules 10%
Calglucon Powder
Calglucon Tablets
Felamine Tablets
Gynergen Ampules
Gynergen Liquid
Gynergen Tablets
Optalidon Tablets
Panthesine Ointment
Sandoptal Tablets
Scillaren Solution
Scillaren Tablets
Scillaren B Ampules
Also Ampules: Intravenous, 2 in 3 forms; Subcutaneous and Intramuscular, 3 in 5 forms; *See Chap.* V

SARGENT'S DRUG STORE, INC. **(Sargent)**
23 N. Wabash Avenue, Chicago, Ill.

Petrobran

SCHERING CORPORATION **(Schering**
75 West Street, New York City

Ludosan (Neutralon)
  Belladonna-Neutralon
Neo-Iopax Ampules
Neo-Iopax Retrograde
Niazo Tablets
Progynon Ampules
Progynon Tablets
Saraka
Also Ampules: Intravenous, 1; Subcutaneous and Intramuscular, 1; *See Chap. V*

SCHERING AND GLATZ, INC.* **(Schering and Glatz)**
113 East 18th Street, New York City

Anusol Suppositories
Arhovin Capsules
Arhovin Liquid
Atophan Powder
Atophan Tablets
Atophan-Urotropin Compound Ampules
Atophanyl Intravenous Ampules
Atophanyl Intramuscular Ampules
Arcanol Tablets
Beta-Eucaine Hydrochloride
Beta-Eucaine Lactate
Brovalol Pearls
Camiofen Ointment
Creosote Carbonate
Euphthalmine
Formalin Disinfector
Formalin Liquid
Formalin Pastilles
Formalin Sterilizer
  Paraform Powder
Hegonon
Icterosan Ampules
Iocamfen
Medinal Elixir
Medinal Powder
Medinal Suppositories
Medinal Tablets
Novatophan Powder
Novatophan Tablets
Orphol
Peralga Powder
Peralga Tablets
Sublamine Powder
Sublamine Tablets

*** The above described products are registered in the U. S. Pat. Office.**

Urotropin Ampules
Urotropin Crystals
Urotropin Tablets
Xeroform

SCHIEFFELIN AND COMPANY (Schieffelin)

16 Cooper Square, New York City

Adrenal Extract Tablets
Adrenal Nucleo-Protein Powder
Adrenal Nucleo-Protein Tablets
Adrenal Residue Fluid
Adrenal Residue Pills
Agar-Agar
Antiseptic Soaps 1 to 10
Atomidine Liquid
Atomidine Ointment
Azinol
Bemax
Bensolyptus
Calcium Granular
Calcium Lactophosphate
Cod Liver Oil "Peter Moller's" Plain
Cod Liver Oil "Peter Moller's" Flavored
Cod Liver Oil "Peter Moller's" Super-D
Colalin Laxative Tablets
Colalin Powder
Colalin Tablets
Colalin and Phenolphthalein Tablets
Enzymatase
Ephedrine Inhalant Compound
Ephedrine Inhalant Compound Jelly
Estivin
Fla-Min-Ol
Gleydig Pills
Glovarian Pills
Glyadrenal Pills
Glycana
Glycortal Pills
Glypectus Plain
Glypectus with Codein
Glystitial Pills
Glythoid Pills
Glytuitary Pills
Hemec Tablets
Hemoquinine
Hepatic Saline
Moller A-B-C-D Vitamine Food
Neurocaine
Neuronidia
Nuzon
Orazin
Ovarian Nucleoprotein Powder
Ovarian Nucleoprotein Tablets
Ovarian Residue Solution
Paraglythoid Pills
Parathyroid Nucleoprotein Tablets
Phenandyne
Pituitary Nucleoprotein Tablets
Salusol
S.A.S.
Steero Cubes
Syl-Agg-Ol
Thyroid Nucleoprotein Powder
Thyroid Nucleoprotein Tablets
Thyroid Residue Ampules
Thyroid Residue Solution
Triton Bath Salts
Uriform
Xeroform
Also Ampules: Subcutaneous and Intramuscular, 1; *See Chap. V*

JULIUS SCHMID, INC. (Schmid)

423–439 West 55th Street, New York City

Ramses Vaginal Jelly

SCHOONMAKER LABORATORIES, INC. (Schoonmaker)

Caldwell, N. J.

Vem
Vem with Boric Acid
Vem with Camphor
Vem with Ichthyol
Zyl

CARL H. SCHULTZ (Schultz)

430–444 First Avenue, New York City

Bilin
Carlsbad
Gleichenberg
Homburg

Hunyadi
Kissingen
Kissingen Bitter Water
Lithia Waters
Marienbad
Obersalzbrunn
Puellna
Pyrmont
Schwalbach
Wildungen

SCOTT AND BOWNE (Scott and Bowne)
Elmira, N. Y.

Emulsion of Cod Liver Oil
Norwegian Cod Liver Oil Flavored
Norwegian Cod Liver Oil Plain
Vitamins A and D Tablets

G. D. SEARLE AND COMPANY, INC. (Searle)
4737 Ravenswood Avenue, Chicago, Ill.

Adrenal Prostate Compound Capsules
Adrenal Spermin Compound Tablets
Alka Carb
Aminophyllin Ampules
Aminophyllin Tablets
Anemollient
Anter-Pituitary Compound Capsules
Arbutin Tablets
Arsphenamine Ampules
Barbenzal Tablets
Bismogen Liquid
Bismuth Sodium Tartrate Ampules
Bismuth Sodium Tartrate Solution 1.5%
Bismuth and Anesthesin Compound Capsules
Bismuth and Anesthesin Compound Tablets
Calcium Benziodoxyl Capsules
Chiniofon Tablets
Cholphenolate Tablets
Corpus Luteum Substance Ampules
Corpus Luteum Substance Tablets
Digitalis Products:
Digitaligen Tablets
Digitaligen Tincture
Digitalis Leaves Capsules
Digitalis Leaves Powder
Epinephrine 1:1,000 Ampules
Expectorant
Gold Sodium Thiosulphate Ampules
Hex-Arbutin Tablets
Intesti-Sols Orchic Compound Pills
Intesti-Sols Ovarian Compound Pills
Iodicalcium Tablets
Iodithesin Lozenges
Iodochlorol
Iodochlorol Emulsion
Islands of Langerhans Capsules
Islands of Langerhans Intesti-Sols
Islands of Langerhans Tablets
Liver Substance Capsules
Mammary-Placenta Compound with Pituitary Capsules
Mancuhemin Elixir
Mancuhemin Tablets
Mercurochrome 220
Minerasal
Neoarsphenamine Ampules
Orchic Substance Tablets
Ovarian Substance Tablets
Parathyroid and Spermin Compound Capsules
Pituitary Solution (Posterior and Middle Lobes) Ampules
Pituitary Substance Whole Capsules
Procaine Borate
Procaine Borate and Epinephrine Tablets
Proteolac Ampules
Silver Nitrate-Anesthesin Compound Tablets
Sodium Morrhuate 5% with Benzyl Alcohol Ampules
Sodium Thiosulphate Ampules
Sulpharsphenamine Ampules
Suprarenal Substance Tablets
Thymo Pitsin Ampules
Thyroid Substance Tablets
Thyroid Substance Tablets Enteric coated
Tinpronate Tablets
Yohimbin Endocrine Compound Capsules
Yohimbin Endocrine Compound Tablets
Also Ampules: Intravenous, 33 in 51 forms; Subcutaneous and Intramuscular, 31 in 40 forms; *See Chap. V*

SEECK AND KADE, INC. (Seeck and Kade)
440 Washington Street, New York City

Pertussin

SEEDOL MFG. CO. (Seedol)
27 W. 20 Street, New York City

Kelpamalt Tablets

SEYDEL CHEMICAL COMPANY (Seydel)
135 Halladay Street, Jersey City, N. J.

Benacol Solution
Benzyl Alcohol
Ethacaine
Mobenate

SHARP AND DOHME, INC. (Sharp and Dohme)
Philadelphia, Pa.

Acetidine Capsules
Acetidine Tablets
Adrin Solution Ampules
Adrin Solution Liquid
Alkanite
Analgine Tablets
Aseptovols
Blandine Compound
B. F. I. Ointment
B. F. I. Powder
Borocaine Powder
Borocaine Tablets
Borocaine Tablets Hypodermic
Borocaine and Epinephrine Tablets
Bronchol Capsules
Caprokol Solution 2½%
Caprokol Capsules
Carbon Tetrachloride Capsules
Cargentos Capsules
Cargentos Ointment 5%, 10%
Cargentos Scales
Cargentos Suppositories
Cargentos Urethral Bougies
Chloro-Calcium
Corpus Luteum Extract Ampules
Corpus Luteum Extract Capsules
Corpus Luteum Extract Tablets
Corpus Luteum Extract Tablets, Chocolate coated
Cremo Carbonates
Cresatine
Cresatin Spray
Cresatin Suppositories Rectal 10%
Cresatin Suppositories Vaginal 10%
Dialkalos
Digitos Ampules
Dihydranol Capsules
Dihydranol Solution
Diurol
Euphorbia Compound Syrup
Ferro-Manganese Peptonated
Ferro-Manganese Peptonated with Arsenic
Gelatin Compound Phenolized
Glucose Ampules
Hepatone
Hexyl-Resorcinol Solution S.T. 37 Liquid
Hexyl-Resorcinol Solution S.T. 37 Sucrates
Hexyl-Resorcinol Solution S.T. 37 Tooth Paste
Hexyl-Resorcinol Sucrates
Hyotole
Ichthorgin
Ichtholdine
Ichthorcin
Insulin Vials 5, 10, 20, 40 Units
Iodo-Casein Tablets, Plain, Chocolated
Lapactic Pills
Linctus Compound
Liquor Diastase
Liquor Santaiva
Lithiated Sorghum Compound
Liver Extract A-5 Capsules
Liver Extract A-5 Liquid
Mercurophen Tablets
Mercurophen Vials
Mercury Succinimide Ampules
Mercury Succinimide Tablets
Methenos

Methylets
Normal Horse Serum Ampules
Ophthalmic Ointments:
- Atropine Sulphate
- Boric Acid
- Conjunctivitis
- Copper Citrate 5 %, 10 %
- Ichthyol
- Mercuric Chloride, Corrosive
- Mercuric Oxide, Yellow
- Mercuric Oxide Yellow with Atropine
- Mercury, Ammoniated

Ovarian Extract Ampules
Ovarian Residue Extract Ampules
Ovarian Substance Capsules
Ovarian Substance Powder
Ovarian Substance Tablets
Ovaritone
Pabutole
Panalgyn
Pancreatin Powder
Pan-Peptic Elixir, Powder, Tablets
Paraffin Compound
Parathyroid Tablets
Pepetal
Phedros
Pine and Somnos Cordial
Pituitary Extract Obstetrical Ampules
Pituitary Extract Surgical Ampules
Pituitary Entire Powder
Protan Compound
Protan Powder
Protan Tablets
Quinarsin
Res-Unguentum
Sedatole
Sennetal
Solmides Tablets Small, Large
Somnos
Surgodine
Tanichthol Suppositories
Thyrocalx 1 Tablets
Thyrocalx 2 Tablets
Thyroid Gland Capsules
Thyroid Gland Powder
Thyroid Gland Tablets
Tissue Extract 568
Utros
Zinc Permanganate Powder
Zinc Permanganate Tablets
Also Ampules: Intravenous, 18 in 37 forms; Subcutaneous and Intramuscular, 36 in 47 forms; *See Chap. V*

G. H. SHERMAN, M.D., INC. (Sherman)

14600 Jefferson Avenue, East, Detroit, Mich.

Acne Vaccine
A-Vee Preparations:
- Sherman A-Vee 51
- Sherman A-Vee 52
- Sherman A-Vee 11
- Sherman A-Vee 12

Bio-Cream
Bronchitis Vaccine
Corpus Luteum Ampules
Endo-Sepsis Vaccine
Epidemic Meningitis Vaccine
Epinephrine Chloride 1:1,000, Ampules,
Epinephrine Chloride 1:1,000 Solution
Erysipelas Vaccine
Exo-Sepsis Vaccine
Furunculosis Vaccine
Gonorrhea Vaccine
Laryngitis Vaccine
Neo-Acidophilus
Orchic Substance Soluble Extract Ampules
Pituitary Extract Obstetrical Ampules
Pituitary Extract Surgical Ampules
Pneumonia Vaccine
Scarlet Fever Vaccine
Tuberculosis Vaccine
Typhoid Vaccine
Typhoid-Paratyphoid Vaccine
Ulcerative Colitis Vaccine
Undulant "Malta" Fever Vaccine
Whooping Cough Vaccine
Whooping Cough Vaccine Combined
Also Ampules: Intravenous, 18 in 25 forms; Subcutaneous and Intramuscular, 16 in 21 forms; *See Chap V*

J. SKLAR MANUFACTURING CO. (Sklar)

133–143 Floyd Street, Brooklyn, N. Y.

Arzol Mercurochrome Applicators
Arzol Silver Nitrate Applicators

S.M.A. CORPORATION (S.M.A.)

Cleveland, Ohio

Alerdex
Caritol
Cod Liver Oil
Concentrated Liquid Form S.M.A.
Concentrated Liquid Skim Milk
Concentrated Liquid Whole Milk
Crystalline Carotene
Hypoallergic Whole Milk
Hypoallergic Skim Milk
Natural Vitamin D
Powdered Skim Milk
Powdered Half Skimmed Milk
Powdered Whole Milk
S.M.A. Powdered Form
Smaco Maltose and Dextrins
Vitamins A and D
Whole Milk Sterilized

CARROLL DUNHAM SMITH PHARMACAL COMPANY (C. D. Smith)

317 East 34th Street, New York City

Aesculol Suppositories
Choleol
Coci-Codeine
Eczol
Fer-Iodine
Hemo-Vitol Tablets
Hemo-Vitol Capsules
Marrow Malt Compound
Ovarian-Suprarenal Compound Capsules
Passiflora Compound
Phenol-Procaine "D.F."
Trillin Tablets

MARTIN H. SMITH COMPANY (M. H. Smith)

150 Lafayette Street, New York City

Ergoapiol
Glykeron

THE SMITH-DORSEY COMPANY, INC. (Smith-Dorsey)

Lincoln, Nebraska

Auraline
Cal-So-Mag
Compound Mercury Ointment 14
Compound Novocaine Ointment
Dentaline
Ephedrine Inhalant Compound
Ephedrinol
Eucalyptus Thymol Compound
Guaia-Camph Ointment
Liver Extract Capsules
Maradol
Ophthalmic Ointments:
- Argyrol
- Atropine Sulphate
- Boric Acid
- Boric Acid and Phenol
- Cocaine Hydrochloride
- Copper Citrate
- Compound Mercury 14
- Compound Novocaine
- Dionin
- Eserine Alkaloid
- Holocaine Hydrochloride
- Holocaine Hydrochloride and Mercury Yellow Oxide
- Ichthyol

Opthalmic Ointments:—(*Continued*)
- Mercurochrome
- Mercury, Ammoniated
- Mercury, Yellow Oxide and Atrophine Sulphate
- Mercury Bichloride
- Mercury Compound 18
- Mercury Oxide Yellow
- Novocaine
- Orthoform
- Pilocarpine Muriate
- Silver Salts, Colloidal
- Thiosinamine
- White's Ointment
- Zinc Acetate
- Zinc Sulphate

Orchi-Himbine Compound Capsules
Ovarian Substance Tablets
Pancrasin
Silver-Sal Crystals
Silver-Sal Suppositories
Storaxin Ointment
Suppositories 2, 8
Tin Oxide Capsules
Thyroid Substance Capsules
Thyroid Substance Tablets

SMITH, KLINE AND FRENCH LABORATORIES
(Smith, Kline and French)
Philadelphia, Pa.

Benzedrine Inhaler
Citrico "Eskay"
Dextrettes "Eskay"
Neurophosphates "Eskay"
Oxo-Ate
Oxo-Ate "B" Capsules
Oxo-Ate "B" Tablets
Pentnucleotide Ampules
Suxiphen "Eskay"
Also Ampules: Subcutaneous and Intramuscular, 1; *See Chap V*

SOCIETÁ ANONIMA FIUGGI
(Societá Anonima Fiuggi)
530 West Broadway, New York City

Fiuggi

THE SODIPHENE CO. **(Sodiphene)**
Kansas City, Mo.

Sodiphene

SPA PRODUCTS **(Spa Products)**
164 Fifth Avenue, New York City

Duerkheim
Franzensbad
Frazensbad Natural Mud Salts
Kissingen
Marienbad
Marienbad Natural Spring Salt
Mergentheim
Neuenahr

SPICER AND COMPANY **(Spicer)**
Glendale, Calif.

Colalactin Plain
Colalactin with Phenolphthalein
Espinol
Panopsin Tablets
Quicamphol Ampules
Quicamphol Liquid
Quiniobine Ampules
Quiniobine Liquid
Solvochin Ampules
Tartro-Quiniobine Ampules
Tartro-Quiniobine Liquid
Also Ampules: Subcutaneous and Intramuscular, 4 in 4 forms; *See Chap V*

SARATOGA SPRINGS COMMISSION **(State of N. Y.)**
551 Fifth Ave, New York City

Hathorn #2 Water
Cœsa Water
Geyser Water

E. R. SQUIBB AND SONS **(Squibb)**
745 Fifth Avenue, New York City

Acne Vaccine
Adex Tablets 10D
Allergens—Bacterials, Epidermals, Foods, Miscellaneous, Pollens—Individual and Groups; Solution and Powder
Amniotin Hypodermic, Oral
Amniotin Pessaries
Antimeningococcic Serum (Polyvalent)
Antipneumococcus Serum (Types I and II)

Antistreptoccic Serum (Polyvalent)
Arsphenamine Ampules
Bacillus Bulgaricus
Bacillus Coli Communis Vaccine
Beverage Acidophilus
Calcium Gluconate Powder
Calcium Gluconate Tablets
Catarrhal Vaccine Combined
Chloramine Powder
Chloramine Tablets
Chocolate Flavored Vitavose
Cinchophen Powder
Cinchophen Tablets
Citabs Tablets
Cod Liver Oil Plain
Cod Liver Oil Mint Flavored
Colon Vaccine
Cupriferrum Elixir
Cupriferrum Syrup
Cupriferrum Tablets
Dextro-Vitavose
Di-Phen
Diphtheria Antitoxin
Diphtheria Immunity Test
Diphtheria Toxin Antitoxin Mixture
Diphtheria Toxin Antitoxin Mixture (Sheep)
Diphtheria Toxoid
Diphtheria Toxin (Schick Test)
Ephedrine Hydrochloride Tablets
Erysipelas-Streptococcic Antitoxin (Concentrated)
Follutein
Gonococcus Vaccine
Gonococcus Vaccine Combined
Influenza Vaccine
Influenza Vaccine Combined
Insulin 10, 20, 40 Units
Iodobismitol Ampules
Ipral Calcium Tablets
Ipral Amidopyrine Tablets
Leucocyte Extract Syringes
Liquid Petrolatum with Agar Plain
Liquid Petrolatum with Agar and Phenolphthalein
Liquid Petrolatum with Agar Compound
Neoarsphenamine Ampules
Normal Horse Serum
Parathyroid Hormone
Pasteur Rabies Vaccine
Pituitary Solution Ampules, Obstetrical and Surgical
Pneumococcus Vaccine
Pneumococcus-Streptococcus Vaccine
Poison Ivy Balm
Poison Ivy Extract
Poison Oak Extract
Polyvalent Staphylococcus Bacteriophage
Rabies Vaccine (Semple)
Radolatum Jelly
Radolatum Liquid
Scarlet Fever Streptococcus Antitoxin
Scarlet Fever (Schultz-Carlton Test)
Scarlet Fever Streptococcus Toxin (Dick Test)
Scarlet Fever Antitoxin
Schick Test Control
Serenium Tablets
Smallpox Vaccine
Solargentum Powder
Solargentum Tablets
Staphylo Acne Vaccine
Staphylococcus Vaccine
Staphylococcus-Streptococcus Vaccine
Staphylococcus Vaccine Combined
Streptococcus Vaccine
Sulpharsphenamine Ampules
Tetanus Antitoxin
Thromboplastin Dental
Thromboplastin Hypodermic
Typhoid Vaccine (Immunizing)
Typhoid Vaccine Combined (Immunizing)
Thyroxin Tablets and Crystals
Van Cott's Vaccine
Viosterol in Oil 250D
Vitavose
Whooping Cough Vaccine
Whooping Cough Vaccine Combined
Also Ampules: Intravenous, 2 in 14 forms; Subcutaneous and Intramuscular, 3 in 10 forms; *See Chap. V*

STANDARD BRANDS, INC. **(Standard Brands)**
595 Madison Avenue, New York City

Yeast "Fleischmann"

FREDERICK STEARNS AND COMPANY **(Stearns)**
Detroit, Mich.

Alphozone Powder
Alphozone Tablets
Codamines
Codamines Tablets

Diastase Powder
Esterol Tablets
Gastric Mucin "Fogelson"
Hemo-Genin Capsules
Insulin (10, 20, 40 100 Units)
Kasagra
Liver Extract Plain Capsules
Liver Extract 100 X Concentrated Capsules
Neo-Synephrin Aqueous Solution ¼%, 1%
Neo-Synephrin Emulsion, Plain
Neo-Synephrin Emulsion, Compound
Neo-Synephrin Elixir
Neo-Synephrin-Procaine Tablets
Stearnize
Susto Capsules
Susto Powder
Synephrin Tartrate Solution 3%, 5%
Synephrin Tartrate Emulsion, Plain
Synephrin Tartrate Emulsion, Compound
Tricotox

STERLING AND JENSEN (Sterling and Jensen)
Rockville Centre, N. Y.

Idozan

G. S. STODDARD AND COMPANY, INC. (Stoddard)
121 East 24th Street, New York City

Am-Phen-Al Tablets
Atrobutin Tablets
Benzyl Aromatic Capsules
Betanaphthol Compound Tablets
Cactus Compound Tablets
Calomel Camphor Compound Tablets
Camphor Compound Tablets
Cannabin Compound Tablets
Cascarine Compound Tablets
Chlorothol Compound
Cholaphen Tablets
Colchicum Compound Tablets
Corpus Luteum Ampules
Corpus Luteum Solution
Corpus Luteum Tablets
Epinephrin Compound
Glyco-Hydrastin
Hemoglobin Compound Tablets
Liporcin Tablets
Liver Extract
Liver Extract Intramuscular
Lozenges Benzocaine Compound
Mentholic Compound Tablets
Orchic Compound Solution
Orchic Compound Tablets
Orchic Solution Ampules
Orthoben
Ovarian Ampules
Ovarian Tablets
Ovarian Compound Tablets
Pancreatin Tablets
Pancreo Cauda Tablets
Pinus-Codeia
Pituitary Sex Hormone Solution (Anterior) Ampules
Pituitary Solution Ampules
Prostate Compound Tablets
Quinine Camphor Compound Tablets
Quinine Camphor Compound with Morphine Sulphate
Salcetol Powder
Salcetol Tablets
Salcetol Caffeine Compound Tablets
Salcetol Calomel Compound Tablets
Salcetol Codeia Tablets
Salcetol Compound Tablets 1, 2
Salcetol-Corrective
Salcetol-Salol
Sanguinaria Compound Tablets
Stanno-Yeast Tablets
Syrup Guaiacol Ammonium Compound
Tablet Theobutin Compound
Thymus Pituitary Solution Ampules
Thyroid Tablets
Also Ampules: Subcutaneous and Intramuscular, 5 in 6 forms; *See Chap. V*

STOMASEPTINE COMPANY (Stomaseptine)
135 West 26th Street, New York City

Stomaseptine

R. J. STRASENBURGH COMPANY (Strasenburgh)
Rochester, N. Y.

Ammoform Compound
Bismuth Thymol Iodide
Bis-Thiodide Ointment
Buchuform Tablets
Caloxidine Tablets
Caloxidine Compound Throat Tablets
Chloroseptine Tablets
Chloroseptine Aromatic Powder
Creothyol
Ferro-Cop Tablets
Haemobuminate
Iodostan
Mar-Phedaco
Muskola
Oxycaine Tablets
Protenzamyl
Saladin Tablets
Saladin Tablets, Jr.
Saladin Improved Tablets
Sedaco
Sulphodine
Terpazone Tablets
Vitamexol

DR. S. LEWIS SUMMERS ESTATE, INC. (Summers)
Morris Road at Wissahickon Creek (P.O.), Ambler, Pa.

Ami-Salox Capsules
Ami-Salox Powder
Ami-Salox Tablets
Befsal Capsules
Befsal Powder
Befsal Tablets
Iodo-Befsal Capsules
Iodo-Befsal Powder
Iodo-Befsal Tablets
Iodomuth Powder
Iodomuth Tablets

SUTLIFF AND CASE COMPANY, INC. (Sutliff and Case)
Peoria, Ill.

A.L.A. Ampules
A.L.A. Liquid
Amylsol Capsules
Calcium Thiocyanate Tablets
Kolagog
Phytosalicyl
Pthalox Tablets
Thiocyan-Elix
Tin-Ox Capsules
Also Ampules: Subcutaneous and Intramuscular, 1; *See Chap. V*

TABLAX COMPANY (Tablax)
32 Union Square, New York City

Marvosan
Quinseptikons

TABLE ROCK LABORATORIES, INC. (Table Rock)
Greenville, S. C.

Bismuth Violet Liquid 0.5%
Bismuth Violet Ointment 1%
Citrin Capsules

TAILBY-NASON COMPANY (Tailby-Nason)
4 Carlton Street, Boston, Mass.

Crutar Ointments "Grossman"
Nason's Palatable Cod Liver Oil
Salamene-X
Thaleocolate Tablets

TAPPAN ZEE SURGICAL COMPANY (Tappan Zee)
Box 13, Nyack, N. Y.

Causticks
Cupricsticks
Mercurosticks
Stypsticks

TERRELL'S LABORATORIES (Terrell)
Medical Arts Bldg., Fort Worth, Texas

Allergens—Pollens, Individual
Rabies Vaccine, Phenolized
Also Ampules: Subcutaneous and Intramuscular, 1; *See Chap. V*

THIOPHENE LABORATORIES, INC. (Thiophene)
Chicago, Ill.

Sulbumin Tablets

THE TILDEN COMPANY (Tilden)
New Lebanon, N. Y.

Danish Ointment
Elixir Iodo-Bromide of Calcium Compound
Elixir Iodo-Bromide of Calcium Compound with Mercury Bichloride
Elixir Maltopepsin
Elixir Maltopepsin with Glycerophosphates
Elixir Maltopepsin with Iron, Arsenic, Quinine and Strychnine
Elixir Maltopepsin with Salicylates Compound
Eupinol
Eupinol Ointment
Firolyptol
Firolyptol with Kresote
Haimased
Liquor Maltopepsin
Mankali
Narkogen
Nepenthe
Pasanol
Zemacide

J. CICERO TISE (Tise)
Vade Mecum, N. C.

Vade Mecum Springs

E. TOSSE AND COMPANY, INC. (Tosse)
33 Thirty-fifth Street, Brooklyn, N. Y.

Bismogenol Ampules
Bismogenol Liquid
Bismogenol Liquid Half Strength
Ekzebrol Ampules
Kavalactol
Nitroscleran Ampules
Nitroscleran Salts

TOWNES AND JAMES (Townes and James)
213 Duffield Street, New York City

Baga Capsules

TOWT-NOLAN LABORATORY (Towt-Nolan)
2588 Grove Street, Oakland, Calif.

Lactobacillus

TUCKER PHARMACAL COMPANY, INC. (Tucker)

221 East 38th Street, New York City

Bromo-Adonis
Me-ox-ol

ULMER LABORATORIES (Ulmer)

412 South 6th Street, Minneapolis, Minn.

Biliposol Ampules
Cal-Zo
Picro Benzyl
Sodium Morrhuate 7% Solution
Vari-Chlor-Ose Ampules
Varitose Ampules
Varitose Liquid

UNITED LABORATORIES, LTD. (United Laboratories)

327 South Fair Oaks Avenue, Pasadena, Calif.

Condensed Acidophilus
Culture Bacillus Acidophilus
Hepaticon
Leucocyte Extract Ampules
Liver Extract Ampules
Orchitic Extract Ampules
Ovarian Extract Ampules
Ovestrumon Ampules
Pituitary Extract (Whole) Solution
Spleen Extract Ampules
Stomachon
"67" Serum

U. S. STANDARD PRODUCTS COMPANY (U. S. Standard)

Woodworth, Wis.

Acne Vaccine
Antimengococcus Serum
Diphtheria Toxin-Antitoxin Mixture
Diphtheria Toxin-Antitoxin Mixture (Goat)
Diphtheria Toxin-Antitoxin Mixture (Sheep)
Diphtheria Toxin for Schick Test and Control
Diphtheria Toxoid
Rabies Vaccine Semple
Typhoid Vaccine
Typhoid-Paratyphoid Vaccine Combined

THE UPJOHN COMPANY (Upjohn)

Kalamazoo, Mich.

Accessorone
Acetonyl
Bromionyl
Bromionyl with Acetylsalicylic Acid
Bromionyl with Barbital
Calamoin
Calcionates
Caripeptic Liquid
Carica Powder
Carica with Glycerophosphate Tablets
Carica Compound Tablets
Cheracol
Chlorhydrionic with Hexamethylene Tetramine
Citro Carbonate
Corpus Luteum Tablets
Colon Streptococcus Mixed Vaccine
Dextrolac 1, 2
Diginfuse
Digitora Tablets
Formohydrion Tablets
Gonococcus Vaccine
Gonococcus Vaccine Mixed
Influenza Vaccine Mixed
Jeculin
Kerolysin
Liver Extract Capsules
Luthorm Ampules
Myeladol
Ophthalmic Ointments:
- Boric Acid
- Mercury Bichloride
- Mercury Oxide
- Mercury Yellow Oxide Compound
- Phenacaine and Epinephrine
- Silloid

Ovarian Extract Ampules

Ovarian Substance Tablets
Pitamin Obstetrical Ampules
Pitamin Surgical Ampules
Pneumococcus Vaccine
Salicionyl
Staphylococcus Mixed Vaccine
Streptococcus Vaccine
Streptococcus Mixed Vaccine
Super D Cod Liver Oil
Super D Cod Liver Oil Concentrate Pearls and Liquid.
Thyroid Gland Tablets
Typhoid Vaccine
Typhoid-Paratyphoid Mixed Vaccine
Also Ampules: Intravenous, 17 in 27 forms; Subcutaneous and Intramuscular, 25 in 31 forms; *See Chap. V*

THE UPSHER SMITH COMPANY **(Upsher Smith)**
529 South 7th Street, Minneapolis, Minn.

Digilutea Capsules
Digilutea Liquid
Digilutea Tablets
Digismith Capsules
Digismith Liquid
Digismith Tablets

UVURSIN **(Uvursin)**
88 First Street, San Francisco, Calif.

Uvursin Capsules

VALENTINE'S MEAT JUICE COMPANY **(Valentine)**
Richmond, Va.

Liver Extract E 29
Liver Extract E 29 with Iron
Meat Juice

CHAS. VAN DER BRUCK, INC. **(Van Der Bruck)**
61 Park Place, New York City

Ems
Ems Mineral Spring Salt
Rhens
Wildungen

THE VASS CHEMICAL COMPANY **(Vass Chemical)**
Danbury, Conn.

Thialion

THE VIBURNO COMPANY, INC. **(Viburno)**
146 Front Street, New York City

Viburno

VITALAIT LABORATORY OF CALIFORNIA, LTD. **(Vitalait)**
327 South Fair Oaks Avenue, Pasadena, Calif.

Culture Bacillus Acidophilus

VITAMIN FOOD COMPANY, INC. **(Vitamin Food)**
122 Hudson Street, New York City

Vegex
Vitafood

WALKER PHARMACAL CO. **(Walker Pharmacal)**
4200 Laclede Avenue, St. Louis, Mo.

Dermocaine

HENRY K. WAMPOLE AND COMPANY, INC. **(Wampole)**
440 Fairmount Avenue, Philadelphia, Pa.

Bismuth Hydrate Compound
Bon-Sol
Creo-Terpin
Hypno-Bromic Compound
Organidin
Perfected Preparation
Phospho-Lecithin
Sodium Glycocholate Compound Tablets

THE WANDER COMPANY **(Wander)**
180 N. Michigan Avenue, Chicago, Ill.

Alucol Powder
Alucol Tablets

WILLIAM R. WARNER AND COMPANY, INC. **(Warner)**
113 West 18th Street, New York City

Agarol
Alka-Zane
Cal-Bis-Ma
Guaiatonic
Iodoformal Powder
Iodoformal Ointment 10%
Iodoformal Suppositories

WATERBURY COMPANY **(Waterbury)**
113 West 18th Street, New York City

Waterbury's Compound

THE WEST BADEN SPRINGS CO. **(West Baden)**
West Baden, Ind.

West Baden Springs

WEST DISINFECTING COMPANY **(West Disinfecting)**
Long Island City, N. Y.

Phenoco

THE WESTERFIELD PHARMACAL COMPANY, INC. **(Westerfield)**
11 St. Marys Street, Dayton, Ohio

Acido-Sodium Tablets
Benzo-Acetate
Calculi-Sol
Cali-Chlorides

Corpus Luteum Tablets
Digicardalis Tablets
Enteri-Drastis Tablets
Gallo-Gogue Tablets
Gastro-Gallate
Ichthyolate Ointment
Low-Tone Tablets
Neuro-Calm Tablets
Menovarian Tablets
Ovarian Tablets
Thymus Tablets
Thyroid Tablets
Yeast Capsules

WHITE ROCK MINERAL SPRING COMPANY (White Rock)

100 Broadway, New York City

White Rock Springs

WHITE SULPHUR SPRINGS, INC. (White Sulphur)

White Sulphur Springs, W. Va.

White Sulphur Springs

WILSON "999" CORP. (Wilson)

138 West 17th Street, New York City

Crockett Arsenic Lithia Springs

WINTHROP CHEMICAL COMPANY, INC. (Winthrop)

170 Varick Street, New York City

Abasin Tablets
Adalin Powder
Adalin Tablets
Adalin-Luminal Tablets
Agurin
Alypin Powder
Alypin Tablets
Amatin Tablets
Antophysin Ampules
Aristol Powder
Avertin Fluid Ampules
Bismutose Powder
Butolan Tablets
Cafumal Tablets
Chaulmestrol Ampules
Chaulmestrol Powder
Chiniofon Tablets
Chiniofon Powder
Chinoplasmin Tablets
Compral Tablets
Coryfin
Creosotal
Curtasal
Cymarin Ampules
Cymarin Tablets
Diatrast (Neoskiodan Ampules)
Duotal Tablets
Duotal Powder
Elarson Tablets
Eldoform Tablets
Ferro Elarson Tabloids
Ferro-Sajodin Tablets
Gono-Yatren
Guaiacose
Helmitol Powder
Helmitol Tablets
Homocamfin Ampules
Hydrastinin Liquid
Hydrastinin Tablets
Iothion
Iothion Oil
Kresival
Kreslumin
Lumalgin Tablets
Luminal Capsules
Luminal Powder
Luminal Tablets
Luminal Elixir
Luminal-Sodium Ampules
Luminal-Sodium Powder
Luminal-Sodium Tablets
Lumodrin Tablets
Mesotan
Mesurol Ampules
Mesurol Powder
Myorgal Tablets
Neofosfan Ampules

Novaspirin Powder
Novaspirin Tablets
Novasurol Ampules
Novocaine Ampules
Optarson Ampules
Padutin Ampules
Pantocain Ampules, Spinal
Pantocain Solution 2%, Surface
Phanodorn Tablets
Phenacetin Powder
Phenacetin Tablets
Piperazine
Plasmochin Tablets
Plasmochin Compound Tablets
Protargol Powder, Granules
Sabromin Powder
Sabromin Tablets
Sajodin Powder
Sajodin Tablets
Salophen Powder
Salophen Tablets
Salophen-Phenacetin Compound Tablets
Salvarsan Ampules
Skiodan Liquid
Skiodan Powder
Solarson Ampules
Spirosal
Sulfonal Powder
Sulfonal Tablets
Tannigen
Tenamin Ampules
Tenamin Liquid
Theocin Powder
Theocin Tablets
Theocin, Soluble Powder
Theocin, Soluble Tablets
Theocin Sodium Acetate
Theominal Tablets
Thyractin Tablets
Trional Powder
Trional Tablets
Tutocaine Tablets 1 to 6
Veronal Elixir
Veronal Powder
Veronal Tablets
Veronal-Sodium Tablets
Viosterol
Yatren-Casein Solution, Strong
Yatren-Casein Solution, Weak
Also Ampules: Intravenous, 20 in 71 forms; Subcutaneous and Intramuscular, 38 in 66 forms; *See Chap V*

JOHN WYETH AND BRO., INC. (Wyeth)

1118 Washington Avenue, Philadelphia, Pa.

Algos (Gynalgos)
Asepticaps
Camolus Spray
Camolus with Ephedrine 0.5%
Cerose
Collyrium
Corpus Luteum Gland Ampules
Corpus Luteum Gland Powder
Corpus Luteum Gland Tablets
Liquenzyme
Neo Sevetol
Ophthalmic Ointments:
  Argenol
  Boric Acid
  Congestive
  Mercuric Chloride, Corrosive
  Mercuric Oxide Yellow
Ovarian Substance Ampules
Ovarian Substance Powder
Ovarian Substance Tablets
Pancreatin Powder
Petrogen Products
Picratol Ointment
Picratol Suppositories Rectal
Picratol Suppositories Urethral
Picratol Suppositories Vaginal
Pituitary Anterior Powder
Pituitary Extract Obstetrical Ampules
Pituitary Whole Powder
Robinol
Siderol
Suprarenal Tablets
Suprarenal Powder
Surgical Powder
Thymus Gland Powder
Thyroid Gland Powder
Thyroid Gland Tablets
Also Ampules: Intravenous, 7 in 8 forms; Subcutaneous and Intramuscular, 22 in 26 forms; *See Chap V*

W. F. YOUNG, INC. (Young)

111 Lyman Street, Springfield, Mass.

Absorbine Jr.

THE ZEMMER COMPANY, INC. (Zemmer)
3943 Sennott Street, Pittsburgh, Pa.

Corpus Luteum Ampules
Corpus Luteum Capsules
Corpus Luteum Tablets
Epinephrine Chloride Solution Ampules (1:1,000)
Ephedrine Hydrochloride Ampules
Ephedrine Hydrochloride Solution 3%
Liver Extract Capsules
Liver Substance Capsules
Liver Substance Tablets
Liver Substance Solution Ampules
Mammary Substance Tablets
Ophthalmic Ointments:
- Acid Boric
- Acid Boric Compound
- Argentum
- Atropine Sulphate, ½%, 1%, 2%
- Butyn
- Cocaine Hydrochloride
- Cupric Citrate
- Cupric Sulphate
- Dionin
- Eserine Salicylate
- Holocaine et Adrenalin
- Hydrargyrum Chloridum Corrosivum
- Hydrargyrum Oxidum Flavum gr 4, gr 8
- Hydrargyrum Oxidum Flavum et Atropin
- Hydrargyrum Oxidum Flavum et Adrenalin Comp.
- Ichthyol 5%

Ophthalmic Ointments:—(*Continued*)
- Lunosol 10%
- Mercurochrome 1%, 2%
- Optochin Hydrochloride 1%, 2%
- Orthoform 1%, 2%
- Pilocarpine Muriate 1%
- Thiosinamine 10%
- Zinc Acetate
- Zinc Ichthyol
- Zinc Sulphate

Orchic Substance Tablets
Ovarian Substance Tablets
Parathyroid Tablets
Phedrolene Inhalant
Pineal Substance Tablets
Pituitary Substance Tablets
Pituitary Substance Anterior Tablets
Pituitary Substance Posterior Tablets
Pituitary Extract Ampules
Pituitary-Ovarian Compound Tablets
Placenta Substance Tablets
Prostate Substance Tablets
Secretin Compound Tablets
Spleen Substance Tablets
Suprarenal Tablets
Thymus Tablets
Thyroid Tablets
Thyroid-Pituitary Compound Tablets
Thyroid-Ovarian Compound Tablets
Also Ampules: Intravenous, 22 in 32 forms; Subcutaneous and Intramuscular, 20 in 21 forms; *See Chap V*

ZONITE PRODUCTS CORPORATION (Zonite)
Chrysler Building, New York City

Zonite Liquid
Zonite Ointment
Zonite Suppositories

THERAPEUTIC INDEX

This Index is intended also as a guide to the drugs of use in each of the disorders enumerated; following each heading are the preparations where such disorders are mentioned under *Uses*.

DRUG INDEX

All Distributors' Names, Pharmaceutical Products and page numbers of principal descriptions are presented in bold type

* Hynson, Westcott and Dunning.